ENDOCRINOLOGY

ENDOCRINOLOGY

Proceedings of the 7th International Congress of Endocrinology, Quebec City, 1–7 July 1984

Editors:

Fernand Labrie, Louise Proulx
Department of Molecular Endocrinology,
Centre Hospitalier de l'Université Laval
Quebec, Canada

1984

Excerpta Medica, Amsterdam - New York - Oxford

International Congress Series No. 655
ISBN 0 444 80637 7

Published by:

Elsevier Science Publishers B.V.
P.O. Box 211
1000 AE Amsterdam
The Netherlands

Sole distributors for the USA and Canada:

Elsevier Science Publishing Company Inc.
52 Vanderbilt Avenue
New York, NY 10017
USA

Library of Congress Cataloging in Publication Data

International Congress of Endocrinology (7th : 1984 : Québec, Québec)
Endocrinology: proceedings of the 7th International Congress of Endocrinology, Quebec City, 1–7 July 1984.
(International congress series; no. 655)
Includes indexes.
1. Endocrinology--Congresses. 2. Clinical endocrinology--Congresses. I. Labrie, Fernand, 1937-
II. Proulx, Louise. III. Title. IV. Series. [DNLM:
1. Endocrinology--congresses. W3 EX89 no. 655 / WK 100 161 1984e]
QP187.154 1984 599'.0142 84-21229
ISBN 0-444-80637-7 (U.S.)

Printed in The Netherlands

Contents

PLENARY LECTURES

SYMPOSIA

1. Clinical Aspects of Hormone-Producing Tumors

5. Pineal Gland and Endocrine Rhythms

6. Adrenergic Receptors

7. Central Nervous System Peptides and Pituitary Function

8. Prolactin

9. Regulation of Aldosterone Secretion

10. Fertility Control

11. Pathogenesis of Type II Diabetes Mellitus

12. Organization and Expression of Hormone Genes

19. The Renin-Angiotensin System and Hypertension

20. Thermogenesis and Body Weight

32. Opioid Peptides in the Brain and Endocrine Tissue

33. Biosynthesis and Processing of Peptide Hormones II

34. Hormonal Control of Electrolyte Balance

41. Regulation of Ovarian Function

42. GRF and Regulation of GH Secretion

43. Receptor Diseases

44. Therapeutic Problems

45. Neurohypophysial Peptides

46. Hormones and Aging

MEET-THE-PROFESSOR

NEW TECHNICAL DEVELOPMENTS

PLENARY LECTURES

Endocrinology
F. Labrie, L. Proulx, eds.

STEROID HORMONES RELIEVE REPRESSION OF THE OVALBUMIN GENE PROMOTER IN CHICK OVIDUCT TUBULAR GLAND CELLS

P. CHAMBON, M.P. GAUB, J.P. LEPENNEC, A. DIERICH and D. ASTINOTTI

Laboratoire de Génétique Moléculaire des Eucaryotes du CNRS,
Unité 184 de Biologie Moléculaire et de Génie Génétique de l'INSERM,
Institut de Chimie Biologique, Faculté de Médecine, 67085 Strasbourg (France)

INTRODUCTION

Control of gene expression by steroid hormones has been extensively studied with the aim of elucidating the molecular mechanisms regulating gene expression in eukaryotes. The chick oviduct is a particularly suitable system, because the synthesis of the major egg-white proteins can be modulated by the administration and withdrawal of estrogens, progestins, glucocorticoids and androgens, each acting through a distinct hormone receptor (1, 2 and refs. therein). Administration of estrogen to immature chicks causes a proliferation and differentiation of the oviduct magnum tubular gland cells; these cells synthesize the major egg-white proteins including ovalbumin, conalbumin, ovomucoid and lysozyme. Arrest of this "primary" stimulation (withdrawal) leads to the cessation of synthesis of these proteins, which can be restimulated by administrations of anyone of the four steroid hormones (secondary stimulation). Following hormonal stimulation, there is an accumulation of the egg-white protein mRNAs, which results from both an increased rate of transcription of the corresponding genes and a decreased rate of degradation of the mRNAs (1-7 and refs. therein).

The molecular mechanisms by which steroid hormones induce transcription are poorly understood, but it is assumed that nuclear steroid hormone-receptor complexes bind to regulatory sequences in the vicinity of the induced genes. With the advent of molecular cloning, direct study of the possible interaction _in vitro_ between steroid hormone-receptor complexes and specific gene fragments became possible, as well as functional analysis of sequence requirements for hormonal induction of transcription of cloned genes after transfer to cells containing steroid hormone-receptors. Preferential _in vitro_ binding of glucocorticoid receptor to 5' flanking region of MMTV DNA (8, 9 and refs. therein), human metallothionein IIA gene (10) and chicken lysozyme gene (11) has been reported. Similarly, preferential binding of progesterone receptor to 5' flanking sequences of the other chicken egg-white protein genes has been observed (12, 13). Concomitantly, functional studies involving transfer of cloned genes to hormone-responsive cells have shown that the DNA sequence which contains these binding sites are important for control of transcription by glucocorticoids (10, 11, 14-17 and refs. therein) and progesterone (18). No similar studies with estrogens have been as yet reported. Furthermore, it is not known whether the interaction between the hormone-receptor complex and the regulatory sequences leads to the activation of promoter elements otherwise intrinsically inactive (positive regulation) or to a relief of repression on promoter elements "constitutively" active unless repressed (negative regulation).

We have previously cloned the ovalbumin gene and determined its structure (19 and refs. therein). We have also shown that it is not accurately or efficiently expressed when transferred into a variety of non-oviduct cells (20, 21), a result which was not surprising, since in the whole animal the ovalbumin gene is transcribed only in oviduct tubular gland cells. Unfortunately there is no permanent chicken cultured cell line derived from oviduct or other chicken tissues which contains estrogen and progestin hormone receptors, and in which the ovalbumin gene could be validly transferred to study its function and the mechanisms of its hormonal induction. We decided therefore to microinject recombinants containing the ovalbumin promoter region into the nucleus of primary cultured oviduct tubular gland cells, a procedure which has allowed Renkawitz et al. (7, 11) to analyze the sequence requirements for activation of transcription from the lysozyme gene promoter by progesterone and dexamethasone. We demonstrate here that in the absence of steroid hormone the ovalbumin promoter is negatively regulated in tubular gland cells by a control element located between 295 and 420 bp upstream from the capsite, and that this repression can be relieved by addition of either estradiol or progesterone.

RESULTS

A) A microinjection assay for ovalbumin promoter activity.

Since the RNA transcribed from an ovalbumin promoter-containing recombinant could not be routinely analyzed after microinjection into cell nuclei, we have studied the ovalbumin promoter function by coupling 5'-flanking fragments of increasing lengths (from position -1 to positions -132, -295, -420 or -1348 upstream to the capsite - Fig. 1, the pTOT series) to the SV40 T-antigen coding sequence in such a manner that T-antigen expression is now under the control of the ovalbumin promoter region. DNAs (approximately 100 molecules per nucleus) of the pTOT series were microinjected into the nuclei of primary cultured oviduct tubular gland cells. 24 hrs later the function of the ovalbumin promoter region was monitored by indirect immunofluorescence against T-antigen as described in ref. 22. The validity of the microinjection immunofluorescence assay to estimate the function of a promoter when linked to the T-antigen coding sequence in a chimeric recombinant has been previously discussed (22). Subsequent comparisons of the results obtained for a given set of recombinants, using either the microinjection immunofluorescence assay or quantitative S1 nuclease analysis of the synthesized RNA after calcium phosphate transfection, have shown that there is a non-linear proportionality between the number of fluorescent nuclei and the relative promoter efficiency as estimated from quantitative RNA determinations (22-24). Since variations of fluorescence intensity cannot be validly measured and are not taken into account, the present assay which scores only the number of fluorescent nuclei rapidly reaches a saturation level as the amount of synthesized RNA increases. Large decreases in the efficiency of a promoter are accompanied by very significant decreases of the number of immunofluorescent nuclei, whereas increases of promoter efficiency above a certain level are reflected by only small increases in this number. In each series of experiments, the wild-type recombinant pSV1 (SV40 control in Tables) was microinjected in parallel to permit normalization of the data. It contains the full SV40 early transcription unit including its promoter which functions in all cell types and is not sensitive to steroid hormones (21). The results obtained with the pTOT series were expressed as per cent relative to the number of immunofluorescent cells obtained with pSV1 taken as 100% [usually 50-60% of the cells microinjected with pSV1 were T-antigen positive - see Tables in which the average percentage of immunofluorescent tubular gland cells after microinjection of a given pTOT recombinant is underlined; the number of independent microinjection experiments and the extreme values for each recombinant are shown in parenthesis and in brackets, respectively].

B) Effect of steroid hormone antagonists on expression of the ovalbumin promoter recombinants.

All four pTOT recombinants were expressed to approximately the same level after microinjection in nuclei of oviduct tubular gland cells, maintained in a medium containing foetal calf serum (MFCS) (Table 1; data for pTOT -1348 are not shown). In contrast, none of the pTOT recombinant was expressed when microinjected into the fibroblasts which were also present in primary cultures of chicken oviduct cells, whereas the SV40 recombinant pSV1 was similarly expressed in both oviduct cell types (not shown, see ref. 21). The reason why on average the number of tubular gland cells expressing the pTOT recombinants was lower than that of the same cells expressing pSV1 is unknown. It may reflect an heterogeneity in tubular gland cells, since doubling the amount of microinjected pTOT DNA molecules did not result in significant increases in the relative number of fluorescent cells. The possible effect of the steroid hormones present in foetal calf serum on expression of the ovalbumin promoter recombinant was then investigated using the anti-estrogen, Tamoxifen, and a new compound, RU486, which is both an anti-glucocorticoid and an anti-progestin in mammals, but which exhibits only anti-glucocorticoid activity in chicken (25 and V. Govindan, personal communication). It is striking that although Tamoxifen and RU486 did not significantly affect the expression of pTOT-132 and pTOT-295, the expression of

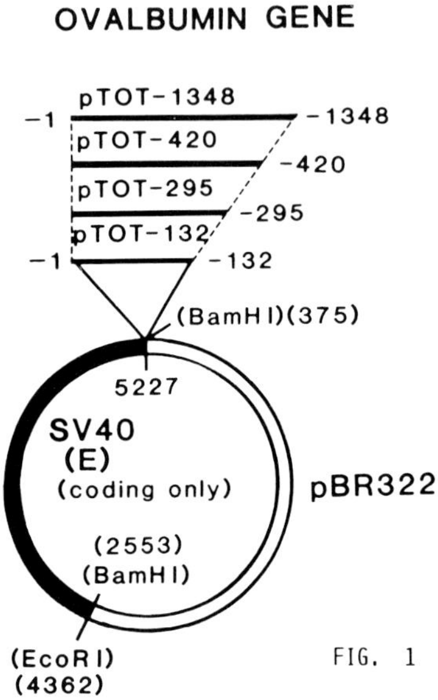

FIG. 1

TABLE 1

EFFECT OF ANTI-ESTROGEN AND ANTI-GLUCOCORTICOID ON THE ACTIVITY OF THE OVALBUMIN PROMOTER IN PRIMARY CULTURE OF CHICKEN OVIDUCT CELLS MAINTAINED IN MEDIUM WITH FOETAL CALF SERUM (MFCS: DNA : 100 COPIES/NUCLEUS, 24 HRS)

		RECOMBINANT		
	CONTROL SV40	pTOT-132	pTOT-295	pTOT-420
MFCS	100% (A)	66%[53-91](4)	53%[36-64](7)	53%[38-77](9)
MFCS + TAMOXIFEN (10^{-6}M)	100% (B)	49%[46-54](3)	47%[33-64](4)	ND
MFCS + RU486 (2×10^{-6}M)	100% (C)	47%[43-52](4)	41%[36-45](3)	ND
MFCS + TAMOXIFEN (10^{-6}M) + RU486 (2×10^{-6}M)	100% (D)	60%[44-84](6)	44%[36-49](4)	8%[0-16](8)

(A) 100% = 53% OF INJECTED CELLS BECAME T ANTIGEN-POSITIVE (8 EXP.: EXTREME VALUES : 43-59)
(B) 100% = 61% OF INJECTED CELLS BECAME T ANTIGEN-POSITIVE (3 EXP.: EXTREME VALUES : 54-67)
(C) 100% = 58% OF INJECTED CELLS BECAME T ANTIGEN-POSITIVE (4 EXP.: EXTREME VALUES : 54-65)
(D) 100% = 55% OF INJECTED CELLS BECAME T ANTIGEN-POSITIVE (6 EXP.: EXTREME VALUES : 46-71)

pTOT-420 (and of pTOT-1348, not shown) was drastically inhibited by these antagonists. The residual level of activity may correspond to the presence of variable amounts of progestins in foetal calf serum (see below).

C) Expression of pTOT-420, but not of pTOT-295 and pTOT-132, is blocked in the absence of steroid hormones.

To demonstrate directly that expression of pTOT-420, but not of pTOT-295 and pTOT-132 is dependent on steroid hormones, primary cultured oviduct cells were maintained in a medium from which these hormones were removed by treatment with dextran-charcoal, which is known to remove most, but not all, of the steroid hormones present in serum (26). When tubular gland cells were maintained in such a stripped medium (SM), the expression of the microinjected pTOT-132 and pTOT-295 recombinants was the same as in cells maintained in the presence of untreated foetal calf serum (compare Tables 1 and 2) and there was no significant effect of addition of either estradiol or progesterone or steroid hormone antagonists (Table 2). On the contrary, microinjection of pTOT-420 into cells maintained in stripped medium, resulted in a lower level of expression (26% in Table 2 instead of 53% in Table 1). The variability of this level (20-42%) is most likely due to variations in residual amounts of estrogens and glucocorticoids in the stripped medium, since addition of both Tamoxifen and RU486 caused a further decrease of expression down to 4% on average, which may reflect a residual amount of progestins in the stripped medium.

That the repression which is exerted on expression of pTOT-420 in the absence of steroid hormones can be relieved by the presence of estradiol or progesterone is shown directly by the data obtained after addition of these hormones to the stripped medium (Table 2). Both of them increased pTOT-420 expression to a level similar to that observed for pTOT-132 and pTOT-295. A similar level was obtained by adding progesterone to the stripped medium in the presence of RU486 (not shown), confirming that this compound has no anti-progestin activity in oviduct tubular gland cells (see above). Similar microinjection experiments with pTOT-1348 gave results identical to those obtained with pTOT-420 (not shown). The effect of glucocorticoids on expression of pTOT-420 has not yet been studied, but the results obtained after addition of the specific glucocorticoid antagonist RU486 suggest that the repression exerted in the absence of steroid hormones can also be relieved by glucocorticoids, a conclusion in agreement with the known effect of these steroid hormones on ovalbumin gene expression _in vivo_ (see Introduction).

CONCLUSIONS

In chicken the ovalbumin gene promoter functions only in tubular gland cells of the oviduct after activation by steroid hormone treatment (see Introduction). We have previously shown that it is not active, when microinjected in the form of any of the pTOT recombinants, into a variety of heterologuous non-chicken or chicken cells, including the fibroblasts present in primary cultured oviduct or liver cells (21). However, anyone of these recombinants was efficiently expressed in primary cultures of chicken embryo hepatocytes (21), irrespective of the presence of steroid hormones, although the ovalbumin gene is never expressed in chicken liver in spite of the presence of estradiol receptor. These results together with those presented here, lead to the following conclusions for the regulation of ovalbumin gene expression (see also Fig. 2):

1. Chicken hepatocytes contain cell-specific factor(s) which permit the constitutive activity of the microinjected ovalbumin promoter in the absence of steroid hormones. The corresponding control element(s) is contained within 132 bp upstream from the capsite.

2. Oviduct tubular gland cells contain similar cell-specific factor(s), which permit the "constitutive" expression of the ovalbumin promoter region up to -295 bp upstream from the capsite, in the absence of steroid hormones. This cell-specific factor(s) is apparently not present in fibroblasts from primary cultures of liver or oviduct cells.

3. A negative control is exerted on the activity of the ovalbumin promoter region in oviduct tubular gland cells and is dependent on sequences located between -295 and -420.

4. Hepatocytes lack the factor responsible for this negative control mechanism.

5. The presence of estradiol and/or progesterone (and most likely of glucocorticoids) relieves the "repression" in oviduct tubular gland cells.

It appears therefore that the inactivity of the ovalbumin promoter in chicken tubular gland cells in the absence of steroid hormones is due to the existence of a negative regulatory element (a blocker), located between -295 and -420 upstream from the capsite. Since there is no repression in hepatocytes, it is most likely that the blocker element is functional only in the presence of a "trans-acting" repressor. Thus the non-expression of the ovalbumin gene in the liver of the whole animal is not due to the absence of cell-specific transcription factor(s) which acts positively on promoter elements contained within 132 bp upstream from the capsite or to the presence of the repressor factor, but must be due to a cis-acting negative mechanism which results from the "developmental history" of the gene (epigenetic information, e.g. "inactive" chromatin structure, DNA methylation, or any other process which results in a permanent "closing" of the gene). This permanent closing mechanism can be bypassed by microinjection of plasmid recombinants. In other chicken cells, like fibroblasts, the cell-specific transcription factor(s) appears to be absent, since pTOT-132 is not expressed.

Our findings raise a number of interesting questions. First, what is the nature of the repres-

TABLE 2

EFFECT OF ESTRADIOL AND PROGESTERONE ON THE ACTIVITY OF THE OVALBUMIN PROMOTER IN PRIMARY CULTURE OF CHICKEN OVIDUCT CELLS MAINTAINED IN STEROID HORMONE-STRIPPED MEDIUM (SM)
(DNA : 100 COPIES/NUCLEUS; 24 HRS)

RECOMBINANT	CULTURE MEDIUM					
	SM	+ ESTRADIOL (10^{-8}M)	+ PROGESTERONE (10^{-9}M)	+TAMOXIFEN (10^{-6}M)	+RU486 (2×10^{-6}M)	+TAMOXIFEN + RU486
CONTROL (SV40)	100% (A)	100% (B)	100% (C)	100% (D)	100% (E)	100% (F)
pTOT-132	60%[42-100](7)	74%[58-84](4)	75%[60-85](5)	75%[58-91](2)	ND	60%[52-71](4)
pTOT-420	26%[10-42](13)	60%[34-91](8)	55%[34-75](7)	12%[8-17](4)	13%[5-20](4)	4%[0-8] (7)
pTOT-295	60%[50-72](3)	64%[44-83](2)	65%[49-81](2)	ND	ND	53%[42-65](2)

(A) 100% = 50% OF THE INJECTED CELLS BECAME T ANTIGEN-POSITIVE (15 EXP.; EXTREME VALUES 43-60)
(B) 100% = 49% OF THE INJECTED CELLS BECAME T ANTIGEN-POSITIVE (9 EXP.; EXTREME VALUES 36-74)
(C) 100% = 53% OF THE INJECTED CELLS BECAME T ANTIGEN-POSITIVE (9 EXP.; EXTREME VALUES 34-68)
(D) 100% = 50% OF THE INJECTED CELLS BECAME T ANTIGEN-POSITIVE (3 EXP.; EXTREME VALUES 45-55)
(E) 100% = 55% OF THE INJECTED CELLS BECAME T ANTIGEN-POSITIVE (4 EXP.; EXTREME VALUES 45-67)
(F) 100% = 48% OF THE INJECTED CELLS BECAME T ANTIGEN-POSITIVE (8 EXP.; EXTREME VALUES 36-68)

FIGURE 2 CONTROL OF OVALBUMIN GENE EXPRESSION

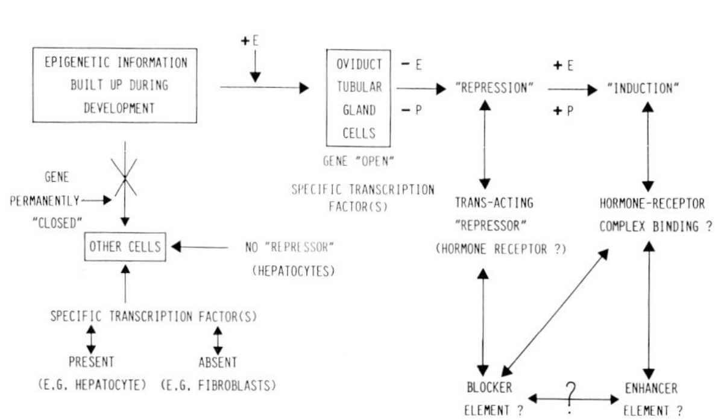

sor and how is its negative effect relieved by steroid hormones. Recent studies indicate that steroid hormone receptor molecules may be permanently located in the nucleus (see 27 for refs.), which suggests that the unfilled receptor molecule may be the repressor. However, this hypothesis is not supported by the lack of repression in hepatocytes which contains estrogen receptor molecules, although perhaps at too low a level to be efficient (28). Second, do the various steroid hormone-receptor complexes bind to the blocker element or to a positive dominant regulatory element(s) when repression is relieved ? Is such a positive regulatory element(s) an enhancer(s), as it has been shown to be the case for regulation of MMTV promoter function by glucocorticoids (see 17 and 29 for refs.)? In any case, it is clear that the sequences responsible for steroid hormone induction are located between positions -295 and -420; this is upstream from the -95 and -222 sequence, which has been identified as responsible for a five-fold activation of the ovalbumin promoter by progesterone (13, 18). It is possible that the effect of this sequence has been missed in our present study, because of the relative insensitivity of the immunofluorescence assay (see above). On the other hand, the blocker effect of the -295 to -420 sequence has not been observed by Dean et al. (18), most likely because their ovalbumin promoter chimeric recombinant contains the SV40 enhancer. We have indeed observed that the effect of the blocker sequence is not seen when the SV40 enhancer is introduced into pTOT-420 or pTOT-1348 (results not shown). Finally, it is puzzling that a blocker element can direct the repression of promoter elements which are located downstream. That such a mechanism may have some generality is however suggested by the recent observation that the prokaryotic AraC repressor interacts with a regulatory element which is located more than 280 bp upstream from the RNA startsite (30). It is worthmentioning that additional regulatory elements modulating the activity of the ovalbumin gene may be present further upstream from the blocker sequence, since nuclease sensitivity studies on oviduct chromatin have revealed the existence of steroid hormone inducible hypersensitive regions at approximately 1, 3 and 6 kb upstream from the capsite (31 and unpublished observations). Obviously the possible regulatory function of these sequences is not revealed by the present microinjection studies.

To our best knowledge, the present results constitue the first clear demonstration of the existence of a far upstream negative regulatory element (a blocker) participating in the regulation of gene expression in a higher eukaryote. Together with enhancers (29), blockers may provide the large number of combinatorial possibilities which are required for multifactorial regulation of gene expression in complex organisms.

ACKNOWLEGEMENTS

We thank Roussel-Uclaf (Paris) for providing RU486.

REFERENCES

1. Palmiter RD, Mulvihill, ER, Shepherd JH, McKnight GS (1981) J Biol Chem 256:7910-7916
2. Shepherd JH, Mulvihill ER, Thomas PS, Palmiter RD (1980) J Cell Biol 87:142-151
3. Swanek GE, Nordstrom JL, Tsai SY, Tsai MJ, O'Malley BW (1979) Proc Natl Acad Sci USA 76:1049-1053
4. Bellard M, Gannon F, Chambon P (1977) Cold Spring Harbor Symp Quant Biol 42:1209-1234
5. Moen RC, Palmiter RD (1980) Developmental Biol 78:450-463
6. McKnight GS, Palmiter RD (1979) J Biol Chem 254:9050-9058
7. Renkawitz R, Beug H, Graf T, Matthias P, Grez M, Schütz G (1982) Cell 31: 167-176
8. Payvar F, DeFranco D, Firestone G, Edgar B, Wrange O, Okret, S, Gustafson JA, Yamamoto KR (1983) Cell:381-392
9. Scheidereit C, Beato M (1984) Proc Natl Acad Sci USA, in press
10. Karin M, Haslinger A, Holtgreve H, Richards RI, Krauter P, Westphal HM, Beato M (1984) Nature 308: 513-519
11. Renkawitz R, Schütz G, von der Ahe D, Beato M (1984) Cell 37:503-510
12. Mulvihill EP, LePennec JP, Chambon P (1982) Cell 24:621-632
13. Compton JG, Schrader WT, O'Malley BW (1983) Proc Natl Acad Sci USA 80:16-20
14. Hynes N, VanOoyen AJJ, Kennedy N, Herrlich P, Ponta H, Groner B (1983) Proc Natl Acad Sci USA 80:3637-3641
15. Buetti E, Diggelmann H (1983) EMBO J 2:1423-1429
16. Majors J, Varmus H (1983) Proc Natl Acad Sci USA 80:5866-5870
17. Chandler Vl, Maler BA, Yamamoto KR (1983) Cell 33:489-499
18. Dean DC, Knoll BJ, Riser ME, O'Malley BW (1983) Nature 305:551-554
19. Heilig R, Murakowsky R, Mandel JL (1982) J Mol Biol 156:1-19
20. Breathnach R, Mantei N, Chambon P (1980) Proc Natl Acad Sci USA 77:740-744
21. Dierich A, Gaub MP, Lepennec JP, Wasylyk, B, Chambon P, in preparation
22. Moreau P, Hen R, Wasylyk B, Everett R, Gaub MP, Chambon P, (1981) Nucleic Acids Res 9:6047-6068
23. Wasylyk B, Wasylyk C, Augereau P, Chambon P (1983) Cell 32:503-514
24. Hen R, Sassone-Corsi P, Corden J, Gaub MP, Chambon P (1982) Proc Natl Acad Sci USA 79:7132-7136
25. Sakiz E, Euvrard C, Baulieu EE (1984) In: Proceedings of the 7th International Congress of Endocrinology (Quebec-Canada) Elsevier, Amsterdam, in press.
26. Vignon F, Terqui M, Westley B, Derocq D, Rochefort H (1980) Endocrinology 106:1079-1086
27. Schrader WT (1984) Nature 308:17-18
28. Lazier CB (1978) Biochem J 174:143-152
29. Chambon P, Dierich A, Gaub MP, Jakowlev S, Jongstra J, Krust A, LePennec JP, Oudet P, Reudelhuber T (1984) In: Greep RO (ed) Recent Progress in Hormone Research. Academic Press, pp 1-42
30. Dunn TM, Han, S, Ogden S, Schleif RF (1984) Proc Natl Acad Sci USA, in press
31. Kaye JS, Bellard M, Dretzen G, Bellard F, Chambon P (1984) EMBO J 3:1137-1144

© 1984 Elsevier Science Publishers B.V.
Endocrinology
F. Labrie, L. Proulx, eds.

RECENT ADVANCES IN THE DIAGNOSIS AND TREATMENT OF PITUITARY DISEASE

LESLEY H. REES
Department of Chemical Endocrinology, St. Bartholomew's Hospital, London, EC1A 7BE, U.K.

INTRODUCTION

Since the last International Congress of Endocrinology, several major advances in neuroendocrinology and radiology have made a considerable impact in our understanding of a variety of pituitary diseases. In particular the discovery of growth hormone releasing hormone (GRH) and corticotrophin releasing factor (CRF) in conjunction with improvements in high resolution CAT scanning have broadened our understanding of hormone deficient states and suggested new therapeutic possibilities. Our increasing understanding of the role of endogenous opioids in pituitary regulation has implicated them in the pathogenesis of hyperprolactinaemic hypogonadism as well as in exercise induced amenorrhoea. Finally, studies on the abnormal processing of pro-opiomelanocortin (POMC) in pituitary disease, as well as the nature of the CRF complex provide fascinating insights into the control and nature of the products of the corticotroph in health and disease.

GRH

Growth hormone-releasing hormone (GRH) was recently isolated from two human pancreatic tumours in patients with acromegaly. The predominant activity in one tumour was related to a 44 residue peptide with smaller amounts of C-terminal shortened forms of 37 and 41 amino acids (1). Whilst in the other tumour only GRH 1-40 was identified (2). It is believed, based on immunocytochemical studies, that human hypothalamic GRH is similar to these peptides. Studies in normal subjects demonstrated that both GRH 1-40 and 1-44 were potent stimulators of GH release (3,4). It then became clear that in most patients with so-called 'isolated GH deficiency', as determined by insulin induced hypoglycaemia, that pituitary GH release could be achieved by GRH (4,5), which would be compatible with a functional defect either of GRH release or its availability. Further studies by Grossman and colleagues (6) comparing three analogues of GRH, demonstrated that the shorter peptide (GRH 1-29 NH_2) was equipotent with GRH 1-40. He also studied 20 children and young adults with growth hormone deficiency and observed that 8 showed a normal or only slightly impaired GH response to GRH. Two of these patients had hypothalamic tumours and the others 'idiopathic GH deficiency' or panhypopituitarism. Furthermore, studies in patients with prolactinomas previously treated by megavoltage radiotherapy who had developed GH deficiency, again revealed the ability of the pituitary to respond to exogenous GRH with GH release (7). These data, again point to a deficiency either in synthesis and/or delivery of endogenous GRH from the hypothalamus to the pituitary as a result of hypothalamo-pituitary irradiation. Despite the fact that megavoltage irradiation was delivered by a 3-field, isolated technique, with a field size rarely exceeding 4 x 4cm, the hypothalamus was inevitably irradiated.

These observations suggest that children with idiopathic GH deficiency as well as those who develop GH deficiency after radioatherapy for the treatment of intracranial tumours (8) may well benefit from long term administration of GRH.

CRF

Although the presence of a corticotrophin releasing factor (CRF) was demonstrated in the hypothalamus as long ago as 1955 it was not until 1981 that a CRF was finally characterised (9). This 41 residue peptide (CRF-41) was extracted from ovine hypothalami and observed to be a potent releaser of ACTH in rat (10) and man (11). Furthermore, Gibbs and Vale (12) demonstrated its release into rat portal blood at levels compatible with stimulation of ACTH release and its presence was also confirmed in rat and human hypothalamic neurones which terminate in the median eminence (13). Thus, CRF-41 satisfied most criteria for a physiological hypothalamic regulatory hormone.

The ACTH response to CRF-41 is inhibited by dexamethasone (14), suggesting that the site of negative feedback control of ACTH secretion is, at least in part at the pituitary level. In patients with hypothalamic and pituitary disorders the use of cortisol measurements during insulin induced hypoglycaemia tests the integrity of the entire hypothalamo-pituitary adrenal axis. For this to occur, endogenous CRF must be released in response to stress, hence releasing ACTH and cortisol. Studies in patients with pituitary and hypothalamic diseases and a normal response to insulin induced hypoglycaemia also showed a normal cortisol response to CRF-41, although interestingly the peak response was significantly less to 100μg CRF-41 than insulin-induced hypoglycaemia (14). Thus, hypoglycaemia provides a more prolonged ACTH stimulus than CRF-41, or it is possible that another ACTH hypothalamic regulating factor is secreted in addition to CRF-41, thus providing a more complex and more intensive stimulus (15).

Most patients with evidence of pituitary ACTH deficiency and absent ACTH responses to hypoglycaemia also show a normal cortisol response to CRF-41 including patients with pituitary tumours and suprasella extensions. Again, as with GRH and GH deficiency this suggests a functional impairment as a result of a defect in synthesis, release or transport of endogenous CRF. In a patient with idiopathic isolated ACTH deficiency, CRF-41 produced an adequate although delayed ACTH response, thus suggesting that the principle defect is hypothalamic <u>not</u>

pituitary and that the correct diagnosis is "isolated CRF deficiency" not ACTH deficiency.

In patients with untreated pituitary dependent Cushing's syndrome an excessive cortisol response to CRF-41 was observed in four out of five patients (14). Thus, this contrasts with the impaired action of CRF-41 observed in normal subjects after dexamethasone (14). Hence, in pituitary dependent Cushing's disease there is an impairment of the inhibitory control of ACTH secretion via corticosteroids which indeed may be the pathogenetic basis of this disorder. In patients with the ectopic ACTH syndrome, variable ACTH responses to CRF are observed and the hope that administration of CRF-41 will provide a test of value in the differential diagnosis of ACTH dependent Cushing's syndrome seems unlikely. Thus, CRF-41 has provided a safe test of pituitary ACTH reserve and although vasopressin probably acts in the same way, directly on the corticotroph, side-effects following its administration may be unpleasant so that non-specific 'stress' becomes a problem. As with GRF, CRF probably causes ACTH secretion from the readily released pool within the corticotroph.

Endogenous Opioids and Pituitary Function

Exogenous administration of opiates has been shown to inhibit both LH and FSH release in man and conversely naloxone, the opiate antagonist increases their secretion (16,17), probably by increasing the pulse frequency of LHRH release (18,19). It has been suggested that changes in endogenous opiate inhibition may be the factor controlling alterations in LH pulse frequency that occur during the menstrual cycle (20,21) as well as for menstrual irregularities that occur in women with hyperprolactinaemia. Furthermore it has been suggested that endogenous opioids might be involved in the regulation of appetite and body weight. Since low, non pulsatile levels of gonadotrophins are characteristic of anorexia nervosa (22), it has been postulated that excess opioid tone might suppress gonadotrophins in this condition (23). However, in a study by Grossman and colleagues (24) the infusion of naloxone into women suffering from weight related amenorrhoea failed to significantly alter their LH and FSH levels. This was in marked contrast to the effect observed in hyperprolactinaemic women where marked rises in LH and FSH occurred in all subjects. Prolactin levels did not change in either groups of subjects. Since the hypogonadism of hyperprolactinaemia is complex and involves not only direct inhibition of gonadal steroidogenesis but also a hypothalamic derangement of LHRH secretion, this latter component may be mediated via altered endogenous opioid tone in the hypothalamus. Likewise, endogenous opioids may be involved in the female hypogonadism associated with excessive exercise training. Since the latter is becoming increasingly popular in many countries for the prevention and treatment of disease, this constitutes an increasingly common problem. Regular strenous physical exercise can result in a number of menstrual disturbances including delay of menarche, amenorrhoea and inadequate luteal phase. As in anorexia, low levels of gonadotrophins are reported, although abnormal pulsatility and an exaggerated response to LHRH also occur (25). Furthermore, infusion of the opiate antagonist naloxone into amenorrhoeic runners can cause a striking increase in the amplitude of LH and FSH pulsation (25). Pronounced release of both β-endorphin and met-enkephalin have been shown to occur during treadmill exercise in a group of normal young American college females, not previously engaging in regular aerobic exercise (26). The release of β-endorphin is to be expected being secreted from the pituitary in response to the 'stress' of exercise. However, we have been unable to confirm the facilitation of its release with exercise training as previously reported. That met-enkephalin is released, albeit in a variable manner, is of considerable interest since exercise is the first known physiological stimulus known to cause alteration in peripheral enkephalin-secretion. Although the source of this peptide remains unclear secretion from the adrenal medulla, sympathetic nerve endings in the gut, decreased degradation or release of met-enkephalin from precursors circulating in plasma are all possibilities. Since opioid receptors in the median eminence of the hypothalamus, outside the blood brain barrier, are known to inhibit pulsatile LHRH release as discussed earlier, it is possible that the release of these opioids into plasma might play a part in the menstrual disturbances of exercise. However, other antigonadotrophic substances are also released during exercise including prolactin and melatonin.

Pro-opiomelanocortin (POMC) and Cushing's Syndrome

Difficulties still exist in establishing the cause of ACTH-dependent Cushing's syndrome and with the use of transsphenoidal surgery as the treatment of choice for pituitary Cushing's disease, exclusion of an occult ectopic source has become even more important. The majority of circulating ACTH in patients with pituitary dependent Cushing's disease comprises ACTH 1-39 whilst in patients with the ectopic ACTH syndrome a larger molecular size ACTH, approximate molecular weight 22,000 kilodaltons (22K) can be found in addition to ACTH 1-39 (27). Occasional patients with pituitary dependent Cushing's disease and large pituitary tumours exhibit clinical and biochemical characteristics of the ectopic ACTH syndrome, in particular profound hypokalaemic alkalosis. Extensive chromatographic characterisation of tumour tissue and plasma from such a patient (28) reveals the presence of a wide array of pro-opiocortin derived products including the normal products ACTH 1-39, N-terminal pro-opiocortin (N-POC) 1-76 as well as a peak of 6-10K ACTH and a heterogeneous peak containing both ACTH and γ-MSH immunoreactivity, indicating it to be the 22K pro-ACTH fragment of POMC after the cleavage of β-LPH. The chromatographic heterogeneity of the 22K fragment suggests variations in the degree of glycosylation of the fragment as

Concanavalin A affinity chromatography of the tumour extract indicates partial glycosylation of the 31K and 22K form. There is clear data suggesting that fragments of N-POC can cause potentiation of ACTH - induced steroidogenesis by adrenocortical cells. This has been demonstrated using the 16K fragment of N-POC and the synthetic peptide γ_3MSH, comprising residues 51-76 of tumour N-POC (29). Others demonstrated the potentiating effect of purified pituitary N-POC 1-76 on perfused isolated adrenal cells, and suggested that the effect is mediated through stimulation of mRNA synthesis (30). It is possible therefore, that such a potentiating effect of unusual N-POC/ACTH fragments might be involved in the appearance of hypokalaemia in patients with the ectopic ACTH syndrome. Since aldosterone levels are normal or low in this condition and marked increases in desoxycorticosterone (DOC) and corticosterone are reported (31) suggesting a partial 17-α-hydroxylase block, such a mechanism might be operative in certain pathological states such as the ectopic ACTH syndrome. Thus, secretion of large molecular weight forms of ACTH, or fragments of N-POC may cause potentiation of steroidogenesis and in conjunction with a 17-α-hydroxylase adrenal block might lead to abnormal mineralocorticoid and glucocorticoid affects and ultimately to hypokalaemia. However at the present time such thoughts must be still regarded as highly speculative.

CRF/Gastrin Releasing Peptide (GRP)

The remission of Cushing's syndrome after the removal of a medullary carcinoma of the thyroid which contained immunoreactive bombesin and very little ACTH had led to an investigation of the ACTH releasing properties of this peptide. The mammalian counterpart of this amphibian skin peptide is gastrin releasing peptide (GRP) (32). An acid extract of the tumour tissue caused ACTH release from isolated rat anterior pituitary cells *in vitro*. Large doses of synthetic C-terminal GRP, GRP(14-27) 10-1000ng/ml also caused ACTH release whereas much lower doses (10-1000pg/ml) were ineffective alone, but potentiated the CRF-41 mediated release of ACTH from the cells (33). The presence of bombesin-like immunoreactivity in the mammalian hypothalamus (34) and the identification of pituitary cell bombesin receptors (35) indicate a possible role for bombesin-like peptides in pituitary regulation. Since the hypothalamic factor responsible for the control of ACTH is a multifactoral complex and not a single substances (15) the possibility exists that GRP, the mammalian counterpart of amphibian bombesin is involved in the CRF complex.

ACKNOWLEDGEMENTS

I gratefully acknowledge the following members of the Chemical Endocrinology and Endocrinology departments at St. Bartholomew's Hospital whose data I have quoted from extensively. G.M. Besser, J.A.H. Wass, M.O. Savage, A. Grossman,

A. Hale, L. McLoughlin, T. Howlett, J. Price, S. Ratter, E. Penny, N. Lytras, J.F. Ackland and S. Tomlin. I also acknowledge with gratitude the collaboration of Dr. J. McArthur.

REFERENCES

1. Guillemin R, Brazeau P, Bohlen P, Esch F, Ling N, Wehrenberg WB (1982) Science 218:585-587
2. Rivier J, Spiess J, Thorner M, Vale W (1982) Nature 300:276-278
3. Thorner MO, Rivier J, Spiess J, Borges JL, Vance VL, Bloom SR, Rogol AD, Cronin MJ, Kaiser DL, Evens WS, Webster JD, MacLeod RM, Vale W (1983) Lancet i:24-28
4. Grossman A, Wass JAH, Sueiras-Diaz J, Savage M, Lytras N, Coy DH, Besser GM (1983) Lancet ii:137-138
5. Borges JLC, Blizzard RM, Gelato MC, Furlanetto R, Rogol AD, Evans WS, Vance ML, Kaiser DL, MacLeod RM, Merriam GR, Loriaux DL, Spiess J, Rivier J, Vale W, Thorner MO (1983) Lancet ii: 119-124.
6. Grossman A, Savage MO, Lytras N, Preece MA, Sueiras-Diaz J, Coy DH, Rees LH, Besser GM (1984) Clin Endoc in press
7. Grossman A, Lytras N. Savage MO, Wass JAH, Coy D, Rees LH, Jones AE, Besser GM (1984) Brit Med J 288:1785-1787
8. Shalet SM (1983) Clin Endoc 18:637-659
9. Vale W, Spiess J, Rivier C, Rivier J (1981) Science 213:1394-1397
10. Turkleson CM, Arimura A, Cullen MD, Fishback JB, Grout K, Kanda M, Lauciano M, Thomas CR, Chang D, Chang JK, Shimizu M (1981) Peptides 2:425-429
11. Grossman A, Nieuwenhuyzen Kruseman AC, Perry L, Tomlin S, Schally AV, Coy DH, Rees LH, Comaru-Schally AM, Besser GM (1982) Lancet i:921-922
12. Gibbs DM, Vale W (1982) Endocrinology 111:1418-1420
13. Paull WK, Scholer J, Arimura A, Meyers CA, Chang JK, Chang D, Shimuzu M (1982) Peptides 1:198-191
14 Lytras N, Grossman A, Perry L, Tomlin S, Wass JAH, Coy DH, Schally AV, Rees LH, Besser GM (1984) Clin Endo 20:71-84
15. Gillies GE, Linton EA, Lowry PJ (1982) Nature 299:355-357
16. Morley JE, Baranetsky NG, Wingert TD, Carlson HE, Hershman JM, Melmed S, Levin SR, Jamison KR, Wertzmann R, Chang RJ, Varner AA (1980) J Clin Endoc Metab 50:251-257
17. Grossman A, Moult PJA, Gaillard RC, Delitala G, Toff WD, Rees LH, Besser GM (1981) Clin Endoc 14:41-47
18. Moult PJA, Grossman A, Evans JM, Rees LH, Besser GM (1981) Clin Endoc 14: 321-324
19. Delitala G, Devilla L, Arata L (1981) Acta Endocrinologica 97:150-156
20. Quigley ME, Yen SSC (1981) J Clin Endoc Metab 51:179-180
21. Ropert JF, Quigley ME, Yen SSC (1981) J Clin Endoc Metab 52:583-585
22. Boyar RM, Katz J, Finkelstein JW, Kapen S, Weiner H, Weitzman ED (1974) New Eng J Med 291:86-805
23. Gillman MA, Lichtigfield FJ (1981) J Roy Soc Med 74:631

24. Grossman A, Moult PJA, McIntyre H, Evans J, Silvestone T, Rees LH, Besser GM, (1982) Clin Endoc 17:379-388

25. McArthur JW, Bullen BA, Bettins IZ, Pagane M, Badger TM, Klibanski A (1980) Endoc R Commun 7:13-25

26. Howlett TA, Tomlin S, Ngahfoong L, Rees LH, Bullen BA, Skrinar GS, McArthur JW (1984) Brit Med J in press

27. Ratter SJ, Lowry PJ, Besser GM, Rees LH (1980) J Endocr 85:359-369

28. Hale AC, Millar JGB, Ratter SJ, Pickard JD, Doniach I, Rees LH (1984) Clin Endoc in press

29. Pedersen RC, Brownie AC (1980) Proc Nat Acad Sci 77:2239-2243

30. Al-Dujaili EAS, Williams BC, Edwards CRW, Salacinski P, Lowry PJ (1982) J Biochem 204:301-305

31. Schambelan M, Slaton PEJ, Biglieri EG (1971) Am J Med 51:299-303

32. McDonald TJ, Jornvall N, Nilsson G, Vagne M, Ghatei M, Bloom SR, Mutt V (1979) Biochem Biophys Res Commun 90:227-233

33. Hale AC, Price J, Ackland JF, Doniach I, Ratter SJ, Besser GM, Rees LH (1984) J Endoc in press

34. Brown MR, Allen R, Villarreal J, Rivier J, Vale W (1978) Life Sci 23:2721-2728

35. Westendorf JM, Schonbrunn A (1983) J Biol Chem 258:7527-7535

© 1984 Elsevier Science Publishers B.V.
Endocrinology
F. Labrie, L. Proulx, eds.

HYBRIDIZATION HISTOCHEMISTRY

COGHLAN, J.P., ALDRED, P., BUTKUS, A., CRAWFORD, R.J., DARBY, I.A., FERNLEY, R.T., HARALAMBIDIS, J., HUDSON, P.J., MITRI,R., NIALL, H.D., PENSCHOW, J.D., ROCHE, P.J., SCANLON, D.B., AND TREGEAR, G.W.

Howard Florey Institute of Experimental Physiology & Medicine, University of Melbourne, Parkville, Australia

R. RICHARDS, BARBARA VAN LEEUWEN,

Australian National University, Canberra,

And

L. RALL, J. SCOTT, G. BELL,

Chiron Corporation, California

INTRODUCTION

A technique we have called hybridization histochemistry has been developed for the location of specific mRNA populations in specially prepared sections of tissue (1,2,3,4,5,6). Later the same approach has been used by others to identify specific neurones in the hypothalamus (7), to study the origin in fate of identified neurones in aphysia (8), location of specific genes in Dosophila embryos (9) and enkephalin in the adrenal (10).

The idea of using the property of base pairing between mRNA/DNA and DNA for tissue localization has been around for some time (3). Indeed in situ tissue hybridization or hybridization histochemistry is simply a logical extension of standard procedures used in molecular biology. HYBRIDIZATION HISTOCHEMISTRY is thus a procedure in which cells or tissue sections are treated so as to immobilize and protect the naturally occurring DNA or mRNA for in situ hybridization while at the same time retaining sufficient cellular morphology for accurate histological location.

MATERIALS AND METHODS

Tissue preparation, including whole animal sections; cDNA labelling and DNA synthesis and other detail have been described extensively elsewhere (1,3,6).

RESULTS AND DISCUSSION

There are certain problems in describing the results of hybridization histochemistry. Although the actual pictures are cardinal to any real appreciation of the technique, space constraints preclude the use of anymore than a few black and white examples here.

Under these circumstances it seems to us that the most realistic way of covering the lecture would be to provide an outline of the major issues, more than anything as an aide memoire.

The historical development of hybridization histochemistry has been reviewed in brief (3). From 1969 onwards, initial progress was slow even though suitable probes were available. ^{3}H or ^{125}I probes were used almost universally in the mistaken belief that other radioactive isotopes would give poor resolutions. This was not the only issue. It was very nearly impossible to establish this complex technique if the results would only be reviewed each 9 month period.

Thus, because there were so many methodological variables we decided to use ^{32}P so as to get "ideal conditions established as quickly as possible. In the event ^{32}P was not the disaster we expected. Appropriate conditions were established quickly, and with fast X-ray film the sections could be "previewed" after overnight exposure to determine the most appropriate exposure time for single coated fine grain X-ray film or emulsion. Examples were used to show that ^{32}P probes of calcitonin, and prolactin cDNA could give good resolution down to single cells with an exposure time of only 7 days or less compared to 3 months at least for tritium.

Rat relaxin cDNA was used to illustrate that the relaxin gene is expressed in the rat ovary at about day 9 of pregnancy, and that "turn off" immediately follows parturition. An important illustration that the technique can detect the "turn on" and "Turn off" of a gene. Human relaxin was shown to be present in the corpus luteum of the pregnant human ovary using human relaxin cDNA.

In collaboration with Chiron Corp. EGF cDNA was used to examine sections of whole mice revealing that the kidney in addition to the salivary gland was a major site where the EGF gene was expressed. At high magnification, examination of the mouse kidney showed that this labelling was in the straight distal tubule and early convoluted distal tubule. Immunoprecipitation studies however, showed that while the salivary gland was rich in EGF and pro-EGF, that EGF was in low concentrations or absent in the kidney. These findings indicated that while the gene for EGF was being expressed in the kidney, there was a high probability of altered processing. Interestingly enough, consistent with the above findings, the gene for EGF-binding protein (type 11) was not expressed at a detectable level when kidney sections were probed with a 30 mer synthetic oligonucleotide, although EGF-BP was being expressed at a high rate in the salivary gland.

cDNA for sheep renin was used to show that in sections of lamb kidney that the sites of renin production are multiple and as well as the modified myo-epithelial cells of the afferent arteriole (JGA) also include cells in the interlobular arteries and in the afferent arterioles distant from the JGA (Fig. 1). These findings confirm earlier EM studies of sheep kidney and establish that the granules reported in these sites remote from the JGA are most likely to be renin (11).

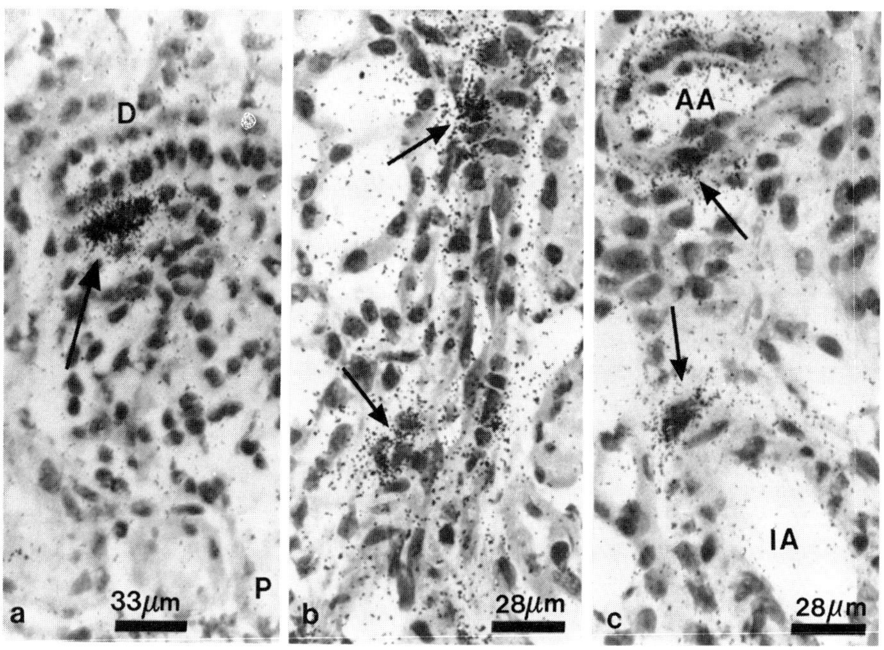

Fig. 1. Lamb kidney sections autoradiographed after hybridization histochemistry with 32P labelled sheep renin probe. (a) 300X Glomerulus with distal convoluted tubule (d) and proximal convoluted tubule (P). Labelling is confined to the afferent arteriole of the juxtaglomerular apparatus. (Arrowed). (b) 350X Segment of afferent arteriole in the renal cortex. Labelling is over smooth muscle cells in the vessel wall (Arrowed). (c) 350X Afferent arteriole (AA) and interlobular artery (IA) in the renal cortex. Renin probe labels cells in the smooth muscle layer of the vessel wall.

Kallikrein had been shown to be expressed in the convoluted distal tubule of the mouse kidney (3). Kallikrein was used to illustrate the use of the whole body sections for screening for sites of specific gene expression and to show that "short" 20 mer synthetic oligonucleotides are suitable - the use of shorter probes is not recommended because of inherent lack of specificity.

Synthetic DNA probes have considerable advantages over cDNA probes, some of which are worth reiterating here. Synthetic probes can be made in a few days. These synthetic probes are much easier to prepare and label in an ordinary laboratory, at once unshackling the technique from its dependence on a first rate biotechnology laboratory. Overall better and more consistent labelling of tissue is achieved because "unlimited" amounts of probes are available. Disadvantages of synthetic probes mainly relate to their "newness", in the sense that a great deal is yet to be learnt about their shelf life, stability in use, labelling and so forth.

A synthetic 30 mer probe for CRF was shown to label the paraventricular complex in brain sections of stressed sheep. This result had been predicted by immunocytochemical studies (12).

Synthetic DNA probes of 30 mer each were made for oxytocin and AVP from sequences from its non coding region. These were selected to have the maximum difference possible (77%) (13). In many hypothalamic serial sections of sheep brain it could be shown that cells which were labelled with AVP did not label with OT. Examples of the use of the 30 mer probe on sheep brain sections are shown in (Fig. 2). Preliminary studies in sheep, rats and the Brattleboro rat have shown high levels of expression of AVP which is not easily altered by physiological manipulation.

SUMMARY

Hybridization histochemistry is a technique to detect cells producing a specific mRNA in sections of functionally complex and morphologically heterogeneous tissues. The resolution even using ^{32}P labelled probes is at the single cell level. The adaption of tissue sections of whole animals for use with the technique allows a quick screening procedure for the anatomical sites where genes are expressed. The potential and widespread applicability of the technique has been improved vastly by the successful use of synthetic DNA. Thus Hybridization Histochemistry should have an important role complementary to existing techniques for evaluation of cell function and as a diagnostic tool.

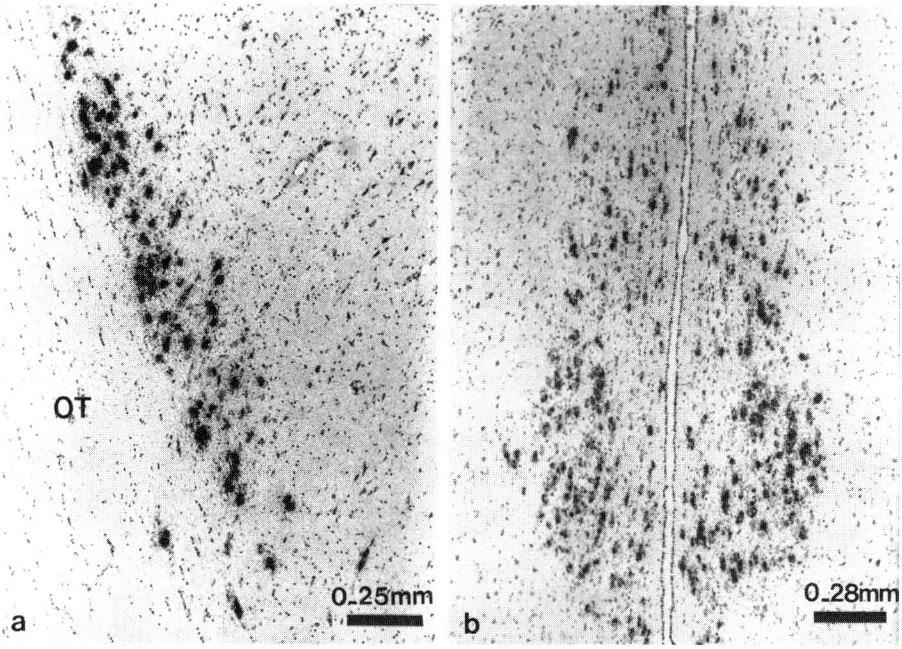

Fig. 2. Autoradiographs of 10μ frozen sections of sheep anterior hypothalamus with a ^{32}P-labelled synthetic oligodeoxyribonucleotide 30 mer in length corresponding to the amino acid sequence (-1 60 + 12) of bovine AVP-Np II.
a) Supraoptic nucleus showing dense labelling over neuronal cell bodies bordering the optic tract (OT). b) Magnocellular neurones of the paraventricular nucleus adjacent to the 3rd ventricle (centre field) are labelling.

ACKNOWLEDGEMENTS

Mr. Bruce Thorley and Ms. Janice Turton provided invaluable assistance with probe labelling and synthesis; Dr. Jack Jacobs of Department of Medicine, University of Texas, provided calcitonin cDNA; Dr. John Shine of the Australian National University, Canberra, now Californian Biotechnology, California, provided m renin cDNA, r growth hormone, mPOMC cDNA's; and prolactin cDNA. Dr. J. Fiddes of Californian Biotechnology, provided h CG cDNA, and Dr. Pierre Corvol, Pathologie Vasculaire et Endocrinologie Renal, INSERM 36 and Dr. Francis Rougeon, Unite Genetique and Biochimie Institute Pasteur, provided a m renin cDNA clone which was instrumental in our obtaining sheep renin cDNA. Although all these probes are not mentioned in the above text they provided crucial data for the oral presentation and are mentioned here as a grateful acknowledgement of generous collaboration.

This work was supported by grants-in-aid from the National health and Medical Research Council of Australia; the Myer Family Trusts; the Ian Potter Foundation; the Howard Florey Biomedical Foundation (USA).

REFERENCES

1. Hudson, P.J., Penschow, J.D., Shine, J., Ryan, G., Niall, H.D. and Coghlan, J.P. (1980) Hybridization Histochemistry. Proc. Endocrine Soc. of Aust., 23: 22

2. Coghlan, J.P., Butkus, A., Hudson, P.J., Niall, H.D., Penschow, J.D., Shine, J., Ryan, G. and Walsh, J. (1981) Hybridization Histochemistry: Use of Recombinant DNA as a "homing probe" for tissue localization of specific mRNA populations. Proc. Aust. Endo. Soc., 24: 58

3. Coghlan, J.P., Penschow, J.D., Hudson, P.J. and Niall, H.D. (1984) Hybridization Histochemistry: Use of Recombinant DNA for tissue localization of specific mRNA populations, Clin. and Exp. Hypertension, A2, 63-78

4. Hudson, P.J., Penschow, J.D., Shine, J., Ryan, G., Niall, H.D. and Coghlan, J.P. (1981) Hybridization Histochemistry: Use of Recombinant DNA as a "homing probe" for tissue localization of specific mRNA populations. Endocrinology, 108: 353-356

5. Jacobs, J.W., Simpson, E., Penschow, J.D., Hudson, P.J., Coghlan, J.P. and Niall, H.D. (1983) Characterization and localization of calcitonin mRNA in rat thyroid. Endocrinology, 113: 1616-1622

6. Coghlan, J.P., Penschow, J.D., Tregear, G.W. and Niall, H.D. Hybridization Histochemistry: Use of complementary DNA for tissue localization of specific mRNA populations, Receptors, membranes and Transport Mechanisms in Medicine, Mendelsohn, F. (ed) Excerpta Medica, in press.

7. Gee, C.E., Chen, C.L.C., Roberts, R.L., Thompson, R. and Watson, S.J. (1983) Identification of propiomelanacortin neurones in rat hypothalamus. Nature (Lond.) 306: 374-376

8. McAllister, L.B., Schiller, R.H., Kandel, E.R. and Richard, A. (1983) In situ hybridization to study the origin and fate of identified neurones. Science, 222: 800-808

9. McGinnis, W., Levine, C.H.S., Hafen, E., Kurowa and W.J. Gehring (1984) A conserved DNA sequence in homoeotic genes of the Drosophila Antennapedia and bithorax complexes. Nature 308: 428-433

10. Block, B., Milner, J.R., Baird, A., Gubber, W., Raymond, C., Bohlen, P., Le Guellec, D. and Bloom, F.E. (1984) Detection of mRNA coding for preproenkephalin-A in bovine adrenal by in situ hybridization. Regulatory Peptides, in press

11. Hill, P.A., Coghlan, J.P., McDougall, J.G. and Ryan, G.B. (1983) Structural studies of the adrenal zona glomerulosa and renal juxtaglomerular apparatus in pregnant sheep. Cell & Tissue Res. 232: 177-187

12. Paull, W.K., Scholer, J., Arimura, A., Myers, C.A., Chang, J.D., Chang, D. and Stimiza, M. (1982) Immunocytochemical localization of CRF in the ovine hypothalamus. Peptides, 1: 183-191

13. Land, H., Grez, M., Ruppert, S., Schmale, H., Rehbein, M., Richter, D., Schutz, G. (1983) Deduced amino acid sequence from the bovine oxytocin-neurophysin I precursor cDNA. Nature (Lond.), 302 (5906): 342-4

Endocrinology
F. Labrie, L. Proulx, eds.

PULSATILE GONADOTROPIN-RELEASING HORMONE (GnRH) - STUDIES OF PUBERTY AND THE MENSTRUAL CYCLE

J.C. MARSHALL, R.P. KELCH, S.E. SAUDER, A. BARKAN, N.E. REAME, S. KHOURY

Divisions of Endocrinology, Departments of Internal Medicine and Pediatrics, University of Michigan, Ann Arbor, MI 48109, USA.

INTRODUCTION

The hypothalamic-pituitary-gonadal axis is functional in the fetus, but GnRH secretion is suppressed in prepubertal children and the onset of puberty is related to increased secretion of GnRH. With the onset of pubertal maturation, gonadotropin secretion is pulsatile (1) suggesting an intermittent pituitary stimulus by hypothalamic GnRH. In addition, the pattern of gonadotropin responses to exogenous GnRH changes during maturation and the initially greater FSH response seen in prepubertal girls diminishes with LH secretion becoming predominant. During the follicular phase of the menstrual cycle, a similar pattern with an initially higher FSH and subsequently higher LH is seen in plasma. In these studies we aimed to determine 1.) whether GnRH secretion is pulsatile in prepubertal children - if so, the onset of puberty would result from augmentation of a pre-existing pulsatile release pattern; 2.) are the changing patterns of FSH and LH responses to GnRH seen during puberty and the menstrual cycle consistent with the effects of a single GnRH; and 3.) is the pulsatile pattern of GnRH secretion important in determining gonadotropin secretion in women, and do changes in GnRH pulse frequency play a role in regulating normal menstrual cyclicity.

METHODS AND SUBJECTS STUDIED

Basal patterns of LH and FSH secretion were measured in blood samples obtained at 10-20 min. intervals over 12-24 hrs. Studies were performed in prepubertal children, patients with isolated GnRH deficiency, and normal women.

Synthetic GnRH was given to subjects in a manner aimed to mimic physiological secretion of GnRH. In these studies we used GnRH in a dose of 25 ng/kg given intravenously every two hours. This regimen produced peak serum GnRH concentrations of approximately 200 pg/ml, which is similar to measured values in pituitary portal blood in animal studies. In addition, in early pubertal children, LH responses to this dose of GnRH during the day were similar to spontaneous nocturnal LH pulses (Fig. 1). This suggests that this dosage of GnRH provides a physiological stimulus to the pituitary (2).

Acknowledgements:
Our thanks are due to the nursing staff of the Clinical Research Center at the University of Michigan for their invaluable help with the clinical studies; to M. Markovs of the Endocrine Laboratory for hormonal assays and to C. Grant for typing the manuscript.

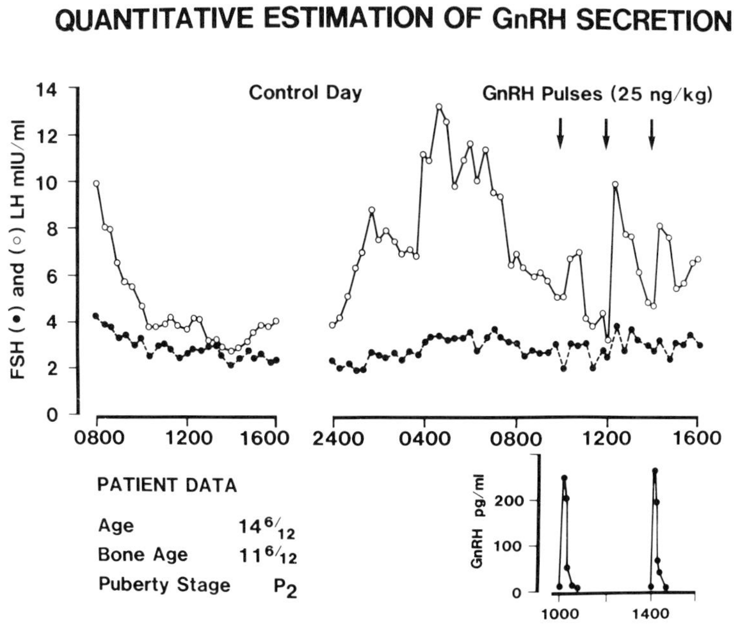

Figure 1. Three pulse injections of GnRH were given during the day to a subject in early puberty. LH responses are comparable to spontaneous nocturnal LH pulses.

RESULTS AND DISCUSSION

1. Studies to determine whether GnRH secretion is pulsatile in prepubertal children;- basal LH and FSH levels measured during the day are low in prepubertal children and the detection limits of the assays preclude assessment of pulsatile secretion. We administered pulsatile GnRH to prepubertal children for four days as a means of augmenting pituitary responsiveness to GnRH. Data from one subject are shown in Fig. 2, and reveal augmentation of LH and FSH secretion following GnRH with evidence of spontaneous pulsatile gonadotropin secretion being present. These data show that GnRH is secreted in an intermittent manner prior to puberty and suggests that puberty results from augmentation of a pre-existing pulsatile mode of GnRH release.

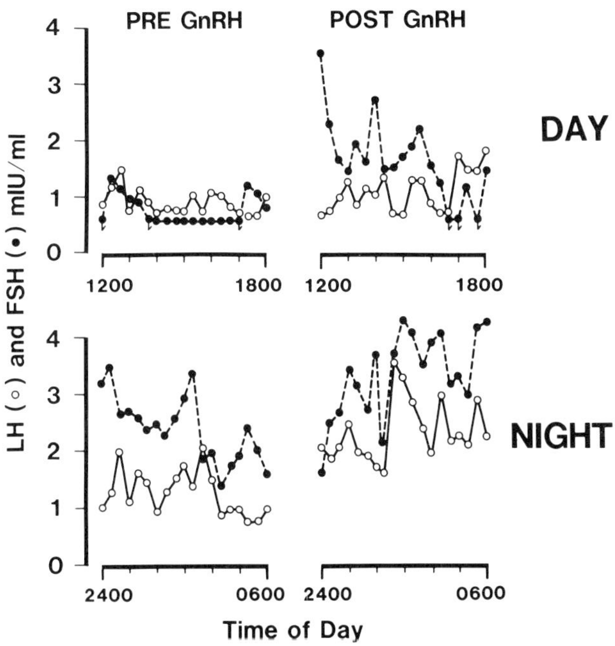

Figure 2. LH and FSH was measured in samples obtained before and after GnRH pulses (25 ng/kg every 2 hrs. for four days). The post GnRH data revealed spontaneous LH and FSH pulsatile secretion during day and pulses are augmented during sleep.

2. Studies to determine the etiology of the changing pattern of gonadotropin responses to GnRH during puberty; - we administered pulsatile GnRH to GnRH deficient women (anorexia nervosa at low body weight and isolated gonadotropin deficiency) to assess the progressive FSH and LH responses to GnRH. Results from two such studies are shown in Fig. 3. Similar response patterns are seen in all patients with GnRH deficiency. The absence of spontaneous GnRH secretion is seen by the lack of pulsatile LH secretion on Day 0. Administration of GnRH elicits release of FSH and LH and the FSH response is greater during the first two days. Thereafter, FSH responses decline as LH responsiveness increases. This pattern of responses is similar to that observed during normal puberty. The decline in FSH occurred when estradiol levels were rising and suggested that FSH responses were inhibited by estradiol.

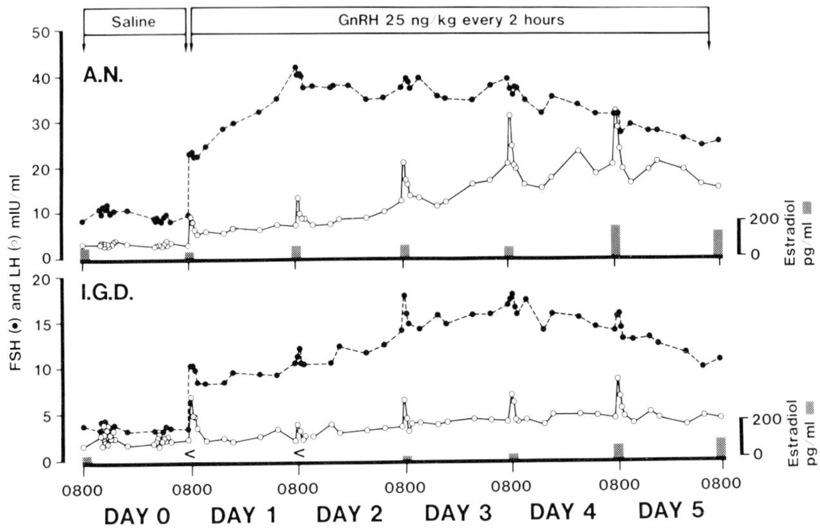

Figure 3. Serum LH, FSH, and estradiol responses to pulsatile GnRH in a patient with anorexia nervosa at low body weight (AN) and in a patient with isolated gonadotropin deficiency (IGD). Data are from samples drawn before GnRH injections and acute responses to the 0800 h GnRH injections are also shown.

In other studies we administered GnRH pulses to GnRH deficient patients, both before and after replacement with estradiol. FSH responses were abolished in the presence of estradiol, while LH responses were only slightly impaired (3). These data show that estradiol selectively inhibits FSH responses to GnRH and estradiol concentrations of 75 pg/ml or higher are effective in reducing FSH secretion. Thus the patterns of FSH and LH responses during pubertal maturation are compatible with the effects of GnRH in the presence of different serum concentrations of estradiol.

3. Assessment of pulsatile GnRH secretion in normal women and the role of GnRH pulse frequency in regulation of the menstrual cycle; - Prolonged administration of pulsatile GnRH injections to GnRH deficient women produces changes in serum FSH and LH which mimic those seen during the follicular phase of the menstrual cycle (4,5). The initial response is one of FSH secretion which declines as serum estradiol rises with follicular maturation. A mid-cycle LH surge occurs in response to the positive feedback effect of estradiol on LH responses to GnRH. Ovulation does not always occur however, suggesting

that the 25 ng/kg dose given every 2 hrs. may not accurately reflect normal GnRH secretion. When GnRH pulses are given to women who have spontaneous pulsatile LH release (and by inference GnRH secretion) the initial FSH response does not occur and follicular development is not seen. Thus pulsatile GnRH produces follicular maturation in GnRH deficient women, and this together with the lack of effect in women with spontaneous GnRH secretion suggests that GnRH secretion has to be reduced or absent, or that serum estradiol has to be low, before pulsatile GnRH injections will induce predominant FSH secretion. To provide data on the patterns of GnRH secretion in normal women, we studied hormonal patterns at different phases of the same ovulatory menstrual cycle in eight normal women. The pattern of response in one woman is shown in Fig. 4 and mean data for the group in Fig. 5.

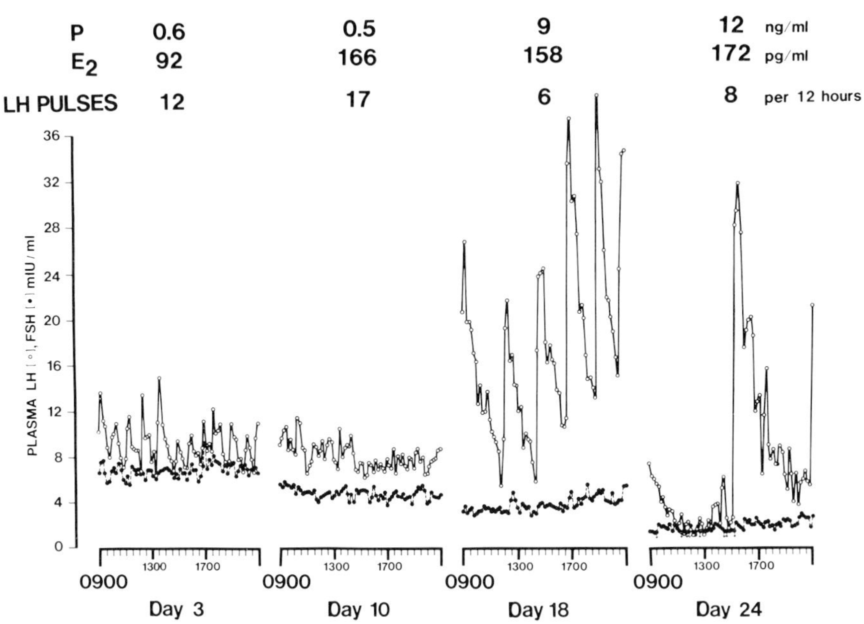

Figure 4. Plasma LH, FSH, estradiol and progesterone during an ovulatory menstrual cycle. Samples were drawn at 10 min. intervals for 12 hrs. on Days 3, 10, 18, and 24 of the cycle.

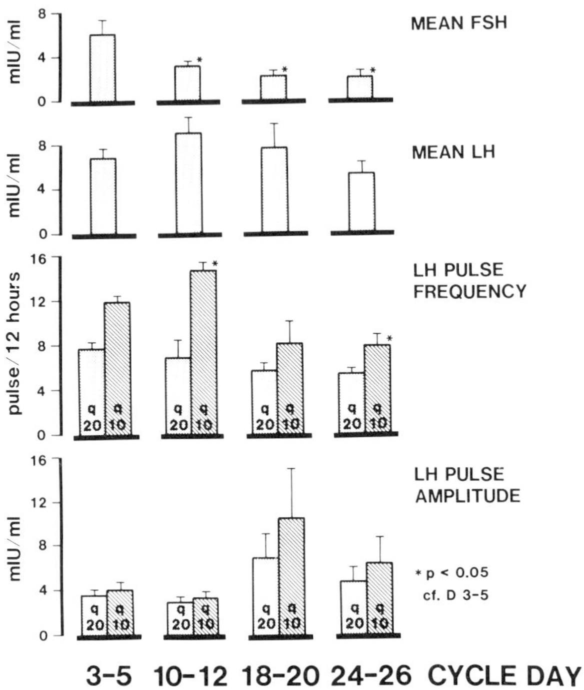

Figure 5. Gonadotropin secretion during eight ovulatory cycles in normal women. Data are from samples drawn every 20 min. for 24 hrs. (q 20) or every 10 min. for 12 hrs. (q 10).

These results show that plasma FSH is decreased when estradiol is elevated and that LH concentrations are unchanged during the cycle. LH pulse frequency increased from 12 to 15.5 pulses/12 hrs. during the follicular phase and decreased to eight pulses/12 hrs. in the luteal phase. LH pulses were regular in frequency and amplitude during the follicular phase but showed marked irregularity in the luteal phase. These data suggest that the initial FSH stimulus is essential for follicular maturation and thereafter FSH release is suppressed by estradiol. The irregular and infrequent LH pulses occur only during the luteal phase and suggest that progesterone acts at the hypothalamus to produce a slow and irregular pattern of GnRH release. These observations have suggested a hypothesis for regulation of the hormonal changes during the menstrual cycle which is outlined in Fig. 6.

Luteal Phase

↑ **Estradiol – Inhibits FSH release**
Progesterone – ↓ GnRH pulse frequency and LH synthesis

↓ **Estradiol – Allows FSH release**
Progesterone – ↑ GnRH pulse frequency

↑ FSH initiates the next cycle

Figure 6. Hypothesis for the role of luteal phase ovarian steroids and changes in GnRH pulse frequency in the initiation of the menstrual cycle.

This hypothesis is supported by other data obtained in GnRH deficient women given pulsatile GnRH. If responses to a single GnRH bolus are observed after stopping pulsatile GnRH, LH responses decline and are less than those of FSH after 14 to 16 days. This suggests that a regular GnRH stimulus is required to maintain LH synthesis and suggests that the reduced GnRH secretion in the luteal phase may impair LH but not FSH synthesis by the pituitary. Also, GnRH pulses produce regular, one-on-one LH responses, in GnRH deficient women pretreated with estradiol and progesterone to mimic luteal phase concentrations. Thus the irregular pulses seen during the luteal phase appear to reflect GnRH secretion. The suggested role of GnRH pulsatile secretion in the normal menstrual cycle is shown in Fig. 7. During the follicular phase GnRH pulse frequency increases and the higher frequency, together with the positive effect of estradiol in an augmenting LH responses to GnRH results in the mid cycle LH surge. After ovulation, FSH responses to GnRH are suppressed by estradiol and the elevated progesterone produces irregular patterns of GnRH secretion. The intermittent release of LH and reduced LH synthesis, leads to depletion of pituitary LH stores.

With the decline of the corpus luteum GnRH pulse frequency increases and the fall in estradiol allows secretion of FSH which initiates the next cycle of follicular maturation. The ability to change GnRH pulse frequency may therefore be important in maintaining normal menstrual cyclicity.

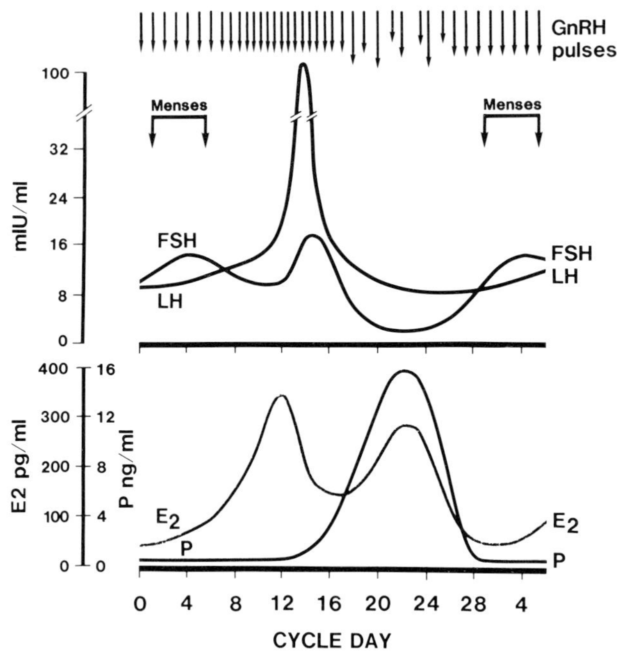

Figure 7. Suggested role of pulsatile GnRH secretion in regulation of the menstrual cycle.

REFERENCES

1. Boyar, RM, Katz J, Finkelstein JW, Kapen S, Weiner H, Weitzman ED, and Hellman L. N. Engl. J. Med. 291:861, 1974.
2. Corley KP, Valk TW, Kelch RP, and Marshall JC. Pediatric Res. 15:157, 1981.
3. Marshall JC, Case GD, Valk TW, Corley KP, Sauder SE, and Kelch RP. J. Clin. Invest. 71:243, 1983.
4. Crowley WF and McArthur JD. J. Clin. Endocrinol. Metab. 51:173, 1980.
5. Valk TW, Marshall, JC, and Kelch RP. Am. J. Obstet. Gynecol. 141:842, 1981.

© 1984 Elsevier Science Publishers B.V.
Endocrinology
F. Labrie, L. Proulx, eds.

MEMBRANE PHOSPHOLIPIDES AND THE MECHANISM OF ACTION OF HORMONES

YASUTOMI NISHIZUKA

Department of Biochemistry, Kobe University School of Medicine, Kobe 650, and Department of Cell Biology, National Institute for Basic Biology, Okazaki 444, Japan

SUMMARY

Information of various hormones, neurotransmitters, growth factors and many other biologically active substances appears to flow from the cell surface into the cell interior through two routes, Ca^{2+} mobilization and protein kinase C activation. Both routes are normally opened by a single ligand-receptor interaction, and act synergistically to elicit full cellular responses such as secretion and exocytosis, and growth promotion. The signal-induced breakdown of inositol phospholipids, particularly phosphatidylinositol bisphosphate is a key event for initiating these processes.

INTRODUCTION

The biochemical basis of the transduction of extracellular signals into intracellular events has been a subject of great interest. Recently, much attention has been paid to the role of inositol phospholipid turnover that is frequently observed immediately after the stimulation of cell surface receptors. This phospholipid turn-

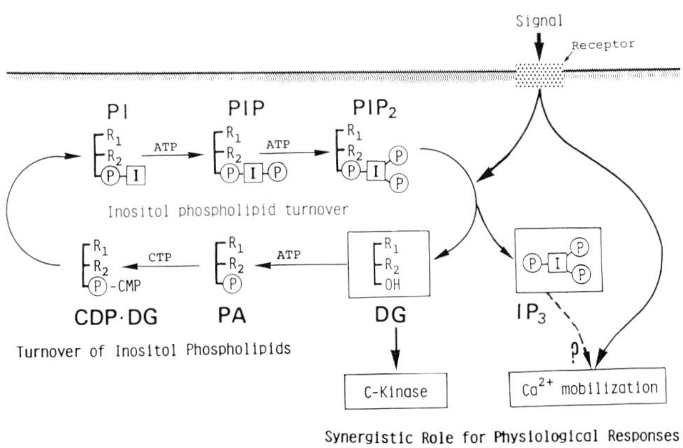

Fig. 1. Inositol phospholipid turnover and signal transduction. PI, phosphatidylinositol; PIP, phosphatidylinositol 4-phosphate; PIP_2, phosphatidylinositol 4,5-bisphosphate; DG, 1,2-diacylglycerol; PA, phosphatidic acid; CDP-PA, CDP-phosphatidic acid; IP_3, inositol 1,4,5-trisphosphate; I, inositol moiety; P, phosphoryl group; C-Kinase, protein kinase C.

over is usually associated with Ca^{2+} mobilization. Initially, phosphatidylinositol (PI) was regarded as the prime target, but recent evidence suggests that phosphatidylinositol bisphosphate (PIP_2) rather than PI is broken more rapidly upon stimulation of receptors (1,2). Diacylglycerol, one of the earliest products of this reaction, is found in this laboratory to serve as the activator of a unique protein kinase that we call protein kinase C. This article will briefly describe the evidence for this enzyme activation and for the importance of that activation for subsequent cellular responses. It will be also described that the activation of cellular functions by this route is separate from and synergistic to that induced by an increase in the intracellular Ca^{2+} (Fig. 1). More recently, inositol 1,4,5-trisphosphate, the other product of PIP_2 hydrolysis is proposed to be a mediator for Ca^{2+} mobilization from the intracellular reservoir (3). Some aspects of protein kinase C have been reviewed elsewhere (4,5).

ACTIVATION OF PROTEIN KINASE C

Protein kinase C absolutely requires Ca^{2+} and phospholipid for its activation. At a physiological concentration of Ca^{2+}, protein kinase C requires diacylglycerol in addition to phospholipid for its activation. Diacylglycerol is normally almost absent from membranes, but is transiently produced from inositol phospholipids in a signal-dependent manner. Kinetically, a small quantity of diacylglycerol dramatically increases the affinity of this protein kinase C for Ca^{2+}, and renders it fully active without a net increase in the Ca^{2+} concentration (6). Evidence to support this view has primarily come from a series of experiments with platelets. When platelets are stimulated by thrombin or collagen, two endogenous proteins having molecular weights of 40,000 (40K protein) and 20,000 (20K protein) are rapidly phosphorylated, and the phosphorylation of these proteins is associated with release reactions (7-9). The 20K protein is myosin light chain, and the calmodulin-dependent phosphorylation of this protein requires mobilization of Ca^{2+} (10). On the other hand, the 40K protein is shown to serve as a substrate specific to protein kinase C, and the signal-induced formation of endogenous diacylglycerol always accompanies the 40K protein phosphorylation (11). Tumor-promoting phorbol esters such as 12-O-tetradecanoyl-phorbol-13-acetate (TPA) and phorbol-12,13-dibutyrate can substitute for diacylglycerol and directly activate protein kinase C in the presence of Ca^{2+} and phospholipid (12).

In cell-free systems various diacylglycerols are equally capable of activating protein kinase C. While, in intact cell systems diacylglycerols having two long fatty acids such as diolein are unable to be intercalated into the membrane. If, however, one long fatty acid is replaced by acetyl group, then the resulting diacylglycerol, 1-oleoyl-2-acetyl-glycerol, obtains detergent-like properties, and can be dispersed into the phospholipid bilayer to activate protein kinase C directly (13,14). In fact, in platelets, this synthetic diacylglycerol induces rapid phosphorylation of 40K protein just as it is observed after stimulation by natural extracellular messengers such as thrombin (Fig. 2). Under the same conditions neither the breakdown of inositol phospholipids nor the formation of endogenous diacylglycerol is observed. The fingerprint analysis of tryptic phosphopeptides of the radioactive 40K protein preparations confirms that protein kinase C is indeed activated. Similar results are obtained with TPA instead of synthetic diacylglycerol (12,15). Thus, it may be concluded that, in platelets, the receptor-mediated breakdown of inositol phospho-

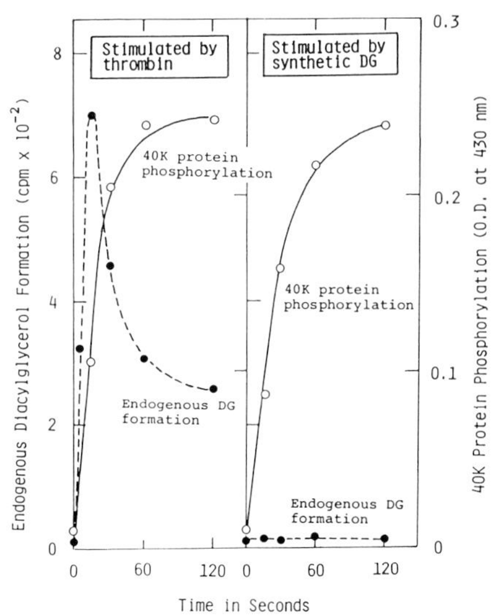

Fig. 2. Direct activation of protein kinase C in intact platelets by synthetic diacylglycerol. Human platelets were labeled with either ^{32}Pi of [^{3}H]arachidonic acid, and then stimulated by thrombin or 1-oleoyl-2-acetyl-glycerol as indicated. The phosphorylation of 40K protein and formation of endogenous radioactive diacylglycerol were determined after various time intervals as described elsewhere (14).

lipids is directly linked with activation of protein kinase C, and that synthetic diacylglycerol as well as tumor-promoting phorbol ester can be used for intact cells to activate this protein kinase directly. It is worth noting that either synthetic diacylglycerol or TPA does not mobilize Ca^{2+}.

SYNERGISTIC ACTION OF PROTEIN KINASE C AND Ca^{2+} FOR RELEASE REACTIONS

The stimulation of receptors which provoke inositol phospholipid breakdown generally mobilizes Ca^{2+}. Experiements with synthetic diacylglycerol and TPA indicate that the activation of protein kinase C alone is a prerequisite and not a complete requirement for causing full physiological cellular responses. Under appropriate conditions, it is possible to induce protein kinase C activation and Ca^{2+} mobilization independently by the addition of synthetic diacylglycerol or phorbol ester for the former, and Ca^{2+} ionophore such as A23187 for the latter (Fig. 3). Platelets are particularly suited for the demonstration because these two events may be selectively quantitated by measuring the phosphorylation of the 40K and 20K proteins mentioned above. By using these procedures it is shown that both protein kinase C activation and Ca^{2+} mobilization are essential and act synergistically to cause full release of serotonin (13,14). The phosphorylation of 40K protein induced by synthetic diacylglycerol is not enhanced further by the addition of A23187, while the overall response of platelets is insufficient by the addition of diacylglycerol alone, and the full platelet response may be observed in the simultaneous presence of diacylglycerol and A23187 (Fig. 4). The Ca^{2+} ionophore alone at the concentration

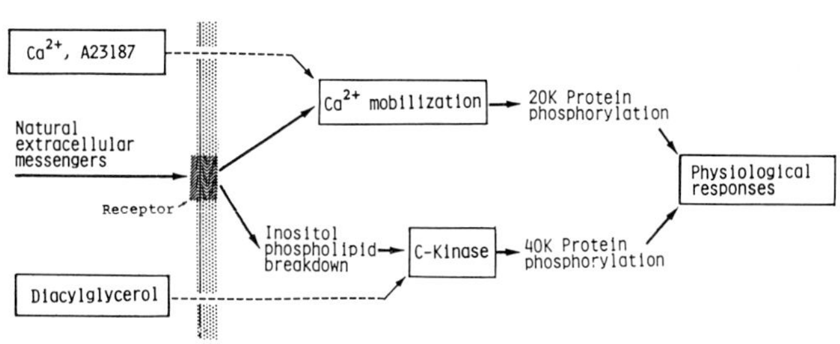

Fig. 3. Synergistic action of Ca^{2+} mobilization and protein kinase C activation for physiological responses. Ca^{2+}-mobilization and protein kinase C activation can be selectively induced by Ca^{2+} ionophore and synthetic diacylglycerol, respectively. C-Kinase, protein kinase C.

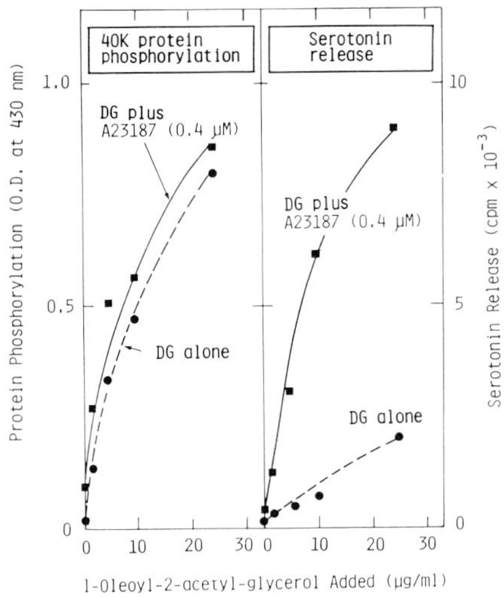

Fig. 4. Effects of synthetic diacylglycerol and Ca^{2+} ionophore on protein kinase C activation and serotonin release. Protein kinase C activation was assayed by measuring the phosphorylation of 40K protein in intact platelets. Detailed conditions were described elsewhere (14). DG, diacylglycerol.

employed shows practically no effect. Similar results are obtained with TPA instead of diacylglycerol (15).

The synergistic effect of synthetic diacylglycerol and Ca^{2+} ionophore is not confined to the serotonin release from platelets but extended to the lysosomal enzyme release from platelets as well as from neutrophils (16), and also to the histamine release from mast cells (17). More recently, this proposal has been supported by the demonstration of similar synergism for several other systems, such as epinephrine secretion from adrenal medullary cells (18), aldosterone secretion from adrenal glomerulosa cells (19), insulin release from pancreatic islets (20), amylase secretion from pancreatic acinar cells (21), and acetylcholine release from the cholinergic nerve endings of ileum (22). It is plausible that the two routes mentioned above are crucially important for the release reactions in a variety of cell types.

SYNERGISTIC ACTION OF PROTEIN KINASE C AND Ca^{2+} FOR GROWTH RESPONSE

Stimulation of the receptors that induce inositol phospholipid breakdown often causes cellular proliferation and differentiation. Protein kinase C appears to be a receptor protein of tumor-promoting

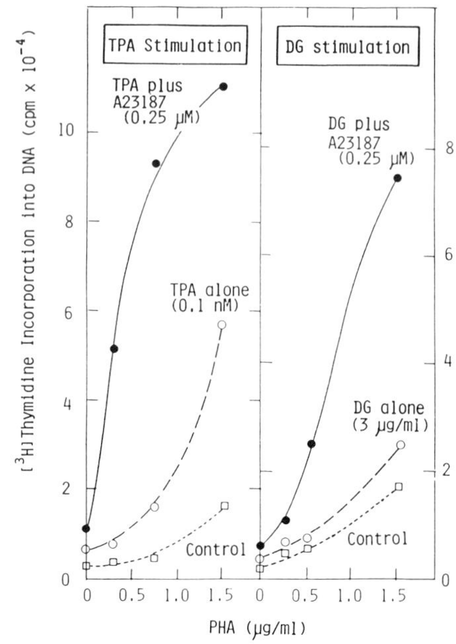

Fig. 5. Effects of Ca^{2+} ionophore and TPA or synthetic diacylglycerol on thymidine incorporation into DNA in human peripheral lymphocytes. Macrophage-depleted peripheral lymphocytes were incubated for 72 hours with phytohemagglutinin in the presence or absence of A23187, TPA, and synthetic diacylglycerol as indicated. [^{3}H-methyl]thymidine was added 16 hours before harvesting. Detailed conditions were described elsewhere (23).

phorbol esters, and many of the pleiotropic actions of the tumor promoter are most likely to be mediated through the action of this enzyme (5). Several mitogens and growth factors such as epidermal growth factor may induce rapid turnover of inositol phospholipids in their target tissues.

Macrophage-depleted peripheral lymphocytes are incubated with A23187 and either synthetic diacylglycerol or TPA in the presence of various concentrations of phytohemagglutinin. Then, the radioactive thymidine that is incorporated into DNA is determined by using a conventional procedure. It is found that either synthetic diacylglycerol or TPA alone is not sufficient, and that the supplement of A23187 may be necessary for causing a rapid incorporation of thymidine into DNA (23) (Fig. 5). The Ca^{2+} ionophore alone shows no effect under the given conditions. The results suggest that protein kinase C activation and Ca^{2+} mobilization may play synergistic roles in phytohemagglutinin-induced proliferation of the peripheral lymphocytes. It is noted that under these conditions at least three soluble proteins having molecular weights of about 82,000, 56,000 and 45,000, and one particulate protein having a molecular weight of 68,000 are phosphorylated in the stimulated lymphocytes, and that all these proteins serve as preferable substrates for a purified preparation of protein kinase C.

CONCLUSION

The experimental results outlined above have been obtained from the studies with limited number of limited tissues. Nevertheless, it is attractive to imagine that protein kinase C plays a crucial role in signal transduction for the activation of cellular functions and proliferation. The evidence thus far available suggests that either the receptor-linked activation of protein kinase C or Ca^{2+} mobilization alone is not sufficient for complete signal transduction, and that their synergistic actions are necessary for the transmembrane control of various cellular processes. Obviously, both Ca^{2+} and protein kinase C may play diverse roles in the biological regulation, and the precise targets of protein kinase C will be clarified by further investigations.

ACKNOWLEDGEMENT

This investivation has been supported in part by research grants from the Research Fund of the Ministry of Education, Science and Culture, the Intractable Diseases Division, Public Health Bureasu, the Ministry of Health and Welfare, a grant-in-aid of New Drug Development from the Ministry of Health and Welfare, and by the Special Coordination Funds from the Science and Technology Agency, Japan.

REFERENCES

1. Downes CP, Michell RH (1982) Cell Calcium 3:467-502
2. Berridge MJ, Dawson RMC, Downes CP, Heslop JP, Irvine RF (1983) Biochem J 212:473-482
3. Streb H, Irvine RF, Berridge MJ, Schulz I (1983) Nature 306:67-69
4. Nishizuka Y, Takai Y, Kishimoto A, Kikkawa U, Kaibuchi K. (1984) Recent Prog Horm Res 40:301-345
5. Nishizuka Y (1984) Nature 308:693-697
6. Kishimoto A, Takai Y, Mori T, Kikkawa U, Nishizuka Y (1980) J Biol Chem 255:2273-2276

7. Lyons RM, Stanford N, Majerus PW (1975) J Clin Invest 56:924-936

8. Haslam RJ, Lynham, JA (1977) Biochem Biophys Res Commun 77:714-722

9. Kawahara Y, Takai Y, Minakuchi R, Sano K, Nishizuka Y (1980) Biochem Biophys Res Commun 97:309-317

10. Hathaway DR, Adelstein RS (1979) Proc Natl Acad Sci 76:1653-1657

11. Sano K, Takai Y, Yamanishi J, Nishizuka Y (1983) 258:2010-2013

12. Castagna M, Takai Y, Kaibuchi K, Sano K, Kikkawa U, Nishizuka Y (1982) J Biol Chem 257:7847-7851

13. Kaibuchi K, Sano K, Hoshijima M, Takai Y, Nishizuka Y (1982) Cell Calcium 3:323-335

14. Kaibuchi K, Takai Y, Sawamura M, Hoshijima M, Fujikura T, Nishizuka Y (1983) J Biol Chem 258:6701-6704

15. Yamanishi J, Takai Y, Kaibuchi K, Sano K, Castagna M, Nishizuka Y (1983) Biochem Biophys Res Commun 112:778-786

16. Kajikawa N, Kaibuchi K, Matsubara T, Kikkawa U, Takai Y, Nishizuka Y, Itoh K, Tomioka C (1983) Biochem Biophys Res Commun 116:743-750

17. Katakami Y, Kaibuchi K, Sawamura M, Takai Y, Nishizuka Y (1984) Biochem Biophys Res Commun, in press

18. Knight DE, Baker PE (1983) FEBS Lett 160:98-100

19. Kojima I, Lippes H, Kojima K, Rasmussen H (1983) Biochem Biophys Res Commun 116:555-562

20. Zawalichi W, Brown C, Rasmussen H (1983) Biochem Biophys Res Commun 117:448-455

21. de Pont JJHHM, Fleuren-Jakobs AMM (1984) FEBS Lett 170:64-68

22. Tanaka C, Taniyama K, Kusunoki M (1984) FEBS Lett in press

23. Kaibuchi K, Sawamura M, Katakami Y, Kikkawa U, Takai Y, Nishizuka, Y. (1984): In: Bleasdale JE, Eichberg J, Hauser G (eds) Inositol and Phosphoinositides, Humana Press, Dallas, in press

Endocrinology
F. Labrie, L. Proulx, eds.

REGULATION OF PANCREATIC B-CELL FUNCTION*

WILLY J. MALAISSE
Laboratory of Experimental Medicine, Brussels Free University, Brussels, Belgium

INTRODUCTION

For the last two decades, the availability of suitable methods for both the immunoassay of insulin (1) and isolation of pancreatic islets (2) have allowed to study the secretory behaviour of the pancreatic B-cell and to compare secretory data to a number of other parameters of islet function. In the course of these investigations, it became soon evident that insulin release is regulated in vivo, in an immediate and direct manner, by nutrients, hormones and neurotransmitters and, in a delayed or chronic fashion, by a number of ontogenic, nutritional and endocrine factors. The functional organization of the pancreatic B-cell thus involves an array of sensor systems capable of identifying suitable insulinotropic agents, the information provided by different sensor systems being eventually integrated to regulate a single and final process of insulin release (3). The present account summarizes some of the current views on the cytophysiology of insulin release.

NUTRIENT-STIMULATED INSULIN RELEASE : THE FUEL CONCEPT

In its most simple description, the process of insulin release can be viewed as a sequence of three major events, respectively the identification of secretagogues, a coupling process connecting the identification site to that of hormonal release, and the activation of the effector system controlling the exocytosis of secretory granules. In the process of nutrient-stimulated insulin secretion, the identification step coincides with an acceleration of oxidative fluxes and respiration. In this respect, the B-cell can be viewed as a fuel-sensor organ. The fuel concept is supported by a number of observations on both the anomeric specificity of the metabolic and secretory response to D-glucose and D-mannose (4) and the mode of action of nonmetabolized or poorly metabolized nutrient analogs (5). The latter observations have clearly indicated that the metabolic response to a given nutrient secretagogue reflects not solely its own catabolism but also its facilitating or sparing action on the utilization of endogenous nutrients. In this respect, the study of metabolic events in islets deprived of exogenous nutrients (Fig. 1) may help to elucidate the regulation of fuel homeostasis in the B-cell when exposed *in vivo* to the heterogenous constellation of

---

*The Berson Memorial Lecture.

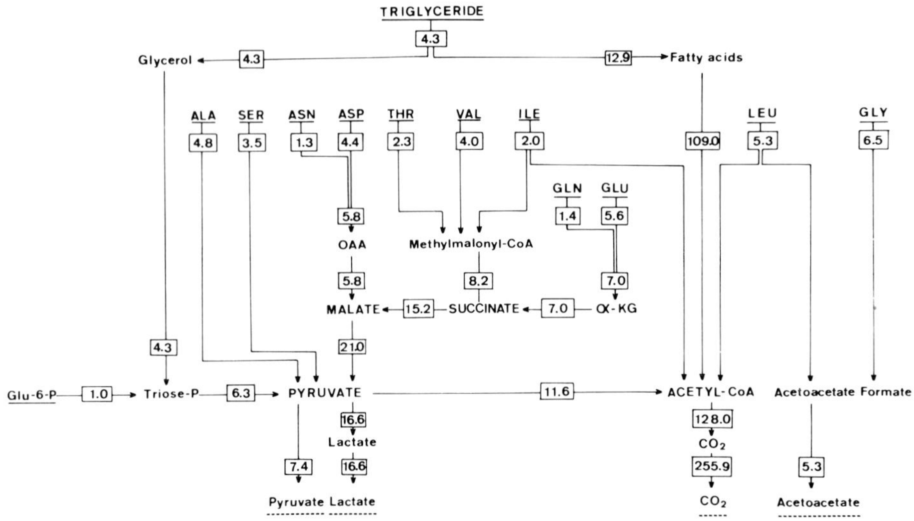

Fig. 1. Schematic view of metabolic events in pancreatic islets deprived of exogenous nutrient. Metabolic flows are expressed as pmol/60 min per islet and refer to the rate of utilization of the metabolite entering into each reaction, except for the production of fatty acids from triglyceride and their conversion to acetyl-CoA in which cases the flow rate refers to the metabolite emerging from the reaction. The parent nutrients and some of their metabolic end-products are underlined by solid and dashed lines, respectively (16, 17).

circulating nutrients.

The concept that the secretory response to nutrient secretagogues reflects their capacity to augment oxidative fluxes, warrants further investigations on the regulation of nutrient catabolism in the islet cells. In the case of glucose, the rapid equilibration of the hexose across the cell membrane and the suppression of hexokinase in intact islets by endogenous glucose 6-phosphate would apparently assign a key role to glucokinase in the regulation of glycolysis. However, in order for the rate of glycolysis to keep pace with the rate of glucose phosphorylation, phosphofructokinase may need to be suitably activated. Such an activation could be mediated, in part at least, by fructose-2,6-bisphosphate. In response to an increase in extracellular glucose concentration, the changes in the fructose-2,6-bisphosphate content of purified B-cells occur rapidly enough and are sufficiently marked (Fig. 2) to account for a quick and fine regulation of phosphofructokinase activity.

Coupling of metabolic to distal events

The nature of the mechanism(s) coupling metabolic events to more distal events

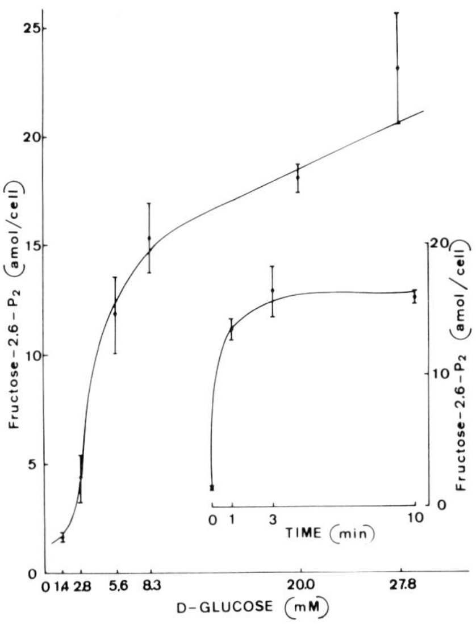

Fig. 2. Dose-response and the time course for the glucose-induced accumulation of fructose 2,6-bisphosphate in purified pancreatic B-cells. In the main graph, measurements were performed after 60 min incubation at the stated concentration of glucose. In the inset, the glucose concentration was raised at time zero from 1.4 to 20.0 mM. Mean values ($\pm$ SEM) refer to 3-8 individual observations (18).

in the secretory sequence remains a matter of debate. Current hypotheses emphasize the possible role of an increase in the generation rate of either ATP, protons or reducing equivalents (6). An increased availability of ATP could favour the active pumping of cytosolic Ca^{2+} into either intracellular organelles or the extracellular fluid and, hence, cause the closing of Ca^{2+}-responsive K^+ channels, the depolarization of the plasma membrane and the gating of voltage-sensitive Ca^{2+} channels (7). Protons, through acidification of the cytosol, could directly inhibit the outflow of K^+ and, possibly, Ca^{2+} (8).The induction of a more reduced redox state could, by changing the thiol-disulfide balance of proteins, alter their participation in ionic movements or other regulatory events (9). Anyhow, glucose causes an extensive remodelling of the fluxes of such ions as Cl^-, inorganic phosphate, H^+, Na^+, K^+ and, obviously, Ca^{2+}.

Cytosolic Ca^{2+} as the trigger for insulin release

It has long been postulated that glucose increases the cytosolic Ca^{2+} concentration in the B-cell. Yet, this was never demonstrated. On the contrary, a recent study conducted in the insulin-producing clonal cell line RINm5F indicates that glucose lowers cytosolic Ca^{2+} activity in these tumoral cells, in which glucose exerts little effect upon insulin release (10). The results illustrated

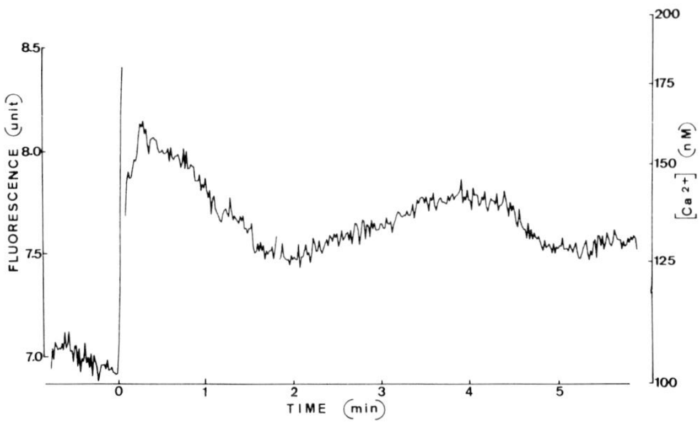

Fig. 3. Time course for the change in fluorescence of a suspension of pancreatic islet cells prelabelled with quin-2 tetraacetoxymethyl ester. At time zero, the glucose concentration was raised from 1.7 to 17.0 mM. The data collected in the test experiment were corrected for those collected in a paired control experiment in which the glucose concentration was maintained at 1.7 mM throughout. The fluorescence is expressed in arbitrary units (left ordinates) and converted to cytosolic Ca^{2+} activity (right ordinates) after calibration of the system.

in Fig. 3 unambiguously demonstrate that glucose increases cytosolic Ca^{2+} concentration in normal islet cells labelled with the membrane-permeable tetraacetoxymethyl ester of the fluorescent Ca^{2+} indicator quin-2. Incidentally in control experiments performed in cells not exposed to the fluorescent indicator, the glucose-induced increment in fluorescence, attributable to an increased content of the islet cells in reduced pyridine nucleotides, did not exceed 20 % of that found in the quin-2-labelled cells.

The glucose-induced increment in cytosolic Ca^{2+} activity results, in part at least, from the gating of Ca^{2+} channels which are blocked by organic calcium-antagonists, e.g. nifedipine. However, another dihydropyridine, Bay K 8644, enhances glucose-stimulated ^{45}Ca net uptake and insulin release (Fig. 4). The latter drug also stimulates ^{45}Ca efflux from prelabelled islets, the latter effect being abolished in the absence of extracellular Ca^{2+} and, hence, reflecting stimulation of a process of exchange between influent $^{40}Ca^{2+}$ and effluent $^{45}Ca^{2+}$ (Fig. 5).

Ultrastructural, secretory and cinematographic data have indicated that cytosolic Ca^{2+} may trigger insulin release, in part at least, by stimulating the contractile activity of the microfilamentous cell web (11). In biochemical term, this may correspond to the presence in islet cells of a Ca-calmodulin-sensitive myosin light chain kinase (12). Calmodulin may also participate in

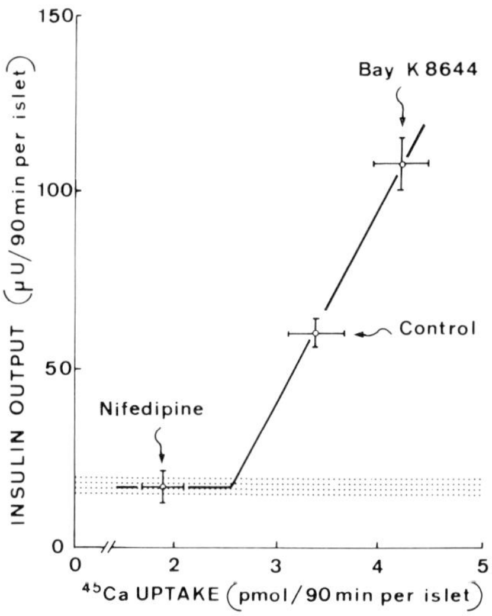

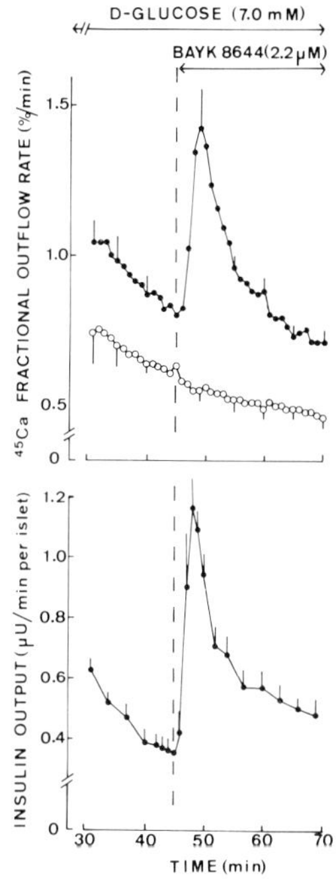

Fig. 4. (left) Relationship between ^{45}Ca net uptake and insulin output by pancreatic islets incubated at 7.0 mM-glucose in the absence (control) or presence of either BAY K 8644 (2.2 μM) or nifedipine (1.0 μM). Mean values (± SEM) refer to 11 or more individual observations. The shaded horizontal area corresponds to the basal insulin release, as measured in the absence of glucose.

Fig. 5. (right) Effect of BAY K 8644 (2.2 μM) upon ^{45}Ca fractional outflow rate and insulin release from islets perifused in the presence of D-glucose (7.0 mM) at normal Ca^{2+} concentration (1.0 mM; closed circles) or in the absence of Ca^{2+} and presence of EGTA (0.5 mM; open circles). Mean values (± SEM) refer to 4 experiments in each case.

the secretory sequence by activating adenylate cyclase (13). Other Ca^{2+}-responsive targets may include, *inter alia*, quinine-sensitive K^+ channels, Ca^{2+}-ATPases located at the plasma membrane and in the endoplasmic reticulum and transglutaminase. A phospholipid-dependent, diacylglycerol-activated and Ca^{2+}-responsive protein kinase C is also present in islet cells. The tumor-promoting agent, 12-0-tetradecanoylphorbol-13-acetate, which is a potent insulin secretagogue, can substitute for diacylglycerol as activator of this enzyme, even at a very low Ca^{2+} concentration (Figs. 6 & 7).

ENVIRONMENTAL MODIFICATION OF NUTRIENT-STIMULATED INSULIN RELEASE

The key role played by the B-cell in fuel homeostasis is quite compatible

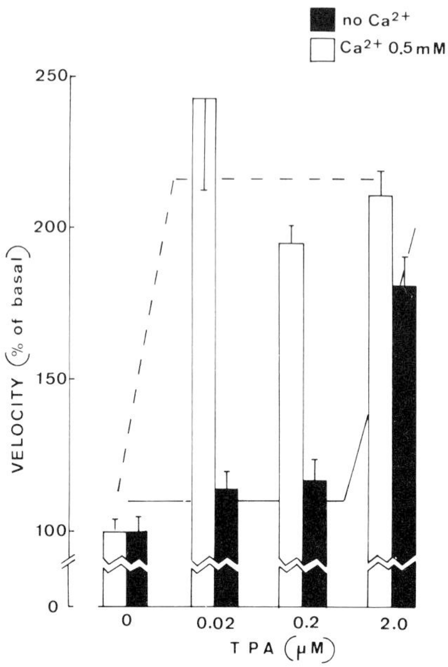

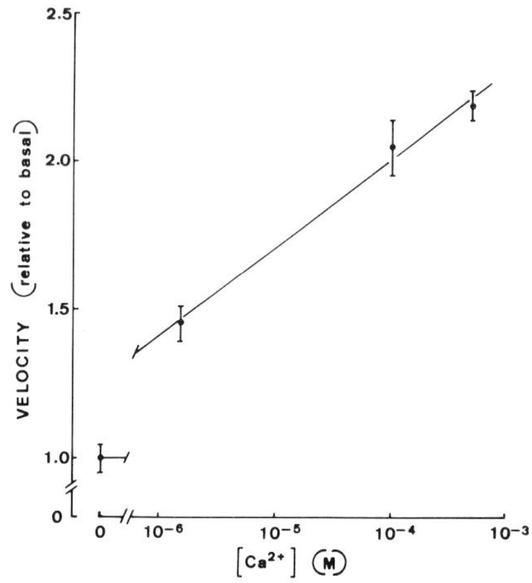

Fig. 6. (left) Effect of increasing concentrations of TPA upon the velocity of histone phosphorylation by islet homogenates in the presence of phosphatidylserine (25 µg/ml), as measured in the absence (solid line) or presence (dashed line) of Ca^{2+}. Mean values (± SEM) refer to 3 or more individual determinations and are expressed in percent of the control value found at the same Ca^{2+} level in the absence of TPA.

Fig. 7. (right) Effect of increasing Ca^{2+} concentrations (logarithmic scale) upon the velocity of histone phosphorylation by islet homogenates in the presence of phosphatidylserine (25 µg/ml) and TPA (0.02 µM). Mean values (± SEM) refer to 6 individual determinations and are expressed relative to the basal value measured in the absence of Ca^{2+}.

TABLE 1

Effect of epinephrine upon insulin release (µU/islet per 60 min) evoked by D-glucose in pancreatic islets removed from control rats or animals pretreated for 48 hours with islet activating protein

Animals	No epinephrine	Epinephrine (0.4 µM)	P
Control	301.1 ± 18.2 (24)*	29.0 ± 9.3 (24)	< 0.001
IAP-treated	337.8 ± 10.5 (12)	333.6 ± 24.1 (12)	> 0.8

*Mean values (± SEM) are shown together with the number of individual observations. In each group, the islets were derived from 3-6 rats.

with the influence of nonnutrient insulinotropic agents which participate *in vivo* in the regulation of insulin release. For instance, the stimulation of insulin release by cholinergic neurotransmitters, associated with food intake, may favour the uptake and storage of nutrients in extrapancreatic tissues. Inversely, in stress or exercise, the inhibition of insulin release by catecholamines may favour the mobilization of nutrients from the liver and adipose tissue.

Cholinergic agents, like nutrient secretagogues, provoke the hydrolysis of phosphatidylinositol and polyphosphoinositides in pancreatic islets (14). By liberating diacylglycerol from membrane phospholipids, these agents could thus cause activation of protein kinase C. This proposal is supported by the finding that exogenous phospholipase C stimulates insulin release (15).

Adrenergic agents, acting through α_2-adrenoceptors, inhibit both adenylate cyclase activity in islet crude homogenates and cyclic AMP production in intact islets. A more distal effect of adrenergic agents, e.g. on the intracellular distribution of Ca^{2+} should not be ruled out. In normal islets, the inhibitory effect of catecholamines upon glucose-stimulated insulin release is abolished in the presence of α_2 blocking agents, e.g. idazoxan. In islets of rat pretreated 48 hours before sacrifice with the islet activating protein isolated from the culture medium of *Bordetella pertussis*, no inhibitory effect of adrenaline upon insulin release can anymore be detected (Table 1). We have recently identified the α-subunit of both the Ns and Ni regulatory proteins in islet membranes exposed to (α-^{32}P)NAD in the presence of cholera toxin and islet activating protein respectively (unpublished data). It thus appears that islet cells, like other tissues, are equipped with suitable receptor/transducer/catalyzer complexes which mediate the response of the pancreatic B-cell to environmental, hormonal or neurotransmitter, regulatory factors.

CONCLUSION

Our present understanding of the cytophysiology of insulin release has reached a high degree of sophistication. Yet, I am convinced that the present knowledge only represents a minor fraction of all that could be learned on the functional organization of the pancreatic B-cell, which remains therefore a field open for further research and progress.

ACKNOWLEDGEMENTS

I am indebted to M. Deleers, C. Hubinont, F. Malaisse-Lagae, P. Mathias and A. Sener for their participation in the original work illustrated in this report. This work was supported by grants from the Belgian Ministry of Scientific Policy and Belgian Foundation for Scientific Medical Research.

REFERENCES

1. Yalow RS, Berson SA (1959) Nature (Lond.) 184:1648
2. Lacy PE, Kostianovsky M (1967) Diabetes 16:35-39
3. Malaisse WJ (1973) Diabetologia 9:167-173
4. Malaisse WJ, Malaisse-Lagae F, Sener A (1983) Physiol Rev 63:773-786
5. Malaisse WJ (1983) Diab Metab 9:313-320
6. Malaisse WJ, Hutton JC, Kawazu S, Herchuelz A, Valverde I, Sener A (1979) Diabetologia 16:331-341
7. Atwater I (1980) Ciênc Biol (Portugal) 5:299-314
8. Malaisse WJ, Herchuelz A, Sener A (1980) Life Sci 26:1367-1371
9. Anjaneyulu K, Anjaneyulu R, Sener A, Malaisse WJ (1982) Biochimie 64:29-36
10. Rorsman P, Berggren P-O, Gylfe E, Hellman B (1983) Bioscience Reports 3:939-946
11. Malaisse WJ, Orci L (1979) Methods Achiev Exp Pathol 9:112-136
12. MacDonald MJ, Kowluru A (1982) Diabetes 31:566-570
13. Valverde I, Vandermeers A, Anjaneyulu R, Malaisse WJ (1979) Science 206: 225-227
14. Best L, Malaisse WJ (1983) Biochim Biophys Acta 750:157-163
15. Hubinont C, Best L, Sener A, Malaisse WJ (1984) FEBS Letters in press
16. Malaisse WJ, Best L, Kawazu S, Malaisse-Lagae F, Sener A (1983) Arch Biochem Biophys 224:102-110
17. Malaisse WJ (1983) IRCS Med Sci 11:540-541
18. Sener A, Van Schaftingen E, Van De Winkel M, Pipeleers DG, Malaisse-Lagae F, Malaisse WJ, Hers H-G (1984) Biochem J 221: in press

Endocrinology
F. Labrie, L. Proulx, eds.

STRUCTURES, EXPRESSION AND PRODUCTS OF NEUROPEPTIDE AND RECEPTOR GENES

SHOSAKU NUMA
Department of Medical Chemistry, Kyoto University Faculty of Medicine, Kyoto 606 (Japan)

INTRODUCTION

A powerful tool for studying neural and hormonal peptides as well as neurotransmitter receptors has recently been provided by recombinant DNA technology. By cloning and sequencing cDNAs, we have elucidated the primary structures of three opioid peptide precursors and the corticotropin-releasing factor precursor (prepro-CRF) and of all four subunits of the nicotinic acetylcholine receptor (AChR). The genes encoding the neuropeptide precursors and the AChR subunits have also been isolated and characterized. Furthermore, we have developed an expression system in which the synthesis of the functional AChR is directed by cloned cDNAs encoding the receptor subunits. These studies on the molecular structures of the neuropeptide precursors and the AChR as well as on the expression of their genes are presented here.

MATERIALS AND METHODS

The mRNA encoding the corticotropin-β-lipotropin precursor (abbreviated as ACTH-β-LPH precursor; designated alternatively as preproopiomelanocortin), which was found to be a major mRNA species in the bovine pituitary intermediate lobe (1), was purified to homogeneity (2), and the purified mRNA was used as template to clone cDNA for this precursor (3,4). cDNAs for bovine prepro-enkephalin A (also referred to as preproenkephalin) (5), porcine prepro-enkephalin B (designated alternatively as preprodynorphin or prepronorphin) (6), ovine prepro-CRF (7) and the four subunits of the *Torpedo californica* electroplax AChR (8-10), whose mRNAs are present in low abundance, were cloned by screening a cDNA library by hybridization with a mixture of oligodeoxyribo-nucleotides synthesized by the triester method; in some cases, a synthetic oligodeoxyribonucleotide was also used for specific priming of the reverse transcription. cDNAs for the calf skeletal muscle AChR subunits were cloned from a cDNA library by hybridization with *T. californica* or calf cDNA probes (11-13). The plasmid pBR322 or the Okayama-Berg vector was used for cloning cDNAs. For the isolation of the genes encoding the neuropeptide precursors and the AChR subunits, genomic DNA libraries were screened with corresponding cDNA or genomic DNA probes (11,14-20). DNA sequencing was carried out by the procedure of Maxam and Gilbert.

RESULTS AND DISCUSSION

Primary structures of opioid peptide precursors deduced from cDNA sequences

Nucleotide sequence analysis of the cloned cDNAs has revealed the primary structures of the three opioid peptide precursors (4-6), which are schematically shown in Fig. 1. All of the endogenous opioid peptides hitherto identified are derived from these three precursors. In addition, some novel neural and hormonal peptides have been discovered from the cDNA sequences. They include N-terminal peptide containing γ-melanotropin (γ-MSH) present in the ACTH-β-LPH precursor (4), [Met]enkephalin-Arg^6-Gly^7-Leu^8 in preproenkephalin A (5) and leumorphin in preproenkephalin B (6); the opioid octapeptide has also been identified by protein sequencing (21). Leumorphin, synthesized chemically (22), exhibits potent opiate-like activity and interacts with the κ-opioid receptor (23), as do the other opioid peptides derived from preproenkephalin B. Evidence indicating the presence of leumorphin in the pituitary has been provided by radioimmunoassay (24). All the peptides known to be biologically active as well as the potentially active peptides contained in the three opioid peptide precursors are each bounded by paired basic amino acid residues, which apparently represent the sites of proteolytic processing.

The structural organizations of the three precursors are strikingly similar (Fig. 1). All of them, having a nearly identical molecular size, contain multiple repeated units of MSH or enkephalin in the carboxy-terminal one- or

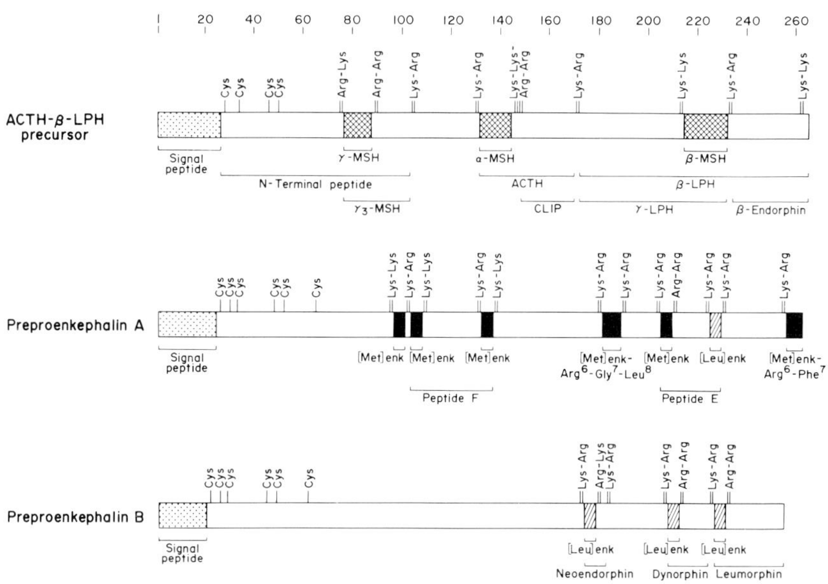

Fig. 1. Structures of opioid peptide precursors. The schemes are based on the data taken from refs. 4-6.

two-thirds of their molecules and an even number of cysteine residues in the amino-terminal region of the prohormones. Furthermore, considerable amino acid sequence homology is noted between preproenkephalin A and preproenkephalin B, extending over the entire molecules (18). This, together with the similarity found between the structural organizations of the genes encoding the two precursors (see below), suggests that the preproenkephalin A and preproenkephalin B genes have been generated from a common ancestor by gene duplication.

The fact that different biologically active peptides are elaborated from a common precursor suggests that their functions may be coordinated with one another (4-6). The biological significance of such multi-hormone precursors may be to effect the simultaneous production of multiple active peptides that perform coordinate functions.

Structures and expression of opioid peptide precursor genes

The structural organizations of the three opioid peptide precursor genes (14-18,20) are strikingly similar (Fig. 2). All of the repeated MSH or enkephalin sequences present in these precursors are encoded by a single large exon. A second small exon mainly encodes the signal peptide. The similarity in structural organization suggests that the preproenkephalin A and preproenkephalin B genes and the ACTH-β-LPH precursor gene may have evolved by an analogous mechanism. The complete nucleotide sequence of the human ACTH-β-LPH precursor gene, composed of 7665 base pairs, has been determined (25).

The cellular content of the mRNA encoding the ACTH-β-LPH precursor is depressed by glucocorticoids, and the effects of various steroids on the mRNA level correlate with the binding specificity of the glucocorticoid receptor (26,27). The promoter region of the human ACTH-β-LPH precursor gene (28,29) and of the human preproenkephalin A gene (30) has been mapped.

Structures of corticotropin-releasing factor precursor and its gene

Figure 3 schematically shows the primary structure of prepro-CRF (7) together with the structural organization of its gene (19). It is noteworthy that the amino-terminal one-third of the pro-CRF molecule is similar in amino

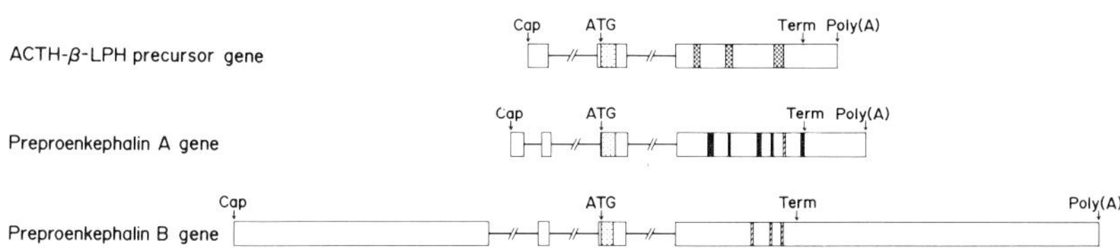

Fig. 2. Structures of opioid peptide precursor genes. Exons are shown by blocks, and introns by lines; the capping site of the preproenkephalin B gene has tentatively been assigned. The coding regions for the MSH and enkephalin sequences and the signal peptide are indicated by boxes. The schemes are based on the data taken from refs. 14, 15, 17 and 18.

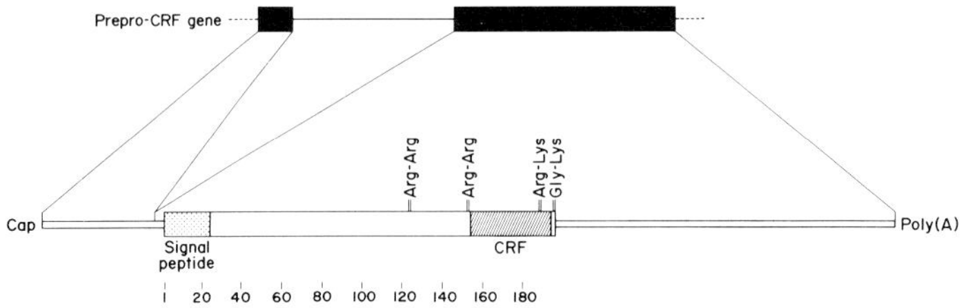

Fig. 3. Structures of prepro-CRF and its gene. The capping site has tentatively been assigned. The scheme is based on the data taken from ref. 19.

acid sequence to the amino-terminal region of the prohormone of the arginine vasopressin-neurophysin II precursor (31), while the carboxy-terminal two-thirds of the pro-CRF molecule are related to the region encompassing ACTH of the ACTH-β-LPH precursor (7). This implies an evolutionary relatedness of the three precursor proteins, which seems conceivable in view of the fact that arginine vasopressin potentiates the ACTH-releasing activity of CRF.

Primary structures of Torpedo electroplax acetylcholine receptor subunits deduced from cDNA sequences

Figure 4 shows the primary structures of the α- (8), β- (9), γ- (10,32) and

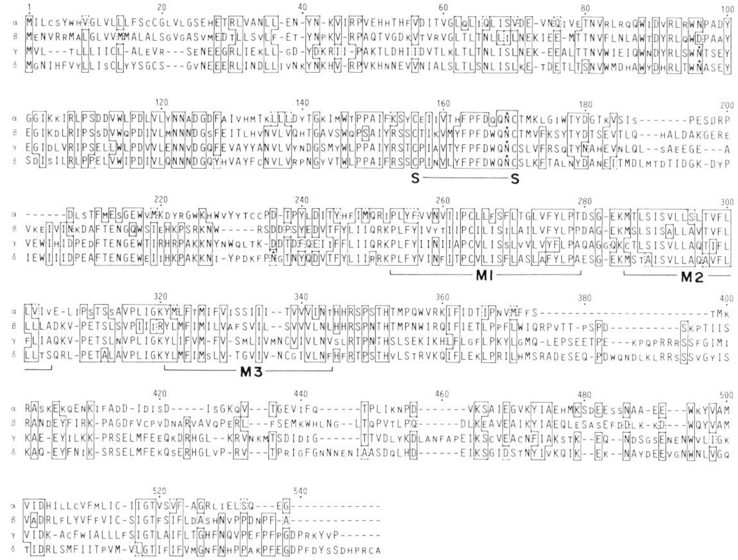

Fig. 4. Alignment of the amino acid sequences of the α-, β-, γ- and δ-subunit precursors of the *T. californica* electroplax AChR. Sets of three or four identical residues at one aligned position are enclosed with solid lines, and the fourth residues regarded as favoured substitutions at the same position with dotted lines. Reprinted from ref. 10.

δ-subunit precursors (9) of the T. californica electroplax AChR deduced from the cDNA sequences. The alignment of the amino acid sequences of the four subunits exhibits marked homology, suggesting that the genes encoding them have been generated from a single common ancestor by gene duplications. The hydrophilicity profiles along the aligned amino acid sequences as well as the predicted secondary structures are similar for the four subunits. This suggests that all subunits are oriented in a pseudosymmetric fashion across the membrane. We have initially identified four strongly hydrophobic regions with predicted secondary structure in the α-subunit molecule and have assumed that they represent transmembrane segments or are involved in inter-subunit interaction (8). Similarly, four markedly hydrophobic regions with predicted secondary structure have been found at equivalent positions in the β- (9), γ- (10,32) and δ-subunits (9). These four hydrophobic regions each correspond to a continuous stretch of 19-27 uncharged amino acid residues including many nonpolar residues (68-93%). These segments, designated as M1, M2, M3 and M4 (Fig. 4), most likely traverse the membrane, forming α-helical structures. Because the amino-terminal half of the mature subunit molecules preceding the transmembrane segment M1 contains potential N-glycosylation sites (marked with asterisks in Fig. 4), the orientation of the transmembrane segments M1-M4 is assigned as shown in Fig. 5. The putative transmembrane segments are presumably involved in the cation channel of the AChR. Interestingly, the polar uncharged side chains present in these

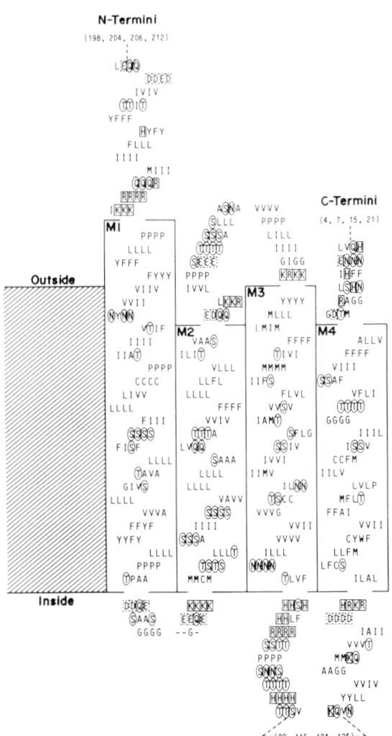

Fig. 5. Proposed orientation of the subunit polypeptides of the T. californica electroplax AChR across the membrane. Sets of four letters indicate the amino acid residues in the aligned α-, β-, γ- and δ-subunit sequences, respectively, from left to right; gaps (-) have been removed, except at position 283 (see Fig. 4), to permit ready identification of the side chains extending toward one side of an α-helix. Sets of four numbers in parentheses indicate the sum of residues in the mature α-, β-, γ- and δ-subunit sequences, respectively (from left to right), that either extend beyond the ends of the displayed sequences or are inserted between them. Uncharged polar residues are enclosed with solid circles, positively charged residues with solid squares, and negatively charged residues with dotted squares. Reprinted from ref. 10.

segments are clustered largely on one side of an α-helix, whereas the opposite side is mostly hydrophobic (Fig. 5). Recently, Guy (33) and Finer-Moore and Stroud (34) have proposed that all four subunits contain a fifth, amphipathic transmembrane segment located between the segments M3 and M4.

It has been shown that the α-subunit of the AChR contains part or all of the acetylcholine (ACh) binding site and that a disulphide bridge is present in close proximity to this site (35). We have proposed that the ACh binding site is located in the region encompassing the cysteine residues at positions 156 and 170 (8). These cysteine residues most likely form a disulphide bridge, although the possible involvement of one of the two remaining extracellular cysteine residues (positions 233 and 234) cannot be excluded. Interestingly, the two cysteine residues at positions 156 and 170 are conserved in all four subunits, and one of them is adjacent to the asparagine residue (position 169) that is the only glycosylation site conserved in all four subunits.

Structures of mammalian muscle acetylcholine receptor subunits and their genes

The primary structures of the α- (11), β- (12), γ- (13) and δ-subunit precursors of the calf skeletal muscle AChR and those of the α- (11) and γ-subunit precursors of its human counterpart have been deduced from the nucleotide sequences of the cloned cDNAs and genomic DNAs, respectively. The mammalian AChR subunits share structural features common to all four subunits of the *Torpedo* AChR, presumably exhibiting the same transmembrane topology as proposed for the *Torpedo* AChR subunits. The protein-coding sequences of the human AChR α- and γ-subunit genes are divided into nine and twelve exons, respectively, as shown schematically in Fig. 6. The protein regions encoded by distinct exons seem to correspond to different structural and functional domains of the subunit precursor molecules, and some regions are more highly conserved between the mammals and fish. The degree of overall sequence homology between the α-subunits

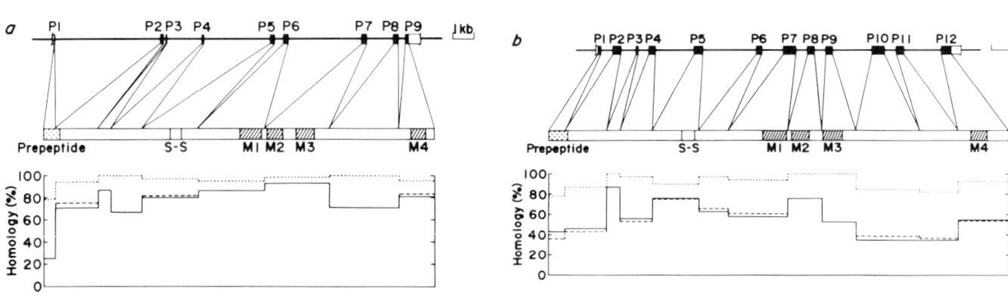

Fig. 6. Arrangement of the protein-coding regions in the human muscle AChR α- (*a*) and γ-subunit genes (*b*) and amino acid sequence homology in the protein regions encoded by different exons. The exons comprising the protein-coding sequence (closed boxes) are shown. The amino acid sequence homology in each protein region is given for the human/calf (dotted lines), human/*Torpedo* (solid lines) and calf/*Torpedo* (dashed lines or solid lines where no dashed lines are shown) pairs. Figure 6*a* has been taken from ref. 11.

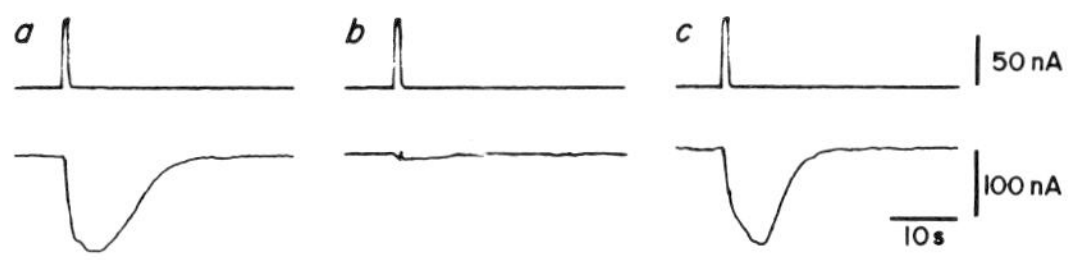

Fig. 7. ACh responses recorded from a Xenopus laevis oocyte. Upper traces, currents used for ionophoresis of ACh; lower traces, ACh currents recorded under voltage clamp (downward deflection indicates inward current). The responses to ACh before (a) and 2.5 min after perfusion with 2.5 μM (+)tubocurarine (b) and 15 min after washing out the antagonist (c) are shown. Reprinted from ref. 36.

of the mammalian and fish AChR is higher than those between the β-, γ- and δ-subunits. This may suggest different rates of evolution for the α- and the three other subunits. We have also isolated the human muscle AChR β- and δ-subunit genes. The human muscle AChR δ- and γ-subunit genes have been shown to be juxtaposed in the same orientation.

Expression of functional acetylcholine receptor from cloned cDNAs

Each of the cDNAs encoding the four subunit precursors of the T. californica AChR, carried by a simian virus 40 vector, was introduced by transfection into COS monkey cells (36). Poly(A)$^+$ RNAs containing the respective subunit-specific mRNAs, isolated from the transfected COS cells, were combined and injected into Xenopus oocytes (36), which were used as a translation system (37). These oocytes, when studied electrophysiologically, exhibited a (+)tubocurarine-sensitive response to ACh (Fig. 7). Thus, the cloned cDNAs direct the synthesis of the functional AChR of the nicotinic type.

Studies on the effect of deletion of each subunit have suggested that all four subunits of the AChR are required to elicit a normal response to ACh, whereas only the α-subunit is indispensable for α-bungarotoxin binding activity (36). In view of the finding that 2-3% of the oocytes injected with all but the γ- or δ-subunit-specific mRNA responded slightly to ACh, the possibility remains that the γ- and δ-subunits can replace each other to some extent for the receptor function (36). The expression system described, in conjunction with site-directed mutagenesis, will be useful for further studies on the question, what roles subunits, domains and specific amino acids play in the operation of the AChR. The antigenic determinants on the AChR molecule, which are causally related to myasthenia gravis, will also be analysed by the same approach.

REFERENCES

1. Taii S, Nakanishi S, Numa S (1979) Eur J Biochem 93:205-212
2. Kita T, Inoue A, Nakanishi S, Numa S (1979) Eur J Biochem 93:213-220
3. Nakanishi S, Inoue A, Kita T, Numa S, Chang ACY, Cohen SN, Nunberg J Schimke RT (1978) Proc Natl Acad Sci USA 75:6021-6025
4. Nakanishi S, Inoue A, Kita T, Nakamura M, Chang ACY, Cohen SN, Numa S (1979) Nature 278:423-427

5. Noda M, Furutani Y, Takahashi H, Toyosato M, Hirose T, Inayama S, Nakanishi S, Numa S (1982) Nature 295:202-206
6. Kakidani H, Furutani Y, Takahashi H, Noda M, Morimoto Y, Hirose T, Asai M, Inayama S, Nakanishi S, Numa S (1982) Nature 298:245-249
7. Furutani Y, Morimoto Y, Shibahara S, Noda M, Takahashi H, Hirose T, Asai M, Inayama S, Hayashida H, Miyata T, Numa S (1983) Nature 301:537-540
8. Noda M, Takahashi H, Tanabe T, Toyosato M, Furutani Y, Hirose T, Asai M, Inayama S, Miyata T, Numa S (1982) Nature 299:793-797
9. Noda M, Takahashi H, Tanabe T, Toyosato M, Kikyotani S, Hirose T, Asai M, Takashima H, Inayama S, Miyata T, Numa S (1983) Nature 301:251-255
10. Noda M, Takahashi H, Tanabe T, Toyosato M, Kikyotani S, Furutani Y, Hirose T, Takashima H, Inayama S, Miyata T, Numa S (1983) Nature 302:528-532
11. Noda M, Furutani Y, Takahashi H, Toyosato M, Tanabe T, Shimizu S, Kikyotani S, Kayano T, Hirose T, Inayama S, Numa S (1983) Nature 305:818-823
12. Tanabe T, Noda M, Furutani Y, Takai T, Takahashi H, Tanaka K, Hirose T, Inayama S, Numa S (1984) Eur J Biochem, in press
13. Takai T, Noda M, Furutani Y, Takahashi H, Notake M, Shimizu S, Kayano T, Tanabe T, Tanaka K, Hirose T, Inayama S, Numa S (1984) Eur J Biochem, in press
14. Nakanishi S, Teranishi Y, Noda M, Notake M, Watanabe Y, Kakidani H, Jingami H, Numa S (1980) Nature 287:752-755
15. Nakanishi S, Teranishi Y, Watanabe Y, Notake M, Noda M, Kakidani H, Jingami H, Numa S (1981) Eur J Biochem 115:429-438
16. Takahashi H, Teranishi Y, Nakanishi S, Numa S (1981) FEBS Lett 135:97-102
17. Noda M, Teranishi Y, Takahashi H, Toyosato M, Notake M, Nakanishi S, Numa S (1982) Nature 297:431-434
18. Horikawa S, Takai T, Toyosato M, Takahashi H, Noda M, Kakidani H, Kubo T, Hirose T, Inayama S, Hayashida H, Miyata T, Numa S (1983) Nature 306:611-614
19. Shibahara S, Morimoto Y, Furutani Y, Notake M, Takahashi H, Shimizu S, Horikawa S, Numa S (1983) EMBO J 2:775-779
20. Notake M, Tobimatsu T, Watanabe Y, Takahashi H, Mishina M, Numa S (1983) FEBS Lett 156:67-71
21. Kilpatrick DL, Jones BN, Kojima K, Udenfriend S (1981) Biochem Biophys Res Commun 103:698-705
22. Yamamoto Y, Yanaihara C, Katsumaru Y, Mochizuki T, Tobe A, Egawa M, Imura H, Numa S, Yanaihara N (1983) Reg Peptides 6:163-168
23. Suda M, Nakao K, Yoshimasa T, Ikeda Y, Sakamoto M, Yanaihara N, Numa S, Imura H (1983) Life Sci 32:2769-2775
24. Nakao K, Suda M, Sakamoto M, Yoshimasa T, Morii N, Ikeda Y, Yanaihara C, Yanaihara N, Numa S, Imura H (1983) Biochem Biophys Res Commun 117:695-701
25. Takahashi H, Hakamata Y, Watanabe Y, Kikuno R, Miyata T, Numa S (1983) Nucleic Acids Res 11:6847-6858
26. Nakanishi S, Kita T, Taii S, Imura H, Numa S (1977) Proc Natl Acad Sci USA 74:3283-3286
27. Nakamura M, Nakanishi S, Sueoka S, Imura H, Numa S (1978) Eur J Biochem 86:61-66
28. Mishina M, Kurosaki T, Yamamoto T, Notake M, Masu M, Numa S (1982) EMBO J 1:1533-1538
29. Notake M, Kurosaki T, Yamamoto T, Handa H, Mishina M, Numa S (1983) Eur J Biochem 133:599-605
30. Terao M, Watanabe Y, Mishina M, Numa S (1983) EMBO J 2:2223-2228
31. Land H, Schütz G, Schmale H, Richter D (1982) Nature 295:299-303
32. Claudio T, Ballivet M, Patrick J, Heinemann S (1983) Proc Natl Acad Sci USA 80:1111-1115
33. Guy HR (1984) Biophys J 45:249-261
34. Finer-Moore J, Stroud RM (1984) Proc Natl Acad Sci USA 81:155-159
35. Karlin A (1969) J Gen Physiol 54:245s-264s
36. Mishina M, Kurosaki T, Tobimatsu T, Morimoto Y, Noda M, Yamamoto T, Terao M, Lindstrom J, Takahashi T, Kuno M, Numa S (1984) Nature 307:604-608
37. Barnard EA, Miledi R, Sumikawa K (1982) Proc R Soc Lond B 215:241-246

Endocrinology
F. Labrie, L. Proulx, eds.

RECEPTOR-MEDIATED ACTIVATION MECHANISMS IN THE HYPOTHALAMIC CONTROL OF PITUITARY-GONADAL FUNCTION

K.J. CATT, E. LOUMAYE, P. WYNN, C. SUAREZ-QUIAN, L. KIESEL, M. IWASHITA, K. HIROTA, R. MORGAN, AND J. CHANG

Endocrinology Reproduction Research Branch, National Institute of Child Health and Human Development, National Institutes of Health, Bethesda, MD 20205

Elucidation of the biochemical mechanisms by which hormone receptors regulate target-cell function in the endocrine system has undergone remarkable advances in the last four years. The concept that highly specific cell-surface receptor sites are responsible for the ability of peptide hormones to activate plasma-membrane "second message" systems based on adenylate cyclase and calcium-calmodulin regulated processes is now well-established. This notion has been extended to include newly-defined effector mechanisms that involve guanyl nucleotide coupling proteins (1), modulation of calcium channels (2), rapid changes in phospholipid metabolism and calcium mobilization (3), and the participation of recently discovered enzymes such as protein kinase C (4), in the cellular response to ligand-activation in numerous endocrine-regulated target tissues. It has become clear that most cells possess a variety of ligand-activated effector mechanisms through which specific target-cell responses can be elicited by locally-produced or systemic hormones, and that the biochemical processes involved in hormonal control include a broad range of enzymatic reactions and evanescent messenger molecules. In the control of pituitary function by hypothalamic neuropeptides, and the regulation of gonadotropin secretion and actions in the testis and ovary, there is a considerable degree of diversity among the mechanisms of hormonal activation of the individual target cells.

While cyclic AMP-dependent processes appear to mediate most or all of the gonadal actions of LH and FSH, the actions of hypothalamic hormones on the pituitary gland involve both cyclic AMP and calcium-dependent mechanisms of which one or other extreme may predominate in the individual cell-types. The occurrence of both forms of response to peptide hormones in closely adjacent cell types is a feature of the anterior pituitary gland. The ability to utilize more than one response pathway is clearly appropriate to cells in which multiple

---

Abbreviations: AA arachidonic acid; CHAPS 3[(3-cholamidopropyl) dimethyl-ammonio]-1-propane sulfonate; GnRH gonadotropin-releasing hormone; GnRHa [D-Ala^6]des-Gly^{10}-GnRH N-ethylamide; TPA (12-0-tetra-decanoylphorbol-13-acetate).

receptor inputs must be accomodated, but it is not yet clear why certain peptide hormones act predominately through one or the other of the two major response pathways. In the case of GnRH, the primary regulator of LH and FSH secretion, calcium and phospholipid-dependent mechanisms are largely responsible for the immediate mobilization of stored gonadotropins (5). The actions of GnRH and other factors upon pituitary receptors for GnRH and release of LH _in vitro_ have been extensively analyzed in cultured rat pituitary cells, of which about 12% are gonadotrophs. For studies on GnRH-induced changes in potential intracellular mediators, none of which are unique to the gonadotroph, the detection of specific responses to ligand stimulation is facilitated by the use of gonadotroph-enriched cell fractions such as those prepared by centrifugal elutriation (6). This discussion will focus on the major mechanisms through which the hypothalamus exerts its control of pituitary-gonadal function, and on the integration of cyclic AMP, calcium, and phospholipid-mediated activation pathways in the gonadotrophs, the target cells through which the neuroendocrine regulation of reproductive processes is expressed and coordinated.

GnRH RECEPTORS: REGULATION BY AGONIST AND ANTAGONIST ANALOGS

The regulation of specific plasma-membrane receptors by changes in the ambient concentration of the homologous hormone is often a notable feature of peptide hormone action, and may lead to altered target-cell sensitivity or responsiveness to subsequent hormonal stimulation. Such regulation may be particularly important in the control of reproductive function, since the secretion of biologically appropriate gonadotropin profiles is determined by the phasic and pulsatile secretion of GnRH from the hypothalamus, acting via specific receptor sites in the pituitary gonadotrophs. Such GnRH receptors, which have been identified and assayed by binding studies with radioiodinated GnRH superagonist analogs (GnRHa), are now known to undergo marked changes in the pituitary gland according to the state of reproductive function (7). Thus, during the rat estrous cycle, there is a two-fold increase in pituitary GnRH receptors at proestrus, followed by a fall around the time of the LH surge. Conversely, GnRH receptors are decreased during lactation, when gonadotropin secretion is reduced due to decreased release of GnRH from the hypothalmus, and after prolactin treatment. These changes, with the enhancing effect of castration on pituitary receptors and its prevention by maneuvers that block GnRH secretion or action, have indicated that pituitary GnRH receptors are regulated by the prevailing rate of GnRH secretion (8).

The ability of GnRH receptors to exhibit up- and down-regulation could modulate pituitary function and responsiveness in various reproductive states. In particular, the down-regulatory mechanism could be relevant to the antifertility effect of long-term treatment with GnRH agonists. When the *in vitro* effects of GnRH and its analogs are analyzed in cultured rat pituitary cells, there is a consistent increase in GnRH receptors at low concentration of GnRH agonists, and a decrease at higher concentrations (9). These concentration-dependent effects of GnRH on its receptors may be responsible for the changes in GnRH receptors during the estrous cycle. In contrast, GnRH antagonists do not cause down-regulation of GnRH receptors, and block the regulatory effect of the agonist ligands on both LH secretion and GnRH receptors. The kinetics of action of GnRH upon its receptors are characterized by an initial loss of sites, followed by a return to the control level and then by an increase in receptors. The early phase of receptor loss or down-regulation depends upon activation of receptor sites by the hormonal ligand, and is not observed after cell stimulation by a depolarizing concentration of potassium or after exposure to GnRH antagonists (10). In cultured gonadotrophs, phorbol esters (11) and cyclic AMP analogs (12) also cause changes in GnRH receptors, suggesting that a phosphorylation event is involved in the regulation of receptor turnover.

The delayed return and up-regulation of receptors following the initial phase of depletion is dependent on protein and RNA synthesis, which are required for the formation of receptors or other protein(s) that are involved in the replenishment process (10). Morphological studies on the turnover and the fate of GnRH receptors have included the use of fluorescent and radioiodinated GnRH analogs. In cultured rat pituitary cells, rhodamine-labeled [D-Lys^{6}]GnRH showed progressive clustering and clumping within 10 to 20 minutes, consistent with processing and uptake of the receptor-bound ligand (13). EM-autoradiographic studies showed initial localization of ^{125}I-labeled GnRH agonists at the gonadotroph plasma membrane, followed by rapid appearance within the cell in association with endocytic vesicles and other organelles (14). Internalization of GnRH agonists occurred via receptor-mediated endocytosis, as in many other ligand-stimulated cells. After binding to specific receptors, which are often located on microvilli, GnRH agonists were rapidly taken up through a coated-pit mechanism which precedes either degradation or recycling to the plasma membrane. In the gonadotroph, much of the internalized GnRH was delivered to lysosomes, and there is probably little or no recycling of receptors to the cell surface. In contrast to the rapid internalization of agonists, a potent GnRH antagonist analog remained bound at the cell surface for a much longer period (15).

The marked difference in rates of internalization of GnRH agonist and antagonist derivatives was also evident in studies with gold-conjugated analogs, which again showed rapid incorporation of agonist-coated particles into multivesicular bodies and secondary lysosomes, whereas the antagonist-coated beads remained at the cell surface for much longer periods. These findings imply that endocytosis of the agonist-receptor complex is stimulated by receptor activation, whereas the non-activating antagonist ligand undergoes much slower cellular processing that is probably more related to plasma-membrane protein turnover than to ligand-stimulated receptor-mediated endocytosis (15). The ability of GnRH super-agonists to desensitize the pituitary gland, and to suppress gonadotropin release when employed for contraception or treatment of precocious puberty and certain steroid-dependent tumors, is related to the marked loss of receptors and activation responses that follow chronic exposure to the agonist ligand. In contrast, potent GnRH antagonists show prolonged binding to the gonadotrophs without true receptor loss, and provide an alternative means of blockade of gonadotropin secretion.

PHYSICO-CHEMICAL PROPERTIES OF THE GnRH RECEPTOR.

Pituitary GnRH receptors have been characterized in several species as specific binding sites with high affinity for GnRH and its potent analogs, either agonist or antagonist. Similar receptors are present in the rat testis and ovary, where the direct actions of GnRH are predominately inhibitory in nature. Although much is known about the binding properties and physiological regulation of GnRH receptors, relatively little information is available about their chemical structure. The recent application of photoaffinity labeling to the GnRH receptor (16) has provided initial characterization of the rat pituitary and ovarian binding sites, and has revealed one receptor component in the pituitary and two in the ovary. Recently, the zwitterionic detergent, CHAPS, has been employed to solubilize pituitary GnRH receptors with retention of binding activity (17). To characterize the pituitary GnRH receptor, we analyzed the membrane receptors by photoaffinity labeling and the CHAPS-solubilized sites by binding studies with GnRH superagonist and antagonist analogs.

Soluble pituitary GnRH receptors extracted with 5 mM CHAPS retained the high binding affinity and specificity of the membrane-bound sites. They were also more stable than the particulate sites, and showed higher binding of the potent GnRH antagonist, ^{125}I-[Ac-D-p-Cl-Phe^{1,2}, D-Trp^{3}, D-Lys^{6}, D-Ala^{10}]GnRH, than of radioiodinated GnRH agonists. During gel filtration under non-denaturing conditions, both free and prelabeled GnRH receptors behaved as high molecular weight species with MW of about 700,000. The CHAPS-solubilized receptor also exhibited a high molecular weight on sucrose density gradient centrifugation, with sedimentation coefficient of about 10S. To compare the holoreceptor with its binding units, and to explore the binding sites in different species, GnRH receptors in rat, mouse, rabbit, ovine and bovine pituitaries were analyzed by photoaffinity labeling using ^{125}I-[N$^{\varepsilon}$-azidobenzoyl-D-Lys^{6}]-des--Gly^{10}-GnRH-N-ethylamide. After photolysis of the specifically-bound photoaffinity ligand, analysis by SDS-PAGE on 5-15% polyacrylamide gels showed major bands of MW 50-60,000 and minor components of 40,000 MW in the rat, mouse, and rabbit pituitaries. Only the lower MW component was observed in ovine and bovine pituitary glands. These results demonstrate that the subunit nature of the GnRH receptors, as well as their biochemical functions, are similar in the various species studied, and that at least two components with binding activity can be detected in the multimeric GnRH receptor.

MECHANISMS OF ACTION OF GnRH.

The secretory response to GnRH is highly calcium-dependent, and does not appear to involve rapid cyclic AMP-mediated processes during the acute phase of gonadotropin release. In these respects, the gonadotroph is similar to many other secretory cells, in which the mechanisms involved in the calcium-mediated response pathway are only now beginning to be defined. GnRH is known to stimulate phospholipid metabolism in the gonadotroph, with increased phosphatidyl inositol (PI) turnover (18) and arachidonic acid (AA) release (7). The products formed after PI (or TPI) hydrolysis by phospholipase C, including diacylglycerol (DG), inositol phosphates, and phosphatidic acid (PA), as well as the arachidonate metabolites produced after cleavage of AA by phospholipase A_2 or diglyceride lipase, are putative intermediates in the action of GnRH upon LH release. Evidence for the potential role of AA metabolites and PA in this process has been previously presented (7,19).

More recently, the potential importance of inositol triphosphate (IP_3) as a mediator of ligand-induced calcium mobilization has been emphasized (20). The extent to which IP_3 acts as a mediator of peptide hormone action is not yet known, but its involvement in the action of TRH has been demonstrated in mammotropic tumor cells (21). In rat gonadotrophs, we observed no release of IP_3 during stimulation with GnRH, under conditions in which prominent increases in inositol monophosphate and biphosphate were readily demonstrable. Given the need to optimize the conditions necessary to detect TPI turnover for individual cell types, such negative findings may not exclude a role of IP_3 in GnRH action. However, as described below, we believe that other mechanisms which do not depend on changes in cytosolic calcium are important components of the secretory response of the gonadotroph to GnRH and its agonist analogs.

It has been well established in several cell types that the DG formed during PI breakdown is a potent activator of the calcium- and phospholipid-dependent enzyme, protein kinase C (4). This enzyme, which is normally present as an inactive form, has increased affinity for calcium in the presence of DG, and is activated to a form that undergoes redistribution from cytosolic to membrane-associated sites. The calcium-dependence and phospholipid turnover associated with GnRH-induced LH secretion suggest the possible involvement of protein kinase C. To analyze the activity of this enzyme in the rat gonadotroph, the stimulatory effects of TPA and GnRH on LH secretion and protein kinase C, and the inhibitory effects of retinal on these responses, were examined in cultured pituitary cells. Protein phosphorylation by rat anterior pituitary cytosol was increased in the presence of Ca^{2+} and was further enhanced by phosphatidylserine (PS) and 1,2-diolein. Also, TPA was found to fully activate kinase C in pituitary cytosol in the presence of Ca^{2+} and PS, and to stimulate LH secretion with about 50% of the efficacy of GnRH. In contrast, retinal inhibited kinase C in the presence of Ca^{2+} and diolein when added at concentrations greater than 10^{-7} M. In cultured pituitary cells stimulated with a maximal dose of GnRH (10 nM), addition of retinal also reduced GnRH-induced LH release in a dose-dependent fashion. The maximum inhibition of GnRH-induced LH release was 47 ± 13% with 10^{-4} M retinal, a concentration at which kinase C activity was also maximally inhibited. The ability of TPA to activate pituitary kinase C and to stimulate LH secretion, and the converse effects of retinal on kinase C and GnRH-induced LH release, suggest that kinase C participates in the action of GnRH upon LH secretion.

This mechanism was further evaluated by analysis of the distribution of protein kinase C activity between cytosol and membrane fractions in cells treated with GnRH. In pituitary cells fractionated by centrifugal elutriation, the greatest change in protein kinase C activity during GnRH stimulation was correlated with the maximal enrichment of gonadotrophs. Stimulation of LH release in gonadotroph-enriched cells by GnRH was accompanied by a rapid and dose-dependent decrease in cytosolic protein kinase C activity, and by a significant increase in protein kinase C associated with the membrane fraction. The ability of GnRH to cause rapid translocation of cytosolic protein kinase C to a membrane-associated form is consistent with the activation of protein kinase C as an early event in the stimulation of LH secretion by GnRH.

The actions of GnRH on LH release in cultured rat pituitary cells are inhibited by certain calcium channel blockers and calmodulin antagonists, and are reproduced by high concentrations of A23187 (22). As noted above, the ability of TPA to stimulate LH release at low concentrations (0.1 nM), and with up to 50% of the efficacy of 10 nM GnRHa, suggests that protein kinase C is also involved in LH release. In analyzing the role of these mechanisms in LH release by cultured rat pituitary cells, we observed two additional findings of interest. First, calmodulin antagonists increased the LH response to TPA: 10 μM pimozide or W7 doubled the LH release elicited by 10 pM to 1 μM TPA, although these antagonists reduced GnRHa-stimulated LH release by 50%. Second, the potent GnRH antagonist (GnRHant) not only completely inhibited GnRHa-stimulated

LH release, but also reduced the effect of TPA by 50%. These results support the involvement of both calmodulin and kinase C pathways in calcium-dependent LH release, and suggest that inhibition of calmodulin binding facilitates the activation of protein kinase C, possibly by preventing calmodulin-dependent phosphatase action. The inhibition of TPA-induced LH release by a GnRH antagonist suggests that protein kinase C causes phosphorylation and activation of the GnRH receptor, possibly via a conformational change that is prevented when the receptor is locked into its inactive state by the tightly bound antagonist.

To pursue the possibility that phorbol esters cause receptor activation, their effects on GnRH receptor sites were analyzed in cultured rat anterior pituitary cells. In addition to causing a dose-related stimulation of LH secretion, TPA markedly inhibited the binding of GnRH to rat pituitary cells. In each of these effects, TPA was the most potent agent among several phorbol esters including phorbol, 12,13-dibutyrate, phorbol 12,13-diacetate, 4α-phorbol and 4α-phorbol 12,13-didecanoate. Scatchard analysis indicated that the TPA-induced reduction in GnRH binding was due to a decrease in the number of GnRH receptors, without any change in the affinity of the receptors for GnRH. Pre-treatment with the potent GnRH antagonist reduced the effect of TPA on LH secretion and inhibition of GnRH binding, but did not prevent the redistribution of protein kinase C between cytosol and membrane fractions. The ability of a GnRH antagonist to block the suppressive effect of TPA on GnRH receptors, as well as the stimulatory effect on LH secretion, supports the proposal that the actions of phorbol esters are at least partially expressed through protein kinase C-dependent phosphorylation of the GnRH receptor or its regulatory proteins.

Arachidonic acid (AA) metabolites of the 5-lipoxygenase (LO) and monooxygenase (MO) pathways have also been implicated as potential mediators of GnRH-induced LH secretion from pituitary gonadotrophs (23,24). In order to characterize these metabolites during conditions of altered LH secretion, the products released from ^{3}H-AA pre-labeled rat gonadotrophs during 3 h culture were analyzed by reverse-phase high-performance liquid chromatography. At least 15 readily measurable ^{3}H-AA metabolites were formed, including several major non-polar products eluting between the monohydroxylated AAs of the LO pathway (5-, 12- and 15-HETEs) and AA itself, possibly representing epoxyeicosatrienoic acids of the MO pathway; at least 8 dihydroxy derivatives and leukotrienes of intermediate polarity were formed from AA via LO or MO activity, in addition to several cyclooxygenase products including PGE_2. Stimulation of LH release by GnRH, phorbol esters, and the Ca^{2+} ionophore A23187, was in general associated with increased production of ^{3}H-AA metabolites. However, GnRH-induced LH secretion and its enhancement by cyclooxygenase inhibitors were accompanied by both quantitative and qualitative changes (including some decreases) among unidentified ^{3}H-AA products of intermediate polarity. The LH secretory response to 10 nM GnRH was attenuated by the LO inhibitor nordihydroguaiaretic acid (40 μM), and by the general AA metabolism inhibitor eicosatetraynoic acid (40 μM), but was augmented by the cytochrome P-450 (MO) inhibitor, SKF 525A. Thus, gonadotrophs biosynthesize 5-LO and MO products, as well as several AA metabolites of intermediate polarity which undergo changes during GnRH-stimulation of LH secretion, and which are potential modulators of GnRH action. Although leukotrienes are the most highly active products of the 5-LO pathway, in pituitary cells the stimulatory actions of leukotrienes B_4 and C_4 on LH release were relatively small. Also, the leukotriene antagonist FPL 55712 had only a minor inhibitory effect on GnRH-induced LH release. Therefore, while AA and 5-HETE consistently stimulate LH release, and epoxy derivatives of AA have been implicated in the release process (24), the quantitative contribution of AA and its oxygenated metabolites to GnRH-induced gonadotropin secretion has yet to be established.

Based on the findings described above, it appears likely that the calcium-dependent activation of gonadotropin-secretion by GnRH involves not one but several inter-related mechanisms. While there is now growing evidence for a long-term role of cyclic AMP in regulating the responsiveness of gonadotrophs to GnRH stimulation (25), the immediate effects of GnRH do not appear to involve cyclic AMP-dependent processes. The acute secretory episodes elicited by pulses of GnRH include a rapid initial release of LH that peaks within one minute, followed by a secondary phase over the ensuing several minutes (14). It is possible that the early rapid component is mediated by calcium-calmodulin dependent mechanisms, while the subsequent phase is related to activation and redistribution of protein kinase C in the gonadotroph. Further analysis of the individual and combined effects of phospholipid turnover, calcium-calmodulin and protein kinase C, arachidonic acid, and cyclic AMP, should clarify the mechanisms responsible for physiological activation of gonadotropin secretion, as well as the steps at which refractoriness of the gonadotroph occurs during agonist-induced desensitization of pituitary function.

REFERENCES

1. Gilman AG (1984) J Clin Invest 73:1-4
2. Reuter H (1983) Nature 301:569-574
3. Farese RV (1984) Mol Cell Endocrinol 35:1-14
4. Nishizuka Y (1984) Nature 308:693-698
5. Naor Z, Catt KJ (1981) J Biol Chem 256:2226-2229
6. Hyde CL, Childs G, Wahl LM, Naor Z, Catt KJ (1982) Endocrinology 111: 1421-1423

7. Clayton RN, Catt KJ (1981) Endocr Rev 2:186-209

8. Clayton RN, Channabasavaiah K, Stewart JM, Catt KJ (1982) Endocrinology 110:1108-1115

9. Loumaye E, Catt KJ (1982) Science 215:983-985

10. Loumaye E, Catt KJ (1983) J Biol Chem 258:12002-12009

11. Hirota K, Hirota T, Aguilera G, Catt KJ (1984) Proc 7th Int Cong Endocrinol (1984) 773 (abs)

12. Young LS, Naik SI, Clayton RN (1984) Endocrinology 114:2114

13. Naor Z, Atlas D, Clayton RN, Forman DS, Amsterdam A, Catt KJ (1981) J Biol Chem 256:3049-3052

14. Catt KJ, Loumaye E, Katikineni M, Hyde CL, Childs G, Amsterdam A, Naor Z (1983) In: McCann SM, Dhindsa D (eds) Role of Peptides and Proteins in Control of Reproduction. Elsevier, Amsterdam, pp 33-61

15. Loumaye E, Wynn PC, Coy D, Catt KJ (1984) J Biol Chem 259 (in press)

16. Hazum E (1983) Endoc Rev 4:352-362

17. Winiger BP, Birabeau MA, Lang U, Capponi AM, Sizonenko PC, Aubert ML (1983) Mol Cell Endocrinol 31:77-91

18. Snyder GD, Bleasdale (1982) Mol Cell Endocrinol 28:55-63

19. Kiesel L, Catt KJ (1984) Arch Biochem Biophys 231:202-210

20. Burgess GM, Godfrey PP, McKinney JS, Berridge MJ, Irvine RF, Putney JW (1984) Nature 309:63-66

21. Gershengorn MC, Geras E, Purrello VS, Rebecchi MJ (1984) J Biol Chem 259:10675-10681

22. Conn PM, Hsueh AJW, Crowley WF (1984) Fed Proc 43:2351-2361

23. Naor Z, Vanderhoek JY, Lindner HR, Catt KJ, (1983) In: Advances in Prostaglandin, Thromboxane, and Leukotriene Research 12:259-263

24. Snyder GD, Capdevila J, Chacos N, Manna S, Falck JR (1983) Proc Natl Acad Sci USA 80:3504-3507

25. Cronin MJ, Evans WS, Hewlett EL, Thorner MO (1984) Am J Physiol 246:E44-51

SYMPOSIA

1. Clinical Aspects of Hormone-Producing Tumors

© 1984 Elsevier Science Publishers B.V.
Endocrinology
F. Labrie, L. Proulx, eds.

IMMUNOHISTOCHEMISTRY OF HUMAN PITUITARY ADENOMAS

KALMAN KOVACS
Department of Pathology, St. Michael's Hospital, 30 Bond St., University of Toronto, Toronto, Ontario, Canada

Although clinical and biochemical findings can establish the underlying endocrine abnormality in the substantial majority of patients with pituitary adenoma, the accurate identification of the cells constituting the tumor can only be undertaken by morphologic techniques (1-4). Immunohistochemical methods are capable of detecting growth hormone (GH), prolactin (PRL), adrenocorticotropic hormone (ACTH), endorphins, thyroid-stimulating hormone (TSH), follicle-stimulating hormone (FSH), luteinizing hormone (LH) and α-subunit of glycoprotein hormones in the cytoplasm of adenoma cells, providing evidence that all known adenohypophysial hormones can be produced by pituitary tumors (5,6). In addition, antibodies raised against non-hormonal markers, such as keratin, neuron specific enolase, S-100 protein, GFA protein, factor 8, chromogranin, etc., can be used to label certain cell types and separate pituitary adenomas from other neoplasms. The immunoperoxidase technique has replaced previously applied immunofluorescence procedures in studies related to the pituitary. It is sensitive, reliable and reproducible; tissue fixed in formalin or embedded in paraffin and stored for a considerable length of time can be immunostained for adenohypophysial hormones. The original procedure was modified by several authors; currently, the avidin-biotin-peroxidase complex method is used by most laboratories (7,8). Immunostaining can be performed at the light microscopic and ultrastructural levels. Immunoelectron microscopy localizes hormones at their subcellular sites and is regarded, at present, the most sensitive approach to cell identification. Immunohistochemical techniques are not quantitative; they demonstrate the presence of hormones, but fail to provide reliable information on the amount of stored hormone, the rate of hormone synthesis and release. Rigorous control studies are necessary to avoid misleading conclusions. In many cases of pituitary adenoma, clinical and biochemical findings can be correlated with immunohistochemical results.

A great variety of tumors occur in the region of the sella turcica. The immunoperoxidase technique can be successfully applied in their differential diagnosis, since it separates tumors which contain adenonypophysial hormones from those which exhibit no immunoreactivity. A positive immunostaining for one or more adenohypophysial hormones supports the diagnosis of pituitary adenoma or carcinoma, with the exception of those extrapituitary tumors which produce hypophysial hormones ectopically. One must keep in mind that negative immunostaining does not exclude the possibility that the tumor consists of adenohypophysial cells, since certain pituitary adenomas are negative for all known adenohypophysial hormones.

Based on the staining affinity of the cell cytoplasm, pituitary adenomas were previously classified as acidophilic, basophilic or chromophobic tumors. This classification is simplistic and has very little value, since it fails to reveal hormone content, subcellular details and cytogenesis, and is of no use in correlating structural features with endocrine activity.

The pituitary adenoma classification, which is used currently, hinges on immunocytologic and ultrastructural features of the tumor cells and takes into consideration hormone content and cellular origin (1-5). On the grounds of this modern classification, pituitary adenomas can be divided into the following entities: 1) growth hormone cell adenomas; 2) prolactin cell adenomas; 3) corticotroph cell adenomas secreting excess ACTH; 4) silent corticotroph cell adenomas; 5) thyrotroph cell adenomas; 6) gonadotroph cell adenomas; 7) null cell adenomas: 8) oncocytomas; 9) plurihormonal adenomas.

Growth hormone cell- prolactin cell- corticotroph cell- thyrotroph cell- and gonadotroph cell- adenomas produce their respective hormones which can be demonstrated by immunocytologic techniques in the cell cytoplasm. The silent corticotroph cell adenomas are unassociated with clinical or biochemical evidence of ACTH overproduction, but contain ACTH or biologically inactive precursors or various fragments of the proopiomelanocortin molecule which can be detected by immunohistochemical methods, but have no biologic activity.

The immunohistochemical investigation plays a major role in the diagnosis of plurihormonal adenomas (9-13). These tumors, capable of producing two or more hormones different in chemical composition, immunoreactivity and biologic action, can be divided into monomorphous and plurimorphous adenomas. The former tumors consist of one cell type and two or more hormones are present in the cytoplasm of the same cell. The latter are composed of two or more cell types and each hormone is present in different cells. The most common variants of plurihormonal adenomas produce GH and PRL. They can be separated into three entities: mixed growth hormone cell- prolactin cell adenomas, acidophil stem cell adenomas and mammosomatotroph cell adenomas. Mixed growth hormone cell-prolactin cell adenomas are bimorphous, bihormonal tumors. They are composed of two morphologically distinct, separate cell types; the growth hormone cells produce growth hormone; the prolactin cells, prolactin. Acidophil stem cell adenomas are monomorphous bihormonal tumors. They consist of one cell type which contains both growth hormone and prolactin, and is assumed to be the common progenitor of growth hormone cells and prolactin cells. Mammosomatotroph cell adenomas are monomorphous, bihormonal, well differentiated tumors producing both growth hormone and prolactin. Occasionally, plurihormonal adenomas produce unusual combinations of hormones, such as GH + TSH, GH + PRL + TSH, GH + PRL + ACTH, GH + PRL + α-subunit, etc. In some plurihormonal adenomas, the hormones are discharged into the circulation leading to various endocrine abnormalities. In other tumors, one or more components are silent and hormone production can only be proven by the application of immunohistochemical techniques.

The study of pituitary adenomas by immunohistochemical methods provides conclusive evidence that all the known adenohypophysial hormones can be synthesized by pituitary adenomas (14). With more widespread availability of a growing number of antibodies, immunohistochemistry will not only play an important role in the diagnostic process, but it will have a profound impact on the better understanding of endocrine function and cytogenesis of pituitary adenomas. Although the introduction of immunohistochemical procedures has resulted in substantial progress during the last decade, many questions remain unresolved, and further studies are required to obtain a deeper insight into the problems which are obscure at present.

ACKNOWLEDGEMENTS

This study was supported in part by Grant MA-6349 of the Medical Research Council of Canada and by a grant of the Physicians' Services Incorporated Foundation of Ontario. The author is greatly indebted to Dr. E. Horvath, Mrs. Gezina Ilse, Mrs. Noemi Losinski, Miss Donna J. McComb and Mrs. Nancy Ryan for their important contributions during this investigation, and to Mrs. Wanda Wlodarski for excellent secretarial work.

REFERENCES

1. Horvath E, Kovacs K (1980) In: Ezrin C, Horvath E, Kaufman B, Kovacs K, Weiss MH (eds) Pathology of the pituitary gland. CRC Press, Boca Raton, pp 1-83
2. Kovacs K, Horvath E (1983) The pituitary. In: Silverberg SG (ed) Principles and practice of surgical pathology. Wiley and Sons, New York, pp 1393-1414
3. Kovacs K, McComb DJ, Horvath E (1983) Subcellular investigation of experimental and human pituitary adenomas. Neuroendocr Perspect 2:251-291
4. Scheithauer BW (1982) Surgical pathology of the pituitary and sella region. In: Laws ERJr, Randall RV, Kern EB, Abboud CF (eds) Management of pituitary adenomas and related lesions with emphasis on transsphenoidal microsurgery. Appleton-Century-Crofts, New York, pp 129-218

5. Kovacs K, Horvath E (1982) Pathology of pituitary adenomas. In: Givens JR (ed) Hormone secreting pituitary tumors. Year Book Med Publ, Chicago pp 97-119

6. Kovacs K, Horvath E, Ryan N (1981) Immunocytology of the human pituitary. In: DeLellis RA (ed) Diagnostic immunohistochemistry. Masson, New York, pp 17-35

7. Hsu SM, Raine L, Fanger H (1981) A comparative study of the peroxidase-antiperoxidase method and an avidin-biotin complex method for studying polypeptide hormones with radioimmunoassay antibodies. Amer J Clin Path 75:734-738

8. Hsu SM, Raine L, Fanger H (1981) The use of antiavidin antibody and avidin-biotin-peroxidase complex in immunoperoxidase technics. Amer J Clin Path 75:816-821

9. Horvath E, Kovacs K, Killinger DW, Smyth HS, Weiss MH, Ezrin C (1983) Mammosomatotroph cell adenoma of the human pituitary: a morphologic entity. Virchows Arch Pathol Anat 398:277-289

10. Horvath E, Kovacs K, Scheithauer BW, Randall RV, Laws ERJr, Thorner MO, Tindall GT, Barrow DL (1983) Pituitary adenomas producing growth hormone, prolactin, and one or more glycoprotein hormones: a histologic, immunohistochemical, and ultrastructural study of four surgically removed tumors. Ultrastruct Path 5:171-183

11. Kovacs K, Horvath E, Ezrin C, Weiss MH (1982) Adenoma of the human pituitary producing growth hormone and thyrotropin. A histologic, immunocytologic and fine structural study. Virchows Arch Pathol Anat 395:59-68

12. Lloyd RV, Gikes PW, Chandler WF (1983) Prolactin and growth hormone-producing pituitary adenomas. An immunohistochemical and ultrastructural study. Amer J Surg Path 7:251-260

13. McComb DJ, Bayley TA, Horvath E, Kovacs K, Kourides IA (1984) Monomorphous plurihormonal adenoma of the human pituitary. A histologic, immunocytologic and ultrastructural study. Cancer 53:1538-1544

14. McComb DJ, Ryan N, Horvath E, Kovacs K (1983) Subclinical adenomas of the human pituitary. New light on old problems. Arch Pathol Lab Med 107:488-491

Endocrinology
F. Labrie, L. Proulx, eds.

SECRETION OF GROWTH HORMONE RELEASING FACTOR (GRF) BY TUMORS

LAWRENCE A. FROHMAN, JENNIFER THOMINET, AND THOMAS DOWNS

Division of Endocrinology and Metabolism, University of Cincinnati College of Medicine, Cincinnati, Ohio 45267

HISTORICAL BACKGROUND

The presence of extrapituitary neoplasms in patients with growth hormone (GH)-secreting pituitary tumors and acromegaly has been recognized for more than 50 years and constitutes, in part, the syndrome of multiple endocrine neoplasia type I. Beginning in 1960, a number of case reports appeared documenting the association of carcinoid tumors, generally of bronchial origin and acromegaly (1). The first suggestion that these tumors exhibited a pathogenic role in GH hypersecretion was by Dabek (2) who reported a patient whose elevated GH levels returned to normal after removal of a bronchial carcinoid which did not contain GH. The first demonstrations of GRF activity occurred in 1978 (3,4) and the increased awareness of this syndrome (5) eventually led to the preoperative identification of two patients with GRF-secreting pancreatic islet tumors from which the sequence of GRF was determined (6,7).

CHARACTERIZATION OF GRF

Although there was for a time considerable interest in the role of carcinoid-derived indoleamines, particularly serotonin, as a mediater of GH secretion, the biologically active principle was found to be a peptide (5). Its mechanism of action was largely characterized before its structure was determined, and was found to resemble that of the other hypothalamic releasing factors, with both cyclic AMP and Ca^{++} serving as second messengers. All of the results obtained with partially purified ectopic GRF have subsequently been confirmed with synthetic peptide. A single peptide, of varying length (37, 40, and 44 residues) has been identified from the tumors studied and the cDNA has been isolated and its structure determined (6-8). The different sequence lengths in the different tumors is not unexpected, given the frequently observed variations in processing enzymes in neoplastic tissue. The 40 and 44 residue peptides exhibit similar biological activity both in vitro and in vivo whereas the 37 residue peptide is less active. Recent studies have indicated that human hypothalamic GRF also exists as a 40 and a 44 amino acid peptide and is identical to ectopic GRF.

QUANTITATION OF GRF IN TUMORS

Measurements of GRF in tumors were performed initially by bioassay and more recently by radioimmunoassay using an assay with a sensitivity of 5 pg (9). The highest levels found, in a pancreatic islet tumor, was 45 pg/mg tissue (more than 100 times the concentration in the hypothalamus). With one exception, all tumors with GRF levels of 100 pg/mg or greater were associated with clinical and/or biochemical evidence of GH hypersecretion. In tumors with moderate to high GRF levels (>10 pg/mg), the activity as measured by the two assays was significantly correlated. Tumors most frequently found to contain GRF are carcinoid tumors of either bronchial or intestinal origin, pancreatic islet tumors, small cell carcinomas, neural crest tumors and endometrial carcinomas. Those tumors associated with manifestations of acromegaly are generally benign, or if malignant, very slow growing, since several years of GRF hypersecretion are required to produce clinical features. GRF-secreting tumors also frequently secrete other hormones, including ACTH, CRF, somatostatin, GH, insulin, and serotonin.

In addition to tumors which release GRF into the systemic circulation, two varieties of GRF-containing tumors associated with acromegaly have been found in the region of the hypothalamus and pituitary. Intrapituitary gangliocytomas (choristomas) have been found in direct contiguity with somatotroph adenomas where GRF presumably exhibits a paracrine action (10) and a GRF-containing hypothalamic hamartoma has also been demonstrated in a patient with a somatotroph adenoma where the GRF was presumably released into hypothalamic portal vessels.

DIAGNOSIS OF THE ECTOPIC GRF SYNDROME

It has been suggested that somatotroph hyperplasia is a characteristic feature of excessive GRF production and that its presence suggests the existence of a GRF-secreting tumor. Although consistent exposure of the somatotrophs to

GRF can lead to hyperplasia, several patients with ectopic GRF production have shown well documented edivence of pituitary tumor formation, so the absence of somatotroph hyperplasia does not argue against the diagnosis. Plasma GH responses to provocative stimuli also fail to distinguish between acromegalic patients with and without ectopic GRF secretion. Almost all patients with GRF-secreting tumors exhibit stimulatory responses to TRH, suppressive effects by dopamine or l-dopa, and absence of glucose suppression (1).

PLASMA IMMUNOREACTIVE (IR)-GRF LEVELS

In patients with ectopic GRF production, plasma IR-GRF levels have ranged from 190 pg/ml to 25 ng/ml (11), with most patients exhibiting levels > 1 ng/ml. The lowest levels observed in patients with clinical evidence of GH hypersecretion are comparable to the threshold levels required during constant infusions in normal subjects (200-300 pg/ml) to elicit a sustained release of GH (12). In patients with acromegaly not suspected of harboring a GRF-secreting tumor, plasma IR-GRF levels rang from undetectable values (<20 pg/ml) to 75 pg/ml (11). IR-GRF levels in most normal subjects are undetectable, though a few subjects exhibit levels comparable to those seen in acromegalics. Determination of the plasma GRF half-life (51 min) and metabolic clearance rate (194 l/m^2/day) (13) has permitted calculation of the GRF secretion rate in patients with GRF-secreting tumors, which has ranged from 50 to 2500 µg/day.

Although no patients with unsuspected ectopic GRF secretion have yet been diagnosed by measurement of circulating IR-GRF levels, the relative infrequency of acromegaly, the ease of measuring the elevated IR-GRF in patients with ectopic GRF-secreting tumors, and the markedly different therapy required for this disease all justify screening acrogemalic patients on one occasion for the presence of elevated plasma IR-GRF levels. Because of the infrequency of the disease, extensive radiologic procedures to search for a clinically inapparent tumor is not warranted unless the diagnosis is suggested by other factors.

THERAPY OF ECTOPIC GRF SYNDROME

Treatment of ectopic GRF-secreting tumors is by complete excision. In all cases of documented total tumor removal, GH hypersecretion has reversed completely. In patients with persistance or recurrence of GH hypersecretion, residual or recurrent tumor must be presumed. GH secretion in some patients has been at least partially controlled by bromocriptine and this therapy should be considered if ectopic GRF secretion cannot be eliminated. It is unknown whether bromocriptine is more effective in this type of acromegaly than in patients without ectopic GRF secretion. On the basis of limited experience, bromocriptine does not appear to suppress ectopic GRF secretion directly. In one patient, ectopic GRF secretion has been suppressed by somatostatin on a short-term basis.

REFERENCES

1. Frohman LA, Thominet JL, Szabo M (1984) In: Raiti S, Tolman R (eds) Human Growth Hormone. Plenum Publishing, New York, (in press)

2. Dabek JT (1974) J Clin Endocrinol Metab 38:329

3. Zafar MS, Mellinger RC, Fine G, Szabo M, Frohman LA (1979) J Clin Endocrinol Metab 48:66

4. Shalet SM, Beardwell CG, MacFarlane IA, Ellison ML, Norman CM, Hughes M (1979) Clin Endocrinol 10:61

5. Frohman LA, Szabo M, Berelowitz M, Stachura ME (1980) J Clin Invest 65:43

6. Rivier J, Spiess J, Thorner M, Vale W (1982) Nature 300:276

7. Guillemin R, Brazeau P, Bohlen P, Esch P, Ling N, Wehrenberg WB (1982) Science 218:585

8. Gubler U, Monahan JJ, Lomedico PT, Bhatt RS, Collier KJ, Hoffman BJ, Bohlen P, Esch F, Ling N, Zeytin F, Brazeau P, Poonian M, Gage LP (1983) Proc Natl Acad Sci USA 80:4311

9. Frohman LA (1984) J Lab Clin Med 103:819

10. Asa SL, Scheithauer BW, Bilbao JM, Horvath E, Ryan N, Kovacs K, Randall RV, Laws ER Jr, Singer W, Linfoot JA, Thorner M, Vale W (1984) J Clin Endocrinol Metab 58:796

11. Thorner MO, Frohman LA, Leong DA, Thominet J, Downs T, Hellmann P, Chitwood J, Vaughn JM, Vale W (1984) J Clin Endocrinol Metab (in press)

12. Webb CB, Vance ML, Thorner MO, Perisutti G, Thominet J, Rivier J, Vale W, Frohman LA (1984) J Clin Invest (in press)

13. Frohman LA, Thominet JL, Webb CB, Vance ML, Uderman H, Rivier J, Vale W, Thorner MO (1984) J Clin Invest 73:1304

Endocrinology
F. Labrie, L. Proulx, eds.

PRODUCTION OF GASTRIN-RELEASING PEPTIDE (BOMBESIN) BY TUMORS

KAORU ABE, KEN YAMAGUCHI, ISAMU ADACHI, MASAFUMI SUZUKI, SATOSHI KIMURA, AKIHIKO SHIMADA, KANAME MARUNO and NOBORU YANAIHARA*
Endocrinology Division, National Cancer Center Research Institute, Chuo-ku, Tokyo 104, and *Shizuoka College of Pharmacy, Shizuoka, 422, (Japan)

INTRODUCTION

It has been reported by our laboratory that immunoreactive bombesin detected in small cell carcinomas of the lung (SCCL) has an amino-acid sequence similar to gastrin-releasing peptide (GRP) rather than bombesin and that immunoreactive GRP (IR-GRP) was produced not only by SCCL but also non-small cell carcinomas of the lung (1). Medullary carcinomas of the thyroid (MCT) were proven to produce IR-GRP as well (2). We have extended these observations further and found that IR-GRP is produced by various other types of tumors and that it is often associated with production of other peptide hormones.

MATERIALS AND METHODS

The tumor tissues examined were 139 lung cancer tissues (38 small cell carcinomas, 44 squamous cell carcinomas, 46 adenocarcinomas and 11 large cell carcinomas), 13 MCTs, 72 pancreatic endocrine tumors (PETs; 21 insulinomas, 10 gastrinomas, 9 vasoactive intestinal peptide-producing tumors, 3 glucagonomas, 3 ACTH-producing tumors and 26 asymptomatic tumors), 33 neuroblastic tumors (NBTs; 13 ganglioneuroblastomas, 1 ganglioneuroma and 19 neuroblastomas), 25 pheochromocytomas (PHEO) and 22 carcinoids. Most of these were obtained surgically and some at autopsy. Immediately after removal, the tumor tissues were stored at -80°C until extraction.

GRP radioimmunoassay (RIA) was carried out as reported previously with slight modifications (1). The antiserum used was produced in a rabbit immunized with synthetic bombesin (provided kindly by Prof. J.H. Walsh, CURE, UCLA, Cal., USA). Synthetic porcine GRP (pGRP) was used as the iodinated antigen and assay standard. This GRP RIA could not discriminate pGRP(1-27) from bombesin or pGRP(18-27). The RIAs of bombesin, calcitonin (CT), vasoactive intestinal peptide (VIP), somatostatin (SRIF) and pancreatic growth hormone-releasing factor (pGRF) were carried out, as previously reported (1, 3-6).

The tumor tissues were extracted by boiling water and acetic acid (1), and the average recovery was 85% for GRP, 65% for CT, 66% for VIP, 70% for SRIF and 100% for pGRF. When assayed, the solution was diluted 20-fold or more by adding the standard diluent, and 0.1 ml of each solution was used for the RIAs. When significant displacement was observed in only one dilution, the substance was considered undetectable.

After an overnight fast, peripheral venous blood was collected in a heparinized test tube containing Trasylol (500 KIU/ml of blood) from 10 normal subjects and 12 patients (5 MCTs, 5 SCCLs and 2 PETs).

RESULTS

Tumor production of IR-GRP. The tumor extracts showed a dose-response parallel to that of pGRP(1-27). As shown in Fig. 1, the frequency of IR-GRP production was highest in MCT (92%), which was followed by SCCL (74%), carcinoids and PHEO (64%), PETs (61%) and NBTs (42%). The number of tumors which produced larger amounts of IR-GRP was increased in those types of tumors in which the frequency of IR-GRP production was higher except for NBTs and PHEO.

Tumor production of other hormones. The frequency of tumor production of IR-CT, IR-VIP, IR-SRIF and IR-pGRF in these tumors is summarized in Table 1. These tumors were found to produce these peptides with variable frequency, and it was higher in SCCL, MCT, PETs, PHEO, NBTs and carcinoids, when compared with those observed in non-small cell carcinomas of the lung. When IR-GRP was detected, one or more other hormones examined here tended to be detectable. IR-bombesin was undetectable in the tumor extracts thus far examined.

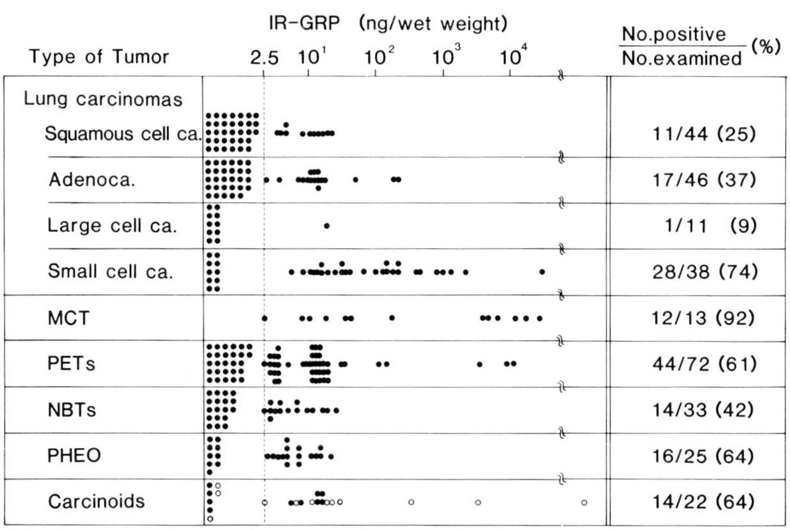

Fig. 1 Incidence of IR-GRP and its quantities in lung carcinomas, medullary carcinoma of the thyroid (MCT), pancreatic endocrine tumors (PETs), neuroblastic tumors (NBTs), pheochromocytoma (PHEO) and carcinoids. Open circles indicate bronchial carcinoid.

Table 1 Frequency of hormone production by tumors
No. detected / No. examined (%)

Type of tumor	CT	VIP	SRIF	pGRF
Lung carcinomas				
small cell ca.	16/24(67)	16/29(21)	10/29(35)	20/45(44)
adenocarcinoma	4/39(10)	5/39(13)	18/39(46)	7/47(15)
squamous cell ca.	3/28(11)	4/28(14)	5/25(20)	1/28(4)
large cell ca.	1/14(7)	1/14(7)	4/14(29)	2/13(15)
Medullary ca. of the thyroid	16/16(100)	8/14(57)	11/13(85)	5/ 7(71)
Pancreatic endocrine tumors	19/45(42)	23/40(58)	34/45(76)	34/74(46)
Neuroblastic tumors	5/26(19)	21/28(75)	23/28(82)	9/21(43)
Pheochromocytoma	8/11(73)	11/16(69)	14/16(88)	6/15(40)
Carcinoids	8/17(47)	6/16(38)	12/16(75)	10/21(48)

Plasma IR-GRP levels. Plasma levels of IR-GRP in some patients whose tumor tissue had been proven to produce larger amounts of IR-GRP are summarized in Table 2. Only 3 patients with MCT and one with PET had an elevated plasma level of IR-GRP, but they showed no signs compatible with peptic ulcer or clinical signs due to plasma GRP excess.

DISCUSSION

In 1978, a peptide composed of 27 amino acids with gastrin-releasing activity was isolated from porcine nonantral tissue and named as GRP (7). Because of its similarity in pharmacological effects and homologous amino-acid sequence to bombesin, GRP is now considered to be a mammalian counterpart of bombesin (7). Our previous data suggest that IR-bombesin produced by SCCL and MCT has a structure similar to GRP rather than bombesin (1,2), and in the tumors examined here IR-bombesin was undetectable. These observations indicate that the substance produced by human tumors is GRP, not bombesin. The data presented here revealed that the tumor production of IR-GRP is not confined to lung carcinomas and MCT, but that carcinoids, PHEO, PETs and NBTs, which could be considered as neuroendocrine tumors, also produce it. Furthermore, the production of GRP is often associated with that of

Table 2 Plasma level and tumor content of IR-GRP

Patient No.	Type of tumor	Plasma (pg/ml)	Tumor (ng/g)
1	MCT	780	1,600
2	MCT	160	3,200
3	MCT	130	9.5
4	MCT	< 100	34,000
5	MCT	< 100	2,000
6	SCCL	< 100	1,200
7	SCCL	< 100	270
8	SCCL	< 100	130
9	SCCL	< 100	93
10	SCCL	< 100	48
11	PET	860	5,500
12	PET	< 100	4.3

MCT, medullary carcinoma of the thyroid
SCCL, small cell carcinoma of the lung
PET, pancreatic endocrine tumors

CT, VIP, SRIF and pGRF in these tumor tissues. These data indicate that GRP-producing tumors are multiple hormone producers.

Although several investigators have examined plasma IR-bombesin or GRP levels in patients with SCCL, their elevation was rarely reported (8-10). In the present study, plasma IR-GRP level was elevated only in 3 MCT and one PET patient, and they did not show any signs due to GRP excess. Further studies will be needed to explain these results.

SUMMARY

Gastrin-releasing peptide, not bombesin, is produced frequently by neuroendocrine tumors including carcinoids, PHEO, PETs and NBTs, and its production is often associated with the production of other hormones such as CT, VIP, SRIF and pGRF.

Acknowledgements

This work was supported in part by Grants-in-Aid for Cancer Research (57-8, 57S, 58-2, 59S-1, 59-1) and Research Grant for the Intractable Diseases from the Ministry of Health and Welfare, and by Grants-in-Aid for Cancer Research from the Ministry of Education, Science and Culture, Japan.

References

(1) Yamaguchi K, Abe K, Kameya T, Adachi I, Taguchi S, Otsubo K, Yanaihara N (1983) Cancer Res 43:3932-3939

(2) Yamaguchi K, Abe K, Adachi I, Suzuki M, Kimura S, Kameya T, Yanaihara N (1984) Metabolism (in press)

(3) Abe K, Adachi I, Miyakawa S, Tanaka M, Yamaguchi K, Tanaka N, Kameya T, Shimosato Y (1977) Cancer Res 37:4190-4194

(4) Yamaguchi K, Abe K, Miyakawa S, Ohnami M, Sakagami M, Yanaihara N (1980) Gastroenterology 79:687-694

(5) Yamaguchi K, Adachi I, Miyakawa S, Abe K, Yanaihara N (1981) In: Japanese Society of Gut Hormones (ed) Proceedings of the Third Gut Hormone Conference. Igaku Tosho Shuppan LTD, Tokyo, pp228-235 (in Japanese)

(6) Yamaguchi K, Abe K, Suzuki M, Adachi I, Kimura S, Shimada A, Ohno H, Kanai A, Kameya T (1983) Gann 74:814-817

(7) McDonald TJ (1981) In: Bloom SR, Polak JM (eds) Gut Hormones, Ed 2. Churchill Livingstone, Inc., Edinburgh, pp407-412

(8) Moody TW, Pert CB, Gazdar AF, Carney DN, Minna JD (1981) Science (Wash. D.C.) 214:1246-1248

(9) Wood SM, Wood JR, Ghatei MA, Lee YC, O'Shaughnessy D, Bloom SR (1981) J Clin Endocrinol Metab 53:1310-1312

(10) Sorenson GD, Bloom SR, Ghatei MA, Del Prete SA, Cate CC, Pettengill OS (1982) Regul Pep 4:59-66

2. Pathogenesis of Type I Diabetes Mellitus

© 1984 Elsevier Science Publishers B.V.
Endocrinology
F. Labrie, L. Proulx, eds.

FAMILIAL MEDULLARY CARCINOMA OF THE THYROID

KENNETH E. W. MELVIN, M.D., F.A.C.P.
Department of Medicine, St. Vincent Hospital and Medical Center
Portland, Oregon, USA

Medullary carcinoma of the thyroid (MCT) may occur as a genetic variant, with dominant inheritance, frequently in association with polyendocrine and/or neuroectodermal neoplasia; or as a sporadic tumor. The genetic form is important for its familial implications, and for the frequent association with pheochromocytoma, parathyroid neoplasia, and less frequently, with multiple mucosal neuromata. Collectively, these elements constitute the medullary carcinoma syndrome.

The sporadic form is neither heritable, nor accompanied by other features of the medullary carcinoma syndrome.

It is the genetic form of MCT and its associated syndromes, either in the context of familial disease, or arising freshly as a new mutation, that is the subject of this report.

Oncogenesis: MCT arises as a tumor of C-cells, which derive from the embryonic neural crest [1,2]. These, together with other cells not necessarily of neural crest origin, but which share the functional characteristics of amine precursor uptake and decarboxylation (APUD), share also the genetic predisposition to hyperplasia and multifocal neoplasia which characterizes the medullary carcinoma syndrome.

Familial MCT is a bilateral tumor, in a setting of diffuse C-cell hyperplasia throughout the thyroid gland. C-cell hyperplasia occurs as the initial, premalignant event, with subsequent transformation to frankly malignant MCT [3]. It is not surprising, therefore, that the tumor is usually multifocal and bilateral. Similar diffuse hyperplasia leading to multifocal tumor formation occurs in the adrenal medulla [4,5]. What is surprising, given this setting, is the observation in a single patient with glucose-6-phosphate dehydrogenase mosaicism, that both the MCT and the pheochromocytoma were of monoclonal origin [6], suggesting that some but not all the C-cells and adrenal neurochromaffin cells participated in the neoplastic process.

It remains to be determined what factors initiate and maintain the hyperplastic/neoplastic changes in the genetically predisposed cells. Interest is currently focussed upon a possible role for circulating growth factors, e.g. nerve growth factor [7], in the pathogenesis of the medullary carcinoma syndrome.

Some investigators have described a chromosomal instability [8], or short arm deletion in chromosome 20p [9], in kindreds affected by familial MCT. Should this be confirmed as a consistent finding, it would be of importance not only in the pathogenesis, but also in providing a cytogenetic marker of the carrier state.

Most medullary carcinomas contain amyloid. This amyloid differs in structure from immune amyloid, containing polymerized calcitonin [10], or calcitonin prohormone [11].

Hormonal and Biosynthetic Activity of MCT: MCT is unique amongst hormone secreting tumors, consistently secreting calcitonin (CT), and frequently given also to the ectopic production of a variety of other peptides, and various bioactive molecules. The latter include ACTH, somatostatin, katacalcin, gastrin releasing peptide, γ-trace, prostaglandins, carcinoembryonic antigen (CEA), histaminase, dopa-decarboxylase, and serotonin.

Hypercalcitoninemia is present universally in affected individuals, either basally or in response to provocative testing with calcitonin-secretagogues such as pentagastrin or calcium. Identification of this circulating tumor-marker by means of a sensitive radioimmunoassay permits the early diagnosis of clinically occult MCT [12], even in the premalignant stage of C-cell hyperplasia, and with the greatest accuracy.

All direct relatives of affected individuals should be screened by means of provocative testing for hypercalcitoninemia. Since peak presentation is in the pediatric age group, and most cases will have declared by the age of 30, screening should have commenced by age 5 and continue annually until at least the age of 35 [13].

Similarly, serum levels of calcitonin provide a means of quantifying the response of MCT to treatment, and of monitoring patients for recurrence following surgery. Currently, the only effective therapy of MCT is surgical; there is some evidence that radiotherapy to the neck postoperatively may reduce the frequency of local recurrence and improve longterm survival.

In patients with MCT, hypercalcitoninemia is usually metabolically silent, but is probably the cause of the severe secretory diarrhea that may complicate disseminated disease and may actually be the presenting symptom.

The relative tumor content of calcitonin and dopa-decarboxylase is of prognostic significance in any given case. Similarly, serum levels of CEA may be of prognostic importance, high levels being associated with more virulent tumors.

In common with other APUD-tumors, MCT shares a propensity for ectopic production of ACTH, and may present initially as Cushing's syndrome [14]. The syndrome is typically fulminant, with severe hypokalemic alkalosis and proximal muscle weakness. Progression may be so rapid as to leave little time for the development of a typical Cushingoid appearance, which is often lacking. The response to thyroidectomy can be dramatic; medical management with aminoglutethamide is also effective.

The Medullary Carcinoma Syndrome: Often referred to as multiple endocrine neoplasia, type II (MEN II), the MCT syndrome presents a genetically based spectrum of (i) MCT alone, (ii) MCT and pheochromocytoma, or (iii) MCT and pheochromocytoma and multiple mucosal neuromata (sometimes referred to as MEN II b). Parathyroid abnormalities, usually hyperplasia but occasionally adenomata, occur frequently in association with (i) and (ii), but only very rarely with (iii). Renal stones occur quite frequently, and are not necessarily accompanied by hypercalcemia. In some affected families there has been a perplexing lack of correlation between levels of serum calcium, serum PTH, and histologic parathyroid hyperplasia. The mechanism whereby the parathyroids are involved in this syndrome remains obscure. A reactive rather than a genetic cause has been considered, but the finding of elevated serum PTH levels in some individuals prior to the development of elevated calcitonin levels argues against this as the cause in all cases. Similarly, the rarity with which parathyroid abnormalities occur in association with MCT and mucosal neuromata, and their absence in cases of sporadic MCT -- all of which exhibit hypercalcitoninemia -- favor a genetic influence.

Adrenal medullary involvement in the medullary carcinoma syndrome may range from diffuse hyperplasia, through nodular hyperplasia, to multiple pheochromocytomas, and is usually bilateral. Pheochromocytomas are usually intra-adrenal; several instances of malignancy have been reported.

Although symptoms are frequently mild, or even absent, catastrophic crises may be precipitated by radiographic or surgical interventions, and patients should be screened for pheochromocytoma before operating upon the neck for MCT. Computered axial tomography and adrenal scintigraphy with iodinated metaiodobenzylguanidine will probably supplant adrenal angiography in localizing adrenal medullary disease. Pre-operative treatment with the tyrosine hydroxylase inhibitor, metyrosine (MSD), offers advantages over adrenergic receptor blockade. Consideration should be given at the time of surgery to the implantation of salvaged adrenocortical tissue in the abdominal (or other) musculature.

A few patients will exhibit the medullary carcinoma phenotype, which includes a characteristic facies and habitus that permit immediate and positive diagnosis [15]. Mucosal neuromata may be evident on the tongue, lips and conjunctivae. A Marfanoid habitus may be present, often associated with other skeletal abnormalities including pes cavus, pectus excavatum, high arched palate, kyphoscoliosis, hyperextensibility of joints, and abnormalities of dental enamel. Hypertrophied corneal nerves can frequently be seen with a slit-lamp. Ganglioneuromatosis may occur extensively throughout the autonomic nervous system, and may present in infancy with megacolon. Most individuals with mucosal neuromata will ultimately develop pheochromocytoma, which are usually bilateral.

Conclusion: The unique genetic and endocrine features of the medullary carcinoma syndrome offer unparalleled opportunities for advancing our understanding of tumor-cell biology and oncogenic mechanisms. The application of this knowledge has already resulted in greatly enhanced patient care, through the development of diagnostic tests which make possible the reliable and early diagnosis of a cancer in its curable stages.

References

1. Williams ED: Histogenesis of medullary carcinoma of the thyroid. J Clin Pathol 19:114-118, 1966.
2. LeDouarin J, Lievre C: Demonstration de l'origine neurale des cellules a calcitonine du corps ultimobronchial chez l'embryon de Poulet. C Hebd Acad Sci, Seanc Paris Serie D 270:2857-2860, 1970.

3. Wolfe JH, Melvin KEW, Cervi-Skinner SJ, Al Saadi AA, Juliar JF, Jackson CE, Tashjian AH Jr: C-cell hyperplasia preceding medullary thyroid carcinoma. N Engl J Med 289:437-441, 1973.
4. Carney JA, Sizemore GW, Sheps SG: Adrenal medullary disease in multiple endocrine neoplasia, Type 2: Pheochromocytoma and its precursors. Am J Clin Pathol 66:279-290, 1976.
5. De Lellis RA, Wolfe JH, Gagel RF, Feldman ZT, Miller HH, Gang DL, Reichlin S: Adrenal medullary hyperplasia: A morphometric analysis in patients with familial medullary thyroid carcinoma. Am J Pathol 83:177-196, 1976.
6. Baylin SB, Hsu SH, Gann DS, Smallridge RC, Wells SA: Inherited medullary thyroid carcinoma: A final monoclonal mutation in one of multiple clones of susceptible cells. Science 199:429-431, 1978.
7. Bigazzi M, Revoltella T, Casciano S, Vigneti E: High level of a nerve growth factor in the serum of a patient with medullary carcinoma of the thyroid gland. Clin Endocrinol 6:105, 1977.
8. Samaan NA, Hsu TC, Pathak S, Saad MF, Ordonez NG, Hickey RC: Chromosomal instability in medullary carcinoma of the thyroid. World Journal of Surgery, in press.
9. VanDyke DL, Jackson CE, Babu VR: Prometaphase chromosomes in cancer families: Multiple endocrine neoplasia 2 syndrome and neurofibromatosis. Clin Res 29:37A, 1981.
10. Tashjian AJ Jr, Wolfe HJ, Voelkel EF: Human calcitonin: Immunologic assay, cytologic localization and studies on medullary thyroid carcinoma. Am J Med 56:840, 1974.
11. Sletten K, Westermark P, Natvig JB: Characterization of amyloid fibril proteins from medullary carcinoma of the thyroid. J Exp Med 143:993, 1976.
12. Melvin KEW, Tashjian AH Jr, Miller HH: Studies in familial (medullary) thyroid carcinoma. Rec Prog in Horm Res 28:399-470, 1972.
13. Gagel RF, Jackson CE, Block MA, Feldman ZT, Reichlin S, Hamilton BP, Tashjian AJ Jr: Age-related probability of development of hereditary medullary thyroid carcinoma. J Pediatrics 101:941-946, 1982.
14. Melvin KEW, Tashjian AH Jr, Cassidy CE, Givens JR: Cushing's syndrome caused by ACTH--and calcitonin--secreting medullary carcinoma of the thyroid. Metab Exp Biol 19:831-838, 1970.
15. Gorlin RJ, Sedano HO, Vickers RA, Cervenka J: Multiple mucosal neuromas, pheochromocytoma and medullary carcinoma of the thyroid -- a syndrome. Cancer 22:293-300, 1968.

© 1984 Elsevier Science Publishers B.V.
Endocrinology
F. Labrie, L. Proulx, eds.

PATHOGENESIS OF THE TYPE I DIABETES MELLITUS OF THE BB RAT

J.-F. YALE, M. GROSE, AND E.B. MARLISS
McGill Nutrition and Food Science Centre, Royal Victoria Hospital, 687 Pine Avenue West, Montreal, Quebec H3A 1A1 (Canada)

The spontaneously diabetic BB rat, since its discovery in 1974, has become a widely-studied "model" of diabetes etiology, pathogenesis, pathophysiology, and complications. It shows many analogies to human Type I diabetes: sudden onset of severe hyperglycemia, glycosuria, ketonuria, and weight loss leading to death in a few days in the absence of insulin therapy, with morphological evidence of insulitis. Peak onset follows the age of sexual maturation (60-120 days), both sexes are affected, and obesity is absent. Sublines with expected high diabetes incidence (BBdp) (40-100% overt diabetes) have been developed, as well as non diabetes-prone BB (BBn) sublines. Though derived from a Wistar strain, and not yet "inbred", it should no longer be referred to as a "Wistar" rat. The proceedings of a symposium on this rat (9) and a review of its immunological aspects (17) have recently been published.

This review describes current understanding of the immunological disorders. A "best estimate" of the chronology of appearance of abnormalities of the BB rat is schematized in figure 1. It is not known whether the beta cell destruction is a single, fulminant process, a progressive subacute process, or the result of repeated minor episodes. Since at least 80-90% of the beta cell mass must be destroyed in association with severe insulitis before overt diabetes occurs, many rats with milder insulitis show impaired glucose tolerance or no metabolic changes, and all other BBdp rats show the typical immune disorders without insulitis. At present, the precipitating factor(s) of diabetes in BBdp rats are unknown. Pancreatic lymphocytic infiltration (PLI) around ducts and acini has been observed as early as 50 days (Seemayer, et al in 9), and may antedate insulitis. Insulitis appears to precede overt diabetes by 2-3 weeks or possibly longer (8,9). The immunological concomitants which precede and accompany diabetes are described below.

MAJOR HISTOCOMPATIBILITY COMPLEX (MHC) ASSOCIATION

The $RT1^u$ haplotype of the rat MHC seems essential for susceptibility to diabetes. Hybrids between BB rats and several inbred strains develop diabetes only when this haplotype is present (Colle et al, in 9). Two groups have recently identified class II gene restriction enzyme fragment polymorphisms, specific to BBdp rats, with one pattern present in homozygous form in BB and crossbred strains with high diabetes incidence.

CELLULAR IMMUNITY

The profound lymphopenia has been a highly reproducible finding in all BBdp rats (2,3,4,9(Naji et al),14). In these rats, the normal rise in lymphocyte counts with age does not occur (17), and counts rarely rise above 50% of normal. Diabetes without lymphopenia has not yet been reported in a significant number of animals. Cross-breeding experiments suggest that the lymphopenia is not $RT1^u$ associated. The peripheral blood lymphopenia is due to a decrease in T (monoclonal antibody W3/13+) lymphocytes (2,4,14), the absolute counts of B cells being normal. Among the T cell subsets, that which includes helper (W3/25+) cells is reduced to less than one-third of normal whereas the non-helper (OX8+)

is less affected (2,4,14). The W3/25 deficit is already present at 5 days of age, while the OX8 deficit appears later (Yale, unpublished). These defects are as severe in the rats that become diabetic as in BBdp siblings that do not. There is no change in lymphocyte subsets at the onset of diabetes. Similar findings have been obtained in lymph nodes and spleen. In the thymus, most lymphocytes are positive for both W3/25 and OX8 determinants, although the total number of lymphocytes is decreased.

Skin allograft rejection is delayed in these nonsyngeneic rats, and transfers from RT1 incompatible donors are rejected more slowly than by an inbred $RT1^u$ strain, Wistar-Furth (WF)(2,11). In contrast, normal WF or BBn islets are destroyed more rapidly when transferred to diabetic BB rats than to BBn or WF rats rendered diabetic by streptozotocin (9,(Naji et al),11). Mixed lymphocyte reactions (MLR) reveal markedly decreased responses in BBdp rats (2,9(Naji et al)), with some variation according to the source of lymphocytes studied. Proliferative responses to Concanavalin A (ConA) of blood lymphocytes from diabetes-prone BB rats are deficient (2,9(Jackson et al)). Elder and Maclaren described the release of interleukin 2 (IL-2) upon exposure to ConA as normal, but with a failure to respond to exogenous IL-2 (2). In contrast, Prud'homme _et al_ found a decreased IL-2 production in all BBdp rats, which was greatly improved by partial depletion of macrophages, while BB splenic macrophages suppressed the response of WF spleen cells to ConA (15). Scott and colleagues showed a good MLR response of T-cell enriched preparations. They also have data from bone marrow irradiation chimeras suggesting a stem cell defect in the defective T cell population(s). Thus, not only numbers but many aspects of lymphocyte function are abnormal.

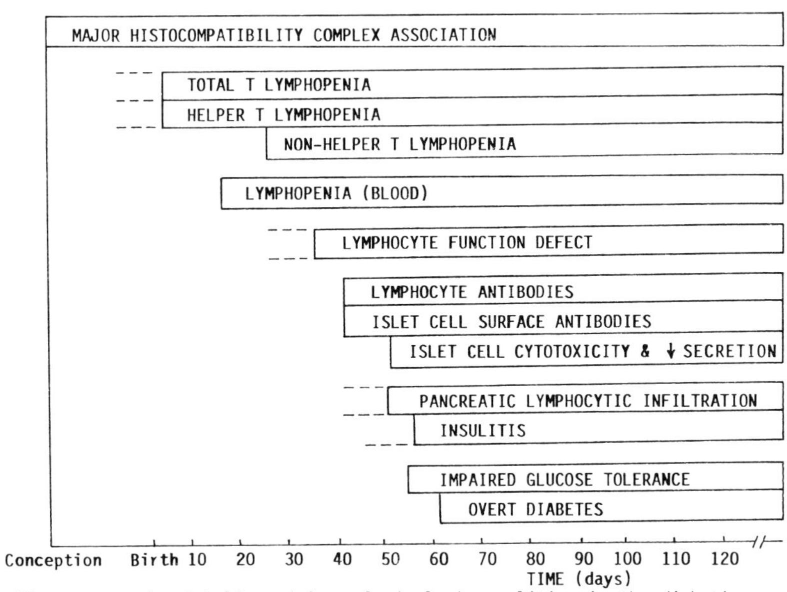

Fig.1: Time course of metabolic and immunological abnormalities in the diabetic syndrome of the BB rat. Dashed horizontal lines signify that onset could be earlier. Commencement of each horizontal bar indicates earliest age for which data are available.

HUMORAL IMMUNITY

Islet cell surface antibodies (ICSA) occur in almost all BBdp rats studied (1). They may appear both before and after onset of diabetes. They induce beta cytotoxicity in vitro, can inhibit insulin secretion (15), and seem to identify antigens of comparable molecular-size on non BB rat islets and rat insulinomas as do human ICSA. Complement fixing islet cell antibodies (10) and lymphocyte antibodies have also been found and the latter show tight correlation with ICSA (10). Antibodies have also been shown against thyroid colloid, gastric mucosa and vascular smooth muscle. Thyroiditis with lymphocytic infiltration has been shown, but not abnormal thyroid function.

PASSIVE TRANSFER OF INSULITIS

The transfer of insulitis to athymic nude mice, with intensity related to dose of transferred lymphocytes has been shown (12), as was the transfer of insulitis to BB rat recipients (11). Earlier than expected appearance of the overt syndrome in BBdp rats by such transfer has been shown by lymphocytes previously incubated with Concanavalin A (5) and diabetes has been induced in immunosuppressed BBn rats. Injection of serum from diabetic rats has not produced insulitis or diabetes in BB recipients (11).

IMMUNE INTERVENTIONS

Many standard approaches to immunosuppression appear to "prevent" overt diabetes, including antilymphocyte serum administration, neonatal thymectomy, total-body irradiation, cyclosporine, and other immunosuppressants alone and in combinations (6,7). Unfortunately, effects of these measures on the immune defects of the BB rat have not generally been reported in these studies. The cyclosporine results are among the most provocative. Doses of 8-10mg/kg to susceptible rats prevented diabetes appearance (untreated incidence was 75%). When the drug was stopped, at 121 days, many developed diabetes by 169 days (6). The mechanism of this effect has not been elucidated. Decreased incidence of diabetes among BB rats was found after neonatal bone marrow transfer from WF donors. Concomitantly, responses to skin grafts, resistance to infection, total T cell numbers and MLR returned toward normal but not the absolute numbers of helper T cells (11,9(Naji et al)). Mordes et al reported decreased diabetes incidence by lymphocyte transfusions from normal rats. The continued function of transplanted islets in immunosuppressed BB rats indicates that the destruction of not only the rats' own islets but those of a donor can be prevented (9,Naji et al). As noted, accelerated destruction of normal islets by diabetic recipients occurs, though this may diminish somewhat with duration of diabetes.

DISCUSSION

The BB rat demonstrates a profound immunodeficiency, and a multi-organ "autoimmune" syndrome in which Type I diabetes is the predominant feature. Reliable associations of the syndrome are the MHC group $RT1^u$, the cellular immune defects (T lymphopenia with dramatic reduction in the helper subset in most lymphoid tissues, functional T cell defects), and insulitis. Each seems essential but not sufficient for diabetes occurence. Common but not yet proven to be essential are the occurence of ICSA, lymphocyte antibodies and PLI. The recognition by ICSA of normal beta cells, the accelerated rejection of transplanted beta cells and the passive transfer of insulitis suggest that abnormal determinants on the beta cell are not a necessary condition. In comparing the rat syndrome with that of man, obvious differences are that man has neither lymphopenia, reproducible subset defects nor the magnitude or reproducibility of functional T cell deficits. Insulitis is present in man and rat, as well as a tendency to show other organ-specific autoimmunity and the MHC association. The one other common finding, ICSA, shows appropriate specificity and functional effects on beta cells to be the critical factor in the pathogenesis of the beta cell destruction, though this is still readily contested in both syndromes. Further enlightement is expected by the development of monoclonal beta cell antibodies from BB rats (13). Elucidation of both the spontaneous process and the mechanisms of the successful interventions in the BB rat could help orient future studies in the human.

ACKNOWLEDGEMENTS

The author's research is supported by a grant from the Medical Research Council of Canada (MA-6540). The technical and secretarial assistance of Mario Boni, Marie Montambault and Suzan Roy-Gasperec are gratefully acknowledged.

1. Dyrberg, T., Poussier, P., Nakhooda, A.F., Marliss, E.B. & Lernmark, A.: Diabetologia **26**: 159-165, 1984.

2. Elder, M.E. & Maclaren, N.K.: J. Immunol. **130**: 1723, 1983.

3. Guttman, R.D., Colle, E., Michel, F., Seemayer, T.: J. Immunol. **130**: 1732, 1983.

4. Jackson, R., Rossi, N., Crump, T., Haynes, B. & Eisenbarth, E.S.: Diabetes **30**: 887, 1981.

5. Koevary, S., Rossini, A., Stoller, W., Chick, W., & Williams, R.M.: Science **220**: 727, 1983.

6. Laupacis, A., Gardell, C., Dupre, J., Stiller, C.R., Keown, P., Wallace, A.C. & Thibert, P.: Lancet **1**: 10, 1983.

7. Like, A.A., Anthony, M., Guberski, D.L., & Rossini, A.A.: Diabetes **32**: 326, 1983.

8. Logothetopoulos, J., Valiquette, N., Madura, E., & Cuet, D.: Diabetes **33**: 33-36, 1984.

9. Marliss, E.B. (Ed.): Metab. Clin. Exptal. **32** (Suppl. 1): 123, 1983.

10. Martin, D.R., Logothetopoulos, J.: Diabetes **33**: 93-96, 1984.

11. Naji, A., Silvers, W.K., Bellgrau, D., Anderson, A.O., Plotkin, S. & Barker, C.F.: Annals of Surgery **194**: 328, 1981.

12. Nakhooda, A.F., Sima, A.A.F., Poussier, P.G. & Marliss, E.B.: Endocrinology **109**: 2264, 1981.

13. Poussier, P., Brogren, C.H., Hirsch, F., & Druet, P.: Diabetes **33**: 158A, 1984.

14. Poussier, P., Nakhooda, A.F., Falk, J.A., Lee, C. & Marliss, E.B.: Endocrinology **110**: 1825, 1982.

15. Poussier, P., Sai, P. & Assan, R.: Diabetes **32** (Suppl. 1): 21A, 1983.

16. Prud'homme, G.J., Fuks, A., Colle, E., Seemayer, T.A. & Guttman, R.D.: J. Exper. Med. **159**: 463-478, 1984.

17. Yale, J.-F., Marliss, E.B.: Altered Immunity and Diabetes in the BB Rat. Clin. & Exp. Immunol., 1984. (in press)

Endocrinology
F. Labrie, L. Proulx, eds.

PATHOGENESIS OF TYPE I DIABETES MELLITUS

Åke Lernmark[1], Steinunn Bækkeskov[1], Thomas Dyrberg[1], Ivan Gerling[1], Birgitte Marner[1], George Papadopoulos[1], Annette Svenningsen[1], Christian Binder[2], Morten Christy[2], Jørn Nerup[2] and Thomas Mandrup-Poulsen[2]. [1]Hagedorn Research Laboratory and [2]Steno Memorial Hospital, DK-2820 Gentofte (DENMARK)

INTRODUCTION

The clinical onset of insulin-dependent (Type I) diabetes mellitus (IDDM) in man is precipitated by the disappearance of pancreatic B-cells in a number sufficient to induce the classical symptoms of insulin deficiency: hyperglycemia, glucosuria and ketonuria. These symptoms are observeable at all ages,and although the incidence of IDDM is highest in adolescence, it is now recognized that the disorder develops irrespectively of age. The incidence of IDDM also show peculiar geographic as well as seasonal variation. IDDM has a tendency to run in families,but the influence of genetic factors is complex and only 50 per cent or less of identical twins are concordant for the disease. Extensive analyses of HLA-types indicate, however, that the HLA-DR specificities 3 and/ or 4 account for more than 98% of IDDM patients compared to about 60% of the background population. This HLA-DR association is of interest, since the HLA-DR antigens of Class II molecules are thought to control the immune response in man.

The complexity of the islet organ has precluded systematic and quantitative investigations, and it was not until recently that the careful studies by Gepts[1], demonstrating the presence of inflammatory cells (insulitis) focused the interest on the pancreatic B cells as the primary target cell in an immune-related pathological process. This hypothesis was supported in subsequent studies demonstrating an increased prevalence of organ-specific autoimmune disorders among IDDM patients[2], the presence of cellular hypersensitivity reactions against pancreatic antigens in IDDM patients of recent onset[3], and, finally, the detection of circulating islet cell antibodies[4].

ISLET CELL ANTIBODIES

The clinical onset of IDDM is associated with the presence of circulating autoantibodies reactive with either intracellular or cell surface determinants (Table 1). The number of assay systems to detect islet cell antibodies are increasing, however, there is a lack of quantitative assays with established reproducibility and precision.

The prevalence of islet cell antibodies (ICA), which in the indirect immunofluorescence assay on frozen sections of the human pancreas are found to induce an immunofluorescence reaction covering all islet cells, among 84 IDDM patients of all ages (8-69 years of age) at the Steno Memorial Hospital was nearly 60%. A prospective analysis of these patients showed that the titre of ICA was highest at the time of onset and decreased thereafter. The ICA titre varied between undiluted to a serum dilution of more than 1: 729. After 30 months follow-up, 32 per cent remained ICA positive due to the fact that these patients had the highest ICA titres (median 1:27) at onset. ICA is usually found among 0.1 - 1% of the background population[5].

Previous cross-sectional studies of ICA in IDDM have failed to demonstrate that ICA is associated with a diminution of the B cell function. Radioimmunoassay of circulating c-peptide, the connecting peptide formed when proinsulin is converted to insulin and secreted in parallel with the hormoned have shown that the residual B-cell function gradually decreases with increasing duration of IDDM. In long-standing IDDM patients c-peptide often remain below the level of detection of the radioimmunoassay while most patients after 1-6 months of insulin therapy have levels of fasting c-peptide well within the normal range. Our prospective analysis indicates that a high ICA titre at diagnosis seemed to predict an increased insulin requirement and a lower fasting c-peptide 30 months later as compared to ICA negative patients. Further studies will be necessary to verify whether titration of ICA qualifies as a predictive test for altered B-cell function.

Table 1. Prevalence of islet cell antibodies at the time of clinical onset of insulin-dependent diabetes mellitus.

Antibody	Abbreviation	Tissue Preparation	Assay	Prevalence
Islet cell cytoplasmic	ICA	Sections of frozen human pancreas	Indirect Immuno-fluorescence	60-80%
Islet cell surface	ICSA	Living islet cells	Indirect immuno-fluorescence	60-80%
		Protein A		30-50%
Cototoxic	CAMC	Living islet cells	^{51}Cr-release Dye exclusion	50-70%

ISLET CELL SURFACE ANTIBODIES

Islet cell surface antibodies (ICSA) are demonstrated with dispersed living rodent or human islet cells by indirect immunofluorescence or in radioligand assay using protein A (Table 1). ICSA were detected among 2-4% of control subjects and among 60-80% of newly diagnosed IDDM patients[5]. The antibodies, which are usually of the IgG class also showed a decreased prevalence with increasing duration of IDDM. In contrast to ICA, there is evidence that ICSA among young onset IDDM patients are pancreatic B-cell specific. The observation that antibodies are capable of binding to living B cells is important, since it allows tests of the possibility that surface-bound antibodies either mediate immune effector mechanisms or directly affects the function of the B cells. Evidence has been obtained that cytotoxic islet cell antibodies (CAMC) correlate well with ICSA[6]. However, our studies indicate that only 60% of IDDM patients are concordant for both ICA and ICSA[7].

Recent experiments with passive transfer to mice followed by _in vitro_ pancreas perfusion[8] or perifusion of isolated rat islet cells[9] with immunoglobulin prepared from the plasma of children with IDDM of short duration suggest that islet cell antibodies binding to intact pancreatic B cells may interfere with the mechanism by which glucose stimulates insulin release. Experiments are in progress to define those determinants reactive with islet cell antibodies which affect the B-cell function.

ISLET CELL AUTOANTIGENS

The presence of antibodies which are able to bind to pancreatic B cells indicate that the immune system in the affected individual has initiated an immune response against either an antigen which is normally present in the target cell or a foreign antigen showing molecular similarities with a pancreatic B-cell antigen. Since the variety of autoantibodies in IDDM patients rather signify a broad abnormal immune response not only against the pancreatic B cells but also other endocrine tissues as well, it might well be that primary lesions to the B-cells result in an out-flow of antigens towards which the immune response reacts but only in individuals carrying the susceptibility to develop IDDM. Immuneprecipitation of extracts of radioactively labelled human pancreatic islets with IDDM sera showed that many patients have antibodies against a M_r 64 000 protein[10]. Antibodies against this cell component, which seems to represent an integral membrane protein, were present in about 80% of IDDM patients of short duration and were primarily detected in sera positive for B-cell specific ICSA[10]. IDDM sera also detected the M_r 64 000 protein in radioactively labelled rodent islets or in a crude plasma membrane preparation from a cloned insulin-islet tumor cell line. The M_r 64 000 antibodies (64 KAg) could be detected in one individual up to two years before his clinical onset of IDDM and before the ICA appeared (Table 2).

Table 2. Prospective analysis of a HLA-DR 3/7 male developing IDDM after the diagnosis of his twin brother in 1980.

Date	Age	Fasting blood sugar	HbA_{1c}	Fasting c-peptide	ICA	64KAg
	(years)	(mmol/l)	(%)	(pmol/ml)		
1980-Nov	24	5.4	4.5	0.38	neg	+
1981-Sept	25	5.7	4.9	0.34	+	+
1982-March	26	5.2	NT	NT	+	+
-June		4.9	NT	0.22	+	+
-Sept		NT	5.8	NT	+	+
-Dec		17.0		IDDM	+	+

These experiments suggest that the M_r 64 000 component represents a major antigenic islet component. Current studies are focused on both cellular and humoral mechanisms which are involved in the development of an immune response against pancreatic B-cell antigens in individuals carrying the susceptibility markers HLA-DR 3 and/or 4.

ACKNOWLEDGEMENT

Supported in part by grants from the National Institutes of Health (AM 26190, AM 33873).

REFERENCES

1. Gepts W (1965) Pathologic anatomy of the pancreas in juvenile diabetes mellitus. Diabetes 14: 619-633.
2. MacCuish AC, Irvine, WJ (1975) Autoimmunological aspects of diabetes mellitus. Clin. Endocr. Metabl. 4: 435-471
3. Nerup J, Andersen OO, Bendixen G, Egebjerg J, Poulsen JE (1971) Antipancreatic cellular hypersensitivity in diabetes mellitus. Diabetes 20: 424-427.
4. Botazzo GF, Florin-Christensen A, Doniach D (1974) Islet cell antibodies in diabetes mellitus with autoimmune polyendocrine deficiencies. Lancet ii: 1279-1283

5. Brogren CH, Lernmark Å (1982) Islet cell antibodies in diabetes. Clin. Endocrinol. Metab. 11: 409-430

6. Dobersen MJ, Scharff JE, Ginsberg-Fellner F, Notkins AL (1980) Cytotoxic autoantibodies to beta-cells in the serum of patients with insulin-dependent diabetes mellitus. N Engl J Med 303:1493-1498

7. Freedman ZR, Feed CM, Irvine WJ, Lernmark Å, Rubenstein AH, Steiner DF, Huen A (1979) Islet-cell cytoplasmic and cell-surface antibodies in diabetes mellitus. Trans.Assoc.Am. Phys.: 64-76

8. Svenningsen A, Dyrberg T, Gerling I, Lernmark Å, Mackay P, Rabinovitch A (1983) Inhibition of insulin release after passive transfer of immunoglobulin from insulin-dependent diabetic children to mice. J Clin Endocrinol Metab 57 (6): 1301-1304

9. Kanatsuna T, Bækkeskov S, Lernmark Å, Ludvigsson J (1983) Immunoglobulin from insulin-dependent diabetic children inhibits glucose-induced insulin release. Diabetes 32: 520-524

10. Bækkeskov S, Nielsen JH, Marner B, Bilde T, Ludvigsson J, Lernmark Å (1982) Autoantibodies in newly diagnosed diabetic children immunoprecipitate specific human pancreatic islet cell protein. Nature 298: 167-169

Endocrinology
F. Labrie, L. Proulx, eds.

VIRUSES AND AUTOIMMUNITY

ABNER LOUIS NOTKINS AND JAVARAIAH SRINIVASAPPA

National Institutes of Health, Bethesda, MARYLAND (USA)

In patients with insulin-dependent diabetes mellitus (IDDM), autoantibodies have been found that react with antigens in the cytoplasm and on the surface of cells in the islets of Langerhans. Autoantibodies to a variety of other tissues and antigens (e.g., thyroid, anterior pituitary, gastric mucosal cells, lymphocytes and nucleic acid) also have been reported. What triggers the production of autoantibodies in IDDM and in the many other human autoimmune diseases is not known. There are a number of theories ranging from genetically programmed immunological abnormalities to environmental insults. The appearance of autoantibodies, albeit of low titer and short-lived, in the sera of animals and humans following certain infections, suggest that viruses may sometimes be involved (1). Recently, considerable information has been obtained about virus-induced autoimmunity from studies with reovirus (2). In newborn mice, this virus triggers an autoimmune polyendocrine disease characterized by a mild and transient form of diabetes and retardation in growth. The virus infects several organs including cells in the anterior pituitary and in the islets of Langerhans. In the sera of reovirus-infected mice, autoantibodies that react with tissue sections (e.g., anterior pituitary, pancreatic islets, gastric mucosa) from normal, uninfected mice have been found. Immunosuppression, at the time of infection, prevents the appearance of these autoantibodies and the development of the clinical syndrome (3). Moreover, by fusing spleen cells from reovirus-infected mice with myeloma cells, monoclonal autoantibodies that react with endocrine cells have been obtained (Figure) (4).

There are several mechanisms by which a virus might trigger the production of autoantibodies (1). The first is that the virus acts on the target cell to which the autoantibody is ultimately directed. The infected cell or some component of it becomes foreign to the host. This may occur if the virus incorporates host antigens into its envelope; inserts, exposes or modifies host antigens on the cell surface; or releases sequestrated antigens, perhaps in a precursor form, which the host's immune system does not ordinarily see.

A second possibility is that the virus acts on effector cells (i.e., the immunoregulatory system), rather than on the target cell to which the autoantibody is ultimately directed. The virus may stimulate or destroy subpopulations of lymphocytes (e.g., helper or suppressor T cells) or macrophages or antigen presenting cells, and this in turn may lead to the generation of autoantibodies. In fact, immunological abnormalities are known to follow certain viral infections.

In the case of Epstein-Barr virus (EBV), the virus infects and transforms human B lymphocytes, which have a limited life span, into lymphoblastoid cell lines that proliferate indefinitely in vitro without need of foreign antigenic stimulation. These immortalized cells are capable of secreting immunoglobulins, and some of the immunoglobulins, which are predominantly of the IgM class, react with antigens in normal cells. By cloning these transformed cells, we have obtained monoclonal autoantibodies that react with a variety of organs including the thyroid, pituitary, stomach and pancreas (5).

A third way by which a virus might trigger an autoimmune response is through what is sometimes referred to as "molecular mimicry." The idea is that an antibody raised against an epitope on a virus may cross-react with a similar epitope on normal host cells. Although this is an old idea, definitive proof has been difficult to obtain. Monoclonal antibodies are now beginning to provide that proof. Recently, we screened several hundred monoclonal antibodies, made specifically against viruses, for their reactivity with normal tissues (J. Srinivasappa et al, manuscript in preparation). Approximately 4% of these monoclonal antibodies reacted with perfectly normal tissues and several reacted with endocrine organs. For example, as seen in the Figure, an antibody to herpes simplex virus was found to react with cells in the islets of Langerhans and an antibody to rabies reacted with cells in the anterior pituitary.

These studies on virus-induced autoimmunity, especially the work with monoclonal antibodies, are revealing some new and unexpected insights into the nature of autoantibodies. We found that many of these monoclonal antibodies react with antigens in more than one organ (e.g., pancreatic islets, pituitary, thyroid and stomach) (6,7). We refer to these multiple organ-reactive antibodies as MOR antibodies (Table). Initially, we thought that these antibodies were unusual and rare, but, as a result of more extensive screening procedures, MOR antibodies are

EXAMPLES OF MONOCLONAL AUTOANTIBODIES SHOWING MULTIPLE-ORGAN REACTIVITY

Antibody	Thyroid	Pancreas	Stomach	Small Intestine	Pituitary
D5-2[a]	Acinar	Islets, Ducts	Smooth Muscle	Negative	Negative
E10-1[a]	Colloid	Basement Membrane of Ducts	Negative	Negative	Negative
MOR-1[b]	Negative	Islets	Mucosa	Mucosa	Anterior Lobe

(a) EBV-transformed cells; (b) Hybridoma from reovirus-infected mouse turning out to be the rule rather than the exception. Even some of the monoclonal antibodies that we initially thought reacted with a single protein (i.e. hormones) show MOR activity (J. Saegusa et al., manuscript submitted). The most likely explanation for multiple organ reactivity is that these autoantibodies are recognizing the same molecule that is present in more than one organ or that they are

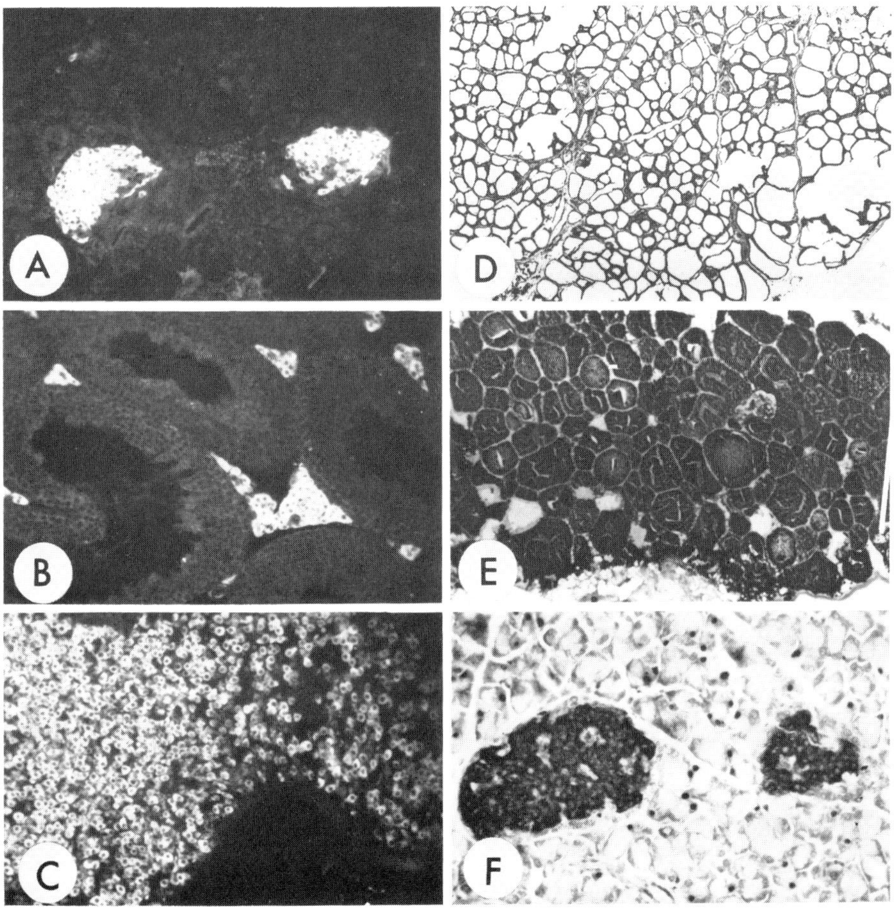

Reactivity of monoclonal antibodies with normal tissues detected by indirect immunofluorescence (A, B, C) or immunoperoxidase (D, E, F). Hybridomas obtained from reovirus-infected mice produce monoclonal autoantibodies that react with mouse (A) pancreatic β cells in the islets of Langerhans and (B) interstitial cells in the testis. (C) Rabies monoclonal antiviral antibody that reacts with mouse anterior pituitary cells. Monoclonal antibodies secreted by EBV-transformed human B lymphocytes that react with (D) acinar cells and (E) colloid of monkey thyroid. (F) Monoclonal antiviral antibody to herpes simplex virus that reacts with hamster pancreatic β cells in the islets of Langerhans.

recognizing similar epitopes on different molecules in multiple organs (6,8). An antibody elicited against a common antigenic determinant in one organ would react with all organs containing that determinant. Thus, MOR antibodies may be a partial explanation for the capacity of sera from patients with certain autoimmune disorders to react with multiple organs.

It should be stressed that the inherent capacity of the individual's B lymphocytes to make autoantibodies exists prior to the viral infection. These lymphocytes are part of the individual's normal B lymphocyte repertoire. We know this because we recently succeeded in making some very similar types of autoantibody-producing hybridomas from the spleens of normal uninfected animals (B. Prabhakar et al., manuscript submitted). Thus, it appears that, in vivo, the virus infection, by one or more of the mechanisms discussed, triggers B lymphocytes to secrete these autoantibodies into the circulation.

Regardless of how these monoclonal autoantibody-producing clones are generated, these antibodies should prove to be useful reagents for diagnostic purposes, for studying development and differentiation, and for preparing immunoaffinity columns. With these columns it is now becoming possible to isolate and characterize human autoantigens (8).

REFERENCES

1. Notkins AL, Onodera T, Prabhakar B (1984) Virus-induced autoimmunity. In: Notkins AL, Oldstone MBA (eds) Concepts in Viral Pathogenesis. Springer-Verlag, New York (in press)

2. Onodera T, Toniolo A, Ray UR, Jenson AB, Knazek RA, Notkins AL (1981) Virus-induced diabetes mellitus. XX. Polyendocrinopathy and autoimmunty. J Exp Med 153:1457-1473

3. Onodera T, Ray UR, Melez KA, Suzuki H, Toniolo A, Notkins AL (1982) Virus-induced diabetes mellitus: Autoimmunity and polyendocrine disease prevented by immunosuppression. Nature 297:66-68

4. Haspel MV, Onodera T, Prabhakar BS, Horita M, Suzuki H, Notkins AL (1983) Virus-induced autoimmunity: Monoclonal antibodies that react with endocrine tissues. Science 220:304-306

5. Garzelli C, Taub FE, Scharff JE, Prabhakar BS, Ginsberg-Fellner F, Notkins AL (1984) Epstein-Barr virus-transformed lymphocytes produce monoclonal autoantibodies that react with antigens in multiple organs. J Virol (in press)

6. Haspel MV, Onodera T, Prabhakar BS, McClintock PR, Essani K, Ray UR, Yagihashi S, Notkins AL (1983) Multiple organ-reactive monoclonal autoantibodies. Nature 304:73-76

7. Satoh J, Prabhakar BS, Haspel MV, Ginsberg-Fellner F, Notkins AL (1983) Human monoclonal autoantibodies that react with multiple endocrine organs. N Engl J Med 309:217-220

8. Satoh J, Essani K, McClintock PR, Notkins AL (1984) Human multiple organ-reactive monoclonal autoantibody recognizes growth hormone and a 35K protein. J Clin Invest (in press)

3. Steroid Receptors and Genomes

Endocrinology
F. Labrie, L. Proulx, eds.

GENE TRANSFER STUDIES TO INVESTIGATE ANDROGEN ACTION

MALCOLM PARKER and MAURICE NEEDHAM
Imperial Cancer Research Fund, Lincoln's Inn Fields, London WC2A 3PX (U.K.)

INTRODUCTION

Androgens regulate the expression of prostatic steroid binding protein (1) partly by effects on transcription but primarily by post-transcriptional events (2). The protein is a tetramer consisting of C1 and C2 polypeptides each encoded by unique genes (3) and two C3 polypeptides. Both C3 polypeptides are expressed by a single gene, C3(1), although there is a second gene C3(2) which is not expressed in any tissue that we have examined (4). In view of this difference in expression, we have selected the genes for C3 to study in detail.

The approach we have taken to study the rôle of androgens in gene expression is gene transfer. The cloned C3 genes have been introduced into S115 cells whose proliferation is stimulated by testosterone showing that they have functional androgen receptors (5). In independent clones of cells, where the C3 genes were stably integrated, both C3(1) and C3(2) were expressed accurately at similar levels and 25% were stimulated up to five-fold by testosterone (6). We have now investigated whether the effect of testosterone is on the C3 promoter by analysing the transient expression of chimaeric genes. In both heterologous mouse cells and homologous prostate cells the C3 promoter was unresponsive to testosterone.

MATERIALS AND METHODS

The following materials were gifts: human β interferon cDNA (W. Fiers, State University of Ghent, Belgium); polyoma MboI DNA fragments which contains poly(A) addition sites (M. Fried, ICRF, London); pSV_2CAT (C.M. Gorman, Imperial College, London).

Vector constructions

Chimaeric genes were constructed by ligating human β interferon to an MboI DNA fragment containing poly(A) addition sites and a putative C3(1) promoter from nucleotide -800 to +20 in the C3(1) gene (7).

Transfection procedures

Cells were transfected using calcium phosphate precipitation (6) followed by a glycerol shock step (8) and an overnight sodium butyrate treatment (9).

Assays

Interferon was quantitated using a cytopathic effect bioassay. Cell culture medium was serially diluted onto 10^4 human embryo fibroblasts in 96 well dishes overnight and then infected with 10^4 pfu of encephalomyocarditis virus. Cells were stained with crystal violet after approximately 30 h.

Chloramphenicol acetyltransferase (CAT) was assayed in cell-free extracts 48-72 h after transfection using ^{14}C chloramphenicol as described (10). Acetylated derivatives of chloramphenicol were separated by thin layer chromatography and identified by autoradiography.

RESULTS

We have investigated the effects of testosterone on the C3(1) gene promoter by analysing the transient expression of the chimaeric gene shown in Fig. 1.

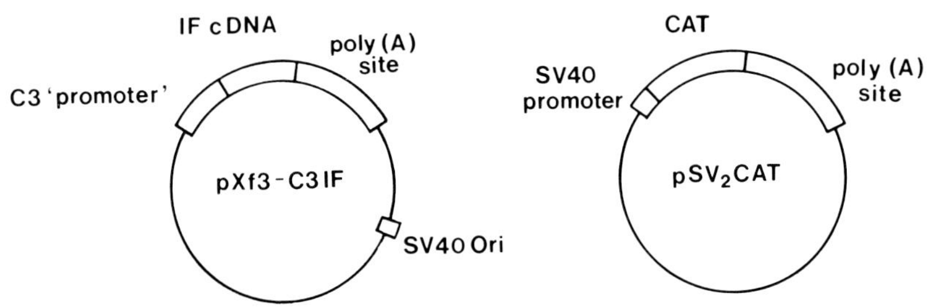

Fig. 1. DNA vectors to study C3 promoter function.
pXF3 C3IF is a chimaeric gene containing the C3 promoter from nucleotide -800 to +20 and pSV_2CAT (10) is a chimaeric gene for use as an internal control.

Initially we introduced the gene into the androgen-responsive S115 cell line. S115 cells were withdrawn from testosterone for 4 days, transfected with DNA and then cultured in the presence or absence of $10^{-8}M$ testosterone for 2-3 days when medium was removed to assay for interferon activity. Since testosterone stimulates S115 cell proliferation (5) and general protein metabolism (11) we included in the transfection a control gene whose promoter was insensitive to testosterone. We used a gene encoding chloramphenicol acetyltransferase with the viral SV40 early promoter. In this way CAT activity could be measured in cells whose culture medium was assayed for interferon.

Interferon activity was apparently stimulated approximately 4-fold by testosterone (Fig. 2, tracks 1-3, minus testosterone versus tracks 4-6 plus testosterone). However, CAT activity was similarly stimulated (Fig. 3) indicating that the hormone was stimulating cell growth or general cell metabolism rather than acting specifically on the C3 gene promoter.

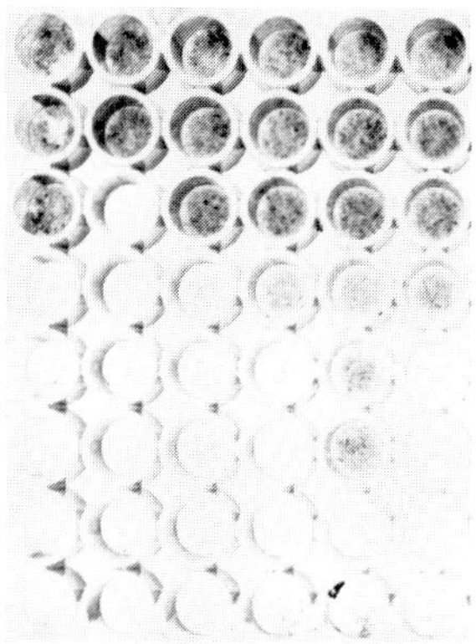

Fig. 2. Effect of testosterone on interferon activity in S115 cells.
Medium from cells grown in the absence (tracks 1-3) or presence (tracks 4-6) of testosterone was diluted 2-fold (A), 4-fold (B), 8-fold (C), 16-fold (D), 32-fold (E), 64-fold (F), 128-fold (G) and 256-fold (H) and assayed for interferon using a cytopathic effect assay. Viable cells were stained with crystal violet.

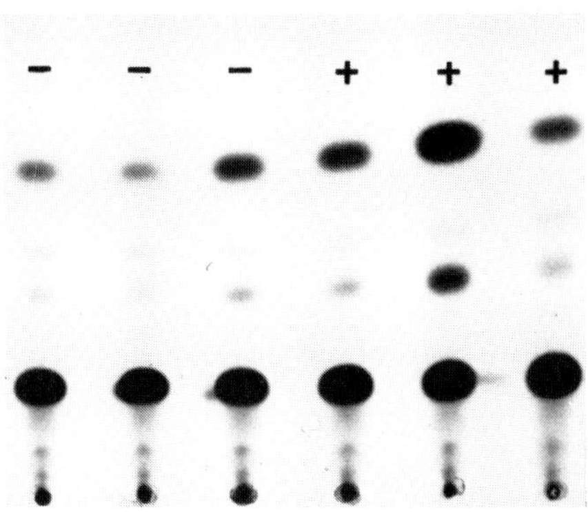

Fig. 3. Effect of testosterone on CAT activity.
CAT activity was assayed in cell-free extracts of S115 cells grown in the absence (-) or presence (+) of testosterone. ^{14}C-chloramphenicol is at the bottom of the autoradiograph and acetylated chloramphenicol products are above it.

Recently we have been attempting similar gene transfer experiments with primary cultures of rat ventral prostate epithelium. The cultures had an epithelial morphology and immunochemical staining for the presence of keratin, a specific marker for cells of epithelial origin, was positive. However, the cells showed no response to testosterone in terms of their proliferation or expression of prostatic steroid binding protein on plastic, dried collagen films or on Swiss 3T3 feeder cells. Likewise, the C3 promoter was insensitive to testosterone after gene transfer experiments, although it was utilised and gave rise to interferon expression.

DISCUSSION

Although androgens regulate gene expression, in part, by stimulating transcription rate (2) the mechanism whereby, directly or indirectly, they modulate gene promoter activity is unknown. We have failed to detect any effect of testosterone on the C3 promoter either in heterologous cells or homologous ventral prostate cells using transient expression assays. It is possible that responsiveness to androgen depends on tissue specific factors as described for the chicken oviduct lysozyme gene (12) which could account for our results with S115 cells. Since we have previously demonstrated that the whole C3 gene is responsive in certain stably transformed cell lines (6) we conclude that such stimulation may have depended on the site of integration of the gene or alternatively the hormone may be acting not on the promoter but on another region of the gene.

Lack of sensitivity of the C3 promoter in ventral prostate cells was not too surprising in view of the failure of testosterone to stimulate the growth of the cultures. It is likely that the regulation of prostatic steroid binding protein expression may depend on the growth of cells on a specific biomatrix or occur only in the absence of cell proliferation. We are investigating these possibilities.

REFERENCES

1. Heyns W, De Moor P (1977) Eur J Biochem 78:221-230
2. Page MJ, Parker MG (1982) Mol Cell Endocrinol 27:343-345
3. Parker MG, Needham M, White R, Hurst H, Page M (1982) Nucleic Acids Res 10:5121-5132
4. Parker MG, White R, Hurst H, Needham M, Tilly R (1983) J Biol Chem 258:12-15
5. Yates J, King RJB (1981) J Steroid Biochem 14:819-822
6. Page MJ, Parker MG (1983) Cell 32:495-502
7. Hurst H, Parker MG (1983) EMBO J 2:769-774
8. Frost E, Williams J (1978) Virology 91:39-50
9. Gorman CM, Howard BH (1983) Nucleic Acids Res 11:7631
10. Gorman CM, Moffat LF, Howard BH (1982) Mol Cell Biol 2:1044-1051
11. Robinson JH, Smith JA, Dee LA (1976) Expl Cell Res 102:117-126
12. Renkawitz R, Beung H, Graf T, Matthias P, Grez M, Schutz G (1982) Cell 31:167-176

Endocrinology
F. Labrie, L. Proulx, eds.

NUCLEAR ACCEPTOR SITES IN STEROID HORMONE ACTION: THE NUCLEAR MATRIX

EVELYN R. BARRACK

Department of Urology, The Johns Hopkins University School of Medicine, Baltimore, Maryland 21205, USA

INTRODUCTION

Steroid hormones regulate differentiation, specific gene expression and cell division, but only in specific target tissues that contain specific receptor proteins. While the detailed molecular mechanisms of these events remain the subject of intensive investigation, the interaction of steroid-receptor complexes with the nucleus of target tissues is widely recognized to be involved in the modulation of the structure and function of DNA. But what is the nature of the effector site (i.e., the acceptor site) for the steroid-receptor complex?

Evidence is mounting that cellular structural proteins are involved in the regulation of biological function. Whereas the cytoskeleton provides structural and functional organization of cytoplasmic components, the nuclear matrix, which is a residual scaffolding of the nucleus, appears to play a fundamental role in the organization of the nuclear DNA and in many dynamic aspects of nuclear function, including DNA replication, and heterogeneous nuclear RNA synthesis and processing (1,2). In addition, several actively transcribed genes have been shown to be associated with the nuclear matrix, whereas inactive genes are not (1,2). Since steroid hormones affect these processes in specific target tissues, we have focused on these nuclear structural proteins as important elements in hormone action.

To isolate the nuclear matrix, nuclei are extracted sequentially with 1% Triton X-100, DNase I, low ionic strength buffer, and 2 M NaCl. This sequence of extractions removes >95% of the total nuclear phospholipid and DNA, >85% of the nuclear protein, and >60% of the nuclear RNA. What remains is the nuclear matrix, which consists predominantly of nonhistone nuclear proteins (1).

Steroid Receptors are Associated with the Nuclear Matrix

The nuclear matrix appears to be a major site of steroid hormone receptor binding in the nucleus. We have demonstrated that in several androgen and estrogen target tissues, the nuclear matrix contains a major proportion (50-90%) of the total nuclear steroid receptor content (1,2). We have also shown directly that the nuclear matrix contains acceptor sites to which steroid-receptor complexes bind with high affinity (2,3).

Using an *in vitro* exchange assay in which nuclear matrix fractions isolated from hormone-treated animals are incubated with radiolabeled steroid, we have identified and characterized androgen and estrogen receptors associated with the nuclear matrix of androgen and estrogen target tissues, respectively (1,2). The nuclear matrix-associated estrogen receptors in rat uterus and hen liver,

*Supported by Grant AM 22000 from the NIH, USPHS.

and androgen receptors in rat and human prostate have all the properties of bona fide steroid hormone receptors, in that the binding of steroids to these sites is saturable, high affinity ($K_d \sim 1$ nM), steroid specific, and tissue specific. In addition, receptors become associated with the nuclear matrix in response to an appropriate hormonal stimulus, not indiscriminately. For example, in response to high blood levels of estrogen, the liver of egg-laying hens synthesizes vitellogenin and its nuclear matrix contains high levels of estrogen receptor. In contrast, roosters do not make vitellogenin, and their liver nuclear matrix contains only 12% as many estrogen receptors. High dose estrogen treatment of roosters induces the synthesis of yolk proteins as well as the association of estrogen receptors with the liver nuclear matrix. Similarly, in an androgen target tissue such as the rat ventral prostate the presence of androgen receptors on the nuclear matrix is associated with androgen stimulation of this gland. Receptors are present on the matrix in intact rats, but not in castrated rats. Administration of androgens, but not of estrogens, results in the association of androgen receptors with the prostate nuclear matrix within 1 hour. All these data are consistent with the conclusion that the specific binding of steroid to the nuclear matrix occurs via receptor proteins that had been translocated to the nucleus *in vivo* by endogenous hormone (1,2).

A major proportion (50-90%) of the total nuclear receptor content is localized to the nuclear matrix, which contains only 10-15% of the total nuclear protein and 1-2% of the DNA (1,2). Per unit amount of protein, nuclear receptors are enriched on the nuclear matrix 4-5 fold compared to total nuclei. The nuclear matrix consists of a peripheral pore complex lamina, residual nucleoli, and an internal residual ribonucleoprotein network. We have studied the localization of receptors within this structure, and find that they are predominantly (75%) associated with the internal RNP network of the matrix (1,2). On a protein basis, receptors are enriched in this component of the matrix more than 8-fold relative to total nuclei (1,2).

Acceptors for these Steroid Receptors are Associated with the Nuclear Matrix

In interpreting the association of receptors with the nuclear matrix, it became important to determine whether this interaction was due simply to spurious binding of receptors occurring during isolation of the matrix, or whether indeed it was due to the presence of specific acceptor sites in the matrix. To address this issue, we have used a cell-free binding assay to test directly for the presence, in the prostate nuclear matrix, of acceptors for androgen receptors (2,3).

In these experiments, androgen receptors in rat ventral prostate cytosol are charged with radiolabeled steroid (^{3}H-R1881) and increasing amounts of these labeled receptors are added to a constant amount of ventral prostate nuclear matrix isolated from castrated rats (to deplete the nuclei and matrix of endogenous androgen receptors). As shown in Fig. 1, androgen receptors bind to a saturable number of sites (acceptors) on the prostate nuclear matrix. Scatchard analysis of these data shows that the interaction is of high affinity ($K_d = 1 \times 10^{-10}$M) (2,3). In addition, the binding of receptors to nuclear matrix is tissue specific, since liver nuclear matrix contains only 15% as many acceptors for androgen receptors as the prostate nuclear matrix (Fig. 1).

Other experiments, summarized in Table I, showed that it is the steroid-receptor complex that binds to the matrix, since free steroid does not bind to the castrate rat prostate matrix. In addition, the binding of androgen receptor to acceptor sites is dependent on the presence of an activated androgen-receptor complex. When cytosol receptors are prepared in the presence of 25 mM sodium molybdate (added to the homogenization buffer) only 13% as many androgen receptors bind to the nuclear matrix as when cytosol prepared without molybdate is used. Because sodium molybdate is known to be an effective inhibitor of steroid receptor activation, these experiments indicate that the binding of androgen receptor to acceptor sites is indeed dependent on receptor activation.

We also determined that the binding of receptors to acceptors on the matrix is steroid-dependent. To show this, prostate matrix was incubated with androgen-free cytosol, pelleted and washed once to remove unbound receptor; the amount of bound receptor was then measured using a labeled steroid binding assay (2,3). This experiment showed that the binding of unoccupied androgen receptors to the matrix is only 20% of the level of binding of activated steroid-receptor complexes to the matrix.

We conclude therefore, that there are indeed specific acceptor sites for androgen receptors in the prostate nuclear matrix, and that receptors do not merely become associated with the nuclear matrix as a result of spurious binding.

The Nature of the Acceptor Sites Associated with the Nuclear Matrix

We have begun studies to elucidate the nature of the acceptor sites on the nuclear matrix. For example, by varying the extent of DNase I digestion, as well as the order of the DNase and high salt treatments, we have obtained prostate nuclear matrix preparations that contain varying amounts of DNA and varying amounts of acceptors for labeled androgen-receptor complexes (Table II). These data indicate that the acceptors are relatively resistant to DNase I digestion, since after removal of 99.1% of the nuclear DNA, 51% of the nuclear acceptors still remain associated with the nuclear matrix. If the acceptor is DNA, then it is enriched on the matrix 57-fold. Additional experiments are underway to determine whether the acceptor is matrix-associated DNA, protein, or a combination of nucleic acid and protein.

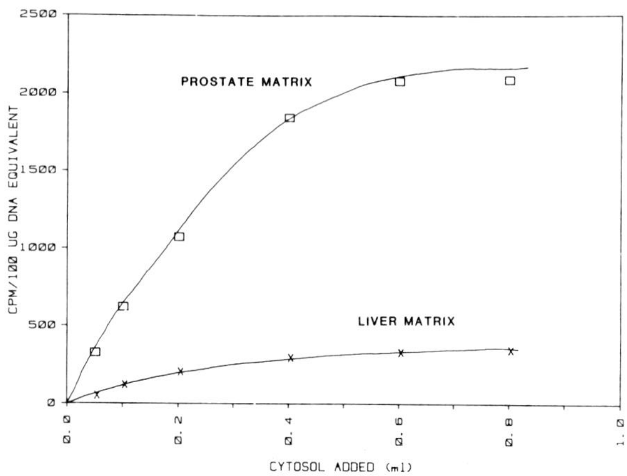

Fig. 1. Cell-free binding of ^{3}H-R1881 labeled androgen-receptor complexes to isolated nuclear matrix of castrate rat prostate and liver. See text and Ref. 3 for details.

TABLE I. BINDING OF VARIOUS LIGANDS TO THE ACCEPTOR ON THE NUCLEAR MATRIX

Addition	Relative Binding To Prostate Matrix of Castrate Rats
Activated Androgen·Receptor Complex (A·R')	100
Unactivated Androgen·Receptor Complex (A·R)	13
Unoccupied Receptor (R)	20
Free Steroid (A)	0

TABLE II. ENRICHMENT OF ACCEPTORS ON THE NUCLEAR MATRIX

Treatment of Nuclei	DNA Remaining (Relative)	Acceptors Remaining (Relative)	Acceptors/ DNA (Relative)
None	100	100	1.0
DNase Only (20 μg/ml)	95	93	1.0
DNase Only (200 μg/ml)	65	80	1.2
HS Only (2 M NaCl)	43	81	1.9
HS → DNase (200 μg/ml)	4	70	18
DNase (20 μg/ml) → HS	3.4	68	20
DNase (200 μg/ml) → HS	0.9	51	57

REFERENCES

1. Barrack ER, Coffey DS (1982) Recent Prog Horm Res 38:133-195
2. Barrack ER (1984) In: Berezney R (ed) The Nuclear Matrix. Plenum Press, In press.
3. Barrack ER (1983) Endocrinology 113:430-432

© 1984 Elsevier Science Publishers B.V.
Endocrinology
F. Labrie, L. Proulx, eds.

A TRANSCRIPTIONAL REGULATION SEQUENCE IN THE LONG TERMINAL REPEAT OF MOUSE MAMMARY TUMOR VIRUS HAS HORMONE INDUCTION AND ENHANCER QUALITIES

HELMUT PONTA[1], URSULA RAHMSDORF[1], PETRA BUTKERAITIS[1], NANCY E. HYNES[2], AND BERND GRONER[2]

[1] Institute of Genetics, Kernforschungszentrum, D-7500 Karlsruhe, F.R. Germany

[2] Ludwig Institute for Cancer Research, Inselspital, 3010 Bern, Switzerland

INTRODUCTION

In vitro recombination of cloned fragments of proviral DNA of mouse mammary tumor virus (MMTV) with heterologous genes has provided important insights into the sequence requirements for glucocorticoid hormone action (1), parameters of the induction process (2) and the molecular interaction of essential components (3). Reintroduction of defined chimeric MMTV LTR - tk gene constructs into cultured cells and their performance in the absence and presence of hormone in the growth medium led to the identification of a 143 nucleotide region in the MMTV LTR (position -59 to -202 with respect to the LTR RNA initiation site) with regulatory potential (1). This fragment confers hormonal inducibility onto heterologous genes when it is located in a 5' syn configuration. It exhibits enhancer properties when it is placed in a 5' anti position or linked at the 3' end of a gene. This enhancer function is also exerted by intact proviral DNA and may play a role in the insertional activation of cellular genes by MMTV in mammary tumors.

MATERIALS AND METHODS

Recombination of the MMTV-HRE (hormone response element) with the mouse globin gene

The mouse α globin gene (4) was inserted into the Eco RI site of the pSV 2 gpt vector (5) shown in Fig. 1, construct 5. A 774 bp Eco RI fragment containing 184 bp of MMTV LTR sequences (-52 to -236, construct 6 in Fig. 1) was inserted into an Eco RI site located 1.1 kb 5' of the α globin cap site (constructs 1 and 2 in Fig. 1) or 1.1 kb 3' of the α globin cap site (constructs 3 and 4 in Fig. 1) in both of the possible orientations. Mouse L cells were transfected with constructs 1 to 5. Stably transfected cell clones were cultured in the absence and presence of dexamethasone (10^{-6}M for 18 hrs). Cellular RNA was extracted and hybridized to a 104 nucleotide Hae III - Pst I fragment in which the Hae III site was 5' end labeled. Upon S1 nuclease digestion accurately initiated α globin mRNA protects a 98 nucleotide fragment.

Recombination of MMTV proviral DNA with the thymidine kinase gene

A molecular clone of intact MMTV proviral DNA was recombined with tk DNA. A 2.4 kb Eco RI fragment of the tk gene (6) was inserted into an Eco RI site located 222 nucleotides 3' of the proviral DNA (constructs 1 and 2 in Fig. 2) or a 3.6 kb Bam Hl fragment of the tk gene was inserted 1 kb 5' of the proviral DNA (constructs 3 and 4 in Fig. 2) in both of the possible orientations. Mouse L cells were stably transfected with constructs 1 to 4 and cultured in the absence and presence of dexamethasone (10^{-6}M for 18 hours). Transcripts originating at the tk cap site were quantitated by the S1 mapping procedure (7). A protected 56 nucleotide signal is indicative of correctly initiated tk mRNA.

RESULTS AND DISCUSSION

The functional delimitation of a regulatory DNA sequence within the MMTV LTR showed that a fragment of 143 nucleotides (-59 to -202) is sufficient to confer hormonal inducibility onto a downstream promoter (1). The hormone regulation element (HRE) can thus be clearly distinguished from the MMTV promoter region which comprises the LTR RNA initiation site and the TATA box. This distinction allowed us to test the dependence of the HRE on position and orientation with respect to the regulated promoter and RNA initiation site. For this purpose the five chimeric gene constructs shown in Fig. 1 were introduced into cultured cells and the effect of the presence of the HRE upon α globin gene transcription was quantitated. The 98 nucleotide signal is indicative of correctly initiated α globin transcripts. Construct 1, in the absence of hormone (lane 1 -), and construct 5 (lane 5), show a constitutive expression of α globin mRNA. Construct 1, in the presence of hormone (lane 1 +), and constructs 2, 3 and 4 show a strongly enhanced expression of α globin. This experiment shows that the HRE fulfills the functional definition of an enhancer (8, relative independence from position and orientation with respect to the enhanced gene) in all but the 5' syn orientation. In this orientation hormone is required for enhancer function. This suggests a functional similarity between hormonal induction and enhancement.

The induction of mammary carcinomas by MMTV is thought to involve proviral integration and the insertional activation of cellular genes (9, 10). The effect of the proviral DNA must be conferred over a distance because the integration sites around the tumor-specific int-1 and int-2 transcripts are scattered over several kilobases. A preferred orientation of the exogenously integrated proviral DNA with respect to the activated cellular gene has been found (Fig. 2A). We tested the influence of proviral DNA upon the expression of an adjacent gene ex-

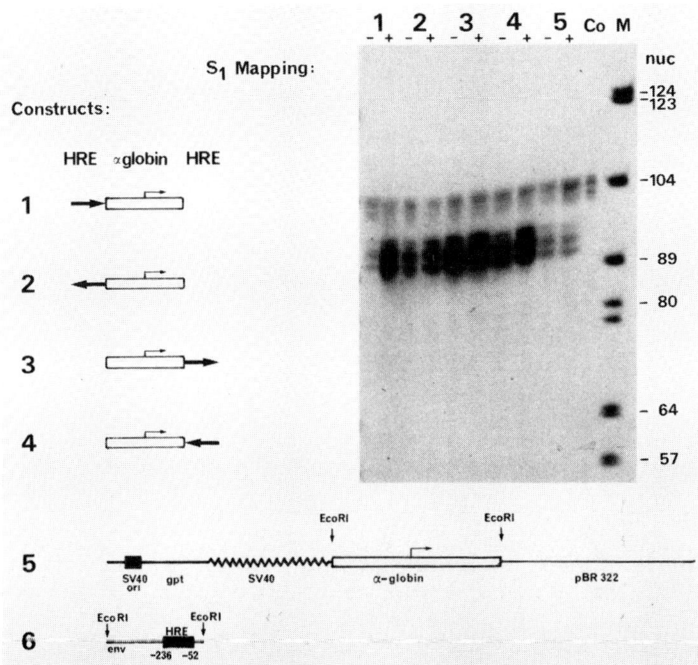

Fig. 1. Constructs of HRE α globin genes and S1 mapping of α globin transcripts in transfected cells grown with (+) and without (-) dexamethasone. The construct number corresponds to the lane in the autoradiograph.

perimentally. Fig. 2B shows the constructs which link the tk gene at the 5' and at the 3' sides of the MMTV gene. After introduction into cultured cells the extent of tk transcription was quantitated in cellular RNA. Fig. 2B shows the indicative signal of 56 nucleotides which characterizes tk mRNA. Constructs 1 and 2 in which the tk gene is located 3' of the MMTV gene support hormonally inducible tk mRNA synthesis. Constructs 3 and 4 in which the tk gene is located 5' of MMTV gene support strongly enhanced tk mRNA synthesis which is independent of hormone. This experiment shows that the enhancer quality found in the HRE is also functional in the context of the intact provirus. The strong enhancement was found in constructs 3 and 4 which are analogous to the relative orientation found between the int loci and proviral DNA in tumors. We therefore suggest that hormone-independent enhancement and not promoter insertion or hormonal induction seems to be important in MMTV-induced mammary tumorigenesis.

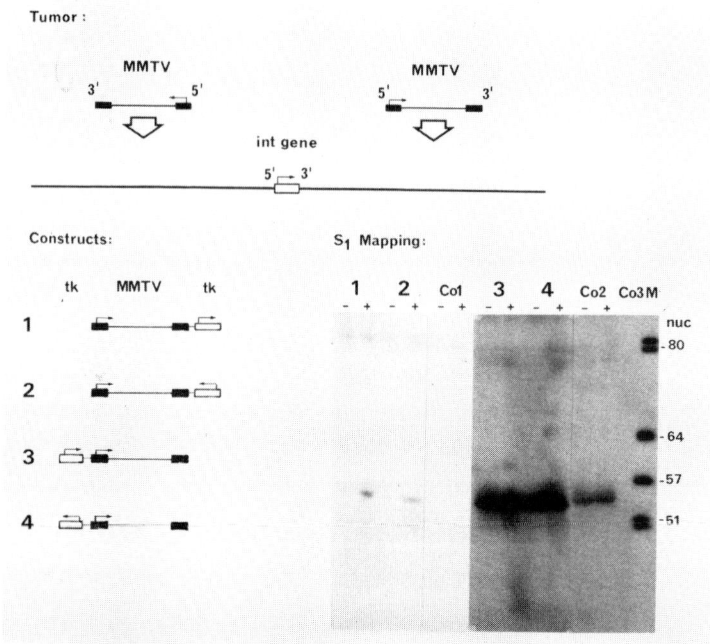

Fig. 2. Integration of proviral MMTV in mammary tumors (9,10) and constructs of MMTV-tk chimeras. S1 mapping of tk transcripts in cells transfected with constructs and grown in the absence (-) and presence (+) of dexamethasone. The construct number corresponds to the lane on the autoradiograph.

REFERENCES

1. Groner B, Kennedy N, Skroch P, Hynes NE, Ponta H (1984) Biochim Biophys Acta 781:1-6
2. Groner B, Hynes NE, Rahmsdorf U, Ponta H (1983) Nucleic Acids Res 11: 4713-4725
3. Scheiderreit C, Geisse S, Westphal HM, Beato M (1983) Nature 304:749-752
4. Nishioka Y, Leder P (1979) Cell 18:875-882
5. Southern PJ, Berg P (1982) J Mol Appl Gen 1:327-341
6. Wilkie NM, Clements JB, Boll W, Mantei N, Lonsdale D, Weissmann C (1978) Nucleic Acids Res 7:859-877
7. Hynes NE, van Ooyen A, Kennedy N, Herrlich P, Ponta H, Groner B (1983) Proc Natl Acad Sci USA 80:3637-3641
8. Gruss P (1984) DNA 3:1-5
9. Nusse R, Varmus HE (1982) Cell 31:99-109
10. Peters G, Brookes G, Smith R, Dickson C (1983) Cell 33:369-377

4. Behavioral Effects of Hormones

© 1984 Elsevier Science Publishers B.V.
Endocrinology
F. Labrie, L. Proulx, eds.

CELLULAR PRODUCTS RELATED TO ESTROGEN EFFECTS ON HYPOTHALAMIC NEURONS AND REPRODUCTIVE BEHAVIOR

R.E. HARLAN, D.W. PFAFF AND B.D. SHIVERS
The Rockefeller University, 1230 York Avenue, New York, NY 10021-6399 USA

INTRODUCTION

Steroid hormones, particularly estrogen, influence certain behavioral, autonomic and endocrine functions regulated by neural circuitries in forebrain and hypothalamic regions. If neuropeptides play key roles in communication among neurons forming these neural circuits, one way in which estrogen may act is by altering the output of specific peptidergic neurons. We review evidence here that two neuropeptides, luteinizing hormone-releasing hormone (LHRH) and a prolactin-like substance (immunoreactive or ir-prolactin), are candidates for mediating particular actions of estrogen on the brain.

Estrogen facilitates the female reproductive behavior, lordosis, by acting on cells in the mediobasal hypothalamus (1,2). Lordosis-facilitating neurons send projections to the dorsal midbrain, especially the central gray (3,4). If estrogen acts to alter the production and/or release of lordosis-facilitating peptides, then these peptides should a) be synthesized in cell bodies in the mediobasal hypothalamus with projections to the midbrain central gray (MCG), b) facilitate lordosis when applied to the MCG, and c) be regulated by estrogen.

LHRH

Behavioral effect

A lordosis-facilitating effect of LHRH (5,6) has been demonstrated in the MCG (7,8). Interestingly, analogs or fragments of LHRH which facilitate lordosis do not necessarily augment release of luteinizing hormone (LH) from the pituitary, and some LHRH analogs that are antagonistic at the pituitary facilitate lordosis (9-11). The mechanisms for these differential responses have not been elucidated, but may include receptor requirements and degradative controls.

Cellular location

Since LHRH has a potent lordosis-facilitating effect when applied to the MCG, it is noteworthy that the MCG contains a small number of LHRH fibers (12-14), which probably terminate there since they do not extend further caudally into the brain stem. We have indirect evidence that estrogen augments release of LHRH from fibers, in the MCG (14). Using a variety of LHRH antisera, we (14) and others (13,15,16) have demonstrated only a small number of LHRH cell bodies in the mediobasal hypothalamus of the rat. The evidence so far thus suggests a greater role for preoptic-to-midbrain than for hypothalamus-to-midbrain circuitry as regards the behavioral effect of LHRH.

Effect of estrogen

Although estrogen is well known to alter LHRH release from the median eminence (17), and thus participates in the neural control of ovulation, we have found that LHRH cells rarely concentrate estradiol in their nuclei (18). Given the prevailing concept that genomic actions of estrogen rely on steroid retention by nuclear receptors (19), our results imply that genomic actions of estrogen on LHRH synthesis and/or release--for example, induction of the LHRH and LH surges (20,21)--must be mediated by another class of estrogen-concentrating neurons.

PROLACTIN-LIKE SUBSTANCE

Cellular location

Looking for chemically-identified neurons with cell bodies in the mediobasal hypothalamus and fibers in the MCG, our attention was drawn to ir-prolactin (22). We have confirmed and extended these observations, and have localized immunocytochemically an estimated 2000-3000 cell bodies containing ir-prolactin in the mediobasal hypothalamus, with extensive projection systems to many brain regions, especially the MCG (23). Specific staining has been found with two anti-prolactin antisera (one from the National Hormone and Pituitary Program, produced by A. Parlow and one from M. Leiberman, Univ. Wisconsin), and is not dependent on the presence of the pituitary. Preliminary evidence, based on ultrastructural immunocytochemistry, suggests that ir-prolactin is found in terminals consistent with a neurosecretory or modulatory role (24).

Behavioral effect

Release of ir-prolactin from presumed terminals in the MCG appears to facilitate lordosis (25). Microinfusion of rat prolactin into the MCG facilitated lordosis in estrogen-treated rats, while microinfusion of anti-prolactin immune serum inhibited lordosis. These behavioral results, combined with the neuroanatomy of ir-prolactin cell bodies and fibers, make ir-prolactin a primary candidate for a lordosis-facilitating neuropeptide produced in cell bodies in the mediobasal hypothalamus and released in the MCG.

Effect of estrogen

By combining immunocytochemistry and steroid autoradiography in the same tissue section, we have found that a substantial portion of cells containing ir-prolactin also concentrate estradiol (26). Of nearly 1700 ir-prolactin cells examined to date, about 30% concentrated estradiol. In some sections, especially near the caudal end of the distribution of ir-prolactin cells, about half the nuclei of ir-prolactin cells concentrated tritiated estradiol. These findings set the stage for rigorous examinations of the effects of estrogen on production of ir-prolactin in the hypothalamus.

Chemical characterization

The exact chemical identity of brain ir-prolactin is not yet known, although evidence suggests that the substance is at least closely related to prolactin. A contaminating antibody in the anti-prolactin immune serum seems unlikely, since (a) the staining is robust even at dilutions of 1:2000; (b) preabsorption of the antibody with purified prolactin eliminated staining; (c) preabsorption with several other peptides and pituitary hormones did not eliminate staining; and (d) staining has been found with two anti-prolactin immune sera, which were prepared against different, highly-purified prolactin preparations (23). These data suggest that brain ir-prolactin shares antigenic sites with pituitary prolactin.

In a partial characterization of brain ir-prolactin, we have immunoprecipitated hypothalamic explant cultures and electrophoresed the immunoprecipitates on SDS polyacrylamide gels to determine apparent molecular weights (27). We have demonstrated synthesis of ir-prolactin in the hypothalamus, and have determined that the antiserum precipitates a protein with an apparent molecular weight indistinguishable from that of pituitary prolactin (about 22,000 daltons).

If prolactin is synthesized in the hypothalamus, then prolactin messenger RNA (mRNA) should be present in this part of the brain. To examine this question, we (28) extracted RNA and purified this to prepare a fraction enriched in polyadenylated RNA. The purified RNA was then electrophoresed on agarose gels, transfered to Gene Screen filters, and probed with a radiolabeled DNA complementary to mature prolactin RNA, using stringent hybridization conditions. The Northern blot autoradiograms revealed a polyadenylated mRNA in the hypothalamus, complementary to the prolactin cDNA probe, and the same size as mature pituitary prolactin mRNA, providing strong evidence for the existence of prolactin mRNA in the rat hypothalamus. To address whether the cells which contain prolactin mRNA also contain ir-prolactin, we are performing *in situ* DNA/RNA hybridization and immunocytochemistry on adjacent tissue sections.

SUMMARY

Two neuropeptides are evaluated as candidates for estrogen-modulated, lordosis-facilitatory, neurosecretory products produced in the mediobasal hypothalamus and released from terminals in the dorsal midbrain. Luteinizing hormone-releasing hormone 1) facilitates lordosis when applied to the dorsal midbrain, 2) is *not* found in cell bodies in the mediobasal hypothalamus and is found in only a few fibers in the dorsal midbrain, 3) is modulated by estrogen, but not directly through nuclear retention of estradiol by neurons producing the peptide. A prolactin-like substance 1) is found in cell bodies in the mediobasal hypothalamus, with strong fiber projections to the dorsal midbrain, 2) facilitates lordosis by acting on midbrain cells, 3) is produced by neurons which concentrate estradiol in their nuclei.

REFERENCES

1. Davis PG, McEwen BS, Pfaff DW (1979) Endocrinol 104: 898-903
2. Rubin BS, Barfield RJ (1980) Endocrinol 106: 504-509
3. Pfaff DW (1980) Estrogens and brain function. Springer-Verlag, New York
4. Morrell JI, Pfaff DW (1982) Science 217: 1273-1275
5. Moss RL, McCann SM (1973) Science 181: 177-179
6. Pfaff DW (1973) Science 182: 1148-1149
7. Riskind P, Moss RL (1979) Brain Res Bull 4: 203-205
8. Sakuma Y, Pfaff DW (1980) Nature 283: 566-567
9. Sakuma Y, Pfaff DW (1983) Neuroendocrinol 36: 218-224
10. Dudley CA, Vale W, Rivier J, Moss RL (1983) Neuroendocrinol 36: 486-488
11. Kastin AJ, Coy DH, Schally AV, Zadina JE (1980) Pharm Biochem Behav 13: 913-914
12. Liposits Z, Setalo G (1980) Neurosci Lett 20: 1-4
13. Witkin JW, Paden CM, Silverman A-J (1982) Neuroendocrinol 35: 429-438
14. Shivers BD, Harlan RE, Morrell JI, Pfaff DW (1983) Neuroendocrinol 36: 1-12
15. Kozlowski GP, Rees WL (1984) J Histo Cyto 32: 83-91
16. Bennett-Clark C, Joseph SA (1982) Cell Tiss Res 221: 493-504
17. Fink G (1979) Ann Rev Physiol 41: 571-585
18. Shivers BD, Harlan RE, Morrell JI, Pfaff DW (1983) Nature 304: 345-347
19. O'Malley BW, Means AR (1974) Science 183: 610-620
20. Jackson GL (1972) Endocrinol 91: 1284-1287
21. Jackson GL (1973) Endocrinol 93: 887-892
22. Toubeau G, Desclin J, Parmentier M, Pasteels JL (1979) J Endocrinol 83: 261-266
23. Shivers BD, Harlan RE, Pfaff DW (1983) Abst Soc Neurosci 9: 1018
24. Nishizuka M, Shivers BD, Pfaff DW, Leranth CS (1984) Abst Soc Neurosci vol 10
25. Harlan RE, Shivers BD, Pfaff DW (1983) Science 219: 1451-1453
26. Shivers BD, Harlan RE, Pfaff DW (1984) Abst Soc Neurosci vol 10
27. Harlan RE, Shivers BD, Kalamaridis M, Pfaff DW (1984) Abst Soc Neurosci vol 10
28. Schachter B, Durgerian S, Harlan R, Pfaff D, Shivers B (1984) Abst 7th Intern Congr Endocrinol; (1984) Endocrinol 114: 1947-1949

Endocrinology
F. Labrie, L. Proulx, eds.

STRUCTURE OF THE COMMANDS FOR NEUROPEPTIDE-MEDIATED BEHAVIORS IN APLYSIA

FELIX STRUMWASSER

Dept. of Physiology, Boston University School of Medicine, 80 E. Concord Street, Boston, MA. 02118

INTRODUCTION

From an evolutionary point of view, the nervous system is a conservative structure, since neurons utilize similar or identical mechanisms to carry out their functions in the simplest (coelenterates) and most complex forms (mammals). We can hope therefore to gain insights into neuroendocrine control of behavior from the study of model systems in simpler forms.

In the opisthobranch mollusc, Aplysia, there are two behaviors that are controlled by discrete and different neurosecretory structures in the nervous system. Egg-laying behavior (extrusion, attachment and winding of the egg-string) is controlled by the approximately 1000 peptidergic bag cell neurons in the abdominal ganglion, while circadian locomotor activity is controlled by a circadian oscillator in each of the two eyes. In this brief paper, I will review the status of knowledge about these two neuroendocrine systems and their control of behavior.

THE PEPTIDERGIC BAG CELL NEURONS AND CONTROL OF EGG LAYING

Structure and target actions of ELH

The command for egg-laying is the peptide ELH (egg-laying hormone), synthesized and released by the bag cells. ELH is a basic peptide (pI 9.1) containing 36 amino-acid residues with a calculated molecular weight of 4385 daltons (1). The structure of ELH is:

H-Ile-Ser-Ile-Asn-Gln-Asp-Leu-Lys-Ala-Ile-Thr-Asp-Met-Leu-Leu-Thr-Glu-Gln-Ile-Arg-Glu-Arg-Gln-Arg-Tyr-Leu-Ala-Asp-Leu-Arg-Gln-Arg-Leu-Leu-Glu-Lys-OH

ELH acts directly on the ovotestis to release eggs into the reproductive tract (2) and also acts back on targets in the nervous system (3) to inhibit feeding (buccal ganglia) and locomotion (pedal ganglia). In the case of the buccal ganglion, one target of ELH is the motoneurons that cause retraction of the buccal mass (3,4).

The command for ELH release (bag cell afterdischarge)

The command for ELH release is a 30 minute program of synchronized activity ("afterdischarge") in the BCs (5), the synchronization being mediated by electrical (gap-junction) coupling between BCs (6). The afterdischarge program is mediated by cyclic AMP-dependent protein phosphorylation changes. The evidence for this includes the demonstration that isolated BCs (in primary culture) contain the program for afterdischarge. Long-lasting afterdischarge, in such isolated BCs, can be released by priming with membrane permeant, phosphodiesterase-resistant, cyclic AMP analogs and directly firing a few calcium action potentials (7). At least two proteins are phosphorylated at an increased rate during afterdischarge, with apparent molecular weights of 21,000 and 33,000 daltons (8).

The precommand for egg-laying

The pre-command for egg-laying is partially worked out. Two peptides in the atrial gland, a part of the reproductive tract near the gonopore, cause egg-laying in a bag cell-dependent manner. These peptides are homologous with one another but share no significant sequences with ELH. Peptides A and B contain 34 amino-acid residues each, have molecular weights of 3924 and 4932 daltons, and pI of 8.0 and 9.1, respectively (9). These peptides induce bag cell afterdischarge, in vitro, and thus resemble releasing factors in their actions. However, the atrial gland has an exocrine structure (10) and it remains to be seen whether peptides A and B have homologs in the CNS. We have recently shown that antibodies to ELH, besides staining bag cells (11), also stain particular small sets of neurons in the pleural and cerebral ganglia (12).

THE CIRCADIAN OSCILLATOR IN THE EYE AND CONTROL OF CIRCADIAN LOCOMOTION

Circadian locomotion is controlled by a neuronal circadian oscillator in each eye. The isolated eye, in darkness, produces a pacemaker discharge, emitted in the optic nerve. The frequency of these action potentials varies smoothly over 24 hours, with peak activity near projected dawn and minimal activity near projected dusk (13, 14). One of the output cells of this retina contains 100 nm dense core granules and, by autoradiographic criteria, is the most active protein synthesizing cell in the retina (15). Radioactive release experiments indicate that at least two peptides are released from the isolated eye with a circadian rhythm. It is likely that these peptides act in the cerebral ganglion, rather than the circulation, for animals with sectioned optic nerves are arhythmic in their free running activity (Strumwasser and Mailheau, unpublished).

ACKNOWLEDGEMENTS

I would like to thank certain of my graduate students (Gerald Audesirk, Arlene Y. Chiu, Kent Jennings, Duncan K. Stuart), research fellows (Eri Heller, Leonard K. Kaczmarek, Jack C. Woolum) and collaborators (Michael Hunkapiller) without whose efforts this work would not have been possible. I would also like to acknowledge support from NIH grants.

REFERENCES

1. Chiu AY, Hunkapiller MW, Heller E, Stuart DK, Hood LE, Strumwasser, F (1979) Proc Natl Acad Sci USA 76:6656-6660
2. Rothman BS, Weir G, Dudek FE (1980) Soc. for Neurosci. Abstracts 6:623
3. Stuart DK, Strumwasser F (1980) J Neurophysiol 43:499-519
4. Ram JL (1983) Brain Research (in press)
5. Stuart DK, Chiu AY, Strumwasser F (1980) J. Neurophysiol. 43:488-498

6. Kaczmarek LK, Finbow M, Revel JP, Strumwasser F (1979) J. Neurobiol. 10:535-550

7. Kaczmarek LK, Strumwasser F (1981) J. Neurosci. 1:626-634

8. Jennings KR, Kaczmarek LK, Hewick RM, Dreyer WJ, Strumwasser F (1982) J. Neurosci. 2:158-168

9. Heller E, Kaczmarek LK, Hunkapiller MW, Hood LE Strumwasser F (1980) Proc. Natl. Acad. Sci. USA 77:2328-2332

10. Beard M, Millecchia L, Masuoka C and Arch S (1982) Tissue & Cell 14:297-308

11. Chiu AY, Strumwasser F (1981) J. of Neurosci. 1:812-826

12. Chiu AY, Strumwasser, F (1984) Brain Research 294:83-93

13. Jacklet JW (1969) Science 164:562-563

14. Rothman BS, Strumwasser F (1976) J Gen Physiol 68:359-384

15. Strumwasser F, Alvarez RB, Viele DP, Woolum JC (1979) In: Suda M, Hayaishi O, Nakagawa H (eds) Biological Rhythms and their Central Mechanism. Elsevier, Amsterdam, pp 41-56

Endocrinology
F. Labrie, L. Proulx, eds.

EFFECTS OF SEX STEROIDS ON BEHAVIORAL AND BRAIN ORGANIZATION

ROGER A. GORSKI

Department of Anatomy and Laboratory of Neuroendocrinology of the Brain Research Institute, UCLA School of Medicine, Los Angeles, California (USA)

INTRODUCTION

The fact that gonadal hormones act on the brain has been thoroughly documented both in the adult and during development. However, the nature of hormone action is thought to differ depending on animal age, at least at the conceptual level, if not in terms of actual biochemical mechanisms. The transient actions of gonadal steroids which typify the adult animal, are called *activational*; whereas the permanent actions which occur during development are called *organizational*. The present discussion will focus on reproductive behavior as an index of the organizational actions of gonadal steroids. Moreover, a specific structural sex difference in the rat brain will be presented as a model system for the study of the mechanism of these actions.

SEX DIFFERENCES IN SEXUAL BEHAVIOR AND THEIR ORIGIN

In the adult female rat, reproductive behavior is dependent upon the sequential activational effects of the ovarian hormones estrogen and progesterone (P). In contrast, masculine sexual behavior is elicited by the testicular hormone testosterone. These hormones appear to act on different neural substrates, the ventromedial hypothalamus[1] for lordosis behavior (an important index of feminine behavior) and the medial preoptic area (MPOA) for masculine sexual behavior[2]. (In both cases, other neural circuitry is also presumably involved[1,3])

Although the hormonal bases for the activation of masculine and feminine sexual behavior differ, it is now clear that the neural mechanisms which subserve these behaviors are themselves sexually dimorphic. Thus, when a male rat is castrated as an adult and treated with exogenous estradiol benzoate (EB) and P, he only rarely exhibits the lordosis reflex. With respect to masculine sexual behavior, especially in terms of mounting activity, the sex dimorphism in rats is less dramatic. It must be emphasized, however, that the obvious functional sexual dimorphism in behavior is imposed on an inherently feminine, or at least bipotential, brain by the hormonal environment perinatally. The genetic male, if castrated within the first few days of birth will, when adult, respond to EB and P with feminine rates of lordosis. On the other hand, if the neonatal female is exposed to exogenous androgen she will display the masculine pattern of low lordosis responsiveness to exogenous EB and P given to her during adulthood. Thus, the sex difference in the behavioral response to gonadal steroids in the adult rat is the consequence of hormone action rather than an inherent genomic difference between the male and female brain.[4,5]

STRUCTURAL SEX DIFFERENCES IN THE RAT BRAIN

Recently, the concept of the sexual differentiation of the brain has been strengthened by the identification of structural sex differences. These range from subtle changes in synaptology[6,7] to relatively gross differences in the histological organization of the brain.[8] In the rat hypothalamus, for example, an area we have called the sexually dimorphic nucleus of the preoptic area (SDN-POA) is 3-5 times larger and is composed of more neurons in the male than in the female.[9,10] The sex difference in SDN-POA volume develops during the first postnatal week,[11] the precise period of the functional differentiation of the brain. Moreover, the ultimate volume of the SDN-POA is hormone dependent: castration of the newborn male rat reduces SDN-POA volume by 50% in the adult,[9] and importantly, prolonged perinatal exposure of the female to testosterone propionate[12] (or to diethylstilbestrol[13]) completely sex reverses SDN-POA volume. We consider the SDN-POA a morphological signature of the organizational action of gonadal hormones on the developing brain.

We have found by tritiated thymidine autoradiography that about one third of the neurons of the SDN-POA become postmitotic several days later than those of the surrounding MPOA. When prenatal rats are exposed to thymidine on day 18 of gestation, one third of the neurons of the SDN-POA are specifically and permanently labeled.[14] We have used this fact to establish the site of origin and pathway of migration of SDN-POA neurons. These neurons appear to be formed in the lateral walls of the third ventricle, then migrate first ventrally to the base of the ventricle and the surrounding neural parenchyma, then upward and laterally to the site of the SDN-POA.[15] Although to date we have not observed a statistical sex difference in this process, it is clear that labeled neurons disappear during the migration process. These neurons either migrate out of the areas analyzed or perhaps more likely, die. It has also been reported that gonadal hormones stimulate the growth of neuronal processes in vitro.[16] It appears, therefore, that gonadal steroids may be trophic factors which promote the growth of neuronal processes and indirectly neuronal survival, or perhaps which directly maintain neuronal survival during the process of migration.

THE FUNCTION OF THE SDN-POA

Clearly, if the SDN-POA can be shown to be related to reproductive behaviors, these studies would provide unique insight into the mechanisms of the sexual differentiation of the neural substrate for these behaviors. At present, however, we cannot prove a relationship between the SDN-POA and sexual behavior. In the adult male rat, small lesions restricted to the SDN-POA do not alter masculine behavior, whereas equally small lesions placed dorsal to the SDN-POA are quite effective in disrupting masculine copulatory behavior.[2] In other studies, however, we have found that the stereotaxic transplantation of the MPOA including the SDN-POA from the newborn male to the MPOA of littermate females results in a potentiation of their masculine behavior as adults.[17] Since feminine reproductive behavior is also facilitated it is difficult to conclude that such transplants truly masculinize the host brain. Since many functional processes are sexually dimorphic the specific function(s) of the SDN-POA remain unknown.

SEX DIFFERENCES IN SEROTONIN DISTRIBUTION

Another approach to the functional significance of the neurons of the SDN-POA is to determine their connectivity particularly in terms of their neurotransmitter input. To this end we have evaluated the distribution of serotonin (5HT) terminals (determined by immunohistofluorescence). A combined approach of the analysis of 5HT distribution and cytoarchitectonics has permitted us to identify the SDN-POA as a 5HT free, cell dense central component of the medial preoptic nucleus (MPN).[18] The MPN itself, can be divided into three subdivisions which differ in 5HT distribution. The medial component (in which the central component is embedded) has a moderate plexus of 5HT terminals, while the lateral component has a rich plexus of 5HT terminals. Each of these components of the MPN is sexually dimorphic, and can be sex-reversed by the prolonged exposure to TP perinatally shown previously to sex-reverse SDN-POA volume.[19]

SUMMARY AND CONCLUSION

The organizational action of gonadal steroids brings about both the functional and structural sexual differentiation of the brain. The SDN-POA, which is larger in volume and comprised of more neurons in the male sex, can be viewed as a morphological signature of the effects of gonadal steroids in the developing brain. The identification of the SDN-POA has provided a model system in which to study the possible effects of gonadal hormones on neurogenesis, neuronal migration and survival, and the existence of sex differences in 5HT distribution. To date the function(s) of the SDN-POA remain unknown, but it is anticipated that the elucidation of the development of the sex difference in this nucleus will ultimately contribute to our fundamental understanding of the sexual differentiation of neurobehavioral mechanisms.

ACKNOWLEDGEMENTS

The research of the author supported by NIH grant HD-01182 and grants from the Ford, Grant and Kroc Foundations and the Tejon Ranch, California.

REFERENCES

1. Pfaff DW (1980) Estrogens and Brain Function. Springer-Verlag, New York
2. Arendash GW, Gorski RA (1983) Brain Res Bull 10:147-154
3. Gorski RA (1974) In: Newton G, Riesen AH (eds) Advances in Psychobiology, Vol II. John Wiley & Sons, New York
4. Goy RW, McEwen BS (1980) Sexual Differentiation of the Brain. MIT Press, Cambridge MA
5. Gorski RA (1983) In: Müller EE, MacLeod RM (eds) Neuroendocrine Perspectives, Vol 2. Elsevier, Amsterdam
6. Raisman G, Field PM (1973) Brain Res 54:1-29
7. Matsumoto A, Arai Y (1980) Brain Res 190:238-242
8. Nottebohm F, Arnold A (1976) Science 194:211-213
9. Gorski RA, Gordon JH, Shryne JE, Southam AM (1978) Brain Res 148:333-346
10. Gorski RA, Harlan RE, Jacobson CD, Shryne JE, Southam AM (1980) J Comp Neurol 193:529-539
11. Jacobson CD, Shryne JE, Shapiro F, Gorski RA (1980) J Comp Neurol 193:541-548
12. Döhler KD, Coquelin A, Davis F, Hines M, Shryne JE, Gorski RA (1982) Neurosci Lett 33:295-298
13. Döhler KD, Hines M, Coquelin A, Davis F, Shryne JE, Gorski RA (1982) Neuroendocrinol Lett 4:361-365
14. Jacobson CD, Gorski RA (1981) J Comp Neurol 196:519-529
15. Jacobson CD, Davis FC, Freiberg E, Gorski RA (1981) Soc Neurosci Abstr 7:286
16. Toran-Allerand CD, Hashimoto K, Greenough WT, Saltarelli M (1983) Develop Brain Res 7:97-101
17. Arendash GW, Gorski RA (1982) Science 217:1276-1278
18. Simerly RB, Swanson LW, Gorski RA (1984) J Comp Neurol 225:151-166
19. Simerly RB, Swanson LW, Gorski RA (1984) Anat Rec 208:166A-167A

© 1984 Elsevier Science Publishers B.V.
Endocrinology
F. Labrie, L. Proulx, eds.

BEHAVIORAL EFFECTS OF NEUROHYPOPHYSEAL HORMONES

TJ.B. VAN WIMERSMA GREIDANUS AND J.P.H. BURBACH
Rudolf Magnus Institute for Pharmacology, Medical Faculty, University of Utrecht, Vondellaan 6, 3521 GD Utrecht (The Netherlands)

In addition to their well known effects on water homeostasis and contraction of smooth muscles the neurohypophyseal hormones vasopressin and oxytocin induce a variety of behavioral effects. A number of recent experiments on these effects of vasopressin and oxytocin incorporating antisera, antagonists and metabolites with potent and selectively central activity has indicated that peripherally and centrally acting vasopressin represent two functionally separate systems.

The first publication on a behavioral effect described the inhibition of extinction of a shuttle box avoidance response of posterior lobectomized rats following administration of pitressin or [Lys^8]vasopressin (LVP). In intact rats administration of pitressin or LVP results in a long lasting resistance to extinction of a conditioned avoidance response (1,2). This inhibitory effect of vasopressin on extinction lasted far beyond the actual presence of the injected material in the organism, suggesting that vasopressin triggers a long term effect on the maintenance of a learned response, probably by facilitating processes involved in memory consolidation (3).

The long-term preservation of an acquired response was also found in a passive avoidance situation (4,5). Administration of vasopressin immediately after the single learning trial is most effective, and if postponed for 3 or 6 hrs. the facilitating influence of the peptide on passive avoidance behavior is markedly reduced or absent. However, if the administration of vasopressin is postponed to shortly before the retention test, passive avoidance latencies are again considerably increased. This suggests that vasopressin improves avoidance behavior by stimulating storage as well as retrieval processes which are related to memory function. Vasopressin also facilitates passive avoidance behavior of mice in a situation where the aversive stimulus is attack by a trained fighter mouse (6). In addition, it increases resistance to extinction of sexually motivated approach behavior (7), of a positively rewarded discrimination task (8), and of conditioned taste aversion (9). These data suggest an effect of vasopressin on processes related to memory (10).

Further evidence for this assumption was obtained from the effects of vasopressin on amnesia. It appeared that vasopressin and its congeners prevent or reverse amnesia induced by puromycin (11), electro-convulsive shock (12), CO_2 inhalation (13) or by pentylene-tetrazol (14,15). Also the finding that vasopressin facilitates the development of tolerance to morphine and ethanol (16,17), a process that is regarded as a form of learning and memory, supports the notion that this peptide hormone affects processes underlying memory function (10).

Although neurohypophyseal hormones or their fragments also affect other types of behavior (electrical selfstimulation (18,19), maternal behavior (20)), far out most of the behavioral effects are found in situations in which processes related to learning and memory are involved (10).

Generally oxytocin has behavioral effects opposite to those of vasopressin. For example oxytocin attenuates passive avoidance behavior. Time gradient studies using this behavioral paradigm reveal that oxytocin impairs storage as well as retrieval processes and it has been considered as an amnesic neuropeptide (4,5).

Reasoning that specific antisera to vasopressin or oxytocin would temporarily bind and therefore neutralize the biological activities of neurohypophyseal hormones, administration of antisera was used to study the role of endogenous vasopressin and oxytocin in brain functions underlying behavior and learning and memory processes (4,21,22). I.c.v. administration of anti-oxytocin serum facilitates passive avoidance behavior (4), whereas i.c.v., but not intravenous (i.v.) administration of anti-vasopressin serum results in a marked deficit in passive avoidance behavior (21). This finding, together with the observation that i.v. administration of anti-vasopressin serum effectively inhibits antidiuresis and reduces vasopressin levels in urine (21), points to the importance of central rather than peripheral vasopressin in processes underlying behavior and memory.

Structure-activity studies with synthetic fragments of vasopressin and oxytocin have shown that the peripheral and central (behavioral) actions of vasopressin can be dissociated: various peptides devoid of antidiuretic, pressor and/or ACTH-releasing activities induce behavioral effects similar to or comparable with those of the parent (vasopressin) molecule (23). Based on these experiments the existence of vasopressin fragments with more selective and/or potent activities has been presumed. The identification of such peptides has been approached by studying the *in vitro* conversion of vasopressin (AVP) by peptidases from rat brain membranes (24). A major component was isolated and characterized as [pGlu^4,Cyt^6]AVP-(4-9). When administered i.c.v. this AVP fragment as well as its des-gly-NH_2 derivative [pGlu^4,Cyt^6]AVP-(4-8) facilitated passive avoidance behavior in extremely low (0.1 pg) doses. Thus, such AVP metabolites, which are devoid of peripheral hormonal activities, constitute highly potent neuropeptides with selective central effects related to memory (24) and appear to be endogenously present in the brain (25). By use of [pGlu^4,Cyt^6]AVP-(4-8) and the vasopressin antagonist d$(CH_2)_5$Tyr(ME)AVP it could be demonstrated that the behavioral effects of vasopressin or its analogues were elicited by central rather than peripheral actions (26). The vasopressor antagonist injected subcutaneously (s.c., 3 μg) prior to s.c. treatment with AVP (3 μg) or AVP-(4-8) (0.3 μg) antagonized the behavioral actions of these peptides and it appeared that the antagonism between the peptides and the antagonist was competitive in nature. The same was found after i.c.v. administration of the antagonist (3 ng) and AVP or AVP-(4-8). These data suggest that the vasopressor antagonist acts directly on the central receptor sites that are activated by AVP and AVP-(4-8) and that mediate the effect of these peptides on passive avoidance behavior. When the antagonist was given s.c. and AVP was administered i.c.v. in a dose of 3 ng, which is inactive upon s.c. injection, the effect of AVP on behavior was completely antagonized. Also, such an antagonism was found when the antagonist was injected i.c.v. and AVP or AVP-(4-8) s.c.. This suggests that the antagonism occurs in the brain following both i.c.v. and s.c. administration of the peptides.

In addition, it appeared that s.c. injection of 3.0 μg AVP, but not AVP-(4-8) induced increase in blood pressure associated with bradycardia. I.c.v. administration of 30 ng AVP or 0.3 ng AVP-(4-8), which exert maximal behavioral effects, did not induce a pressor response or bradycardia. The vasopressor antagonist prevented AVP-induced pressor response and bradycardia following s.c. injection of 3.0 μg. However, i.c.v. administration of the antagonist (3 ng) which can block the behavioral action of s.c. or i.c.v. injected AVP or AVP-(4-8) had no effect on the pressor response to s.c. administration of 3.0 μg AVP. Thus, it is suggested (26) that AVP exerts its effect on blood pressure and heart rate by activation of peripherally located receptor systems, which can be blocked by the used vasopressor antagonist. Apparently these receptor systems cannot be activated by AVP-(4-8) and appear not to be involved in mediating the behavioral effects of vasopressin or its derivative. Thus, the receptors mediating the behavioral effects are situated in the brain and differ in specificity from the peripheral (blood pressure) vasopressin receptors. Both the pressor and the behavioral receptor can be blocked by the used vasopressor antagonist.

In conclusion, vasopressin facilitates, improves or maintains behavior in which brain processes related to memory function are involved; it facilitates storage as well as retrieval of information. Oxytocin is regarded as an amnesic peptide. The behavioral effects are centrally mediated as appeared from lesion studies (27), local application of the neurohypophyseal hormones (27) and studies with antagonists and metabolites with exclusively central activity. Structure-activity and biotransformation studies suggest that vasopressin and oxytocin serve as precursor molecules of neuropeptides with more specific and potent effects on behavior in the brain. These studies also distinguish the peripheral (classical endocrinological) and central (behavioral) actions of vasopressin and oxytocin and recognize two functionally separate vasopressin and oxytocin systems.

REFERENCES

1. De Wied D, Bohus B (1966) Nature 212: 1484-1486.
2. De Wied D (1971) Nature 232: 58-60.
3. De Wied D, Bohus B, van Wimersma Greidanus TjB (1974) Progr Brain Res 41: 417-428.
4. Bohus B, Urban I, van Wimersma Greidanus TjB, De Wied D (1978) Neuropharmacology 17: 239-247.
5. Bohus B, Kovács GL, De Wied D (1978) Brain Res 157: 414-417.
6. Leshner AI, Roche KE (1977) Physiol Behav 18: 879-883.
7. Bohus B (1977) Horm Behav 8: 52-61.
8. Hostetter G, Jubb SL, Kozlowski GP (1977) Life Sci 21: 1323-1328.
9. Rigter H, Popping A (1976) Psychopharmacology 46: 255-261.
10. van Wimersma Greidanus TjB, Van Ree JM, De Wied D (1983) Pharmacol Ther 20: 437-458.
11. Lande S, Flexner JB, Flexner B (1972) Proc Natl Acad Sci USA 69: 558-560.
12. Pfeifer WD, Bookin HB (1978) Pharmacol Biochem Behav 9: 261-263.
13. Rigter H, Van Riezen H, De Wied D (1974) Physiol Behav 13: 381-388.
14. Bookin HB, Pfeifer WD (1977) Pharmacol Biochem Behav 7: 51-54.
15. Bohus B, Conti L, Kovács GL, Versteeg DHG (1982) In: Marsan CA, Matthies H (eds) Neuronal Plasticity and Memory Formation. Raven Press, New York, pp. 75-87.
16. Krivoy WA, Zimmerman E, Lande S (1974) Proc Natl Acad Sci USA 71: 1852-1856.
17. Hoffman PL, Ritzmann RF, Walter R, Tabakoff B (1978) Nature 276: 614-616.
18. Schwarzberg H, Hartmann G, Kovács GL, Telegdy G (1976) Acta Physiol Acad Sci Hung 47: 127-131.
19. Dorsa DM, Van Ree JM (1979) Brain Res 172: 367-371.
20. Pedersen CA, Ascher JA, Monroe YL, Prange AJ Jr (1982) Science 216: 648-649.
21. van Wimersma Greidanus TjB, Dogterom J, De Wied D (1975) Life Sci 16: 637-644.
22. van Wimersma Greidanus TjB, De Wied D (1976) Behav Biol 18: 325-333.
23. De Wied D, Greven HM, Lande S, Witter A (1972) Brit J Pharmacol 45: 118-122.
24. Burbach JPH, Kovács GL, De Wied D, Van Nispen JW, Greven HM (1983) Science 221: 1310-1312.
25. Burbach JPH, Wang X-C, Ten Haaf JA, De Wied D (1984) Brain Res 306: 384-387.
26. De Wied D, Gaffori O, Van Ree JM, De Jong W (1984) Nature 308: 276-278.
27. van Wimersma Greidanus TjB, Bohus B, Kovács GL, Versteeg DHG, Burbach JPH, De Wied D (1983) Neurosci Biobehav Rev 7: 453-463.

5. Pineal Gland and Endocrine Rhythms

© 1984 Elsevier Science Publishers B.V.
Endocrinology
F. Labrie, L. Proulx, eds.

THE MAMMALIAN MELATONIN RHYTHM GENERATING SYSTEM

DAVID C. KLEIN, DAVID SUGDEN, PIERRE VOISIN, and JIRI VANECEK
Section on Neuroendocrinology, Laboratory of Developmental Neurobiology, National Institute of Child Health and Human Development, National Institutes of Health Bethesda, Maryland 20205

There is a daily rhythm in circulating melatonin in all vertebrates, with high values occurring at night. The pineal gland is the major source of melatonin. The mammalian pineal gland has evolved from a tissue complex in lower vertebrates which both responds directly to light and has the capacity to make and release melatonin (1). During evolution this "third eye" system has lost the capacity to respond directly to light, but has retained the ability to make and release melatonin. Despite the loss of photosensitivity, light still remains the most important environmental factor regulating the mammalian pineal gland. Photic regulation in mammals involves the lateral eyes and a complex neural circuit having both central and peripheral components. The pineal gland and this neural circuit constitute the mammalian melatonin rhythm generating system (Figure 1).

I. THE NEURAL CIRCUIT

The neural circuit regulating the mammalian pineal gland appears to be: retina->retinohypothalamic projection->suprachiasmatic nucleus (SCN)-> paraventricular nucleus->intermediolateral cell column of the spinal cord-> superior cervical ganglia->inferior carotid nerve->nervi conarii->pineal gland. The SCN is the key to circadian rhythmicity in the pineal gland, because it is a master circadian clock regulating many physiological rhythms. The involvement of the SCN in this circuit may indicate that there was survival advantage to having the pineal gland turned on and off by an endogenous clock, rather than by environmental lighting. The SCN, which had no known function 10 years ago, has been studied extensively in the intervening years. It functions autonomously to drive circadian rhythms indefinitely, even in constant darkness or blind animals. Evidence that it, and not another part of the brain is the source of circadian rhythmicity comes from electrophysiological investigations of hypothalamic islands containing the SCN: circadian rhythmicity is retained in these islands, but is lost elsewhere (3).

The period of the endogenous clock in the SCN varies from animal to animal and is not exactly 24-hours, but can be up to 30 minutes longer or shorter. However, light acts to reset the clock each day, ensuring that it

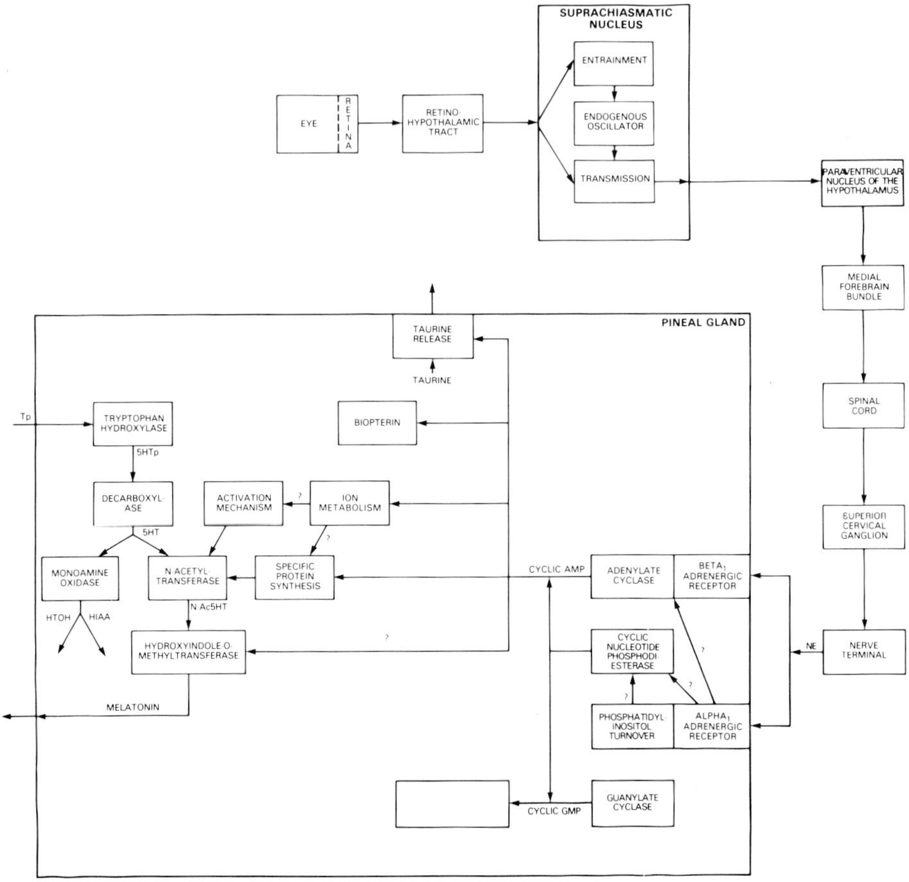

Figure 1. Melatonin rhythm generating system (from ref. 2).

is entrained to the environmental lighting cycle (4). Another important effect of light is to terminate neural stimulation of the pineal gland by the pineal and circulating melatonin (2). Light acts on the SCN *via* the retinohypothalamic tract, a monosynaptic projection from the retina which passes through the optic nerve and merges at the level of the optic chiasm (2).

II. TRANSSYNAPTIC AND CELLULAR REGULATION OF MELATONIN PRODUCTION

At night activation of the sympathetic fibers to the pineal occurs and results in the release of norepinephrine from terminals in the gland. Three adrenergic receptors which influence melatonin production are present in the pineal gland: one on presynaptic structures and two on pinealocytes. The presynaptic adrenoceptor belongs to the alpha$_2$-subclass, and serves to modulate transmitter release, as occurs generally in adrenergic nerves. Alpha$_1$- and beta$_1$-adrenoceptors are located on pinealocytes and act to regulate melatonin production (2).

In many tissues, alpha$_1$- and beta$_1$-adrenoceptors have opposite effects. In contrast, in the pineal gland alpha$_1$-adrenoceptors act synergistically with beta$_1$-adrenoceptors. Their action is expressed through both cyclic AMP and cyclic GMP. The former nucleotide is clearly involved in the regulation of melatonin synthesis, and will be discussed in detail here. The function of cyclic GMP remains unknown. Following denervation the cyclic AMP response increases and the cyclic GMP response decreases, a phenomenon described as see-saw signal processing (5).

Cyclic AMP production is stimulated by norepinephrine acting at both alpha$_1$- and beta$_1$-adrenoceptors (2,6,7). Beta$_1$-adrenergic activation is required for cyclic AMP to increase; beta-adrenergic agonists activate adenylate cyclase. However, pure beta$_1$-adrenergic activation produces only partial elevation of cyclic AMP. Full elevation of cyclic AMP, such as occurs with norepinephrine, occurs with isoproterenol, a beta-adrenergic agonist, only if an alpha$_1$-adrenergic agonist, such as phenylephrine, is also present. The mechanism of action of alpha$_1$-adrenergic agonists has not been revealed. Earlier studies had clearly indicated that norepinephrine stimulates phospholipid turnover in the pineal gland through an alpha$_1$-adrenergic mechanism (2). It may be possible that this effect is in some way linked to the potentiating effects of alpha$_1$-adrenergic agonists on the beta$_1$-adrenergic stimulation of cyclic AMP. The precise mechanism might promote a more efficient beta$_1$-adrenergic activation of adenylate cyclase, an inhibition of phosphodiesterase activity, or both.

Cyclic AMP acts to stimulate melatonin production each night primarily by stimulating the activity of one enzyme involved in melatonin synthesis, serotonin N-acetyltransferase. This stimulation is 70-fold in the rat, appears to involve both induction and activation mechanisms, and requires hyperpolarization of the pinealocyte membrane. The increase in N-acetylation increases the production of the melatonin precursor N-acetylserotonin, leading to an increase in melatonin production by a mass-action effect. The second enzyme in the conversion of serotonin to melatonin, hydroxyindole-O-methyltransferase, exhibits little or no daily rhythm. However, it also is neurally regulated, but changes slowly after interruption of neural stimulation, with a 70% decrease apparent following ten days of constant light (2).

Melatonin appears to be released from the pineal gland as a function of production. There is no evidence of a mechanism controlling the release of this highly lipophilic molecule. It is rapidly metabolized in the liver to 6-hydroxy-conjugates, and more than 85% of circulating melatonin is excreted as 6-sulfatoxy melatonin (8). Removal of the pineal gland reduces urinary 6-hydroxymelatonin to undetectable or nearly undetectable levels in the rat and monkey, indicating that essentially all melatonin comes from the pineal gland in these and probably other species (2).

REFERENCES

1. Meissl H., Dodt E. (1981) in Oksche A and Pevet P (eds) The Pineal Organ. Elsevier/North-Holland, New York, pp 61-80.
2. Klein DC (1985) In: Weiner N, Trendelenberg U, (eds) Catecholamines II, Springer Verlag, New York (in press).
3. Inouye St, Kawamura H. (1979) Proc Nat Acad Sci USA 76:5962.
4. Illnerova H., Vanecek J. (1982) J comp Physiol 145:539.
5. Klein DC, Auerbach DA, Weller JL (1981) Proc natl Acad Sci USA 78:4625.
6. Klein DC, Sugden D, Weller JL (1983) Proc natl Acad Sci USA 80:599.
7. Vanecek J, Klein DC (unpublished data).
8. Klein DC, Auerbach DA, Namboodiri MAA, Wheler GHT (1981) In: Reiter R, (ed) Pineal Gland: Anatomy and Biochemistry. CRC Press, Boca Raton, pp 199-228.

Endocrinology
F. Labrie, L. Proulx, eds.

IMPORTANCE OF DURATION OF THE NOCTURNAL INCREASE IN MELATONIN SECRETION IN DETERMINING THE REPRODUCTIVE RESPONSE TO PHOTOPERIOD

FRED J. KARSCH, NANCY L. WAYNE, AND ERIC L. BITTMAN
Reproductive Endocrinology Program, Department of Physiology, The University of Michigan, Ann Arbor, Michigan, 48109 (USA)

INTRODUCTION

Melatonin is a hormone which mediates the effects of daylength on seasonal reproduction in both long- and short-day breeding mammals (1-3). The pineal gland secretes this hormone in a circadian fashion and the properties of this rhythm are such that elevated secretion occurs only at night (1,2,4). In the ewe, pinealectomy abolishes the reproductive response to both stimulatory (short) and inhibitory (long) photoperiods; replacement of physiological melatonin patterns reinstates both of these responses (1-2). While the importance of the pineal and melatonin to seasonal reproduction in sheep are established, the specific feature of the melatonin pattern which encodes the photoperiodic message is not. Those characteristics which have been considered include amplitude, duration and time course of the elevated secretion at night, and the phase of this elevation relative to the 24-hour light-dark cycle (1,2,5-7). In this report, we summarize our studies to examine the importance of one feature of the melatonin pattern, the *duration* of the nighttime rise, in transmitting the photoperiodic message to the hypothalamo-hypophyseal axis of a short-day breeder, the female Suffolk sheep.

DURATION OF THE NIGHTTIME MELATONIN RISE

For this feature to be crucial, it must be strictly controlled by photoperiod. We have examined the nature of the melatonin pattern in 3 types of studies, each of which indicates that the period of increased melatonin secretion is essentially equivalent to the length of the night. *First*, at the day-night transitions, serum concentrations of melatonin rose rapidly within 15 minutes after lights off and then plummeted to baseline within 15 minutes of lights on (Fig. 1, data obtained on 14.5L:9.5D). *Second*, throughout the dark period, serum melatonin, although variable, remained greater than the low baseline observed during the day. Thus,

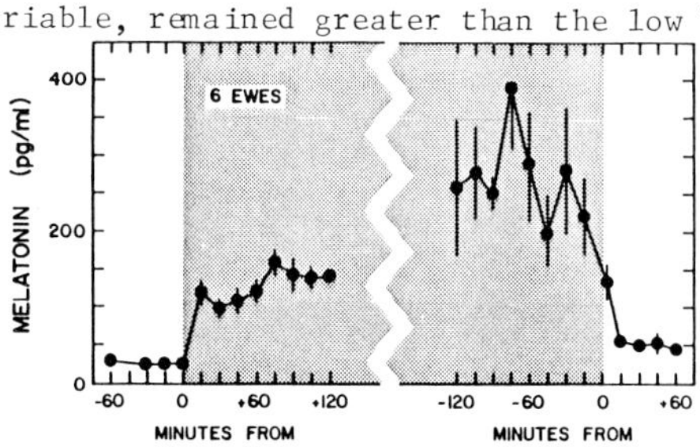

Fig. 1. Mean ± SEM serum melatonin concentration in 6 ewes sampled every 15 min for 3 hr at the day-night transitions during the same 24-hr period. Shaded area depicts dark phase of artificial light-dark cycle of 14.5L:9.5D. When no SEM is shown, it fell within the data point.

the duration of heightened melatonin secretion equalled that of darkness, at least for photoperiods as diverse as 8 and 16 hours of light/day (Fig. 2).

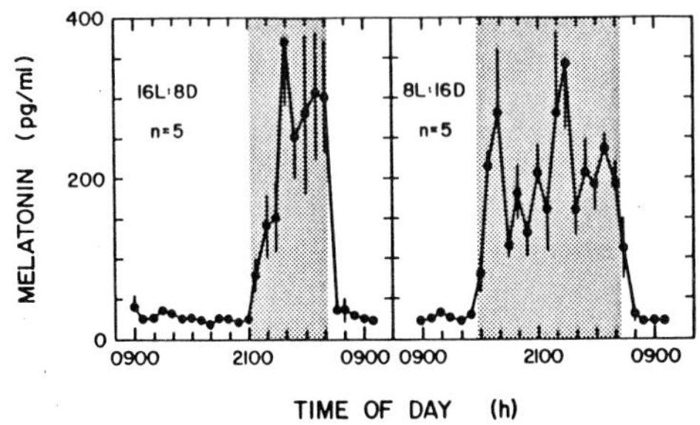

Fig. 2. Mean ± SEM serum melatonin concentration in samples obtained hourly from 5 ewes maintained in artificial inhibitory (16L:8D) or inductive (8L:16D) daylength. Shaded areas depict dark period. When no SEM is shown, it fell within the data point.

Third, during a series of stepwise changes in artificial photoperiod, the duration of elevated melatonin secretion matched the length of the night regardless of whether daylength was increasing or decreasing (Fig. 3). As the light cycle changes, therefore, the pattern of melatonin secretion seems to be largely independent of the *direction* of that change in daylength.

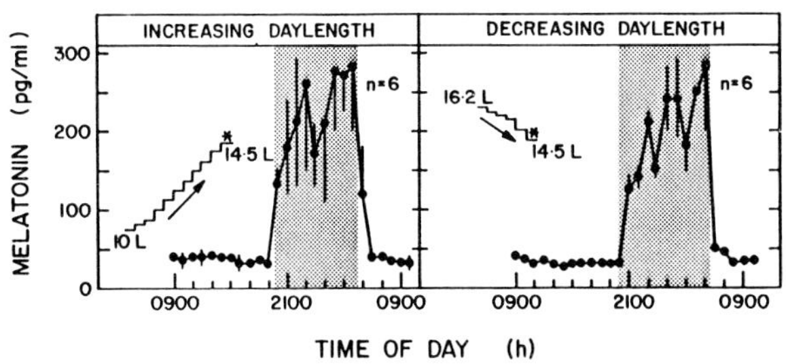

Fig. 3. Mean ± SEM serum melatonin level in 6 ewes in same artificial photoperiod of 14.5L:9.5D which was either increasing (left) or decreasing (right) by 15-30 min approximately every 2 weeks (arrows show nature and direction of change). Data obtained (asterisks) 10-14 days after last light shift. Further details in Fig. 2.

The above observations were made in ewes that were ovariectomized and treated with constant-release estradiol implants. This eliminated any variation in melatonin that may result from changes in endogenous ovarian steroids (8). Our results lead to the conclusion that daylength sets the duration of the nighttime melatonin rise in the Suffolk ewe, a conclusion consistent with the notion that duration determines the reproductive response to photoperiod in this short-day breeder.

REPRODUCTIVE RESPONSE TO EXOGENOUS MELATONIN

Our approach here has been to produce a physiological melatonin increment by its nightly infusion into pinealectomized ewes housed in artificial photoperiods. The duration of the melatonin increment either matched or mismatched the length of the night. Two types of mismatches were used, a long-day pattern of melatonin (8-hr infusion) in ewes maintained in short days and a short-day pattern of melatonin (16-hr infusion) in long days. Our rationale was as follows: If duration provides the code for photoperiod, the reproductive state generated by such melatonin infusions must be appropriate to the duration of the melatonin infusion, independent of the daylength. Reproductive state was assessed from the capacity of constant-release estradiol implants to inhibit tonic LH secretion in ovariectomized ewes. This photoperiodically sensitive marker of reproductive condition is known to mediate the photo-sexual response of the ewe (2,9).

In one such study, two groups of pinealectomized ewes were first reproductively suppressed by infusion of the long-day pattern of melatonin in long days. The ewes were then transferred to short days. At the time of this transfer, the duration of the nightly melatonin infusion in one group was switched to match the increased period of darkness; this stimulated reproductive induction (Fig. 4A, LH increased). In the other group (mismatch), the long-day pattern of melatonin was maintained following transfer to short days; this maintained reproductive arrest (Fig. 4B, LH remained low). In another mismatch experiment, two groups of pinealectomized ewes

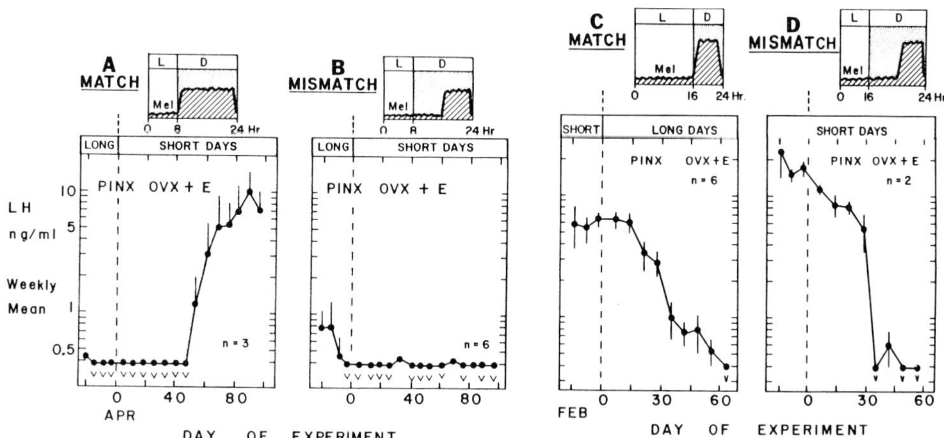

Fig. 4. Mean ± SEM serum LH concentrations in pinealectomized ovariectomized ewes bearing estradiol implants (PINX OVX + E) maintained in long or short days (16L:8D or 8L:16D, respectively) as indicated at top of big boxes. From day 0, the ewes received the nightly melatonin (MEL) treatments, depicted on top, which either matched (A,C) or mismatched (B,D) the photoperiod. Number of ewes given by n. Further details and control data in reference 10; from references 2 and 10.

were initially reproductively induced by infusion of a short-day pattern of melatonin in short days. In both groups, the duration of the melatonin infusion was switched to the long-day pattern. This precipitated reproductive suppression (fall in LH) whether the daylength was concurrently switched to long days (Fig. 4C) or whether it remained short (Fig. 4D).

In still another such experiment, the converse mismatch was used - a short-day pattern was infused under long days. Again the response was appropriate to the duration of the nightly melatonin infusion and LH increased (11). The salient finding of all these experiments is that the reproductive state invariably conformed to the length of time that melatonin was elevated in a 24-hour period.

CONCLUSION

Our description of the patterns of endogenous melatonin secretion and the responses to various patterns of exogenous melatonin provide a strong inference that the *duration* of the nighttime rise in circulating melatonin encodes the photoperiodic message which governs seasonal reproduction in the short-day breeding Suffolk ewe. Recent observations in the male Djungarian hamster demonstrate this feature of the melatonin rhythm is also crucial in that long-day breeder (3). It should be stressed, however, that our studies in sheep do not exclude a role for other aspects of the melatonin pattern. Of those alternatives which have been considered, the possible importance of phase of the melatonin rise relative to the 24-hour light-dark cycle is of special interest. Although evidence in the Djungarian hamster is inconsistent with a circadian phase of responsiveness to melatonin (3), observations in another long-day breeding rodent, the Syrian hamster, have been interpreted as demonstrating that phase is important (but the dose and pattern of melatonin provided in those studies were not shown to be physiological) (12). In current experiments, we are testing whether circadian rhythms contribute to the post-pineal processing of the photoperiodic message in the ewe, or whether the involvement of such rhythms is restricted to the generation of the circadian rhythm of melatonin secretion.

ACKNOWLEDGEMENTS

Supported by grants from NIH (HD-11311; HD-05914; HD-07048; HD-18337) and the Michigan Society of Fellows.

REFERENCES

1. Bittman EL (1984) In: Reiter RJ (ed) The Pineal Gland. Raven Press, New York, pp 155-192
2. Karsch FJ, Bittman EL, Foster DL, Goodman RL, Legan SJ, Robinson JE (1984) Rec Prog Horm Res 40:185-232
3. Carter DS, Goldman BD (1984) Endocrinology 113:1261-1267
4. Rollag MD, Niswender GD (1976) Endocrinology 98:482-489
5. Lincoln GA, Almeida OFX, Arendt J (1981) J Reprod Fert, Suppl 30:23-31
6. Arendt J, Symons AM, Laud C (1981) Experentia 37:584-586
7. Almeida OFX, Lincoln GA (1982) Biol Reprod 27:1062-1075
8. Arendt J, Laud CA, Symons AM, Pryde SJ (1983) J Reprod Fert 68:213-218
9. Legan SJ, Karsch FJ (1979) Biol Reprod 20:74-85
10. Bittman EL, Karsch FJ (1984) Biol Reprod 30:585-593
11. Yellon SM, Bittman EL, Robinson JE, Olster DH, Karsch FJ (1984) Abstr 76th Ann Mtng, Am Soc An Sci
12. Watson-Whitmyre M, Stetson MH (1983) Endocrinology 112:763-765

© 1984 Elsevier Science Publishers B.V.
Endocrinology
F. Labrie, L. Proulx, eds.

BIOLOGICALLY ACTIVE COMPOUNDS IN PINEALS AND RETINAS OF ANIMALS, EXPOSED TO DIFFERENT LIGHT CONDITIONS

I. EBELS[1] and G. CREMER-BARTELS[2]

1) Department of Organic Chemistry, State University of Utrecht, P.O. Box 5055, 3502 JB Utrecht, The Netherlands.

2) Eye Hospital of the Westphalian Wilhelms University, 4400 Münster (Westf.) Federal Republic of Germany

INTRODUCTION

Different biologically active compounds have been isolated, purified and identified from pineal glands in the last ten years. Besides the well-known melatonin, other methoxy- and hydroxyindoles were studied. Another group of compounds, the very light-sensitive pteridines were isolated and characterized, e.g. the natural cofactor for three aromatic amino acid mono-oxygenases: 6-L-erythrobiopterin (6-L-B). Reduced 6-L-B is very important for the biosynthesis of hydroxy- and methoxyindoles and catecholamines (1-4).

Cremer-Bartels (5) showed that a pteridine-like substance is present in mammalian retina (6). Cremer-Bartels et al. (7) were the first authors who showed that synthetic pteridines can influence the activity of retinal hydroxy-indole-O-methyltransferase (HIOMT). This last enzyme of melatonin biosynthesis occurs in the pineal gland and in the visual cells of the mammalian retina, but not however, in the photoreceptor outer segments (8).

Hudson and Menaker (9) stressed that: "the photoreceptors that supply environmental information to the mammalian circadian system are located within the eye, however the properties of these circadian "photoreceptors" differ markedly from the properties of those involved in vision".

In this paper a survey will be given of the influence of pteridines and partially purified, yet unknown, low molecular weight pineal and retinal compounds on the activity of HIOMT, isolated by a flat-bed gelectrophoresis technique.

MATERIALS AND METHODS

The methods and materials, which were used for the experiments described in this paper are described in detail by: Cremer Bartels (10), Cremer-Bartels and Ebels (11), Cremer-Bartels et al. (12), Ebels and Cremer-Bartels (13) and Cremer-Bartels et al. (14).

EXPERIMENTAL RESULTS

Cremer-Bartels et al.(7) were the first authors who demonstrated that synthetic pteridines affected the retinal HIOMT in dependence of the seasons.

Further experiments with partially purified pineal HIOMT confirmed that phenomenon (10,11). We did not understand at that time, why synthetic pteridines decreased HIOMT-activity significantly at low N-acetylserotonin (NAS) concentrations and increased that activity at higher NAS concentrations. HIOMT catalyzes the methylation of NAS; S-adenosyl-methionine (SAM) is the methyl-donor, which is converted into S-adenosyl-homocysteine (SAH). The latter is a potent inhibitor of HIOMT. So the enzyme is inhibited by one of the products formed during the reaction. Very recently Cremer-Bartels et al. (unpublished results) examined the effect of synthetic pteridines in dependence of different SAM-concentrations, on a highly purified HIOMT preparation, inhibited by SAH.

It was found in 5 independent experiments, that the addition of synthetic pteridines antagonized the inhibitory effect of SAH, as is illustrated in Fig. 1.

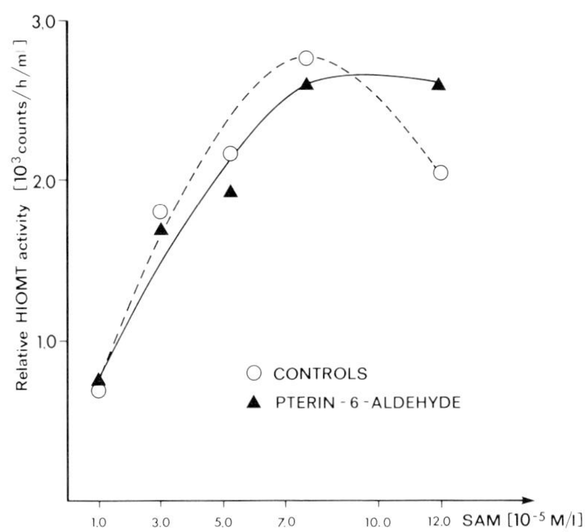

Fig. 1. Effect of pterin-6-aldehyde on SAH-inhibition of HIOMT-activity *in vitro*.

At high SAM-concentrations the addition of pteridines increased the HIOMT-activity. Therefore it is possible that the inhibition of high amounts of SAH, formed when higher concentrations of NAS are used, can be antagonized by pteridines. This effect may be a mechanism to stimulate melatonin biosynthesis. It may be that in different months of the year, the detection of HIOMT-activity is influenced by this mechanism.

Another compound, which can influence HIOMT activity is the synthetic peptide scotophobin, originally isolated from the brain of animals trained with shock to avoid the dark (15,16).

In the last years, it was tried to isolate and characterize the compound(s) in the ovine pineal ultrafiltration fraction UM05F (MW < 500), which influence(s) the activity of isolated HIOMT *in vitro*. This active ovine pineal fraction UM05F, separated on a Sephadex G-15 column, is eluted just before the high fluorescence peak, from which 6-L-B has been isolated and identified (3). When the active Sephadex G-15-fraction was re-filtrated on a Sephadex G-10 column, the activity was eluted in two fractions approximately in the same region as Cl^--ions, which indicates that the unknown HIOMT-suppressor(s) are not retarded on the Sephadex G-10. High performance liquid chromatography (HPLC) -experiments show that the main activity of one of those active fractions is located in one peak which shows an UV-absorbance at 210 nm. No other chemical characteristics could be specified so far. After HPLC-experiments of the other active Sephadex G-10-fraction, the activity, with a maximum UV absorption at 258 nm, was located approximately in the same region where synthetic SAH is eluted under the same experimental conditions.

Both active HPLC-fractions are unstable and loose their effect after some months, even if stored at -20°C in darkness.

DISCUSSION

In the experiments described above it was demonstrated that the biosynthesis of melatonin by HIOMT is a complicated mechanism. Not only NAS, SAH and SAM-concentrations probably influence the capacity of the retina and pineal in synthesizing melatonin, but the light-sensitive pteridines may also play an important role. It seems that pteridines are bound by preference to HIOMT, so that SAH cannot inhibit HIOMT-activity. That may be a mechanism to keep the melatonin biosynthesis going, especially in the dark period of the year. The experimental results point to a seasonal dependence of the effects of pteridines on HIOMT-activity (7). Not only pteridines but also low molecular weight retinal- and pineal compounds, which are yet unknonwn, can also influence HIOMT-activity *in vitro*, which makes the regulation of melatonin-biosynthesis more complicated. Therefore our first aim in future research will be to purify and characterize the above described natural HIOMT-suppressors, with the aim to obtain a better understanding about how pineal- and retinal compounds are involved in the regulation of melatonin biosynthesis. Afterwards, it has to be studied whether these, yet unknown, substances play a role in circadian- and seasonal rhythmicities.

REFERENCES

1. Ebels I, Benson B (1978) In: Reiter RJ (ed) The Pineal and Reproduction S Karger, Basel, pp 51-89.
2. Benson B, Ebels I (1981) In: Reiter RJ (ed) The Pineal Gland, Vol. II, CRC Press Inc., Boca Raton, Florida, pp 165-187.

3. Ebels I (1981) In: Oksche A, Pévet P (eds) The Pineal Organ. Elsevier/ North Holland, Amsterdam, pp 281-302.

4. Ebels I, Balemans MGM, Benthem J van, Noteborn HPJM, Morée A de (1983) In: Axelrod J, Fraschini F, Velo GP (eds) The Pineal Gland and its Endocrine Role. Plenum Press, pp 151-178.

5. Cremer-Bartels G (1962) v Graeves Archiv. Für Ophthalmologie 164:391-398

6. Cremer-Bartels G, Balazs EA (1973) Exp. Eye Res. 17:313-320.

7. Cremer-Bartels G, Hollwich F, Kotulla, W (1975) Klin. Mbl. Augenheilkunde 165:88-93.

8. Wiechmann AF, Bok D, Horwitz J (1984) Investigative Ophthalmology & Visual Sciene (Suppl) 25:242.

9. Hudson DJ, Menaker M (1984) Investigative Ophthalmology & Visual Science (Suppl) 25:242.

10. Cremer-Bartels G (1979) Progr. Brain Res. 52:231-239.

11. Cremer-Bartels G, Ebels I (1980) Proc. Natl. Acad. Sci. U.S.A. 77:2415-2418.

12. Cremer-Bartels G, Küchle HJ, Liedtmann W, Malten K (1981) In: Birau N, Schloot W (eds) Melatonin - Current Status and Perspectives. Pergamon Press, Oxford, New York, Toronto, Sidney, Paris, Frankfurt, pp 57-54.

13. Ebels I, Cremer-Bartels G (1982) Life Sciences 30:1369-1377.

14. Cremer-Bartels G, Ebels I, Sykes JEC, Morée A de (1983) J. Neural Transm. 58:107-119.

15. Satake N, Morton BE (1979) Pharm. Biochem. & Behav. 10:449-456.

16. Satake N, Morton BE (1979) Pharm. Biochem. & Behav. 10:457-462.

Endocrinology
F. Labrie, L. Proulx, eds.

REGULATION OF CIRCULATING MELATONIN AND N-ACETYLSEROTONIN

G.M. BROWN, A.K. HO, T.G. BURNS, L. HARVEY, L.J. GROTA* and J. SEGGIE
Department of Neurosciences, McMaster University, Hamilton, Ontario L8N 3Z5 (Canada) and *Department of Psychiatry, University of Rochester Medical Centre, Rochester, N.Y. 14642 (U.S.A.)

INTRODUCTION

In all species studied serum melatonin (MT) and pineal N-acetyltransferase (NATase) show a distinct circadian rhythm with higher night than day levels (1,2). In the synthesis of MT, serotonin in the pineal is acetylated to N-acetylserotonin (NAS) by the enzyme NATase (3) and NAS is further converted to MT by hydroxy-indole-O-methyltransferase (HIOMT) (4). NATase is particularly responsive to light showing a 15 to 70 fold increase in the dark phase (5) and displaying differences in its rhythm under different artificial and natural photoperiods (6). Because of this responsiveness to light it is generally assumed that the pineal and serum MT rhythms are a result of the rhythm in NATase activity.

Recent findings suggest that this assumption warrants re-examination. Dissociation of the serum rhythms of NAS and MT is observed under short photoperiods (7,8). Since NAS is the immediate product of NATase in the pineal, dissociation of MT and NAS in serum could indicate that alterations in pineal NATase may not always be associated with altered pineal and serum MT. Moreover there are conflicting reports on effects of long and short photoperiods on NATase. Illnerova and Vanacek (6) report that reducing hours of light alters the timing of elevated NATase activity while Shivers and Yochim (9) report no alterations. Furthermore, MT and the enzyme HIOMT are present in the retina and other tissues (10-14) and conceivably could give rise to serum MT and contribute to its rhythm.

Based on the above considerations the following questions were addressed. Does NATase reflect serum MT? Does pineal MT reflect serum MT? Does serum NAS reflect pineal NAS?

REGULATION OF CIRCULATING MELATONIN

In earlier studies we had shown that under a 12 h of light and 12 h of darkness (LD 12:12) photoperiod, rats fed ad libitum showed close parallelism between serum and pineal MT rhythms (15). Moore and Traynor (16) had shown that the pineal NATase rhythm was unaltered in rats given 1 hour access to water each morning and we had shown that the blood melatonin rhythm is also unaltered when rats were given 2 h access to food and water in the morning despite a change in the corticosterone rhythm (15).

In order to re-examine this issue, pineal NATase, pineal MT and serum MT were examined in rats exposed to four artificial light regimens: a) LD 16:8 for 2 weeks; b) LD 12:12 for 2 weeks; c) LD 4:20 for 2 weeks and d) LD 4:20 for 4 weeks. Under all conditions close parallelism of serum MT and pineal MT measured by radioimmunoassay (17) and pineal NATase rhythms was established. These findings support the idea that pineal NATase accurately represents melatonin synthesis and that rhythms of pineal and serum MT content are in phase under short and long photoperiods.

To examine the issue of possible extra pineal sources of circulating MT, we have examined serum MT in two groups of pinealectomized rats sacrificed at 4 h intervals after 3 and 7 weeks under LD 2:22. In both studies groups of pinealectomized rats had non-detectable serum MT at all times studied, while intact rats had measurable levels during the dark period (18). These findings are in accord with other studies showing virtual disappearance of serum MT in the pinealectomized rat (19) and support the concept that under these conditions serum MT is almost entirely derived from the pineal. Having reached this conclusion regarding serum MT the question of the factors regulating the serum NAS was unresolved.

RELATIONSHIP OF SERUM NAS TO SERUM AND PINEAL MELATONIN

There is evidence from studies of acute immobilization (20) and ether administration (21) that acute stimulation activates pineal NATase in the rat. We have performed studies comparing the serum corticosterone, melatonin and N-acetylserotonin responses to stimulation (22,23). Corticosterone and melatonin levels rose in response to three minutes of each of four different stimuli: ether, cold exposure, noise and novel environment. All stimuli led to a rise in melatonin by the end of the three minute stimulus and cold exposure produced a prolonged rise peaking at 30 min. NAS showed a prompt drop with stimulation, followed by a rebound to pre stimulus levels. As expected, the direction of NAS and MT responses differed. However, cold exposure did not have a more potent or prolonged effect on serum NAS as it did on MT and immobilization stress reduced both NAS and MT levels in the pineal (27). These findings provide additional evidence that serum MT and serum NAS are regulated separately. The mechanism underlying the transient drop in NAS is not known.

One possibility, that of increased conversion of circulating NAS to MT, is unlikely as levels of MT achieved following stimulation would be much higher than observed, given that serum NAS levels are approximately 200 fold higher than serum melatonin levels at rest. Another possibility, decreased output of NAS from the pineal into the blood is equally unlikely. Although melatonin in serum is essentially eliminated by pinealectomy, N-acetylserotonin levels are relatively unaffected (24). The latter observation has recently been confirmed in our laboratory (Harvey et al) using a more specific assay system (25). Thus the source of the majority of circulating NAS is not the pineal.

In earlier studies on regulation of serum NAS under altered photoperiodic conditions, a rhythm in NAS which was not correlated with the rhythm in serum MT was observed (7,8). As scheduled feeding is capable of cuing several rhythms including the corticosterone rhythm (15) we have examined the possibility that the serum NAS rhythm might also be regulated by time of feeding. Two groups of rats were studied on LD 14:10, one with access to food between 2 and 5 hours after lights on and the second with access between 2 and 5 hours after lights off (26). As expected, the serum corticosterone rhythm differed on the two feeding cycles. Pineal NATase, pineal MT, pineal NAS and serum MT all showed peaks during the dark phase under both feeding conditions and showed no evidence of synchronization by scheduled feeding. In contrast, the serum NAS rhythm was significantly influenced by scheduled feeding showing a rise in level just before as well as following feeding. Actual food intake was not necessary for the rise to occur. One group of animals, not fed on the day of study, showed a very similar rise at the expected time of feeding. These studies provide direct evidence that serum NAS is regulated independently of pineal NAS. Moreover, the serum NAS rhythm, like the serum corticosterone rhythm, is influenced by the time of feeding.

CONCLUSION

These studies provide evidence that under a wide variety of photoperiodic conditions, rat pineal and serum MT rhythms are a result of the pineal NATase rhythm, and that the photoperiod is the critical determinant of these rhythms. In contrast, the serum NAS rhythm is not rigidly coupled to the photoperiod and can be influenced to a marked extent by the time of feeding. The majority of serum NAS does not originate in the pineal but possibly from a wide variety of other tissues, including retina, Harderian gland, brain and liver, which were known to contain NATase. The source(s) of circulating NAS and its possible role(s) in physiologic function are currently unknown.

REFERENCES

1. Brown GM, Niles LP (1982) In: Martini L, Besser GM (eds) Clinical Neuroendocrinology, Vol 2, Academic Press, New York, pp 205-264.
2. Klein DC (1979) In: Krieger DC (ed) Endocrine Rhythms. Raven Press, New York, pp 203-223.
3. Weissbach H, Redfield BG, Axelrod J (1960) Biochem Biophys Acta 43: 352-353.

4. Axelrod J, Weissbach H (1960) Science 131:1312.
5. Klein DC, Weller JL (1972) Science 177:532-326.
6. Illnerova H, Vanacek J (1980) Neuroendocrinology 31:321-326.
7. Grota LJ, Brown GM, Pang SF (1981) Abstracts, Soc Neurosc 7:717.
8. Brown GM, Grota LJ, Harvey L, Tsui HW and Pang SF (1983) In: Axelrod J, Fraschini F, Vels GP (eds) The Pineal Gland and its Endocrine Role. Plenum Press, New York, pp 257-276.
9. Shivers BD, Yochim JM (1979) Biol Reprod 21:385-392.
10. Bubenik GA, Brown GM, Grota LJ (1976) Brain Res 118:417-427.
11. Bubenik GA, Brown GM, Grota LJ (1976) J Histochem & Cytochem 2411:1173-1177.
12. Bubenik GA, Brown GM, Grota LJ (1977) Experientia 33:662-663.
13. Gern WA, Ralph CL (1979) Science 104:183-184.
14. Cardinali DP, Rosner JM (1971) Endocrinology 89:301-303.
15. Holloway WR, Tsui HW, Grota LJ, Brown GM (1979) Life Sci 25:1837-1842.
16. Moore RY, Traynor ME (1976) Neuroendocrinology 20:250-259.
17. Grota LJ, Snieckus V, deSilva SO, Tsui HW, Holloway WR, Lewy AJ, Brown GM (1981) Progress in Neuro-Psychopharmacol 5:523-526.
18. Brown GM, Grota LJ, Pulido O, Burns TG, Niles LP, Snieckus V (1983) In: Reiter RJ (ed) Pineal Research Reviews 1, Alan R. Liss, New York, pp 207-246.
19. Lewy AJ, Tetsuo M, Markey SP, Goodwin FK, Kopin I (1980) J Clin Endocrinol Metab 50:204-205.
20. Lynch HJ, Ho M, Wurtman RJ (1977) J Neural Transmission 40:87.
21. Vaughan GM, Allen JP, Tussil W, Sackman JW, Vaughan MK (1978) Neuroscience Letter 9:83.
22. Seggie J, Brown GM, Campbell L, Grota LJ (1982) Abstracts Soc Neurosc 8:550.
23. Seggie J, Brown GM, Grota LJ (1983) Clin Invest Med 6:45.
24. Yu HS, Pang SF, Tang PL, Brown GM (1981) Neuroendocrinology 32:262-265.
25. Pang SF, Brown GM, Campbell L, Snieckus V, deSilva S, Young S, Grota LJ (1981) J Immunoassay 2:263.
26. Ho AK, Burns TG, Grota LJ and Brown GM (1983) Abstracts Soc Neuroscience 9:1074.
27. Yocca F, Friedman EJ (1984) Neurochemistry 42:1427.

6. Adrenergic Receptors

Endocrinology
F. Labrie, L. Proulx, eds.

BIOCHEMICAL CHARACTERIZATION OF THE ADRENERGIC RECEPTORS: PURIFICATION, AFFINITY LABELLING AND RECONSTITUTION STUDIES

MARC G. CARON, RICHARD A. CERIONE, L.M. FREDRIK LEEB-LUNDBERG, JEFFREY L. BENOVIC, JOHN W. REGAN, KENNETH E.J. DICKINSON, SARAH L. HEALD and ROBERT J. LEFKOWITZ
Howard Hughes Medical Institute, Depts. of Physiology, Medicine and Biochemistry, Duke University Medical Center, Durham, North Carolina 27710 U.S.A.

INTRODUCTION

Catecholamines mediate their diverse physiological effects by initially interacting with specific membrane-bound receptors on their target tissues. Both β_1- and β_2-adrenergic effects are mediated via activation of the enzyme adenylate cyclase (AC) whereas the response to α_2-adrenergic agonists is translated via an inhibition of AC. Catecholamine responses of α_1-adrenergic specificity are brought about by a different biochemical signal transfer mechanism, i.e. rapid turnover of membrane phospholipids and mobilization of calcium.

Because of their ubiquity and clinical relevance catecholamine receptors have been used as models to understand the biochemical mechanisms of signal transduction across the plasma membrane. Toward this end we have used two main approaches in an attempt to characterize these various catecholamine receptors. The development of specific probes (1-3) to label the ligand binding site of these receptors as well as affinity chromatography supports for each of these receptors (4-5) has provided insights into the molecular properties of these proteins. For the β-adrenergic receptor (βAR), the availability of the purified receptor protein has allowed the functional reconstitution of the interactions of the receptor with the other components of the system, the pure guanine nucleotide binding protein (N_s) (6) and the resolved AC (7). The results of these studies will be briefly summarized below.

AFFINITY AND PHOTOAFFINITY LABELLING OF THE ADRENERGIC RECEPTORS

Irreversible probes designed to identify the ligand binding subunit of the βAR and α_1AR have been developed (1,2). These ligands display a high degree of selectivity and specificity. They bind to these receptors with high affinity and can be radioactively labelled with a high specific activity radionuclide such as iodine. These probes, which are photosensitive, are far superior in their selectivity to simple affinity probes because of the ease with which their reactivity can be controlled.

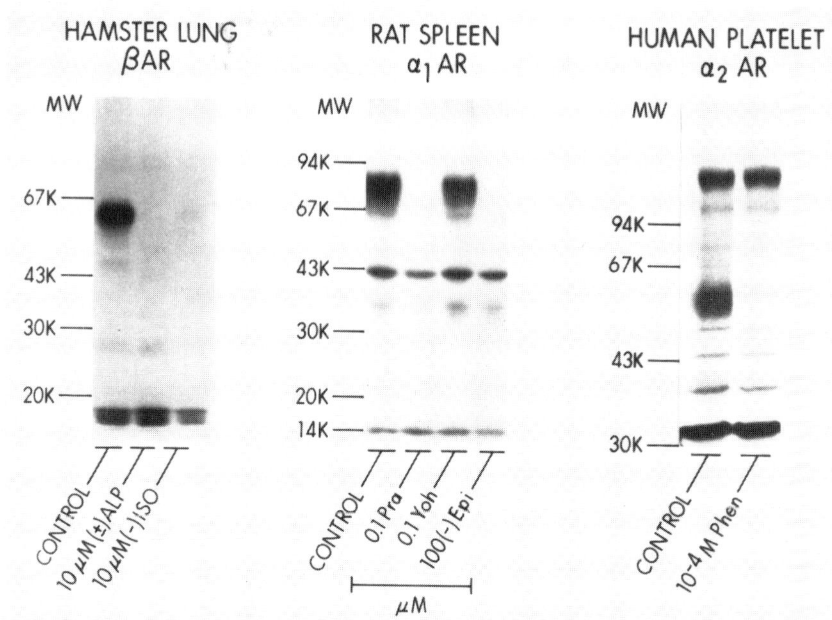

Fig. 1. Identification of the binding subunit of the various AR subtypes by affinity and photoaffinity labelling. (A) Labelling of hamster lung membranes with the β-adrenergic photoaffinity probe [^{125}I]p-azidobenzylcarazolol. (B) Labelling of rat spleen membranes with the α_1 selective photoaffinity probe [^{125}I]APDQ (taken from Leeb-Lundberg et al., 1984 (2)). (C) Affinity labelling of partially purified α_2AR preparation with [^{3}H]phenoxybenzamine (taken from Regan et al., 1984 (3)).

Fig. 1A represents an autoradiogram of an SDS-PAGE of hamster lung membranes labelled with the β-adrenergic probe [^{125}I]p-azidobenzylcarazolol. A single peptide of M_r = 64,000 is revealed and the incorporation of the probe can be blocked with an appropriate β-adrenergic specificity. Other studies from our laboratories have shown that although β_1 and β_2 receptors appear to reside on peptides of similar size (M_r 62-64,000) these peptides are probably distinct proteins as evidenced by distinct peptide maps (8). Fig. 1B shows the incorporation of the photoaffinity probe [^{125}I]APDQ, an analog of the α_1 antagonist prazosin, into plasma membranes derived from rat spleen, a tissue which contains α_1AR (2). An M_r = 80,000 peptide is evidenced with appropriate α_1-adrenergic specificity. Fig. 1C shows that in a partially purified preparation of α_2AR obtained by affinity chromatography (5) of a solubilized preparation of human platelet membranes, [^{3}H]phenoxybenzamine specifically labels a peptide of M_r = 61,000. To date, no specific photoaffinity probe is yet available for the α_2AR. Thus, the various receptors for adrenergic catecholamines appear to reside on distinct polypeptides.

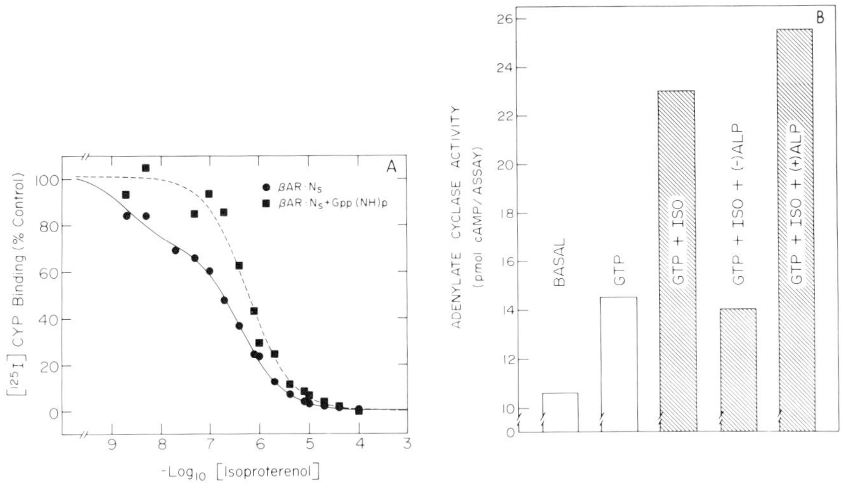

Fig. 2. Reconstitution of the interactions of the resolved components of an AC system. (A) Isoproterenol competition curve for the binding of [^{125}I]cyano-pindolol to phospholipid vesicles containing pure guinea pig lung βAR and pure human erythrocyte N_s (taken from Cerione et al., 1984 (6)). (B) AC activity in phospholipid vesicles containing in addition to βAR and N_s as in (A) a resolved AC catalytic subunit from caudate nucleus (taken from Cerione et al., 1984 (7)).

THE PURE β-ADRENERGIC RECEPTOR: FUNCTIONAL RECONSTITUTION OF ITS INTERACTIONS

The βAR has been purified to apparent homogeneity from several sources (reviewed in 9,10) using a combination of affinity and size exclusion chromatography. In every tissue from which the βAR has been isolated the same peptide which was evidenced by photoaffinity labelling could be isolated and shown to bind ligands with an appropriate β-adrenergic specificity (9,10). Other components of the hormone responsive AC system have also been characterized. The guanine nucleotide binding protein (N_s) has been isolated in pure form and is a heterotrimer of M_r 45,000 (α subunit); 35,000 (β subunit) and 5-10,000 (γ subunit) (11). The AC moiety on the other hand has not been completely purified yet. However, the AC from bovine caudate nucleus can be resolved from N_s by a chromatographic procedure (12). The availability of these isolated components makes it possible to study their interactions in a well defined environment. AC coupled-receptors perform several functions which can be demonstrated using isolated components reinserted into an artificial lipid milieu. As shown in Fig. 2A, when pure βAR and pure N_s are reconstituted into phospholipid vesicles, a guanine nucleotide sensitive high affinity state of the receptor for the agonist isoproterenol can be established (6).

The interactions of βAR with N_s can also be monitored by an increased guanine nucleotide binding to N_s or the establishment of a GTPase activity in the N_s protein (6,13). As shown in Fig. 2B when all the components of the system, βAR, N_s and AC (resolved from caudate nucleus) are incorporated into the phospholipid vesicles, a β-adrenergic stimulation of the enzyme which is specifically blocked by antagonists can be established (7). Under these experimental conditions the GTPase elicited by the interaction of βAR and N_s is not further increased upon interaction with the catalytic moiety of AC (data not shown) (7).

Thus, these results indicate that the isolated βAR peptide carries all of the expected functions of an AC coupled-receptor: binding of ligands; interaction with N_s and ability to mediate a β-adrenergic stimulation of AC. Moreover, these data indicate that the GTPase activity of the N_s protein which presumably serves as the turnoff mechanism for AC activation does not depend upon the interaction of AC with N_s as had been commonly assumed, but rather results from the interaction of βAR with N_s. Presumably the turnover of the GTPase activity is slow enough (0.5-2.0 min.$^{-1}$) to allow efficient interaction of N_s with and activation of AC. Examination of the interactions of these various isolated components at the molecular level will undoubtedly lead to the ultimate understanding of this class of mechanism of signal transfer through biological membranes.

REFERENCES

1. Lavin TN, Nambi P, Heald SL, Jeffs PW, Lefkowitz RJ, Caron MG (1982) J Biol Chem 257:12332-12340
2. Leeb-Lundberg LMF, Dickinson KEJ, Heald SL, Wikberg JES, Hagen P-O, DeBernardis JF, Winn M, Arendsen DL, Lefkowitz RJ, Caron MG (1984) J Biol Chem 259:2579-2587
3. Regan JW, DeMarinis RM, Caron MG, Lefkowitz RJ (1984) J Biol Chem, 259:7864-7869
4. Caron MG, Srinivasan Y, Pitha J, Kociolek K, Lefkowitz RJ (1979) J Biol Chem 254:2923-2927
5. Regan JW, Barden N, Lefkowitz RJ, Caron MG, DeMarinis RM, Krog AJ, Holden KJ, Matthews WD, Hieble JP (1982) Proc Natl Acad Sci USA 79:7223-7227
6. Cerione RA, Codina J, Benovic JL, Lefkowitz RJ, Birnbaumer L, Caron MG (1984) Biochemistry, in press
7. Cerione RA, Sibley DR, Benovic JL, Caron MG, Lefkowitz RJ, Winslow J, Neer, EJ, Codina J, Birnbaumer L (1984) J Biol Chem, in press.
8. Stiles GL, Strasser RH, Caron MG, Lefkowitz RJ (1983) J Biol Chem 258:10689-10694
9. Lefkowitz RJ, Stadel JM, Caron MG (1983) Annu Rev Biochem 52:159-186
10. Benovic JL, Shorr RGL, Caron MG, Lefkowitz RJ (1984) Biochemistry, in press
11. Codina J, Hildebrandt JD, Sekura RD, Birnbaumer M, Bryan J, Manclark CR, Iyengar R, Birnbaumer L (1984) J Biol Chem 259:5871-5886
12. Strittmatter S, Neer EJ (1980) Proc Natl Acad Sci USA 77:6344-6348
13. Brandt DR, Asano T, Pedersen SE, Ross EM (1983) Biochemistry 22:4357-4362

Endocrinology
F. Labrie, L. Proulx, eds.

ROLE OF N PROTEIN IN COUPLING OF ADRENERGIC RECEPTORS AND ADENYLATE CYCLASE

MICHIO UI, TOSHIAKI KATADA, TOSHIHIKO MURAYAMA and HITOSHI KUROSE

Department of Physiological Chemistry, Faculty of Pharmaceutical Sciences, Hokkaido University, Sapporo (Japan)

INTRODUCTION

Adrenergic receptors are classified into four subtypes of α_1, α_2, β_1 and β_2. α_1-Adrenergic receptors are not, but other subtypes are, linked to adenylate cyclase. The linkage of the receptors (R) to the adenylate cyclase catalytic protein (C) is mediated by the guanine nucleotide regulatory protein which is usually termed N, G or G/F. Stimulation of β_1- or β_2-receptors leads to activation of C via a kind of N (N_s), while α_2-receptors are coupled to C in an inhibitory fashion via another kind of N (N_i). N_s mediates β-receptor-induced adenylate cyclase activation as follows. In the absence of agonists (A), GDP is bound to N_s which exists in the plasma membrane in a state separated from R and C. Occupation of R by A leads to formation of a ternary complex, A-R-N_s, on which GDP is replaced by GTP. The GTP-bound N_s is an active form (and hence the GTP-GDP exchange is a "turnon" reaction) in the sense that it activates C after dissociation from R. Simultaneously, A is dissociated from R, since the affinity of A for R is lower than for R-N_s. Activation of C continues until GTP is hydrolyzed to GDP on N_s as a "turnoff" reaction. Cholera toxin has contributed to the current knowledge about the N_s/R coupling mechanism, since it is a specific modifier of N_s.

The other bacterial toxin produced by *Bordetella pertussis* is a promising probe for N_i studies (1). The pertussis toxin was termed by Ui an islet-activating protein (IAP), since he first found that exposure of rat pancreatic islets to the toxin resulted in reversal of α_2-adrenergic inhibition of insulin secretion from the islets. Further studies from his laboratory have revealed that IAP interacts with a variety of other cell types; receptor-mediated inhibitions of membrane adenylate cyclase (or decreases in the cellular content of cAMP) were abolished by prior treatment of these cells with a low concentration of IAP (2-8). IAP is an A-B toxin composed of an A-protomer and a B-oligomer. The A-protomer is inserted into the plasma membrane as a result of binding of the B-oligomer moiety to a particular site on the cell surface (9). Inside the membrane, the sulfhydryl bonds in the molecule of the A-protomer are reduced to afford its active form, an ADP-ribosyltransferase (10) the specific substrate of which is the membrane M_r= 41,000 protein (11). This IAP substrate is the GTP-binding subunit of N_i (12). The mechanism whereby IAP-sensitive N_i mediates R-linked inhibition of C is very similar to the above-mentioned mechanism for N_s-mediated activation as will be shown below.

AGONIST-INDUCED GTP-GDP EXCHANGE DIFFERENTIALLY OCCURRING ON N_s AND N_i

Membranes from rat adipocytes were first labeled with [^{3}H]GTP in the presence of isoproterenol. The labeled membranes were then washed with the medium containing a β-adrenergic antagonist and GTP for the purpose of cessation of the β-receptor-induced activation of N_s and minimizing non-specific radioactivity labeling. [^{3}H]GTP bound to N_s was hydrolyzed to [^{3}H]GDP during this washing procedure and then released in response to the second addition of isoproterenol and GTP (or Gpp(NH)p). [^{3}H]GDP release was promoted not only by isoproterenol but also by agonists (e.g., glucagon and secretin) of other receptors that stimulate adenylate cyclase in the same membranes. No [^{3}H]GDP release occurred in response to these agonists, however, unless the medium for the final release assay contained GTP (or Gpp(NH)p), indicating that it reflected the GTP-GDP exchange reaction occurring on R-coupled N_s. Thus, a common pool of N_s is linked to multiple receptors (R_a) that are involved in adenylate cyclase activation in rat adipocyte membranes (13).

Membranes that had been labeled with [^{3}H]GTP in the presence of isoproterenol was exposed to the active component of cholera toxin and NAD during the next washing procedure. [^{3}H]GDP was released from these toxin-treated membranes spontaneously but slowly, in exchange for added GTP, even without addition of receptor agonists to the release assay medium. The toxin was without effect unless NAD was simultaneously added, indicating that ADP-ribosylation was involved. Thus, no receptor stimulation is needed for GTP to displace GDP from the N_s that has been ADP-ribosylated by cholera toxin; N_s is stabilized in its active state by the toxin. In sharp contrast, exposure of the similarly labeled membranes to the preactivated A-protomer of IAP and NAD failed to induce spontaneous release of [^{3}H]GDP under the same conditions. Nor was the agonist-induced [^{3}H]GDP release altered by the IAP treatment; IAP does not interact with N_s (13).

There are α_2-adrenergic receptors, in addition to β_1-receptors, in hamster adipocyte membranes. Membrane adenylate cyclase is inhibited via α_2-receptors in a GTP-dependent manner. When the hamster adipocyte membranes were labeled with [^{3}H]GTP in the presence of a β-agonist, the subsequent release of [^{3}H]GDP in exchange for newly added GTP was promoted by β-agonists but was not by α-agonists or the agonists (e.g., prostaglandin E_1 and nicotinic acid) of other receptors involved in cyclase inhibition. In another series of experiments in which α_2-receptors, rather than β-receptors, were stimulated during the first [^{3}H]GTP labeling of membranes, much more [^{3}H]GDP was subsequently released from these membranes when an α-agonist was again added than when a β-agonist was added to the release assay medium. Prostaglandin E_1 or nicotinic acid was also effective in releasing [^{3}H]-GDP from these membranes. Thus, a common pool of N_i is coupled to multiple receptors (R_i) that are involved in the inhibition of adenylate cyclase and are not linked to β-receptors in membranes (13).

Hamster adipocyte membranes labeled with [^{3}H]GTP in the presence of an α-agonist were then exposed to the A-protomer of IAP and NAD during the washing procedure for 3 min. Essentially no [^{3}H]GDP was subsequently released in response to α-agonists or prostaglandin E_1 from these IAP-treated membranes. The membrane M_r=41,000 protein was ADP-ribosylated during the IAP treatment. When IAP was replaced by cholera toxin, however, there was no interference with the action of α-agonists or prostaglandin E_1 to promote [^{3}H]GDP release. Neither IAP nor cholera toxin provoked spontaneous [^{3}H]GDP release from the membranes labeled with [^{3}H]GTP via α_2-adrenergic stimulation. Thus, N_i is uncoupled from R_i after IAP-catalyzed ADP-ribosylation of its α-subunit with M_r=41,000.

AFFINITY FOR AGONIST BINDING TO RECEPTORS AS AN INDEX OF N/R COUPLING

If N_i is coupled to R_i in a fashion similar to the above-mentioned N_s/R_a coupling (see INTRODUCTION), GTP or its analogue will lower the affinity of agonists for R_i as a result of conversion of A-R_i-N_i to A-R_i. Such was actually the case; α-adrenergic (norepinephrine), muscarinic (carbachol) and opiate (morphine) receptor agonists were bound to NG108-15 cell membranes with lower affinities in the presence of Gpp(NH)p than in its absence (6). These binding experiments were repeated with membranes from IAP-treated cells. The affinities of norepinephrine, carbachol and morphine for the respective receptors in the IAP-treated cell membranes were one-order of magnitude lower than their affinities for the control (non-treated) membranes in the absence of Gpp(NH)p. The affinities were not further

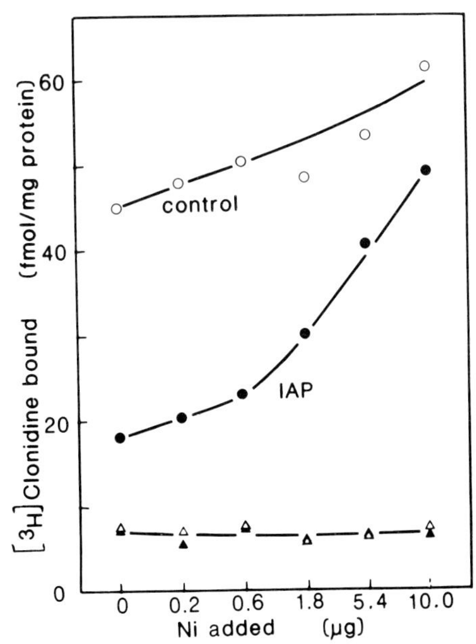

Fig. 1. IAP-induced inhibition of agonist binding to α_2-adrenergic receptors and its reversal by N_i. NG108-15 cell membranes were incubated with 1 mM NAD in the presence (●,▲) or absence (○,△) of 20 μg/ml of the preactivated A-protomer of IAP. These membranes (2 mg of protein/200 μl) were first incubated at 30°C for 10 min with N_i in the amount indicated. N_i used were purified from rat brain by the method of Katada and Ui (unpublished). Specific binding of an agonist to α_2-receptors was then measured with 4 nM [^{3}H]clonidine in the presence (△,▲) or absence (○, ●) of 100 μM GTPγS.

reduced by the addition of the GTP analogue to the IAP-treated cell membranes (6). Thus, no association product is formed between N_i and R_i, when N_i has been ADP-ribosylated by IAP.

In order to comfirm the participation of N_i in the increase in the affinity of agonists for α_2-adrenergic receptors, we have tried to insert purified N_i to IAP-treated membranes as shown in Fig. 1. Membranes from NG108-15 cells were incubated with $[^3H]$clonidine, an α_2-agonist, at a concentration as low as 4 nM. The amount of the agonist bound to membranes was smaller in IAP-treated membranes than in control membranes in the absence of GTPγS due to the agonist's lower affinity for receptors. The addition of increasing amounts of N_i to the membrane preparation resulted in progressive increases in the amount of the agonist bound. The increase was greater in IAP-treated membranes than in control membranes; IAP-induced inhibition of binding was mostly reversed by the addition of 10 μg of N_i. The agonist binding in the presence of GTPγS, however, was very small and was not altered by IAP treatment or by the addition of N_i.

These results in Fig. 1 clearly indicate that N_i increases the affinity of agonists for α_2-adrenergic receptors as a result of the formation of the ternary complex (A-R_i-N_i) and that no ternary complex is formed either when the GTP analogue exchanges for GDP on N_i or when N_i is ADP-ribosylated by IAP. Thus, N_i is coupled to R_i in a manner very similar to N_s/R_a coupling, and IAP-catalyzed ADP-ribosylation of N_i blocks the signal transduction from α_2-adrenergic (or other inhibitory) receptors to adenylate cyclase.

REFERENCES

1. Ui M (1984) Trend Pharmacol Sci 5: in press
2. Katada T, Ui M (1979) J Biol Chem 254: 469-479
3. Katada T, Ui M (1980) J Biol Chem 255: 9580-9588
4. Hazeki O, Ui M (1981) J Biol Chem 256: 2856-2862
5. Katada T, Ui M (1981) J Biol Chem 256: 8310-8317
6. Kurose H, Katada T, Amano T, Ui M (1983) J Biol Chem 258: 4870-4875
7. Murayama T, Ui M (1983) J Biol Chem 258: 3319-3326
8. Murayama T, Katada T, Ui M (1983) Arch Biochem Biophys 221: 381-390
9. Tamura M, Nogimori K, Yajima M, Ase K, Ui M (1983) J Biol Chem 258: 6756-6761
10. Katada T, Tamura M, Ui M (1983) Arch Biochem Biophy 224: 290-298
11. Katada T, Ui M (1982) Proc Natl Acad Sci USA 79: 3129-3133
12. Katada T, Ui M (1982) J Biol Chem 257: 7210-7216
13. Murayama T, Ui M (1984) J Biol Chem 259: 761-769

Endocrinology
F. Labrie, L. Proulx, eds.

THYROID HORMONES: REGULATORS OF ALPHA- AND BETA-ADRENERGIC RESPONSES

CRAIG C. MALBON, ANA CUBERO, MICHAEL GRAZIANO, TOM MANGANO, AND CARY MOXHAM

Dept.Pharmacological Sciences, Health Sciences Center, The State University of New York at Stony Brook, Stony Brook, New York 11794 USA

Thyroid hormones modulate the responsiveness of many tissues to the actions of catecholamine hormones. The signs and symptoms of hyperthyroidism and hypothyroidism in man graphically illustrate the ability of thyroid hormones to regulate adrenergic sensitivity. Research during the past 5 years has focused on elucidating the biochemical basis for the changes in catecholamine responsiveness observed in altered thyroid states(for reviews see Refs.1,2). The catecholamine-sensitive adenylate cyclase system provides a useful model for such studies. In spite of many recent advances in the biochemical description of the hormone-sensitive adenylate cyclase system, the question of how thyroid hormones exert their "permissive" effects on alpha- and beta-adrenergic hormone action remains unanswered.

Heart, liver and fat tissue have proven to be useful models for the investigation of the interactions between thyroid hormones and beta-adrenergic catecholamines (1,2). In heart and fat tissue, hyperthyroidism potentiates, while hypothyroidism impairs, beta-adrenergic sensitivity. The amount of beta-adrenergic receptor (R) in heart has been shown to increase in the hyperthyroid state and decrease in the hypothyroid state. In liver, unlike the situation in the heart, hypothyroidism potentiates rather than impairs beta-adrenergic sensitivity. The steady-state number of R increases 3-fold in hepatocytes from the hypothyroid rat. These models demonstrate that the expression of the permissive effects of thyroid hormones on adrenergic action can vary considerably from one tissue to another. Regulation of receptor number appears to be at least one mode by which thyroid hormones modulate beta-adrenergic sensitivity. How thyroid hormones modulate R number remains to be established.

Thyroid hormones regulate beta-adrenergic sensitivity in rat fat cells without altering beta-adrenergic receptor number (1,2). Current information suggests that the catecholamine-responsive adenylate cyclase system is composed of at least three separable units: the beta-receptor (R), a guanine nucleotide-binding stimulatory regulatory component (Ns), and a catalytic moiety (C) (3). In order to investigate the basis for the impaired activation of adenylate cyclase by beta-agonists in the hypothyroid rat fat cell, a strategy designed to probe each of these components was developed. The nature and abundance of R, Ns, and C in the fat cell were investigated with a variety of probes and were found to be largely unaltered in the hypothyroid state. The plant diterpene forskolin activates C in cells and membranes (4). The activity of C in both intact fat cells and membranes prepared from these cells was not altered by hypothyroidism (5). Ns can be covalently radiolabeled in the presence of cholera toxin and (32P)NAD+ or assayed for function via reconstitution with membranes from S49 mouse lymphoma _cyc_- mutant cells which lack functional Ns (3). The major substrate for cholera toxin-catalyzed ADP-ribosylation in fat cell membranes from euthyroid and hypothyroid rats is the 42,000-Mr, alpha-subunit of Ns. The amount of label incorporated into the alpha-subunit of Ns by the toxin and the amount of Ns activity assayed in the _cyc_- reconstitution system are equivalent in euthyroid and hypothyroid states (6). Analysis of R in the hypothyroid state reveals no change in the character (beta-1), abundance, or affinity for beta-antagonists of R from hypothyroid rat fat cells (7).

The observation that hypothyroid rat fat cell R does not display an agonist-specific shift in affinity in the presence of guanine nucleotides (8) focused our attentions on R-Ns interactions. Recent studies reveal that the R of the hypothyroid rat fat cell interacts ineffectively with Ns and that implanting R from euthyroid rat fat cells, liver cells, or S49 _cyc_- cells into hypothyroid rat fat cells reconstitutes the beta-adrenergic responsiveness of the cells (6). The reconstitution is blocked by prior treatment of the donor R with a beta-adrenergic antagonist covalent affinity label(6).

Definition of the mechanisms responsible for thyroid hormone regulation of receptor number (as observed in heart and liver) and receptor function (as observed in fat) will require the development of new strategies and probes. Structural studies may elucidate the basis for the impaired function of R from the hypothyroid rat fat cell. We have purified R from rat fat cells to apparent homogeneity and determined that it is a 67,000-Mr peptide (lane 1, Fig.1 and Ref. 9). R of hypothyroid rat fat cells has also been purified (10) and it appears to be very similar to its euthyroid counterpart (lane 2, Fig.1). Peptide mapping and isoelectric focusing of R from hypothyroid rat fat cells may reveal a structural basis for its altered ability to interact with Ns. Antibodies specific for R should provide the immunochemical means with which to study the dynamics of R metabolism in heart, liver, and fat cells. We have succeeded in raising antibodies against fat cell R using hybridoma technology (11). Whether or not these monoclonal antibodies will prove useful in our investigations of the mechanisms responsible for thyroid hormone regulation of

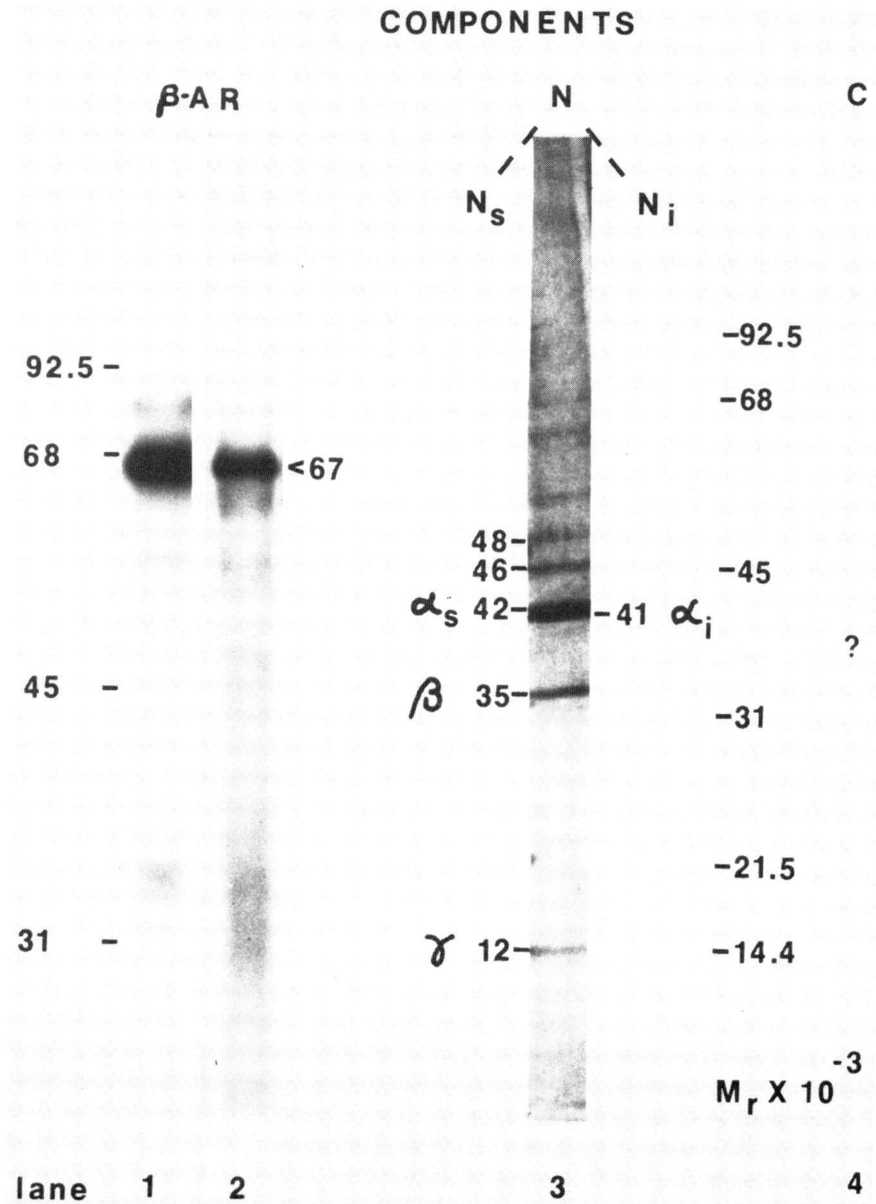

Fig. 1 Structural studies of the components of β-adrenergic sensitive-adenylate cyclase systems. Autoradiogram of SDS-PAGE of purified, iodinated fat cell R from euthyroid (lane 1) and hypothyroid (lane 2) rats. Silver-stained SDS-PAGE of purified N proteins of rabbit heart (lane 3).

R number and function remains to be established.

Thyroid hormones appear to regulate the activity of the guanine nucleotide-binding inhibitory regulatory component of adenylate cyclase (Ni) in fat cells of the rat (12). The effects of thyroid status on alpha-adrenergic responses are unclear. Since alpha-2 receptors appear to act via Ni the data from the fat cell system again underscore the need to examine each of the components of the system when evaluating the influence of thyroid hormones on adrenergic responses. In order to pursue a more comprehensive approach to these questions we have purified Ns and Ni from rabbit heart (lane 3, Fig. 1) and are currently raising antibodies against the alpha subunits of Ns (42,000-Mr) and Ni (41,000-Mr) and the beta- (35,000-Mr) and gamma(12,000-Mr)subunits common to Ns and Ni. These antibodies should prove valuable as probes of N protein structure and metabolism and of the influence of thyroid hormones on these parameters. Difficulties associated with the purification of C has limited progress in the biochemical characterization of this component of the system. It seems likely that exciting new information as to the mechanisms responsible for thyroid hormone regulation of adrenergic hormone action is just on the horizon.

ACKNOWLEDGEMENTS

This work was supported by USPHS grants AM25410, AM 30111, K04-AM00786 from the NIH.

REFERENCES

1. Kunos, G (1981) In: Kunos G (ed) Adrenoceptors and Catecholamine Action, Part A. Wiley, New York, pp 297-334
2. Stiles GL, Caron MG, Lefkowitz RJ (1984) Physiol Rev 64:661-743
3. Ross EM, Gilman AG (1980) Annu Rev Biochem 49:533-564
4. Seamon KB, Daly JW (1981) J Cyclic Nucleotide Res 7:201-224
5. Malbon CC, Graziano MP (1983) FEBS Lettr 155:35-38
6. Malbon CC, Graziano MP, Johnson GL (1984) J Biol Chem 259:3254-3260
7. Malbon CC, Moreno FJ, Cabelli RJ, Fain JN (1978) J Biol Chem 253:671-678
8. Malbon CC (1980) Mol Pharmacol 18:193-198
9. Cubero A, Malbon CC (1984) J Biol Chem 259:1344-1350
10. Moxham C, Malbon CC, Manuscript in preparation
11. Malbon CC, Brandwein H, Moxham C, Cubero A, Manuscript in preparation
12. Rapiejko PJ, Malbon CC, Garcia-Sainz JA (1984) Fed Proc 43:1584

Endocrinology
F. Labrie, L. Proulx, eds.

BETA- AND ALPHA$_2$-ADRENOCEPTORS INTERPLAY IN THE REGULATION OF HUMAN FAT CELL LIPOLYSIS

MAX LAFONTAN* AND MICHEL BERLAN**
Institut de Physiologie*, Laboratoire de Pharmacologie Médicale**, Université Paul Sabatier, ERA 412 CNRS, Rue François Magendie, 31400 TOULOUSE (France)

INTRODUCTION

It is now well accepted that lipid mobilization is modulated by the sympathetic nervous system and that catecholamines (CA) control the lipolytic activity of the adipose tissue in various species. Physiological amines (PA) are the most potent stimulators of lipolysis in human fat cells, the lipolytic effect is exerted through beta$_1$-adrenoceptors stimulation as demonstrated in " in vivo " and " in vitro " studies. Over the past few years, evidence has also been presented that antilipolytic effects are achieved by alpha$_2$-adrenoceptor stimulation [1,2,3]. However, the alpha$_2$-component of the response to PA has been questioned concerning its biological significance. Since both beta$_1$- and alpha$_2$- sites are intimately associated with the adenylate cyclase complex of the plasma membrane, the purpose of the present study is to work out the mechanism whereby PA occupancy of both receptor sites triggers the biological response (lipolysis or antilipolysis). Investigations were carried out to demonstrate the role and even the advantages of the two antagonistic adrenoceptor populations in the regulation of human fat cell activity. Such a set up could offer a better flexibility for the modulation of fat cell activity as compared with systems based on exclusive beta-adrenergic control of cell activation.Insights on human fat cell adrenoceptor properties from ligand binding studies were associated with biological assays to clarify the functional status of this double signalling system.

MATERIALS AND METHODS

The experimental conditions for lipolysis studies and binding assays have been reported in previous papers from our group[4,5,6]. Isolated fat cells from subcutaneous adipose tissue of women undergoing surgical lipectomy were used in these experiments. The patients were fasted overnight before tissue removal, they had no identified metabolic or endocrinological disorder. Lipolysis studies were compared with binding parameters defined on the same fat cell batch.

Insights on fat cell membrane adrenoceptors from ligand binding studies:

Alpha$_2$- and beta$_1$- sites have been identified with ^{3}H-yohimbine (^{3}H-YOH) and ^{3}H-dihydroalprenolol (^{3}H-DHA) or ^{3}H-CGP respectively. Kinetics and equilibrium experiments, performed at 25°C and 37°C indicate that both alpha$_2$- and beta$_1$- ^{3}H-ligands bind to a single population of sites with the same affinity over the 0.5-15 nM concentration range. Binding parameters revealed two major points: 1)- The beta$_1$- adrenoceptor sites labeled by ^{3}H-DHA and ^{3}H-CGP are at most a third or a quarter less numerous than the alpha$_2$ sites labeled by ^{3}H-YOH (180 ± 40 fmol /mg vs 550 ± 90 fmol/mg protein respectively). 2)- Equilibrium dissociation constants (K_D) estimated from direct radioligand binding to plasma membranes revealed that epinephrine (EPI) and norepinephrine (NEPI) exhibit a higher affinity for alpha$_2$- than for beta$_1$-sites. EPI has an even higher affinity than NEPI for alpha$_2$-sites (K_D's: 240 ± 40 vs 820 ± 110 nM respectively) while the amines are equipotent at the beta$_1$-sites (K_D's: 2500 ± 700 vs 1750 ± 600 nM). Competition curves yielded shallow binding isotherms with a reduced slope factor suggesting the presence of heterogenous binding sites.

Can ligand binding data help to give any explanation of the efficacy of the two PA on the adipocyte ? A cursory examination of binding results suggests that they do not correlate with receptor-mediated cellular response since, classically, it is the beta$_1$-dependent lipolytic action which has always been observed (Fig.1A.). If it is postulated that the efficacy of the amines is a function of their relative affinity for alpha$_2$- and beta$_1$-sites and receptor number, a better convergence between lipolysis responses and receptor properties would be expected.

Re-evaluation of catecholamine effects on lipolysis in human adipocytes:

The binding results prompted us to re-evaluate the effects of CA on lipolysis with precise dose-response studies using different approaches summarized in the Fig.1. As shown in Fig. 1A., the "classical" response of isolated human subcutaneous fat cells reveals the relative order of potency of CA commonly described: ISO > NEPI > EPI; the pure beta-agonist being far more efficient than the PA.

Incubated human fat cells release small amounts of adenosine which accumulate in fat cell suspensions over the incubation period. Adenosine is known to act as an inhibitory modulator of cyclic AMP production and lipolysis through interaction with adenosine receptors of the "R_i" type and through inhibition of adenylate cyclase[7,8,9]. When adenosine was prevented from accumulating in the incubation medium by addition of adenosine deaminase (ADA)(2µg/ml), *EPI alone and to a lesser extent, NEPI alone initiated an inhibition of lipolysis at lower contrations (Fig.1B.)* while the efficacy of ISO was increased. *The antilipolytic action was reversed at higher doses which correspond to the classical lipolytic ones "in vitro" (Fig.1A.).* This rebound was suppressed by propranolol(10^{-5}M); moreover, the antilipolytic action of EPI was suppressed by yohimbine(10^{-5}M) and the lipolytic effect of EPI and NEPI was thus revealed. It is not exclusively the lowered adenosine level which explains the ocurrence of the biphasic effect of the PA since it also occurs when basal lipolysis is increased by lower doses of beta-adrenergic agonist (ISO; 10^{-7}M) or even theophylline (1.6 mM).

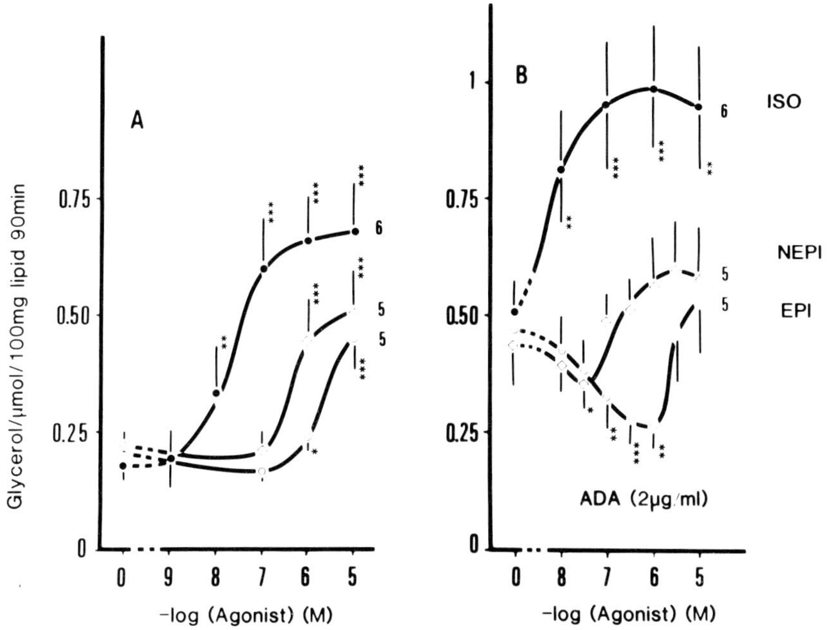

Fig.1. Effect of epinephrine (○), norepinephrine(□) and isoproterenol (●) on lipolysis in human isolated fat cells from subcutaneous adipose tissue. Incubations were done in Krebs-Ringer-Bicarbonate buffer[4,5] containing bovine serum albumin(35mg/ml), glucose(6µmol/ml) and ascorbic acid(0.1mM)

- A. Incubations were done using the standard "classical" method.
- B. Adenosine deaminase (2µg/ml) was included in the incubation medium.

Values are means ± SEM; ( ) number of experiments; * $p<0.05$; ** $p<0.02$ and *** $p<0.001$ indicates a significant difference between basal and stimulated value. *Epinephrine alone is lipolytic or antilipolytic depending on the incubation technique; isoproterenol is always lipolytic.*

However, it is noticeable that the alpha$_2$-effect of EPI does not counteract the lipolysis of fat cells overstimulated by higher doses of ISO(10^{-5}M).

It is now clear that the binding parameters fit with receptor-mediated cellular responses in human fat cells. The most striking fact is that, in isolated subcutaneous fat cells *EPI and to a lesser extent NEPI can inhibit lipolysis before exerting their lipolytic action.* Alpha$_2$-adrenoceptors, with their higher number and higher affinity for PA, are the adrenoceptor population first involved at the lowest concentration of the amines, the beta$_1$-sites with a lower number and weaker affinity for PA are involved when higher concentrations of the amines reach the plasma membrane. These studies have allowed the dissociation of the effect of PA on each kind of human fat cell adrenoceptor involved in the control of lipo lysis; they focus on the interest of associating reliable receptor studies and accurate measurements of receptor-mediated cellular responses.

To conclude, this clear definition of the relationships between CA and $beta_1$- and $alpha_2$-adrenoceptors of human fat cells opens new perspectives in the understanding of the physiology and probably the pathology of human adipose tissue. There is now no doubt that, as already suspected, the adrenergic response of the adipocyte results from the functional balance between $alpha_2$- and $beta_1$- adrenoceptor stimulation. The differential recruitment of both sites, based on different affinities for the CA seems to be a mechanism able to modulate the effects of the CA in a tissue possessing both antagonistic adrenoceptors regulating the same metabolic event. Further studies should be undertaken to assess the status of such interactions in conditions which are known to alter CA responsiveness of fat cells(e.g. caloric restriction, fasting, site differences and hypothyroidism) $Alpha_2$-adrenoceptors seem to play a major role in human fat cells, they are mainly involved in the control of the state of activity of the cell, to prevent physiological increments of lipolysis. It can be proposed that they represent a modulating system of fat cell activity or even a sort of"buffer" or stabilising process against variations of CA levels. In support of this point of view,it can be noted that $alpha_2$-adrenergic stimulation does not counterregulate overstimulated fat cells which are probably in a state which is far from that encountered in physiological conditions. The importance of this system as opposed to the other inhibiting mechanisms controlling lipolysis(e.g, adenosine, prostaglandins,insulin) remains to be more precisely investigated.

Numerous questions are still unanswered. What is the physiological relevance of these "in vitro" studies? Is EPI, the major physiological agonist of fat cell $alpha_2$-adrenoceptors, able to reach the $alpha_2$-sites under physiological conditions if the vasoconstrictor tonicity of the vascular bed is modified by the physiological amine?

REFERENCES

1. Lafontan M, Berlan M. (1981) Trends Pharmacol.Sci. 2: 126-129
2. Kather H. (1981) Triangle 20: 131-143
3. Fain JN, Garcia-Sainz A. (1983) J. Lipid Res. 24: 945-966
4. Lafontan M, Berlan M. (1980) Eur. J. Pharmacol. 66: 87-93
5. Berlan M, Lafontan M. (1982) J. Physiol.(Paris) 78: 279-287
6. Lafontan M, Berlan M, Villeneuve A. (1983) J.Lipid Res. 24: 429-440
7. Schwabe U, Ebert R, Erbler HC. (1975) Adv.Cycl.Nucl.Res. 5: 569-584
8. Fredholm BB. (1981) Int.J.Obesity 5: 643-649
9. Wolff J, Londos C, Cooper DMF (1981) Adv.Cycl.Nucl.Res. 14: 199-214

The investigations are supported by CNRS and INSERM (CRL 82705;PRC 12 8003) and ATP CNRS"Pharmacologie des recepteurs des Neuromediateurs"

7. Central Nervous System Peptides and Pituitary Function

Endocrinology
F. Labrie, L. Proulx, eds.

LOCALIZATION OF PEPTIDES AND INTERACTIONS OF RF NEURONS IN THE CENTRAL NERVOUS SYSTEMS

GEORGES PELLETIER

MRC Group in Molecular Endocrinology,
CHUL, 2705, boul. Laurier, Ste-Foy, Québec G1V 4G2, Canada

INTRODUCTION

During the last fifteen years, a large number of peptides have been found in the central nervous system. Some of these neuropeptides have been isolated from the hypothalamus because of their direct action on the anterior pituitary function. These are thyrotropin-releasing hormone (TRH), luteinizing hormone-releasing hormone (LHRH), somatostatin, corticotropin-releasing factor (CRF) and growth hormone-releasing factor (GRF).

In order to investigate the site(s) of action of these neuropeptides, it is important to determine their exact localization in the brain and their interactions with other neuronal systems. In this chapter, we have tried to summarize what is known about the localization in the hypothalamus of the neuropeptides which are directly involved in the regulation of pituitary secretion and the anatomical connection of these peptidergic systems with other systems.

LOCALIZATION OF HYPOTHALAMIC REGULATORY PEPTIDES.

LHRH. In the guinea pig, mouse and rat, neuronal cell bodies containing immunoreactive LHRH were only observed in the septopreoptic area and the suprachiasmatic areas (1-5). These neurons project to the capillaries of the organum vasculosum of the lamina terminalis and of the external zone of the median eminence. In these two areas of projection, immunostaining was detected in the dense core vesicles of endings located close to the fenestrated capillaries (2, 4). In man and monkey, most LHRH-containing perikarya were found in the infundibular nucleus and premamillary bodies (6-8).

Somatostatin. In the rat hypothalamus, somatostatin-containing cell bodies were only found in the periventricular nucleus from the level of the suprachiasmatic nucleus adjacent to the third ventricle, extending as far caudal as the level of the rostral margin of the ventromedial nucleus (9-13). A few scattered somatostatin-perikarya have also been detected in the anterior pituitary nucleus and the lateral hypothalamus. The cell bodies present in the periventricular nucleus are projecting to the external zone of the median eminence. Immunoelectron microscopy performed in the periventricular nucleus and the median eminence has revealed that the reaction product is restricted to the large dense core vesicles (90-130 nm in diameter) in both cell bodies and endings (11, 13).

CRF. Like TRH and somatostatin (9), CRF has been found to be widely distributed throughout the central nervous system (14, 15). In the hypothalamus, a large number of CRF-stained fibers are located in the external zone of the median eminence (14-16). These fibers appear to originate from the parvocellular division of the paraventricular nucleus which contain a large number of CRF-containing cell bodies. Using immunoelectron microscopy, CRF was observed in dense core vesicles of endings located close to the fenestrated capillaries in the external zone of the median eminence (16), supporting the hypothesis that the recently discovered CRF is a peptide of physiological importance in the regulation of ACTH secretion.

TRH. It was certainly a surprise when TRH, the first hypophysiotropic peptide characterized from the hypothalamus, was shown to be present not only in the hypothalamus but also in several brain areas, suggesting a possible extrahypothalamic role for this peptide (17). For technical reasons, the immunocytochemical studies on localization of TRH in the hypothalamus have been remarkedly limited (18, 19). A great density of immunoreactive cell bodies have been demonstrated in the preoptic nucleus, parvocellular subdivision of the paraventricular nucleus, perifornical region, dorsomedial nucleus and basolateral hypothalamus. On the basis of previous electrophysiological and histophysiological works, it appears reasonable to postulate that TRH neurons located in the paraventricular nucleus are projecting to the external zone of the median eminence.

GRF. Very few immunocytochemical studies about the localization of the newly-discovered GRF have so far reported (20, 21). Using antibodies against hpGRF-1-40, Merchentaler et al. (21) and Smith et al. (22) have been successful in localizing neurons containing immunoreactive GRF in the rat hypothalamus. The great majority of stained perikarya were located in the arcuate nucleus and the medial perifornical region of the lateral hypothalamus. On the basis of neuroanatomical studies, it seems likely that these two groups of neurons are projecting to the external zone of the median eminence which contains high concentration of GRF terminals.

ANATOMICAL INTERACTIONS OF NEUROPEPTIDERGIC SYSTEMS

Although the influence of neurotransmitters on the release of hypophysiotrophic factors from the hypothalamus have been extensively studied, the anatomical interactions existing between different systems involved in neuroendocrine regulation are still almost completely unknown. This probably pertains to technical difficulties of analyzing the anatomical connections between two or more systems at the ultrastructural level.

Recently, we have developed a double labeling technique involving a combination of radioautography and immunocytochemistry applied to the same ultrathin section (23). This relatively easy approach can be used for the simultaneous localization of biogenic amines and neuropeptides. We have recently studied at the electron microscopic level the anatomical connections of the LHRH and somatostatinergic systems with other systems.

LHRH system. Although close spatial association between LHRH-containing cell bodies and fibers staining for serotonin or norepinephrine have been shown by light microscopy, the existence of these postulated connections were not demonstrated at the electron microscopic level. Using immunoelectron microscopy for localization of LHRH, we have recently been able to demonstrate that stained nerve terminals can make asymmetrical synaptic contacts with labeled dendrites and cell bodies in the preoptico-septal area. In the external zone of the median eminence, close opposition between dopaminergic endings and LHRH-containing endings were shown, suggesting that the influence of dopamine on LHRH secretion is exerted via involvement of the dopaminergic tuberoinfundibular system.

Somatostatinergic system. Using immunocytochemistry at the light microscopic level, we had previously demonstrated that somatostatin-containing endings were in close association with immunoreactive cell bodies in the periventricular nucleus. Very recently, using immunoelectron microscopy, we have shown that stained endings were making symmetrical synaptic contacts with positive cell bodies and dendrites.

These recent findings indicate that neurons producing the same peptides can have contacts between themselves. These recent observations about the LHRH and somatostatinergic systems coupled to the previous description of contacts between POMC neurons (24) provide morphological evidence for autoregulation of neuropeptide systems.

REFERENCES

1. Barry J, Dubois MP, Poulain P (1973) Z Zellforsch 146:351-366
2. Pelletier G, Labrie F, Puviani R, Arimura A, Schally AV (1974) Endocrinology 95:314-317
3. Pelletier G (1976) In: Labrie F, Meites J and Pelletier G (eds) Hypothalamus and Endocrine Functions, Plenum Press, New York, pp. 433-450
4. Pelletier G, Leclerc R, Dubé D (1976) J Histochem Cytochem 24: 864-871
5. Setalo G, Vigh S, Schally AV, Arimura, A. (1976) Acta Biol Acad Sci Hung 27: 75-77
6. Pelletier, G (1979) In: Collu R, Barbeau A, Ducharme J, Rochefort JG (eds), Central Nervous System and Other Peptides, Raven Press, New York, pp 325-344
7. Barry J, Carette B (1975) Cell Tiss Res 164: 163-178
8. Pelletier G (1982) In: Besser GM, Martini L (eds), Clinical Neuroendocrinology, Academic Press, New York, pp 397-428
9. Brownstein MJ, Arimura A, Sato H, Schally AV, Kizer JS (1975) Endocrinology 96: 1431-1441
10. Elde RP, Parsons JA (1975) Am J Anat 144:541-548
11. Pelletier G, Leclerc R, Dubé D, Labrie F, Puviani R, Arimura A, Schally AV (1975) Am J Anat 142: 397-405
12. Dubé D, Leclerc R, Pelletier G (1976) Am J Anat 147: 103-108
13. Pelletier G, Dubé D, Puviani R (1977) Science 196: 1469-1470
14. Cummings S, Elde R, Ells J, Lindall A (1983) J Neurosci 3: 1355-1368
15. Swansson LW, Swachenko PE, Vale WW (1983) Neuroendocrinology 36: 165-186.
16. Pelletier G (1982) Neuroendocrinology 35: 402-404
17. Jackson IMD, Reichlin S (1974) Endocrinology 95: 854-860
18. Hökfelt T, Fuxe K, Johansson O, Jeffcoate S, White N (1975) Eur J Pharmacol 34: 389-396
19. Johansson O, Hökfelt T (1980) J Histochem Cytochem 28:364-372
20. Lechan RM, Jackson JMD (1982) Endocrinology 111:55-65
21. Merchenthaler I, Vigh S, Schally AV, Petrusz P (1984) Endocrinology 114:1082-1085
22. Smith RM, Howe PRC, Oliver JR, Willoughby JO (1984) Neuropeptides 4:109-115
23. Pelletier G (1983) J Histochem Cytochem 31:562-564
24. Chen YY, Pelletier G (1983) Neurosci Lett 43:271-276

Endocrinology
F. Labrie, L. Proulx, eds.

REGULATION OF PITUITARY HORMONE SECRETION BY VIP AND RELATED PEPTIDES

YUZURU KATO, AKIRA SHIMATSU, NORIO MATSUSHITA, HIKARU OHTA, KATSUYOSHI TOJO, YASUHIRO KABAYAMA, TATSUHIDE INOUE AND HIROO IMURA

Second Medical Clinic, Department of Medicine, Kyoto University Faculty of Medicine, Sakyo-ku, Kyoto 606 (Japan)

INTRODUCTION

Vasoactive intestinal polypeptide (VIP), first discovered in the digestive tract (1), has been detected in the hypothalamus. We first demonstrated that VIP stimulates prolactin secretion in the rat (2). Subsequent studies suggest that VIP is secreted into the hypophysial portal blood (3) and acts directly at the pituitary level to evoke prolactin release (4,5), suggesting a potential role of VIP as a prolactin releasing factor (PRF).

It is suggested that prolactin secretion induced by serotonergic stimulation in the brain is mediated by hypothalamic PRF (6,7). We have previously reported that serotonin and 5-hydroxytryptophan (5-HTP), a precursor of serotonin, stimulates VIP release from the hypothalamus into the hypophysial portal blood (8,9).

PHI, first isolated from porcine intestinal tissue (10), has been shown in nerve fibers in the rat median eminence and hypothalamus (11). The structural similarities between VIP and PHI suggest a possible role of PHI in the hypothalamo pituitary function. It is also suggested that VIP and PHI may be synthesized from the common precursor molecule (12).

In the present study, we report the role of VIP and PHI in regulating the pituitary function, especially prolactin secretion in rats and man.

MATERIALS AND METHODS

Effects of VIP and PHI on plasma prolactin levels were examined in Wistar male rats anesthetized with urethane (2) or in conscious rats chronically implanted with intraatrial and intraventricular catheters (13).

We further examined by the passive immunization method the role of hypothalamic VIP in serotonin (5HT)-induced prolactin secretion in urethane-anesthetized rats. Anti-VIP serum was generated in rabbits against VIP-PVP mixture (R501, R502) and VIP-bovine thyroglobulin conjugate (KRV-1). Kd and Bmax were 4.9×10^{-12}M and 0.8 nmol/ml (R501), 7.7×10^{-12}M and 0.9 nmol/ml (R502), and 2.4×10^{-10}M and 7.2 nmol/ml (KRV-1), respectively.

In human, the intramuscular injection of VIP on plasma prolactin and growth hormone (GH) levels were examined in normal women and patients with prolactinoma or acromegaly.

Blood samples were obtained every 5 to 30 min after the injection of test substances.

Prolactin release from dispersed anterior pituitary cells was studied in rats and man by the superfusion method described previously (5,14). The perfusate was collected every 5 min.

Prolactin concentrations in the plasma and the effluent were measured by specific radioimmunoassays as described previously (2,6). Statistical analysis was performed by Duncan's new multiple range test.

RESULTS

Prolactin secretion was dose-relatedly stimulated in the rat *in vivo* by VIP injected intravenously (iv) at a dose of 0.3 to 3 nmol/100 μl/100 g BW or intraventricularly (icv) at a dose of 0.06 to 3 nmol/10 μl/rat in the urethane-anesthetized rat. Either icv or iv injection of VIP (3 nmol/rat) also raised plasma prolactin levels in conscious rats.

Intramuscular injection of VIP (60 nmol) resulted in a significant increase in plasma prolactin levels in normal women (peak values 28.1±6.7 *vs* control 11.4±1.6 ng/ml, $p<0.05$), whereas plasma GH and cortisol levels were not affected. VIP injection slightly raised plasma prolactin levels (more than 120 % of the basal value) in most patients with prolactinoma and plasma GH levels (more than 150 % of the basal value) in a part of acromegalic patients.

Prolactin release from superfused rat anterior pituitary cells was stimulated by VIP (10^{-9}- 10^{-6}M) in a dose-related manner, and the stimulating action of VIP

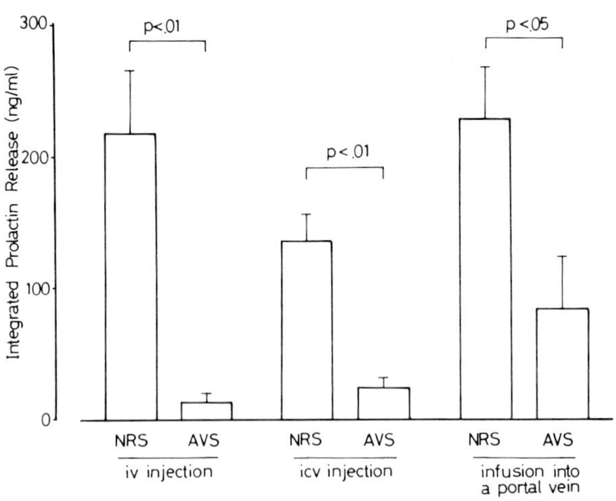

Fig. 1. Effect of anti-VIP rabbit serum (AVS) on prolactin release induced by serotonin (5HT). AVS or normal rabbit serum (NRS) was injected iv or icv 30 min before icv injection of 5HT (10 μg/rat). AVS or NRS was also infused into a single hypophysial portal vein at a rate of 2 μl/min and 5HT was injected icv 10 min after the start of infusion. Mean (±SE) values of integrated prolactin release are shown.

(10^{-7}M) was shown in the presence of dopamine (10^{-7}M) or GABA (10^{-5}M), a possible prolactin inhibiting factor.

VIP stimulated GH release from superfused pituitary adenoma cells obtained from acromegalic patients and prolactin secretion from prolactinoma cells.

Either icv injection of 5HT (10 μg/rat) or iv injection of 5HTP (5 mg/100 g BW) increased plasma prolactin levels in the anesthetized rats. Plasma prolactin levels raised by 5HT were suppressed in animals in which anti-VIP serum was injected icv or iv, and infused into a single hypophysial portal vein as shown in Fig. 1. Prolactin release induced by 5HTP was also blunted by anti-VIP serum compared with normal rabbit serum (integrated prolactin release 493±82 _vs_ 304±37 ng/ml, $p<0.05$).

Intraventricular injection of PHI (0.06, 0.6 and 6 nmol/rat) raised plasma prolactin levels in a dose-related manner in urethane-anesthetized rats. In conscious animals, either icv or iv injection of PHI (3 nmol/rat) also raised plasma prolactin levels as shown in Fig. 2.

In _in vitro_ experiments, prolactin release from superfused rat anterior pituitary cells was stimulated by PHI (10^{-9}, 10^{-8} and 10^{-7}M). Prolactin responses to PHI were dose-dependent and the mean(±SE) maximum percent changes of prolactin release were 146±12, 161±13 and 182±19 %, respectively. The maximum changes of prolactin release by VIP (10^{-7}M) was 196±16 % in the same experiments.

As shown in Fig. 3, PHI (10^{-8}M) as well as hpGRF (10^{-9}, 10^{-8} and 10^{-7}M) stimulated prolactin release from superfused pituitary adenoma cells obtained at the surgery of a patient with acromegaly who had showed hypersecretion of both GH

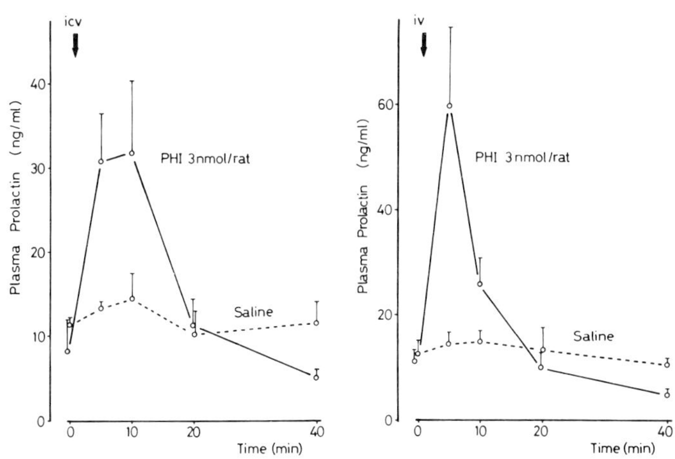

Fig. 2. Effects of either icv or iv injection of porcine PHI-27 (3 nmol/rat) on plasma prolactin levels in conscious rats. Mean(±SE) values are shown. Saline was injected in a control group.

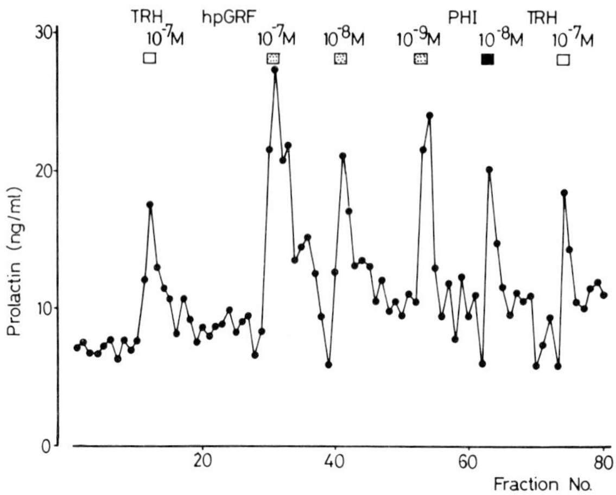

Fig. 3. Effects of hpGRF-44-NH_2 (10^{-9}-10^{-7}M), PHI (10^{-8}M) and TRH (10^{-7}M) on prolactin release from superfused pituitary adenoma cells obtained from a patient with acromegaly.

and prolactin. PHI also stimulated GH release from pituitary adenoma cells *in vitro* in some acromegalic patients.

DISCUSSION

VIP is now accepted as a putative prolactin releasing factor since it is present in the hypophysial portal blood in high concentrations (3) sufficient to stimulate prolactin release from the pituitary cells *in vitro* (4,5). However, the physiological role of VIP remains to be elucidated.

Serotonin stimulates prolactin secretion by acting in the central nervous system to stimulate PRF release (6,7). We have previously reported that serotonin stimulates VIP release from the median eminence into rat hypophysial portal blood *in vivo* (8) and from the hypothalamic fragments perifused *in vitro* (9). We have demonstrated that prolactin release induced by serotonergic stmulation is blunted by anti-VIP rabbit serum in the rat.

It is suggested, therefore, that prolactin secretion induced by brain serotonin is mediated, at least in part, by hypothalamic VIP release into the hypophysial portal vein.

We have recently reported that PHI-like immunoreactivity is highly concentrated in the hypophysial portal blood, correlated with VIP concentrations at the molar ration of 1:1 (15). In the present study, PHI stimulated prolactin release from superfused rat anterior pituitary cells *in vitro*. These findings are on the same line of other previous reports (16,17). We further demonstrated that PHI stimulated prolactin secretion in the rat *in vivo*.

GH and prolactin release from pituitary adenoma cells obtained from patients with acromegaly and prolactinoma were also stimulated by PHI and VIP. These results may indicate that PHI as well as VIP have a role in regulating the pituitary function by acting, at least in part, directly in rats and man. However, interrelation between VIP and PHI remains to be further elucidated.

ACKNOWLEDGEMENTS

This study was supported in part by grants from the Ministry of Education and the Ministray of Health and Welfare, Japan.

REFERENCES

1. Said SI, Rosenberg RN (1976) Science 192:907-908
2. Kato Y, Iwasaki Y, Iwasaki J, Abe N, Yanaihara N, Imura H (1978) Endocrinology 103:554-558
3. Shimatsu A, Kato Y, Matsushita N, Katakami H, Yanaihara N, Imura H (1981) Endocrinology 108:395-398
4. Ruberg M, Rosztejn WH, Arancibia S, Besson J, Enjalbert A (1978) Eur J Pharmacol 51:319-320
5. Matsushita N, Kato Y, Shimatsu A, Katakami H, Yanaihara N, Imura H (1983) Life Sci 32:1263-1269
6. Kato Y, Nakai Y, Imura H, Chihara K, Ohgo S (1974) J Clin Endocrinol Metab 38:695-697
7. Ohgo S, Kato Y, Chihara K, Maeda K, Imura H (1976) Endocrinol Jpn 23:485-491
8. Shimatsu A, Kato Y, Matsushita N, Katakami H, Yanaihara N, Imura H (1982) Endocrinology 111:338-340
9. Shimatsu A, Kato Y, Matsushita N, Katakami H, Ohta H, Yanaihara N, Imura H (1983) Brain Res 264:148-151
10. Tatemoto K, Mutt V (1981) Proc Natl Acad Sci USA 78:6603-6607
11. Hökfelt T, Fahrenkrug J, Tatemoto K, Mutt V, Werner S (1982) Acta Physiol Scand 116:469-461
12. Itoh N, Obata K, Yanaihara N, Okamoto N (1983) Nature 304:547-549
13. Kato Y, Hiroto S, Katakami H, Matsushita N, Shimatsu A, Imura H (1982) Proc Soc Exp Biol Med 169:95-100
14. Matsushita N, Kato Y, Katakami H, Shimatsu A, Yanaihara N, Imura H (1982) J Clin Endocrinol Metab 54:773-779
15. Shimatsu A, Kato Y, Inoue T, Christofides NS, Bloom SR, Imura H (1983) Neurosci Lett 43:259-262
16. Werner S, Hultimg A-L, Hökfelt T, Eneroth P, Tatemoto K, Mutt V, Maroder L (1983) Neuroendocrinology 37:476-478
17. Samson WK, Lumpkin MD, McDonald JK, McCann SM (1983) Peptides 4:817-819

Endocrinology
F. Labrie, L. Proulx, eds.

OPIOID PEPTIDES AND ANTERIOR PITUITARY HORMONE SECRETION

ASHLEY GROSSMAN
Department of Endocrinology, St. Bartholomew's Hospital, London, EC1A 7BE, UK.

The endogenous opioid peptides, endorphins and enkephalins, are now well-established as important modulators of neuroendocrine function. Rather than reviewing all the literature on this enlarging subject (1-4), this brief review will attempt to summarise and synthesize our current knowledge, with special reference to the situation in man.

Early studies clearly demonstrated that exogenous opioid peptides could stimulate the release of serum prolactin and GH in man (5), compatible with data in the rat. However, it is not possible to stimulate GH release with synthetic β-endorphin, while there is a dissociation in the effects of various opiate alkaloids in their ability to release prolactin or GH (6). This suggests that the stimulatory pathways for these two hormones are distinct. In the rat, opioid peptides decrease the turnover of newly-formed dopamine in the hypothalamus, and suppress the secretion of dopamine into the hypophyseal portal blood. Most studies have excluded a direct effect of opioid peptides on the pituitary lactotrophs themselves, and these data taken together indicate that the principal mode of action of opioids is to stimulate prolactin release through disinhibition of hypothalamic dopamine. Recent work in our laboratory, in association with Prof. G. Delitala, suggests that a similar mechanism operates in man (7). However, a role for a 5HT-VIP system is also likely, according to other studies in the rat. Opioid-stimulated GH release is separated functionally and anatomically from prolactin release (8), and is probably mainly dependent on the stimulation of growth hormone-releasing hormone (9). However, a disinhibition of somatostatin release by exogenous opiates has been shown by ourselves and others in vitro, although it is likely to be of lesser importance than changes in GHRH. In man, there is evidence that opioid modulation occurs via a cholinergic, and possibly a histaminergic, linking interneuron (10,11): dopaminergic, serotoninergic, and noradrenergic receptors appear not to be involved.

What is the functional significance of these putative opioid receptors for prolactin and GH release? While in the rat, the opioid antagonist naloxone has generally been found to lower basal prolactin and GH and blunt stress-induced elevations, and i.c.v. β-endorphin antiserum blocks the stress-induced prolactin increase, the evidence in man is mostly against endogenous opioid peptides playing any significant role in the pathophysiological control of these hormones. In one interesting study, naloxone blocked the rise in serum prolactin and GH seen in athletes undergoing intense exercise (12), but no effect of naloxone has been seen in studies employing similar protocols in untrained subjects. It is possible that the process of physical training activates an endorphinergic modulatory system, but this remains speculative at present. What is clear is that either the endogenous opioids are not important regulators of prolactin and GH secretion in man, or that we have not as yet defined the situations in which they are activated.

Similar considerations apply to TSH release. Exogenous opioids directly suppress the release of hypothalamic TRH in the rat, and may modulate the TSH response to cold-stress. However, in man opiates are stimulatory, probably at μ-receptors. A slight suppression of basal TSH by naloxone has been shown in some studies, but both stimulatory and inhibitory effects are of such a small magnitude as to be of minor clinical significance.

In the case of the gonadotrophins, endogenous opioids appear to be much more relevant in both rat and man. In both species, applied opioids and opiates suppress gonadotrophin release, almost certainly via an inhibition of the pulsatile delivery of GnRH into the portal blood. In the rat, part of the feedback effect of gonadal steroids may operate through this mechanism, which may in turn involve mediating dopaminergic and noradrenergic receptors. In one model proposed by Bhanot and Wilkson, the process of pubertal maturation is conceived as involving the diminishing ability of an endogenous opioid to inhibit the increasing noradrenergic stimulation of GnRH release (13). However, such a complex interaction appears not to operate in man, in whom opiate-GnRH interactions do not involve dopamine or noradrenaline (14). Endogenous opioids also do not appear to be involved in the initiation of human puberty. Nevertheless, naloxone administration increases the frequency, and possibly the amplitude, of LH pulsatility in normal man, and demonstrates a varying opioid tone throughout the menstrual cycle. Maximal opioid inhibition probably appears during the luteal phase (15), and may mediate the progesterone-dominated low-frequency LH pulsatility seen at this time. The naloxone-sensitivity of these responses (2) suggests that the endogenous modulator is β-endorphin. Of great interest is the discovery that short-term naloxone infusion can counteract the absent LH pulsatility usually seen in hyperprolactinaemic amenorrhoea, leading to a return of a normal (or supranormal) LH pulse frequency and amplitude (16). In studies in our laboratory, Dr. Ana-Maria Lengyel has shown that in vivo prolactin administration to the rat diminishes the in vitro release of GnRH from the mediobasal hypothalamus, and that this can be overcome by naloxone (Fig. 1). Thus, at least part of the inhibition of GnRH release seen in hyperprolactinaemia is mediated via endogenous β-endorphin.

Short-term delivery of opiates produces an immediate stimulation of ACTH release in the rat; this has been shown to occur via the stimulation of endogenous CRF. However, long-term administration leads to a suppression of ACTH and related

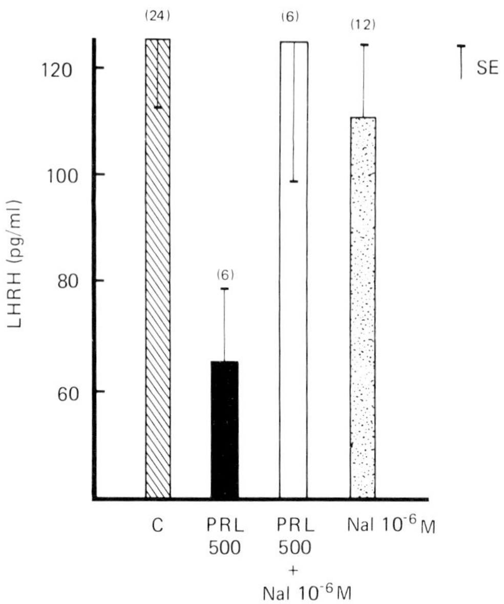

Fig. 1. The effect of naloxone (10^{-6}M) on the inhibition of LHRH release from rat hypothalami in vitro induced by prolactin 500ng/ml.

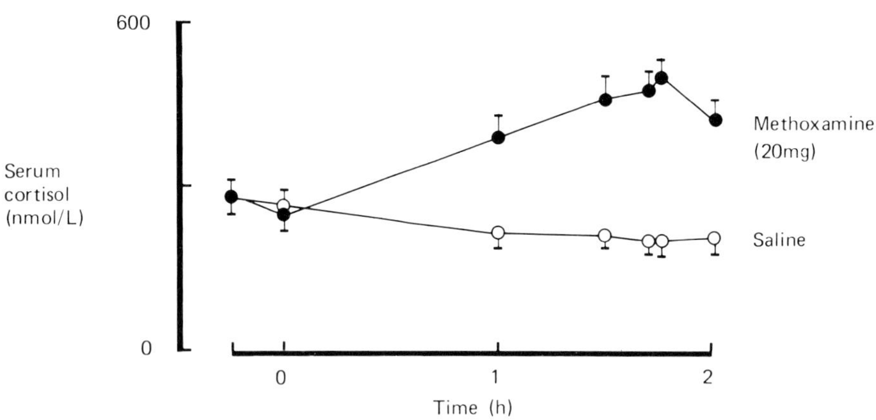

Fig. 2. The effect of the α_1-agonist methoxamine, or saline, on mean serum cortisol in six normal subjects.

peptides, probably (though not certainly) via inhibition of CRF. High-dose naloxone in both man and rat leads to an elevation in circulating ACTH, LPH, β-endorphin, and cortisol/corticosterone, suggesting the dominant control of CRF release by an inhibitory opioid peptide (17). This occurs at relatively naloxone -insensitive opioid receptors (K or δ ?) (18). This is particularly important in man, in whom exogenous opiates only inhibit cortisol release, without any preceding stimulation. This inhibitory control of CRF release is present throughout the day and night (19). The α_1-adrenoceptor agonist methoxamine stimulates ACTH and cortisol release in man, according to recent studies in our department by Dr. Saad Al-Damluji (Fig. 2). This response is blocked by the α_1-antagonist thymoxamine, as is the rise in cortisol induced by naloxone (20). This implies that opioids inhibit CRF release through the (?presynaptic) modulation of an excitatory noradrenergic input from the brain-stem, similar to the model put forward to explain the control of GnRH release in the rat. As the release of ACTH (and related peptides) is the principal neuroendocrine correlate of the "stress" response, this further implies that endogenous opioids act to dampen down or attenuate this response. In studies with Dr. Pierre Bouloux, we have recently shown that opioids also block the sympathoadrenal activation characteristic of stress, and furthermore, an intrinsic opioid inhibition of catecholamine release is only revealed when the organism is first stressed (21,22). It currently remains uncertain as to whether there is an 'integrated' opioid system, welding together the disparate neuroendocrine changes involving the endogenous opioids. However, I would like to suggest that, in man, one of the most important functions of the endogenous opioid system is to react whenever the homeostasis of the organism is perturbed by an overwhelming stimulus. By suppressing the activity of CRF and the sympathoadrenal system, inhibiting sensory input, inducing analgesia and, at least in animals, decreasing sexual activity, an integrated opioid system could isolate the organism from the perturbing environment, and allow it to recuperate. According to Selye's original theory, disturbances in this adaptive process may have long-term pathophysiological consequences.

In summary, opioid peptides stimulate prolactin, GH, and TSH release in man, but do not appear to be of great physiological significance. GnRH secretion is modulated by an endogenous opioid, probably β-endorphin, with increasing tonic inhibition in the luteal phase of the menstrual cycle, and especially in hyperprolactinaemia. An endogenous opioid peptide, possibly met-enkephalin or dynorphin, inhibits the sympathoadrenal system and the noradrenergic stimulation of CRF release in man, and it is postulated that this represents part of the organisms' ability to terminate the endocrine changes characteristic of the acute stress response.

ACKNOWLEDGEMENTS

I am grateful to Miss Fenella Moore for secretarial assistance, to my research nurses over the years (particularly Julia Williams), and to Prof. Michael Besser for valuable support.

REFERENCES

1. Morley JE (1981) Metabolism 30: 195
2. Grossman A (1983) In: Scanlon MF (ed) Clinics in Endocrinology and Metabolism 12 (3). WB Saunders, London, pp725-746
3. Grossman A, Rees LH (1983) Brit Med Bull 39: 83
4. Morley JE (1983) Psychoneuroendocrinol 8: 361
5. Stubbs WA, Delitala G, Jones A et al (1978) Lancet ii: 1225
6. Delitala G, Grossman A, Besser GM (1983) Neuroendocrinol 37: 275
7. Delitala G, Grossman A, Besser GM (1983) Clin Endocrinol 19: 437
8. Belchetz PE (1981) Life Sci 28: 2961
9. Wehrenberg WB, Brazeau P, Luben R, Ling N, Guillemin R (1983) Neuroendocrinol 36: 489
10. Delitala G, Grossman A, Besser GM (1983) Clin Endocrinol 18: 401
11. Penalva A, Villanueva L, Casanueva F et al (1983) Psychopharmacol 80: 120
12. Moretti C, Fabbri A, Gnessi L et al (1983) Clin Endocrinol 18:135
13. Bhanot R, Wilkinson M (1983) Endocrinol 113: 596
14. Veldhuis JD, Rogol AD, Williams FA, Johnson ML (1983) J Clin Endocrinol Metab 57: 1292
15. Quigley ME, Yen SSC (1980) J Clin Endocrinol Metab 51: 179
16. Grossman A, Moult PJA, McIntyre H et al (1982) Clin Endocrinol 17: 379
17. Volavka J, Cho D, Mallya A, Bauman J (1979) N Eng J Med 300: 1056
18. Grossman A, Clement-Jones V (1983). In: Clayton RC (ed) Clinics in Endocrinology and Metabolism 12 (1). WB Saunders, London, pp31-56
19. Grossman A, Gaillard RC, McCartney P et al (1982) Clin Endocrinol 17: 279
20. Grossman A, Besser GM (1982) Clin Endocrinol 17: 287
21. Grossman A, Bouloux P, Price P et al (1984) Clin Sci, in press
22. Bouloux P, Grossman A, Lytras N, Besser GM (1984) Clin Endocrinol, in press

Endocrinology
F. Labrie, L. Proulx, eds.

INTERACTIONS OF BRAIN PEPTIDES WITHIN THE HYPOTHALAMUS TO ALTER ANTERIOR PITUITARY HORMONE SECRETION

S.M. MC CANN, M.D. LUMPKIN, N. ONO, O. KHORRAM, A. OTTLECZ, J. KOENIG, J. BEDRAN DE CASTRO, L. KRULICH AND W.K. SAMSON
Department of Physiology, University of Texas Health Science Center at Dallas, Dallas, Texas 75235

INTRODUCTION

A host of peptides have been found to be resident within the hypothalamus. Among them are the characterized peptidic hypothalamic releasing and inhibiting hormones, the neurohypophyseal peptides, the opioid peptides, α-MSH, and a series of peptides thought previously to reside solely within the gut. We review here our studies on the possible interactions amongst these peptides to control the release of pituitary hormones. Space limitations prohibit examination of the effects of some of these peptides (1).

RESULTS AND DISCUSSION

1) Characterized peptidic hypothalamic hormones:

Corticotropin Releasing Factor (CRF). Injection of CRF into the ventricle stimulated ACTH release in a dose-related manner presumably by uptake of the peptide into portal vessels and direct activation of the corticotrophs. When the dose was further reduced, no effect was seen on plasma ACTH. Under these resting conditions, intraventricular CRF resulted in a decline in plasma GH and LH in ovariectomized females. Since stress in general inhibits LH and GH release in the rat, it appears that CRF released in the hypothalamus may act to suppress release of LHRH and GRF or stimulate SRIF release (2) and thereby reproduce the stress pattern of release of these pituitary hormones.

To determine if CRF could alter the release of ACTH in stress by a hypothalamic action, the peptide was injected intraventricularly in doses too low to stimulate a release of ACTH. Following injection of these doses and the imposition of ether stress for one minute, plasma ACTH levels were elevated further by ether in the CRF-injected animals than in the saline-injected controls. We postulate that this may be an example of a positive ultra-short loop feedback of the peptide to augment its own release in stress. This appears reasonable since a negative ultra-short loop feedback under these conditions would tend to suppress the stress response. The situation appears analagous to the already demonstrated positive feedback effect of gonadal steroids to augment the preovulatory release of gonadotropins.

Growth Hormone Releasing Factor. Intraventricular injection of GRF resulted in stimulation of the release of GH as evidenced by significant increases in plasma GH levels. Presumably this action is via uptake of the GRF by portal capillaries and delivery to pituitary where it exerts a stimulatory action on the somatotrophs. When the dose was reduced so that there was no stimulation of the release of GH directly, the action was opposite and plasma GH levels fell at low doses of intraventricular GRF. We postulate that the GRF is taken up from the ventricle by the periventricular tissue and acts there to inhibit the release of GRF and/or to stimulate somatostatin release.

Somatostatin. We had previously concluded that somatostatin acts within the hypothalamus to bring about the stimulation of GH release either via stimulation of release of GH-releasing factor (GRF) or by inhibition of the release of somatostatin itself (3). At the same time it would appear that somatostatin has an inhibitory effect on the release of TRH and also LHRH to account for the decline in release of these hormones.

2) Neurohypophyseal Hormones

Oxytocin. Oxytocin can stimulate prolactin (Prl) release from male rat pituitary cells incubated *in vitro* (4). More recently we have found a dramatic stimulation of Prl release from dispersed pituitary cells of lactating rats perifused in a column, with 7-8 fold stimulations of release with a minimal effective dose of 10^{-9}M oxytocin. Following the intraventricular injection of oxytocin there was a suppression of Prl release as evidenced by declines in plasma Prl. This is indicative of a possible ultra-short loop feedback whereby oxytocin taken up from the ventricle suppresses the firing of PRF-containing neurons which are stimulatory to Prl. Removal of the stimulation via oxytocin results in a fall in Prl release.

3) Gastrointestinal Hormones:

Secretin Family of Peptides. Various members of the secretin family of peptides such as vasoactive intestinal polypeptide (VIP), secretin, and porcine intestinal peptide (PHI) can directly stimulate the lactotrophs to release Prl *in vitro*; however, when secretin is injected into the third ventricle Prl release is inhibited (5). This may be another example of an inhibitory ultra-short loop feedback since secretin has been found to exist in the hypothalamus.

Gastric Inhibitory Polypeptide (GIP). GIP is another member of the secretin family of peptides which has yet to be demonstrated conclusively in the brain. We anticipate that it ultimately will be found there and consequently have evaluated this peptide. It has a relatively high potency to stimulate release of pituitary FSH and LH from dispersed pituitary cells incubated *in vitro* and also from perifused pituitary cells. Following its injection into the third ventricle there is a selective decrease in plasma FSH but no effect on LH. These results again suggest a possible ultra-short loop feedback mechanism whereby GIP inhibits its own release. The fact that the inhibition is limited to FSH secretion is suggestive of the possibility that it has a selective inhibitory effect on the release of a FSH-releasing factor (FSHRF) but not on the release of LHRH. We have obtained recently further evidence for the existence of FSHRF.

Motilin. Motilin, another peptide found in the hypothalamus has been shown by us to be capable of stimulating GH release by direct action on pituitary cells incubated *in vitro* with a minimal effective dose of 10^{-9} M (6). It is less effective, however, than GRF yet has an additive action with GRF to stimulate GH release *in vitro*. That it may play some role as a GRF is indicated by the ability of antisera directed against motilin to suppress GH release. Injection of motilin into the third ventricle produced the opposite action, namely a depression in plasma GH levels. This is probably accomplished by either an inhibition of the release of motilin or GRF or by a stimulation of the release of somatostatin or by a combination of these actions. Since motilin has been found in the brain, these results may have physiological significance.

Neuropeptide Y (NPY). NPY is structurally similar to the pancreatic polypeptides (PP) and is present in the rat hypothalamus. Intraventricular injection of NPY in doses ranging from 0.02 to 5 µg resulted in a significant depression of LH and GH levels. Plasma FSH levels were unaffected (7). Similar effects were observed with avian and bovine PP. We have observed recently significant stimulation of LH and GH release by NPY from perifused, dispersed cell columns.

4) Proopiomelanocortin-derived peptides.

β-Endorphin. Many opioid peptides have now been discovered in the brain including the hypothalamus. It is clear that opiates and the various opioid peptides are capable of stimulating Prl and GH secretion while inhibiting LH secretion by an action on the hypothalamus. The actions of the opiates on the release of the various pituitary hormones can be blocked by the opiate receptor blocker, naloxone. The inhibitory action of opiates on LH secretion appears to have physiologic signficance since injection of the opiate antagonist, naloxone, results in an elevation of plasma LH under most circumstances. We believe that the opioid peptide involved is β-endorphin since intraventricular injection of antisera specifically directed against β-endorphin resulted in elevation of LH presumably by removing the tonic inhibition via β-endorphin.

α-MSH. α-MSH is found in the same neurons which contain β-endorphin. These have their cell bodies predominantly in the arcuate nucleus and axons projecting to various regions of the brain. Recently another population of cells in the dorsal hypothalamus has been found to contain only α-MSH and to have projections to the median eminence. We have evaluated the actions of α-MSH injected intraventricularly and have found that relatively small doses of the peptide can inhibit the release of both LH and Prl in ovariectomized females. The action appears to be via dopamine receptors since these actions are blocked by pimozide, a dopamine receptor blocker, or by inhibition of dopamine synthesis by the administration of α-methyl-p-tyrosine (8). Injection of specific antisera directed against α-MSH resulted in significant and lasting elevations of plasma Prl and LH. Furthermore, there was a failure of Prl to increase further following ether anesthesia, whereas in the normal rabbit serum-injected controls an elevation of Prl followed induction of ether anesthesia.

In conclusion, it is apparent that there are complex interactions amongst the various peptides found in the hypothalamus to bring about alterations in the release of various anterior pituitary hormones. In many instances we have found that peptides which have an action on the pituitary directly have an opposite action when injected into the third ventricle. We postulate that these are examples of ultra-short loop negative feedback originally postulated many years ago by Martini and co-workers. We have uncovered also what appears to be one example of a positive ultra-short loop feedback of CRF to augment its own release during stress. Additionally, other peptides which appear to have no action at the pituitary level, have powerful effects to alter pituitary hormone secretion by intrahypothalamic actions and these actions appear to be physiologically significant in the case of β-endorphin and α-MSH.

REFERENCES

1. McCann SM (1982) In: Muller EE, MacLeod RM (eds) Neuroendocrine Perspectives. Elsevier, Amsterdam, pp. 1-22

2. Ono N, Lumpkin MD, Samson WK, McDonald JK, McCann, SM (1984) Life Sciences: In Press

3. Lumpkin MD, Negro-Vilar A, McCann SM (1981) Science 211:1072

4. Lumpkin MD, Samson WK, McCann SM (1983) Endocrinology 112:1711

5. Samson WK, Lumpkin MD, McCann SM (1984) Life Sciences 34: 144

6. Samson WK, Lumpkin MD, Nilaver G, McCann SM (1984) Brain Res. Bull 12: 57

7. McDonald JM, Lumpkin MD, Samson WK, McCann SM (1984) submitted.

8. Khorram O, DePalatis LR, McCann SM. (1984) Endocrinology 114:227

8. Prolactin

Endocrinology
F. Labrie, L. Proulx, eds.

ALTERATION IN DISTRIBUTIONS OF PROLACTIN IN LACTOTROPHS UNDER VARIOUS PHYSIOLOGICAL CONDITIONS: IMMUNOELECTRON MICROSCOPIC INVESTIGATIONS

ROBERT Y. OSAMURA*, KEIICHI WATANABE* AND PAUL K. NAKANE**
Departments of Pathology(*) and Cell Biology(**), Tokai University School of Medicine, Bohseidai, Isehara, Kanagawa, 259-11 (Japan)

INTRODUCTION

The concept that a given physiological state reflects upon the morphology and visa versa has been well established at tissue and cell levels. The association has also been recognized with some benign and neoplastic tumors as the morphology of the tumors often reflects their environment. The cell ultrastructure reflects the physiological state of the cell as well, although a little is documented about the sub-cellular distribution of a specific secretory product in various organelles at a given functional state. Because of its well defined affecter and effect, endocrine cells are best suited to study the subcellular morphological changes in response to environment. The lactotrophs and prolactin secreting pituitary adenomas which may be stimulated to produce and secrete prolactin (PRL) by estrogen (1) and may be suppressed by either the removal of estrogen or the injections of bromocriptine (2) were used to investigate immunohistochemically the alterations in the sub-cellular distribution of PRL under various physiological states. It was found that the normal lactotrophs and adenomas both undergo similar changes in the sub-cellular distribution of PRL under the hyper- and hypo-functional states.

MATERIALS AND METHODS

Adult female Wistar rats were divided into five groups; a) untreated, b) received 5 mg estradiol depot intramuscularly every four weeks for the maximum of six months, c) received estradiol as in the (b) and followed by daily subcutaneous injection of 1 mg bromocriptine (Sandoz) for one week, d) castrated for the maximum of three weeks, e) castrated for three weeks followed by an injection of 5 mg estradiol depot and kept alive for four days. Human PRL secreting pituitary adenomas were obtained at the time of surgery in hospitals of the metropolitan and suburban Tokyo. Anterior pituitary glands of the rat and human pituitary adenomas were fixed in the solution of picric acid and formaldehyde (3) for overnight. The fixed tissues were frozen and sectioned at 4-6 μM in thickness. The sections were mounted on glass slides and were reacted with antisera. Rabbit antiserum against ovine PRL which cross reacts specifically with rat and human PRL was used as the first antibody and horse-radish peroxidase labeled Fab' of goat anti-rabbit IgG was used as the second antibody. The immunostained sections were processed for light and electron microscopy using the pre-embedding method (4). This procedure was used because it could define the intracellular sites of PRL in every cell organelle involved in protein synthesis (5). The serum level of PRL was determined by radioimmunoassay.

RESULTS

In the normal female rat with the serum PRL level of 0.3-0.4 μg/ml, the lactotrophs contained PRL in peri-nuclear space, cisternae of rough endoplasmic reticulum (RER), Golgi saccules (GA) and secretory granules(SG). Four weeks after castration, the serum level of PRL was 0.1 μg/ml. The cytoplasm of lactotrophs was filled with PRL-positive condensed SG. RER and Golgi saccules were reduced in size and contained little or no PRL. Four days after administration of estrogen to the castrated rats, the serum level of PRL was 0.3-0.5 μg/ml. The cytoplasms of lactotrophs were filled with lamellar or whorling RER with PRL. GA and SG were less in number and contained little PRL. At the periphery of the cytoplasm, PRL positive RER were found frequently in juxtaposition to the inner surface of plasm membrane. When the estrogen-induced rat prolactinoma (serum PRL level of over 1 μg/ml) and human prolactinoma (serum PRL level of 0.1-10 μg/ml) were treated with bromocriptine, the serum PRL level was less than 0.1 μg/ml in rats and to 0.01-0.3 μg/ml in some human. With some human sera, the levels of PRL were unchanged following the bromocriptine administration. In the rat prolactinoma and in the human adenoma which responded to the bromocriptine treatment, the sites of PRL was shifted from the cisternae of RER and GA (Figs. 1 and 3) to condensed SG as the number of SG increased and RER and GA atrophied (Figs. 2 and 4). In those human adenomas which did not respond to the bromocriptine treatment, the prolactin containing RER were abundant and the SG were sparse.

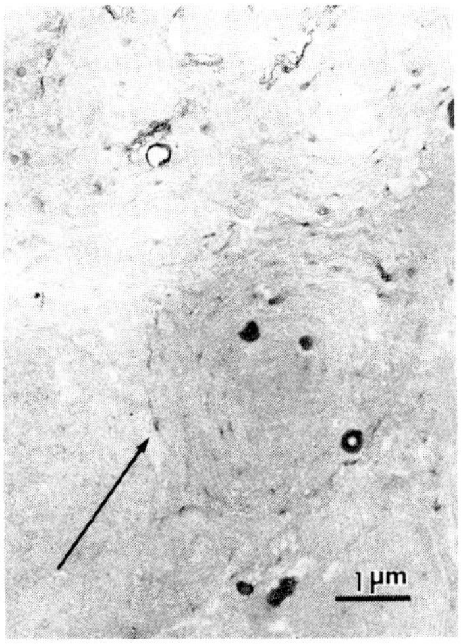

Fig. 1. Estrogen induced rat prolactinoma. (↗) indicates RER.

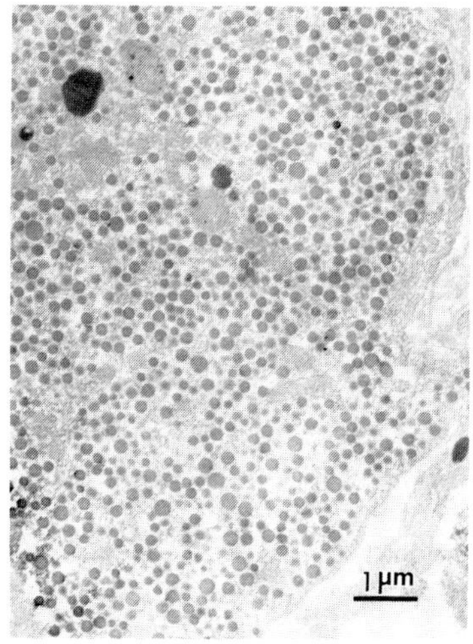

Fig. 2. Bromocriptine treated rat prolactinoma.

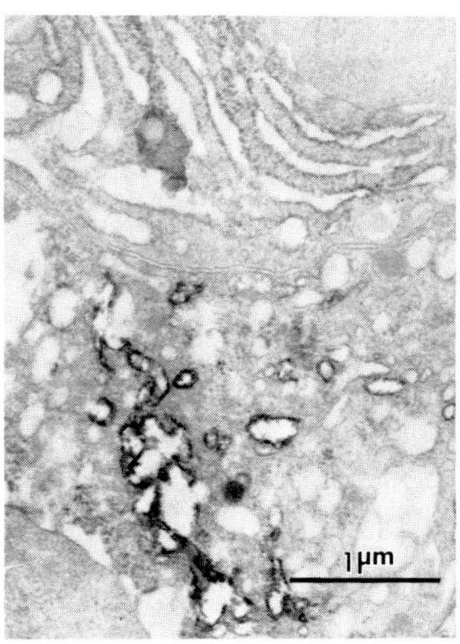

Fig. 3. Human prolactinoma.

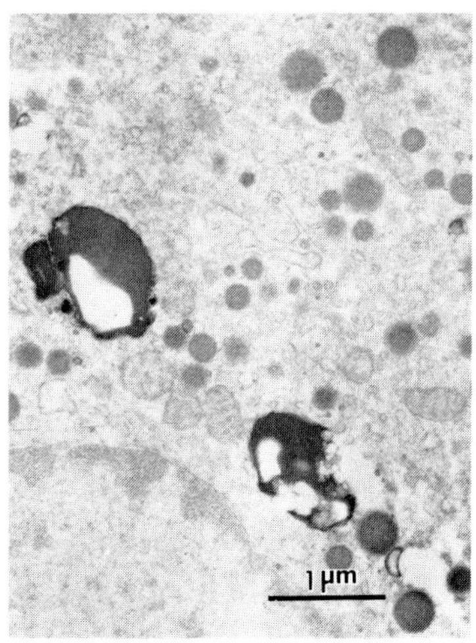

Fig. 4. Bromocriptine treated human prolactinoma.

DISCUSSION

At the ultrastructural level, the hyper-functional state of the lactotrophs induced by the estrogen administration was characterized by the well developed PRL containing RER and reduction in the numbers of SG. On the other hand, the hypo-functional state of the lactotrophs induced by the castration or by the administration of bromocriptine was characterized by the atrophy of RER and accumulation of SG. Depending upon the functional phase of lactotrophs, the size, shape and number of SG and possibly the content of PRL in each SG varied considerably and it was difficult even to define the cell types without the aid of immunoelectron microscopy.

The prolactin secreting rat pituitary adenomas underwent the alterations identical with the hyper- and hypo-functional changes associated with the normal lactotrophs. With the prolactin secreting human pituitary adenomas of those responded to the bromocriptine treatments, the cells entered the hypo-functional state similar to that seen with the rat. However, of those failed to respond, the hyper-functional state persisted. These observations suggested that the bromocriptine treatment shifts the hyper-functional state to the hypo-functional state of the lactotrophs. The differences in the response to the bromocriptine treatment may have resulted from the quantitative differences of dopamine receptors on the adenomas, since the bromocriptine is a potent dopamine agonist (6), although the receptors were not quantitated in this study.

REFERENCES

1. Chen C, Meites J (1970) Endocrinology 86: 503-505
2. Del Pozo E, Brun Del Re R, Varga L, Friesen H (1972) J Clin Endocrinol Metab 35: 768-771
3. Zamboni L, De Marino C (1967) J Cell Biol 25:148A
4. Nakane PK (1973) In: Wisse E, Daems WT, Molenaar I, van Duijn P (eds) Electron microscopy and Cytochemistry. North-Holland, Amsterdam, 129-143
5. Osamura RY, Komatsu N, Izumi S, Yoshimura S, Watanabe K (1982) J Histochem Cytochem 30: 919-925
6. Pasteels JL, Danguy A, Frerotte M, Ectors F (1977) Ann Endocrinol 32:188-192

Endocrinology
F. Labrie, L. Proulx, eds.

THE ROLE OF PHOSPHOLIPID HYDROLYSIS IN THE RELEASE OF PROLACTIN FROM ANTERIOR PITUITARY CELLS

R.M. MacLEOD, A.M. JUDD, K. KOIKE, P.L. CANONICO, AND I.S. LOGIN
University of Virginia School of Medicine, Charlottesville, Virginia 22908 USA

INTRODUCTION

An important function is being recognized for phospholipids and long-chain fatty acids, particularly arachidonate (AA), in regulating hormone release from secretory cells including the anterior pituitary (1-5). The phosphatidylinositol (PI) cycle consists of the enzymatic metabolism of PI and/or polyphosphoinositides to diacylglycerol (DG), subsequently transformed into phosphatidic acid, and finally reconverted to PI. Acceleration of this process is associated with the release of hormones from several tissues (1,2,4). A series of intermediate products are produced via the PI cycle that may have important functions in hormone release (6). Among these products is AA, that can be released from phospholipids directly by phospholipase A_2 or that can be released from intermediates of the PI cycle (2,3,5).

In this overview we present data on the effects of TRH and dopamine on pituitary phospholipid turnover and AA release. The role that DG and AA may play in prolactin release will also be examined.

RESULTS

TRH-induced prolactin release is associated with an increased turnover of pituitary phospholipids (4). Dopamine inhibits the in vivo and in vitro release of prolactin and we designed studies to determine whether this effect is associated with changes in pituitary lipid metabolism. The data in Table 1 demonstrate that dopamine decreases basal and TRH-stimulated ^{32}P-incorporation into PI. Hence the TRH-induced increase in prolactin is associated with an increase in PI turnover while dopamine decreases basal and TRH-induced increases in PI turnover and prolactin release.

AA is released from actively secreting tissues (2,3,5). The data presented in Table 1 show that AA is released from the phospholipids of pituitary cells preincubated with ^{3}H-AA. The presence of TRH stimulates AA release while dopamine has little effect on basal, but inhibits the TRH-stimulated release of the fatty acid. This increase in AA release promoted by TRH occurs within one minute of exposing the cells to TRH and TRH increases arachidonate release over the same concentration range that the peptide increases prolactin release (data not presented). Dopamine inhibits TRH-induced arachidonate and prolactin release over a similar concentration range.

TABLE 1

Effects of TRH and dopamine on hemipituitary incorporation of ^{32}P into phosphatidylinositol and on release of 3H-arachidonic acid from primary cultured pituitary cells

Hemipituitary Glands		Primary Cultured Cells	
Treatment	cpm ^{32}P-phosphatidylinositol	Treatment	dpm ^{3}H-arachidonate
Vehicle	312 ± 13	Vehicle	600 ± 20
TRH 100 nM	427 ± 20[a]	TRH 1 uM	920 ±40[a]
Dopamine 500 nM	176 ± 10[a]	Dopamine 1 uM	545 ± 10
TRH + dopamine	303 ± 14[b]	TRH + dopamine	583 ± 35[b]

[a] $p < 0.01$ vs. vehicle [b] $p < 0.01$ vs. TRH

AA appears to be an important component in the process of prolactin release because agents that reduce AA metabolism also decrease prolactin secretion; conversely, addition of exogenous AA or the release of endogenous AA by phospholipase-A_2 stimulates prolactin secretion (Table 2).

Specifically quinacrine, an inhibitor of phospholipase A_2 activity (3), and RHC 80267, an inhibitor of the lipase that promotes the release of AA from DG (7), both inhibit basal and TRH-induced prolactin release. The AA-induced prolactin release may be mediated via AA metabolites because BW755c, an inhibitor of AA metabolism (5), decreases basal, TRH-, AA-, or phospholipase A_2-induced prolactin secretion. AA is metabolized by numerous enzymatic pathways including the cyclooxygenase pathway to prostaglandins and the lipoxygenase pathway to leukotrienes (8). We propose that AA metabolites responsible for the effects on prolactin secretion are lipoxygenase products because the cyclooxygenase blocker indomethacin has no effect on basal or TRH-induced and potentiates the AA-induced release of prolactin. Furthermore, nordihydroguaiaretic acid (NDGA), a lipoxygenase blocker (5) inhibits basal, TRH-, AA-, and phospholipase A_2-induced prolactin release. A second lipoxygenase inhibitor, nafazatrom (8), also inhibits basal prolactin release.

Diacylglycerol is a product of PI hydrolysis and is a potent activator of protein kinase C (PKC), an important factor in the secretory activity of several cells (9,10). Addition of synthetic DG, 1-oleoyl-2-acetyl-glycerol, or the potent PKC activator phorbol myristate acetate (PMA, ref.9) to cultured pituitary cells stimulates prolactin release (Table 3). Dopamine not only

TABLE 2

Effect on prolactin release of agents that modify arachidonate metabolism

	Prolactin release from hemipituitary (% of control)			
	Vehicle	TRH 100 nM	Phospholipase-A_2 10 mU/ml	Arachidonate 100 uM
Control	100 ± 15	183 ± 17	200 ± 12	156 ± 20
Quinacrine 50 uM	14 ± 07[a]	18 ± 05[b]	----	----
NDGA 50 uM	43 ± 05[a]	29 ± 06[b]	55 ± 08[c]	36 ± 06[d]
BW755c 250 uM	43 ± 10[a]	30 ± 12[b]	48 ± 06[c]	39 ± 07[d]
Indomethacin 50 uM	111 ± 15	185 ± 10	----	189 ± 12[e]
RHC 80267 60 uM	14 ± 03[a]	40 ± 05[b]	----	----
Nafazatrom 60 uM	40 ± 5[a]	----	----	----

$p < 0.01$ vs control (a), TRH (b), A2 (c), AA(e) $p < 0.05$ vs AA (d)

reduces basal prolactin release but abolishes DG- or PMA-stimulated hormone release. We speculate that DG released during phospholipid hydrolysis increases prolactin release by activating PKC and that dopamine decreases prolactin release by decreasing phospholipid turnover, thereby subsequently decreasing the availability of intracellular DG. Dopamine also inhibits prolactin release at some point distal to PKC activation by DG.

Calcium (Ca^{2+}) is required for basal and TRH-induced prolactin release (4) and may interact with the phospholipid-arachidonate system at several points. Although Ca^{2+} is not requisite for the TRH-induced increase in PI turnover (4), extracellular Ca^{2+} is necessary for TRH to stimulate AA release (data not presented). Therefore Ca^{2+} mobilization by TRH may cause AA release that in turn may increase prolactin release.

Calcium interacts with PKC to increase the secretory activity of several cells (10). In the pituitary, the presence of calcium ionophore A23187, ineffective by itself, potentiates the prolactin releasing effects of synthetic DG or PMA (Table 3). Therefore small changes in cellular Ca^{2+} concentration may enhance activation of PKC by DG to increase prolactin release. Dopamine may act distal to PKC activation and calcium mobilization since it blocks prolactin secretion induced by ionophore, PMA, or DG (Table 3).

SUMMARY

Phospholipid hydrolysis may play a major role in regulating prolactin

TABLE 3

Effect of synthetic diacylglycerol (DG), phorbol myristate acetate (PMA), and A23187 on prolactin release from cultured pituitary cells

	ng prolactin/well		
	Vehicle	Synthetic DG 100 ug/ml	PMA 100 uM
Control	1116 ± 38	1550 ± 152[c]	2101 ± 108[c]
Dopamine 1 uM	543 ± 102[a]	621 ± 47[a]	528 ± 86[a]
A23187 400 nM	1264 ± 99	2282 ± 104[d]	2951 ± 149[d]
A23187 + dopamine	579 ± 34[b]	795 ± 94[b]	1004 ± 49[b]

[a] $p < 0.01$ vs. control [b] $p < 0.01$ vs. A23187
[c] $p < 0.01$ vs. vehicle [d] $p < 0.01$ vs. control + diacylglycerol or phorbol

release because TRH stimulates while dopamine inhibits PI turnover. In addition to any direct effect of phospholipid hydrolysis, phospholipid metabolites, including arachidonate through its lipoxygenase products and diacylglycerol by activating protein kinase C, may regulate prolactin release. Calcium interacts with phospholipid hydrolysis in that it is requisite for TRH-induced prolactin and arachidonate release and potentiates prolactin release induced by protein kinase C activators. Dopamine inhibits prolactin release by interacting with the phsopholipid system at multiple points including phospholipid turnover and arachidonate release and may have effects late in the stimulus-secretion coupling process.

REFERENCES

1. Berridge MJ (1981) Mol Cell Endocrinol 24:115
2. Marshall PJ, Dixon JF, Hokin LB (1980) Proc Natl Acad Sci USA 77:3292
3. Naor Z, Catt KJ (1981) J Biol Chem 256:2226
4. Sutton CA, Martin TFJ (1982) Endocrinology 110:1273
5. Naor Z, Vanderhoek JY, Lindner HR, Catt KJ (1983) In: Samuelsson B, Paoletti R, Ramwell P (eds) Advances in Prostaglandin, Thromboxane, and Leukotriene Research, Vol. 12. Raven Press, New York, pp 259-63
6. Thomas AP, Alexander J, Williamson JR (1984) J Biol Chem 259:5574
7. Sutherland CA, Amin D (1982) J Biol Chem 257:14006
8. Honn KV, Busse WD, Sloane BF (1983) Biochem Pharmacol 32:1
9. Castagna M, Takai Y, Kaibuchi K, Sano K, Kikkawa U, Nishizuka Y (1982) J Biol Chem 257:7847
10. Kaibuchi K, Takai Y, Sawamura M, Hoshijima M, Fujikura T, Nishizuka Y (1983) J Biol Chem 258:6701

© 1984 Elsevier Science Publishers B.V.
Endocrinology
F. Labrie, L. Proulx, eds.

REGULATORY SEQUENCES IN THE HUMAN PROLACTIN GENE

J.A. MARTIAL, A.T. TRUONG, P. ELIARD*, M. MATHY-HARTERT, G.G. ROUSSEAU*, and A. BELAYEW

Laboratoire de Génie Génétique (B6) Université de Liège B-4000 Sart Tilman,Belgium.
*Unité Hormones et Métabolisme, International Institute of Cellular and Molecular Pathology, 75, avenue Hippocrate, B-1200 Brussels, Belgium

INTRODUCTION

Prolactin (PRL), growth hormone (GH) and placental lactogen (CS) are polypeptide hormones which have evolved from a common ancestor protein. They share not only sequence homologies but also several biological and immunological properties.

Despite their homologies, the genes coding for these hormones are expressed and regulated in their own way. CS is constitutively expressed in the placenta. PRL and GH are expressed in different cells of the anterior pituitary where they are regulated, generally in opposite direction, by a variety of hormones. As an example, glucocorticoids stimulate GH and inhibit PRL synthesis. These regulations could be mediated at the transcriptional level, although definite evidence has not been obtained yet.

As it is well know now, glucocorticoid action is mediated by specific intracellular receptors which, upon association with the steroid, interact with DNA containing nuclear sites. These sites could be the DNA itself since, using the murine mammary tumor virus (MMTV) system, it has been shown that purified hormone receptor complexes selectively associate *in vitro*, with pure MMTV DNA (Scheideret *et al*, 1983; Payvar *et al*, 1983). It has furthermore been shown in this system, that one of the binding regions, which was located near the transcription start site, was in fact, *in vivo*, a glucocorticoid dependent transcriptional enhancer element (Hynes *et al*, 1983)

In this paper, we are going to : first, review the characteristics of the hPRL gene; second, analyse the first experiments which show that there is a specific region within the hPRL gene which interacts with the human glucocorticoid receptor; and third, present data analysing the "enhancer" activity of the various regions of the hPRL gene. Putting all these results together might suggest that the glucocorticoids inhibit PRL expression because the glucocorticoid-receptor complex, by binding on the hPRL gene, would interfere with the activity of its endogenous enhancing elements.

THE HUMAN PROLACTIN GENE

A few years ago, we cloned in bacteria the DNA copy (cDNA) of the messenger RNA coding for hPRL (Cooke *et al*, 1981). Recently, we used this cloned cDNA to screen a human genomic DNA library in phage lambda and we isolated a recombinant phage containing the whole hPRL gene. We characterized this gene (Truong *et al*, 1984) by restriction endonuclease mapping, DNA heteroduplex analysis at the electron microscope and by nucleotide sequencing. Figure 1 shows a very simplified restriction map of the hPRL gene where only EcoRI sites are represented. The gene is about 10 Kb long and contains 4 introns. It is located on chromosome 6 as a single copy per haploid genome. We also determined its origin of transcription by S1 nuclease mapping.

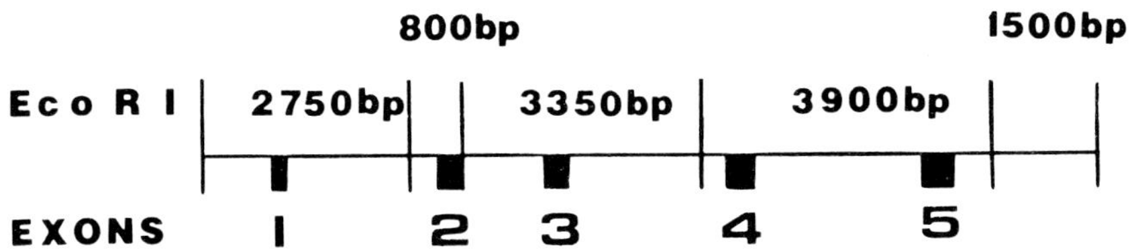

Fig. 1. EcoRI restriction map of the human prolactin gene.

When the 5'sequences of the hPRL gene are compared to their rat counterpart, several non coding regions of significant length show more than 90% homology whereas the average homology of the coding regions is only 73%.

This sequence conservation in non coding regions strongly suggests that some DNA regions are of great importance for the regulation of the gene expression.

SEARCH FOR SPECIFIC INTERACTION BETWEEN THE PURIFIED HUMAN GLUCOCORTICOID RECEPTOR AND THE CLONED hPRL GENE

The first approach we choose to characterize more precisely these DNA regions involved in the gene regulation was to look at the *in vitro* interaction between the gene and a purified regulatory protein.

The human glucocorticoid receptor was purified from a spleen homogenate by sequential chromatography on a phosphocellulose and an affinity column. After these two steps, the receptor was about 30 to 50% pure as estimated by electrophoresis on SDS-polyacrylamide gel.

Once activated, the purified hormone-receptor complex did bind MMTV LTR DNA (Kindly provided by B. Groner) with about ten times higher affinity than unspecific DNA, represented in our nitrocellulose binding assay by the plamid pBR325 (Figure 2). When the EcoRI fragments of the hPRL gene were compared to the MMTV LTR and pBR325 DNA one of them definitely singled out by showing at least 5 times more affinity than the others for the activated hormone-receptor complex. This fragment is the most upstream in the gene, containing the promoter region, the first exon and two thirds of the first intron. We are currently focusing on the exact binding site.

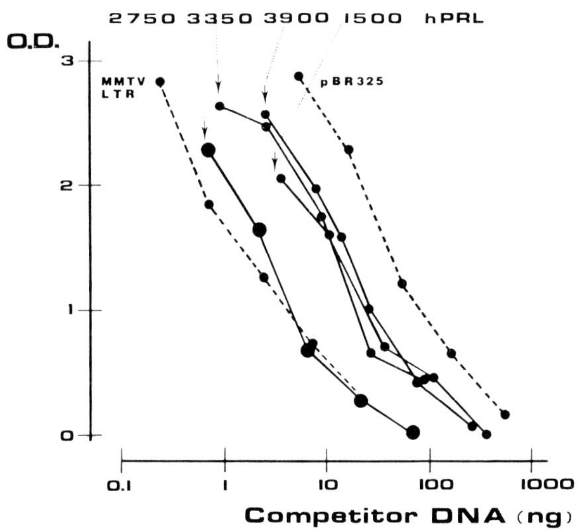

Fig. 2. Nitrocellulose retention of radioactive MMTV LTR DNA bound to activated human glucocorticoid receptor complex in the presence of increasing concentrations of the unlabelled competitor DNA fragments indicated. Autoradiographies of radioactive nitrocellulose filters were scanned in a densitometer to give optical density values.

SEARCH FOR DNA REGIONS WITHIN THE hPRL GENE DISPLAYING ENHANCER ACTIVITY

To answer this question, we used a pSV2CAT transfection assay. In the pSV2CAT (kindly provided by P. Gruss) vector constructed by Gorman *et al* (1982), the structural part of the bacterial chloramphenicol acetyl transferase gene is under the control of the SV40 early promoter and the SV40 72bp repeat enhancers. 24 hours after transfecting the pSV2CAT DNA in HeLa cells the CAT enzymatic activity is assayed according to Gorman *et al* (1982).

We estimated the enhancing activity of the EcoRI fragments of the hPRL gene by substituting each of them for the 72 bp repeat SV40 enhancers in the pSV2CAT vector and measuring the CAT enzymatic activity 24 hours after transfection in HeLa cells. The results are shown in table 1. Four out of five fragments display an enhancing activity in our assay.

This positive result could be correlated with the naturally high level of expression of the hPRL gene in the absence of physiological negative regulations such as that provided by dopamine, etc...

We are currently checking that these 4 hPRL fragments are *bona fide* "enhancer" (*i.e.* function in either orientation, upstream or downstream from the promoter; reviewed by Gruss, 1984) before focusing on the precise DNA regions which display this activity.

TABLE 1.

ENHANCING ACTIVITY OF EcoRI FRAGMENTS FROM THE hPRL GENE

	Controls		5'		hPRL		3'
Fragment assayed for enhancing activity	SV40 72bp repeat	None	2750	800	3350	3900	1500
CAT enzymatic activity in transfected cells	++++	-	+	++	++	-	+++

CONCLUSIONS

The hPRL gene, whose expression is negatively regulated by the glucocorticoids has at least one high affinity binding site for the glucocorticoid-receptor complex located in its 5' region. It comprizes also several enhancing sequences which are mainly located within the structural part of the gene. A possible interpretation of these results is that glucocorticoids down regulate the transcription of the hPRL gene by physically interfering with the natural enhancing activity of the gene itself.

ACKNOWLEDGEMENTS

This work was supported by a grant "Actions concertées génie génétique 81/86" from the Belgian Government. We thank B. Groner and P. Gruss for providing MMTV LTR and pSV2CAT plasmids, as well as T.Vissers for typing assistance.

REFERENCES

- Cooke, N.E. *et al* (1981) J. Biol. Chem. 256, 4007-4016.
- Gorman, C. *et al* (1982) Mol. Cell. Biol. 2, 1044-1051.
- Gruss,P. (1984) DNA 3, 1-5.
- Hynes, N.E. *et al* (1983) Proc. Natl. Acad. Sci. USA. 80, 3637-3641.
- Payvar, F. *et al* (1983) Cell, 35, 381-392.
- Scheideret, C. *et al* (1983) Nature, 304, 749-752.
- Truong, A.T. *et al* (1984) EMBO J. 3, 429-437.

Endocrinology
F. Labrie, L. Proulx, eds.

THE MECHANISM OF ACTION OF PROLACTIN ON CASEIN GENE EXPRESSION

LOUIS-MARIE HOUDEBINE, JEAN DJIANE, PAUL A. KELLY[+], MASAO KATOH[+], ISABELLE DUSANTER-FOURT, PAULE MARTEL

Laboratoire Physiologie de la Lactation, INRA-CNRZ-78350 Jouy-en-Josas, France.
+ Laboratoire d'Endocrinologie Moléculaire, Hopital Royal Victoria,Montréal,Canada

Prolactin has many known functions but its mechanism of action is studied essentially in the mammary gland. In this tissue, prolactin induces cell multiplication it stimulates milk protein gene expression and it provokes the hypertrophy of the epithelial cells. The first two effects can be obtained at physiological concentrations in organ culture, at least in the rabbit. These effects are thus mediated via a direct action of the hormone on the mammary cells.

Prolactin induces casein synthesis and accumulation of casein mRNAs. This accumulation results in part from a stimulation of casein gene transcription (1,2). These effects are amplified by glucocorticoids and inhibited by progesterone. Insulin has also recently been shown to be indispensable in mouse for prolactin to induce casein synthesis (3). In rabbit and ewe, a low but significant induction takes place in the absence of insulin (Fig.1), which is never active alone. Prolactin is therefore the inducer and insulin an amplifier. The maximum stimulation in rabbit and ewe is obtained with concentrations of insulin as high as 5µg/ml and it is coincident with the accumulation of casein mRNA (Fig.2). This suggests that a large part of the stimulation is not due to a strictly physiological insulin effect. Both rabbit and ewe are also stimulated in the absence of glucocorticoids which appear somewhat more active in the ewe than in the rabbit (Fig.1). The mouse which requires both insulin and glucocorticoids to be stimulated by prolactin appears therefore rather poorly sensitive to prolactin. Moreover, ewe requires about 1000 ng/ml ovine prolactin and rabbit only 100 ng/ml to be fully stimulated. Interestingly, the affinity of the receptors for ovine prolactin is ten times higher in the rabbit than in the ewe whereas, the level of circulating prolactin is about ten times higher in the ewe than in the rabbit.

In attempts to understand the mechanism of action of prolactin on the induction of DNA synthesis and of casein gene expression, the effects of various chemical compounds were studied. The results of these experiments are summarized in table 1. Among the conclusions which can be drawn from these data, it appears that 1°) cAMP and cGMP cannot be considered as mediators, 2°) mechanisms involving the action of calmodulin, kinase C or phospholipases do not seem to be involved, 3°) the down-regulation of prolactin receptors is not necessary, 4°) several drugs altering microtubule integrity are inhibitory whereas others are not, which suggests that microtubules integrity is not strictly required but tubulin might participate to the transfer of the prolactin information into the mammary cell.

TABLE I

Effect of various chemical compounds on the induction of casein and DNA syntheses and on down-regulation of prolactin receptors. The essential of these data have been published in various papers not referenced here.

Drugs	DNA Synthesis	Casein Synthesis	Receptor Down-Regulation	Possible Conclusions
dB cAMP	-	slight inhibition	-	cAMP and cGMP
dB cGMP	-	slight stimulation	-	no mediators
Trifluoperazine	no effect	no effect	-	Calmodulin not involved Kinase C not involved
A 23187	no effect	no effect	no effect	Ca^{++} not involved
Bromophenacyl bromide	no effect	no effect	no effect	Phospholipase not involved
Chlorpromazine	no effect	no effect	no effect	Kinase C not involved
Chloroquine NH_4Cl	no effect	no effect	inhibition	Down-regulation not involved
Bacitracin	no effect	no effect	inhibition	Transglutaminase
Ethylamine	"	"	"	
Dansyl cadaverine	"	"	no effect	not involved
Cytochalasin B	no effect	no effect	no effect	Microfilaments not involved
Microtubule destabilizers	inhibition or no effect	inhibition or no effect	slight inhibition or no effect	-Microtubules not involved - Tubulin possibly involved
Tunicamycin	no effect	no effect	-	Glycosylation not involved
Con A	no effect	no effect	-	some carbohydrates not involved in receptor-PRL recognition
Phorbol esters	inhibition	inhibition	no effect	Kinase C not involved
Butyrate	inhibition	inhibition	no effect	?
Isobutyrate	no effect	no effect	no effect	
Amiloride	inhibition	inhibition	no effect	?
Indomethacin	inhibition	no effect	-	Prostaglandins not involved

Polyclonal antibodies raised against prolactin receptors partially purified from rabbit mammary gland mimic prolactin action on casein and DNA synthesis at low concentration and they provoke the accumulation of casein mRNAs (4). They inhibit prolactin actions and their own actions at high concentrations (Fig.2) (4). $F(ab')_2$ fragments prepared from the anti-receptor antibodies act as the

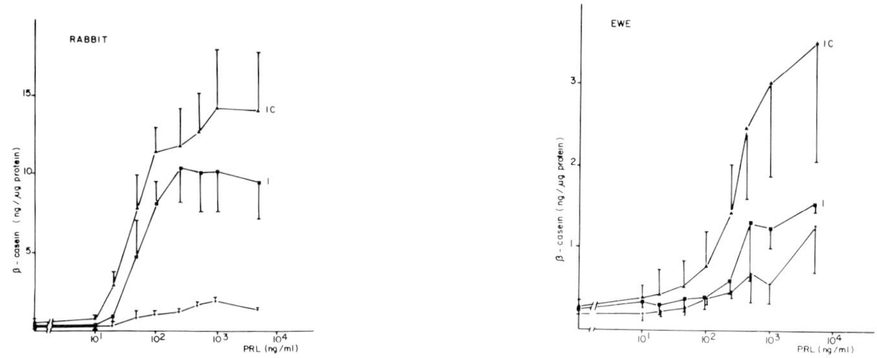

Fig.1. Effect of insulin (5 μg/ml) prolactin and cortisol (500 ng/ml) on the induction of β-casein synthesis.

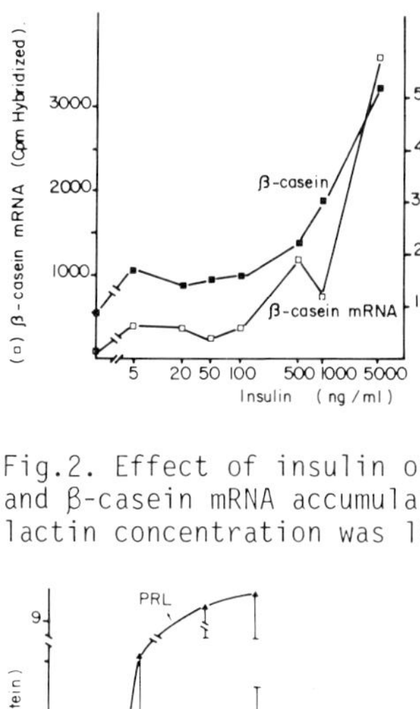

Fig.2. Effect of insulin on β-casein and β-casein mRNA accumulation. Prolactin concentration was 100 ng/ml.

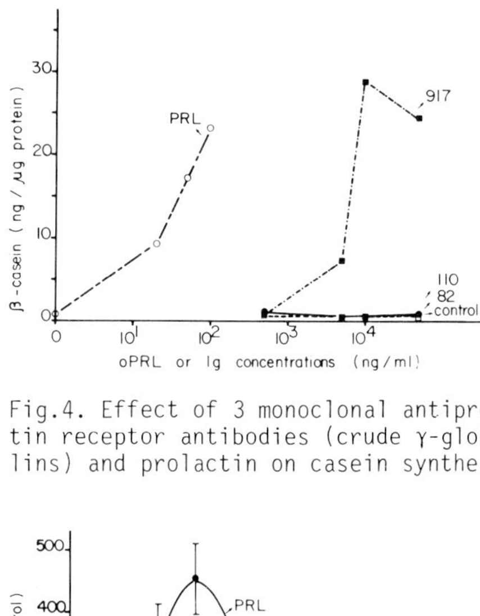

Fig.4. Effect of 3 monoclonal antiprolactin receptor antibodies (crude γ-globulins) and prolactin on casein synthesis.

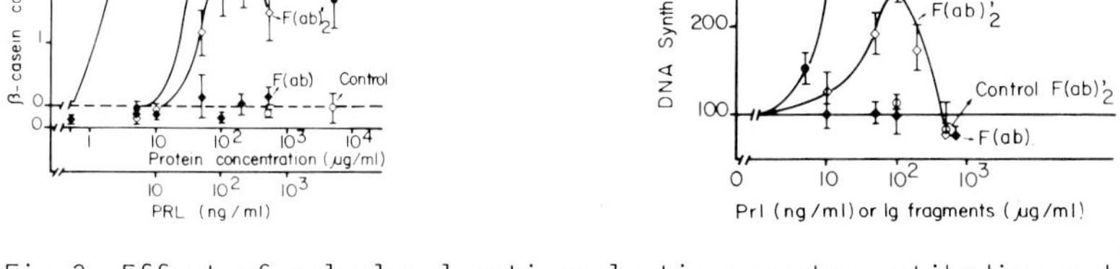

Fig.3. Effect of polyclonal anti-prolactin receptor antibodies and their derivatives on rabbit casein and DNA synthesis.

unmodified immunoglobulins whereas the monovalent Fab derivatives are devoid of activity (Fig.2) (5) although the three forms of antibody are equally active to inhibit the binding of prolactin to its receptors and to provoke their down-regulation (5). The exact meaning of these observations is not known. A clear comparison with prolactin effect is not simple since the hormone is generally considered as acting in monomeric form. Monoclonal antibodies against prolactin receptors compete with prolactin for the binding to receptors from mammary gland, testis, ovary and adrenal. Two of these antibodies cross-react with receptors from sow and but not from ewe and rat. The three monoclonal antibodies inhibit prolactin action on casein synthesis but only one of them has a marked prolactin like activity (Fig.3). These observations clearly demonstrate 1°) that the prolactin molecule is not necessary beyond the receptor, 2°) that an information starts from the receptor to genes, as soon as the receptor is properly stimulated by a ligand having a high specificity and a high affinity. Moreover, the various monoclonal antibodies allow to discriminate binding from active sites in the prolactin receptor.

All these data support the view that a mediator is formed or that a mechanism is activated at the membrane level when the receptor is occupied. Results of table 1 suggest that none of the classical mechanisms known for protein hormone can account for prolactin action in the mammary cell. Several years ago, we have suggested that the prolactin intracellular mediator which acts on casein genes might be a small peptide which is released from membranes under the influence of the hormone. Experimental data supporting this hypothesis have been published (6) A recent reevaluation of the problem has shown that many of these data cannot be reproduced by all members of both laboratories. The existence of the identified prolactin mediator must therefore be considered as not strictly established until new experiments have been carried out. It remains our major working-hypothesis.

REFERENCES

1. Guyette WA, Matusik RJ, Rosen JM (1979) Cell 17:1013-1023.
2. Teyssot B, Houdebine LM (1980) Eur. J. Biochem. 110:263-272.
3. Bolander FF, Nicholas KR, Vanwyck JJ, Topper YJ (1981) Proc. Natl. Acad. Sci. USA 78:5682-5684.
4. Djiane J, Houdebine LM, Kelly PA (1981) Proc. Natl. Acad. Sci. USA 78:7445-7448.
5. Dusanter-Fourt I, Kelly PA, Houdebine LM, Teyssot B (1984) Endocr. 114:1021-1027.
6. Teyssot B, Houdebine LM, Djiane J (1981) Proc. Natl. Acad. Sci. USA 78:563-568.

9. Regulation of Aldosterone Secretion

Endocrinology
F. Labrie, L. Proulx, eds.

REGULATION OF ALDOSTERONE PRODUCTION BY A NEW ALDOSTERONE-STIMULATING FACTOR

EMMANUEL L. BRAVO
Research Division, Cleveland Clinic Foundation, 9500 Euclid Avenue, Cleveland, OH 44106 (United States)

SUMMARY

Clinical and experimental studies suggest the presence of an "unidentified" compound that stimulates aldosterone production. The glycoprotein fraction (26,000 daltons) isolated from normal human urine appears to be an excellent candidate. In the last three years, we have accumulated evidence which strongly indicates that this compound is a true aldosterone secretagogue and that its steroidogenic properties are readily distinguishable from those of ACTH, Ang II, and β-LPH. However, major questions remain as to how it is regulated and its significance in man and his disease.

INTRODUCTION

The secretion of aldosterone by the adrenal zona glomerulosa is controlled by a complex set of regulators that includes the renin-angiotensin system, extracellular sodium and potassium, pituitary peptides and other less well-defined factors. Although angiotensin II appears to be the main regulator of zona glomerulosa function, there are several clinical and experimental conditions in which angiotensin II cannot explain the changes in aldosterone secretion. Of particular relevance is the inability of angiotensin II to reproduce the levels of aldosterone secretion observed during sodium restriction (1, 2). Furthermore, increases in aldosterone secretion during progressive sodium loss have been observed under conditions in which renin production is inhibited by infusion of angiotensin II into the renal artery (3), and when plasma angiotensin II levels are maintained at a constant level by systemic infusion of the peptide.

In 1977, Sen et al (4) reported the isolation of a glycoprotein fraction from normal human urine, which when injected chronically over a period of 10-15 days in a normal rat produced sustained hypertension. The hypertension was accompanied by expansion of plasma volume, retention of sodium, suppression of renin, hypertrophy of the adrenal cortex and increased circulating aldosterone. It had no effect on adrenalectomized animals, suggesting it is not directly pressor and that its hypertensive action is mediated through the adrenal cortex. Since that initial description, the compound has been more fully purified and characterized. It has now been determined to be a glycoprotein of anterior pituitary origin with a molecular weight of about 26,000 daltons; its chromatographic and electrophoretic mobilities are distinguishable from those of ACTH, Ang II, or β-LPH (4). This report summarizes the steroidogenic properties of this new aldosterone stimulating factor (ASF).

METHODS

Studies were performed in collagenase-dispersed adrenal capsular cells harvested from male, New Zealand white rabbits that were on either regular or low sodium diets for 7-10 days. Adrenal capsular cell suspensions were prepared by the method described by Fredlund et al (5).

Incubation studies were performed in polyethylene scintillation counting vials at 37°C under 95% O_2 and 5% CO_2 for 2 hours in a Dubnoff metabolic shaker. Diluent for test substances was medium 199 containing BSA (2 mg/ml) and potassium (4 mEq/L). Approximately 200,000 cells in medium 199 and 0.1 ml of diluent with or without the test substance was added to each vial for a final volume of 1.0 ml and the incubation run in duplicate. After incubating, the medium was transferred to plastic tubes.

Aldosterone was measured by a commercially available radioimmunoassay kit. The interassay and intraassay variability is 10% and 7%, respectively.

The agonist concentrations required to elicit the half maximum aldosterone responses (ED_{50}) were determined by computer analysis using a four parameter logistic function. The data are expressed as mean ± SEM. Statistical evaluation of the results was performed by Student's t-test and analysis of variance.

RESULTS AND DISCUSSION

In initial studies (6) we found that ASF produced dose-related increases in aldosterone and cortisol production following incubation at 37°C for 2 hours. However, its effect was not as potent as either angiotensin II or III. In addition, its steroidogenic effect was not associated with increases in cyclic AMP, could not be inhibited by specific competitive antagonist of angiotensin II and could be prevented by the absence of potassium in incubation media. These preliminary results suggested that the compound initiates steroidogenesis by mechanisms similar to that of angiotensin II; however, the inability to block its effect on steroidogenesis with a specific competitive antagonist of angiotensin II provides evidence of its action on a separate receptor site. We also found that while a specific competitive antagonist of ACTH, (Ile^9) ACTH inhibited the response to both ACTH and beta-lipotropin, it had no effect on ASF-induced increases in aldosterone production. This strongly suggested that the new ASF interacts with receptor sites distinct from those of either ACTH or beta-lipotropin.

In more recent studies (7), the requirements for its in vitro steroidogenic activity have been more clearly defined. We found that urinary ASF is less potent (ED_{50} = 10^{-9}M) than either angiotensin II (ED_{50} = $8x10^{-11}$M) or ACTH (ED_{50} = $4x10^{-11}$M). Increases in cyclic AMP accompanied the steroidogenic response to ACTH but not to either urinary ASF or Ang II. Deprivation of potassium or calcium in incubation media or the addition of ouabain (1 mM) during incubation completely inhibited the steroidogenic response to either urinary ASF, ACTH, or Ang II. However, the aldosterone-stimulating activity of ASF did not appear to be as dependent on potassium concentration in media as that of angiotensin II. Whereas the aldosterone response to angiotensin II did not reach maximal until the potassium concentration was at least 4.0 mM, urinary ASF produced maximal responses with potassium concentrations of 2.0 mM. At potassium concentrations of 8.0 mM, the increase in aldosterone achieved was not different from that produced when combined with maximal doses of either Ang II, ACTH or urinary ASF.

Thus the mechanisms by which urinary ASF stimulate aldosterone production are readily distinguishable from ACTH. In the first place, ASF-induced steroid responses are not associated with increased generation of cAMP, while those of ACTH are. Secondly, and more importantly, its ability to stimulate aldosterone production could not be inhibited by (Ile^9) ACTH, a specific competitive antagonist of ACTH. Although it shares some similarities with Ang II, the inability of a specific angiotensin II antagonist to inhibit its steroidogenic activity indicates that it acts at a separate receptor site. Finally, like Ang II and ACTH, urinary ASF is highly dependent on potassium for its steroidogenic action.

More recently we have defined the interaction of ASF with angiotensin II and ACTH during variations of dietary sodium (8). In cells from sodium-replete rabbits, the concentration required to elicit the half maximum response (ED_{50}) was 2.2 ± 0.3 (SE) x 10^{-11}M, 7.2 ± 1.1 x 10^{-10}M and 3.4 ± 0.5 x 10^{-8}M for ACTH, AII, and ASF, respectively. Sodium depletion increased maximal responses but not sensitivity to Ang II and ACTH; responses to ASF were essentially unchanged. Large concentrations of ASF (10^{-7}M) potentiated AII-induced aldosterone responses of adrenal capsular cells from sodium depleted, but not sodium-replete, rabbits. In marked contrast, similar concentrations of ASF inhibited ACTH-induced aldosterone production of adrenal capsular cells from both sodium-replete and sodium-depleted rabbits.

It is concluded that ASF has its own intrinsic steroidogenic activity. Furthermore, although large concentrations of ASF potentiate AII responses in sodium-depleted animals, it inhibits the aldosterone-stimulating activity of ACTH in both sodium-replete and sodium-deplete animals.

REFERENCES

1. Aguilera G, Catt KJ (1983) J Steroid Biochem 19:525-530
2. Boyd GW, Adamson AR, Arnolds M, James VHT, Peart WS (1972) Clin Sci 49:91-104
3. Blair-West JR, Coghlan JP, Denton DA, Scoggins BA (1974) In: Page IH, Bumpus FM (eds) Angiotensin. Springer-Verlag, New York, pp 337-368
4. Sen S, Bravo EL, Bumpus FM (1977) Circ Res 40 (Suppl I):5-10
5. Fredlund P, Saltman S, Catt KS (1975) Endocrinology 97:1577
6. Bravo EL, Saito I, Zanella MT, Sen S, Bumpus FM (1981) J Clin Endocrinol Metab 51:176-178
7. Saito I, Bravo EL, Zanella T, Sen S, Bumpus FM (1981) Hypertension 3:300-305
8. Hata T, Bravo EL, Sen S, Bumpus FM (1984) Endocrinology; submitted for publication.

Endocrinology
F. Labrie, L. Proulx, eds.

PHYSIOLOGICAL REGULATION OF ALDOSTERONE SECRETION IN THE RAT

G.P. VINSON, *B.J. WHITEHOUSE, J.P. HINSON AND P.W. RAVEN

Department of Biochemistry, Medical College of St Bartholomew's Hospital, Charterhouse Square, LONDON EC1M 6BQ and *Department of Physiology, Queen Elizabeth College, Campden Hill Road, LONDON W8 7AH

INTRODUCTION

The control of aldosterone secretion has been widely studied over a period of many years, using a variety of *in vivo* and *in vitro* techniques, including adrenal vein and peripheral plasma sampling, incubation *in vitro* of whole tissue or slices or cell suspensions of varying degrees of purity (1-4). Although it seems likely that dispersed cells may well respond *in vitro* to physiological concentrations of known stimulants, little attention has been paid to the possibility that the nature of the preparation may itself affect the nature of the secretory response, but some evidence suggests that the secreted steroid profile may be different under different conditions (5-7). For these reasons it seemed desirable to develop methods for studying the gland under conditions in which the supply of stimulant can be carefully controlled but in which also the architecture of the gland, including its vasculature, is preserved. This paper describes the function of such a system, the in situ perfused rat adrenal gland, and compares its responses with those of whole tissue and dispersed cells *in vitro*, with particular regard to the actions of the more recently recognised zona glomerulosa effector, α-MSH (8).

MATERIALS AND METHODS

In vitro methods

Using male rats (250-400g), the left adrenal gland was perfused according to the method of Sibley et al (9). Briefly perfusate was introduced through a cannula in the coeliac artery. With other vessels ligated as required, perfusate was thus introduced into an isolated segment of the aorta, from which the adrenal arteries were supplied. A pocket in the renal vein was cannulated to allow collection of the adrenal venous drainage. The gland thus receives only administered perfusate, and is not subject to stimulation by the animals' hypothalamus-pituitary or renin-angiotensin systems. Stimulants were added in 200μl boluses via a syringe attached to the coeliac cannula. Steroids were estimated using glc and RIA techniques as previously described (10,11).

RESULTS AND DISCUSSION

The actions of α-MSH and ACTH in the perfused gland are illustrated in Figs 1 and 2. The results show quite clearly that at low concentrations α-MSH is a specific glomerulosa stimulant and only at higher concentrations behaves like ACTH in stimulating corticosterone as much as aldosterone secretion. Comparison with *in vitro* data emphasises that aldosterone output varies considerably with the nature of the preparation. In general it appears that the more the tissue is dispersed, and the more cells lose contact with one another, the lower the capacity for aldosterone production becomes. In contrast corticosterone is greatly stimulated by specific glomerulosa stimulants in dispersed cells and whole tissue *in vitro* but hardly at all in the intact perfused gland. In these respects, the dispersed cells, intact tissue in vitro, and intact perfused gland, form a series with increasing aldosterone/corticosterone ratios (6,7).

Figure 1.

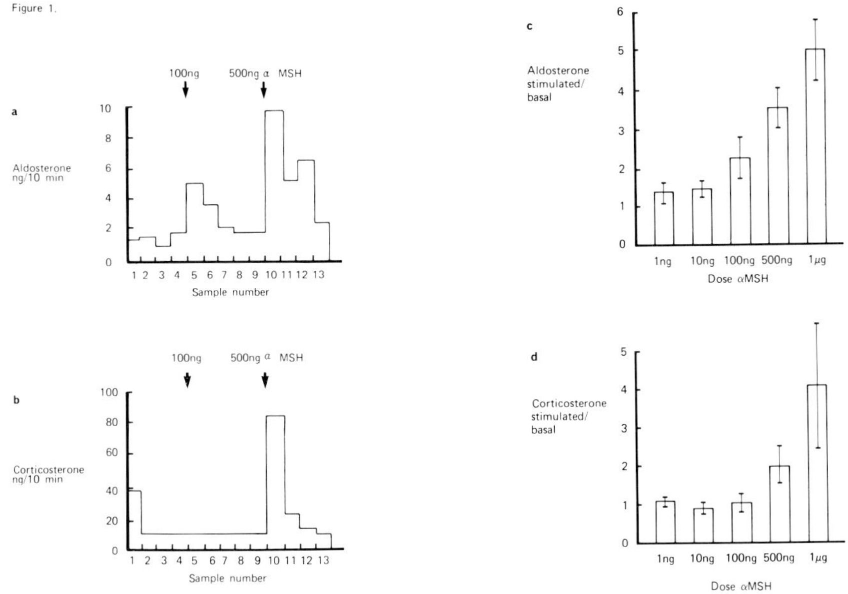

Fig. 1. Response of the perfused rat adrenal gland to stimulation by α-MSH. (a) and (b) represent data from a typical perfusion for aldosterone and corticosterone responses, (c) and (d) represent pooled data from different perfusions for the same two steroids. Data in (c) and (d) are expressed as stimulation ratios. For the different doses, starting at 1ng, numbers of experiments were 6,9,9,4,7 respectively. Aldosterone is more strongly stimulated than corticosterone, especially at lower concentrations of α-MSH; corticosterone is not stimulated at all by 100ng or less of α-MSH, whereas aldosterone invariably is.

From the point of view of studying aldosterone production, it is clearly desirable to retain tissue in as intact a form as possible. The importance of this is demonstrated strongly by the contrast between the actions of α-MSH on dispersed cells from the rat adrenal capsule fraction, and in the intact gland. Peptides of the α-MSH series, as well as other MSH's have recently been shown to be specific effectors acting on the zona glomerulosa at low concentrations, and only

Figure 2.

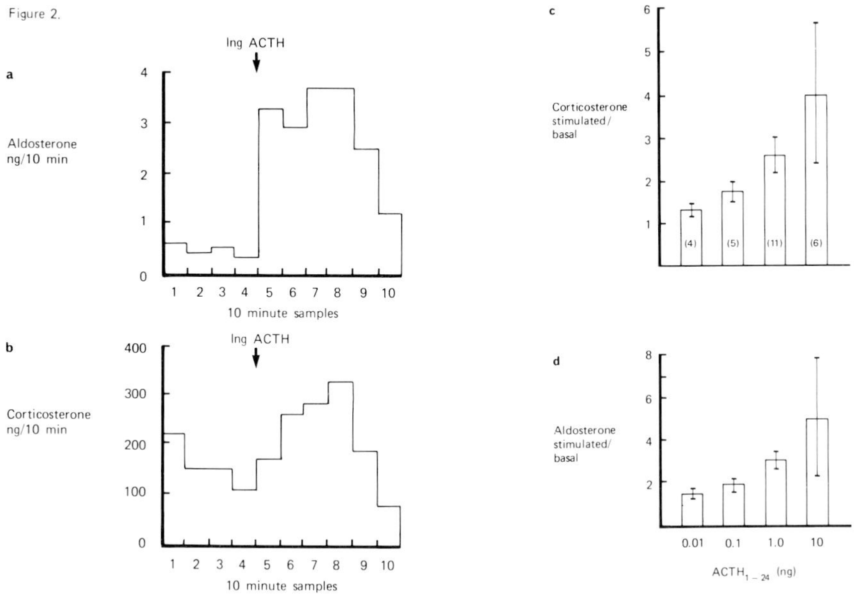

Fig. 2. Responses of perfused rat adrenals to $ACTH_{1-24}$ stimulation. Typical data from a single experiment are shown for aldosterone and corticosterone in (a) and (b); and (as for Fig. 1) pooled data from different experiments are shown in (c) and (d). Numbers in brackets are numbers of experiments. Both steroids are stimulated at all levels of ACTH.

interacting with the fasciculata cells (presumably through the ACTH receptors), at higher concentrations (8,12). Even in zona glomerulosa cells however, these interactions are best shown in corticosterone production values, since corticosterone is stimulated much more strongly. This belies the potential physiological importance of these peptides however, and in the intact perfused gland it is quite clear that only aldosterone is produced in response to α-MSH stimulation at low concentration (Fig. 1). In the intact gland therefore the production of aldosterone is a characteristic of glomerulosa function whereas corticosterone production is not. The increase in corticosterone seen at higher concentrations of α-MSH in the intact perfused gland is similar to the effect of ACTH (Fig. 2) and can be attributed to the interaction of the peptide with fasciculata cells at higher concentrations. In this respect, the function of the perfused gland reflects responses to α-MSH *in vivo* whereas dispersed cells do not (13).

In conclusion, the most important product of the intact zona glomerulosa is aldosterone, and not corticosterone. A reason why this may not appear to be the case in *in vitro* incubation systems, particularly of dispersed cells, is that sequestered, protease-sensitive, stores of aldosterone may be lost during the process of tissue preparation for incubation (6,7,14,15).

ACKNOWLEDGEMENTS

We are most grateful to Drs DM Burley, PA Desaulles and K Scheibli for the provision of ACTH (Synacthen) and α-MSH used in these studies. We are also most grateful to the MRC for project grant support for GPV and BJW.

REFERENCES

1. Vinson GP, Whitehouse BJ (1970) In: Briggs MH (Ed) Advances in steroid biochemistry and pharmacology. Academic Press, New York and London, Vol I, pp 163-342.
2. Muller J (1971) Regulation of aldosterone biosynthesis. Springer Verlag Berlin.
3. Fraser R, Brown JJ, Lever AF, Mason PA, Robertson JIS (1979) Clin. Sci. 56: 389.
4. Tait JF, Tait SAS, Bell JBG (1980) Essays in Biochemistry 16:99.
5. Redmond AF, Bell CC (1974) Endocrinology 94:822.
6. Vinson GP, Whitehouse BJ, Goddard C, Sibley CP (1979) J. Steroid Biochem. 11:175
7. Raven PW, McCredie E, McAuley M, Vinson GP (1983) Cell Biochem. Funct 1:17.
8. Vinson GP, Whitehouse BJ, Dell A, Etienne T, Morris HR (1980) Nature, Lond. 284:464.
9. Sibley CP, Whitehouse BJ, Vinson GP, Goddard C, McCredie E (1981) J. Endocr. 91:313.
10. Vinson GP, Goddard C, Whitehouse BJ (1978) J. Steroid Biochem. 9:657.
11. Vazir H, Whitehouse BJ, Vinson GP, McCredie E (1981) Acta Endocr. (Kbh) 97: 533.
12. Vinson GP, Whitehouse BJ, Dell A, Bateman A, McAuley ME (1983) J. Steroid Biochem. 19:537.
13. Villareal JZ, Shenker Y, Sider RS, Grekin RJ (1983) Proc. 5th Annual Meeting The Endocrine Soc. pp 95.
14. Raven PW, McAuley ME, Vinson GP (1983) J. Endocr. 99:13
15. Raven PW, McCredie E, Vinson GP, Goddard C, Whitehouse BJ, (1982) Biochem. Biophys. Res. Comm. 104:1247.

© 1984 Elsevier Science Publishers B.V.
Endocrinology
F. Labrie, L. Proulx, eds.

INTERACTION OF POTASSIUM AND THE RENIN-ANGIOTENSIN SYSTEM IN THE CONTROL OF ALDOSTERONE SECRETION IN NORMAL AND PATHOPHYSIOLOGIC STATES

MORRIS SCHAMBELAN, ANTHONY SEBASTIAN, EDWARD G. BIGLIERI, AND ROSEMARY HERNANDEZ
General Clinical Research Centers, San Francisco General Hospital and Moffitt Hospital, and the Department of Medicine, University of California, San Francisco, California 94110 (USA)

INTRODUCTION

Aldosterone secretion is controlled by a complex interaction of multiple regulatory factors, that include such diverse influences as the pituitary gland (ACTH, other pro-opiomelanocortin derived peptides, aldosterone stimulating glycoprotein), biogenic amines (dopamine, serotonin), the renin-angiotensin system (both angiotensin II and III) and the circulating and/or intracellular concentrations of various ionic species (Na^+, K^+, Ca^{++}). Of these, the renin-angiotensin system and K^+ appear to be the predominant influences, a dual regulatory mechanism that has been appreciated for at least the past decade (1,2). The purpose of the present study was to determine the relative influences of and interaction between K^+ and the renin-angiotensin system on aldosterone secretion in chronic metabolic balance studies conducted in normal volunteers and in patients with clinical disorders of electrolyte balance.

MATERIALS AND METHODS

All studies were carried out in the General Clinical Research Centers at Moffitt and San Francisco General Hospitals, University of California. The studies were approved by the institutional Committee on Human Research, and informed consent was obtained from each subject.

Effect of Chronic Experimentally-Induced Potassium Depletion

Sixteen normal male volunteers ingested a constant amount of a liquid synthetic diet supplemented with electrolytes, vitamins and essential trace minerals (3). Three separate protocols were utilized in these subjects:

K^+ deprivation on a normal NaCl intake (Group I, N=6)

Throughout this study the constant amount of sodium chloride in the supplement was 1.8 mmoles/kg body wt/day. During the pre-control (4-9 days) and control (6 days) period, K^+ (1.5 mEq/kg) was provided as the neutral phosphate salt. Potassium deprivation was effected by reduction of potassium phosphate and substitution of neutral sodium phosphate in an equimolar amount. The period of K^+ deprivation varied from 6 to 15 days.

K^+ deprivation on a low NaCl intake (Group II, N=6)

This protocol was identical to that in group I except that the constant amount of sodium chloride given throughout the control and experimental periods was $\leq$ 0.1 mEq/kg. All subjects underwent 15 days of K^+ deprivation.

Concomitant deprivation of K^+ and Cl^- (Group III, N=4)

In this protocol Na^+ was administered as the neutral phosphate salt in an amount equal to 1.8 mEq/kg body weight per day. During the control period K^+ was provided as the chloride salt (1.8 mEq/kg) and during the experimental period (12-15 days) this was withheld completely.

Effect of Potassium Retention

For these protocols normal subjects ingested a constant whole food diet which, for each individual protocol, was identical in composition. All subjects ingested the same amount of diet per kg of body weight. The following maneuvers were done in an attempt to produce K^+ retention and hyperkalemia:

Administration of amiloride (N=5)

Dietary Na^+ (1.8 meq/kg) and K^+ (1.2 meq/kg) were constant throughout. After a steady-state control period (7 days) amiloride, 30-40 mg/day, was administered for 10 days.

Administration of indomethacin (N-3)

These subjects ingested a low Na^+ diet (<0.2 mEq/kg) throughout; K^+ intake in all subjects was 1.2 mEq/kg. After a steady state control period (5 days) indomethacin, 150 mg/day, was administered for 11-12 days.

Administration of captopril (N=3)

Dietary Na^+ (1.8 meq/kg) and K^+ (1.2 meq/kg) were constant throughout. After a steady state control period (5 days) captopril, 450 mg/day, was administered for 7 days.

Studies in Patients with Chronic Electrolyte Disorders

All measurements were obtained after the patients had equilibrated on a constant whole food diet. Fourteen patients had chronic hypokalemia due to idiopathic renal potassium wasting (so-called Bartter's syndrome). Eleven patients had chronic hyperkalemia as a consequence of isolated hyporeninemic hypoaldosteronism in the setting of mild to moderate chronic renal insufficiency (4).

Analytical Methods

Urine and plasma samples were obtained every 2-3 days throughout the control and experimental periods. The excretion rate of aldosterone-18-glucuronide was used as an index of aldosterone production inasmuch as this metabolite is a valid index of aldosterone production even in patients with chronic renal insufficiency (4). Samples obtained in fasting subjects after 2 hours of upright activity (following overnight recumbency) were used for measurement of PRA and K^+ levels.

RESULTS AND DISCUSSION

Potassium restriction resulted in the prompt development of hypokalemia that was sustained at similar levels in the three subgroups (Table I) by adjustment of the relative amounts of Na^+ and K^+ phosphate. In groups I and II, in which K^+ was restricted without a change in dietary anion intake, PRA decreased. This suppression of PRA was associated with an increase in renal Cl^- reabsorption as evidenced by a reduction in urinary Cl^- excretion despite an unchanged dietary Cl^- intake. Body Na^+ content also increased. As a consequence of concomitant decreases in plasma K^+ and PRA, aldosterone excretion was decreased markedly in these paradigms. In group III concomitant reduction in K^+ and Cl^- intakes prevented Cl^- retention. PRA levels were unchanged or increased despite Na^+ retention but aldosterone excretion was still suppressed. Thus chronic hypokalemia blunts the aldosterone secretory response to renin and may reduce aldosterone secretion further by stimulating renal Cl^- reabsorption which in turn suppresses renin secretion. With marked degrees of hyperreninemia (30.4± 4.6 ng/ml/hr) such as occurs in Bartter's syndrome, aldosterone levels may be frankly elevated (21.4±2.3 μg/24h) despite similar degrees of hypokalemia (2.7+0.1 meq/L).

TABLE I.
EFFECT OF ALTERED ELECTROLYTE BALANCE IN NORMAL SUBJECTS

	N	PLASMA K^+		PRA_{UP}		$U_{ALDO}V$	
		CONT	EXPT	CONT	EXPT	CONT	EXPT
		mEq/L		ng/ml/hr		μg/24h	
GROUP I	6	4.0	3.0†	4.6	0.4†	15.1	2.0‡
		±0.1	±0.1	±1.1	±0.2	±1.8	±0.4
GROUP II	6	4.2	2.8‡	24.2	14.9*	98.9	9.3‡
		±0.1	±0.1	±2.7	±2.8	±8.7	±2.1
GROUP III	4	4.4	2.8‡	3.2	6.8	15.5	5.1*
		±0.1	±0.1	±0.8	±0.8	±3.0	±1.8
AMILORIDE	5	4.2	5.4†	10.5	71.1†	12.6	240*
		±0.1	±0.3	±1.8	±11.5	±2.2	±56
INDOMETHACIN	3	4.2	4.3	5.9	3.9†	33.9	23.5*
		±0.1	±0.1	±1.7	±1.6	±3.4	±3.9
CAPTOPRIL	3	4.3	4.4	3.3	35.4*	10.2	9.0
		±0.2	±0.2	±0.4	±5.2	±1.0	±0.5

*, †, and ‡ = $p<0.05$, <0.01, and <0.001, respectively, in comparison to control values (Student's t-test for paired variables). Data are mean ± SEM.

In normal subjects a successful model of chronic hyperkalemia was achieved only by administration of amiloride; aldosterone excretion was stimulated profoundly as a consequence of concomitant hyperreninemia (Table I). Neither indomethacin nor captopril resulted in sustained hyperkalemia although PRA and aldosterone levels decreased significantly with the former as did presumably angiotensin II levels with the latter. Patients with hyporeninemic hypoaldosteronism have marked reductions in aldosterone levels (2.6$\pm$0.4 μg/24h) despite hyperkalemia (5.4$\pm$0.2 meq/L) as a consequence of hyporeninemia (0.4$\pm$0.1 ng/ml/hr). These findings accord with the observations that captopril suppresses the acute aldosterone secretory response to K^+ infusions in the dog (5) and results in reduction in urinary aldosterone levels despite hyperkalemia in patients with chronic renal insufficiency (6). Taken together with the results obtained in subjects with hypokalemia our studies support the concept that aldostserone is under dual regulation by K^+ and angiotensin II. The predominant regulatory factor in these chronic studies appear to be the renin-angiotensin system.

ACKNOWLEDGEMENTS

This work was supported in part by NIH grants HL-11046, AM-06415, AM-21605, RR-00083 and RR-00079.

REFERENCES

1. Williams GH, Dluhy RG (1972) Aldosterone biosynthesis: interrelationship of regulatory factors. Am J Med 53:595-605.
2. Laragh JH (1973) Letter to editor: Potassium, angiotensin and the dual control of aldosterone secretion. N Engl J Med 289:745-746.
3. Kurtz I, Maher T, Hulter HN, Schambelan M, Sebastian A (1983): Effect of diet on plasma acid-base composition in normal humans. Kidney Intern 24:670-680.
4. Schambelan M, Sebastian A, Biglieri EG (1980): Prevalence, pathogenesis, and functional significance of aldosterone deficiency in hyperkalemic patients with chronic renal insufficiency. Kidney Intern 17:89-101.
5. Pratt JH (1982) Role of angiotensin II in potassium-mediated stimulation of aldosterone secretion in the dog. J Clin Invest 70:667-672.
6. Textor SC, Bravo EL, Fouad FM, Tarazi RC (1982) Hyperkalemia in azotemic patients during angiotensin-converting enzyme inhibition and aldosterone reduction with captopril. Am J Med 73:719-725.

© 1984 Elsevier Science Publishers B.V.
Endocrinology
F. Labrie, L. Proulx, eds.

SIGNALLING TRANSMISSION PROCESS OF ANGIOTENSIN II AND POTASSIUM IN ADRENAL GLOMERULOSA PLASMA MEMBRANE

ELISA T. MARUSIC AND MARIA V. LOBO
Dept. Physiology and Biophysics, Sch. Medicine, Univ. of Chile
Santiago, Chile

The requirement to transduce an extracellular signal into an intracellular action is implicit in all endocrine cells. Although there is a vast number of hormones that respond to a single specific physiological stimulus, as is the case of ACTH-cortisol, there are examples of multiple control signals involved in hormonal secretion. Studies related to aldosterone reveal that there are several extracellular stimuli involved in its secretion: the renin-angiotensin system, potassium and sodium ions, and ACTH. Also serotonin, β-MSH, β-endorphin nnd enkephalin seem to participate in aldosterone regulation. It is not clear how these extracellular messengers trigger the signalling process for glomerulosa cell activation. That cAMP acts as the mediator for at least some of these stimuli is indicate indirectly by the ability of exogenous cAMP and elevated endogenous cAMP, as induced by ACTH, to increase significantly the aldosterone output. However, the mechanisms by which angiotensin II (A II) and potassium ions (K^+) regulate aldosterone production are not clear.- A II has no effect on adenylcyclase and there is conflicting evidence about the role of cAMP in the action of K^+. The lack of additivity between steroid responses to A II and K^+ has been thought to suggest that these factors could share a common mechanism of action on steroidogenesis. In an attempt to clarify the action of A II and K we have done several studies related to ion movements and steroidogenesis.

Early studies with adrenal quarters and slices suggested that the ionic makeup on the incubation medium, specially with regard to the K^+ content, influenced the release of aldosterone in response to A II and ACTH. The addition of ouabain to the incubation medium inhibited the release of aldosterone under several stimuli. However, we have measured intracellular K under different conditions and found no correlation between tissue K and aldosterone release (1). Furthermore, we have recently induced K depletion in glomerulosa cells down to 10-20 mM K, by low temperature, without changing the aldosterone response to A II. Therefore, intracellular K^+ seems to be less important for aldosterone output than it was thought in the past. We also studied the role of sodium on the aldosterone response and found that the steroidogenic response to A II or K is completed abolished when Na^{+} is absent from the incubation medium. This suggest that a working Na, K-ATPase is necessary in the mechanism of aldosterone secretion.

In view of the ubiquitous role of calcium ions in cell functions, a great deal of work has been directed to study the involvement of Ca^{2+} on steroidogenesis in the adrenal gland. Early work by Birmingham showed that extracellular Ca^{2+} was required in the adrenal response to ACTH. The first criterion fulfilled to implicate Ca^{2+} in the mechanism of action of A II or K^{+} was the demonstration that these two agents do not stimulate aldosterone biosynthesis in the absence of extracellular Ca^{2+} or in the presence of drugs that block Ca^{2+} entry from the extracellular medium (2,3). In fact, expetiments with verapamil, D-600 and La^{3+} block the stimulation of aldosterone. Studies from Catt's group (2) concluded that Ca^{2+} is not necessary for the binding of A II to glomerulosa cells, suggesting that the specific action of Ca^{2+} occurs at a locus after the initial recognition of angiotensin II by its receptors.

The second criterion for a role of Ca^{2+} as an intracellular mediator for the action of A II or K^{+} required demonstration of movements of Ca^{2+} into an active site prior to aldosterone output. By pre-loading cells with $^{45}Ca^{2+}$ and by measurements of the efflux of this isotope to evaluate channel activity, it was demonstrated that opening of a Ca^{2+} channel could be seen at an early time following administration of A II (4,5). On the other hand, we have shown increased $^{45}Ca^{2+}$ uptake with A II, under steady-state conditions and by measurement of the fluxes in the presence of 1.3 mM $^{40}Ca^{2+}$ (3). An enhaced uptake of $^{45}Ca^{2+}$ was also observed by us in the presence of potassium-stimulated aldosterone production (3). The effect of K on the $^{45}Ca^{2+}$ efflux was minimal and not significant (4).- It has been demonstrated that Ca^{2+} Sr^{2+}, and Ba^{2+} may use the same channel to enter chromaffin cells and that this channel is blocked by D-600. We have studied the effect to these divalent cations on steroidogenesis under basal and stimulated conditions. We found a depressed basal production of aldosterone with Sr^{2+} and Ba^{2+} (6). ACTH and A II elicited a minimal response in the presence of Ba^{2+}, but with Sr^{2+} a significant stimulation was observed. Nevertheless, the response obtained was smaller than that with Ca^{2+}. However, K enhacement of aldosterone production was completely blocked in the presence of Sr^{2+} or Ba^{2+}.- Again, these results suggest a dissociation between the mechanisms of action of A II and K on aldosterone stimulation.

The third requirement that involved intracellular Ca^{2+} as a mediator on the action of angiotensin II was the observation that compounds that increase Ca^{2+} levels in the cytosol also stimulate aldosterone. We showed that this occurs when cytosolic Ca^{2+} is increased by the addition of the ionophore A 23187 (Lilly). This response is dose-dependent, and only a narrow range of ionophore concentration (10^{-7} - 10^{-8} M) has a significant effect on steroidogenesis. Higher doses of the ionophore are inhibitory of aldosterone production. Similarly K-stimulate aldosterone release is inhibited by elevated extracellular concentrations of Ca^{2+}. Thus, it appears that a Ca-mediated on-off system is present in the cytosol of glomerulosa cells.

In order to explore possible routes of ion entry into glomerulosa cells we used drugs that exert a direct effect on ion channels. Veratridine, an activator of the Na channel of electrically excitable cells that allows the entrance of extracellular Ca^{2+} upon depolarization, stimulated aldosterone release in static incubations. This stimulus was blocked by tedrotoxin (TTX, 10^{-5} M). However, the stimulation of aldosterone with A II or K was not blocked by TTX. These results and previous data about the requirement of extracellular Na and K plus the inhibitory action of ouabain suggest the need of an electrogenic Na-pump in order to obtain stimulation of aldosterone by different stimuli.- Our data suggest that there is a remarkable functional homology between glomerulosa cells and neural tissue.

Although it is know that large increases in extracellular K^{+} induce cells membrane depolarization in nerve and muscle cells the unique feature of the adrenal glomerulosa cells is that minimal changes in extracellular K^{+} lead to activation of the cell. We have studied the effect that such changes of external K may have on the distribution of the potential-sensitive lipophilic cation, tetraphenyl-phosphonium, both in the presence and in the absence of Ca^{2+}. The results obtained show that small changes in extracellular K^{+} lead to a calcium-dependent depolarization of the membrane (7). We found that the marked depolarization observed with small changes on external K^{+} was specific of glomerulosa tissue. In contrast, no effect was seen in fasciculata cells. These data raise the possibility that an increase in extracellular K^+ activates a specific Ca^{2+} channel in the plasma membrane of these cells. When similar experiments were done in the presence of A II a biphasic response was obtained: a short hyperpolarization of the cells was followed by depolarization (submitted for publication). The observed hyperpolarization suggest that A II could lead either to an activation of the Na, K-ATPase with a concomitant increase in K uptake, or that a change in the membrane conductance for K could occur. The first possibility was studied in our laboratory some time ago and we were not able to detect any change in the enzyme activity, nor in the uptake of Rb^{86} under the effect of A II (8). We have recently found that angiotensin II induces a change in K conductance that is Ca-dependent and that this increased efflux of K from A II-stimulated cells could account for the initial hyperpolarization of the cells.-

Obviously, our knowledge of the role of different ions in the action of steroidogenic agents on glomerulosa cells is currently incomplete. Nevertheless, it now seems clear that Ca^{2+} plays an important role in the activation of aldosterone production. It is of interest to know that A II and K, the two most potent agents, have different signals at the membrane level. It is hopeful that their role will be more fully defined in the near future.

ACKNOWLEDGMENTS

This work was supported by grants from the Univ. of Chile and CONICYT.

REFERENCES

1. Lobo M V, Marusic E T & Aguilera G (1978) Endocrinology 102: 1061-1068
2. Fakunding J L, Chow R & Catt K J (1979) Endocrinology 105: 32--333
3. Foster R, Lobo M V, Rasmussen H & Marusic E T (1981) Endocrinology 109: 2196 - 2201
4. Williams B C, Mc Dougall J G, Tait J F & Tait S A S (1981) Clin Sci 61: 541-551
5. Foster R & Rasmussen H (1983) Amer J Physiol 245: E281-E287
6. Lobo M V & Marusic E T (1982) J Steroid Biochem 16: 629-632
7. Foster R, Lobo M V, Rasmussen H & Marusic E T (1982) FEBS Lett 149: 253-256
8. Foster R, Lobo M V & Marusic E T (1979) Imer J PKysiol 237: E 363-E366

10. Fertility Control

Endocrinology
F. Labrie, L. Proulx, eds.

CLINICAL TRIAL OF GOSSYPOL AS A CONTRACEPTIVE AGENT FOR MAN

GUO-ZHEN LIU*, KATHERINE CH"IU LYLE**, JIAN CAO*
* Capital Hospital, Beijing, China
**Rockefeller Foundation, New York, New York

INTRODUCTION

Gossypol, a pigment from the cotton plant, was found in the 50's as an accidental cause of male infertility in many rural communes in China where ingestion of raw cotton seed oil was common. Since then, efforts have been made by the China National Coordinating Group on Male Antifertility Agents to develop this compound as a possible pill for men, which could be a valuable supplement to the existing method of contraception. Studies were undertaken in the late 1960's and early 1970's to determine the toxic effects of gossypol, first in animals and then in a few human being. In 1972, a multicenter study, involving 14 centers and 8806 volunteers, was carried out on the use of gossypol as a male contraceptive agent to gather data on efficacy, side-effects and clinical pharmacology.

To answer some of the questions unanswered in the multicenter study in the 70's, a double-blind, randomized, controlled clinical trial supported by a Rockefeller Foundation Contraceptive Development Grant, was initiated in December 1981 and concluded in September 1983 and this paper gives the results of this study.

SUBJECTS AND METHODS

Gossypol contraception in men involves 2 phases: the initial 75-day loading phase using 20 mg daily pill and the maintenance phase using 50 mg weekly pill immediately following the loading. For the loading phase, it was a double-blind, randomized controlled study involving 152 participants in 2 groups: one group of 75 received gossypol pill and another group of 77 received placebos. After the decoding of the double-blind scheme, the treatment group started his maintenance phase and the placebo group started on his gossypol treatment of 20 mg/day pill to initiate the loading phase. Therefore, for the maintenance phase, it was basically a one-year continuation study of gossypol use.

Comparability of the 2 groups was ensured by randomization (Table 1).

TABLE 1

COMPARABILITY OF GOSSYPOL AND PLACEBO GROUPS

Characteristics	Gossypol (75)	Placebo (77)
Age	31.7	31.0
Education		
1 - 9	68	66
>10	7	11
Occupation		
Worker	70	71
Others	5	6
Sexual Intercourse (Weekly)	1.5	1.6
Body Weight (kgs)	64.6	62.6
Blood Pressures		
Systolic (mm Hg)	116.1	114.1
Diastolic (mm Hg)	92.1	80.5
Hemoglobin (gm/100ml)	15.7	15.5
Serum Potassium (mEq/L)	4.25	4.32
Sperm Count (m/cc)	79.9	87.9

RESULTS

Loading phase

A 92 percent efficacy rate was achieved at the end of loading (Table 2). Sperm count for the placebo group remained unchanged.

TABLE 2

SPERM COUNT AT END OF LOADING PHASE

Sperm Count (m/cc)	No. of Participants
0	20 (31 %)
1 - 4	39 (61 %)
5 - 9	2 (3 %)
10 - 125	3 (5 %)

Incidence rates for fatigue, decrease of libido and appetite between the 2 groups showed no differences. No differences were observed for laboratory measurements of hemoglobin, serum potassium, body weight, or blood pressures.

Maintenance phase

Efficacy rates (in terms of sperm count less than 4 m/cc) of 87, 97, 95, 92 and 98 percent were achieved at the end of loading, 3, 6, 9, and 12 months of maintenance phase, respectively (Table 3).

TABLE 3

SPERM COUNT AT VARIOUS TREATMENT INTERVALS

Sperm count (m/cc)	End of Loading	3 Mo.	6 Mo.	9 Mo.	12 Mo.
0	60	111	99	81	77
1 - 4	48	4	4	7	7
5 - 9	6	1	0	3	0
>10	10	2	5	4	2
Total	124	118	108	95	86

No differences were found for incidence of appetite and libido decreases. However, for the incidence of fatigue, our statistical testing showed differences in the occurrence of fatigue among the various intervals of treatment as well as that fatigue occurred more frequently during the loading than during the maintenance phase (Table 4).

TABLE 4

INCIDENCE OF FATIGUE AT VARIOUS TREATMENT INTERVALS

Length of use	Number	No. & Prop of Fatigue	
End of loading	126	11 (0.0873)	
3 months	119	2 (0.0168)	$\chi^2 = 16.4898$ with 4 df
6 months	108	1 (0.0093)	($P < 0.05$)
9 months	93	3 (0.0313)	
12 months	86	0 (0.0000)	

$\chi^2 = 18.0780$ with 4 df ($P < 0.05$)

No differences among the mean for various measurements data were found except that serum potassium level showed significantly differences among various intervals (Table 5). Using Newman-Kreuls test, it was found that serum potassium level at the end of one-year maintenance was significantly lower than the mean value at admission.

TABLE 5

SERUM POTASSIUM LEVELS (mEq/L) AT VARIOUS TREATMENT INTERVALS

Length of use	Number	Mean ($\bar{x}$)	SE ($\bar{x}$)	95% CI
Admission	152	4.29	0.03	4.23 - 4.35
End of loading	124	4.06	0.04	3.99 - 4.14
3 months	118	3.93	0.04	3.85 - 4.01
6 months	108	3.82	0.04	3.74 - 3.90
9 months	95	3.86	0.04	3.78 - 3.94
12 months	86	3.75	0.04	3.67 - 3.83

$F = 30.0305$ ($P < 0.05$)

Using life-table analysis, the continuation rates were 74.3 and 61.2 percent at 6 and 12 months of gossypol use. The net cumulative termination rates for various reasons are presented in Table 6.

TABLE 6

NET CUMULATIVE TERMINATION AND CONTINUATION RATES AFTER 6 and 12 MONTHS OF USE

Reason	6 months	12 months
Pregnancy	0.0 ± 0.0	0.0 ± 0.0
Medical reasons		
Fatigue	1.3 ± 0.13	3.3 ± 0.06
Appetite decrease	4.0 ± 0.07	4.6 ± 0.09
Libido decrease	0.7 ± 0.004	1.3 ± 0.014
Other medicals	2.6 ± 0.04	5.3 ± 0.11
Method-related	10.5 ± 0.29	15.8 ± 0.57
Personal reasons	5.3 ± 0.11	6.6 ± 0.15
Technical	1.3 ± 0.01	2.0 ± 0.02
Total termination	25.7	38.3
Continuation	74.3 ± 3.52	61.2 ± 4.07
Man/months	771.5	1393.5
Lost to follow-up	0	0
Total enrolled	152	

Note: The cut off date was 30 June 1983.

This work is supported by Rockefeller Foundation Grant 80029 to the Chinese Academy of Medical Sciences. We gratefully acknowledge the guidance given to us from Dr. Sheldon J. Segal.

Endocrinology
F. Labrie, L. Proulx, eds.

GnRH ANALOGUES FOR FERTILITY CONTROL IN MAN

SVEN JOHAN NILLIUS
Department of Obstetrics and Gynaecology, University Hospital, S-751 85 Uppsala (Sweden)

INTRODUCTION

Peptide contraception is a fundamentally new lead to birth control based on superactive analogues of the hypothalamic gonadotrophin-releasing hormone GnRH. More than 1000 analogues have been synthesized following the isolation and structural elucidation of the decapeptide GnRH by Schally and his co-workers in 1971. The purpose of this intense activity was to develop potent stimulatory analogues of GnRH for use in the treatment of infertility caused by hypothalamic-pituitary dysfunction and to develop inhibitory analogues of GnRH for contraception (1).

ANTAGONISTIC ANALOGUES OF GnRH

The concept of synthetic peptides acting as competitive inhibitors to endogenous GnRH at the pituitary receptor site was at first met with scepticism but is now clearly proven to be valid (2). Antagonistic analogues of GnRH have been synthesized but until recently they have not had sufficient biological activity for meaningful clinical trials. The lack of long-term toxicity studies on the recent more potent penta-substituted GnRH antagonists have so far prevented contraceptive trials in the human.

AGONISTIC ANALOGUES OF GnRH

The superactive stimulatory GnRH analogues which originally were synthesized to facilitate GnRH therapy of infertility due to hypogonadism, paradoxically proved to be anti-reproductive by nature. Repeated administration of highly potent and long-acting agonists of GnRH results in pituitary desensitization with suppression of the gonadotrophin secretion followed by reversible inhibition of gonadal function. The paradoxical anti-reproductive effects of superagonists of GnRH have been utilized not only for development of new approaches to contraception (3) but recently also for application in management of sex hormone dependent tumours (4).

GnRH Agonists for Female Contraception

Inhibition of ovulation in women by continous superagonist administration was the first new approach to peptide contraception described. It was later demonstrated that mid-luteal phase administration of GnRH agonists could exert a luteolytic effect in women. Early follicular phase administration to induce luteal phase defects was suggested as yet another model for fertility control by superagonists

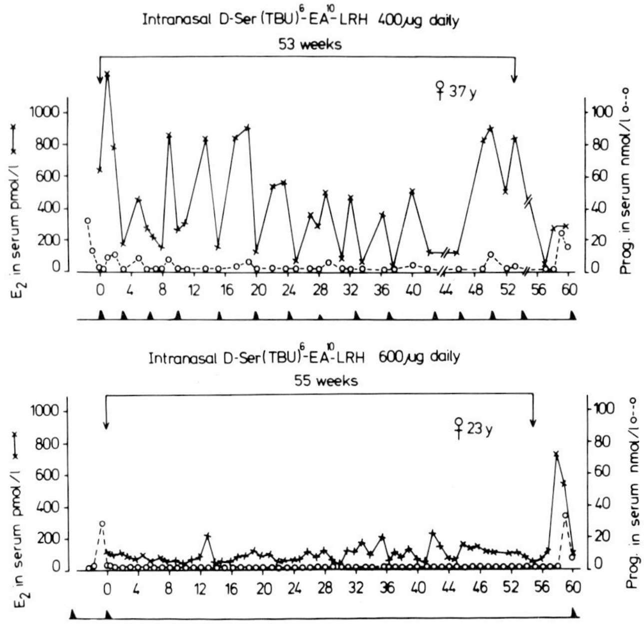

Fig. 1 Serum oestradiol, progesterone and bleeding patterns during prolonged GnRH agonist therapy. One of the volunteers had fairly regular menstrual-like bleedings during 53 weeks of treatment (top) while the other volunteer had amenorrhoea throughout 55 weeks of treatment. Note the rapid return of normal ovulation after cessation of the long-term treatments. From Bergquist C, Nillius SJ, Wide L: Long-term intranasal luteinizing hormone-releasing hormone agonist treatment for contraception in women. Fertil Steril 38:190, 1982. Reproduced by permission of the publisher, The American Fertility Society, Birmingham, Alabama.

of GnRH. The contraceptive effectiveness of these two "luteolytic" approaches to peptide contraception remains to be established in women. Attempts at inducing early abortion by superactive GnRH agonists in women have so far been unsuccessful. The new leads to fertility control in women by GnRH superagonists have recently been reviewed in detail (3). This paper will therefore focus on the most extensively investigated approach to peptide contraception, namely continous intranasal GnRH agonist treatment for inhibition of ovulation in women.

Ovulation in normal women can readily be inhibited by single daily intranasal doses of superactive GnRH agonists. A long-term contraceptive study on 71 healthy female volunteers, who were given continous intranasal superagonist treatment has recently been completed (5). They were treated with 200, 400 or 600 μg daily of the superagonist buserelin (D-Ser(TBU)^{6}-EA^{10}-GnRH, Hoechst AG, FRG) over 3-26 months. Only three of the 628 treatment months were normal ovulatory, according to weekly assessments of progesterone in serum. No pregnancy occurred.

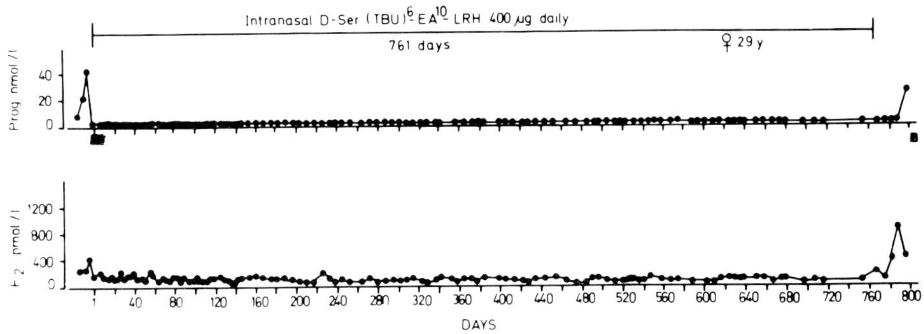

Fig. 2. Serum progesterone and oestradiol concentrations before, during and after more than 2 years of continous intranasal GnRH agonist therapy of a 29-year-old woman with amenorrhoea throughout the prolonged treatment. Ovulation rapidly returned after discontinuation of the long-term therapy. □ = Menstrual bleeding. Reproduced from (5), with permission.

No side effects, except for bleeding disturbances caused by the induced anovulation, occurred during the prolonged GnRH therapy. The bleeding pattern during the chronic superagonist treatment varied from fairly regular menstrual-like bleeds (37%) to oligomenorhoea (38%) or amenorrhoea (25%). There was a tendency to a prolongation of the intervals between the uterine bleedings in the course of the long-term treatment. Only five volunteers experienced spottings of short duration. None had clinical symptoms of dysfunctional uterine bleeding.

Hormone and bleeding patterns in three women under long-term intranasal buserelin treatment are shown in Figs. 1 and 2. The mean oestradiol concentration during the therapy was in the range of the early to mid-follicular phase of the menstrual cycle. The serum progesterone concentrations were slightly raised (e.g. Fig. 1, top) during 53 treatment months (mean 8 nmol/l), indicating luteinization of ovarian follicles or defective corpus luteum function. None of the women had any clinical symptoms or signs of oestrogen deficiency.

Concern about possible adverse effects on the endometrium by unopposed oestrogen secretion has arisen. There were, however, no histopathological signs of hyperproliferative changes in 57 endometrium biopsies obtained. The predominant picture consisted of inactive or weakly proliferative glands with slightly atrophic stroma.

After cessation of the prolonged superagonist treatment, ovulation rapidly returned. The first menstrual bleeding occurred after 41 days, on average. Fertility also returned and the few women, who had a desire of pregnancy after discontinuation of therapy conceived and gave birth to healthy children.

GnRH Agonists for Male Contraception

Chronic treatment with superactive stimulatory GnRH analogues result in pituitary desensitization also in men. However, to acheive enough suppression of the gonadotrophin secretion to affect spermatogenesis a ten-fold higher dose than is required in women to inhibit ovulation has to be given. Such a profound gonadotrophin suppression is unfortunately accompanied by a depression of the testosterone secretion with loss of libido and impotence (6). Superagonists of GnRH therefore have to be administered in combination with long-acting testosterone preparations to induce oligo- or azoospermia without impotence. Testosterone not only obviates the undesirable side effects on potency but also has additive or synergistic inhibitory effects on the pituitary gonadotrophin secretion. Such a combined therapeutic regimen with a GnRH superagonist and testosterone seems to be a promising strategy for male contraception (7).

SUMMARY

Superactive stimulatory analogues of GnRH with their paradoxical anti-fertility effects have up to now almost exlusively been studied in clinical trials of peptide contraception in man. The only new model for fertility control based on GnRH analogues, which has proved to provide acceptable, safe, effective and rapidly reversible contraception in man so far is intranasal superagonist treatment for inhibition of ovulation. This method of birth control clearly merits further investigation. To date, it seems to be the most promising approach to peptide contraception in man.

REFERENCES

1. Schally AV, Kastin AJ, Arimura A (1972) The hypothalamus and reproduction. Am J Obstet Gynecol 114:423-442.
2. Schally AV (1983) Current Status of Antagonistic Analogs of LH-RH as a Contraceptive Method in the Female. Research Frontiers in Fertility Regulation. PARFR (Northwestern University) 2:1-16.
3. Nillius, S.J. (1984) LH-RH Analogues for Contraception. In: Newton JR (ed) Update on contraception. Clinics in Obstetrics and Gynaecology. 11 (3).
4. Waxman J (1984) Analogues of gonadotrophin releasing hormone. Br. Med. J. 288:426-427.
5. Bergquist C, Nillius SJ, Wide L (1984) Peptide contraception in women. Inhibition of ovulation by chronic intranasal LRH agonist therapy. Ups J Med Sci 89:99-106.
6. Linde R, Doelle GC, Alexander N, Kirchner F, Vale W, Rivier J, Rabin, D (1981) Reversible inhibition of testicular steroidogenesis and spermatogenesis by a potent gonadotropin-releasing hormone agonist in normal men. N Engl J Med 305:663-667.
7. Swerdloff RS, Heber D, Bhasin S, Rajfer J (1983) Effect of GnRH superactive analogs (alone and combined with androgen) on testicular function in man and experimental animals. J Steroid Biochem 19: 491-497.

Endocrinology
F. Labrie, L. Proulx, eds.

THE IMMUNOLOGICAL DISRUPTION OF FERTILIZATION

J. AITKEN, Z FARZAD, M.J. HULME, D.W. RICHARDSON
MRC Reproductive Biology Unit, Centre for Reproductive Biology,
37 Chalmers Street, Edinburgh EH3 9EW

INTRODUCTION

The fertilization process involves a complex sequence of highly specific interactions between male and female gametes which, by the very nature of their interdependence and specificity, constitute an ideal point of attack for future contraceptive agents. The fact that many of these gamete-specific components are also highly immunogenic has focused attention on the possible development of fertility-regulating vaccines which would disrupt fertilization through an action on either the spermatozoon or the ovum.

THE OVUM

With respect to the ovum, the most appealing antigenic target for the development of a contraceptive vaccine is the zona pellucida. This structure is an acellular glycoprotein shell which is synthesized by the oocyte during folliculogenesis and serves a number of important functions during fertilization and the early stages of embryonic development (1,2). The notion of using the zona pellucida as the target for an immunological approach to contraception stems from the results of *in vitro* studies, conducted largely with murine gametes, indicating that the preincubation of ova in anti-zona antisera subsequently blocks their fertilization, by disrupting the binding of spermatozoa to specific receptor sites on the zona surface. The mechanism by which this disruption is achieved appears to involve the formation of an immune-precipitate on the outer surface of the zona which occludes the sperm binding sites through a process of steric hindrance (1,2).

The efficacy of anti-zona antibodies *in vivo* was first indicated by passive immunization experiments employing the γ-globulin fraction of antisera raised against either cumulus free mouse ova or mechanically isolated zonae pellucidae (3). Active immunization studies employing heterologous, isolated zonae as the immunogen subsequently confirmed the contraceptive potential of anti-zona antibodies *in vivo* by demonstrating that reversible infertility without adverse side effects could be consistently induced by such means (1,2). Recent studies of this type have indicated that glycoproteins derived from either bovine and porcine zonae pellucidae will also induce infertility in primates such as the common marmoset (Callithrix jacchus) and might therefore have some potential as the basis of a vaccine for human use (1,2). The feasibility of this approach in the human is further suggested by the results of clinical studies indicating that the development of autoimmunity against the zona pellucida may be associated with the induction of infertility in certain groups of patients (3,4).

Mechanism of action studies in actively immunized animals indicate that the disruption of fertilization is, predictably, the major factor behind the induction of infertility. Ova recovered from the tubal ampullae of such animals were found to be surrounded by abnormal, perforated zonae pellucidae exhibiting a pronounced immunoprecipitate on the outer surface. In some immunized animals however, fertilized oocytes were recovered, which were competent to develop as far as the late morula-early blastocyst stage but no further. It is possible that such fertilizations occur when the zonae pellucidae become so perforated that they are unable to prevent spermatozoa from gaining access to the oocyte. The poor structural integrity of such zonae might then be responsible for the subsequent demise of the embryos as a result of the inadequate physical protection they would afford. Whatever the nature of this post-fertilization mechanism its existence must be recognised as a serious flaw in an otherwise promising approach.

THE SPERMATOZOON

The feasibility of directing a contraceptive vaccine against antigenic targets on the surface of the spermatozoon is suggested by a wealth of clinical data indicating that the development of auto- or isoimmunity against sperm antigens is associated with infertility in men and women respectively.

In men, antibodies may be detected in serum and/or seminal plasma, but it is their titre in the latter compartment which is the significant factor in terms of fertility. Pregnancies are rarely observed when the concentration of spermagglutinating antibodies in seminal plasma exceeds 1:64 and seminal antibody titres above this level are generally associated with spontaneous tail-to-tail autoagglutination of the spermatozoa (5). The anti-sperm antibodies present in seminal plasma are the result of both a local lgA-mediated immune response and the transudation of circulating lgG through the prostate gland. The probable importance of local immune responses in the genesis of infertility by anti-sperm antibodies poses a major problem in terms of contraception, since the sites where such immunity becomes established (the epididymis, rete testis and prostate gland) are all linked by their common lack of accessability. Hence with any future male-orientated approach we shall have to induce a systemic immune response against a selected sperm antigen and hope that sufficient antibody enters the male reproductive tract to induce infertility. Since only about 1% of circulating lgG reaches seminal plasma by transudation, this hope may be rather forlorn.

The contraceptive potential of anti-sperm antibodies is significantly more promising in women since, in the female partner, circulating antibodies can gain direct access to the spermatozoa as they progress through the reproductive tract. Active isoimmunization of female guinea pigs, rabbits and mice with sperm or testicular antigens has been shown to suppress fertility, even in the absence of adjuvant stimulation. Direct evidence of the contraceptive potential of isoimmunization protocols in our own species, has come from studies in which women have been immunized against whole semen or isolated human spermatozoa. In such patients the anti-sperm antibody titres were found to remain elevated for up to 12 months and no pregnancies were recorded as long as antibody titres remained high. Further evidence supporting this approach has come from clinical studies indicating the existence of a relationship between the presence of circulating sperm agglutinating antibodies in women and both the duration of infertility and the cumulative probability of conception per year.

In addition to a systemic immune response the induction of local immunity against sperm antigens at the level of the cervix may also be a significant factor in the genesis of female infertility. Both sperm agglutinating and sperm immobilising antibodies have been detected in the cervical secretions of a small percentage of infertile women and the existence of such responses has been correlated with the incidence of pregnancy. The competence of the cervix to generate local immune responses to antigens presented to its external surface suggest that a combined approach, involving the induction of both local and systemic immunity, might be an effective contraceptive strategy.

The mechanisms by which fertility is disrupted by anti-sperm antibodies include the inhibition of sperm transport through the female reproductive tract, the suppression of fertilization and a direct action in the embryo. The screening of monoclonal or polyclonal antibodies in order to identify those capable of blocking fertilization is the most feasible avenue at the present time, as a result of the availability of interspecific *in vitro* fertilization systems for assessing the fertilizing capacity of human spermatozoa. Polyclonal antibodies obtained from infertile patients are currently being evaluated in order to correlate the nature of the sperm antigens involved in the immune response with the capacity of the antisera to block fertilization. These results are revealing a surprisingly simple assortment of antigens responsible for generating auto- and isoimmune responses against human spermatozoa, the dominant antigens having molecular weights of around 90 (6) and 20 x 10^6 Daltons.

Further definition of sperm antigens with contraceptive potential is also being obtained through the use of monoclonal antibodies. Monoclonals capable of disrupting the fertilizing potential of hamster spermatozoa have been identified (7) and we have recently produced a monoclonal antibody directed against the equatorial segment of human spermatozoa which exhibits similar properties. The continuation of these studies should serve to identify components of the spermatozoon suitable for further consideration as the basis for an antifertility vaccine, as well as elucidating the nature of those auto- and isoimmune conditions responsible for the generation of idiopathic human infertility.

REFERENCES

1. Aitken RJ, Richardson DW (1980) In: Hearn JP (ed) Immunological Aspects of Reproduction and Fertility Control. MTP Press, Lancaster, pp 173-201.
2. Aitken RJ, Richardson DW, Hulme M (1984) In: Crighton DB (ed). Immunological Aspects of Reproduction in Mammals. Butterworths, London. (in press)
3. Mori T, Nishimoto T, Kohda H, Takai I, Nishimura T, Oikawa T (1979) Fertil Steril 32: 67-72.
4. Mhaskar A, Buchshee K, Talwar GP (1984) Contraception 29: 75-82.
5. Aitken RJ (1982) In: Jeffcoate SL, Sandler M (eds) Progress towards a Male Contraceptive. John Wiley, Chichester, pp. 109-134.
6. Lee C-YG, Lunn V, Wong E, Menge AC, Huang Y-S (1983) Amer. J. Immunol. 3: 183-187.
7. Moore HDM, Hartman TD (1984) J. Reprod. Fertil 70: 175-183.

© 1984 Elsevier Science Publishers B.V.
Endocrinology
F. Labrie, L. Proulx, eds.

THE ANTIPROGESTERONE ACTIVITY OF RU 486, A CONTRAGESTIVE AGENT IN THE HUMAN

E. SAKIZ*, C. EUVRARD*, E.E. BAULIEU+, *Roussel-Uclaf, 35 bd des Invalides, 75007 Paris and +INSERM U33, Lab Hormones, 94270 Bicêtre, France

RU 486 (17β-hydroxy-11β-(4-dimethylaminophenyl 1)-17α (prop-1-ynyl)-estra-4, 9-dien-3-one), is a $\Delta_{9(10)}$ 17α-propynyl derivative of 19-nortestosterone with a large dimethyl-amino-phenyl substitution at the C11β-position.

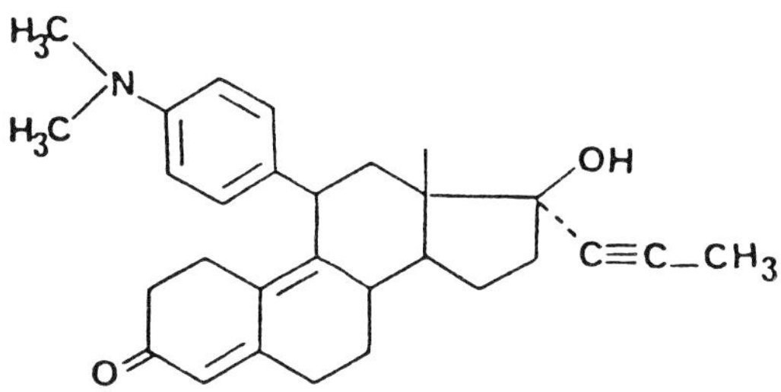

RU 486

It may be visualized as a derivative of the progestagen norethindrone with 1. at the 11β-position, an aromatic nucleus showing some analogy with the third cycle of triphenyl-ethylene antiestrogens, and likely responsible for antagonistic properties ; and 2. a 17α side chain increasing affinity to the progesterone receptor (PR). Indeed its affinity for PR in all mammalian species so far tested is > to that of progesterone itself (but nil for the chick PR). Furthermore, it also shows very high affinity for the glucocorticosteroid receptor (including in avian), some affinity for the androgen receptor, but no measurable affinity for estradiol receptor and mineralocorticosteroid receptor. Orally administered, RU 486 has no progesterone-like activity in laboratory animals, but on the contrary antiprogesterone effects : this was demonstrated 1. at the endometrium level in estrogen primed rabbit uterus after systemic or intrauterine administration (Clauberg test), 2. in measuring LH levels in rats in vivo and in cultured pituitary cells, and 3. in antagonizing formation of progesterone dependent trauma-induced deciduoma in the rat uterus. When RU 486 was given to pregnant rats, castrated on the 8th day and supplemented with progesterone, no implantation was anymore observed on the 12th day. When it was administered for 3 successive days at any period of pregnancy in intact rats, no implantation or developping pregnancy was observed with a dose of 10 mg/kg/d. Pregnancy interruption was not due to a decrease of circulating progesterone level, and indeed RU 486 provoked abortion more rapidly than castration and more efficiently than administration of the progesterone biosynthesis inhibitor aminogluthetimid (150 mg/kg). Similar results were obtained in a variety of other laboratory animals (mice, guinea pig, dog). In cynomolgus monkeys (1, 2), studies in hormone-supplemented castrated females confirmed the antiprogesterone activity of RU 486 (administered s/c), and in intact animals there also was interruption of pregnancies and of the menstrual cycle during the luteal phase and of pregnancies.

On the basis of the receptor mechanism of action of RU 486 and of toxicological studies, the compound was administered to human beings.

Non-pregnant women

During the luteal phase, when RU 486 was given "late" (50 mg/d x 4 d, on the 22nd-25th days (3)), there was uterine bleeding, luteolysis and decrease of LH/FSH. When it was administered "early" (32 cases) : (100, 50 or 25 mg/d x 4 d on the 18th-21st days), there was immediate decrease of LH and bleeding on the 3rd day of administration, in a dose dependent manner. However, and interestingly, there was luteolysis only in (approximately) 50 % of the women, including at the 100 mg/d/dosage (Schaison et al., in preparation). In absence of luteolysis, a second bleeding took place at the expected time of menses. This result confirm the early contention (3) of direct effect at the levels of pituitary and endometrium, while luteolysis appears to be a secondary event. When given before ovulation, RU 486 did not provoke uterine bleeding ; preliminary studies of Herrmann et al. suggest that it can delay ovulation in a dose-dependent manner (a result which may due to the postulated progesterone effect upon ovulation).

In post-menopausal women pretreated with estrogen, RU 486 alone displayed some progesterone-like activity in the endometrium and, however full antiprogesterone effect when administered together with progesterone.

Early medical interruption of pregnancy

RU 486 was given to 94 5-10 week pregnant women that could be studied rigorously. 50-200 mg/d were given orally, usually in 2 intakes per day, orally for 3 or 4 days. Patients were treated in Geneva, Paris, Stockholm, Szegreb,

Upsala, and Utrecht. 55 complete abortions were obtained (∿ 60 %), bleeding starting on the 3rd-4th day of administration. Until expulsion, progesterone and estradiol did not go down, nor did β-hCG. It is only after expulsion of the conceptus that there was a brutal decrease of these hormones, suggesting that luteolyis occured likely as a consequence of the suppression of the chorial hormone. After this medical abortion, return to normal ovulation was observed in the next cycle. In 23 cases, pregnancy also was arrested, but spontaneous uterine evacuation was not complete, and in 16 cases, pregnancy was not stopped. No clearcut dose-dependent effect was observed within the range of doses used . In all cases, including failures, a remarkable softening of the cervix was observed. Heavy bleeding had to be stopped in 2 cases. No significant clinical and biological side-effects were observed (see action on the pituitary-adrenal system in a next paragraph). Trials in 4-10 week pregnancies using different doseages, number of days of administration, and intramuscular injections are in progress, as also studies of RU 486 as a 2nd trimester abortifacient (to be compared or in conjunction with prostaglandin or other treatment).

Other effects

No androgen, estrogen or gluco- and mineralo-corticosteroid activity was observed Antiandrogenic effect was tested in laboratory animals and found moderate. No antiestrogen activity was observed, even at high doses. The remarkable antiglucocorticosteroid properties of the compound was studied in depth. Besides in vivo (rat, monkey) and in vitro (many cultured cell systems) laboratory experiments, the ACTH/lipotropin/β-endorphin/cortisol system was studied in women receiving RU 486 for pregnancy or cycle interruption, and in normal male volunteers. A dose dependent activity ascribable to antiglucocorticosteroid activity at the receptor level was observed, desinhibiting the pituitary-adrenal system at doses > 100 mg/d. It amplified the early morning rise of hormones of the circadian rhythm (4). Easy reversal of the antiglucocorticosteroid activity was obtained by giving dexamethasone. Metabolic studies indicated that water transit and glucid metabolism were not perturbated, even when cortisol was increased after RU 486, as if the antiglucocorticosteroid activity of RU 486 was compensated by the regulatory homeostatic mechanism of the adrenal pituitary system. These results confirmed the lack of observed side-effects when RU 486 was used for cycle interruption and pregnancy.

Conclusions

Fulfilling the requirements indicated by Djerassi (5) and presently the only efficient antiprogesterone steroid available, RU 486 appears to be a very promissing compound for human fertility control : its use for interrupting pregnancy as well as a mense inducer deserves further studies. In addition several endocrine-reproductive pathological problems may become accessible to its antiprogesterone properties.

The data reported here have been obtained with Pr W. Herrmann, Dr R. Wyss, Dr A. Riondel and Dr R. Gaillard (Geneva) ; Dr L. Kovacs (Szeged) and Pr M. Bygdeman (Stockholm), within the frame of WHO's Special Programme of Research in Human Reproduction ; Drs W. Bardin and I. Spitz (New York), in a Population Council programme ; Drs G. Hodgen and D. Healy (Bethesda), thanks to the National Institute of Child Health and Human Development ; Pr Haspels (Utrecht) ; Dr D. Elia (Paris) and Pr G. Schaison (Bicêtre), and our colleagues.

References

1. Healy DL, Baulieu EE, Hodgen GD (1983) Induction of menstruation by antiprogesterone steroid (RU 486) in primates : site of action, dose-response relationships and hormonal effects. Fertility and Sterility 40:253-257.
2. Healy DL, Chrousos GP, Schulte HM, Williams RF, Gold PW, Baulieu EE, Hodgen GD (1983) Pituitary and adrenal responses to the antiprogesterone and antiglucocorticoid steroid RU 486 in primates. J Clin Endocr Metab 57:863-865.
3. Herrmann W, Wyss R, Riondel A, Philibert D, Teutsch G, Sakiz E, Baulieu EE (1982) Effet d'un stéroïde anti-progestérone chez la femme : interruption du cycle menstruel et de la grossesse au début. CR Acad Sci 294:933-938.
4. Gaillard RC, Riondel A, Muller MF, Herrmann W, Baulieu EE (1984) RU 486 : a steroid with antiglucocorticosteroid activity that only disinhibits the human pituitary-adrenal system at a specific time of day. Proc Natl Acad Sci USA, in press, July issue.
5. Djerassi C (1970) Birth control after 1984. Science 169:941-951.

11. Pathogenesis of Type II Diabetes Mellitus

Endocrinology
F. Labrie, L. Proulx, eds.

INSULIN GENE POLYMORPHISM AND TYPE II OR NON-INSULIN DEPENDENT DIABETES MELLITUS (NIDDM)

M.A. PERMUTT, T. ANDREONE, J. CHIRGWIN, S. ELBEIN, W. KNOWLER*, P. ROTWEIN

Washington University School of Medicine, St. Louis, Missouri 63110 and NIADDKD, Phoenix, AZ 85014*

USE OF RECOMBINANT DNA METHODOLOGY TO DEFINE THE GENE DEFECT(S)

The importance of inheritance in NIDDM has been emphasized by the finding of a very high concordance in monozygotic twins, yet the genetic factors involved remain undefined. Because NIDDM is invariably associated with relative insulin lack, the defect(s) may involve any number of genes. One can imagine many causes of impaired insulin production and/or action. Since B cell mass may be reduced in NIDDM, a gene which regulates replication might be defective. Any genes which regulate biosynthesis and/or secretion are obvious candidates. Similarly, genes controlling insulin action might be involved, or any combination of the above.

Restriction enzyme site polymorphism has been used as a genetic marker in clinical medicine. An example is the restriction enzyme site polymorphism on chromosome 4 which is linked with a mutation in the Huntington's disease gene (1). The nature of the gene defect is completely unknown, yet the linked polymorphism provides a useful genetic marker.

Since the human insulin gene has been cloned, one might use the "likely candidate gene approach" (2) to investigate its possible role in NIDDM. One hypothesis which is being tested by our labs is the hypoinsulinemia of NIDDM may be due to mutations in regulatory regions of the insulin gene. Southern blot analysis of DNA from diabetics has been used to test this hypothesis.

INSULIN GENE POLYMORPHISM IN THREE RACIAL GROUPS

A highly polymorphic region in the 5' flanking portion of the human insulin gene was identified (3,4), approximately 500 bp from the transcription initiation site. This region is composed of a family of tandemly repeating oligonucleotides (5) producing insulin gene fragments in individuals which vary according to size. A common size allele accounted for approximately two-thirds, and variant alleles both larger and smaller were present in the remaining one-third. Within the group of variant alleles, a 1.6 kb larger allele was by far the most frequent, accounting for 90% of the variants.

Three racial groups have been studied, including American Blacks and Caucasians from St. Louis, and Pima Indians. To facilitate analysis, we have adopted the classification of polymorphic alleles of Bell et al (6).

The 5' flanking region of the insulin gene in American Blacks exhibited the most polymorphism (Table I). In Blacks 56%, in Pimas 40%, and in Caucasians 36% were heterozygous at the insulin locus (i.e. genotypes 1/3, 1/2, or 2/3). This classification provides a minimal estimate of heterozygosity since on a single gel electrophoretic analysis, alleles of the same class which differ by only 50-100 bp can often be distinguished. Allelic frequencies differed significantly between Blacks and Caucasians, and Blacks and Pimas (Table II). The frequency of the class 2 allele (Table II) was 1.9% in Caucasians, 9.2% in Blacks and 0 in Pimas. The frequency of the class 3 allele was the same in Caucasian and Pimas (23%), and increased in Blacks to 28%. The observed genotypic frequencies in the racial groups did not deviate from the expected when tested for Hardy-Weinberg equilibrium.

RELATIONSHIP OF THE 5' FLANKING POLYMORPHISM TO DIABETES

In a study of approximately 200 individuals we noted a significant association of the 1.6 kb larger allele with NIDDM but not IDDM (7). Since that report we have analyzed more than 400 individuals. Within the Caucasian and Pima groups the frequency of the class 3 allele was approximately 23%, and not significantly different in non-diabetics and NIDDM (Table II). However, only 4 Pima individuals were noted to be homozygous for the class 3 allele (Table I), and all four were diabetic. The insulin gene polymorphism does not seem to play a role in the pathogenesis of NIDDM in Pima Indians, nor does it influence glucose or insulin concentrations (manuscript submitted).

In the Blacks there may be an increase in homozygosity for the class 3 allele in the NIDDM group. Even in this group the data do not support this conclusion at the present time. Because of the potential importance of this observation, and the small number of homozygous individuals in this population, this population analysis is being extended.

COMPARISON WITH OTHER STUDIES

Owerbach et. al. found a positive association of class 3 alleles within NIDDM in Danish Caucasians (8). Bell et. al. (6) reported an association of class 1 alleles with IDDM in Caucasians but found no association with either type of diabetes in Asians or American Blacks. Combining these results (Table III), the aggregate data for Caucasians shows no difference in the allelic frequencies of NIDDM and non-diabetics. As previously noted (6), there is a significant increase of class 1 alleles in the IDDM group. A similar trend can be seen in the aggregate data for Blacks but the sample size is smaller. In view of our more recent findings in Pimas and Caucasians, it appears that with the possible exception of Black subjects, class 3 alleles do not directly predispose to NIDDM.

An association between class 3 alleles and atherosclerosis, independent of diabetes (9), and with diabetic hypertriglyceridemia have been reported (10). In both of these studies the population size was very small.

FAMILY STUDIES

Family studies provide an important alternative approach to population studies since the latter are complicated by heterogeneity. In collaboration with Dr. Stefan Fajans (Ann Arbor, MI) we have established lack of linkage in one large pedigree with maturity onset diabetes of the young (manuscript submitted). Whether defects at the insulin locus represent a significant contributor to the genetic component of NIDDM in other families remains to be determined.

TABLE I

THE DISTRIBUTION OF GENOTYPES AT THE INSULIN GENE LOCUS BY 5'-FLANKING REGION POLYMORPHISM AND DIABETES STATUS

	Genotype Frequency						
	1/1	1/2	1/3	2/2	2/3	3/3	Total
Caucasian							
Non-diabetic	30	2	18			4	54
IDDM	11		4			2	17
NIDDM	35	2	21		1	3	62
	76(.571)	4(.030)	43(.323)		1(.008)	9(.068)	133
Black							
Non-diabetic	24	7	33	1	6	2	73
IDDM	4	1	2				7
NIDDM	33	10	30	1	2	7	83
	61(.370)	18(.110)	65(.399)	2(.012)	8(.049)	9(.055)	163
Pima							
Non-diabetic	30		27				57
NIDDM	35		19			4	58
	65(.565)		46(.400)			4(.035)	115

Class 1 alleles are the common size allele previously described (4,7), or the L allele of Owerbach et. al. (8), class 3 alleles include a polymorphic region and are at least 1.6 kbp larger than class 1 alleles (U allele of Owerbach et. al. (8)), and class 2 alleles are intermediate in size.

TABLE II

POLYMORPHISM AT THE INSULIN GENE LOCUS: ALLELIC FREQUENCIES

	Number of alleles (frequency)		
	Class 1	Class 2	Class 3
Caucasian			
Non-diabetic	80 (.741)	2 (.019)	26 (.241)
IDDM	26 (.765)	0	8 (.235)
NIDDM	93 (.750)	3 (.024)	28 (.226)
	199 (.748)	5 (.019)	62 (.233)
Black*			
Non-diabetic	88 (.603)	15 (.103)	43 (.295)
IDDM	11 (.786)	1 (.071)	2 (.143)
NIDDM	106 (.639)	14 (.084)	46 (.277)
	205 (.629)	30 (.092)	91 (.279)
Pima			
Non-diabetic	87 (.763)	0	27 (.237)
NIDDM	89 (.767)	0	27 (.233)
	176 (.765)	0	54 (.235)

*3 x 2 analysis vs Caucasian, $x^2 = 18.1$, df = 2, $p < .001$
3 x 2 analysis vs Pima, $x^2 = 24.9$, df = 2, $p < .001$

TABLE III

POLYMORPHISM AT THE INSULIN GENE LOCUS IN CAUCASIANS: RESULTS OF POPULATION ANALYSIS FROM ST. LOUIS, SAN FRANCISCO (6), AND COPENHAGEN (8)

	Allelic frequency			Genotypic frequency		
	1	2	3	1/1	1/3	3/3
Caucasian						
Nondiabetic						
St. Louis	.74 (80)	.02 (2)	.24 (26)	.56 (30)	.37 (20)	.07 (4)
San Francisco	.67 (112)	.01 (1)	.32 (53)	.45 (37)	.46 (38)	.10 (8)
Denmark	.73 (76)		.27 (28)	.50 (26)	.46 (24)	.04 (2)
	.61 (268)	.01 (3)	.28 (107)	.49 (93)	.43 (82)	.07 (14)
IDDM*						
St. Louis	.77 (26)	0	.24 (8)	.65 (11)	.24 (4)	.12 (2)
San Francisco	.88 (199)	0 (1)	.12 (26)	.76 (86)	.24 (27)	0 (0)
Copenhagen	.85 (63)		.5 (11)	.73 (27)	.24 (9)	.03 (1)
	.84 (288)	0 (1)	.14 (45)	.74 (124)	.24 (40)	.02 (3)
NIDDM						
St. Louis	.75 (93)	.02 (3)	.23 (28)	.57 (35)	.39 (24)	.05 (3)
San Francisco	.79 (120)	0	.21 (32)	.63 (48)	.32 (24)	.05 (4)
Copenhagen	.65 (61)		.35 (33)	.47 (22)	.36 (17)	.17 (8)
	.74 (274)	.01 (3)	.25 (930)	.57 (105)	.39 (65)	.09 (15)

*Allelic frequencies of IDDM vs non-diabetic, 3 x 2 analysis, $x^2 = 23.95$, $p<.001$

REFERENCES

1. Gusella, J.F., Wexler, N.S., Conneally, P.M., Naylor, S.L., Anderson, M.A., Tanzi, R.E., Watkins, P.C., Ottina, K., Wallace, M.R., Sakaguchi, A.Y., Young, A.B., Shoulson, I., Bonilla, E., and Martin, J.B.: A polymorphic DNA marker genetically linked to Huntington's disease. Nature 306:234-238, 1983.
2. White, R.L., Barker, D., Holm, T., Berkowitz, J., Lepert, M., Cavenee, W., Leach, R., and Drayna, D.: Approaches to linkage analysis in the human. In: Banbury Report 14. Recombination DNA Applications to Human Disease. Caskey, C.T., and White, R.L., eds., Cold Spring Harbor Laboratory, 1983, pp. 235-250.
3. Bell, G.I., Pictet, R., and Rutter, W.J.: Analysis of the regions flanking the human insulin gene and sequence of an Alu family member. Nucleic Acids Res. 8:4001-4008, 1980.
4. Rotwein, P., Chyn, R., Chirgwin, J., Cordell, B., Goodman, H., and Permutt, M.A.: Polymorphism in the 5'-flanking region of the human insulin gene and its possible relation to Type 2 diabetes. Science 213:1117-1120, 1981.
5. Bell, G.I., Selby, M.J., and Rutter, W.J.: The highly polymorphic region near the human insulin gene is composed of simple tandemly repeating sequences. Nature 295:31-35, 1982.
6. Bell, G.I., Horita, S., and Karam, J.H.: A polymorphic locus near the human insulin gene is associated with insulin-dependent diabetes mellitus. Diabetes, Feb., 1984.
7. Rotwein, P.S., Chirgwin, J., Province, M., Knowler, W.C., Pettitt, D.J., Cordell, B., Goodman, H.M., and Permutt, M.A.: Polymorphism in the 5' flanking region of the human insulin gene: A genetic marker for non-insulin-dependent diabetes. New Engl. J. Med. 308:65-71, 1983.
8. Owerbach, D., and Nerup, J.: Restriction fragment length polymorphism of the insulin gene in diabetes mellitus. Diabetes 31:275-277, 1982.
9. Mandrup-Poulsen, T., Owerbach, D., Mortensen, S.A., Johansen, K., Meinertz, H., Sorensen, H., and Nerup, J.: DNA-sequences flanking the insulin gene on chromosome 11 confer risk of atherosclerosis. Submitted to Lancet.
10. Jowett, N.I., Williams, L.G., Hitman,G.A., Galton, D.J.: Diabetic hypertriglyceridaemia and related 5' flanking polymorphism of the human insulin gene. Br. Med. J. 288:96-99, 1984.

© 1984 Elsevier Science Publishers B.V.
Endocrinology
F. Labrie, L. Proulx, eds.

THE ROLE OF INSULIN RECEPTOR KINASE ACTIVITY IN INSULIN ACTION: IMPLICATIONS FROM INSULIN RESISTANT STATES

C. RONALD KAHN, MARCO CRETTAZ, FLORIN GRIGORESCU, SUMIKO TAKAYAMA, OM P. GANDA, and JEFFREY S. FLIER

Joslin Diabetes Center and Harvard Medical School, One Joslin Place, Boston, MA 02215

Insulin binds to specific receptors on the plasma membrane of the cell and thus initiates a chain of events which leads to its characteristic biological effects on cells. Over the past several years, considerable progress has been made in elucidating the structural features of the insulin receptor, and in determining some of the early steps in insulin action. Since alterations in the insulin receptor and insulin action occur in many diabetic states, particularly non-insulin-dependent forms of diabetes, an understanding of these processes is of critical importance.

STRUCTURE OF THE INSULIN RECEPTOR

The insulin receptor is a high molecular weight glycoprotein composed of two distinct subunits (Figure 1) (1,2). The α-subunit of the receptor has a molecular weight of 135,000 and appears to be the insulin binding subunit. The α-subunit can be labeled using bifunctional cross-linking reagents and ^{125}I-insulin or photoaffinity insulin analogues. In intact cells, the α-subunit is sensitive to trypsin treatment, suggesting a major extracellular domain for this subunit. The β-subunit of the insulin receptor has a molecular weight of 95,000 and appears to be transmembrane in nature, suggesting that it is likely to be involved in the signal transduction function of the receptor (see below). Both subunits of the receptor are glycoproteins with complex carbohydrate side chains; however, the β-subunit appears to be richer in terminal sialic acidic residues and has a more acidic pI.

Under non-reducing conditions, the α and β subunits of the receptor form disulfide-linked oligomers. The most commonly depicted model is one with a β-α-α-β structure (Figure 1). In studies in which biosynthetically-labeled or surface-labeled receptors are analyzed using non-reduced gels, multiple forms are observed. At present, the functional significance of these various redox-states of the receptor is unclear, but studies in our laboratory have suggested that the highest molecular weight forms may have a lower affinity for insulin and be more actively involved in insulin action (3).

THE INSULIN RECEPTOR AS TYROSINE-PROTEIN KINASE

Since our initial observation (4), considerable evidence has been accumulated that the insulin receptor is a tyrosine-specific protein kinase. This was first demonstrated by using intact cultured lymphocytes and hepatoma cells, but now has been extended to a wide variety of intact and broken cell preparations (reviewed in reference 5). These studies have shown that the tyrosine-specific protein kinase activity is intrinsic to the receptor itself and co-purifies with the receptor; insulin stimulates the kinase activity of the receptor by increasing the V_{max} for ATP (Figure 2); *in vitro*, the kinase activity requires divalent cations, in particular Mn^{++}; the isolated receptor actively phosphorylates itself, as well as exogenous substrates; this kinase activity is probably present in the β-subunit of the receptor since this subunit has an ATP binding site and is the subunit which is most heavily autophosphorylated; in the intact cell, there is also serine phosphorylation of the receptor; the kinase involved in the phosphorylation is as of yet unknown.

Although the function of the kinase activity of the receptor is unknown, it seems quite likely that it is involved in insulin action, since it is intrinsic to the receptor itself and stimulated by insulin. Recently, Simpson and Hedo challenged this notion, since serum taken from a patient with anti-receptor antibodies mimicked insulin's effect on glucose transport without stimulating receptor phosphorylation (6). There are several potential explanations for this observation. First, the serum used is polyclonal and contains a mixture of antibodies which may have variable potency for inhibition of insulin binding, stimulation of phosphorylation, and activation of glucose transport. Secondly, the

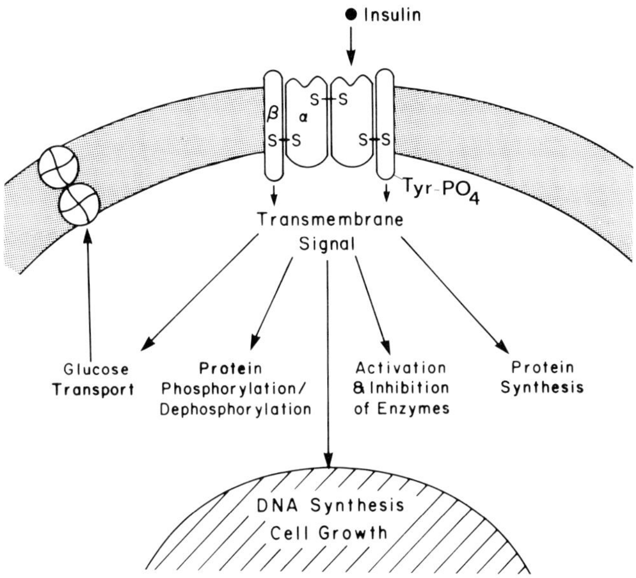

Figure 1. Current Model of the Insulin Receptor and Insulin Action

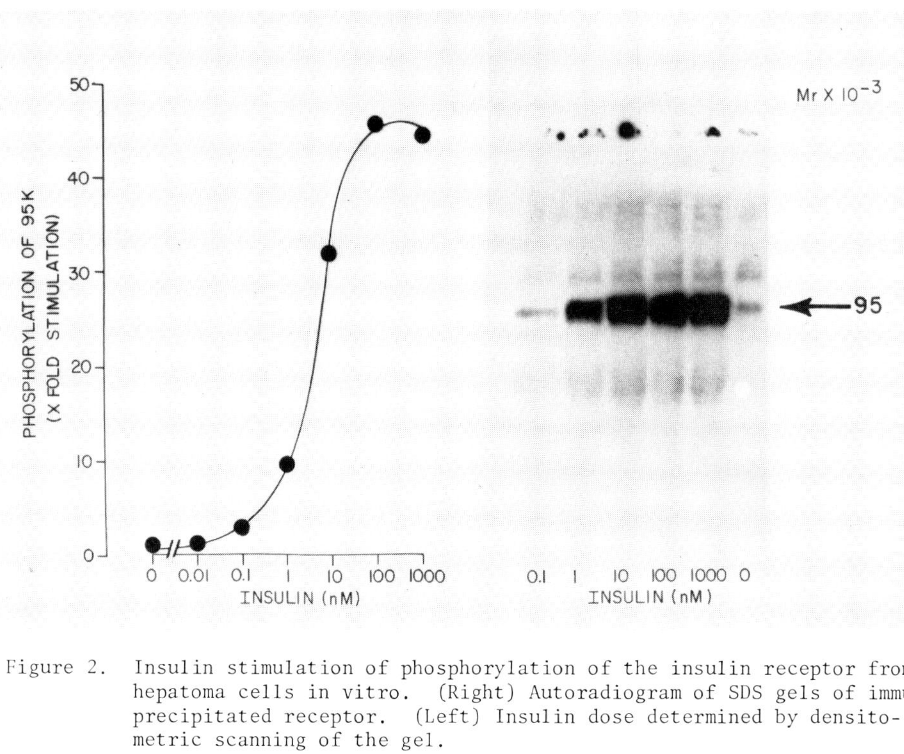

Figure 2. Insulin stimulation of phosphorylation of the insulin receptor from hepatoma cells in vitro. (Right) Autoradiogram of SDS gels of immunoprecipitated receptor. (Left) Insulin dose determined by densitometric scanning of the gel.

concentration of anti-serum used was probably insufficient to see an effect if it existed. Third, the phosphorylated receptor appeared to be internalized and was found in an intracellular membrane fraction. Finally, it is quite possible that the anti-receptor antibody stimulates glucose transport in a manner which is not identical to that of insulin. For example, anti-receptor antibodies stimulate transport only when they are bivalent, whereas insulin presumably acts as a monovalent ligand (7). Obviously, more studies are needed on this point.

ALTERATIONS IN RECEPTOR AUTOPHOSPHORYLATION IN INSULIN RESISTANT STATES

One approach to determining the role of the receptor kinase activity in insulin action is to study this aspect of receptor function in states of altered insulin action. In this regard, we have studied insulin binding and autophosphorylation in both cells in culture and freshly isolated cells in which there are acquired or genetic defects in action.

Down-regulation and desensitization

Prolonged exposure of hepatoma cells to insulin produces both a marked decrease in receptor number (down-regulation) and a total desensitization of the cells to the action of the hormone on glycogen synthase and tyrosine aminotransferase (3). The decrease in receptor number could account for only a part of this decrease in biological response. To know whether receptor phosphorylation was involved in this process, intact cells were labeled with ^{32}P and exposed to 10^{-7} M insulin (15 mU/ml) for various time periods. A 30 minute incubation with hormone produced a 6-fold increase in receptor phosphorylation. Longer incubations were associated with a progressive decrease in this effect, and after 24 hr exposure, a time at which total desensitization occurred, no insulin effect on receptor phosphorylation could be detected. When receptors were partially purified from control and desensitized cells and assayed in a cell-free system, phosphorylation was decreased in desensitized cells, when expressed per mg of protein. However, when expressed per receptor, receptors of desensitized cells were phosphorylated to the same extent as those of control cells. Thus, the decrease in receptor phosphorylation observed in desensitized cells reflects the decrease in receptor number.

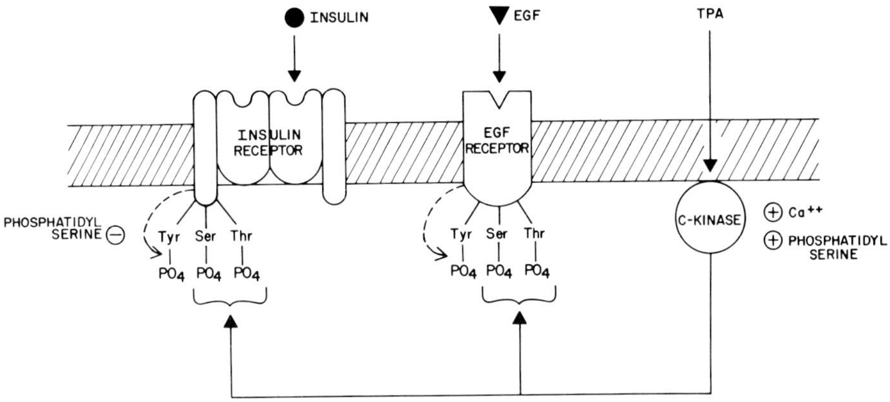

Figure 3. Model of TPA Effect on Insulin Receptor Phosphorylation

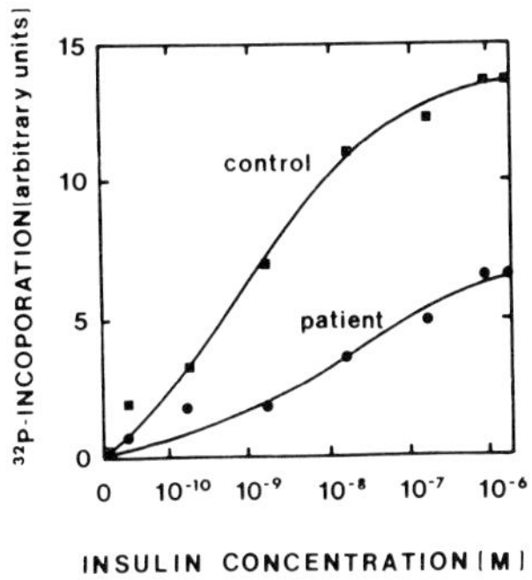

Figure 4. Phosphorylation of the erythrocyte insulin receptor from a normal control and an insulin resistant patient.

This is not surprising, since we have previously shown that both the α and β subunits are lost proportionally during down-regulation.

Phorbol esters, on the other hand, produce a desensitization of insulin action in hepatoma cells without producing a change in insulin binding (8). When hepatoma cells are exposed to TPA, a potent phorbol diester, there is a marked decrease in the ability of insulin to activate glycogen synthase and stimulate tyrosine aminotransferase. This effect occurs within 30 min and is dependent on the concentration of TPA.

When cells were labeled with ^{32}P-orthophosphate, we found that TPA stimulated the phosphorylation of the insulin receptor by 32%, while reducing insulin stimulated phosphorylation by 50%. Phosphoamino acid analysis revealed that TPA alone increased both phosphoserine and phosphothreonine while producing a decrease in insulin-stimulated phosphorylation of tyrosine. Thus, TPA stimulates phosphorylation of the insulin receptor on serine, presumably through activation of a calcium and phospholipid dependent kinase, C-kinase, and this results in a decrease in insulin-stimulated tyrosine phosphorylation and development of an insulin resistant state (Figure 3). These data suggest that while tyrosine phosphorylation may "activate" the insulin receptor kinase, serine and/or threonine phosphorylation may serve to inactivate the kinase.

Altered insulin receptor phosphorylation in disease states

The syndrome of insulin resistance and acanthosis nigricans Type A is characterized by severe insulin resistance due to a primary defect in insulin action at the cellular level. The receptor defect in Type A patients is heterogenous. In some patients, the primary defect consists of a major decrease in insulin binding which is observed in several different cellular systems derived from the patients including erythrocytes, monocytes, and fibroblasts. This defect is also trained in the solubilized form of the receptor. To define possible defects in receptor kinase activity in this disease, we have developed methods to study receptor phosphorylation using human erythrocytes and fibroblasts (9). Using these techniques, we found that the kinase activity of the receptor is also markedly decreased in

Type A patients, as evidenced by a decrease in insulin-stimulated receptor phosphorylation (Figure 4). Interestingly, in one of our patients, and in a patient reported by Grunberger et al. (10), a significant reduction in kinase activity was observed in the presence of unaltered insulin binding. Thus, in these patients, there is "post-binding" defect in insulin action located at the level of the receptor kinase activity.

We have also studied insulin binding and kinase activity in monozygotic twin pairs discordant for Type II diabetes. Thus far, three twin pairs, discordant for diabetes for 10-20 years, have been studied. In all three pairs, insulin binding to circulating erythrocytes and monocytes was lower in the diabetic patient than in the non-affected twin mate. The decrease in insulin binding in the erythrocytes was small, and thus in most cases, data on both twins actually fell within the normal range. Quantitative analysis of the binding data revealed that this decrease in binding was due to a decrease in receptor affinity in erythrocytes and a decrease in receptor number in monocytes. Insulin receptor autophosphorylation was studied using receptors extracted from the erythrocytes of one pair of twins. Although autophosphorylation was similar at maximal insulin concentrations, the dose-response curve for the diabetic twin was shifted to the right, consistent with the lower receptor affinity.

In summary, the insulin receptor is an insulin-stimulated, tyrosine-specific protein kinase. In genetic and acquired forms of insulin resistance in which there is a decrease in total receptor number, there is a proportional decrease in both the binding and kinase activity of the receptor. Selective decreases in tyrosine kinase activity may also occur, for example after phorbol ester treatment or in some Type A patients. In these situations, the decrease in autophosphorylation correlates with the presence of an insulin-resistant state. These data suggest an important role of the insulin action, and also provide a potential mechanism for post-binding receptor defects in insulin resistant states.

REFERENCES

1. Czech M (1981) Amer J Med 70:142

2. Kasuga M, Hedo, JA, Yamada KM, Kahn CR (1982) J Biol Chem 257:10392

3. Crettaz M, Kahn CR (1984) Diabetes 33:472

4. Kasuga M, Karlsson FA, Kahn CR (1982) Science 215:185

5. Kahn CR, White M, Grigorescu F, Haring HU, Crettaz M In: Czech M (ed) Molecular Basis of Insulin Action. Plenum Press, in press.

6. Simpson I, Hedo JA (1984) Science 223:1301

7. Kahn CR, Baird KL, Jarrett DB, Flier JS (1978) Proc Natl Acad Sci USA 75: 4209

8. Takayama S, White MF, Lauris V, Kahn CR (1984) Proc Natl Acad Sci USA, in press

9. Grigorescu F, White MF, Kahn CR (1983) J Biol Chem 258:13708

Endocrinology
F. Labrie, L. Proulx, eds.

DETERMINANTS AND PATHOGENESIS OF NON-INSULIN-DEPENDENT DIABETES IN THE PIMA INDIANS

PETER H. BENNETT, CLIFTON BOGARDUS, JAMES FOLEY, WILLIAM C. KNOWLER, AND DAVID J. PETTITT
National Institute of Arthritis, Diabetes, and Digestive and Kidney Diseases, Phoenix, Arizona, U.S.A.

INTRODUCTION

The Pima Indian population of Arizona has the highest frequency of diabetes yet recorded. The disease appears to be exclusively of the non-insulin-dependent type (NIDDM) and is associated with the development of the usual characteristic vascular complications (1). As the Pima are a well circumscribed, stable and relatively homogeneous population, longitudinal epidemiological, genetic, and clinical research among them has led to knowledge of some aspects of the determinants and pathogenesis of NIDDM.

CHARACTERISTICS AND DETERMINANTS OF NIDDM IN THE PIMA

Development of NIDDM in the Pima is related to interactions of age, degree of obesity and preexisting evidence of glucose intolerance, as well as the presence of diabetes in one or both parents (2). Evidence of the importance of genetic determinants includes familial aggregation of the disease, such that the incidence after adjustment for other factors is dependent on the presence or absence of diabetes in the parents; the association of a decreasing frequency of the disease in those with non-Indian admixture; and an association of the disease with a specific genetic marker (3). Bimodal frequency distributions of plasma glucose levels in the adult population suggest that a single major gene may be the most important determinant of susceptibility (4), and analyses of kindreds indicate that, if so, a dominant mode of inheritance with variable penetrance, to account for the variations seen with age and obesity, etc., is the most likely mechanism.

Obesity and diabetes are also more common in the offspring of diabetic pregnancies than in offspring whose mothers developed diabetes only later (5). Thus, non-genetic factors, even those operating before birth, may influence the expression of the disease.

Hyperinsulinemia is a characteristic of Pima Indians who are at high risk of developing the disease, and among diabetics of recent onset fasting insulin levels are high. In those with normal and impaired glucose tolerance insulin levels rise proportionately with increasing glucose intolerance, and are greater in the obese than the nonobese, but do not diminish at the onset of diabetes (6). As no structural abnormality of insulin has been detected among the Pima, insulin resistance appears to be an important feature in the development of the disease.

THE ROLE OF DIMINISHED INSULIN-MEDIATED GLUCOSE DISPOSAL

Insulin sensitivity assessed by *in vivo* insulin-mediated glucose disposal and measured using the euglycemic clamp techniques, shows a sharp decline with increasing glucose levels over the range of normal fasting glucose concentrations in the Pima, whereas in diabetics the disposal rates are consistently very low (7). Severe impairment of insulin-mediated glucose disposal is, therefore, pathognomonic of NIDDM in the Pima.

The decline in insulin-mediated glucose disposal seen over the nondiabetic range of glucose tolerance in subjects at high risk of developing diabetes indicates that this defect is a critical component in the development of NIDDM.

THE CELLULAR BASIS OF DIMINISHED INSULIN ACTION

The cellular basis of the abnormal insulin action has been investigated in adipocytes and in muscle. The capacity of insulin-mediated glucose transport is reduced in adipocytes from Pima diabetics and the insulin concentration required for half-maximal glucose transport is increased (8). The maximal transport capacity, however, can be increased appreciably by insulin treatment to maintain normoglycemia for several weeks (9), whereas the sensitivity to insulin-mediated glucose transport remains unchanged.

Examination of the fate of metabolized glucose in subjects with different degrees of impairment of glucose disposal *in vivo* indicates that the amount of glucose oxidized remains relatively unchanged, but that the amount processed by non-oxidative pathways, and which is stored, is markedly diminished in those with impaired disposal (10). As most of the glucose processed by non-oxidative pathways is taken up by muscle to form glycogen, the relationship between *in vivo* insulin-mediated glucose disposal and muscle glycogen synthase activity was examined (11). Glucose storage correlated well (r=0.78) with glycogen synthase activity measured in muscle biopsies, suggesting that activation of glycogen synthase by insulin was impaired and may account for the decreased storage of infused glucose observed in those with impaired glucose disposal.

As both glucose transport and the activation of glycogen synthase depend on intracellular events, and as no evidence of any abnormality in the binding of insulin to its receptor has been found among the Pima (8), the basis of impaired *in vivo* insulin-mediated glucose disposal appears to be a post-binding defect in insulin action. This leads to abnormalities in at least two important effects of insulin action, glucose transport and glucose storage.

CONCLUSIONS

NIDDM is extraordinarily frequent among the Pima Indians and genetic susceptibility, possibly due to a single major dominant gene, is probably necessary for its development, although other factors, such as age, degree of obesity and exposure to other environmental factors, determine whether or not, and when it becomes manifest. Impairment of insulin-mediated glucose disposal appears to be a critical component in the development of the disease. The mechanism of impaired glucose disposal appears to be a post-binding defect in insulin action. Whether or not this post-binding coupling defect is directly related to the primary inherited abnormality of NIDDM is unknown, but longitudinal studies of the development of NIDDM among the Pima may ultimately lead to understanding of the relationship between the genetic determinants and the defect in insulin action which is associated with the development of NIDDM.

REFERENCES

1. Bennett PH, Rushforth NB, Miller M, LeCompte PM (1976) Recent Prog Horm Res 32:333-376
2. Knowler WC, Pettitt DJ, Savage PJ, Bennett PH (1981) Am J Epidemiol 113: 144-156
3. Williams RC, Knowler WC, Butler WJ, Pettitt DJ, Lisse JR, Bennett PH, Mann DL, Johnson AH, Terasaki PI (1981) Diabetologia 21:460-463
4. Rushforth NB, Bennett PH, Steinberg AG, Burch TA, Miller M (1971) Diabetes 20:756-765
5. Pettitt DJ, Baird HR, Aleck KA, Bennett PH, Knowler WC (1983) N Engl J Med 308:242-245
6. Bennett PH, Knowler WC, Pettitt DJ, Carraher MJ, Vasquez B (1982) In: Eschwege E (ed) Advances in Diabetes Epidemiology. Elsevier, Amsterdam, pp 65-74
7. Bogardus C, Lillioja S, Howard BV, Reaven G, Mott D (1984) J Clin Invest 73: (in press)
8. Kashiwagi A, Verso MA, Andrews J, Vasquez B, Reaven G, Foley JE (1983) J Clin Invest 72:1246-1254
9. Foley JE, Kashiwagi A, Verso MA, Reaven G, Andrews J (1983) J Clin Invest 72:1901-1909
10. Bogardus C, Lillioja S, Mott D, Reaven GR, Kashiwagi A, Foley JE (1984) J Clin Invest 73:800-805
11. Bogardus, C. Lillioja S, Stone K, Mott D (1984) J Clin Invest 74:1185-1190

12. Organization and Expression of Hormone Genes

Endocrinology
F. Labrie, L. Proulx, eds.

STRUCTURE AND EXPRESSION OF THE HUMAN PARATHYROID HORMONE GENE

HENRY M. KRONENBERG, JAMES HELLERMAN, TETSUYA IGARASHI, MASON FREEMAN, STEPHEN BRAND, WILLIAM BORNSTEIN, LIONEL IVASHKIV, AARON RAPOPORT, RICHARD C. MULLIGAN*, ALEXANDER RICH**, AND JOHN T. POTTS, JR

Endocrine Unit, Massachusetts General Hospital and Harvard Medical School, Boston Mass., *Whitehead Institute, and **Department of Biology, Massachusetts Institute of Technology, Cambridge, Mass.

INTRODUCTION

Parathyroid hormone (PTH) is the major regulator of the level of ionized calcium in the blood of all animals more evolutionarily advanced than fish. Calcium, in turn, tightly regulates the secretion of PTH. While the homeostatic system controlling the secretion of PTH is understood, little is known about the regulation of the biosynthesis of PTH. PTH is first synthesized as a larger precursor, preproPTH. This precursor is cleaved in the parathyroid cell, first to an intermediate precursor, proPTH, and then to PTH, as the protein travels from the cisternae of the rough endoplasmic reticulum, to the Golgi apparatus, and then to the secretory granule. Here we shall describe our studies of two aspects of the biosynthesis of PTH: first, the structure of the PTH gene and the regulation of the gene's transcription, and, second, the mechanism of intracellular transport of PTH and the function of precursor sequences.

PARATHYROID HORMONE GENE

Using standard approaches, we first isolated cDNA clones representing the bovine PTH mRNA (1). This probe, in turn, was used to identify human PTH cDNA clones in a cDNA library generated from a parathyroid adenoma removed from a patient with primary hyperparathyroidism (2). Then the human cDNA was used to screen a human genomic DNA lambda phage library. The library was screened both by the plaque-hybridization method and by the use of the ΠVX recombination vector of Seed (3). By comparing the sequence of the genomic DNA with the sequence of the cDNA, it was possible to localize the gene's intervening sequences. We found that the human PTH gene is interrupted by two intervening sequences. The first intervening sequence is 3200 base pairs in length and comes just five base pairs before the start of the gene's coding region. The second intervening sequence is 103 base pairs in length and comes near the end of the "pro" sequence, which connects the "pre" or signal sequence to PTH.

Southern blot analysis showed that the haploid human genome contains only one copy of the PTH gene. By examining a series of human-mouse cell hybirds, each containing different human chromosomes, for the presence of the human PTH gene,

Naylor et al (4) localized the human PTH gene to the short arm of the chromosome 11. Antonarakis et al (5) then found a restriction enzyme site polymorphism closely linked to the human PTH gene. By examining the patterns of inheritance of this polymorphism and of similar polymorphisms associated with the β-globin and insulin genes, these workers demonstrated that the PTH gene is closely linked to the β-globin gene on the short arm of chromosome 11. This sort of genetic analysis is now being extended to follow the inheritance of specific PTH genes in families with disorders of calcium metabolism.

Recently, we have introduced the human PTH gene into cultured cells, in order to analyze the regulation of the gene's transcription. Permanent lines of parathyroid cells are unavailable. Consequently, we have introduced the PTH gene into rat pituitary GH4 cells. These cells have vitamin D receptors and respond to a variety of stimuli with a modulation of intracellular calcium levels. In these ways GH4 cells resemble parathyroid cells and may prove to be acceptable surrogates for determining the effects of vitamin D and calcium on PTH gene transcription.

We introduced the PTH gene into GH4 cells using an electroshock technique developed by Hunt Potter. To assure that the introduced gene would be transcribed, we inserted the *E. coli* gene encoding aminoglycoside resistance (*neo*) into the 5'-non-coding region of the PTH gene. The resultant plasmid also contained 600 base pairs of DNA upstream from the PTH gene. After electroshock, we selected GH4 cells resistant to G418, an aminoglycoside toxic to mammaliam cells. The resultant cell lines all transcribed the *neo* gene, using the same two clusters of transcription start sites used by the PTH gene in human parathyroid cells. These cell lines can now be used to examine the effects of changes in intracellular calcium and vitamin D levels on PTH gene transcription.

INTRACELLULAR TRANSPORT OF PTH

The precursor of PTH, preproPTH, is cleaved to proPTH during the transport of the protein across the membrane of the rough endoplasmic reticulum. The "pre" sequence contains a sequence of hydrophobic residues and resembles other signal sequences usually found at the amino terimini of the precursors of secreted proteins. These signals are thought to direct polysomes synthesizing the precursors to the membrane of the rough endoplasmic reticulum. In order to analyze this process in detail, we have expressed the preproPTH cDNA in two systems that allow us to examine aspects of the secretory process. To follow PTH through the entire secretory pathway, we have expressed the PTH cDNA in cultured GH4 cells (6); to focus on the early steps of the processing of prepro-PTH, we have used an *in vitro* linked transcription-translation system (7).

To express human preproPTH cDNA in GH4 cells, we introduced the cDNA into a retroviral vector containing regulatory sequences from Moloney murine leukemia virus. The cDNA was inserted in place of the viral *gag-pol* sequence. The selectable marker, *E. coli gpt*, was inserted in place of the viral *env* gene. By preserving viral splice sites, we expected that the retroviral provirus would be transcribed into two RNA species: a genome-length RNA that would be translated into preproPTH, and a spliced RNA that would be translated into xanthine-guanine phosphoribosyl transferase, the product of the *gpt* gene. Since we were interested in studying the secretory pathway, which might be affected by the packaging and budding of viral particles, we wanted to package the PTH-retroviral genome into virus without subsequently introducing viral structural genes into GH4 cells. Toward this end, we first transfected the recombinant PTH-retroviral provirus into Psi 2 cells. Psi 2 cells are an NIH 3T3 fibroblast line containing a mutant Moloney leukemia viral provirus in its genome. Because of a small deletion in its "psi" or packaging sequence, the provirus encodes all the normal viral proteins, but these proteins cannot encapsidate the defective viral genomic RNA produced in the cells. When these cells were transfected with the recominant PTH-retrovirus, they then could produce infectious virus containing only the genome of the PTH-retrovirus. This virus was used to infect GH4 cells, and successfully infected cells were selected by the use of a medium that requires the functioning of the *E. coli gpt* gene. As expected, the recombinant PTH-retroviral provirus was inserted into the host cell's genome via the long terminal repeats demarcating the ends of the proviral sequence. Also as expected, the cells produce two retroviral RNA species: a full-length genomic sequence, and a smaller spliced mRNA. These cells were pulse-labeled with [^{35}S]-methionine for 15 minutes and then chased with cold methionine for various times. PTH-related peptides were immune-precipitated from cell extracts and media and subjected to polyacrylamide gel electrophoresis. At the earliest time, proPTH and PTH were found in the cell. Subsequently, the proPTH was converted to PTH, and the PTH was secreted into the medium.

Thyrotropin releasing hormone (TRH), which caused a doubling of the secretion of prolactin from these cells, also caused a doubling of PTH secretion. This result strongly supports the hypotheses that PTH is secreted from GH4 cells via a normal secretory pathway. It also suggests that TRH does not cause the secretion of prolactin specifically, but rather causes the secretion of whatever proteins are transported to an appropriate secretory compartment.

Recently, we have constructed a series of mutant PTH cDNAs encoding modified preproPTHs, missing portions of the precursor-specific region. These mutant cDNAs have been inserted into retroviral vectors and then into GH4 cells.

Using the methodology described above, we have found that different deletions cause characteristically different defects in the secretory pathway. We have also used a linked transcription-translation system to analyze in some detail the early steps of the secretory pathway. To use this system efficiently, we placed the *lac* promoter upstream from the preproPTH cDNA. The plasmid DNA was then transcribed into RNA using *E. coli* RNA polymerase, and the RNA was then translated into protein using either a rabbit reticulocyte lysate or a wheat germ cell-free extract. In both cases addition of microsomes from canine pancreas allowed the cleavage of preproPTH to proPTH and the transport of proPTH into the microsomal vesicular space. As expected, mutant cDNAs display characteristic dysfunction in this system, thus allowing us to analyze the biochemical underpinnings of the mutant phenotypes in greater detail.

CONCLUSION

The cDNA and genomic DNAs encoding preproPTH are reagents that allow us to express the PTH gene and its transcription products in cultured cells and in cell-free extracts. These expression systems are now allowing us to characterize the regulation of gene transcription and the control of the secretory pathway in detail.

REFERENCES

1. Kronenberg HM, McDevitt BE, Majzoub JA, Nathans J, Sharp PA, Potts JT JR, Rich A (1979) Proc Natl Acad Sci USA 76:4981-4985

2. Hendy GN, Kronenberg HM, Potts JT JR, Rich A (1981) Proc Natl Acad Sci USA 78:7365-7369

3. Vasicek T, McDevitt B, Hendy G, Freeman M, Potts JT JR, Rich A, Kronenberg H (1983) Proc Natl Acad Sci USA 80:2127-2131

4. Naylor SL, Sakaguchi AY, Szoka P, Hendy GN, Kronenberg H, Rich A, Shows TB (1983) Somatic Cell Genetics 9:609-616

5. Antonarakis SE, Phillips JA, Mallonee RL, Kazazian HH JR, Fearon ER, Waber PG, Kronenberg HM, Ulrich A, Meyers DA (1983) Proc Natl Acad Sci USA 80:6615-6619

6. Hellerman JG, Cone RC, Segre GV, Potts JT JR, Rich A, Mulligan RC, Kronenberg HM (1984) Proc Acad Sci USA in press

7. Kronenberg HM, Fennick BJ, Vasicek TJ (1983) J Cell Biol 96:1117-1119

Endocrinology
F. Labrie, L. Proulx, eds.

EXPRESSION OF METALLOTHIONEIN-GROWTH HORMONE FUSION GENES IN TRANSGENIC MICE

R. E. HAMMER[1], R. D. PALMITER[2], and R. L. BRINSTER[1]
[1]Laboratory of Reproductive Physiology, School of Veterinary Medicine, University of Pennsylvania, Philadelphia, PA 19104
[2]Department of Biochemistry, Howard Hughes Medical Institute, University of Washington, Seattle, WA 98195

Gene expression and regulation have been studied by utilizing transfected cell lines and more recently transgenic mice. While both methods can provide insight into the nature of gene expression only the transgenic model can provide information on the physiological consequences of such expression. A number of genes have now been successfully introduced into mice and in some cases expression has been demonstrated[1-4]. We have been particularly interested in using fusion genes containing the mouse metallothionein I promoter/regulator sequence (MT) because the metallothionein gene is expressed in a number of tissues, is induced by heavy metals and functions when fused to the herpes simplex viral thymidine kinase (TK) structural gene[5]. The demonstration of MT-TK expression raised the possibility of using this promoter to regulate the transcriptional activity of a growth hormone (GH) gene and thereby control growth. For this purpose we fused the MT promoter to the rat[6] and human[7] GH structural genes.

Linear DNA fragments containing MT human GH (MT-hGH)[8] or rat GH (MT-rGH)[9] genes were microinjected into the male pronuclei of fertilized mouse eggs. The resulting 122 animals that developed from these eggs were analyzed for the presence of the foreign gene by DNA dot hybridization. Forty mice contained from 1 to 455 copies of the fusion gene and the majority (29) grew significantly larger than their littermates. This enhanced growth was correlated with a high level of GH mRNA production in the liver and to a lesser degree in testis, heart and intestine. Superimposed on this hierarchy of tissue expression were striking departures from this pattern which may be attributable to the influence of chromosomal location[9].

High GH mRNA levels correlated with the presence of large quantities of serum GH (Table 1). Although serum GH levels in most MT-hGH mice could be increased by chronic zinc treatment, growth rates were not affected. Apparently the constitutive level of GH present from MT-hGH gene expression (~100ng) was sufficient to stimulate insulin-like growth factor-I (IGF-I) production and thereby accelerate growth maximally.

Transgenic mice carrying MT-rGH or MT-hGH fusion genes start growing faster than littermates a few weeks after birth, enter an accelerated growth phase between 5 and 11 weeks of age and at about 14 weeks begin growing at a rate resembling controls (Fig. 1). Fusion gene mRNA transcripts are present both before and after this growth period (unpublished) and therefore we suspect the lack of accelerated growth at these times reflects the changing developmental responsiveness to GH and/or IGF-I.

TABLE 1

EXPRESSION OF MT-hGH IN TRANSGENIC MICE

Animal	Gene Copy number/cell	Serum hGH ng/ml -Zn	Serum hGH ng/ml +Zn	Growth ratio
184-1♀	2.0	250	11,900	2.37
184-5♂	10.4	520	18,000	1.70
186-4♀	18.0	8,200	143,000	2.14
182-3♂	45.0	3,700	14,600	1.67

Copy number was determined by DNA dot hybridization. Serum samples were taken before (-Zn) or during 25mM $ZnSO_4$ (+Zn) water treatment (17 to 21 weeks of age) and GH determined by RIA.

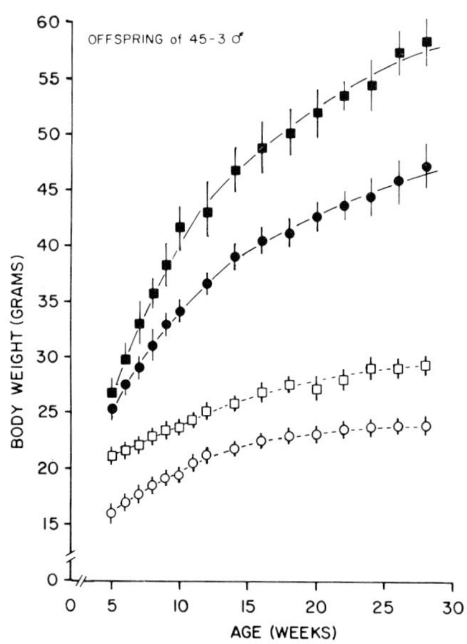

Fig. 1. Comparative growth of transgenic progeny (solid symbols) of 45-3 (MGH 10) expressing MT-rGH fusion genes and control littermates (open symbols). Transgenic mice (weights of males-squares, females-circles) are already larger than controls at 5 weeks of age, enter an accelerated growth phase between 5 and 11 weeks and by 17 weeks of age are double normal size. N ≥ 5 at each point.

Pedigree analysis of transgenic mice indicates that foreign genes are commonly inherited as though they were integrated into a single chromosome, even when there are multiple copies of the gene. The MT-rGH fusion gene has now been transmitted into the 6th generation with continued expression in every offspring that carries the foreign gene. Growth rates remain accelerated with the average increase in adult size being about 2 fold.

As a result of the demonstration that the mouse MT promoter/regulator functions when fused to GH structural genes from two different species we attempted to correct the growth disorder of the GH deficient mutant lit/lit mouse by introducing MT-rGH genes into mutant eggs[10]. Forty-one animals developed from microinjected eggs; seven carried the foreign gene.

Transgenic little mice were twice mutant size by 6 weeks of age and grew to approximately 1.5 times the size of normal heterozygous animals. Restored growth correlated with elevations in serum GH which ranged between 5 to 120 times higher than +/+ controls.

To determine if the fusion gene was stably integrated into the host chromosome making the gene and new phenotype heritable, a male (54-1) containing 8 copies of the MT-rGH gene was outbred (Fig. 2). The fusion gene has been passed into the 3rd generation with every transgenic mutant offspring surpassing mutant and normal size. In addition MT-rGH expression improved the suboptimal fertility of mutant males; however female fertility was impaired.

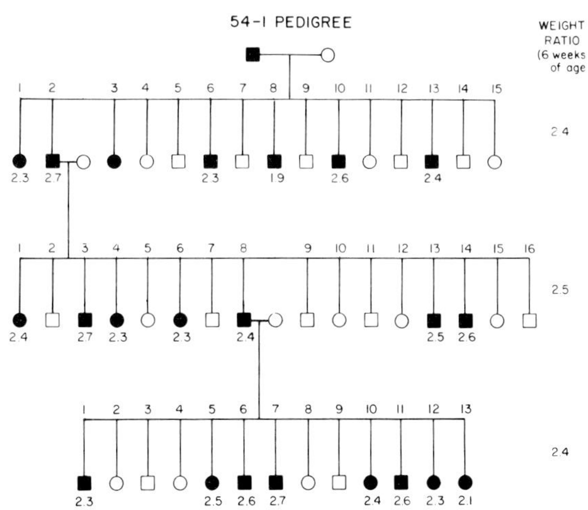

Fig. 2. Pedigree of transgenic mutant male 54-1 showing inheritance and expression of the MT-rGH gene. Approximately 50% of the offspring in three generations carry the fusion gene (solid symbols). All of the transgenic offspring were more than twice mutant size by 6 weeks of age.

Thus we have demonstrated that the effects of a single gene defect can be partially overcome by the introduction of a foreign replacement gene into mutant eggs. Although germ line therapy does not represent a feasible remedy to genetic disorders, it does provide a unique opportunity to examine the etiologies of a variety of hereditary diseases.

ACKNOWLEDGEMENTS

We thank our colleagues for their contributions which made these studies possible. We are grateful to M. Trumbauer and M. Yagle for valuable assistance in the experiments. This work was supported by grants from NIH: HD-07155, HD-09172, HD-17321, AM31322, NSF: PCM-81-07172 and the American Heart Association: 80-728.

REFERENCES

1. Wagner TF, Stewart TA, and Mintz B (1981) Proc Nat Acad Sci USA 78:5016-5020
2. Lacy E, Roberts S, Evans EP, Burtenshaw MD, and Constantini FD (1983) Cell 34:343-358
3. McKnight GS, Hammer RE, Kuenzel EA, and Brinster RL (1983) Cell 34:335-341
4. Brinster RL, Ritchie KA, Hammer RE, O'Brien RL, Arp B, and Storb U (1983) Nature 306:332-336
5. Brinster RL, Chen HY, Trumbauer M, Senear AW, Warren R, and Palmiter RD (1981) Cell 27:223-231
6. Doehmer J, Barinaga M, Vale W, Rosenfeld MG, Verma IM, and Evans RM (1982) Proc Nat Acad Sci USA 79:2268-2272
7. Barsh GS, Seeburg PH, and Gelinas RE (1983) Nucleic Acids Res 11:3939-3958
8. Palmiter RD, Brinster RL, Hammer RE, Trumbauer M, Rosenfeld MA, Birnberg NC, and Evans RM (1982) Nature 300:611-614
9. Palmiter RD, Norstedt G, Gelinas RE, Hammer RE, and Brinster RL (1983) Science 222:809-814
10. Hammer RE, Palmiter RD, and Brinster RL (1984) Nature, in press

Endocrinology
F. Labrie, L. Proulx, eds.

ORGANIZATION AND EXPRESSION OF LUTROPIN SUBUNIT GENES

William W. Chin and Joel F. Habener
Laboratory of Molecular Endocrinology, Massachusetts General Hosp., and Howard Hughes Medical Institute Labs., Harvard Medical School, Boston, MA 02114, USA

INTRODUCTION

Lutropin (LH) is a glycoprotein hormone consisting of two different non-covalently associated subunits, designated α and LHβ, that is synthesized by the gonadotrope of the anterior pituitary gland. LH and the structurally related pituitary thyrotropin and follitropin, and placental chorionic gonadotropin (CG) constitute the glycoprotein hormone family. The apoprotein of the α subunit is identical among hormones within a species whereas the β subunits are dissimilar and, as such, confer specific biological activities to the assembled dimers (1). In addition, the production of LH is regulated by hypothalamic factors and gonadal sex steroid hormones (2). However, little is known about the regulation of the biosynthesis of LH at the pre-translational level. Using new techniques in molecular biology, we have determined the structures of the genes encoding the subunits (α and LHβ) of rat LH and how the genes are organized in the genome. In addition, the cloned cDNAs representing the α and LHβ mRNAs have permitted the assays of steady-state subunit mRNA levels by blot hybridization techniques. In this manuscript, we describe (a) the structure of the rat LHβ gene, (b) the chromosomal localization of the LH subunit genes, and (c) regulation of the steady-state levels of α and LHβ mRNAs by gonadal sex steroids.

MATERIALS AND METHODS

Isolation and characterization of the rat LHβ gene. Cloned DNA encoding the rat LHβ gene was isolated by screening a bacteriophage λ library containing rat genomic DNA with a [^{32}P]-labeled cDNA encoding rat LHβ (3). A bacteriophage clone containing the putative LHβ gene was then subjected to restriction enzyme digestion and DNA sequence analysis (4).

Chromosomal localization of the LH subunit genes in mouse and man. The chromosomal constitution of human-mouse and mouse-Chinese hamster somatic cell hybrids were determined by karyotype and enzyme markers (5). DNAs from these cell lines were subjected to blot hybridization studies using cloned cDNAs encoding human α (6), human CGβ (7), and mouse α (8). Correlation of the presence of a subunit gene in a cell line with the presence or absence of the various human or mouse chromosomes allowed localization of the gene to a particular chromosome (5).

Blot hybridization analysis of subunit mRNAs. Steady-state levels of LH subunit mRNAs in pituitary glands were determined by RNA blot hybridization techniques (3) using cDNAs encoding rat α (9) and LHβ (3).

Radioimmunoassay of rat LH. The serum LH was determined by a sensitive double-antibody radioimmunoassay (RIA) as previously described (10).

RESULTS AND DISCUSSION

Structure of the LH subunit genes. The α and LHβ subunits of rat LH are encoded by separate genes (11). In addition, blot hybridization analyses of rat genomic DNA with rat α and LHβ cDNAs indicate that these subunits are represented by unique genes. We have isolated and characterized the rat LHβ gene (Fig. 1). Of note, in exon 1, is the 5'-untranslated region (5'-UT) which

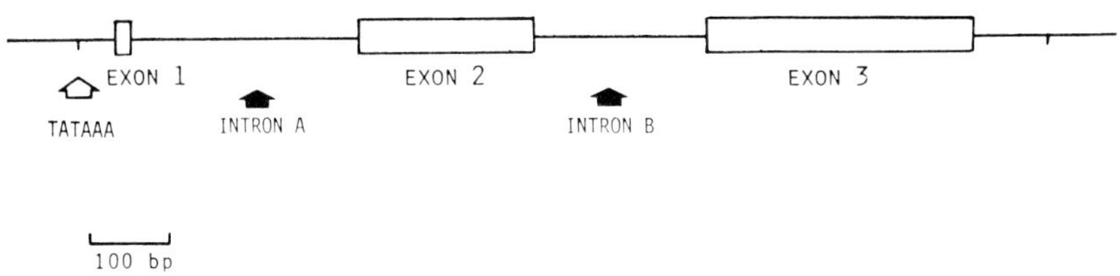

Figure 1. Schematic diagram of the gene encoding the β subunit of rat LH. Eucaryotic genes, in general, are comprised of two types of DNA: exons which contain coding sequences representing the mature mRNA, and introns which are dispersed between exons and presumably contain "extraneous" information. The rat LHβ subunit gene is 0.98 Kb in size and contains 3 exons and 2 introns (solid arrows). The open arrows point to the sequence TATAAA which represents the Goldberg-Hogness promoter region (12).

is short and contains only 7 bases. A comparison of the structure of the rat LHβ gene with those of the human LH and CGβ genes (13) shows that they are conserved. In fact, a computer-assisted analysis of the DNAs representing the 5'-flanking regions of these genes for 200--250 base pairs reveals that the level of homology is high. In this light, it is interesting that the start of transcription for the rat gene is considerably different than the presumed start of transcription for the hCGβ gene [the 5'-UT of the hCGβ gene is >300 bases (13)]. Thus, subtle alterations in these regions of these genes may result in altered starts of transcription. In addition, since the two genes are apparently regulated in different ways by gonadal sex steroids, these differences may shed light on the DNA sequence(s) responsible for the control of transcription of the rat LHβ gene by estrogen and testosterone.

Chromosomal localization of the LH subunit genes. Using well-characterized human-mouse and mouse-Chinese hamster somatic cell hybrids, we have localized the human α and all of the human LH/CGβ [there are 7 CGβ genes in man (13)] genes to chromosomes 6 and 19, respectively, and mouse α and LHβ genes to chromosomes 4 and 7, respectively (5). Therefore, α and LHβ/CGβ are not only encoded by separate genes but genes located on different chromosomes.

Hormonal regulation of the steady-state levels of LH subunit mRNAs. We have studied the effect of gonadectomy on the steady-state levels of LH subunit mRNAs in the pituitary gland and serum LH in rats. Oophorectomized female rats were sacrificed at various times after castration. The pituitary glands were removed for subunit mRNA determinations by blot hybridization methods, and trunk blood was recovered for serum LH by RIA. Serum LH increased >10-fold at 21d after castration. Over the same period, the steady-state levels of mRNAs for the LH subunits also increased 8—10-fold with the major changes occurring after 7d (Fig. 4). Figure 4 also illustrates that there are greater amounts of α than of

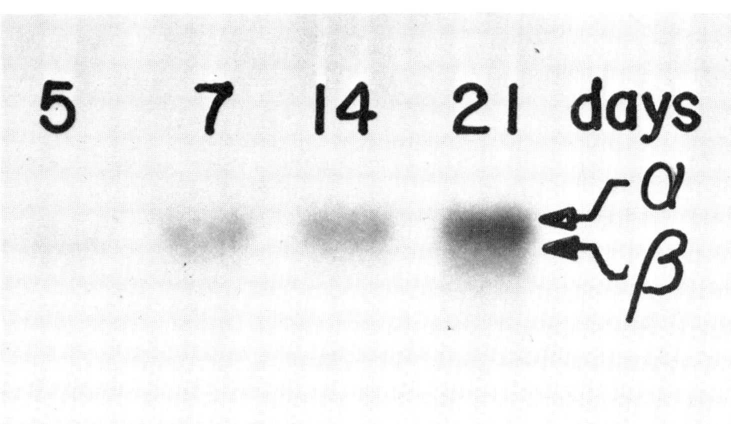

Figure 2. Effect of ovariectomy on the steady-state levels of subunit mRNAs: time course. Rats (Sprague-Dawley; 200--225g) were oophorectomized and sacrificed at various times post-operatively. Total RNA isolated from the pituitary glands of these rats were subjected to RNA blot hybridization analysis using labeled α and LHβ cDNA probes in the same hybridization experiment. Note the gradual increase in the bands corresponding to α and LHβ subunit mRNAs. In addition, it is observed that the ratio of α/LHβ mRNA is >1. The arrows indicate the positions of migration of the α (α) and LHβ (β) mRNAs.

LHβ mRNA at all time points after castration. Similar results have been obtained for the gonadectomized male rat. In addition, in data not shown, we have performed experiments in which gonadectomized rats were replaced with physiologic doses of estrogen and testosterone. The steady-state levels of subunit mRNAs decline in a coordinate fashion in parallel with the serum LH levels. These changes occurred rapidly so that the mRNA and LH levels had reached ~30--40% of control levels by 24h. These results are consistent with those of previous studies (14, 15, 16). However, it is not known whether this control is exerted at the transcriptional and/or RNA stability levels.

SUMMARY

We have cloned and characterized cDNAs and natural genes encoding the α and β subunits of rat LH. In particular, the structure of the rat LHβ subunit gene has been examined in detail. The genes representing the subunits of LH in mouse and man are located on different chromosomes. Finally, the steady-state levels of the subunit mRNAs are regulated by the gonadal sex steroid hormones in a coordinate and rapid (sex-steroid replacement) fashion. The availability of these clones DNAs will permit detailed studies in the molecular mechanisms involved in the regulation of the expression of the LH subunit genes by gonadal steroids.

ACKNOWLEDGEMENTS

We thank Susan Naylor, Larry Jameson, Soheyla Gharib, and Stephen Bowers for their major contributions to these studies.

REFERENCES

1. Pierce JG, Parsons TF (1981) Ann Rev Biochem 50:465
2. Vaitukaitis JL, Ross GT, Braunstein GD, Rayford PL (1976) Rec Prog Horm Res 32:289
3. Chin WW, Godine JE, Klein DR, Chang AS, Tan LK, Habener JF (1983) Proc Natl Acad Sci USA 80:4649
4. Jameson JL, Chin WW, Hollenberg AN, Chang AS, Habener JF (1984) J Biol Chem (submitted).
5. Naylor SL, Chin WW, Goodman HM, Lalley PA, Grzeschik KH, Sakaguchi AY (1983) Somat Cell Genet 9:757
6. Fiddes JC, Goodman HM (1979) Nature 281:351
7. Fiddes JC, Goodman HM (1980) Nature 286:684
8. Chin WW, Kronenberg HM, Dee PC, Maloof F, Habener JF (1981) Proc Natl Acad Sci USA 78:5329
9. Godine JE, Chin WW, Habener JF (1982) J Biol Chem 257:8368
10. Ross DS, Downing MF, Chin WW, Kieffer JD, Ridgway EC (1983) Endocrinology 112:187
11. Godine JE, Chin WW, Habener JF (1980) J Biol Chem 255:8780
12. Benoist C, O'Hare K, Breathmach R, Chambon P (1980) Nucl Acids Res 8:127
13. Talmadge K, Vamvakopoulos NC, Fiddes JC (1984) Nature 307:37
14. Landefeld TD, Kepa J, Karsch FJ (1983) J Biol Chem 258:2390
15. Counis R, Corbani M, Jutisz M (1983) Biochem Biophys Res Commun 114:65
16. Nilson JH, Nejedlik MT, Virgin JB, Crowder ME, Nett TM (1983) J Biol Chem 258:12087

Endocrinology
F. Labrie, L. Proulx, eds.

GROWTH HORMONE AND PLACENTAL LACTOGEN GENES

JOHN S. PARKS
Division of Pediatric Endocrinology, Emory University School of Medicine, Atlanta, Georgia 30322 (U.S.A.)

INTRODUCTION

The growth hormone family of genes consists of five structural genes located over a distance of 55 kilobases (kb) on the long arm of human chromosome 17 (1). These genes are oriented in the same direction in the order 5' hGH-N, hCS-L, hCS-A, hGH-V, hCS-B 3' (2). The organization of each of the five related genes is quite uniform (3). Each contains five coding sequences or exons designated I-V. Four intervening sequences or introns designated A-D occur at identical positions relative to amino acid codons. Transcription results in a premessenger RNA approximately 1,650 nucleotides in length. RNA sequences corresponding to introns are excised and those corresponding to exons are spliced together to form mRNA molecules coding for 217 amino acid prehormones. Proteolytic removal of a 26 residue signal peptide yields mature hormones containing 191 amino acids. The hGH and hCS peptides show 85% homology of amino acid sequence and their messenger RNA's show 94% homology of base sequence (3). In fact, there is greater than 90% sequence homology among the five genes in their 5' flanking, 5' non-translated, coding, intervening and 3' non-translated regions. The hGH and hCS genes begin to show class differences approximately 100 base pairs beyond the polyadenylation sites, where the two hGH genes have a longer extension of middle repetitive, _Alu_ I-type sequences.

Sequencing of cloned genomic DNA fragments has clarified the roles of each of the five hGH and hCS genes. The hGH-N gene works overtime to produce two different growth hormones, while hGH-N has the potential for producing an interesting variant growth hormone. Although the hCS-L gene is disabled through a single base mutation, hCS-A and hCS-B share in the production of human placental lactogen. The hGH-N gene is responsible for production of normal pituitary 22K human growth hormone (hGH). Through alternative splicing of premessenger RNA, it also specifies a second pituitary growth hormone (4). In 90% of hGH-N gene transcripts, intron B is removed and the 3' end of codon 32 is spliced to the 5' end of codon 32. In the remaining 10%, codon 31 is spliced to codon 47 of hGH. The codons for residues 32 to 46 are treated as part of a longer intron B' and the result is an mRNA for a shorter, 176 amino acid peptide. This 20K peptide has somatogenic and lactogenic potencies similar to those of standard hGH, but it is deficient in lipolytic activity. There is no information at present about physiologic modulation of the splicing choice.

The hGH-V gene codes for a variant peptide which differs from hGH at 13 of 191 residues (3). Loss of two acidic and gain of three basic residues yields a more basic peptide with a predicted isoelectric point of 8.9 as compared to 5.5 for standard hGH. An *Eco* RI fragment containing the hGH-V gene has been ligated to SV 40 viral DNA and expressed in cultured monkey kidney cells (5). The hGH-V peptide which is expressed in a transgenomic system cross-reacts weakly with antibodies to hGH, but shows considerable activity in radioreceptor assays which measure either the somatogenic or the lactogenic activities of hGH (6). This gene is not known to be expressed *in vivo*. It is possible that certain somatotrophic pituitary tumors express the gene and give rise to clinical manifestations of acromegaly which are out of proportion to low immunoassayable levels of hGH. Testing of this hypothesis will require development of specific radioimmunoassays for the hGH-V gene product.

The hCS-A and hCS-B genes each code for placental lactogen or human chorionic somatomammotropin (hCS). They specify the same mature hormone, but exhibit one amino acid difference in the signal peptide and several silent base differences (7). The two genes are expressed at roughly equivalent levels in fetal synctiotrophoblasts at term. The hCS-L gene appears to be an unexpressed pseudogene. A single base substitution at the beginning of the second intron destroys a consensus splice sequence and precludes normal processing of the premessenger RNA (2). The predicted consequence of this change would be a mRNA which continues in the same reading frame beyond codon 31, specifies a novel amino acid sequence, and may never re-enter a reading frame appropriate for hCS. No mRNA species for this gene has been identified in term placenta (7) and it is not known whether there is a second gene modification which signals that this gene should not be expressed in pituitary or placental tissue.

Despite their close structural relatedness, there is nearly complete tissue specificity of expression for hGH and hCS genes. There have been several attempts to determine why hGH genes are transcriptionally active in pituitary cells and hCS genes are active in placental cells. Expressed genes tend to show a lesser degree of methylation of cytosine residues and a greater sensitivity to digestion with small quantities of DNase. Members of the hGH gene cluster are hypomethylated in DNA prepared from pituitary and placental tissue as compared to DNA prepared from white blood cells (8). However, it has not been possible to discriminate with certainty between methylation of hGH and hCS genes in the producing tissues. Similar preliminary results have been obtained with respect to DNase sensitivity of sites related to the hGH and hCS genes (2).

One interesting aspect of hGH and hCS production is that the genes are expressed very efficiently, with hGH accounting for 10-20% of pituitary mRNA and hCS accounting for a similar percentage of placental mRNA. Each hormone is produced at a rate of approximately 2 mg/gm tissue/24 hr. A term placenta weighs approximately 500 gm or 1,000 times as much as the anterior pituitary and it produces circulating levels of hCS which are 1,000 times as high as hGH levels. Fortunately, the somatogenic potency of hCS is only 1/1,000 as great as hGH and pregnancy does not produce the clinical syndrome of acromegaly.

Deletions within the hGH gene cluster have contributed to our understanding of hGH and hCS gene function. Homozygosity for 5' deletions involving loss of the hGH-N gene results in a severe form of hGH deficiency (9). No hGH is detectable by RIA in serum specimens and these children tend to develop high titres of antibodies to administered hGH, consistent with a lack of immune tolerance to hGH. Correlation of genotype and phenotype shows that the hGH-N gene is solely responsible for immunoreactive hGH and that the hGH-V gene does not support normal growth when the hGH-N gene is absent. Deletions at the 3' end of the cluster result in loss of hCS-A, hGH-V and hCS-B genes (10). When a fetus is homozygous for this type of deletion, no hCS is detectable in maternal serum and maternal serum levels of IGF-1 do not rise during pregnancy. Nevertheless, there is no impairment of fetal growth, postpartum lactation, or postnatal growth. These observations lead to the conclusion that neither hCS nor a hGH-V gene product is required for normal fetal or postnatal development. Structural studies suggest that the hCS-L gene is not expressed and imply that deletion would have no discernible effect on phenotype. There are currently no published examples of hCS-L gene deletion.

The next objective in relating hGH gene structure to disease is to detect more subtle gene abnormalities which are responsible for deficiency or biological inactivity of hGH. There are five known pairs of restriction fragment length polymorphisms within the hGH gene cluster. Linkage analysis has been used to trace hGH genes through families and to demonstrate that most mutations responsible for recessive deficiency of growth hormone are not linked to hGH genes (11). This category of disease may well be heterogenous, with some families expressing mutations in the hGH gene, some expressing somatocrinin gene mutations and some expressing mutations which impair differentiation of somatotrophic cells. Bioinactivity of hGH has been proposed as a hypothesis to explain some forms of short stature. Heterogeneity for polymorphic hGH gene markers among children with this phenotype implies that their disorders cannot be explained by a single type of hGH gene mutation. Confirmation of the hypothesis of a primary gene alteration will require cloning and sequencing of an abnormal hGH-N gene.

ACKNOWLEDGEMENTS

This work was supported in part by a National Foundation for Birth Defects Clinical Research Grant 6-354, by NIH AM 31149 and by a grant from the Human Growth Foundation.

REFERENCES

1. George DL, Phillips JA III, Francke U, Seeburg PH (1982) Hum Genet 57:138
2. Barsh GS, Seeburg PH, Gelinas RE (1984) Nucleic Acids Res 11:3939
3. Seeburg PH (1982) DNA 1:239
4. DeNoto FM, Moore DD, Goodman HM (1981) 9:3719
5. Pavlakis GN, Hizuka N, Gorden P, Seeburg PH, Hamer DH (1981) Proc Nat Acad Sci ((USA) 78:7398
6. Hizuka N, Hendricks CM, Pavlakis GN, Hamer DH, Gorden P (1982) J Clin Endocrinol Metab 55:545
7. Barrera-Saldena HA, Seeburg PH, Saunders GF (1983) J Biol Chem 25;8:3787
8. Hjelle BL, Phillips JA III, Seeburg PH (1982) Nucleic Acids Res 10:3459
9. Phillips JA III, Hjelle BL, Seeburg PH, Zachmann M (1981) Proc Nat Acad Sci (USA) 78:6372
10. Wurzel J, Parks JS, Hjelle BL, Herd JE, Nielsen PV (1982) DNA 1:251
11. Phillips JA III, Parks JS, Hjelle BL, Herd JE, Plotnick LP, Migeon CJ, Seeburg PH (1982) J Clin Invest 70:489

13. Clinical Aspects of Calcium Metabolism

Endocrinology
F. Labrie, L. Proulx, eds.

INHERITANCE OF DEFICIENT N_s ACTIVITY AND PSEUDOHYPOPARATHYROIDISM, TYPE I

HENRY R. BOURNE

Departments of Pharmacology and Medicine and the Cardiovascular Research Institute, University of California, San Francisco, CA 94143 (USA)

Hormone-sensitive adenylate cyclase in vertebrate cells is composed of three distinct protein components: Hormone receptors, catalytic adenylate cyclase, and a GTP-binding protein, called N_s, that couples receptors to stimulation of cyclase activity. N_s activity is reduced in erythrocytes and other cells and tissues of patients with pseudohypoparathyroidism, Type I (PHP-I), an inherited syndrome of resistance to parathyroid hormone (PTH) and other hormones that act *via* stimulating cAMP synthesis (1,2). Many PHP-I patients exhibit hypocalcemia and its sequelae, including tetany and convulsions. The hypocalcemia is associated with resistance to the metabolic effects of PTH and elevated concentrations of PTH in serum. Most PHP-I patients also exhibit a typical body habitus called Albright's hereditary osteodystrophy (AHO), which includes round face, short stature, and short fingers and toes. (For references, see [3,4].)

The resistance of many PHP-I patients to hormones other than PTH, including thyrotropin, suggested that their biochemical defect should be distal to the hormone receptor, and that it would be generalized. To test this prediction, two assays were used to measure N_s activity in cells from PHP-I patients: 1. Assessment of the ability of membrane extracts to complement the genetic N_s deficiency of membranes from mouse S49 *cyc*$^-$ cells *in vitro*; 2. Quantitation of incorporation of radioactive ADP-ribose from NAD^+ into the N_s protein's α subunit, a reaction catalyzed by cholera toxin. Using these assays, N_s activity was found to be reduced by about 50% in erythrocytes (1,2), platelets (5), cultured skin fibroblasts (6), and virus-transformed lymphoblasts (7) obtained from PHP-I patients. The observation of N_s deficiency in cultured fibroblasts and lymphoblasts indicates that N_s deficiency is coded directly in the genome of individual cells of PHP-I patients.

While none of the cell types we tested exhibits any obvious endocrine abnormality in PHP-I, N_s activity was reportedly (8) decreased in an important target tissue, the kidney, of a PHP-I patient. This patient's erythrocytes also showed decreased N_s activity. For obvious reasons, confirmation of N_s deficiency in kidneys of additional PHP-I patients will be difficult. Nonetheless, it is reasonable to conclude that the N_s deficiency of PHP-I not only involves erythrocytes, platelets, fibroblasts, and lymphoblasts, but also includes endocrine target cells in the organs that exhibit resistance to cAMP-stimulating hormones *in vivo*. These include kidney, thyroid, liver, gonad, and probably bone and anterior pituitary (3,4).

We have found (9) both autosomal dominant and autosomal recessive inheritance of N_s deficiency and the PHP-I phenotype in different kindreds. This genetic heterogeneity surely indicates that more than one kind of molecular defect can cause N_s deficiency. The autosomal dominant disorder probably results from mutational loss of one of two alleles that encode a polypeptide subunit of the N_s protein. This would be consistent with a 50% loss of N_s activity. (We suspect that the α subunit of N_s is affected in PHP-I, because both the *cyc*$^-$ complementation and ADP-ribosylation assays measure activities of the α subunit.) The recessive pattern of inheritance, of course, cannot be explained in this way.

From the PHP-I phenotype we can infer that normal regulation of calcium by PTH requires all or most of the available N_s protein in important target tissues, because a 50% deficiency causes clinically obvious disturbance of calcium homeostasis. By the same reasoning, N_s activity is not limiting -- in most patients -- for functionally adequate regulation of target cells by other hormones. Sufficiently sensitive and subtle endocrine testing can detect subnormal responsiveness to certain hormones in PHP-I, even when no clinical abnormality is obvious (for references see [3,4]). In addition, some N-deficient PHP-I patients do not suffer from hypocalcemia and have only minimally elevated serum PTH, but nonetheless exhibit decreased urinary cAMP responses to PTH. Thus, some individuals apparently do not require all or most of the normal complement of N_s to regulate calcium homeostasis.

Finally, patients in some families with PHP-I do not have detectable N_s deficiency (3). These patients have a lower incidence of AHO and endocrine disorders such as hypothyroidism. At present the molecular basis of this variant of PHP-I is unknown. Isolation of the genes that encode polypeptide subunits of the N_s protein and the catalytic unit of adenylate cyclase will eventually contribute to understanding the molecular pathophysiology of the various subtypes of PHP-I.

ACKNOWLEDGEMENTS

This work was supported in part by grants from the National Institutes of Health (GM 27800 and GM 28310) as well as a grant from the March of Dimes.

REFERENCES

1. Farfel Z, Brickman AS, Kaslow HR, Brothers VM, Bourne HR (1980) New Engl J Med 303:237
2. Levine MA, Downs RW Jr, Singer M, Marx SJ, Aurbach GD, Spiegel AM (1980) Biochem Biophys Res Comm 94:1319
3. Farfel Z, Bourne HR (1982) Mineral Electrolyte Metab 8:227
4. Spiegel AM, Levine MA, Aurbach GD, Downs RW Jr, Marx SJ, Lasker RD, Moses AM, Breslau NA (1982) Am J Physiol 243:E37
5. Farfel Z, Bourne HR (1980) J Clin Endocrinol Metab 51:1202
6. Bourne HR, Kaslow HR, Brickman AS, Farfel Z (1981) J Clin Endocrinol Metab 53:636
7. Farfel Z, Abood ME, Brickman AS, Bourne HR (1982) J Clin Endocrinol Metab 55:113
8. Downs RW Jr, Levine MA, Drezner MK, Burch WM Jr, Spiegel AM (1983) J Clin Invest 71:231
9. Farfel Z, Brothers VM, Brickman AS, Conte F, Neer R, Bourne HR (1981) Proc Natl Acad Sci USA 78:3098

Endocrinology
F. Labrie, L. Proulx, eds.

THE PATHOGENESIS OF PSEUDOHYPOPARATHYROIDISM

CHARLES NAGANT de DEUXCHAISNES

Arthritis Unit, Louvain University in Brussels, St-Luc University Hospital, avenue Hippocrate 10, B-1200 Brussels (Belgium)

Pseudohypoparathyroidism (PHP) is characterized by the existence of the clinical and biochemical findings as seen in hypoparathyroidism (HP). However, unlike HP, the cause of PHP is not a lack of parathyroid hormone (PTH) secretion, but an ability of the end-organs to respond to it in a proper fashion. This was shown by Albright et al. (1) four decades ago, when they administered parathyroid extract (PTE) and found the patients to be resistant to it. Therefore, one of the distinguishing features between HP and PHP is that rather than being atrophic or absent, the parathyroid glands are usually hyperplastic, as reviewed elsewhere (2). With the possibility of measuring immunoreactive PTH (iPTH), observation of elevated levels of circulating iPTH has been an integral part of the diagnosis in the untreated patient for the last 15 years. On the other hand, the finding of Chase et al. (3) that patients with PHP where unable to respond to the administration of PTE with an increase of urinary cyclic AMP (cAMP), one of the messangers of PTH action, has considerably facilitated the diagnosis of PHP, since this test is easily performed and since the cAMP output in the urine upon PTE administration is immediate and striking in the normal person (in the order of a twenty-fold increase), in contrast to the modest phosphaturic response (a 2.5-fold increase) expected with the classic Ellsworth-Howard test. The latter test, however, should not be abandoned, since some patients do not properly excrete phosphate when PTE is administered, whereas cAMP output is normal. The term PHP type II has been coined for this rare entity (4). The more common form of PHP is therefore called PHP type I, or PHP-I (cfr. fig.). Only PHP-I has a familial incidence and the typical somatotype of "classical PHP", often referred to as Albright's hereditary osteodystrophy (AHO), which includes short stature, round face, obesity, brachymetacarpia, brachymetatarsia and/or brachyphalangia, accompanied by mental retardation and ectopic ossifications.

There is no question that the PTE-induced urinary output of cAMP is the most specific defect which characterizes PHP-I, provided it is performed under ideal conditions, i.e. when no other abnormalities such as vitamin D deficiency or hypomagnesemia are present, as outlined elsewhere (2). Primary and secondary (vitamin D-deficient) hyperparathyroidism (HPT) *may* blunt the response towards exogenous PTH as far as cAMP is concerned, by down regulation of the receptors. The latter mechanism has also been suggested as an explanation for the lack of response in patients with PHP towards the administration of PTH. Whereas this undoubtedly plays some role as far as the urinary output of phosphate and cAMP is concerned (2), this is less true for the hypercalcemic response towards PTH. If the best way to *diagnose* PHP-I is to test the renal responsiveness of cAMP versus PTE, the best way to *test* the end-organ responsiveness towards PTE is to administer PTE in a "three-day test" (600 U/d intramuscularly) and to follow the hypercalcemic, the hypophosphatemic and the hyperphosphaturic response (the latter under a constant diet). As shown elsewhere (5), there was no significant down regulation of receptors in bone in 7 patients with primary HPT whose initial serum calcium level was 11.9 (range = 10.8-13.7) mg/dl. After only 48 h of PTE administration (600 U/d), the average serum Ca level had risen to 13.7 mg/dl (+ 1.8 mg/dl). This increase contrasts with the average maximal 0.9 mg/dl increment we obtained with the same dosage in patients with PHP (cfr. Table), with no overlap between the two conditions. As far as serum P is concerned, no decrease could be observed in the already diminished value which is typical of primary HPT. Yet, the phosphaturic response was significantly more pronounced, but there was some overlap with the PHP population. These data demonstrate that there is another factor, besides down regulation of the receptors, which intervenes in determining the resistance towards PTH in PHP.

The easiest way to account for the additional factor of resistance is to explain it by the defect in the adenylcyclase system so well illustrated in the kidney by the acute test of Chase et al. (3). And indeed, this has been the explanation universally accepted. That this could not be so was evident from our experience with PHP patients who had undergone parathyroid surgery (2). In the early sixtees, we tested in the classical way ("the three-day test") two identical twin sisters with PHP. Whether treated or not, one sister behaved like a proper PHP, whereas the other (always tested simultaneously and with the same batch of PTE) responded each time normally. Her cervical area had been explored in 1950 by Dr. O. Cope and the only parathyroid gland that was found was biopsied. It was considered that this exploration could have led to parathyroid insufficiency through interference with the blood supply of the other parathyroid glands. Whatever the explanation, both patients, when later tested with PTE, did not respond as far as cAMP urinary output was concerned. Therefore, we did not consider that the cAMP response, albeit pathognomonic of PHP-I, was of crucial importance for end-organ responsiveness. The alternative hypothesis was considered that the parathyroid glands secreted an abnormal, partially inactive, PTH molecule, that bound to the receptors, preventing exogenously added PTE to exert its action. This was studied prospectively by performing total parathyroidectomy (PTX) in one of the cases of the original Albright paper (1), i.e. case n°3 (R.M.). The case had been resistant to PTH administration at the age of 3 and on three occasions at the age of 25, whether untreated, fully treated, or partially treated (serum Ca : 7.4, 9.4 and 9.0 mg/dl, respectively) with vitamin D. After PTX, whether untreated, partially treated, or fully treated (serum Ca : 7.1, 7.8

and 9.2 mg/dl, respectively), he always responded to PTE. He later was shown to be unable to excrete cAMP in the urine when given PTE. This reinforced our conclusion that it is the PTH (or at least the parathyroid glands) that was of importance as far as the end-organ responsiveness to PTH is concerned, and not cAMP, despite the fact that the latter is undoubtedly a mediator of PTH action and that the dibutyryl derivative can reproduce the action of PTH. It, however, from our experience could not be *the essential mediator* as far as hypercalcemic and hyperphosphaturic action is concerned (2). Other authors have obtained similar results of restored end-organ responsiveness after correction of serum Ca by adequate therapy (6-8). We were unable to do so (2), including when serum Ca and iPTH were normalized with calcitriol (5). However, we were able to achieve a normal response to PTE (5) after a 12 h Ca infusion ("chemical PTX").

The Table shows a summary of our experience of the three-day tests performed on 7 occasions in PHP patients, on 5 occasions in PHP patients who had their glands either removed (3 times in R.M.), or explored (twice in the twin sister), on 4 occasions in a patient with surgical hypoparathyroidism (SHP), and in the 7 patients with primary HPT. The patients with operated PHP have results corresponding more closely to those of the patient with SHP (who has always been our best responder) than to those with PHP. Patients with primary HPT are intermediate. If the hyperphosphaturic and hypophosphatemic responses are less in the patients with operated PHP than in the patient with SHP, this is due either to the exceptional responsiveness of the patient with SHP, or perhaps because part of the phosphaturic action of PTE, albeit a clinically unimportant one, is mediated by cAMP. Therefore, the adenyl cyclase system is of marginal importance as far as mineral metabolism is concerned. On the other hand, it may be more important for some of the endocrine functions which are impaired, but usually have little practical implications. They have been mentioned by the previous speaker (Prof. H.R. Bourne).

When a reliable, sensitive, and specific bioassay for PTH became available in Professor Chayen's laboratory in London, the possibility arose to bring to the

TABLE : EFFECT OF THREE-DAY ADMINISTRATION OF PARATHYROID EXTRACT

		1800 U PTE IM over 3 days			
		PHP (n = 7)	SHP (n = 4)	operated PHP (n = 5)	primary HPT (n = 7)
Maximal Increase Serum Ca (mg/dl)	Av.	0.9	4.1	3.3	2.0
	Range	0.5-1.1	2.8-6.1	2.1-4.6	1.2-2.9
Maximal Decrease Serum P (mg/dl)	Av.	0.2	2.0	1.1	none
	Range	0-0.8	1.3-2.6	0.5-1.6	
Ratio Peak Ur. P/Av. Ur.P	Av.	1.3	2.6	1.8	1.7
	Range	1.0-1.5	2.3-3.1	1.3-2.5	1.1-3.1

"parathyroid theory" versus the "receptor theory" dilemma more than an indirect answer by means of PTE responsiveness under various circumstances. The results of a joint project between this laboratory in London, Professor Fischer's laboratory in Zurich and our Center, were complemented by the studies of N protein activity in the red cell membranes by Professor Bourne's laboratory in San Francisco. In summary, PHP is characterized by a *relative* bioinactive PTH molecule when its activity is compared with iPTH levels (amino-terminal and carboxy-terminal). The *absolute* amounts of bioactive material in the plasma of PHP patients are either low (at times very low), normal, or even high (9). This is not surprising in view of the findings that some patients with PHP may be or may tend to be normocalcemic, and that histologically (and sometimes radiologically) hyperparathyroid bone disease may be the salient feature (2). This is even less surprising when considering that the bioassay is based on the measurement of PTH-induced stimulation of glucose 6-phosphate dehydrogenase activity in the distal convoluted tubules of guinea pig *kidney* cortex incubated with the patient's plasma. So far the relative bioinactivity found only holds for that system, but contrasts to the consistent simultaneous elevations of bio-PTH and iPTH in primary HPT, and decreases in SHP (9). More dramatic are the results of incubating the plasma of PHP patients with bovine PTH-(1-84), and measuring how much of the activity of added PTH is recovered in the cytochemical bioassay (10). In normal plasma, and in plasma of patients with primary HPT or SHP, the recovery amounts to 50-100 %. In PHP (n = 17), this average recovery of biological activity amounts to some 5%, without any overlap with the other categories of plasma tested. Thus in all cases (100 %), there is a circulating factor in the plasma of PHP patients which inhibits the biological activity of PTH in the cytochemical bioassay system, either an abnormal PTH molecule, as anticipated (2), or perhaps more likely an inhibitor of PTH activity. That this factor most probably originates in the parathyroid glands was shown by testing the recovery of PTH added to the plasma of patient R.M. who had undergone total PTX in 1965. The recovery was 84 %. The circulating inhibitor has indeed been removed. This also can be achieved by Ca infusions during several days. Under these circumstances, the inhibitor disappears from the plasma.

The studies of N protein activity showed that, as was known, not all PHP patients had a reduced N protein activity (cfr. Fig.), but pointed to a very interesting finding in the genetic transmission of some abnormalities (11-12). Whereas the PHP patients in a family may or may not have diminished N protein activity, siblings, and most often the mothers of affected patients, who are normal as far as serum biochemistries and PTE-induced cAMP output are concerned, may have a reduced N protein activity (cfr. Fig.). Other abnormalities in "normal" siblings may consist of diminished recovery of added PTH in the bioassay system

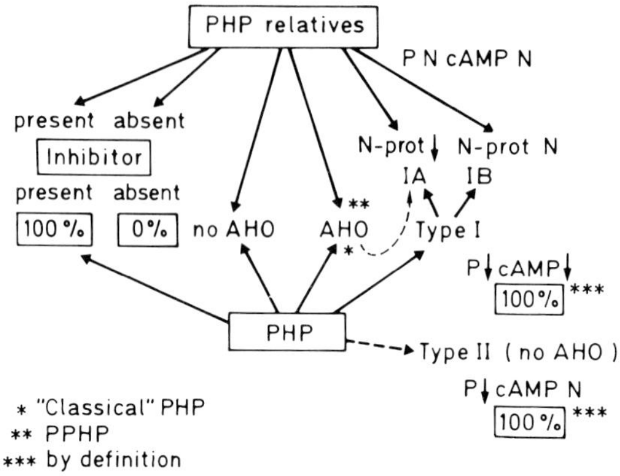

Fig. Different types of pseudohypoparathyroidism (PHP) with or without Albright's hereditary osteodystrophy (AHO), all having the "inhibitor" present. The "normal" PHP relatives may or may not have AHO, diminished N protein activity or an inhibitor present (as well as some other abnormalities).

(although not as pronounced as in the typical PHP patient), increased iPTH levels, and increased TSH concentrations upon TRH administration. When these siblings have the typical somatotype of AHO, they represent cases of pseudo-pseudohypoparathyroidism (PPHP). The latter thus becomes a much more complicated and heterogeneous group of patients as hitherto recognized.

A new era of biochemical research has begun as far as PHP is concerned. It will only come to an end with the isolation and full characterization of the putative inhibitor of PTH activity. Whether or not, or how this inhibitor relates to the adenyl cyclase abnormality, remains to be investigated.

REFERENCES

1. Albright F, Burnett CH, Smith PH, Parson W (1942) Endocrinology 30 : 922-932
2. Nagant de Deuxchaisnes, C, Krane SM (1978) In : Avioli LV, Krane SM (eds) Metabolic Bone Disease, Vol.II. Academic Press, New York, pp 217-445
3. Chase LR, Melson GL, Aurbach GD (1969) J Clin Invest 48 : 1832-1844
4. Drezner MK, Neelon FA, Lebovitz HE (1973) N Engl J Med 289 : 1056-1060
5. Devogelaer JP, Huaux JP, Docquier C, Crabbé J, Nagant de Deuxchaisnes C (1984) Acta Clin Belg (In Press)
6. Suh SM, Fraser D, Kooh SW (1970) J Clin Endocrinol Metab 30 : 609-614
7. Stögmann W, Fischer JA (1975) Am J Med 59 : 140-144
8. Drezner MK, Neelon FA, Haussler M, McPherson HT, Lebovitz HE (1976) J Clin Endocrinol Metab 42 : 621-628
9. Nagant de Deuxchaisnes C, Fischer JA, Dambacher MA, Devogelaer JP, Arber CE, Zanelli JM, Parsons JA, Loveridge N, Bitensky L, Chayen J (1981) J Clin Endocrinol Metab 53 : 1105-1109
10. Loveridge N, Fischer JA, Nagant de Deuxchaisnes C, Dambacher MA, Tschopp F, Werder E, Devogelaer JP, De Meyer R, Bitensky L, Chayen J (1982) J Clin Endocrinol Metab 54 : 1274-1275
11. Fischer JA, Bourne HR, Dambacher MA, Tschopp F, De Meyer R, Devogelaer JP, Werder EA, Nagant de Deuxchaisnes C (1983) Clin Endocrinol(Oxf) 19 : 747-754
12. Fischer JA, Nagant de Deuxchaisnes, C, Loveridge N, Dambacher MA, Tschopp F, Werder E, Bitensky L, Chayen J (1983) In : Frame B, Potts JT, Jr (eds) Clinical Disorders of Bone and Mineral Metabolism. Excerpta Medica, Amsterdam, pp 459-462

Endocrinology
F. Labrie, L. Proulx, eds.

VITAMIN D RESISTANT STATES

URI A. LIBERMAN, CHARLES EIL, STEPHEN J. MARX
Metabolic Diseases, Beilinson Medical Center, Sackler Faculty of Medicine, Tel-Aviv University, Petah-Tikva, Israel. Endocrinology Branch, National Naval Medical Center, Bethesda, MD, U.S.A. and Metabolic Diseases Branch, NIADDK, NIH, Bethesda, MD, U.S.A.

We define resistance to vitamin D (calciferol) as a state where normal levels of the vitamin are associated with subnormal bioeffects; the bioeffects relevant to this discussion are its effect on serum calcium and/or on bone matrix mineralization. Defective mineralization may occur in the growing bone and preosseous cartilage, and along trabeculae in sites of endosteal remodeling, the former is defined as rickets and the later as osteomalacia. Vitamin D may be considered as a prohormone that must undergo two distinct processes in order to become biologically active: a) a series of hydroxylations to active forms, the most potent natural metabolite being 1,25-dihydroxyvitamin D ($1,25(OH)_2D$) that may be considered as a true hormone, and b) signalling by active metabolites in target tissues through a steroidal type receptor mechanism. Normal mineralization of bone matrix is dependent on concentrations of calcium, phosphorus in extracellular fluid and on local cellular factors. A complex interrelationship exists among serum (and presumably tissue) levels of $1,25(OH)_2D$, calcium and phosphorus: $1,25(OH)_2D$ through its effects on mineral transport and particulary upon calcium transport across intestinal mucosa will affect serum concentrations of calcium; changes in serum calcium through modulation of parathyroid gland function will affect serum phosphorus; circulating parathyroid hormone, phosphorus and calcium concentration, among other factors, will affect renal production of $1,25(OH)_2D$.

Based on this information and the availability of assays for measurements of serum levels of vitamin D and its metabolites, vitamin D resistance can be classified as: a) defects in biosynthetic activation of the vitamin (type I D resistance usually with low or inappropriately low circulating concentrations of $1,25(OH)_2D$), b) defects in target tissue response to the hormone (type II D resistance usually with normal or high circulating levels of $1,25(OH)_2D$), and c) defects in bone matrix mineralization due to local tissue factors (type III D resistance with normal circulating levels of $1,25(OH)_2D$, calcium and phosphorus). Each type could be subclassified according to the primary disturbance as a hypocalcemic or hypophosphatemic state, with further subdivision as a hereditary or acquired state. (Table 1). Because of space limitations the rest of this paper will be focused on vitamin D resistance type II-2 (Table 1).

TABLE 1

CLASSIFICATION OF VITAMIN D RESISTANT STATES

Type I: Decreased or inappropriately low circulating levels of $1,25(OH)_2D$.	
1. Hypocalcemic	
a. Hereditary	
i. Primary	e.g. 1-alpha hydroxylase deficiency
ii. Secondary	e.g. primary hypoparathyroidism pseudohypoparathyroidism 25-hydroxylase deficiency?
b. Acquired	e.g. chronic renal failure acquired hypoparathyroidism
2. Hypophosphatemic	
a. Hereditary	e.g. x-linked hypophosphatemia
b. Acquired	e.g. tumor induced osteomalacia
Type II: Increased circulating levels of $1,25(OH)_2D$	
1. No abnormality in target cells	
a. Hypocalcemic	e.g. calcium deficiency; hungry bone syndrome; low birth weight infants
b. Hypophosphatemic	
i. Hereditary	e.g. hypophosphatemic rickets and hypercalciuria
ii. Acquired	e.g. antacid abuse
2. Abnormalities in target cell effector system	
a. Hereditary	e.g. end organ resistance to $1,25(OH)_2D$
b. Acquired?	
Type III: Normal circulating levels of $1,25(OH)_2D$, calcium and phosphorus	
1. Hereditary	e.g. hypophosphatasia
2. Acquired	e.g. intoxication by: fluoride, diphosphonate, aluminum?

TYPE II D RESISTANCE WITH INCREASED CIRCULATING LEVELS OF $1,25(OH)_2D$

2. Abnormalities in target cell effector system.

a. <u>Hereditary</u> (End organ resistance to $1,25(OH)_2D$).

Clinical and biochemical features: There are only 16 kindreds or a total of 21 patients described in the literature with this syndrome (1-15). These patients do not respond to physiological doses of vitamin D, 25(OH)D or $1,25(OH)_2D$ and serum levels of $1,25(OH)_2D$ are high before/or during treatment with high doses of bioactive calciferol preparations. The family pattern in these kindreds is consistent with autosomal recessive inheritance. The syndrome is hetrogenous in its clinical and biochemical presentation (Table 2).

TABLE 2.
CLINICAL AND BIOCHEMICAL FEATURES OF PATIENTS WITH HEREDITARY AND ORGAN RESISTANCE TO $1,25(OH)_2D$ (MODIFIED FROM LIBERMAN ET AL (16).

No. of Kindreds	Total Alopecia	Age of Onset	Remission on High Calciferols	Serum Concentrations of	
				Pi	$24,25(OH)_2D$
3	No	Late	Yes	Low	Normal
3#	No	Early	Yes	Low	Normal
4	Yes	Early	Yes+	Low	Normal
5	Yes	Early	No$	Low	Normal
1	Yes	Early	No≠	High	Low

*Age of onset is considered to be at first recognition of metabolic bone disease.
#In one kindred with a mild form of the disease, fracture diathesis was recognized at the age of 2 years in one sibling and the age of 9 years in the other (4).
+Remission was transient in one patient.
$Spontaneous healing in teen years reported.
≠No response to vitamin D or 1-alpha hydroxylated calciferol metabolites but normocalcemia achieved on $24,25(OH)_2D_3$.

The following summarizes some of this hetrogeneity. Age of onset: Late onset was reported in three sporadic cases, in other patients metabolic bone disease was recognizable prior to 2 years of age (one exception see footnote in Table 2). Ectodermal anomalies: Total alopecia was present prior to one year of age in 10 kindreds. Parental consanguinity when reported was observed only in kindreds with total alopecia. Serum biochemistry: All patients demonstrate secondary hyperparathyroidism with hypophosphatemia, except one patient who had hyperphosphatemia (6). Serum levels of $24,25(OH)_2D$ ranged from low to elevated, depending on treatment with the exception of one patient where serum levels of $24,25(OH)_2D$ were below the lower limit of the assay (less than 0.39 ng/ml versus normal 1.5 - 2.5) (6). Remission of hypocalcemia and metabolic bone disease with moderate to very high doses of bioactive calciferol analogs, was achieved in 10 kindreds. These included all patients with normal hair growth and only 4 kindreds with total alopecia (see footnotes Table 2).

Cellular basis for resistance to $1,25(OH)_2D$: *in vitro* studies with fibroblasts cultured from patient's skin biopsies. Soluble extracts ("cytosol"[a]) of fibro-

[a]The high ionic strength buffer used in this procedure probably solubilizes receptor components from all cell compartments.

blasts cultured from normal human skin demonstrate binding of $[^3H]1,25(OH)_2D_3$ with affinity, capacity and specificity suggestive of a receptor; when intact fibroblasts are incubated with $1,25(OH)_2D_3$ they exhibit high affinity nuclear uptake of $1,25(OH)_2D_3$ with analogous features suggestive of receptor mediation (17-19). We evaluated cultured skin fibroblasts from affected members of 11 kindreds with end organ resistance to $1,25(OH)_2D$. Five distinct patterns were observed _in vitro:_ I. Whole cell nuclear uptake and cytosol binding unmeasurable. II. Normal capacity and affinity of cytosol binding but unmeasurable whole cell nuclear uptake. III. Decreased capacity and normal affinity of both parameters. IV. Normal capacity and decreased affinity, and V. Normal capacity and affinity of both measurements. Patients with pattern II and IV have responded to treatment with high doses of calciferol analogs (18), thus representing deficient sensitivity to the hormone (defined as a state where the level of vitamin D required to obtain a half maximal bioeffect is increased). Patterns I and V may be associated with either a full therapeutic response to very high doses of bioactive vitamin D analogs or a total unresponsiveness (defined as a state where the maximal bioeffect attainable in normals is not attainable with any level of the vitamin) (3,12,17). Thus the data obtained _in vitro_ indicate that resistance to $1,25(OH)_2D$ may reflect five distinct types of abnormality in the effector system for the hormone. Considerations of clinical data as the presence or absence of ectodermal anomalies and the response to treatment may point to additional variation within the five subtypes.

The recent observation of a biochemical response in cultured fibroblasts to the addition _in vitro_ of $1,25(OH)_2D_3$ (stimulation of 25-hydroxyvitamin D-24 hydroxylase (20) may be used as a correlate with bioeffect _in vivo_. Fibroblasts from affected members of seven kindreds with end organ resistance to $1,25(OH)_2D$ showed defective or absent effect of $1,25(OH)_2D_3$ _in vitro_ (12,15,21,22).

Thus, _in vitro_ studies with cultured skin fibroblasts unveiled a multiplicity of intracellular defects in end organ resistance to $1,25(OH)_2D$. The different genetic defect observed may explain in part the clinical hetrogeneity of the syndrome. Finally, a biochemical response of the fibroblasts to $1,25(OH)_2D_3$ _in vitro_ may be used to predict the biological response of patients _in vivo_ to treatment with bioactive calciferol analogs.

REFERENCES

1. Brooks MH, Bell NH, Love L et al (1978) New Engl J Med 298:996
2. Marx SJ, Spiegel AM, Brown EM et al (1978) J Clin Endocrinol Metab 47:1303
3. Zerweck JE, Glass K, Jowsey J, Pak CYC (1979) J Clin Endocrinol Metab 49:171
4. Adams JS, Wahl TO, Moore WV, Horton WA, Lukert BP (1979) 61st Annual Meeting of the Endocrine Society 767 (Abstract)

5. Rosen JF, Fleischman AR, Finberg L, Hamstra A, DeLuca HF (1979) J Pediat 94:729

6. Liberman UA, Samuel R, Halabe AZ et al (1980) Lancet 1:504

7. Fujita T, Normura M, Okajima S, Suruya H (1980) J Clin Endocrinol Metab 50:927

8. Sockalosky JJ, Westrom RA, DeLuca HF, Brown DM (1980) J Pediat 96:701

9. Tsuchiya Y, Matsuo N, Cho H et al (1980) J Clin Endocrinol Metab 51:685

10. Beer S, Tieder M, Kohelet D et al (1981) Clin Endocrinol 14:395

11. Kudoh T, Kumagai T, Uetsuji N et al (1981) Europ J Pediat 137:307

12. Feldman D, Chen T, Cone C et al (1982) J Clin Endocrinol Metab 55:1020

13. Balsan S, Garabedian M, Liberman UA et al (1983) J Clin Endocrinol Metab 57:803

14. Castells S, Greig F, Fusi M et al (1984) Pediat Res 18:291 E (Abstract)

15. Hirst M, Hochman H, Feldman D (1984) 6th Annual Meeting of the American Society for Bone and Mineral Research. AG7 (Abstract)

16. Liberman UA, Eil C, Marx SJ (1983) In: Frame B, Parfitt AR et al (eds) Clinical problems in mineral metabolism. Elsevier Science Publication, Amsterdam pp 441-446

17. Liberman UA, Eil C, Marx SJ (1983) J Clin Invest 71:192

18. Marx SJ, Liberman UA, Eil C et al (1984) Rec Prog Horm Res 40: In press

19. Eil C, Liberman UA, Rosen JF, Marx SJ (1981) N Engl J Med 304:1588

20. Chandler JJ, Chandler SK, Pike JW, Haussler MR (1984) J Biol Chem 259:2214

21. Griffin JE, Chandler JS (1983) J Clin Invest 72:1190

22. Gamblin GT, Liberman UA, DeGrange DA et al (1983) Clin Res 31:693A (Abstract)

Endocrinology
F. Labrie, L. Proulx, eds.

REGULATION OF BONE (TYPE I) COLLAGEN SYNTHESIS

DAVID ROWE, KAREN RUBIN, BARBARA KREAM
Departments of Pediatrics and Medicine, University of Connecticut Health Center, Farmington, CT.

INTRODUCTION

Type I collagen is the primary structural protein of skin, ligament, tendon, and bone. It is one of a family of structural proteins composed of three polypeptide chains arranged in a triple helix (1). Although there is great similarity in gly-pro-hypro sequence found in the helix, the α chains which compose each specific collagen type are unique gene products.

Different tissues are composed of specific collagen types. This implies that the process of differentiation selects for expression of a few members of the collagen gene family. For type I collagen this requires that two specific genes (the α_1(I) and α_2(I) collagen gene) must be activated and regulated in a coordinated manner. Thus a high degree of control is required of these genes which may be unique to specific cell types to meet the specialized requirements of growth, remodeling and repair. This paper will illustrate the complexity of hormone regulation of the type I collagen gene in bone and fibroblastic-like cells and speculate on a mechanism to account for these properties.

MATERIALS AND METHODS

Cell culture. 21 day old fetal rat calvaria were maintained in organ culture in BJG media and incubated in the presence or absence of 1,25 dihydroxyvitamin D ($1,25(OH)_2D_3$) or PTH (2,3). Two hours prior to termination, the tissue was labeled with [5-^{3}H]-L-proline. After the calvaria were washed free of culture media, the periosteum was stripped from the central bone region (4). The two portions were analyzed separately for total collagen synthesis (5) and type I collagen mRNA content (6). Human diploid fibroblasts were grown to confluency in the presence or absence of hydrocortisone (7). The cells were radiolabeled for 6 or 24 hours and analyzed for total collagen synthesis or for the relative proportion of type I and type III synthesis (8). Cells, grown under identical culture conditions were taken for measurement of the type I collagen mRNA content.

Collagen mRNA was analyzed by dot-blot hybridization. In this assay, total RNA is serially diluted and fixed to a nitrocellulose membrane (4). The filter is then hybridized with an α_1 and α_2 specific cDNA probe. The rat mRNA is hybridized with cloned cDNA constructed in this laboratory (4); it is identified as pα1R1 and pα2R2. The human RNA is hybridized with probes synthesized by F. Ramierz of Rutgers University (9,10): Hf404 (alpha 1) and Hf32 (alpha 2). Collagen mRNA is expressed in relative OD units obtained from an autoradiogram of the dot hybridization dilution curve (4).

RESULTS

Both PTH and 1,25 $(OH)_2D_3$ have previously been shown to inhibit type I collagen synthesis in mRNA levels in intact fetal rat calvaria (2,3). When this tissue was dissected such that the osteoblasts-containing central bone region was analyzed separately from the more fibroblastic appearing periosteal cells, it became apparent that inhibitory effects of these hormones are specific on the osteoblastic cell population. For example, in calvaria incubated in 10^{-9}M PTH, collagen production in the osteoblastic cell layer is reduced from 1613 dpm/μg (17.3%) to 273 dpm/μg (4.7%) while in the periosteal component there is no significant change: 488 to 227 dpm/μg (7.8 to 6.1%). Figure 1 is a dot-blot hybridization which shows a relative depletion of α_1 and α_2 mRNA sequences in the central bone but not the periosteal cells.

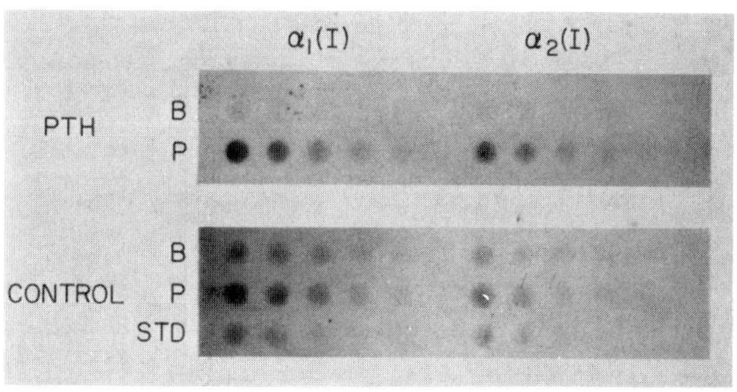

Fig. 1. Dot-blot hybridization of type I collagen mRNA extracted from the central bone (B) and periosteum (P) of control and PTH-treated fetal rat calvaria. The standard RNA (STD) is derived from freshly dissected fetal rat calvaria.

In a similar manner 1,25 $(OH)_2D_3$ exerts a tissue-specific effect on type I col-

TABLE I

RELATIVE COLLAGEN mRNA CONTENT IN 1,25$(OH)_2D_3$-TREATED RAT CALVARIA*

Tissue	Treatment	$\alpha_1(I)$	$\alpha_2(I)$
Bone	Control	360	200
	1,25$(OH)_2D_3$	80	50
Periosteum	Control	120	55
	1,25$(OH)_2D_3$	110	60

*Data expressed in arbitrary absorption units per μg of DNA.

lagen synthesis in osteoblastic cells. The table demonstrates that the osteoblastic cells contain a 3-fold higher content of collagen mRNA per μg of DNA than do the periosteal cells. Upon addition of 1,25 $(OH)_2D_3$ the mRNA content falls in the osteoblasts to the same level as found in the periosteal cells.

In contrast to these two bone-specific hormones, glucocorticoids (GC) have effects on collagen synthesis in fibroblastic cells. Prolonged incubation of human diploid fibroblasts to hydrocortisone (5-7 days) results in an increase in the ratio of type III to type I collagen and a reduction in total collagen production. This data indicate that GC inhibit the production of type I collagen without a similar effect on the type III collagen. The fall in type I collagen synthesis is paralleled by equivalent fall in the content of type I collagen mRNAs (data not shown).

DISCUSSION

The α_1(I) and α_2(I) collagen genes are present as a single copy per haploid set of chromosomes (11). Thus, both bone and fibroblastic cells must utilize the same gene but regulate it in different manners. Both PTH and 1,25 $(OH)_2D_3$ appear to be bone-specific since their inhibitory effect is seen only in osteoblastic cells. Since this tissue makes type I collagen exclusively (2), the effect of these hormones are type I collagen specific. There is no change in the ratio of type I to type III collagen in periosteal cells incubated in the presence of these two hormones (2). In contrast GC do change the ratio of type I to type III collagen due primarily to a fall in type I collagen content. Thus, these studies may explain why PTH and 1,25 $(OH)_2D_3$ limit their connective tissue effect to bone whereas GC affect all connective tissues that are rich in type I collagen.

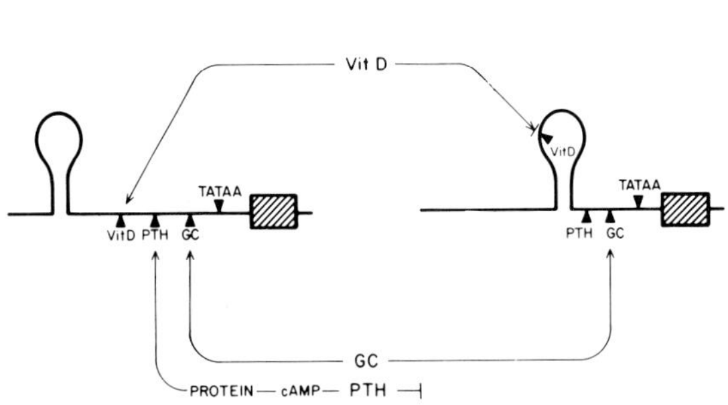

Fig. 2. A model for the tissue specific effects of PTH and 1,25 $(OH)_2D_3$ and generalized effect of GC of type I collagen synthesis. TATAA is the transcription recognition sequence and the filled box represent the first exon.

The mechanisms that are responsible for the tissue-specific regulation of type I collagen are as yet not understood. Figure 2 schematizes one hypothesis that could account for these observations. It has been previously shown that the α_2 (I) promoter region contains three mutually exclusive stem-loop structures which can place the TATA box in different orientations to the other upstream nucleotide sequences. Since this region probably binds the hormone-mediating proteins that alter the transcriptional activity of the gene, the conformation of this region might determine whether such a protein could influence the activity of the promoter. In the model, only hormone-binding domains downstream from the stem-loop structure influence the activity of the promoter. Thus, the structure of the promoter in bone might permit 1,25 $(OH)_2D_3$ binding to alter gene activity whereas the orientation in the fibroblast is unable to influence the transcriptional activity. The same might be true for PTH although the other explanation for PTH effect might be the lack of a PTH-receptor in fibroblastic-like cells. Finally, in this model a GC binding protein would be able to bind and regulate the gene in either conformation. Recent advances in determining nucleotide sequence that interact with DNA binding proteins (12) and gene transfer technology (13) now make testing this type of hypothesis an exciting possibility.

ACKNOWLEDGEMENTS

This work is supported by NIH grants AM29983 and AM29850. David Rowe and Barbara Kream are recipients of RCDA HD00330 and AM01017, respectively.

REFERENCES

1. Bornstein P, Sage A (1980) Ann Rev Biochem 49:957-1003.
2. Rowe DW, Kream BE (1982) J Biol Chem 257:8009-8015.
3. Kream B, Rowe DW, Raisz LG (1980) Proc Natl Acad Sci 77:5654-5658.
4. Genovese C, Rowe D, Kream D (1984) Biochemistry, in press.
5. Peterkofsky B, Diegelmann D (1971) Biochemistry 6:988-994.
6. Sykes B, Puddle B, Francis M, Smith R (1976) Biochem Biophys Res Comm 72:1472-1480.
7. Rowe DW, Starman B, Fujimoto WY, Williams RW (1977) In Vitro 13:824-830.
8. Rowe DW, Poirier M, Shapiro JR (1981) In: Veis A, (ed) The Chemistry and Biology of Mineralized Connective Tissues. Elsevier North-Holland, Inc., New York, pp 155-162.
9. Chu M-L, Myers JC, Bernard MP, Ding JL, Ramierz F (1982) Nuc Acid Res 10:5915-5932.
10. Bernard MP, Myers JC, Chu M-L, Ramirez F, Eikenbery EF, Prockop DJ (1983) Biochemistry 22:1139-1145.
11. Dalgelish R, Trapnell B, Cyrstal R, Tolstoshev P (1982) J Biol Chem 257: 13816-13822.
12. Weintraub H (1983) Cell 32:1191-1203.
13. Karin M, Cathala G, Nguyen-Huu MC (1983) Proc Natl Acad Sci 80:4040-4044.

14. Steroids and the Brain

Endocrinology
F. Labrie, L. Proulx, eds.

INTERACTION OF ADRENAL STEROIDS WITH MONO-AMINE SYSTEMS

E.R. DE KLOET
Rudolf Magnus Institute for Pharmacology, Medical Faculty, University of Utrecht, Vondellaan 6, 3521 GD Utrecht, The Netherlands

INTRODUCTION

Environmental challenges involving a traumatic, toxic, infectuous or psychological event result in autonomous, behavioural, and neuroendocrine responses aimed to maintain homeostasis. In the endocrine chain of events the pituitary-adrenal system plays an important role. ACTH not only stimulates corticosterone (CS) secretion, but has together with the peptides necessary for its own release (vasopressin, CRH) also a direct action on the central nervous system. The peptides act on central mechanisms involved in aspects of adaptation as do the adrenal steroids which feedback on brain and pituitary (1,2). Recently, the importance of adrenal catecholamines for retention of learned behavioural patterns has been reemphasized (3).

CS, which is the naturally occurring glucocorticoid of the rat, feeds back on the brain via receptor sites with a predominant localization in neurons of limbic brain structures e.g. hippocampus, septum and amygdala. The receptors retain CS in cell nuclei. Aldosterone (ALDO) is also retained very well, but displays *in vitro* in cytosol a tenfold lower affinity to the CS receptor. Dexamethasone (DEX) is poorly retained and displays a twentyfold lower affinity to these sites *in vitro*. The CS receptor system in limbic neurons, thus, displays some similarity with mineralocorticoid receptors, but is clearly different from glucocorticoid receptors found in pituitary corticotrophs and presumably in glial cells (2). The latter glucocorticoid receptors display highest affinity to potent synthetic glucocorticoids such as DEX. Binding specificity, capacity and anatomy of the CS receptor system in limbic brain has provided criteria to study interaction of CS with peripheral and central mono-amine systems.

INTERACTION OF CORTICOSTERONE WITH ADRENOMEDULLARY CATECHOLAMINES

Adrenaline (A) has a direct stimulatory action on pituitary ACTH release (4) and glucocorticoids are required for maintenance of the activity of phenylethanolamine-N-methyltransferase (PNMT) in the adrenal, which is the enzyme involved in adrenaline synthesis (5). Interactions between A and glucocorticoids have been found in the periphery, where the steroids appeared to potentiate cardiovascular effects of A (6). In contrast, to this potentiating effect, we found recently that CS reduced the efficacy of A to affect a fear-motivated behavioural response (passive avoidance behaviour).

Rats trained to enter a dark compartment received upon entrance a weak electric shock (learning trial). When the rats were tested 24 hours later in the same situation, the animals will show a latency to reenter the dark compartment. This latency (sec) or passive avoidance is a measure for retention of learned behaviour and is motivated by fear for the previous aversive experience. Passive avoidance behaviour evokes a severe psychological stress and leads to rapid activation of the pituitary-adrenal system.

The passive avoidance response was deficient up to five days after bilateral removal of the adrenals (ADX). Replacement with CS failed to normalize the avoidance response, but administration of A immediately after the learning trial in a dose range of 0.005 - 5 μg/kg resulted in a dose-dependent recovery of the behavioural deficit of ADX rats (7). However, higher doses of A were required to restore the behaviour of adrenomedullectomized (ADXM) rats. ADXM rats have still an intact adrenal cortex and circulating CS. Accordingly, replacement of ADX rats with CS resulted in a shift of the dose-response curve and a tenthousand fold higher dose of A was necessary to restore the deficit in the passive avoidance response. The effect of CS is specific, since DEX and ALDO did not reduce the efficacy of A to affect behaviour (8).

INTERACTION OF CORTICOSTERONE WITH CENTRAL MONO-AMINE SYSTEMS

In our studies we focussed on the principal mono-amine systems that innervate the CS receptor containing structures in the brain. These systems are the noradrenergic (NA) neurons of the locus coeruleus and serotonergic (5-HT) raphe neurons, that project from the brain stem to the hippocampus. ADX did not affect NA turnover in the coeruleo-hippocampal NA system as judged from the disappearance rate of NA after α-methyltyrosine (α-MPT) treatment of the rats (9). An effect of CS on NA receptor sites in the hippocampus has, however, been reported; the steroid reduced NA receptor capacity induced after ADX and neurotoxic lesioning of the NA neurons (10).

5-HT turnover was found reduced in the raphe-hippocampal system after ADX (11). Turnover was based on an index of 5-HT synthesis rate measured after pargyline blocked mono-amine oxydase (MAO) activity. CS replacement in a behaviourally active dose restores this index for 5-HT turnover, while again DEX and ALDO were not active in this respect (12). Simultaneous changes were found in 5-HT receptor density in hippocampal subregions as shown by *in vitro* labelling of frozen tissue sections with ^{3}H-5-HT and quantitative evaluation of the autoradiographical film images by computer-assisted densitometry. It thus appears that the activity of the 5-HT neuron is under the stringent control of CS and probably involves a transsynaptic CS-receptor-mediated mechanism.

In view of the interaction between CS and 5-HT in the brain our present experiments are designed to investigate whether CS action on behaviour requires a functionally active 5-HT system; the effect of CS is studied in rats, that have the 5-HT neurons destroyed with a neurotoxic drug (5.6 dihydroxytryptamine). During these studies we noticed that changes in the 5-HT input to the hippocampus resulted in an altered CS receptor capacity in the hippocampus depending on time and location of the lesion (13). At ten days after the neurotoxic lesion, applied in such a way that only the hippocampal innervation and not other forebrain structures were affected, CS receptor capacity was found increased. These results suggest a feedback loop in interaction of CS with the raphe-hippocampal 5-HT system. CS increases the 5-HT activity of this system, while a reduced 5-HT activity results in increased hippocampal CS receptor activity.

CONCLUDING REMARKS

Stressors lead to a rapid adrenal catecholamine release and a slower neuroendocrine activation of CS secretion. The findings suggest that CS protects the brain against deleterious influences of high circulating A levels. The interaction between CS and peripheral catecholamines may be explained in terms of increased resistance to stressful events, since CS reduces tenthousand fold the efficacy of A to reinforce learned fear-motivated behavioural patterns. However, in view of the temporal relationship in release one cannot exclude that CS "switches off" stress mechanisms by decreasing the efficacy of A action.

The CS action likely takes place via the CS receptor system in neurons of the limbic brain. Neuronal processes taking place in the limbic structures are assumed to control interpretation of sensory stimuli and expression of the type of behaviour analyzed with the passive avoidance paradigm. Moreover, the CS receptor system in limbic brain displays a high degree of specificity for CS, which corresponds to the stringent specificity and dose required to elicit CS effects on behaviour. Behavioural specificity of CS action has been found in other paradigms such as forced extinction, exploration and extinction of a food rewarded runway response of ADX rats (2,14).

A 5-HT- CS feedback loop in the limbic brain seems implicated in the underlying mechanism of CS action on brain function. The CS receptor in the hippocampal neurons responds to CS and informs the brain of ongoing peripheral endocrine events, while the 5-HT neuron activated by CS seems to control via negative feedback the hippocampal CS receptor capacity.

REFERENCES

1. De Kloet ER, De Wied D (1980) In: Martini L, Ganong WF (eds) Frontiers in Neuroendocrinology, vol. 6. Raven Press, New York, pp. 157-201.
2. De Kloet ER, Veldhuis HD (1984) In: Lajtha A (ed) Handbook of Neurochemistry, vol. 8. Pergamon Press, New York, pp. 47-91.
3. McGaugh JM (1983) Ann Rev Psychol 34: 297-243.
4. Long CNH (1951) Rec Progr Horm Res 7: 75-95.
5. Wurtman RJ, Axelrod J (1966) J Biol Chem 241: 2301-2304.
6. Besse JC, Bass AD (1966) J Pharmacol Exp Ther 154: 224-238.
7. Borrell J, De Kloet ER, Versteeg DHG, Bohus B (1983) Behav Neural Biol 39: 241-258.
8. Borrell J, De Kloet ER, Bohus B (1984) Life Sci 34: 99-105.
9. Versteeg DHG, Van Zoest I, De Kloet ER (1984) Experientia 40: 112-114.
10. Roberts DCS, Bloom FE (1981) Eur J Pharmacol 74: 37-41.
11. De Kloet ER, Kovács GL, Szabo G, Telegdy G, Bohus B, Versteeg DHG (1982) Brain Res 239: 659-663.
12. De Kloet ER, Versteeg DHG, Kovács GL (1983) Brain Res 264: 323-327.
13. Angelucci L, Patacchioli FR, Bohus B, De Kloet ER (1982) In: Costa E, Racagni G (eds) Typical and Atypical Antidepressants: Molecular Mechanisms. Raven Press, New York, pp. 365-370.
14. McEwen BS (1982) In: Ganten D, Pfaff D (eds) Current Topics in Neuroendocrinology, vol. 2. Springer Verlag, Berlin, pp. 1-22.

© 1984 Elsevier Science Publishers B.V.
Endocrinology
F. Labrie, L. Proulx, eds.

METABOLISM OF ANDROGENS IN THE RAT AND HAMSTER NEUROENDOCRINE STRUCTURES

FABIO CELOTTI, ROBERTO MAGGI, COSIMO ROBERTO MELCANGI, PAOLA NEGRI- CESI and LUCIANO MARTINI

Department of Endocrinology, University of Milano, 21, Via A. del Sarto, Milano, Italy

I. Localization of the 5alpha-reductase in selected hypothalamic areas

In previous studies from this and other laboratories it has been shown that testosterone can be transformed in the CNS of the rat, and particularly in the hypothalamus, into 5alpha-dihydrotestosterone (5alpha-DHT) and into 5alpha-androstane-3alpha,17beta-diol (3alpha-diol) (see 1 for references). Minute amounts of 5alpha-androstane-3beta,17beta-diol (3beta-diol) and of delta-4-androstenedione (delta-4-A) are also formed (1). The conversion of testosterone into the 5alpha-reduced metabolites is a key step in the mechanism of action of the hormone in its peripheral target tissues, (e.g. prostate, etc.) and is probably of importance for explaining several of the effects exerted by androgens on the CNS both pre- and post-natally (1).

The 5alpha-reduction of testosterone in the hypothalamus, at variance with what happens in the peripheral androgen-sensitive structures and in the anterior pituitary, does not seem to be modulated by endocrine manipulations, as castration or gonadal steroid administration (2,3). Even total or frontal hypothalamic deafferentations, or the "in vivo" treatment with neuroactive drugs such as reserpine, parachlorophenylalanine, atropine, morphine and naloxone have been shown not to produce any significant modifications in the activity of the hypothalamic 5alpha-reductase (4).

Since the hypothalamus is not an homogeneous structure and the testosterone-metabolizing enzymes have been shown to be unevenly distributed (5), it was decided to investigate whether the 5alpha-reductase activity could be modulated in some specific hypothalamic nuclear areas by castration. The selected areas were punched off under a stereomicroscope from frozen brain sections using calibrated needles, according to the technique of Palkovits (6) and utilizing the König and Klippel rat brain atlas (7). The areas so far tested are those including the medial and lateral preoptic nuclei (MPA, LPA), the anterior, lateral and posterior hypothalamic nuclei (AHA, LHA, PHA). Superficial layers of the frontal cerebral cortex were also punched off for comparison.

Table 1 shows the results of "in vitro" incubations performed with 10.000 DPM of C^{14}-testosterone for 2 hrs. at 37°C in presence of a NADPH generating system of the above mentioned areas taken from normal male rats and from animals castrated since 12 days.

TABLE I

"In vitro" formation of 5α-DHT and 3α-DIOL in selected hypothalamic nuclei and in the cerebral cortex of normal and castrated male rats.

	MPA	LPA	AHA	LHA	PHA	CORTEX
CASTRATED						
5α-DHT	173.5 ± 19.7 (10)	290.9 ± 16.6 (9)*	147.0 ± 16.0 (9)	349.1 ± 34.4 (10)*	195.9 ± 58.6 (4)	176.0 ± 23.4 (12)
3α-DIOL	18.0 ± 3.9 (10)	41.0 ± 7.3 (9)	5.9 ± 2.1 (6)	31.5 ± 8.2 (7)	22.6 ± 10.5 (3)	20.6 ± 3.2 (8)
NORMAL						
5α-DHT	169.5 ± 7.6 (10)	276.0 ± 27.0 (10)*	142.7 ± 11.0 (10)	297.0 ± 27.0 (10)*	202.0 ± 31.5 (4)	154.4 ± 23.5 (13)
3α-DIOL	12.8 ± 2.6 (10)	21.8 ± 8.0 (10)	13.9 ± 5.1 (7)	19.3 ± 4.8 (8)	10.9 ± 2.2 (3)	26.4 ± 6.8 (13)

Means ± SEM (number of incubation in brackets - each incubation consisted of a pool of two rats)

* $P < 0.05$ VS the corresponding cortex (one way analysis of variance)

The results are expressed in terms of pg of steroid formed / mm^3 of tissue / 2hrs of incubation

It is apparent that only the lateral preoptic and the lateral hypothalamic nuclei, both from normal and castrated rats, possess a higher converting ability than the cerebral cortex. These two nuclei are also significantly more active than the corresponding medial ones (medial preoptic and anterior hypothalamic nucleus). No effect of castration could be seen in any area considered. The formation of 3alpha-diol does not seem to be significantly different in the various areas considered; also this parameter is not affected by castration. However, it should be noted that the small amounts of 3alpha-diol formed are at the limit of the sensitivity of the assay, and therefore subjected to considerable estimation errors.

II. Is the 5alpha-reductase localized in the neurones or in the glial cells?

In the CNS testosterone metabolism has always been studied in tissue fragments or in homogenates; no attempts have been made so far to clarify whether the neuronal or the glial component is specifically involved in the formation of the 5alpha-reduced compounds. Some indirect evidence suggesting that the 5alpha-reductase activity in the brain is preferentially located in the neuronal component will be presented here. A direct confirmation is expected from cell separation experiments now being performed.

Table 2 shows that the formation of 5alpha-DHT and 3alpha-diol is significantly decreased in frontal cortical areas punched off from frozen sections where a glial proliferation has been induced by means of stereotaxically-placed mechanical lesions.

TABLE II

Formation of 5α-DHT and 3α-DIOL in the rat frontal cerebral cortex, in the cortex after stimulation of neuroglial cell proliferation, in the corpus callosum and in the optic chiasm.

	CORTEX	CORTEX + LESION	CORPUS CALLOSUM	OPTIC CHIASM
5α-DHT	152.0 ± 4.5 (8)	34.4 ± 9.7 (5)*	492.0 ± 24.6 (4)*	873.5 ± 15.5 (4)*
3α-DIOL	26.7 ± 2.0 (8)	2.8 ± 1.1 (3)*	44.3 ± 6.2 (3)	269.0 ± 24.2 (4)*

Means ± SEM (number of incubation in brackets - each incubation consisted of a pool of two rats)

* $P < 0.01$ VS cortex

The results are expressed in terms of pg of steroid formed / mm^3 of tissue / 2hrs of incubation

Moreover, the corpus callosum and the optic chiasm, two structures mainly composed of myelinated axons, have a much higher 5alpha-reductase activity than the cerebral cortex. It is unlikely that the formation of the 5alpha-reduced metabolites might be attributed to the myelin sheath, since in the brain of the developing rat a peak of 5alpha-reductase activity is found, both in the hypothalamus and in the cerebral cortex (8), clearly before the beginning of the myelination process which begins in this species 10 days after birth (9).

III. Effect of the photoperiod on brain and pituitary metabolism of testosterone in the golden hamster

Testosterone metabolism in the nervous structures and in the anterior pituitary of non mammalian photoperiodic species is substantially different from that of mammals. For instance, in birds testosterone is mainly transformed into 5beta-reduced metabolites and into delta-4-androstenedione (1). This metabolic pattern has been associated, at least in birds, with the presence of a photoperiodically-regulated reproductive activity. A single previous study by Callard et al. (10) reports the formation of substantial amounts of 5beta-androstane-3,17-dione after the bulk incubation of 180 mg of the hypothalamus and of the anterior limbic cortex of the golden hamster (Mesocricetus auratus), a photoperiodic mammal. It was therefore felt of interest to analyze in more detail the testosterone metabolic pattern in the central structures of this species. Animals were exposed to long (14 hrs. light; 10 hrs. dark) or short (8 hrs.

light; 16 hrs dark) photoperiods for 15, 30 and 60 days. After 60 days of short photoperiod, but not at earlier intervals, there was a clearcut involution of the testes (0.36 + 0.03 g _vs_ 2.47 + 0.05 in long days), and a decrease of serum testosterone to non detectable values. Tissue fragments from the hypothalamus, the cerebral cortex and the anterior pituitary of single animals were incubated with C^{14}-testosterone as precursor for 2 hrs. at 37°C in the presence of a NADPH generating system. The same tissues of male rats have been used for comparison.

The results so far obtained indicate that no one of the tissues considered produces measurable amounts of the 5beta-reduced metabolites of testosterone. The data regarding the formation of 5alpha-DHT, 3alpha-diol and delta-4-androstenedione are shown in Table 3.

TABLE III

"In vitro" 5α-DHT, 3α-DIOL and Δ_4-ANDROSTENEDIONE (Δ_4-A) formation in the hypothalamus, anterior pituitary and cerebral cortex of adult male rats and adult male hamsters. Hamsters were kept in long photoperiod (14hrs light-10hrs dark) or in short photoperiod (8hrs light-16hrs dark) for 15 (SD 15), 30 (SD 30) and 60 (SD 60) days.

	RATS	HAMSTERS LONG DAYS	HAMSTERS SD 15	HAMSTERS SD 30	HAMSTERS SD 60
HYPOTHALAMUS					
5α-DHT	288.8 ± 25.6 (11)	20.3 ± 9.3 (14)	15.6 ± 1.4 (5)	30.8 ± 3.5 (5)	7.4 ± 0.7 (6)
3α-DIOL	151.6 ± 10.2 (11)	16.1 ± 2.6 (14)	10.7 ± 5.0 (5)	20.9 ± 1.5 (5)	5.1 ± 0.8 (6)
Δ_4-A	13.5 ± 4.0 (8)	104.2 ± 12.3 (10)	103.9 ± 3.9 (5)	–	91.7 ± 14.6 (6)
ANTERIOR PITUITARY					
5α-DHT	416.3 ± 29.6 (11)	34.6 ± 7.9 (15)	48.7 ± 18.2 (4)	47.0 ± 18.9 (5)	57.7 ± 18.7 (6)
3α-DIOL	408.2 ± 45.8 (11)	32.1 ± 8.2 (15)	7.7 ± 2.1 (5)	36.2 ± 16.9 (5)	32.0 ± 16.9 (6)
Δ_4-A	108.9 ± 22.6 (8)	600.0 ± 47.5 (10)	474.1 ± 57.4 (5)	–	837.5 ± 52.9 (6).*
CEREBRAL CORTEX					
5α-DHT	181.7 ± 21.1 (11)	14.5 ± 3.3 (15)	18.4 ± 1.7 (5)	35.7 ± 4.8 (5)	10.3 ± 5.1 (6)
3α-DIOL	148.6 ± 18.5 (11)	3.9 ± 1.0 (15)	–	12.0 ± 4.2 (5)	2.9 ± 0.9 (6)
Δ_4-A	32.0 ± 9.2 (8)	79.1 ± 7.1 (10)	72.6 ± 2.6 (5)	–	74.1 ± 10.7 (6)

Means ± SEM (number of animals in brackets)

* $P < 0.05$ _VS_ anterior pituitary of hamsters in long days.

The results are expressed in terms of pg of streoid formed / mg of tissue / 2hrs of incubation

It appears that the amounts of 5alpha-DHT and 3alpha-diol formed by the three structures considered are significantly lower in the hamster than in the rat. No modification of the 5alpha-reduction of testosterone between long and short photoperiods could be observed. The hypothalamus, the cerebral cortex, and particularly the anterior pituitary of the hamster are able to metabolize testosterone to delta-4-androstenedione in higher quantities than the corresponding structures of the rat. It is worthwhile noting that in the hamster, after 60 days of exposure to a short photoperiod, a significant increase in the formation of delta-4-androstenedione occurs at pituitary level. A similar effect has been shown to occur in birds (11). The possible physiological significance of this observation is presently under investigation.

ACKNOWLEDGEMENTS

The work described in this paper has been supported by the Consiglio Nazionale delle Ricerche, under the project "Preventive and Rehabilitative Medicine" and "Gruppo Nazionale di Endocrinologia".

REFERENCES

1. Martini L (1982) Endocr Rev 3: 1-25

2. Denef C, Magnus C, McEwen BS (1973) J Endocr 59:605-621

3. Celotti F, Farina J M S, Santaniello E, Martini L, Motta M (1979) J Steroid Biochem 11: 215-219

4. Celotti F, Negri-Cesi P, Limonta P, Melcangi C, (1983) J Steroid Biochem 19: 229-234

5. Selmanoff M K, Brodkin L D, Weiner R I, Siiteri P K (1977) Endocrinology 101:841-848

6. Palkovits M (1973) Brain Res 59:449-450

7. König J F R, Klippel R A (1963) The Rat Brain, Williams and Wilkins, Baltimore

8. Massa R, Justo S, Martini L (1975) J Steroid Biochem 6: 567-571

9. Norton W T, Poduslo S E (1973) J Neurochem 21:759-773

10. Callard G V, Hoffman R A, Petro Z, Ryan K J (1973) Biol Reprod. 21:33-38

11. Davies D T, Massa R, James R (1980) J Endocrinol 84:211-222

Endocrinology
F. Labrie, L. Proulx, eds.

NEURO-STEROIDS : 3β-HYDROXY-Δ5-DERIVATIVES IN THE RODENT BRAIN

E.E. BAULIEU and P. ROBEL

INSERM U33 and CNRS ER 125. Lab Hormones, Faculté de Médecine, 94270 Bicêtre, France

Pregnenolone (P) and dehydroepiandrosterone (D) have been detected, characterized, and measured in the rat brain (1, 2). They have been found as unconjugated free (F) steroids, sulfate esters (S) and fatty acid esters (lipoidal derivatives, L). In the following sections, the combined amounts (FP + PS) or (FD + DS) will be designated by the symbols [P] and [D], respectively. Values for PL and DL corrected for recovery, are not yet available.

The quantitation of brain D and P appeared to depend on several environmental and methodological factors. Some have been partly documented, as lighting schedule, food intake, housing conditions (number of animals per cage, rats of the other sex in the same room), and stress (after orchidectomy (orx) plus adrenalectomy (adx), or the corresponding sham operation). We also realized that the work up conditions for the removal and initial processing of brain tissue were critical. Therefore all physiological and pharmacological experiments were conducted under strictly defined condition, with appropriate internal controls, and their statistical significance evaluated. With these restrictions in mind, [D] concentration in the brain of adult male rats (Sprague-Dawley, 11-12 week old), was about 10 pmol per g of tissue, whereas [P] was about 50 pmol per g of tissue. PS concentration was always lower than that of P, whereas DS concentration was greater than that of D. Although we found differences in [P] and [D] concentrations between selected brain areas, the variability between different experiments precluded any definitive statement. However, [P] and [D] were constantly higher in hypothalamus and olfactory bulbs than in any other brain structure.

THE ACCUMULATION OF BRAIN PREGNENOLONE AND DEHYDROEPIANDROSTERONE IS NOT RELATED TO PERIPHERAL ENDOCRINE GLANDS

The rat adrenal secretes P, but not D, as reflected by the measurement of [P] and [D] in adrenals and in plasma. This led us to assume independent mechanisms for the formation/accumulation of brain 3β-hydroxy-Δ5-steroids. The relevant findings have been reported previously (1, 2). Neither [D] nor [P] disappeared or even decreased (compared to sham operated controls) in brain 15 to 45 d after combined adx + orx. Brain [D] was also unchanged after administration of corticotropin or dexamethasone for 3 d, or after an acute nociceptive stimulation. In contrast, stress conditions prevailing 2 d after adx + orx or the corresponding sham operation resulted in a significant increase of brain [D] concentration. The results were less clear cut with [P], because of significant adrenal contribution to acute changes of brain P concentrations.

Since neither D nor P disappeared from the blood of adx + orx animals, brain results may be explained by large accumulation of D and P arising from extra-adrenals source(s). We have tried to check this possibility by injecting radioactive P and D to intact rats. Although the concentrations of steroids were severalfold larger in brain than in plasma, both radioactive steroid were not retained for any longer time than in plasma (2). We concluded that brain P and D were either produced locally or released from still undefined storage forms. Attempts to demonstrate the side-chain cleavage of cholesterol or pregnenolone by brain slices, total homogenates or subcellular fractions were inconclusive (3).

VARIATIONS OF BRAIN PREGNENOLONE ACCORDING TO PHYSIOLOGICAL CONDITIONS

Ontogenesis. [P] and (F + S) corticosterone [B] were measured in rat brain between birth and d 22. In newborns of both sexes, [P] was high at delivery (27 ± 13 ng/g, mean ± sd, n = 12) and decreased steadily during the 1st d (7 ± 2 ng/g, at 6 h, n = 6 and 8 ± 5 ng/g, at 24 h, n = 15). On the following days, [P] was in the 8-22 ng/g range. The high concentrations of [P] and [B] (99 ± 71 ng/g, n = 6) at birth in brain seemed correlated with high levels of [P] and [B] in plasma of fetuses, and mothers. However, brain [P] was always much larger than plasma [P] , contrary to [B]. Brain and plasma [B] decreased to insignificant levels between d 1 and d 10, a period of adrenal inactivity in the rat (4, 5), suggesting that brain P during this period is accumulated through a selective mechanism unrelated, at least in part, to adrenal activity.

Circadian variations. Male adult rats were housed in triads for 2 weeks. Lights were on between 7 am and 8 pm. The levels of [B] in the brain showed a daily trough and crest with timing similar to that observed previously in plasma and brain (6). Brain [P] underwent a similar circadian rhythm, with a trough between 6 and 9 am (8.9 ± 0.3 ng/g at 9 am, n = 3) and a crest between 3 and 12 pm (26 ± 7 ng/g at 9 pm, n = 3). The increase of brain [P] preceeded that of [B] : 21 ± 4 and 7.2 ± 4.2 ng/g, respectively at 12 am. Brain [D] did not vary significantly. The variations of brain [P] were not related to concomittant changes of plasma steroid. Definitive conclusion should await measurements on a much larger number of animals.

ATTEMPTS TO DEMONSTRATE THE BIOLOGICAL ROLES OF PREGNENOLONE AND DEHYDROEPIANDROSTERONE IN BRAIN

P and D as precursors of sex hormones. Incubation of rat brain minces with ^{3}H-P yielded ^{3}H-progesterone and ^{3}H-PL. The yield of progesterone and PL formed per 100 mg tissue was in the ∿ 1 % range in hypothalamus, amygdala, olfactory bulb and other regions of the brain, with the exception of cerebellum and the frontal cortex, where very little metabolism was observed (3). Similarly, ^{3}H-D gave small amounts of ^{3}H-androstenedione and ^{3}H-DL in hypothalamic slices, but no radioactive Δ5-androstenediol or testosterone were found. ^{3}H-PL was also formed ^{3}H-P by the rat glioma C6 line (5-8 % per 10^7 cells per 24 h), whereas no such metabolite could be demonstrated in L 929 mouse fibroblasts.

P and D and sexual behavior. 1. D inhibits aggressive behavior of castrated male mice. Group-housed triads of castrated male mice attack lactating female intruders (7). Five to 6 weeks after castration or sham operation, Swiss male mice received D or vehicle SC for 15 d. Lactating females were introduced in the cages, and the latency and number of attacks recorded for 15 min. D inhibited the aggressive behavior of castrated males in a dose dependent manner, maximally at 80 µg/d. This dose of D resulted in a very small increase of testosterone in brain (from 0.04 ± 0.02 ng/g to 0.13 ± 0.06 ng/g), remaining well below the level in intact males (3.1 ± 1.1 ng/g), whereas brain FD was much increased (8). Results were compatible with an inhibitory effect of D itself, or of another undefined metabolite. The estrogenic Δ5-androstenediol (9) was not active. P injected in equimolar amount to the fully effective dose of D tended to be inhibitory. 2. P and D vary in limbic structures of male rats exposed to female siblings. Eleven week old male rats were exposed to the scent of virgin adult females or of control young adult males, for one week. [P] and [D] were measured in olfactory bulbs, amygdala and hypothalami of exposed males (10). [P] decreased very markedly in the olfactory bulb while augmenting in the amygdala and to a lesser degree in the hypothalamus in response to female scent (no change was recorded in the plasma and peripheral organs). [D] content also decreased in the olfactory bulb, and augmented in the amygdala and even more in the hypothalamus.

Changes in the firing rate of single neurons induced by direct application of D(S) and P(S). The experiments were performed in adult female guinea pigs (400 g), anesthetized with urethane. When FD, DS and PS were applied iontophoretically or by pressure to neurons in the septo-preoptic area, an excitatory effect was observed (11). DS and PS, applied on the same neurone, always produced a similar effect. When DS and D were tested, some neurones were excited by both steroids whereas others responded to DS only. DS, PS and FD-induced responses displayed a short latency in onset and offset, suggesting an action at the membrane level.

CONCLUSION

Contrary to the classical steroid hormones, the 3β-hydroxy-Δ5 steroids pregnenolone (sulfate) and dehydroepiandrosterone (sulfate) are accumulated in rat brain in concentrations far in excess of those found in plasma. Although their functions are still poorly understood, they may affect the brain by metabolism to sex steroid hormones, and they may be functionnaly related to sexual behavior (possibly through direct modulation of the firing rates of neurons). This new chapter of steroid regulation of the brain may not be particular to rodent, since we have preliminary evidence for the presence of P and D in other mammalian species, including primates.

ACKNOWLEDGEMENTS

The work is due to the collaborative efforts of C. Corpéchot, M. Synguelakis, and C. Clarke in our laboratory. We thank R. Guillemin for its hospitality at the Salk Institute (La Jolla, CA). Contributing experiments were performed by J. Sjövall and M. Axelson (Stockholm) for GLC-MS analysis, J. Pedersen (Oslo), P. Brazeau (La Jolla and Montréal), M. Haug and M.L. Schlegel (Strasbourg), J. Roffi (Orsay), B. Carette and P. Poulain (Lille), and S. Tahla (Bicêtre). This work was supported in part by Inserm contract PRC 120048, by the MIR contract n°83.C.0924, by the R.J. and H.C. Kleberg Foundation and by the Philippe Foundation.

REFERENCES

1. Corpéchot C, Robel P, Axelson M, Sjövall J, Baulieu EE (1981) Proc Natl Acad Sci USA, 78:4704-4707.
2. Corpéchot C, Synguelakis M, Tahla S, Axelson M, Sjövall J, Vikho R, Baulieu EE, Robel P (1983) Brain Res 270:119-125.
3. Clarke C, Groyer A, Baulieu EE, Robel P (1984) 7th International Congress of Endocrinology, Quebec, Canada, July 1-7 1984. Abstract.
4. Corbier P, Roffi J (1978) Biol Neonate 33:72-79.
5. Allen C, Kendall JM (1967) Endocrinology 80:926-930.
6. Butte JC, Kakihana R, Noble EP (1976) J Endocr 68:235-239.
7. Haug M, Brain PF (1978) Physiol Behavior 21:549-552.
8. Haug M, Spetz JF, Schlegel ML, Robel P (1983) C R Acad Sci Paris 296:975-977.
9. Seymour-Munn K, Adams J (1983) Endocrinology 112:486-491.
10. Corpéchot C, Baulieu EE, Brazeau P (1983) 65th Annual Meeting of the Endocrine Society, Abstract n°207, and in preparation.
11. Carette B, Poulain P (1984) Neuroscience Letters 45:205-210.

Endocrinology
F. Labrie, L. Proulx, eds.

HYPOTHALAMIC mRNA AND ITS ROLE IN SEXUAL DIFFERENTIATION

HELEN F. STANLEY* AND GEORGE FINK
MRC Brain Metabolism Unit, Dept. of Pharmacology, 1 George Square, Edinburgh, Scotland, U.K.

INTRODUCTION

The rodent brain undergoes sexual differentiation during a 'critical period' of development which ends at approximately postnatal day 10 (1,2). Testicular androgens, largely through their central conversion to oestrogen, have a permanent organising effect on neurons within brain regions controlling reproductive functions and several sexually dimorphic features have been described(3,4). Inhibitors of DNA, RNA and protein synthesis can block or partially protect against the masculinising effects of testosterone in the neonatal rat(5) indicating that hormone-induced changes in gene expression are important in the differentiation process.

To investigate whether sex differences in specific proteins occur during or as a result of sexual differentiation, an electrophoretic analysis of soluble proteins and the *in vitro* translation products of poly (A)+ mRNA extracted from the hypothalamus-preoptic area(H-POA) of male, female and androgenised female rats was carried out.

MATERIALS AND METHODS

Male(M), female(F) and androgenised female(4 day F injected with 1.25mg testosterone propionate;TP F) Wistar Cob rats were used in these studies. Rats were killed by decapitation(6h after testosterone injection) and the H-POA dissected out by incisions extending from the rostral edge of the optic chiasm to the caudal edge of the mamillary body. A soluble protein extract was prepared by centrifuging the tissue homogenate at 120,000g for 1h at 4°C. Protein concentration was determined by the method of Lowry et al(6). Total RNA was extracted by the guanidinium thiocyanate procedure(7). Preparations were enriched for poly (A)+ containing mRNA by oligo-dT cellulose chromatography(8). The mRNA samples were translated in an amino-acid depleted rabbit reticulocyte lysate system(Amersham International) supplimented with either ^{35}S-methionine or ^{3}H-amino-acid mixture. Electrophoresis was carried out according to the method of O'Farrel(9) using 8 - 20% SDS polyacrylamide gradient slab gels with a 4.75% stacking gel. Gels were stained with Coomassie Brilliant Blue R250 or flourographed(10). Proteins were quantified by scanning densitometry.

* Present address: Centre for Reproductive Sciences, Columbia University, New York, NY.

RESULTS

As assessed by scanning densitometry, the H-POA content of a soluble protein (s) of molecular weight (mol. wt.) 55-58,000 was found to be approximately 30% greater in the male than the female at birth (day 0 : see Figure 1).

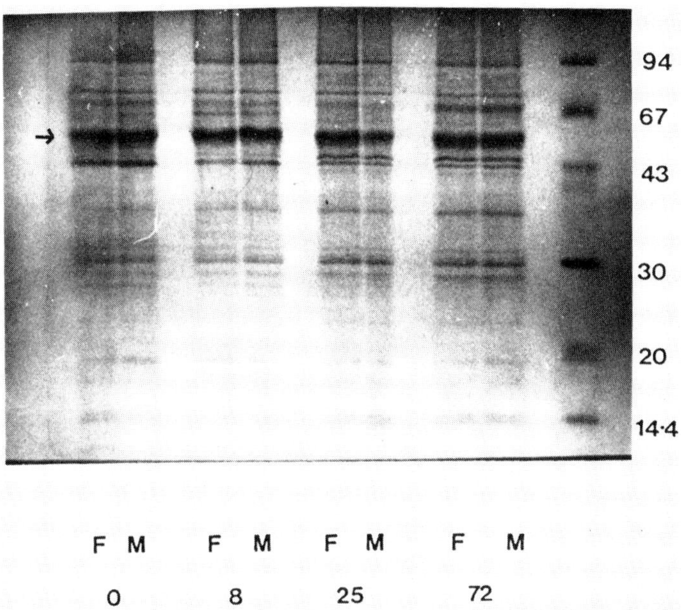

Fig. 1. Soluble H-POA Proteins Throughout Development (Age in days, mol. wt. markers x 10^{-3}).

Translation of mRNA *in vitro* using either ^{35}S-methionine (Fig. 2.) or ^{3}H-amino-acid mixture (Fig. 3.) to label protein, showed that 4 and 12 day androgenised female and male rat H-POA had the capacity to synthesise greater amounts of a 55-58,000 mol. wt. protein(s) than the respective control female H-POA. Sex differences in a number of other proteins were also detected. Two-dimensional analysis of the 4 day H-POA translation products (Figs. 4.) showed what appears to be an androgen-dependent inhibition of a 20,000 mol. wt. protein in the androgenised female with a greater inhibition occurring in the male.

The results from the mRNA studies suggest that the sex difference in content of the 55-58,000 mol. wt. protein(s) in the H-POA detected at day 0 by staining soluble proteins may be due to higher levels of mRNA coding for the protein(s) in the male. The 55-58,000 mol. wt. protein(s) was found to migrate with the same R_f value as a standard preparation of tubulin.

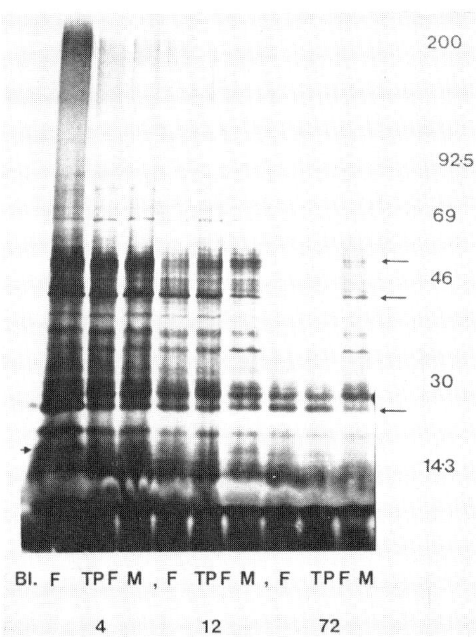

Fig. 2. Translation Products Labelled With ^{35}S-methionine.
Bl= no message blank

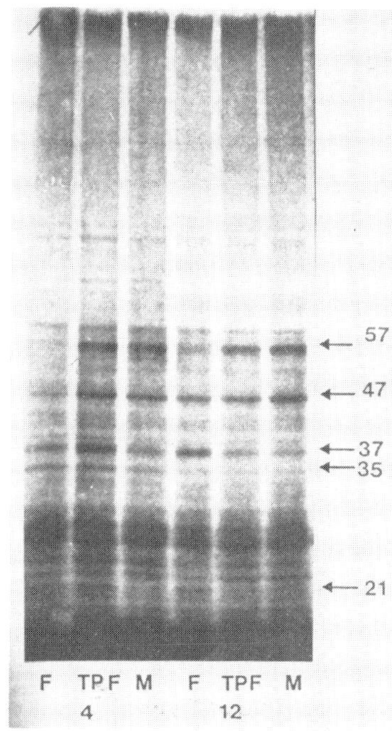

Fig. 3. Translation Products Labelled With ^{3}H-amino-acid Mixture.

These findings indicate that the synthesis of specific proteins appears to be influenced by androgen (or oestrogen) at the mRNA level in the neonatal rat H-POA. Of particular interest is the suggestion of a sex difference in synthesis of a protein with the electrophoretic characteristics of tubulin. Sexual differentiation of the brain, in a number of species, is known to be associated with changes in synapse formation and possibly the patterns of neuritic outgrowth in specific brain areas. The results presented here may support the theory that the structural changes occuring at this time could involve enhanced neuronal outgrowth in the male.

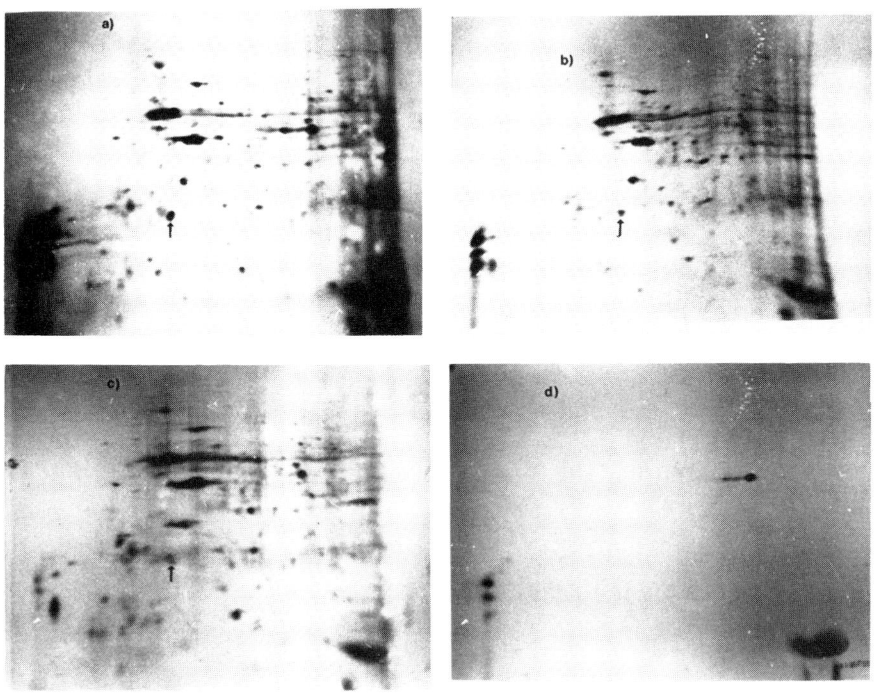

Fig. 4. Two-dimensional Analysis Of 4 Day Translation Products.
a) = F , b) = TP F , c) = M, d) = no-message blank.

ACKNOWLEDGEMENTS

H. Stanley was in receipt of a grant from the MRC.

REFERENCES

1. Barraclough CA (1961) Endocrinology 68:62-67

2. Harris GW (1964) Endocrinology 75:627-648

3. Jacobson CD, Gorski RA (1981) J Comp Neurol 196:519-529

4. Raisman G, Field PM (1973) Brain Res 54:1-29

5. Salaman DF, Birkett S (1974) Nature 247:109-112

6. Lowry OH, Rosebrough NJ, Farr AL, Randall RJ (1951) J Biol Chem 193:263-275

7. Chirgwin JM, Przybyla AE, McDonald RJ, Rutter WJ (1979) Biochemistry 18: 5294-5298

8. Aviv H, Leder P (1972) Proc Natl Acad Sci USA 69:1408-1412

9. O'Farrel PH (1975) J Biol Chem 250:4007-4021

10. Bonner WM, Laskey RA (1974) Eur J Biochem 46:83-88

15. Prostaglandins in Hormone Action

© 1984 Elsevier Science Publishers B.V.
Endocrinology
F. Labrie, L. Proulx, eds.

PROSTAGLANDINS AND OVULATION

KAZUO SATOH, KATSUYUKI KINOSHITA and OSAMU TSUTSUMI
Department of OB & GYN, University of Tokyo, Hongo, Tokyo (Japan)

Prostaglandins(PGs) are 20 carbon membered monocarboxylic acid and consist of nine members designated PGA to I in alphabetical order, including thromboxane (TX) as another member of PG family. PGs are biosynthesized cyclooxygenase (PG synthetase) in the microsome from arachidonic acid to PGsE_2, I_2 and TXsA_2 and B_2 via PGsH_2 and G_2. Nonsteroidal antiinflammatory agents such as aspirin and indomethacin block PG biosynthesis. PGsE_2 and $F_{2\alpha}$ called primary PG are applied clinically for induction and augmentation of labor because of their potent activity to contract uterine muscle. PGI_2 has a strong effect to inhibit platelet aggregation. On the contrary, TXA_2 is a platelet aggregating factor. Ovulation is a phenomenon in which oocyte is expelled out by LH from Graafian follicle matured by FSH, followed by formation of corpus luteum. How is PG involved in the chain reaction to cause ovulation?

I. Levels of PGs in ovulation

Unlike estradiol-17β and progesterone of which levels changed characteristically corresponding to BBT, $PGF_{2\alpha}$ metabolites in blood and urine were not demonstrated to have a specific changing pattern, whereas measurement of $PGF_{2\alpha}$ in the human ovarian vein blood indicated a significant elevation in the side of the ovary with the ovulating follicle within two days before ovulation. Furthermore, the contents of PGsE and F in the Wistar immature rat superovulating ovaries with pregnant mare's serum gonadotropin (PMS) and human chorionic gonadotropin (hCG) increased markedly 12 hrs after hCG injection. The concentrations of PGsE and F and 6-keto $PGF_{1\alpha}$ in gilt ovarian follicles under induced superovulation were elevated exponentially after about 20 hrs lag time as ovulation approached. The preovulatory increases of PGs in the follicular fluid and ovarian vein blood indicate that PGs play an important role in the process of ovulation.

II. PG biosynthesis in the ovarian follicle

Organ culture of the immature rat ovarian follicle primed with 10 iU of PMS for 48 hrs revealed that hCG had dose-dependent stimulatory effects on the production of PCs and progesterone after a time lag of 2 hrs subsequently to the addition of hCG. Indomethacin blocked production of PGs but not of progesterone and, on the contrary, puromycin and actinomycin D inhibited formation not only of PGs but also of progesterone dose-dependently, suggesting the action of LH on the matured follicle results in stimulation of cyclooxygenase through activation of protein biosythesis. Bioconversion of ^{14}C-arachidonic acid in homogenate of Wistar immature rat ovaries revealed that PGE_2 and 6-keto $PGF_{1\alpha}$ were produced at 3, 6 (maximal conversion rates: 7.62 and 2.31%), 8, 16 and 24 hrs after hCG injection subsequently to 48 hrs' PMS priming but not at 1 and 2 hrs. Homogenates of human Graafian follicles were shown to convert ^{14}C-arachidonic acid to PGE_2 at 0.34% but not to 6-keto $PGF_{1\alpha}$, while the stromal tissue produced not only PGE_2 at 0.09% but mainly 6-keto $PGF_{1\alpha}$ at 0.26%. These results suggest that stimulation of PG production in the matured follicle may be more likely due to induction of cyclooxygenase by LH (hCG) than to production of the stimulatory factors. Histochemical study of the subcellular localization of cyclooxygenase in the ovarian follicle cells using the antiserum to the solubilized cyclooxygenase from bovine seminal vesicle revealed that some of the granulosa cells examined were stained light microscopically (the ratio of the stained and unstained was roughly 1/15-20), indicating there may be heterogeneity of granulosa cell population regarding production of PGs. Investigation on phospholipase A_2 activity, the changes in *de novo* synthesis of phospholipids and the incorporation of ^{14}C-arachidonic acid into phospholipids under induced superovulation in Wistar immature rats showed LH inhibited phospholipase A_2 to decrease the release of arachidonic acid from phospholipids and, on the contrary, enhanced the incorporation of it into phospholipids. Therefore, the rate-limiting step of PG biosynthesis in rat ovary stimulated by LH is assessed to be no activation of phospholipase A_2 but cyclooxygenase.

III. Block of ovulation

Cyclooxygenase inhibitors such as indomethacin and mefenamic acid have been well-known to block superovulation induced with PMS and hCG in rats and gilts. Since such inhibitors are potent in blocking not only cyclooxygenase but also other enzymes, it is somewhat prenature to conclude that the action of the inhibitors in supressing ovulation can be solely attributed to their inhibition of PG production. Therefore, the antiserum to cyclooxygenase was used to compare its action with that of indomethacin. The intravenous administration of the antiserum inhibited superovulation in immature rats dose-dependently at doses of 0.1, 0.2 and 0.4 ml at which complete suppression was achieved. Decreased production of PGs was confirmed by 6 hrs' incubation using the follicles excised from the immature rats injected with the antiserum.

IV. Recovery of ovulation

It will be a conclusive proof that ovulation inhibition by suppression of PG production is recovered by the administration of PGs. Two hundred μg/rat of PGsE_2 and $F_{2\alpha}$ recovered superovulation significantly in the immature rats injected intravenously with 100 μg/rat of indomethacin. PGI_2 administered intraperitoneally at a dose of 100 μg/rat restored superovulation almost completely in case of intravenous injection of 100 μg/rat of indomethacin.

V. Steroidogenesis in block of ovulation

Indomethacin was reported to block cyclic AMP-dependent protein kinase purified from the jejunal serosa of rabbits (ID_{50}:0.017-0.048 μM) (ID_{50} of indomethacin 0.17-38 μM) and ornithine decarboxylase (500 μM). These reports suggest that ovulation suppression is more likely due to indomethacine's blocking of the protein kinase rather than of cyclooxygenase. Furthermore, the antibodies to progesterone and testosterone inhibited superovulation in rats. Measurement of progesterone, 17α OH-progesterone, estradiol-17β and testosterone in the peripheral blood in inhibition of superovulation in rats and gilts by indomethacin showed that no differences were observed in the levels of all the steroids measured between control and the group treated with indomethacin. Besides, the activities of mitochondrial cholesterol side chain-cleavage enzymes and microsomal 17α-hydroxylase were changed in the ovulation-blocking group in the same fashion as control. These results indicate inhibition of ovulation by indomethacin does not affect luteinization and steroidogenesis and the action of PGs in ovulation is independent of that of steroid hormones. It is now clear that both PGs and steroids are intrinsically involved in ovulation. The pathological state of the follicle in which no ovulation occurs in spite of luteinization is designated "the luteinized unruptured follicle". Ovulation is usually followed by luteinization of the follicular cells, formation of corpus luteum. Therefore, ovulation and production of progesterone have been considered two sides of the same coin. But the present study suggests that it is possible to isolate the process of steroidogenesis and ovulation and consequently offers a broad, new methodological direction for investigating pathogenesis of the luteinized unruptured follicle syndrome.

VI. Maturation of oocytes

Oocytes in matured follicles resume meiosis by a hormonal stimulus such as LH and complete the first meiotic reductive division at metaphase II prior to ovulation. Indomethacin inhibited meiotic maturation dose-dependently (100 to 500 μg/rat). The inhibition by indomethacin (100 μg/rat) was recovered by the intravenous administration of $PGsE_2$ and $F_{2\alpha}$ (250 μg/rat at 0, 2 and 4 hrs after hCG injection) but not by PGI_2. $PGsE_2$ and $F_{2\alpha}$ were demonstrated to be involved in cytoplasmic maturation during meiotic progression prior to ovulation in terms of activation of phosphofructokinase, a rate-limiting enzyme in glycolysis. Bioconversion of ^{14}C-arachidonic acid to $PGsE_2$ and $F_{2\alpha}$ and 6-keto $PGF_{1\alpha}$ was detected in the cumulus-oocyte complex but not in oocytes. It was revealed by the enzyme cycling method that the activity of 15OH PG dehydrogenase in oocytes decreased from 1.85 to 14.3 pmol/oocyte/hr during meiotic maturation. LH and PGs were demonstrated to activate plasminogen activator in the oocyte probably to facilitate dissociation of cumulus cells from the oocyte.

VII. Action mechanism of PGs

The receptors for $PGsE_1$ and E_2 were indicated to be present in ovarian follicle cells. A marked increase in specific binding of PGE occurs around the time of ovulation. Fibrinolytic system is activated by PGs correspondingly to the time of ovulation. PGs are involved in increases of plasminogen and plasminogen activator in the follicles.

In conclusion, the effect of LH on the follicle matured by FSH results in increasing PG production through the induction of cyclooxygenase in the follicle. The increased PGs act on the receptor for PGs, especially PGE and activate proteolytic enzymes such as plasmin to rupture the apex of the follicle and discharge oocyte.

REFERENCES

1. Satoh K, Mitsuhashi N, Fukuoka H, Shibata J, Nakabayashi M, Kawai Y, Yasumizu T, Kaneko Y, Kinoshita K, Sakamoto S (1977) Obst Gynecol 44:1559 (in Japanese)
2. Satoh K, Fukuoka H, Wu T, Mitsuhashi N, Kinoshita K, Sakamoto S (1981) Prostaglandins Med 7:29
3. Kawai Y, Satoh K, Mitsuhashi N, Hasumi K, Sakakibara K, Knoshita K, Wu T, Sakamoto S (1981) Folia Endocrinol Jap 57:1475
4. Satoh K (1979) Acta Ob Gyn Jap 31:975

Endocrinology
F. Labrie, L. Proulx, eds.

PROSTAGLANDINS AND BONE CELL BIOLOGY

T.J. MARTIN and N.C. PARTRIDGE

Department of Medicine, University of Melbourne, Repatriation General Hospital, Heidelberg, 3081, Australia

The experiments which first demonstrated that prostaglandins were able to resorb bone directly (1) were based on the observation (2) that PGs, like parathyroid hormone (PTH), were capable of stimulating adenylate cyclase activity in bone cell membranes. Of all the arachidonic acid metabolites tested in the bioassay systems, PGE_2 is the most potent bone resorber (3-5). Although prostacyclin (PGI_2) has been shown to resorb cultured fetal rat long bones (6), those experiments required repeated additions of PGI_2, and therefore did not allow an accurate estimate of the potency of this prostanoid. However it seems likely that PGI_2 is less potent in this respect than PGE_2. Although inhibition of bone resorption by imidazole has been demonstrated (7), we have been unable to produce any such inhibition in experiments in which we used more selective thromboxane synthesis inhibitors, dazoxiben and 7-imidazolyl-hydroxyproprionic acid (8). Thromboxane analogues have been found to be have no significant effect on resorption (4) nor have any products of the lipoxygenase pathway of arachidonic acid metabolism.

Bone resorption

In many tissues, PGs act as locally important regulators of biological activities, and this is so also in bone. The actions of certain bone resorbing factors, notable phorbol esters (9), epidermal growth factor (10), melittin (9), complement replete serum (11) and thrombin, require the synthesis within bone of prostanoids, although EGF is also capable of causing resorption by a PG-independent mechanism (12). Mouse bone *in vitro* treated with arachidonic acid or EGF produces substantial amounts of the metabolites of PGE_2 and PGI_2, and smaller amounts of thromboxane (13). Indeed, the studies of Voelkel et al (13) show that the major resorption product is 6,15 diketo $PGF_{1\alpha}$, the metabolite of PGI_2. Thus certain agents can clearly stimulate resorption by PG-requiring pathways, and furthermore there is good evidence (14) that basal (i.e. unstimulated) bone resorption by mouse calvaria in culture is the result of endogenous PG production in bone.

Bone formation

The processes of bone formation and resorption are linked, with several hormonal agents capable of acting on both. This is the case with PGE_2, which can increase proline incorporation into collagen of embryonic chick bone (15), but inhibit collagen synthesis at high concentrations in mouse calvaria (16).

When fetal rat calvaria were treated with cortisol to decrease endogenous PG production a consistent stimulation of collagen synthesis was observed in response to PGE_2 (17), which also prevented the decrease in DNA produced by prolonged exposure to cortisol. Several *in vivo* observations are consistent with the possibility that PGs are capable of stimulating bone formation (8), and thus PGs might be regarded as participating in the regulation of both resorption and formation.

Cellular origin of endogenous PGs of bone

Most mammalian cells have the capacity to produce PGs. The cyclo-oxygenase products of arachidonic acid metabolism have been characterized in osteoblast-rich cultures derived from normal rat bone and in clonal malignant osteoblasts (18). In each case, both PGE_2 and 6-keto-$PGF_{1\alpha}$ are found in the medium, suggesting that the osteoblast is a source of PGs, whatever other cells in bone produce them. There was no evidence obtained for thromboxane production by osteoblasts. Osteoclasts have not been isolated in sufficient numbers or purity to determine whether they produce PGs, but as will be discussed below, there is some evidence that isolated osteoclasts can respond to PGs.

PG action in bone

In organ culture experiments, PGE_2 enhances bone resorption and increases the number and activity of osteoclasts, an action similar to that produced by other bone-resorbing agents. The effect of PGE_2 on bone is similar to that of PTH and appears to require cyclic AMP generation. Studies with osteoblast-rich cultures from rat calvaria, and with clonal malignant osteoblasts, have shown that cells of the osteoblast series have a PG-responsive adenylate cyclase similar to that responsive to PTH (19). The next step in cyclic AMP action, i.e. activation of cyclic AMP-dependent protein kinase, also takes place in these cells in response to PGs, with PGE_2 being the most potent of all the prostanoids, including PGI_2. Indeed it was the observation that the relative potencies of the prostanoids in elevating cyclic AMP in osteoblasts paralleled their relative potencies in stimulating bone resorption (20) which first led us to the view that the primary target of bone resorbing hormones might be the osteoblast and to the hypothesis that osteoclast function might be directed by the hormone-responsive osteoblast (21).

Although PGE_2 and PTH both activate adenylate cyclase and total cyclic AMP-dependent protein kinase, the detailed response mechanisms differ, in that in rat calvarial osteoblasts-like cells, PTH activates both isoenzyme I and II of cyclic AMP-dependent protein kinase, whereas PGE_2 activates isoenzyme II only (22). This difference would lead us to expect that these two hormones might exert different physiological affects on bone, since different phosphorylation patterns would be expected to occur in the target cells.

Certain differences have been noted between PTH and PGE_2 action on bone *in vitro* (e.g. failure of PGE_2 to decrease collagen synthesis at 24 hours, unlike PTH; failure of PGE_2 to be an "inducer" of resorption).

Although the emphasis in this discussion is on the action of PGE_2 on osteoblasts, evidence has been produced that PGE_2 and PGI_2 have a direct effect on isolated osteoclasts, of decreasing their motility, i.e. a calcitonin-like action (23). This intersting observation requires confirmation in other study systems, but indicates another potentially important aspect of intercellular communication in bone.

SUMMARY AND CONCLUSIONS

The prostaglandins can be regarded as important local regulators of bone cell function. It is unlikely that they act on bone as circulating hormones, but rather perhaps represent locally generated modulators whose action resembles closely (but is not identical with) that of the circulating hormone, PTH. They contribute to basal bone resorption *in vitro*, and may even be important physiologically in bone remodelling, e.g. contributing to the bone remodelling which can proceed apparently normally in a total absence of PTH - as in hypoparathyroidism. It is not certain what is the function of the considerable quantity of PGI_2 produced in resorbing bone. It is possible that it is concerned with the maintenance of potency of vascular channels. Finally, PGs can be generated in bone in response to certain stimuli, some physiological and some pathological. In certain disease states in man (e.g. cancer, arthritis), their generation in or near bone by foreign cells can result in pathological bone loss.

ACKNOWLEDGEMENTS

This work was supported by grants from the Anti-Cancer Council of Victoria and the National Health and Medical Research Council of Australia.

REFERENCES

1. Chase LR, Aurbach GD (1970) J Biol Chem 245:1520-1526.
2. Klein DC, Raisz LG (1970) Endocrinology 86:1436-1440.
3. Tashjian AH Jr, Tice JE, Sides K (1977) Nature 266:645-646.
4. Raisz LG, Dietrich JW, Simmons HA, Seyberth HW, Hubbard W, Oates JA (1977) Nature 267:532-534.
5. Greaves M, Ibbotson KJ, Atkins D, Martin TJ (1980) Clin Sci 58:201-210.
6. Raisz LG, Vanderhoek JY, Simmons HA, Kream BF, Nicolau KC (1979) Prostaglandins 17:905-914.
7. Heersche JNM, Jez DH (1981) Prostaglandins 21:401-411.

8. Raisz LG, Martin TJ (1984) In: Peck WA (ed) Bone and Mineral Research, Annual 2. Elsevier, Amsterdam, pp 286-310.

9. Tashjian AH Jr, Ivey JL, Delclos B, Levine L (1978) Prostaglandins 16:221-232.

10. Tashjian AH Jr, Levine L (1978) Biochem Biophys Res Comm 85:966-975.

11. Raisz LG, Sandberg AL, Goodson JM, Simmons HA, Mergenhagen SE (1977) Science 185:789-791.

12. Raisz LG, Simmons HA, Sandberg AL, Canalis E 91980) Endocrinology 107:270-273.

13. Voelkel EF, Tashjian AH Jr, Levine L (1980) Biochim Biophys Acta 620:418-428.

14. Katz JM, Skinner SJM, Wilson T, Gray PH (1983) Prostaglandins 26:545-553.

15. Blumenkrantz N, Sondergaard J (1972) Nature New Biol 239:246.

16. Raisz LG, Koolemans-Beynen AR (1974) Prostaglandins 8:377-385.

17. Chyun YS, Raisz LG (1982) Clin Res 30:387A.

18. Nolan RD, Partridge NC, Godfrey HM, Martin TJ (1983) Calc Tiss Int 35:294.

19. Partridge NC, Alcorn D, Michelangeli VP, Kemp BE, Ryan G, Martin TJ (1981) Endocrinology 108:213-219.

20. Crawford A, Atkins D, Martin TJ (1978) Biochem Biophys Res Comm 82:1195-1201.

21. Rodan GA, Martin TJ (1981) Calc Tiss Int 33:349-351.

22. Livesey SA, Kemp BE, Re C, Partridge NC, Martin TJ (1982) J Biol Chem 257: 14983-14988.

23. Chambers TJ, Magnus CJ (1982) J Path 136:27-29.

Endocrinology
F. Labrie, L. Proulx, eds.

PROSTAGLANDINS AND KIDNEY FUNCTION

D. SCHLONDORFF, M.D.

Nephrology Division, Department of Medicine, Albert Einstein College of Medicine, Bronx, New York, U.S.A.

In the kidney, prostaglandins (PG) can influence such diverse parameters as blood flow and glomerular filtration as well as solute and water excretion by the tubules. The pattern of prostaglandin synthesis varies along the nephron with the locally produced PGs affecting cellular function at the site of their generation.

In the renal cortex PGs are predominantly produced by arterioles and glomeruli (1,2). The role of the PG generated by these structures i.e., PGI_2 and PGE_2 seems to be geared towards maintenance of renal blood flow and glomerular filtration rate during conditions that cause activation of vasoconstrictors (3). The smooth muscle constrictor effect of e.g. angiotensin II, vasopressin and 1 alkyl 2 acetyl glycero -3- phosphocholine, a lipid mediator of inflammation (also known as platelet activating factor; (PAF)) can be demonstrated in vitro using isolated glomeruli or cultured glomerular mesangial cells (4,5). The constrictor effect of these agents can be partially antagonized by exogenous PGE_2 or by PGE_2 generated by glomeruli or mesangial cells, while inhibition of PG synthesis results in enhanced contraction (5,6). Concomitantly the vasoconstrictors cause a rapid increase of PGE_2 synthesis by mesangial cells (5,6,7). The increase in PGE_2 production by angiotensin and PAF is caused by activation of phospholipase C and A_2 (6,7). This causes release of arachidonic acid from phospholipids into a specific pool tightly coupled to cyclooxygenase and results in enhanced PGE_2 synthesis. Thus in the glomerulus, vasoconstrictors increase the production of vasodilatatory PGs, which in turn attenuate the vasoconstriction closing a negative feed-back loop. In this manner glomerular-mesangial PG production tends to preserve glomerular function during activation of vasoconstrictor systems.

In the renal medulla collecting tubules are major sites of PG production (1). Ever since the original observations that PGE_1 inhibits the effect of antidiuretic hormone in mammalian isolated collecting tubules (8) and their analogue, the toad urinary bladder (9) the interaction of ADH with PG has attracted much interest. Multiple studies have confirmed that PGE_1 and PGE_2 antagonize the antidiuretic effect of ADH both in vivo and in vitro (10). Isolated collecting tubules (11), cultured collecting tubular cells (12) and the toad bladder produce predominantly PGE_2 (13). In all of these preparations ADH can stimulate PGE_2 synthesis, though this depends somewhat on the experimental conditions (14,15). While the hydroosmotic effect of ADH is mediated by cAMP, its stimulation of PGE_2 synthesis via activation of phospholipase is not (13). The PGE_2 generated in response to ADH seems to inhibit cAMP generation (8,9). Thus, a negative feed-back loop exists whereby ADH stimulates PGE_2 synthesis which in turn inhibits ADH's action (13).

On the other hand, cAMP generated in response to ADH may inhibit the activation of phospholipase by ADH. This would cause a decrease in arachidonate release and PGE_2 synthesis. Using isolated epithelial cells from toad urinary bladder we were able to provide evidence for this hypothesis (16). Increasing cAMP levels by either 8 bromo cAMP or the phosphodiesterase inhibitor methylisobutylxanthine (MIX) decreased

PGE_2 production under basal and ADH stimulated conditions. This inhibitory effect could be overcome by the addition of exogenous arachidonic acid indicating that cAMP decreased PGE_2 synthesis by inhibiting phospholipase activation and the resulting release of arachidonate. This was further supported by experiments using [^{32}P] labeling of cellular phospholipids. MIX attenuated the ADH-induced changes in [^{32}P] phospholipid turnover, consistent with inhibition of phospholipase by cAMP. Thus a double reciprocal feed-back mechanism may exist whereby ADH stimulates PGE_2 production in a <u>cAMP-independent</u> fashion but also inhibits PGE_2-synthesis in a <u>cAMP-dependent</u> manner. Such an interlocked system would prevent an overshoot of both ADH and PGE_2 response in either direction and maintain PGE_2 production close to a set point appropriate for the physiological condition i.e. elevated during antidiuresis and lower during water diuresis.

As a unifying hypothesis the role of PG in different nephron segments can be visualized as that of local modulators for hormonal responses with the goal of maintaining local cell homeostasis which may be challenged by the changes occurring in response to the hormones.

REFERENCES

1. Smith WL, Bell TG (1978) Am J Physiol 235: F451-F457.

2. Schlondorff D, Roczniak S, Satriano JA, Folkert VW (1980) Am J Physiol 239: F486-F495.

3. Henrich WL, Berl T, McDonald KM, Anderson RJ, Schrier RW (1978) Am J Physiol 235: F46-F51.

4. Ausiello DA, Kreisberg JI, J Clin Invest 65: 754-760.

5. Schlondorff D, Satriano JA, Hagege J, Perez J, Baud L (1984) J Clin Invest 73: 1756-1764.

6. Scharschmidt LA, Dunn MJ (1983) J Clin Invest 71: 1756-1764.

7. Schlondorff D, Perez J, Satriano JA Am J Physiol. In Press.

8. Grantham JJ, Orloff J (1968) J Clin Invest 47: 1154-1161.

9. Orloff J, Handler JS, Bergstrom S (1965) Nature (London) 205: 397-398.

10. Stokes, JB Am J Physiol 240: F471.

11. Kirschenbaum MA, Lowe AG, Trizna W, Fine LG (1982) J Clin Invest 70: 1193-1204.

12. Garcia-Perez, J, Smith WL (1983) Am J Physiol 244: C211-C220.

13. Zusman RM, Keiser HR, Handler JS (1977) J Clin Invest 60: 1339-1347.

14. Burch RM, Halushka PV (1982) Am J Physiol 243: F593-F597.

15. Schlondorff D, Satriano JA, Schwartz GA. Am J Physiol In Press.

16. Schlondorff, D. Adv Prostaglandin, Thromboxane and Leukotriene Res. In Press.

Endocrinology
F. Labrie, L. Proulx, eds.

SEMINAL PROSTAGLANDINS AND SPERM FUNCTION

R W KELLY, R J AITKEN AND J CROSBY
MRC Reproductive Biology Unit, University of Edinburgh Centre for Reproductive Biology, 37 Chalmers Street, Edinburgh, EH3 9EW, UK

Primate spermatozoa, at the time of ejaculation, are presented with the highest concentration of prostaglandin so far recorded. In humans the concentrations of PGE_1 and PGE_2 are seven orders of magnitude higher than those found in peripheral plasma and there are even higher concentrations of 19-OH PGE present. Although it has been suggested that these high PG levels are present to act on the female reproductive tract, possibly to enhance passive migration of spermatozoa, evidence for this hypothesis is still not forthcoming. The obvious possibility that PGs may act on the spermatozoa has been tested in several experiments to investigate the effect of PGs on sperm motility but the conditions of sperm incubation have not always been adequate and the results have generally been inconclusive. However, several observations in the last few years suggest an association between spermatozoa and prostaglandins. Both in human (1,2) and bull(3) semen high sperm counts are associated with low seminal PG levels and studies by Schlegel et al (4) have shown that both antibodies to PGs and prostaglandin metabolizing enzymes cause a reduction in sperm motility. Despite these findings it is difficult to reconcile an effect of PGs on sperm motility with the many studies which have shown that the addition of exogenous prostaglandins has no marked effect on sperm motility and secondly with the absence of high PG levels in many species of mammals.

One function of prostaglandins, which has been widely recognised in the last decade, has been the effect of PGs on the immune system and in particular the action of PGs on various leukocytes. Human seminal plasma exhibits a marked immunosuppressive activity (5) which may be necessary to prevent the sensitization of the female tract to spermatozoa. There are, however, many compounds other than the PGs present in human semen which could fulfil the immunosuppressive role. Moreover, inhibition of the immune response by seminal plasma is found in species such as the mouse (6) which has little prostaglandin present in its semen.

An alternative action of seminal PGs may be sought by studying the direct action of the E series PGs on leukocytes. Such actions on leukocytes have a direct relevance to the spermatozoon since the acrosome, an important organelle of the sperm head, resembles a lysosome embryologically, morphologically and functionally (7). An alternative view that the acrosome more closely resembles a secretory granule makes little difference to the comparison of the acrosome with other secretory organelles since enzyme release in both is preceded by membrane fusion which is calcium dependent and can be stimulated by the calcium ionophore A 23187. The secretion of the acrosomal enzymes of the spermatozoon is followed by the loss of the acrosomal cap, and by the development of a fusogenic ring on the equatorial portion of the spermatozoon. These steps are essential preliminaries to sperm-oocyte fusion and are themselves preceded by the process of capacitation, which probably involves changes in membrane phospholipids. If the comparison between the secretory organelles of the leukocytes and the acrosome of the spermatozoon could be taken further then the clear action of high concentrations of PGE in inhibiting enzyme release from both macrophages (8) and polymorphonuclear leucocytes (9) would suggest that PGE in seminal plasma might regulate acrosomal enzyme release by affecting either the capacitation process or the acrosome reaction. We have tested this possibility by observing the effect of PGs on the *in vitro* fertilization of zona-free hamster oocytes by human spermatozoa. Spermatozoa from a fertile donor were washed (3x) and diluted to a fixed density of 10×10^6/ml in a modified BWW medium (10) containing PGs (4.2 to 270 ug/ml) for a period of three hours and then exposed to zona-free hamster eggs for a further three hours. After this time the oocytes were examined by phase contrast microscopy for the presence of decondensing sperm heads within the vitellus. Poisson distribution theory was then used to correct the results of the *in vitro* fertilization experiments for the number of motile spermatozoa in the incubation media. Paradoxically, PGE_2 stimulated fertilization by 200% ($P<0.005$) at all dose levels studied. Increasing concentrations of PGE_1 gave a typical bell-shaped dose-response curve with highly significant stimulation at lower doses but at 270 ug/ml no stimulation was observed. 19-OH PGEs isolated from semen stimulated oocyte penetration but the effect was weaker than that of PGE. PGF_2 was without effect at all doses studied. In these experiments analysis of variance demonstrated that the effects of prostaglandins was to stimulate motility although the effect was moderate and did not account for the increased capacity for fertilization.

The participation of cAMP in these effects has been studied by the measurement of cAMP present in spermatozoa after exposure to caffeine (a phosphodiesterase inhibitor) with and without prostaglandins. The effect of PGE was to stimulate cAMP content of the sperm 3 to 4 fold almost immediately (<5 min) followed by a gradual decline over a 3 hour period. Such a time curve does not accord with the effects of the prostaglandins in fertilization since the introduction of the PGs for one hour followed by 2 hours incubation without PG was not effective in raising the fertilization rate. However, the increase in cAMP might well be responsible for the small rise in motility found in these studies.

These results indicate that certain prostaglandins are capable of stimulating the fertilizing capacity of human spermatozoa *in vitro* by influencing the ability of these cells to either capacitate or acrosome react. Such a stimulatory action is not observed in semen since one of the principle biological functions of seminal plasma is to inhibit the premature capacitation of the spermatozoa through the action of poorly defined decapacitation factors.

The possibility that the interaction of several seminal components serves to prevent the acrosome reaction can best be studied by the identification of the site(s) of action of PG on the sperm. The existence of binding sites for PGs in the sperm is not fully established. One report of binding of PGE and PGF to the human sperm used the technique of fluorescence quenching but this has not been confirmed using radiolabelled ligand. The reason for this may well be that the high concentrations of PGs in semen allow an interaction with high capacity, low affinity binding sites which would be difficult to detect by more conventional techniques.

A possibility that PGs might interact with the phospholipase enzymes of spermatozoa is attractive because of the important role of the phospholipases (in association with calcium and calmodulin) in the fusogenic events and secretory processes of other cells (11). Recent reports have also suggested a direct interaction between PGs and phospholipase A_2 (12). We have studied the effects of PGE_1 on a phospholipase isolated from human semen and found an inhibitory effect at the PG concentrations found in semen. Thus the PGs in seminal plasma may be acting to inhibit the phospholipases of the plasma or outer acrosomal membrane from producing fusogenic lipids such as lysophosphatidylcholine until the appropriate time when the spermatozoa have ascended the female reproductive tract; once sperm transport has been achieved the generation of such fusogens could initiate capacitation and the acrosome reaction.

The acrosome reaction would release further phospholipases which might assist in the preparation of the fusogenic zone in the equatorial segment of the spermatozoa, which is essential if fertilization of the oocyte is to be achieved.

REFERENCES

1. Svanborg K, Bendvold E, Bygdeman M, Eneroth P (1983) In Samuelson B, Paoletti R, Ramwell P (eds) Advances in Prostaglandin, Thromboxane and Leukotriene Research Vol 12. Raven Press, NY pp 455-459
2. Kelly RW, Cooper I, Templeton AA (1979) J Reprod Fertil 56:195-199
3. Mai J, Kinsella JE (1980) Prostaglandins 20:187-199
4. Schlegel W, Fischer B, Beier HM, Schneider HPG (1983) J Reprod Fertil 68:45-50
5. Lord EM, Sensabaugh GF, Stites DP (1977) J Immunol 118:1704-1711

6. Anderson DJ, Tarter H (1982) J Immunol 128:535-539

7. Green DPL (1978) In: Johnson MH (ed) Development in Mammals. North Holland Publishing Co, Amsterdam Vol 3 pp 65-81

8. Lim LK, Hunt NH, Weidmann MJ (1983) Biochem Biophys Res Commun 114:549-555

9. Zurier RB, Weissmann G, Hoffstein S, Kammerman S, Tai HH (1974) J Clin Invest 53:297-309

10. Aitken RJ, Wang Y-F, Liu J, Best F, Richardson DW (1983) Int J Androl 6:180-193

11. Rubin RP (1984) In: Spiro G (ed) Calcium in Biology. John Wiley, NY pp 175-199

12. Moskowitz N, Shapiro L, Schook W, Puszkin S (1983) Biochem Biophys Res Commun 115:94-99

16. Membrane Receptors and Post-Receptor Events

Endocrinology
F. Labrie, L. Proulx, eds.

STRUCTURE AND BIOSYNTHESIS OF THE INSULIN RECEPTOR

MASATO KASUGA,[*°], JOSE-ANTONIO HEDO[+], C. RONALD KAHN[*], MARCO CRETTAZ[*], OSAMU EZAKI[°], AND TAKASHI KADOWAKI[°]

[*]Research Division, Joslin Diabetes Center and Department of Medicine, Brigham and Women's Hospital, Harvard Medical School, Boston, MA 02215, USA, [+]Diabetes Branch, NIADDK, National Institutes of Health, Bethesda, MD 20205, USA, and [°]The Third Department of Internal Medicine, School of Medicine, University of Tokyo, Bunkyo-ku, Tokyo, JAPAN 113

Insulin receptors have been studied intensively by direct binding techniques and have been identified on cells of all vertebrates examined thus far. Although the binding interaction between the receptor and insulin is well-characterized, its molecular basis is poorly understood. Recently some progress has been made toward elucidating the subunit structure of the receptor using photoreactive insulins or affinity chemical cross-linking techniques.

We have developed a technique to identify the insulin receptor subunits using immunoprecipitation with antibodies to the insulin receptor after either biosynthetic or surface labeling of intact cells. Cells, usually cultured human lymphocytes, were surfaced labeled with $Na^{125}I$ and lactoperoxidase (1,2) or with sodium borohydrite and galactose oxidase (3). For the biosynthetic labeling, the lymphocytes were cultured in the presence of several kinds of tritiated sugars (3), $[^{35}S]$-methionine (4) or $[^{32}P]$-orthophosphate (5). After labeling, the cells were solubilized in Triton X-100. For the methionine or phosphate labeled material, because of high background after immunoprecipitation, the insulin receptor was enriched by chromatography on a wheat germ agglutinin-agarose column. This step is known to produce 20-fold enrichment of insulin binding activity with more than 80% recovery. The insulin receptors were immunoprecipitated with anti-receptor autoantibodies from patients with insulin resistance and acanthosis nigricans. The immunoprecipitates are then analyzed by sodium dodecyl sulfate polyacrylamide gel electrophoresis (SDS-PAGE) after reduction of disulfide bonds by 100 mM dithiothreitol and the labeled bands visualized by autoradiography.

Using this technique, two major subunits of the insulin receptor can be identified (1-5). These have molecular weights of 135,000 and 95,000 and have been referred to as the α and ß subunits, respectively. Both subunits label biosynthetically with either [^{3}H]-sugars or [^{35}S]-methionine and can be identified by surface labeling, indicating that both are glycoproteins and expressed on the external surface of the cell. The ß subunit can also be labeled biosynthetically with [^{32}P]-orthophosphate, indicating that the ß subunit is a phosphoprotein.

When the immunoprecipitates from biosynthetic labeling are analyzed in SDS-PAGE without reduction of disulfide bonds, six specific bands are found. These have apparent molecular weights of 520,000, 350,000, 230,000, 190,000 120,000 and 90,000. To characterize these six bands more carefully, the effect of reduction of disulfide bonds was studied using a two-dimensional gel technique. In the first dimension, the immunoprecipitates were analyzed in SDS-PAGE without reduction. Then, the entire lane was cut out, placed horizontally on a second SDS-polyacrylamide gel and analyzed after reduction of disulfide bonds with dithiothreitol. By this kind of two-dimensional analysis (2), the highest molecular weight band of ^{35}S-methionine labeled 520K was separated into three spots of 210K, 135K, and 95K, with the relative intensity of the label being 210K > 95K > 135K. The 210K appears to be a single chain precursor of the α and ß subunits, i.e., a pro-receptor (2). The 350K band yielded two spots of 135K and 95K, although a small spot was apparent with an M_r = 210,000. The 230K band on reduction yielded only the 135K, suggesting that this is an α_2 disulfide dimer. The 190K, 120K, and 90K spots migrated as the 210K pro-receptor, and α and ß subunits, respectively. These data suggest the existence of free subunits and proreceptor. In addition, one increase in apparent molecular weight after reduction suggests that the α and ß subunits may contain intra-chain disulfide bonds, as well as the inter-chain bonds.

Although the precise role of these disulfide-linked oligomers of α and ß subunits is not clear, we have found that the affinity of the insulin receptor correlates with the proportion of the oligomeric forms present; the greater the proportion of the oligomeric forms, the lower the receptor affinity (6). Thus, surface labeling of hepatoma (Fao) cells after down-regulation of the insulin receptor, hepatoma (Fao) cells revealed a marked decrease of the four oligomeric forms of the receptor with the increased affinity of the receptor. A similar decrease of the oligomeric forms of the insulin receptor and an increase in the affinity of the receptor was also observed when normal Fao cells were treated with 7 mM dithiothreitol. In contrast to Fao cells, down-regulation of the insulin receptor in IM-9 lymphocytes occurs without a change in receptor affinity. In these cells, no change in the proportion of the oligomeric forms to the free subunits of the receptor was found.

Another approach to the structure of the insulin receptor using antibodies is "Western" blotting (7,8). In this type of study, the protein fractions containing the insulin receptor protein are analyzed by SDS-PAGE, after which the proteins are transferred to nitrocellulose paper and the insulin receptor identified by incubation with antibodies to the receptor and ^{125}I-protein A. A serum containing polyclonal antibodies to the insulin receptor made by injecting the purified insulin receptor (kindly provided by Dr. Steve Jacobs) was able to recognize the 135K and 95K protein. On the other hand, most of the autoantibodies from the patients did not recognize the denatured subunits.

Taking advantage of the convenience of this method, we have identified the insulin receptor in the subcellular fractions of rat adipocyte separated on a sucrose gradient technique. The amounts of both subunits of insulin receptor in the "Golgi" fractions were increased after insulin treatment of the cell, followed by the decrease in the amounts of the insulin receptor in the plasma membrane fractions. These data suggest that insulin stimulates the internalization of both subunits of the insulin receptor. Using this "Western" blotting technique, we have also found that increased ^{125}I-insulin binding to the solubilized fraction obtained from streptozotocin-induced diabetic rats is due to the increased amounts of the insulin receptor (7). Since it is difficult to determine accurately the number of insulin receptor by Scatchard plot analysis, "Western" blotting may be a useful method for measurement of the amount of "immunoreactive" insulin receptor.

In order to test the possibility of the involvement of another component of the insulin receptor in the biosynthetic process, the time course of labeling of the receptor by tritiated mannose was studied using the immunoprecipitation technique. Since many cell surface glycoproteins are synthesized via precursors containing high mannose type of carbohydrate chains, the cell were pulse labeled for 15 min and subsequently chased in medium containing unlabeled mannose and glucose for periods of up to 8 hours (9). The earliest labeled receptor component had a molecular weight of 190K and was already apparent after the pulse at 0 minutes. The radioactivity in this band increased during the first hour of the chase and thereafter decreased rapidly and progressively while that in the 210K, 135K and 95K increased steadily. The 190K component is not expressed in the plasma membrane, since this component cannot be labeled by surface labeling technique and is resistant to trypsin treatment. The 190K component probably represents a "high mannose type" of pro-receptor, because this component is not labeled by [^{3}H]-galactose of fucose and sensitive to endoglycosidase H treatment (9). The 210K "pro-receptor" component, is expressed in plasma membrane, contains "complex" type oligosaccharide, and has peptides of both the 135K and 95K subunits.

To account for these two forms, we have proposed the following working hypothesis: After translation and core glycosylation, the 190K high mannose precursor is formed. Some of the high mannose chains are then converted into complex type chains leading to the 210K component. This component may then generate α and β subunits by proteolytic cleavage. Alternatively, the 190K may be cleaved first and fully glycosylated later, since partially glycosylated subunits with M_r = 115,000 and 80,000 are found following monensin-treatment of cells. Some of the 210K component may escape proteolytic cleavage and be inserted into plasma membrane. Thus, the insulin receptor appears to be synthesized via a single polypeptide chain which is cleaved to yield two disulfide-linked subunits. This implies the existence of a single mRNA and a single gene coding for the receptor. In this sense, the pathway of insulin receptor biosynthesis is similar to the pathway of insulin biosynthesis.

REFERENCES

1. Kasuga M, Kahn CR, Hedo JA, Van Obberghen E, Yamada KM (1981) Proc Natl Acad Sci USA 78:6917

2. Kasuga M, Hedo JA, Yamada KM, Kahn CR (1982) J Biol Chem 275:10392

3. Hedo JA, Kasuga M, Van Obberghen E, Roth J, Kahn CR (1981) Proc Natl Acad Sci USA 78:4791

4. Van Obberghen E, Kasuga M, Le Cam A, Itin A, Hedo JA, Harrison LC (1981) Proc Natl Acad Sci USA 78:1052

5. Kasuga M, Karlsson FA, Kahn, CR (1982) Science 215:185

6. Crettaz M, Jialal I, Kasuga M, Kahn, CR J Biol Chem, in press.

7. Kadowaki T, Kasuga M, Akanuma Y, Ezaki O, Takalen F, submitted for publication

8. Maron R, Kahn CR, Jacobs S, Fujita-Yamaguchi Y Diabetes, in press.

9. Hedo JA, Kahn CR, Hayashi N, Yamada KM, Kasuga M (1983) J Biol Chem 258:10020

Endocrinology
F. Labrie, L. Proulx, eds.

THE INSULIN RECEPTOR KINASE

E. VAN OBBERGHEN, H. GAZZANO, R. BALLOTTI, M. FEHLMANN, B. ROSSI, S. GAMMELTOFT*, J.L. SADOUL and Y. LE MARCHAND-BRUSTEL
I.N.S.E.R.M. U 145, Faculté de Médecine, Nice, France, and *Department of Clinical Chemistry, Rigshospitalet, Copenhagen, Denmark

I. INTRODUCTION

The native insulin receptor is a high molecular weight complex and appears to be minimally composed of two M_r 130,000 (α-subunit) and two M_r 95,000 (β-subunit) glycoproteins linked together by disulphide bonds. Binding of insulin to its cell surface receptors on target cells initiates an elaborate program of biochemical processes eventuating in the final hormonal effects. The molecular basis of insulin action is poorly comprehended, but recently a promissing progress has been achieved by demonstrating that the insulin receptor is an insulin-activatable protein kinase (1-11). This novel observation is of interest for our understanding of insulin-regulated processes, since it is now widely accepted that hormone-modulated protein phosphorylation-dephosphorylation reactions play a crucial role in the regulation of cellular events, including those mediated by insulin. We will summarize here our own data on insulin receptor phosphorylation, and discuss its possible role in transmembrane hormone signalling.

II. RESULTS

II.1. Phosphorylation of insulin receptors in intact hepatocytes

When solubilized lectin purified glycoproteins obtained from isolated rat hepatocytes incubated with ^{32}P-orthophosphate were precipitated by anti-receptor antibodies a major labeled band was found with M_r 95,000 (3). We recognise this molecular species as the insulin receptor β-subunit for th e following reasons. First, nonimmune serum did not precipitate a labeled band with a similar electrophoretic mobility. Second, using biosynthetic and affinity labeling methods, we have identified the β-subunit of the insulin receptor with identical electrophoretic mobility (12 - 16). Insulin induced an increase in the labeling of its own receptor β-subunit. This insulin effect is specific, since EGF, which binds to, and increases the phosphorylation of, its own receptors in these cells, was without effect on insulin receptor phosphorylation. Phosphoamino acid analysis of the insulin receptor β-subunit revealed the presence of phosphothreonine and phosphoserine when the cells were labeled in absence of insulin. Further, the stimulatory action of insulin on receptor phosphorylation was accounted for by an increase in phosphoserine (6).

II.2. Phosphorylation of insulin receptors in cell-free systems.

To further characterise the molecular basis of insulin receptor phosphorylation we have used a cell-free phosphorylation assay in which partially purified insulin receptors were incubated with (γ-^{32}P)ATP in absence or presence of insulin. Thereafter, the insulin receptors were precipitated with antireceptor antibodies. SDS-PAGE analysis of the immune precipitates under reducing conditions revealed a major band of M_r 95,000 phosphorylated in the basal state (3). This M_r 95,000 phosphoprotein was identified as the insulin receptor β-subunit by its specific immunoprecipitation by antireceptor antibodies and by its electrophoretic mobility. Similar to its effect in intact cells, insulin increased the phosphorylation of its receptor β-subunit. The dose-relationship of insulin effect on phosphorylation of the hepatic receptor β-subunit was remarkably similar to that previously described for insulin binding to the high affinity component in these hepatocytes (17). Further, different insulin analogues were able to stimulate receptor phosphorylation in accordance of their respective affinity for receptor (in preparation). Finally, this stimulation by insulin is specific, since EGF and glucagon had no effect. The stimulatory action of insulin on its receptor phosphorylation is therefore characterized by the typical affinity and specificity of a receptor-mediated insulin effect. Receptor phosphorylation appears to be a general feature of insulin receptors as it was found in all tissues we studied thus far including lymphocytes (B and T), hepatocytes, fibroblasts, skeletal muscle, brain cortex (11), and erythrocytes. Insulin effect on its receptor phosphorylation is dependent on Mn^{2+}, whereas it is independent of cAMP and calcium. Further, in cell-free systems the insulin receptor is phosphorylated on tyrosine residues, and insulin stimulatory action on its receptor phosphorylation is largely accounted for by an increase in phosphotyrosine (6).

Insulin receptors isolated by specific immunoprecipitation can be phosphorylated and insulin increased several-fold their phosphorylation (4). This indicates that antireceptor antibodies precipitate a functional insulin-stimulatable kinase activity, which is contained in, or closely associated with the receptor. Note that an insulin-independent phosphatase activity is purified with the insulin receptor on lectin chromatography. This activity was no longer found in immunoprecipitated receptors (18).

II.3. Identification of an ATP binding site on the insulin receptor.

Using covalent affinity labeling with oxidized (α-^{32}P)ATP we found a specific ATP binding site on a polypeptide with M_r 95,000 under reducing conditions. This polypeptide was specifically immunoprecipitated by antibodies to insulin receptor, indicating that the insulin receptor is likely to be a protein kinase capable of autophosphorylation (4).

II. 4. Insulin receptor kinase activity towards exogenous protein substrates.

Protein substrates such as histone and casein were found to be phosphorylated by both lectin purified or immunoprecipitated insulin receptors (6). More important, insulin enhanced the insulin receptor kinase activity, resulting in a several-fold increase in ^{32}P-incorporation in the protein substrates. Concerning the aminoacids phosphorylated in the substrates, we observed differences depending on the nature of the receptor preparation used as a protein kinase source. Thus, when partially purified insulin receptors were used, we found under basal phosphorylation conditions (absence of insulin), phosphoserine, phosphothreonine, and phosphotyrosine. Insulin induced a several - fold increase in ^{32}P-incorporation in phosphotyrosine, and has in addition a smaller, but consistent stimulating effect on the labeling of phosphoserine. In contrast, with immunoprecipitated insulin receptors and in absence of insulin, the major labeling of the substrates occurred on phosphotyrosine; only minute amounts of phosphoserine and phosphothreonine were found. However, the stimulating action of insulin on ^{32}P-incorporation was limited to an increase in phosphotyrosine (6).

III. Summary and conclusion.

Hormone-modulated protein phosphorylation-dephosphorylation reactions are known to play a crucial role in the control of cellular processes (19, 20). Recently, attention has been paid on phosphorylation of receptors for hormones, neurotransmitters and growth factors, but very rapidly numerous reports have appeared indicating that receptors can be phosphorylated including those for insulin (1-11), EGF (21), steroid hormones (22), acetylcholine (23), and catecholamines (24).

Our data summarized here allow us to conclude that the insulin receptor is an insulin-activatable protein kinase. We reached this conclusion based on the observation that the receptor β-subunit isolated by immunoprecipitation is a substrate for insulin-stimulated phosphorylation, and that an ATP binding site on this same receptor subunit can be identified. The insulin receptor is not only a kinase capable of self-phosphorylation, but it is also able to catalyse phosphorylation of exogenous substrates.

Taken together the data on receptor and substrate phosphorylation, we have proposed the following model for the insulin receptor and its associated kinase activities (6). We envisage an insulin receptor-kinase complex with two separate protein kinases, a tyrosine and a serine specific kinase. The tyrosine kinase would be a constituent of the insulin receptor, and supported by the existence of an ATP binding site on the receptor β-subunit, this kinase would be contained in the receptor β-subunit itself. In contrast, the serine kinase would be associated with the insulin receptor in the cell membrane, but would not form an integral part of the receptor.

The biological relevance of insulin receptor phosphorylation is not known. It is possible that it plays a role in biologically relevant phenomena such as receptor affinity modulation, hormone and receptor internalisation, and signal transmission. We favour the concept that this insulin-regulated covalent receptor modification is an early step in insulin action, and that the insulin receptor is an integrated system for transmembrane hormone signalling. Thus, the increased kinase activity of the insulin receptor evoked by hormone binding would lead to phosphorylation-dephosphorylation of other cellular proteins, and through the generation of a cascade of reactions this would result in the final effects of insulin. The relationship between the two protein kinase activities associated with the insulin receptor, and their role remain to be established. At least two situations are possible, one in which both kinases serve separate cellular functions, and another one with sequential activation of the kinases. In regards to the first possibility, tyrosine kinases have been implicated in cellular responses to growth factors, such as EGF (21), PDGF (25), TGF (26) and in cell transformation induced by oncogenic viruses (27). It is therefore an appealing idea to conceive that this tyrosine specific enzyme activity is involved in generation of signals regulating insulin's mitogenic action. In contrast, the serine kinase would play a role in metabolic processes controled by insulin. All the known enzymes playing a role in cellular intermediary metabolism and whose activity is modulated by insulin through phosphorylation-dephosphorylation reactions are indeed modified on serine residues. Alternative to this model, implying separate functions for the kinases exists the possibility where one kinase activates the other, and this last one accounts for the generation of the cellular responses to insulin. As the tyrosine kinase is likely a constituent of the insulin receptor, in this model with sequential activation of kinases, insulin binding to its receptor would lead to activation of the tyrosine kinase, which then induces activation of the receptor-associated serine kinase. In conclusion, the data available are consistent with the idea that the insulin receptor fulfills the requirements for a system regulating transmembrane hormone signalling. A major advance for the relevance of this contention will be the demonstration that receptor phosphorylation is necessary and sufficient for insulin to act.

ACKNOWLEDGEMENTS

We gratefully acknowledge the excellent secretarial assistance of A. Rainaud and the superb technical assistance of A. Kowalski and T. Gremaux.

REFERENCES

1. Kasuga M, Karlsson FA, Kahn CR (1982) Science 215: 185
2. Kasuga M, Zick Y, Blithe DL, Crettaz M, Kahn CR (1982) Nature 298: 667
3. Van Obberghen E, Kowalski A (1982) FEBS Lett. 143: 179
4. Van Obberghen E, Rossi B, Kowalski A, Gazzano H, Ponzio G (1983) Proc. Natl. Acad. Sci. USA 80: 945
5. Kasuga M, Fugita-Yamaguchi Y, Blithe DL, Kahn CR (1983) Proc. Natl. Acad. Sci. USA 80: 2137
6. Gazzano H, Kowalski A, Fehlmann M, Van Obberghen E (1983) Biochem. J. 216: 575
7. Avruch J, Nemenoff RA, Blackshear PJ, Pierce MW, and Osathanondh (1982) J. Biol. Chem. 257: 15162
8. Petruzelli, L.M., Ganguly, S., Smith, C.J., Cobb, M.H., Rubin, C.S., Rosen, O.M. (1982) Proc. Natl. Acad. Sci. USA 79: 6792
9. Roth RA, Cassell DJ (1983) Science 219: 299
10. Shia MA, Pilch PF (1983) Biochemistry 22: 717
11. Gammeltoft S, Kowalski A, Fehlmann M, Van Obberghen E (1984) FEBS Lett., in press.
12. Van Obberghen E, Kasuga M, Le Cam A, Hedo JA, Itin A, Harrison LC (1981) Proc. Natl. Acad. Sci. USA 78: 1052
13. Hedo JA, Kasuga M, Van Obberghen E, Roth J, Kahn CR (1981) Proc. Natl. Acad. Sci. USA 78: 4791
14. Kasuga M, Van Obberghen E, Yamada KM, Harrison LC (1981) Diabetes 30: 354
15. Van Obberghen E, Kahn CR (1981) Mol. Cell. Endocrin. 22: 277
16. Van Obberghen E (1984) Biochemical Pharmacology 33: 889
17. Fehlmann M, Morin O, Kitabgi P, Freychet P (1981) Endocrinology 109: 253
18. Kowalski A, Gazzano H, Fehlmann M, Van Obberghen E (1983) Biochem. Biophys. Res. Commun. 117: 885
19. Cohen P (1982) Nature 296: 613
20. Denton RM, Brownsey RW, Belsham GJ (1981) Diabetologia 21: 347
21. Ushiro H, Cohen S (1980) J. Biol. Chem. 255: 8363
22. Migliaccio A, Lastoria S, Montcharmont B, Rotondi A, Auricchio F. (1982) Biochem. Biophys. Res. Commun. 109: 1002
23. Teichberg VI, Sobel A, Changeux JP (1977) Nature 267: 540
24. Stadel JM, Nambi P, Shou RGL, Sawyer DF, Caron MG, Lefkowitz, R.J. (1983) Proc. Natl. Acad. Sci. USA 80: 3173
25. Ek B, Westermark B, Wasteson A, Heldin CH (1982) Nature 295: 419
26. Reynolds FH, Todaro GJ, Fryling C, Stephenson JR (1981) Nature 292: 259
27. Hunter T, Sefton BM (1980) Proc. Natl. Acad. Sci. USA 77: 1311

© 1984 Elsevier Science Publishers B.V.
Endocrinology
F. Labrie, L. Proulx, eds.

MORPHOLOGICAL ASPECTS AND PHYSIOLOGICAL RELEVANCE OF INSULIN RECEPTOR INTERNALIZATION AND RECYCLING

J.-L. CARPENTIER*, M. FEHLMANN+, E. VAN OBBERGHEN+, P. GORDEN°, and L. ORCI*,
*Institute of Histology and Embryology, Geneva, Switzerland, +INSERM U 145, Nice, France and °Diabetes Branch NIADDK, NIH, Bethesda, Md., USA.

It is now clear that after binding to a specific cell surface receptor, insulin as many other polypeptide hormones and growth factors redistributes in the plane of the plasma membrane and is progressively internalized (1). While there are quantitative differences in internalization depending on the ligand and the cell, the qualitative nature of surface redistribution and internalization of polypeptide hormones and many other ligands appears to be similar. Early events include preferential localization on microvillous structures followed by concentration in coated pits (2,3,4). Later the ligands are internalized by an absorptive endocytotic process and sequestered into a series of intracellular compartments: first coated vesicles (4), second endosomes, third multivesicular bodies and fourth typical lysosomes (dense bodies) (5,6).

The implication of this intracellular pathway of the hormone on its biological activities remains unknown. By contrast these morphological observations together with biochemical studies, showing that drugs known to affect lysosomal proteolytic activities (i.e. NH_4Cl, chloroquine, leupeptine, ...) also inhibit intracellular insulin degradation, suggest that internalization and lysosomal association of insulin is involved in the degradation of the hormone (7-11). The observation that the internalization process is time-, temperature- and energy-dependent led us to postulate that ligand removal from the cell surface is linked to the process whereby cell surface receptors are lost, i.e. homotropic receptor regulation or "down-regulation". The concordance of ligand internalization and down-regulation in systems where the ligand is, at least, partially irreversibly bound strengthened this argument (12,13); these studies as well as others (14,15) remained however mostly indirect and lack the prerequisite demonstration of internalization of the receptor together with insulin.

RECEPTOR INTERNALIZATION AND RECYCLING

Recently, we have been able to specifically label the insulin receptor "in situ" using a photoreactive analogue of insulin covalently coupled to the insulin receptor (16-17). Freshly isolated rat hepatocytes were first incubated with ^{125}I-labeled photoreactive insulin in the dark at 15°C, a temperature at which only minimal insulin internalization occurs. When the binding attains a steady state (2-3 hours) the cells were irradiated at 4°C using a water-cooled high pressure mercury lamp. After washings, the cells were incubated for up to 6 hours at 37°C in the absence of labeled ligand. The cell-associated radioactivity was then analyzed by direct solubilization in boiling SDS followed by polyacrylamide gel electrophoresis under reducing condition. When freshly isolated hepatocytes were labeled following this procedure three radioactive bands were revealed: a major band with Mr 130,000 and two minor bands with Mr 125,000 and 23,000 (16). The Mr 130,000 band labeled with the photoreactive ^{125}I-insulin analogue corresponds to the structure identified as the α-subunit of the insulin receptor (18-20). As a function of incubation time at 37°C the polyacrylamide gel electrophoresis pattern of cell associated radioactivity did not change, suggesting that the insulin-receptor complex remained undegraded.

At each time point the distribution of the cell associated radioactivity was analysed by quantitative EM autoradiography. At the end of the 3 hr association period at 15°C about 80 % of the autoradiographic grains were associated with the plasma membrane of hepatocytes. By 60 min. of incubation at 37°C most of the

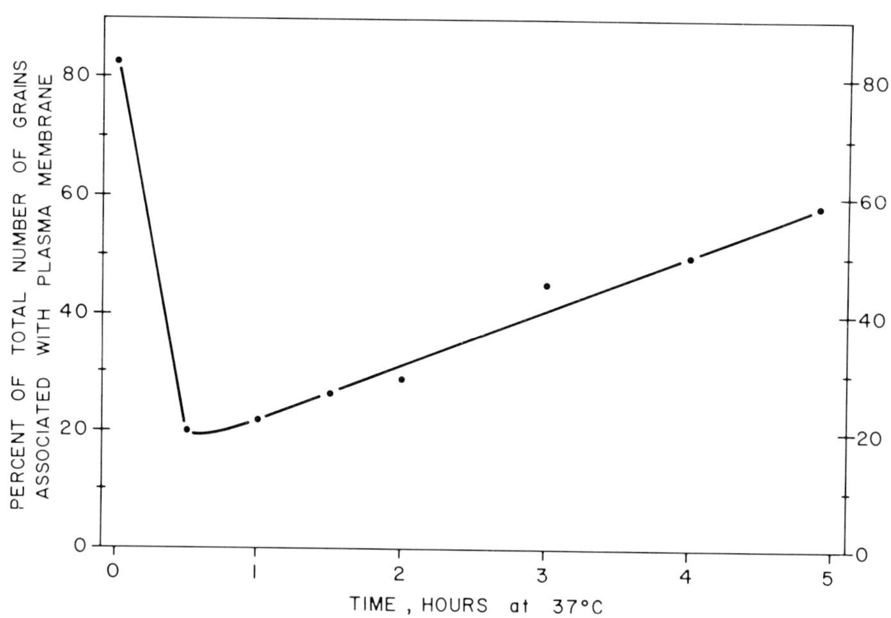

Fig. 1. Relationship of autoradiographic grains with the plasma membrane of isolated rat hepatocytes following 2 hours of incubation at 15°C in the dark with ^{125}I-photoreactive insulin, exposition to U.V., washing and resuspension in buffer in the absence of labeled material for 0 to 5 hours at 37°C. Adapted from (21).

labeled material was internalized since only 20 % of the autoradiographic grains remained associated with the cell surface; later (between 1h and 5hs) the percentage of grains associated with the plasma membrane increased to reach ∿ 60 % by 5 hours of incubation (Fig. 1). These data indicate a progressive recycling of the labeled insulin-receptor complex back to the cell surface. A similar fate for the insulin receptor was found when the surface localization of the ^{125}I-photoreactive insulin-receptor complex was studied by measuring the accessibility of labeled receptors to trypsin (21).

INTRACELLULAR PATHWAY FOLLOWED BY RECEPTOR

The intracellular distribution of the radioactivity was determined at the EM level by the "hypothetical grain" method. Two major intracellular compartments were labeled at all time points studied: electronlucent vesicles and lysosome-like structures. As a function of time at 37°C labeling of small vesicles decreased until 30 to 60 minutes of incubation and then slightly increased in a manner parallel to the reappearance of ^{125}I-photoreactive insulin receptor com-

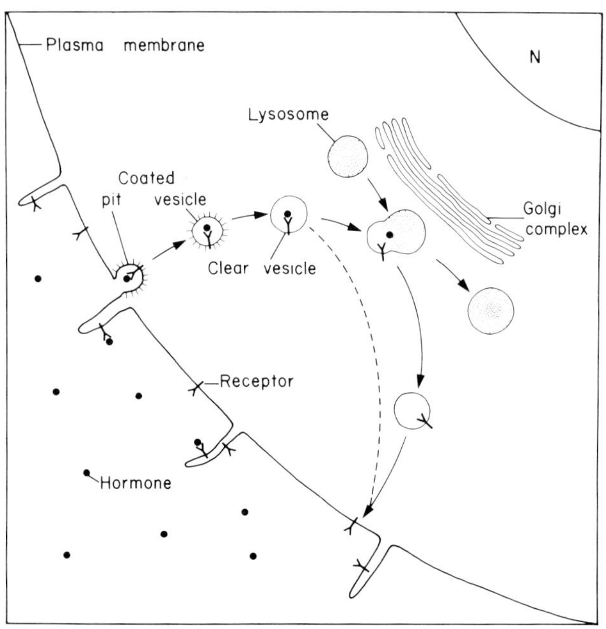

Fig. 2. Schematic drawing illustrating the main morphologic events underlying binding, internalization and recycling of the insulin receptor in a target cell.

plexes on the cell surface. An inverse labeling pattern was observed for lysosome-like structures including both multivesicular bodies and dense bodies (22). When incubations were carried out in the presence of NH_4Cl ($2x10^{-2}M$) insulin receptor recycling was inhibited and the labeled material accumulated intracellularly within lysosome-like structures (mostly multivesicular bodies) (22). These results provide evidence for the involvement of a vesicular compartment in the shuttling of the insulin receptor between the plasma membrane and lysosome-like structures (Fig. 2).

FUNCTIONAL IMPLICATIONS OF INSULIN RECEPTOR INTERNALIZATION AND RECYCLING

It is now clear that one of the first consequences of binding of insulin to its cell surface receptor is endocytosis of the ligand. This provides a mechanism to terminate the signal generated at the cell surface by the hormone receptor complex. Further, it is clear that the receptor is internalized with the ligand. This provides a mechanism for "down regulation" of cell surface receptors. In addition, several lines of evidence shows that the internalized receptor may return to the cell surface. In cells with a quantitatively large internalization rate the receptor recycling rate is therefore an important event regulating cell surface receptors. For instance in U-937 monocytes, cells with a high degree of internalization, monensin, a drug known to inhibit recycling, markedly augments insulin induced down regulation. By contrast in IM-9 lymphocytes, cells with a low degree of internalization, monensin does not augment insulin induced down regulation (23). At present there is no evidence that insulin receptor biosynthesis is altered by down regulation. It would, therefore, appear that insulin receptors on the cell surface are regulated by the rate of internalization, the rate of degradation of internalized receptors and the rate of recycling of non-degraded receptors. Since receptor degradation and recycling depend on the initial internalization event, it would appear that receptor occupancy is the initial rate controlling step ie in the presence of high insulin concentration receptor occupancy is high initiating down regulation.

An interesting correlation of this is suggested by preliminary studies in hypoinsulinaemic states ie streptozotocin diabetes in the rat. Under these conditions receptor concentration is increased on the cell surface and internalization is significantly impaired (24). This suggests a mechanism whereby the cell senses a diminished cell surface signal and attempts to compensate by prolonging that signal or hormone receptor complex on the cell surface.

ACKNOWLEDGEMENTS

This work was supported by grant 3.460.83 from the Swiss National Science Foundation.

REFERENCES

1. Gorden P, Carpentier JL, Freychet P, Orci L (1980) Diabetologia 18:263-274.
2. Carpentier JL, Van Obberghen E, Gorden P, Orci L (1981) J Cell Biol 91:17-25
3. Carpentier JL, Gorden P, Anderson RGW, Goldstein JL, Brown MS, Cohen S, Orci L (1982) J Cell Biol 95:73-77.
4. Fan JY, Carpentier JL, Gorden P, Van Obberghen E, Blackett NM, Grunfeld C, Orci L (1982) Proc Natl Acad Sci USA 79:77-88.
5. Fan JY, Carpentier JL, Van Obberghen E, Blackett NM, Grunfeld C, Gorden P, Orci L (1983) J Histochem Cytochem 31:859-870.
6. Carpentier JL, Gorden P, Freychet P, Le Cam A, Orci L (1979) J Clin Invest 63:1249-1261.
7. Gorden P, Freychet P, Carpentier JL, Canivet B, Orci L (1982) Yale J Biol Med 55:101-112.
8. Marshall ST, Olefsky JM (1979) J Biol Chem 254:10153-10160.
9. Suzuki K, Kono T (1979) J Biol Chem 254:9786-9794.
10. Hammons GT, Jarett L (1980) Diabetes 29:475-486.
11. Terris S, Hoffmann C, Steiner DF (1979) Can J Biochem 57:459-468.
12. Barazzone P, Lesniak MA, Gorden P, Van Obberghen E, Carpentier JL, Orci L (1980) J Cell Biol 87:360-369.
13. Hizuka W, Gorden P, Lesniak MA, Van Obberghen E, Carpentier JL, Orci L (1981) J Biol Chem 256:4591-4597.
14. Marshall S, Olefsky JM (1981) Diabetes 30:746-753.
15. Gorden P, Carpentier JL, Van Obberghen E, Barazzone P, Roth J, Orci L (1979) J Cell Sci 39:77-88.
16. Fehlmann M, Carpentier JL, Le Cam A, Thamm P, Saunders D, Brandenburg D, Orci L, Freychet P (1982) J Cell Biol 93:82-87.
17. Gorden P, Carpentier JL, Moule ML, Yip CC, Orci L (1982) Diabetes 31:659-662.
18. Yip CC, Yeung CWT, Moule ML (1978) J Biol Chem 253:1743-1745.
19. Pilch PF, Czech MP (1979) J Biol Chem 254:3345-3381.
20. Kasuga M, Van Obberghen E, Yamada KM, Harrison LC (1981) Diabetes 30:354-357.
21. Fehlmann M, Carpentier JL, Van Obberghen E, Freychet P, Thamm P, Saunders D, Brandenburg D, Orci L (1982) Proc Natl Acad Sci USA 79:5921-5925.
22. Carpentier JL, Fehlmann M, Van Obberghen E, Gazzano H, Freychet P, Brandenburg D, Orci L (1983) J Cell Biol 97:409a
23. Carpentier JL, Dayer JM, Lang U, Silverman R, Gorden P, Orci L, submitted for publication.
24. Carpentier JL, Robert A, Van Obberghen E, Grunberger G, Gorden P, Orci L, Diabetologia, abstract in press.

Endocrinology
F. Labrie, L. Proulx, eds.

USE OF THE HEAVY ISOTOPE DENSITY-SHIFT METHOD TO INVESTIGATE INSULIN RECEPTOR METABOLISM

M. DANIEL LANE
Department of Biological Chemistry, The Johns Hopkins University School of Medicine, Baltimore, MD 21205 (USA)

INTRODUCTION

The first point at which insulin can interact with, and thereby affect the metabolism of a target cell, is at its specific receptors on the cell surface. Hence, the responsiveness of a cell to insulin depends upon the number of functional insulin receptors on its plasma membrane. There is compelling evidence to indicate that cells have the capacity to modulate the number of cell-surface receptors they possess in response to specific physiological stimuli.

The number of functional insulin receptors in a cell is dependent upon the rates of receptor synthesis, processing, transit to and out of the plasma membrane, and inactivation/degradation. To ascertain which of these processes are affected by physiological stimuli that alter cellular receptor level, we have made use of the heavy isotope density-shift technique (1-6). In this report I will describe how this technique was applied to investigate the mechanisms by which insulin receptor level is altered during preadipocyte differentiation and insulin-induced receptor down-regulation.

THE HEAVY ISOTOPE DENSITY-SHIFT METHOD

With this method newly-synthesized and "old" receptor populations can be distinguished after shifting cells to medium containing "heavy" (>95% ^{15}N, ^{13}C and ^{2}H) amino acids (2,8). Accordingly, newly-synthesized "heavy" and previously-synthesized "light" receptors, solubilized in Triton X-100, can be separated by isopycnic banding on CsCl density gradients and then active light and heavy receptor quantitated by ^{125}I-insulin binding assays. By following changes in the relative amounts of heavy and light receptors after the shift to heavy amino acids, rates of synthesis and inactivation/decay of active receptor can be determined. It should be emphasized that the density-shift method follows the rate at which insulin binding activity of the receptor is produced or lost, and thus, measures the physiologically relevant rate-limiting step(s) in the formation or inactivation of functional receptor.

DIFFERENTIATION-INDUCED INCREASE IN RECEPTOR LEVEL

3T3-L1 preadipocytes from mouse late-embryo cells, differentiate in culture into cells that exhibit morphological and biochemical characteristics of adipocytes. Accompanying differentiation, these cells exhibit a 20-fold rise in insulin receptor level, fully differentiated 3T3-L1 adipocytes acquiring 200,000 receptors per cell (1,2). With the heavy isotope density-shift method, the alteration in insulin receptor metabolism responsible for the dramatic differentiation-induced rise in receptor level was characterized. It was demonstrated (2) that the increase in steady-state receptor level was accompanied by a 20-fold increase in the rate of receptor synthesis. No change in the first-order rate constant for receptor inactivation/degradation accompanied differentiation. Hence, the rise in insulin receptor level induced by adipose conversion is solely the result of an increased rate of receptor synthesis.

INSULIN INDUCED DOWN-REGULATION OF RECEPTOR LEVEL

Chronic (>10 h) exposure of most cell types to insulin causes a 60-65% decrease in the steady-state level of functional insulin receptors, i.e. both cell-surface and total cellular receptor level. This process enables a cell to buffer its responsiveness to insulin when the ambient concentration of the hormone increases. With 3T3-L1 adipocytes and preadipocytes and with 3T3-C2 fibroblasts, the $t_{1/2}$ for down-regulation of the insulin receptor is 3-4 h, the process being complete within 10-12 h (3,4). Scatchard analysis revealed that the insulin-induced decreases in cell-surface and total cellular insulin binding capacity are due to a decrease of receptor number and not insulin binding affinity.

To clarify the mechanism by which down-regulation of insulin receptor occurs, rates of receptor synthesis were determined by the heavy isotope density-shift method (3,4). No change in the rate of receptor synthesis occurred as a consequence of ligand-induced down-regulation (or of up-regulation due to removal of ligand). Down-regulation, however, caused a decrease in the half-life of the receptor from about 15 h to 6-7 h. These results show that in the down-regulated steady-state, the first-order rate constant for receptor inactivation/degradation is increased by about 2.5-fold.

To determine whether down-regulation affects the rate of receptor transit to the cell-surface or the rate of inactivation of surface receptor, the heavy isotope density-shift method was used in combination with covalent labeling of cell-surface receptors (5). The surface labeling procedure involved: cooling the cells to 2°C to prevent further exo- or endocytosis, binding of ^{125}I-insulin to the cell-surface receptors, crosslinking of surface-bound ^{125}I-insulin to receptors with the bifunctional reagent, disuccinimidyl suberate, and then separation and quantitation of heavy and light ^{125}I-labeled receptors by isopycnic banding on CsCl. Thus, when cells are shifted to medium containing "heavy" amino acids (>95% ^{13}C, ^{15}N, ^{3}H) heavy receptor will appear at the cell surface where it can be labeled with ^{125}I-insulin only after the processing pipe-line has been cleared of "light" receptor. Conversely, the kinetics of clearance of light receptors from the cell-surface can be determined. The results revealed that only after 2.5-3 h did newly-synthesized "heavy" receptors reach the plasma membrane after their synthesis in the rough endoplasmic reticulum; following this additional heavy receptors accrue at the cell surface. A decline in the amount of light receptor at the cell surface occurred only after 3 h, i.e. when the pipe-line of light receptor arriving at the cell surface had cleared. Insulin-induced down-regulation had no effect on the time required for newly-synthesized receptors to reach the cell-surface. Down-regulation however, increased the first-order rate constant for the inactivation of cell-surface insulin receptors by 2.2- to 2.5-fold.

Although the results described above indicate that the ultimate cause for the decrease in steady-state receptor level in the down-regulated steady-state is an increased rate of cell-surface receptor inactivation (i.e. loss of insulin binding activity), they do not identify the transitional event(s) which leads to accelerated receptor decay. Two mechanisms for initiating the down-regulation process seemed most probable. First, binding of insulin to the receptor could trigger its translocation (via endocytosis) into an intracellular compartment where receptor inactivation could occur. Alternatively, binding of insulin to its receptor may render the receptor a more susceptible target for inactivation while still on the cell surface. Surface inactivation of the receptor would then be followed by internalization and degradation.

To examine the kinetics of receptor decay during the transition from the basal to the down-regulated steady-state, 3T3-C2 cells were shifted from insulin-free medium to medium containing both insulin and heavy (^{15}N, ^{13}C and ^{2}H) amino acids (6). The rates of light (^{14}N, ^{12}C, and ^{1}H) receptor decay and heavy receptor synthesis were then followed with time by quantitating heavy and light receptors separated by isopycnic banding on CsCl density gradients. Experiments were carried out with both control and down-regulated cells in the steady-state. Within two hours after insulin addition, receptor decay increased abruptly for several hours then gradually declined until the "down-regulated" rate was achieved. The abrupt increase in receptor decay induced by insulin was preceded by a more rapid ($t_{1/2}$ < 10 min) translocation of surface receptors to an "intracellular" trypsin-resistant compartment. Thus, upon exposure to ligand, insulin receptor rapidly redistributes from the cell-surface to an intracellular compartment, without an initial net loss of cellular receptors. Translocation was rapidly reversed ($t_{1/2}$ < 20 min) upon removal of insulin. With prolonged exposure to insulin, the initial rapid translocation of receptor was followed by a slower inactivation of receptor in the intracellular compartment.

Taken together our results indicate that the following sequence of events occurs during insulin-induced down-regulation of its receptor. Upon exposure to ligand, insulin receptors are translocated from the cell-surface to an intracellular site which results in accelerated receptor decay and ultimately to a lower steady-state cellular receptor level.

SUMMARY

Studies on the synthesis, processing, and turnover of the insulin receptor reveal that the receptor is in a dynamic state. In many cell types, cellular insulin receptor turns over with a half-life of 7-8 h. This enables the cell to rapidly adjust its functional insulin receptor level and thereby alter its responsiveness to insulin. For example, during the differentiation of 3T3-L1 preadipocytes into adipocytes, a large increase in receptor level and sensitivity to insulin is caused by a marked increase in receptor synthesis. In a different physiological context, down-regulation of insulin receptor level induced by its ligand is caused by rapid translocation of cell surface receptors into an intracellular compartment not accessible to insulin; this process usually leads to an increased rate of receptor degradation.

REFERENCES

1 Reed, B.C. and Lane, M.D. (1980) Proc. Natl. Acad. Sci. USA, 77, 285-289.
2. Reed, B.C., Ronnett, G.V., Clements, P.R. and Lane, M.D. (1981) J. Biol. Chem., 256, 3917-3925.
3. Ronnett, G.V., Knutson, V.P. and Lane, M.D. (1982) J. Biol. Chem. 257, 4285-4291.
4. Knutson, V.P., Ronnett, G.V. and Lane, M.D. (1982) Proc. Natl. Acad. Sci. USA, 79, 2822-2826.
5. Ronnett, G.V., Tennekoon, G., Knutson, V.P. and Lane, M.D. (1983) J.Biol. Chem., 258, 283-290.
6. Knutson, V.P., Ronnett, G.V. and Lane, M. D. (1983) J. Biol. Chem., 258, 12139-12142.
7. Ronnett, G.V., Knutson, V.P., Kohanski, R., Simpson, T. L. and Lane, M. D. (1984) J. Biol. Chem., 259, 4566-4575.
8. Krupp, M. N., Knutson, V.P., Ronnett, G.V., and Lane, M.D. (1983) Methods in Enzymol., 96, Biomembranes Part J, 423-433.

17. Regulation of Gonadotropin Secretion

Endocrinology
F. Labrie, L. Proulx, eds.

THE LHRH PRECURSOR IS THE SAME SIZE IN HUMAN, RAT AND MOUSE HYPOTHALAMUS

ANN CURTIS, VALERIE LYONS AND GEORGE FINK
MRC Brain Metabolism Unit, University Department of Pharmacology,
1 George Square, Edinburgh EH8 9JZ, Scotland

INTRODUCTION

Many biologically active peptides are synthesized as part of larger precursor molecules, and, recently, we demonstrated the presence in rat hypothalamus of a $28000M_r$ precursor of LHRH (1). Here we demonstrate that the *in vitro* translation products of hypothalamic mRNA extracted from human (post-mortem) and mouse brain also contain a $28000M_r$ polypeptide which incorporates an amino acid sequence immunologically similar to that of biologically active LHRH (2). In addition, we studied mRNA extracts from the hypothalamus of hypogonadal (*hpg*) mice, a mutant strain totally deficient in LHRH, and have shown that the large LHRH immunoreactive polypeptide is absent from the *in vitro* translation products.

MATERIALS AND METHODS

Total RNA was extracted from the hypothalami of 60 adult female rats (Wistar-Cob), 60 adult normal mice (both sexes), 60 adult *hpg* mice (both sexes) and one human female aged 67 (three hours post-mortem) and one human male aged 72 (12 hours post-mortem) by the guanidinium thiocyanate procedure (3). Poly A^+ enriched fractions were isolated by oligo (dT)-cellulose chromatography (4). Neither the human female nor male suffered from a neurological or psychiatric disorder. All hypothalamic dissections were carefully carried out to ensure the incorporation of most of the hypothalamic cell bodies. The mRNA samples were translated in an amino-acid depleted rabbit reticulocyte lysate system as described previously (5). 70000 acid precipitable counts of each sample were electrophoresed on 12.5% polyacrylamide gels according to O'Farrell (6). The gels were fluorographed and exposed to film (Kodak X-omat R) for 10 days.

Aliquots of the translation mixes from all four sources, containing a minimum of 10^6 acid precipitable counts, were immunoprecipitated as described previously (1) with the specific LHRH antiserum using donkey anti rabbit 1gG as the second antibody. The LHRH antiserum (HC6) was raised in rabbits against a LHRH-haemocyanin conjugate and did not cross react with either nine different analogues of LHRH modified at either the N or C terminus, or pituitary hormones, but did cross react 100% with the free acid of LHRH. In a second immunoprecipitation procedure, applied to the rat hypothalamic translation

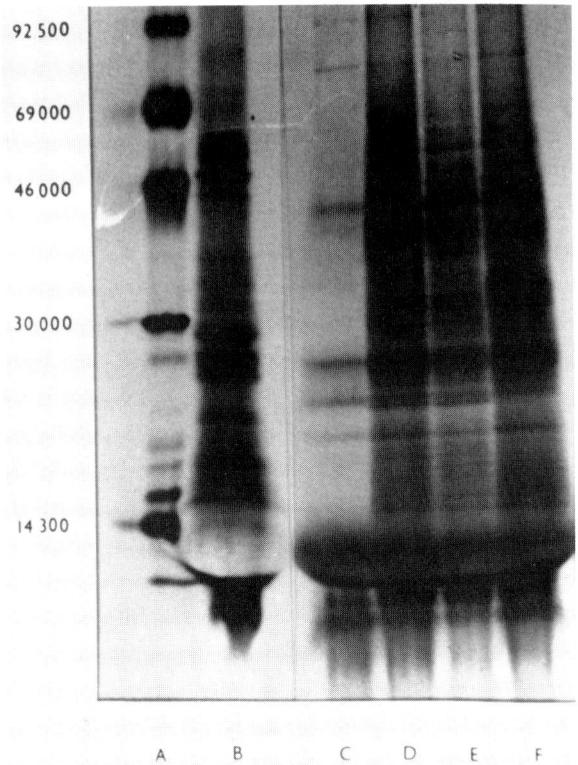

Fig. 1 Autoradiograph of ^{3}H-labelled translation products of hypothalamic messenger RNA samples of human (lane B), normal mouse (lane D) hpg mouse (lane E) and rat (lane F) following polyacrylamide gel electrophoresis. Lane C shows a translation mix to which no exogenous mRNA was added and lane A shows a series of ^{14}C molecular weight standards.

products, Staphylococcal protein A replaced the second antibody in the precipitation of antigen-antibody complexes. The final precipitates were electrophoresed as described above, fluorographed and exposed to film for up to 6 weeks. Autoradiograms from separate gels were aligned according to the positions of the ^{14}C-molecular weight standards which were electrophoresed in parallel.

RESULTS AND DISCUSSION

The translation products of human hypothalamic mRNA spanned a similar molecular weight range to those of the rat and mouse and were of comparable specific activity despite the delay between death and RNA extraction (Fig. 1).

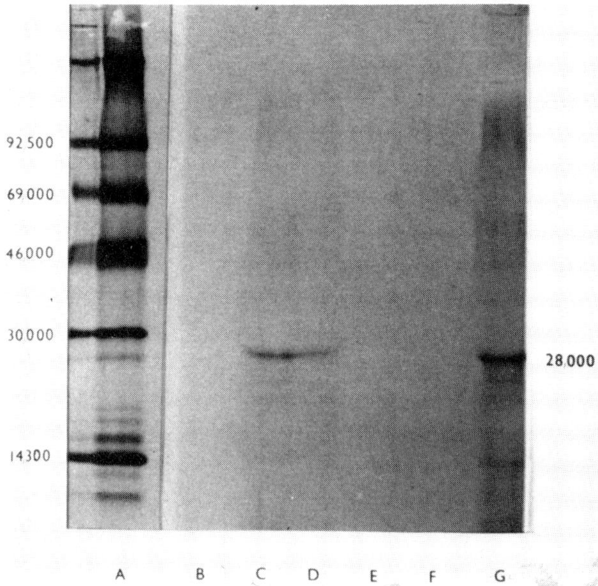

Fig. 2 Autoradiograph of rat and human hypothalamic mRNA translation products following immunoprecipitation with an anti-LHRH serum. The rat hypothalamic translation products were immunoprecipitated in the presence of excess cold LHRH (lane B), using either the second antibody (lane C) or the Staphylococcal protein A immunoprecipitation technique (lane D). A $28000M_r$ polypeptide was immunoprecipitated by both methods. No polypeptides were immunoprecipitated when a translation mix without exogenous mRNA was treated in an identical manner (lane E). The main immunoprecipitation product in the human translation mix was a $28000M_r$ polypeptide (lane 9); no immunoprecipitation was seen in the presence of excess cold LHRH (lane F). Lane A shows a series of ^{14}C molecular weight standards.

Among the translation products of the human, normal mouse and rat hypothalamic mRNA was a single major band with an apparent molecular weight of 28000, which was detected by immunoprecipitation of the radioactively labelled translation products with a specific anti-LHRH serum (Figs. 2 and 3). This polypeptide was immunoprecipitated from the rat hypothalamic mRNA translation products using both second antibody and protein A immunoprecipitation techniques (Fig. 2). It could not be detected, however, amongst the translation products of the rat, human (Fig. 2) or normal mouse (Fig. 3) mRNA when an excess of cold LHRH was added before immunoprecipitation, showing that the decapeptide is able to compete for the antiserum and block its binding with the precursor completely. The $28000M_r$ band was also not detected by the identical immunoprecipitation of a translation mix to which no exogenous mRNA was added or in which normal rabbit serum replaced the anti-LHRH serum (1).

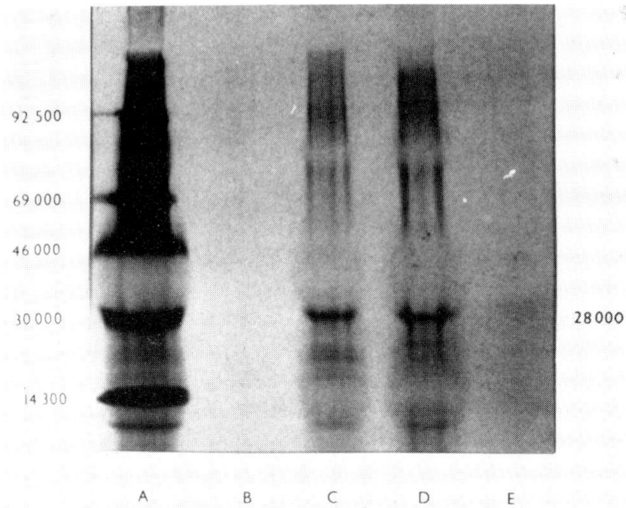

Fig. 3 Autoradiograph of normal mouse and hpg mouse hypothalamic mRNA translation products following immunoprecipitation with an anti-LHRH serum. A $28000M_r$ polypeptide was immunoprecipitated from the normal mouse (lane C) and rat (lane D) hypothalamic translation products. Lane E shows the hpg mouse translation products immunoprecipitated by an identical procedure and demonstrates the absence of any immunoprecipitate. Lane B shows a no-message blank. Lane A shows the ^{14}C molecular weight standards.

When the translation products of the hpg mouse hypothalamic mRNA were treated in an identical manner, no polypeptides were immunoprecipitated (Fig. 3). Though the primary inherited defect of the hpg mouse is unknown, these results suggest that it is unrelated to the processing mechanism of a large precursor molecule since the precursor is either completely absent, or present in a mutated form which is not recognised by the anti-LHRH serum. It is unlikely to be present at levels below our detection limits since the genetics of the hpg defect clearly represents an 'all or none' condition (2). The presence of a defective, non-translateable mRNA, or its complete absence due to a transcriptional defect remains to be determined with the aid of specific LHRH nucleic acid probes.

The identification of a large $28000M_r$ LHRH immunoreactive polypeptide within the hypothalami of three mammalian species, and the demonstration of its absence from the hpg mouse hypothalamus shows that LHRH is initially synthesized by way of a precursor molecule which is twenty times larger than the active peptide in a manner similar to other hypothalamic peptides. Gel filtration studies of hypothalamic extracts suggest that the precursor is processed to LHRH via intermediates which range in size from 26000 to 1800 (7),(8). The precursor may contain several sequences of LHRH and/or other biologically active peptides. However, unless the _hpg_ condition is due to a point mutation, the fact that the _hpg_ mouse is free of any other obvious abnormalities suggests that active components of the precursor, other than LHRH, are unlikely to be crucial for the normal function of the animal.

ACKNOWLEDGEMENTS

We thank Dr. Michael Szelke of the Royal Postgraduate Medical School for providing the LHRH haemocyanin conjugate, Dr. A.J. Harmar for advice on the immunoprecipitation procedures, Dr. Celia Yates for helping us to obtain human post-mortem brain, and Academic Press Inc. by whom this manuscript was originally published.

REFERENCES

1. Curtis, A., and Fink, G. (1983) Endocrinology 112, 390-392.
2. McDowell, I.F.W., Morris, J.F., Charlton, H.M., and Fink, G. (1982) J. Endocr. 95, 331-340.
3. Chirgwin, J.M., Przybyla, A.E., Macdonald, R.J., and Rutter, W.J. (1979) Biochemistry 18, 5294-5298.
4. Aviv, H., and Leder, P. (1972) Proc. Natl. Acad. Sci. U.S.A. 69, 1408-1412.
5. Curtis, A., Lyons, V. and Fink, G. (1983). Biochem. Biophys. Res. Commun. 117, 872-877.
6. O'Farrell, P.H. (1975) J. Biol. Chem. 250, 4007-4021.
7. Millar, R.P., Aehnelt, C., and Rossier, G. (1977) Biochem. Biophys, Res. Commun. 74, 720-731.
8. Gautron, J.P., Pattou, E., and Kordon, C. (1981) Mol. Cell. Endocrinol. 24, 1-15.

Endocrinology
F. Labrie, L. Proulx, eds.

THE RELATIONSHIPS BETWEEN GnRH AND LH SECRETION

IAIN J. CLARKE

Medical Research Centre, Prince Henry's Hospital, St. Kilda Road, Melbourne, Australia 3004

Direct hypothalamic control of the anterior pituitary gland via the neurohumoral route of the hypophyseal portal blood vessels has been appreciated since the experiments of Harris in the late 1940's. Since then various methods have been developed to sample the hypophyseal portal blood and monitor hypothalamic secretions in anaesthetized animals (1,2,3,4). Recently, we described a method for sampling portal blood in conscious sheep (5). This methodology has allowed us to examine the relationships between the secretion of gonadotropin releasing hormone (GnRH) from the hypothalamus and gonadotropins from the pituitary gland. Based on these relationships, we developed an *in vivo* model to study the action of GnRH on the pituitary gland: the pituitary gland was 'disconnected' from the hypothalamus, removing endogenous GnRH inputs to the gland (6). We were then able to administer exogenous GnRH in a controlled manner and restore gonadotropin secretion. Our hypothalamo-pituitary disconnection (HPD) procedure is somewhat analogous to the arcuate nucleus-lesioned monkey model developed by Knobil's group (7). In this paper I will outline the relationships between GnRH and LH that we have defined using our 2 *in vivo* models.

THE RELATIONSHIP BETWEEN GnRH AND LH SECRETION

In ovariectomized (OVX) ewes (5) we were able to establish that the pulsatile pattern of LH secretion, evident by peripheral blood sampling, is the direct consequence of major pulsatile secretory discharges of GnRH into the hypophyseal portal blood. Peak values for the pulses of GnRH that are evident in the portal blood of OVX ewes range from 3-1216 pg/ml (n=7 sheep). Between animal variation may be due to our sampling from different vessels in different sheep; a difficult variable to control since the vascular anatomy on the anterior face of the pituitary gland varies considerably. After taking account of the portal blood flow rate into the sampling cannula, which can vary quite markedly, the pulsatile nature of GnRH secretion is still apparent. Various 'small' GnRH pulses are also apparent between the major GnRH pulses that provoke LH release. The significance of these small pulses is not yet clear but they may be important in sensitizing the gland to the larger pulses (8) and/or promoting synthesis of gonadotropins without release.

There is no clearly pulsatile pattern for the release of FSH in OVX ewes and we have not been able to demonstrate a relationship between GnRH and FSH secretion.

EFFECTS OF ESTROGEN ON GnRH SECRETION

To examine the effect of estrogen on the pattern of GnRH secretion, we sampled OVX ewes following i.m. injections of 50 µg oestradiol benzoate. This treatment causes a biphasic pattern of LH secretion (a decrease followed by an increase) (9). During the negative feedback phase, pulsatile LH secretion ceased but pulsatile GnRH secretion continued (10). During the positive feedback phase the frequency of GnRH pulses increased and the interpulse interval was reduced to 10 min in some sheep. GnRH interpulse intervals for OVX sheep treated with estrogen are given in Table 1. During the positive feedback phase, we measured very high levels (up to 3000 pg/ml) of GnRH in the portal blood of some sheep (10). Sustained GnRH concentrations of this magnitude have never been encountered in untreated OVX sheep.

TABLE 1

MEAN (± s.e.m.) INTERPULSE INTERVALS (MIN) IN OVX EWES DURING THE NEGATIVE AND POSITIVE FEEDBACK PHASES OF LH SECRETION FOLLOWING INJECTIONS OF ESTRADIOL BENZOATE (50 µg i.m.) COMPARED TO OVX CONTROLS (UNTREATED).

Group	n	GnRH Interpulse Interval (Min)
Control	7	54.4 ± 8.4
Negative feedback phase	4	46.2 ± 6.3
Positive feedback phase	6	29.5 ± 4.1*

*P < 0.025 compared to control

In spite of the fact that GnRH concentrations vary depending on the site and extent of cuts in the portal circulation, our data strongly suggest that the estrogen-induced LH surge depends upon an increase in GnRH pulse frequency (Table 1) which raises the overall mean portal concentrations of GnRH. The limitations of our model prevent us from analysing effects of estrogen on GnRH pulse amplitude. Karsch et al. (11) have recently reported that continuous estrogen treatment can increase the LH pulse frequency in OVX ewes which supports our findings regarding the hypothalamic effect of estrogen on GnRH interpulse interval.

EFFECTS OF PROGESTERONE ON GnRH SECRETION

Goodman & Karsch (12) have shown that exogenous progesterone given to ewes immediately after ovariectomy to achieve plasma levels of 10-15 nmol/l will reduce LH pulse frequency. Using a lower dose, giving plasma levels of 4-5 nmol/l, Martin et al. (13) found that progesterone would act synergistically with estrogen to reduce LH pulse frequency in ewes sampled during autumn (breeding season) but not in ewes sampled during spring (non-breeding season). Since LH pulses reflect GnRH pulses (5), it may be deduced that progesterone has a hypothalamic action to reduce GnRH pulse frequency. Also, we have found that GnRH pulses are less frequent during the luteal phase of the estrous cycle than during the follicular phase (I.J. Clarke, unpublished).

EFFECTS OF ESTROGEN ON GnRH ACTION

Earlier studies by Coppings & Malven (14) showed that estrogen could have a direct pituitary action so that, following an estrogen injection to OVX ewes, the sensitivity of the gonadotropes was first decreased and then increased. To obtain more definitive information regarding this pituitary effect we have used our HPD model (15). In OVX-HPD ewes receiving hourly intra-atrial pulses of 500 ng GnRH, a single i.m. injection of 50 µg estradiol benzoate caused a biphasic alteration in the pattern of LH secretion. This result reinforced our belief that the negative feedback effect of estrogen seen in hypothalamo-pituitary intact ewes was the result of a pituitary action, not a reduction of GnRH secretion (see above).

The enhanced responsiveness to GnRH pulses that followed the negative feedback phase could increase LH levels by 2-3 fold in OVX-HPD, GnRH pulsed, estrogen-treated ewes. This was not a sufficient increase to account for LH surges in the hypothalamo-pituitary intact estrogen treated OVX ewe and further points to an action of estrogen at the hypothalamic level to increase GnRH secretion at this time.

EFFECTS OF PROGESTERONE ON GnRH ACTION

Given alone, progesterone is not able to affect GnRH action on the pituitary gland (14). With a background of progesterone, the effects of a single i.m. injection of 50 µg estradiol benzoate on LH secretion are enhanced (15) leading to lower plasma LH levels during the negative feedback phase and higher levels during the positive feedback phase. Thus, progesterone may have a positive influence at the pituitary level.

THE RELATIONSHIP BETWEEN PULSE FREQUENCY AND AMPLITUDE

In the arcuate-nucleus lesioned monkey, Wildt et al. (16) showed that there was an inverse relationship between the frequency of exogenous GnRH pulses and the amplitude of endogenous LH pulses. We have achieved similar results in OVX-HPD ewes (17).

In an effort to understand the basis of the relationship between GnRH pulse frequency and LH pulse amplitude, we conducted experiments in which OVX-HPD ewes were given hourly or 2-hourly pulses of GnRH and then given high-dose infusions of GnRH to measure the releasable pool of pituitary LH (18). With the hourly pulse frequency, the response to the high dose infusions was significantly lower than in those animals pulsed 2-hourly. It remains to be determined whether or not this effect of GnRH pulse frequency on the releasable LH pool is due to an alteration in GnRH receptors or post-receptor events.

CONCLUSION

Using our unique *in vivo* model to collect hypophyseal portal blood from sheep, we have defined the relationships that exist between GnRH and LH secretion. We have also delineated the feedback effects of estrogen and progesterone on GnRH and LH secretion. The amplitude of LH pulses has been found to depend upon GnRH/LH pulse frequency and the releasable pool of pituitary LH, as well as GnRH pulse amplitude (17). Further studies are in progress to determine the cellular mechanisms involved in generating pulsatile secretion of these hormones.

REFERENCES

1. Porter JC, Jones JC (1956) Endocrinology 58:62
2. Worthington WC (1966) Nature Lond 210:710
3. Porter JC, Smith KR (1967) Endocrinology 81:1182
4. Carmel PW, Antunes JL, Ferin M (1979) J Neurosurg 50:75
5. Clarke IJ, Cummins JT (1982) Endocrinology 111:1737
6. Clarke IJ, Cummins JT, de Kretser DM (1983) Neuroendocrinol 36:376
7. Plant TM, Krey LC, Moossy J, McCormack JT, Hess DL, Knobil E (1978) Endocrinology 102:52
8. Hoff JD, Lasley BL, Yen SSC (1979) J Clin Endocrinol Metab 49:8
9. Scaramuzzi RJ, Tillson SA, Thorneycroft IH, Caldwell BV (1971) Biol Reprod 88:1184
10. Clarke IJ, Cummins JT (1985) Endocrinology; submitted
11. Karsch FJ, Foster DL, Bittman EL, Goodman RL (1983) Endocrinology 113:1333
12. Goodman RL, Karsch FJ (1980) Endocrinology 107:1286
13. Martin GB, Scaramuzzi RJ, Henstridge JD (1983) J Endocr 96:181
14. Coppings RJ, Malven PV (1976) Neuroendocrinol 21:181
15. Clarke IJ, Cummins JT (1984) Neuroendocrinol; In Press
16. Wildt L, Hausler A, Marshal G, Hutchison JS, Plant TM, Belchetz PE, Knobil E (1981) Endocrinology 109:376
17. Clarke IJ, Cummins JT, Findlay JK, Burman KJ, Doughton BW (1984) Neuroendocrinol; In Press
18. Clarke IJ, Cummins JT (1985) J Reprod Fert; Submitted

Supported by Australian National Health and Medical Research Council.

© 1984 Elsevier Science Publishers B.V.
Endocrinology
F. Labrie, L. Proulx, eds.

REGULATION OF PITUITARY GnRH RECEPTORS *IN VIVO* AND *IN VITRO*

R.N. CLAYTON, S.I. NAIK, A. DETTA, L.S. YOUNG, H.M. CHARLTON*
Department of Medicine, University of Birmingham, and *Human Anatomy, University of Oxford, U.K.

INTRODUCTION

Pituitary GnRH receptor (GnRH-R) regulation has been extensively studied in different physiological circumstances in rats, and to a lesser extent in hamsters, sheep, and monkeys (1 and Table 1). A positive correlation exists between GnRH-R and serum LH in rats, and with changes in pituitary responsiveness to exogenous GnRH. Recent evidence in rats indicates that GnRH induces homologous receptor up-regulation *in vivo*. We presumed that similar GnRH-R regulation would apply in other rodent species. Thus, we examined GnRH-R changes in different physiological situations in normal mice, and the effect of exogenous GnRH and hypothalamic transplantation on the pituitary-gonadal axis of mice with GnRH deficiency (hpg). Our *in vitro* studies have defined some of the cellular biochemical requirements for the induction of GnRH-R by a variety of agents, including GnRH.

GnRH-R regulation in normal mice (C3H/HeH/101H intercrosses)

Within 24 hrs of gonadectomy (GDX) GnRH-R fall briskly (50%↓) then return towards intact values, before declining to low values (50%↓) which persist for up to 3 mths in both sexes (2,3). Despite the fall in GnRH-R serum LH and FSH show the expected elevation (10-fold). In male mice GDX consistently depletes pituitary LH and FSH (50%↓), while in female mice pituitary gonadotrophin content increases to above intact control values. The GnRH-R fall post-GDX cannot be ascribed to decreased receptor affinity. Thus, post-GDX of mice no positive correlation exists between GnRH-R and serum gonadotrophins as in rats, hamsters, and sheep (Table 1). However, in common with rats, GnRH-R fall by 50% in lactating mice (3). The post-GDX GnRH-R fall in mice cannot be prevented by GnRH antiserum (GnRH-AS) treatment, though the serum LH and FSH rise is abolished. Indeed, GnRH-AS reduces GnRH-R in intact mice, as in rats, and accentuates the post-GDX receptor fall. Moreover, exogenous GnRH cannot prevent the post-GDX GnRH-R fall (4).

These data imply that the post-GDX GnRH-R changes in mice are related primarily to the removal of a stimulatory factor(s) from the gonads, rather than changes in endogenous GnRH secretion

TABLE 1 GnRH RECEPTOR REGULATION IN DIFFERENT SPECIES

	Rat	Mouse	Hamster	Sheep	Cow	Monkey
Oestrous cycle	↑	?	↑	?	↑	?
E_2-induced LH surges	↑	?	?	<——>	?	↑
Lactation	↓	↓	?	?	?	?
Gonadectomy	↑	↓	↑	↑	↑	?

↑ = increased ? = not known ↓ = decreased <——> = unchanged

<u>per se</u>. Thus, E_2 or T treatment partially restores the GnRH-R fall post-GDX. Combined E_2 and GnRH treatment of OVX mice increases GnRH-R values 30% above intact female controls. Single or multiple injections of GnRH (60 ng s.c.) increases GnRH-R in intact female mice, but not in males, an action dependent on protein synthesis (4). E_2 alone reverses the inhibitory effect of GnRH-AS on GnRH-R values in intact and OVX female mice, though serum gonadotrophin values are further suppressed. Collectively, these data indicate that the major factor responsible for the GnRH-R fall post-OVX of mice is removal of oestrogen acting directly on the pituitary to maintain GnRH-R. Additive effects of GnRH and E_2 suggest a synergistic action at the pituitary level, and GnRH-R up-regulation in mice cannot occur in the absence of gonadal steroids. The clear suppressive effect of sex steroids on serum LH and FSH levels, despite stimulation of GnRH-R, provides further evidence for separate mechanisms regulating these processes. Further evidence for an E_2 stimulation of GnRH-R is shown by the 100% increase seen in E_2-treated <u>hpg</u> female mice (5).

<u>GnRH-R regulation in GnRH-deficient (hpg) mice</u>

Since the hypothalami of <u>hpg</u> mice contain no GnRH these animals provide a model for study of the interaction between exogenous GnRH and other hormones acting only at the pituitary level. Thus, a single injection of GnRH (60 ng s.c.) is followed 8-12 hours later by a 100% rise in GnRH-R in intact and castrated <u>hpg</u> mice of both sexes, which is blocked by cycloheximide (6). The time-course and protein synthesis dependence of GnRH-R up-regulation <u>in vivo</u> are identical with that observed <u>in vitro</u> (10), supporting the physiological relevance of <u>in vitro</u> studies. Pulsatile GnRH treatment of male <u>hpg</u> mice normalises GnRH-R within 3 days (7), this rise preceding that of pituitary and serum FSH. Foetal hypothalamic tissue placed into the IIIrd ventricle of <u>hpg</u>

recipients also induce a time-dependent increase in GnRH-R, pituitary and serum gonadotrophins, gonadal weight and LH receptors, though there is more individual variation in response than with exogenous pulsatile GnRH. GnRH-containing axons emanate from the grafts in the direction of the median eminence (8). The ovaries of implant-bearing hpg female mice contain mature ovarian follicles and appear to ovulate on coitus. Long-term stimulation of the hpg pituitary-gonadal axis indicates the central role for GnRH in sexual development.

GnRH-R regulation in vitro

GnRH receptors in intact cultured pituitary cells increase 70-100% after GnRH treatment (10^{-9}M) in a time and dose-dependent manner (9,10). Non-specific LH secretagogues (58mM KCl, Ca ionophore) and cAMP derivatives (1mM), produce similar 100% rises in GnRH-R. Increased endogenous cAMP as a consequence of forskolin (1µM) activation of adenylate cyclase produces a 100% increase in GnRH-R and LH release albeit somewhat later (24h) than after exogenous dbcAMP (Table 2). These receptor increases are prevented by protein synthesis inhibitors, Ca channel blockers and by disruption of microtubule function with vinblastine (11). Coincubation with a GnRH antagonist prevents GnRH and DbcAMP-induced receptor up-regulation, but not that with 58 mM KCl or forskolin, indicating the receptor mediation of the up-regulation by the former. DbcAMP (1mM) inhibits the binding of ^{125}I-GnRH-A to intact pituitary cells (11). GnRH-R increases are observed when there is little or no LH release (DbcAMP and 0.1µM A23187). This data indicates that the 'new' receptors are not originating from insertion of LH secretory granule GnRH-R into the plasma membrane. Further, the intra-cellular mechanism by which these agents up-regulate GnRH-R are distinct from that for LH release, or require a smaller magnitude of change e.g. only a small mobilisation/influx of calcium. Subsequent responsiveness of cells with increased GnRH-R shows that the ED_{50} for stimulation of LH release is unchanged, though the maximum LH release is reduced where the receptor-inducing pre-treatment agent has depleted cellular LH content. Lower LH release in response to A23187 indicates that it is not merely the 'GnRH-releasable' LH pool which is depleted. Hence, acute GnRH-R up-regulation is not paralleled by enhanced pituitary responsiveness to GnRH, implying that the additional receptors are not coupled to the secretory machinery of the cell.

TABLE 2 GnRH RECEPTOR REGULATION AND LH RELEASE IN VITRO

Agent	GnRH-R	LH Release
GnRH (1nM)	↑	+++
KCl (58mM)	↑	+++
DbcAMP (1mM)	↑	+
Forskolin (1μM)	↑	+++
A23187 (10-100nM)	↑	-
A23187 (10μM)	↓	+++

CONCLUSIONS

GnRH receptor changes both *in vivo* and *in vitro* can be dissociated from LH release in a number of circumstances, and the GnRH-R increases do not always sensitise pituitary gonadotrophin responses. GnRH-R increases can be induced by oestrogen acting directly on the pituitary *in vivo*, and other agents *in vitro* which do not always induce gonadotrophin secretion. It is likely that GnRH-R changes in response to GnRH provide another, longer-term, marker of GnRH action in the gonadotroph, the precise physiological relevance of which is not yet fully understood.

REFERENCES

1. Clayton RN (1983) In: P.G. Strange (Ed) Cell Surface Receptors Ellis Horwood, Chichester pp 184-206.
2. Naik SI, Young LS, Charlton HM, Clayton RN (1984a) Endocrinol, 115:
3. Naik SI, Young LS, Charlton HM, Clayton RN (1984b) Endocrinol, 115:
4. Naik, SI, Young LS, Saade G, Kujore A, Charlton HM, Clayton RN (submitted).
5. Naik SI, Young, LS, Charlton HM, Clayton RN.(submitted)
6. Detta A, Naik SI, Charlton HM, Young LS, Clayton RN (1984) Mol. Cell. Endocrinol (in press)
7. Young LS, Speight A, Charlton HM, Clayton RN (1983) Endocrinol 113: 55-61
8. Young LS, Detta A, Clayton RN, Jones A, Charlton HM. (1984) Endocrinol (submitted)
9. Loumaye E, Catt, KJ. (1982) Science 215: 983-985
10. Young LS, Naik, SI, Clayton RN (1984a) Endocrinol (in press)
11. Young LS, Naik SI, CLayton RN (1984b) Mol Cell Endocrinol (submitted)

Endocrinology
F. Labrie, L. Proulx, eds.

THE ROLE OF ENDOGENOUS OPIOID PEPTIDES IN THE CONTROL OF GONADOTROPIN SECRETION IN PRIMATES

MICHEL FERIN

Department of Obstetrics and Gynecology, and Institute for the Study of Reproductive Sciences, Columbia University, New York City, NY 10032

Opiates are known to modify the secretion of several hypophyseal hormones, such as prolactin, ACTH, growth hormone, gonadotropins, vasopressin and oxytocin. In this conference, the evidence which supports a physiological role for endogenous opioid peptides, and β-endorphin in particular, in the control of gonadotropin secretion in the female rhesus monkey will be summarized. A more detailed review was presented at the Laurentian Hormone Conference (1).

1. Intravenous administration of morphine or intraventricular injection of β-endorphin results in a decrease in circulatory LH concentrations, an effect which appears to be the result of a decrease in pulse frequency. FSH release is also inhibited, but to a lesser degree (2).

2. Neuronal cell bodies containing proopiomelanocortin-derived peptides, including β-endorphin, are preferentially clustered in the arcuate area of the medial basal hypothalamus (3), a region in the primate which is also rich in gonadotropin-releasing hormone (GnRH) cell bodies and fibers (4). This anatomical overlap suggests possible interactions between the two peptides.

3. Antagonism of opiate activity by naloxone increases circulatory LH levels. However, a rapid and significant LH response to naloxone is seen only during the luteal phase of the menstrual cycle, suggesting that while there is an interaction between the endogenous opioid peptides and LH release, this regulatory mechanism involves gonadal hormones (5). Similar differential LH responses at different times of the cycle were observed in the human (6).

4. Although β-endorphin concentrations in peripheral blood do not appear to fluctuate with the endocrine milieu, we were able to demonstrate that hypothalamic β-endorphin secretory activity parallels gonadal hormone secretion. β-endorphin release by the hypothalamus was monitored in hypophyseal portal blood (7, 8). Changes in hypophyseal portal blood β-endorphin following ovarian sex steroid modifications were striking. β-endorphin was undetectable following ovariectomy, but increased after estrogen and progesterone replacement. Highest β-endorphin release was found during the luteal phase of the cycle. Naloxone's effectiveness in modifying LH release appears to parallel β-endorphin activity in the hypothalamus.

This research was supported by NIH Grants HD-05077 and 10873.

The above evidence suggests that β-endorphin may play a significant role in the control of the menstrual cycle. It is known that LH pulse frequency varies throughout the menstrual cycle. During the luteal phase, there is an impressive deceleration of pulse frequency (mean: 1 pulse/6 hr vs 1 pulse/1 hr during the early follicular phase). We believe that the observed increase in opiate activity during the luteal phase participates in this decrease in LH pulse frequency: naloxone infusion reverses this process and accelerates pulsatile LH release to a frequency similar to that observed during the early follicular phase, at a time when little or no β-endorphin activity is present (9).

These observations have led us to conclude that in the primate, endogenous opioid peptides are important determinants of gonadotropin secretion during the menstrual cycle, and that they exert their effects by modulating the activity of the GnRH pulse generator. We postulate that the alternation of high and low β-endorphin hypothalamic activity during the menstrual cycle is an important phenomenon in cyclicity. Preliminary data have now indicated that counteraction of the effects of opiates on pulse frequency during the luteal phase by GnRH pulsatile infusions has profound effects on the next menstrual cycle, which is delayed significantly (1).

Our results raise the possibility that amenorrhea may, in certain cases, reflect abnormal hypothalamic β-endorphin activity, leading to an abnormal function of the GnRH pulse generator and hence to pulse frequencies which may be deleterious to cyclicity (10). This hypothesis finds support in clinical studies in which naloxone was shown to amplify pulse patterns of release in certain patients (11).

REFERENCES

1. Ferin M, Van Vugt DA, Wardlaw SL (1984) Recent Prog Horm Res (in press)
2. Ferin M, Wehrenberg WB, Lam NY, Alston EF, Vande Wiele RL (1982) Endocrinology 111:1652-1656
3. Abrams GM, Nilaver G, Hoffman D, Zimmerman EA, Ferin M, Krieger DT, Liotta AS (1980) Neurology 30:1106-1110
4. Silverman AJ, Antunes JL, Abrams G, Nilaver G, Thau R, Robinson JA, Ferin M, Krey LC (1982) J Comp Neurol 211:309-317
5. Van Vugt DA, Bakst G, Dyrenfurth I, Ferin M (1983) Endocrinology 113: 1858-1864
6. Quigley ME, Yen SSC (1980) J Clin Endocr Metab 51:179-181
7. Wehrenberg WB, Wardlaw SL, Frantz AG, Ferin M (1982) Endocrinology 111:879-881
8. Wardlaw SL. Wehrenberg WB, Ferin M, Antunes JL, Frantz AG (1982) J Clin Endocr Metab 55:877-881

9. Van Vugt DA, Lam NY, Ferin M (1984) Endocrinology (in press)

10. Pohl CR, Richardson DW, Hutchison JJ, Germak JA, Knobil E (1983) Endocrinology 112:2076-2080

11. Grossman A, Moult PJ, McIntyre H, Evans J, Silverstone T, Rees LH, Besser GM (1982) Clin Endocr 17:379-382

18. Biosynthesis and Processing of Peptide Hormones I

Endocrinology
F. Labrie, L. Proulx, eds.

INITIAL EVENTS IN PEPTIDE SECRETION: THE DOCKING PROTEIN OF ROUGH ENDOPLASMIC RETICULUM

MICHAEL HORTSCH, DANIELA AVOSSA and DAVID I. MEYER
Cell Biology Program, European Molecular Biology Laboratory, 6900 Heidelberg, West Germany

The pathway by which proteins pass through the cell from their site of synthesis in the cytoplasm to the extracellular milieu has been characterized in general terms (1). Secretory proteins have been sequentially localized in rough endoplasmic reticulum (ER), smooth membranes including those of the Golgi complex, and storage vesicles where they are sequestered until released by fusion of these vesicles with the cell membrane. The first step in this process is the transfer of the peptide, during its synthesis, from the cytoplasmic compartment of the cell across the membrane of the rough ER (2). Two aspects of this process pose interesting questions to the cell biologist: How is a selection made between proteins to be exported and those destined to remain in the cytoplasm; and how does a hydrophilic macromolecule, such as a protein, traverse the hydrophobic barrier posed by the membrane of the rough ER. Although little is known in molecular terms regarding the latter question, the process of sorting secretory from cytoplasmic proteins is becoming increasingly clear.

Much of the progress that has been made has come from the effective use of *in vitro* systems. In 1975 Blobel and Dobberstein (3) demonstrated that rough microsomal vesicles derived from canine pancreas were capable of selecting, translocating and processing nascent secretory proteins synthesized in a cell free system. These microsomes, therefore, contained all of the machinery needed to carry out the aforementioned processes. Subsequent biochemical manipulations and reconstitutions have led to an understanding, in molecular terms, of the recognition and initial membrane interaction of nascent secretory proteins (4).

The signal recognition particle (SRP) is a cytoplasmic ribonucleoprotein which binds to the trademark of nascent secretory peptides, the signal sequence (5). This N-terminal extension of amino acids is, in virtually all cases, the *sine qua non* for recognition and transfer across the membrane. SRP, originally isolated from microsomes (6,7), is in fact cytoplasmically localized where it functions by *arresting* the translation of the nascent peptide as soon as it can be recognized as such by virtue of accessibility of its signal sequence. The arrest is maintained until the ER membrane is contacted, at which point the arrest is released and transfer can thus take place through the correct membrane (8,9). An obvious advantage of this mechanism is its efficiency; it guarantees that secretory proteins, some of which could be harmful intracellularly in even the slightest quantity, are never completed in the cytoplasm.

The initial interaction of the arrested synthetic complex with the rough ER is a binding of the SRP to an integral membrane protein, the Docking Protein (DP) (8). It is via this interaction that the synthetic block is released and the actual translocation can commence. A considerable amount of data has been gathered regarding the Docking Protein and its functions and will be the focus of this article.

One of the most interesting aspects of Docking Protein is that a large cytoplasmically-disposed domain of about 60,000 daltons can be proteolytically cleaved and washed off of the membrane with high salt. This results in the membrane losing its translocation activity. Readdition of this fragment (DPf) under low salt conditions allows the ER to regain activity (10). The isolation and purification of the DPf allowed polyclonal antibodies to be produced which were subsequently used to characterize the intact DP, an integral ER protein of about 72,000 daltons (11). Such antibodies were also successful in blocking Docking Protein's interaction with SRP (8).

Through the use of monoclonal antibodies prepared against the intact docking protein, in combination with limited proteolysis, further characterization of this molecule has been carried out. Using the technique of immunoblotting, we have determined that Docking Protein exists as a 72,000 dalton integral membrane protein in all mammalian species examined including mouse, rat, dog and human. Moreover, when rough and smooth microsomes from rat liver were examined, Docking Protein was found to be localized exclusively in the rough membranes. Although this finding is consistent with its role in translocation, it is significant in that it is the first ER protein of known function to be restricted to the rough form and totally absent from smooth.

By combining limited proteolysis with immunoblotting a rough map of the antigenic determinants of Docking Protein could be drawn up (see figure). Four out of five monoclonals, specific for DP bind to a domain of about 6000 daltons. These antibodies are not identical as they exhibit differing species specificities, and thus one can assume several determinants to be present in this region. The polyclonals recognize a fragment of 7000 daltons closer to the membrane anchoring domain as well as sites on the most protease resistant portion of the 60 kd cytoplasmic domain, a tryptic fragment of 46 kd.

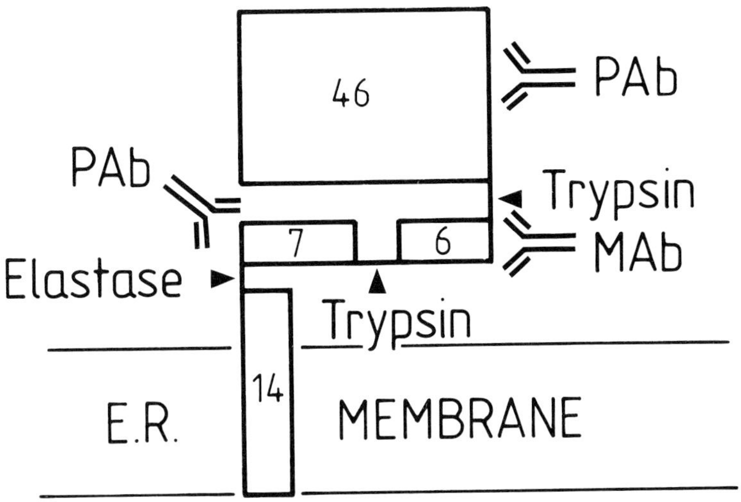

Structural and Antigenic Domains of Canine Docking Protein. Four major regions can be defined by limited proteolysis in conjunction with immunochemical techniques. Numbers refer to apparent molecular weights in kd as determined by SDS polyacrylamide gel electrophoresis. Pab refers to polyclonal, or Mab to monoclonal antibody binding ability of the given domain. Proteolytic cleavage sites are indicated by arrows.

Immunoaffinity chromatography using one of the monoclonals has enabled the isolation of pure 72 kd DP in an active state. In addition, a residual membrane integrated fragment of 27 kd (the membrane anchor of 14 kd plus the 7 and 6 kd domains) which arises through endogenous proteolytic activity of pancreatic tissue was purified. Elastolytic cleavage of the 27 kd fragment resulted in the production of the 14 kd membrane anchoring segment and a 13 kd piece representing the 6 kd plus the 7 kd domains. The latter species was immunoreactive, the membrane anchor contained no antibody binding sites. This type of affinity purification coupled with proteolysis will allow production of an antibody against the membrane anchor, the only major uncharacterized domain of DP. Moreover, the isolation of anti-DP antibodies and large quantities of individual pieces of DP will facilitate the determination of its primary structure by protein and nucleic acid sequencing techniques.

Docking Protein is a "multifunctional" protein. It not only serves as a receptor for SRP, but releases the SRP induced block. Additionally, when removed from the membrane, the 60 kd cytoplasmic domain can recombine with DP-depleted membranes. This implies that at least three functional regions exist: The SRP binding site, a region participating in block release and a site which enables DPf to recombine with DP-depleted microsomes. By the techniques mentioned above, we are in a position to examine the role of specific domains of DP in each of these functions. Preliminary evidence suggests that recombination of DPf with DP-free membranes is mediated by the 6000 dalton fragment, a peptide with a relatively basic pI.

REFERENCES

1. Palade G (1975) Science 189:347-358
2. Redman CM, Siekevitz P, Palade GE (1966) J Biol Chem 241:1150-1158
3. Blobel G, Dobberstein B (1975) J Cell Biol 67:852-862
4. Meyer DI (1982) Trends Biochem Sci (TIBS) 7:320-321
5. Walter P, Blobel G (1981) J Cell Biol 91:551-556
6. Dobberstein B (1978) Hoppe Seyler's Z Physiol Chem 359:1469-1470
7. Walter P, Blobel G (1980) Proc Natl Acad Sci USA 77:7112-7116
8. Meyer DI, Krause E, Dobberstein B (1982) Nature 297:647-650
9. Gilmore R, Blobel G, Walter P (1982) J Cell Biol 95:463-469
10. Meyer DI, Dobberstein B (1980) J Cell Biol 87:503-508
11. Meyer DI, Louvard D, Dobberstein B (1982) J Cell Biol 92:579-583

Endocrinology
F. Labrie, L. Proulx, eds.

ULTRASTRUCTURAL AND BIOCHEMICAL ASPECTS OF BIOSYNTHESIS AND SECRETION OF HORMONES

HARVEY B. POLLARD, RICHARD ORNBERG, MARK LEVINE, ELI HEIDMAN, KYOJI MORITA, PETER LELKES AND JUDITH HELDMAN

Laboratory of Cell Biology and Genetics, NIADDK, National Institutes of Health, Bethesda, Md. 20205 U.S.A.

INTRODUCTION

Chromaffin cells secrete catecholamines by exocytosis from secretory granules packaged in the Golgi. The process of exocytosis depends on the presence of external calcium, which must enter the cell upon stimulation by a physiological secretagogue such as acetylcholine. The increased calcium appears to cause fundamental changes in the interaction of the secretory granule with cytoskeletal elements, and seems to introduce close contacts between the granule and the plasma membrane or between granule membranes, as during compound exocytosis. Then, upon fusion of these membranes exocytosis occurs. We have been particularly interested over the past few years in what these calcium induced processes might be (1), and more recently we have been using new fast freeze fixation techniques to clearly delineate the different morphologic events during exocytosis (2).

Ultrastructure by Fast Freeze Fixation

Using the milli-second fast freeze methods we have begun following the secretion process from the earliest time intervals. However, these new methods, not involving chemical fixation, have also yielded unexpected new information on the structure of the secretory granule. Cultured bovine chromaffin cells contain at least three kinds of secretory granules: two large granule types, within the same cell, distinguished by the texture of the core, and smaller dense cored granules which are destroyed during chemical fixation of cells. The larger conventional granules have also been observed to contain an intragranular vesicle (IGV) of approximately 50 nm diameter, the contents of which are not known at present. Some granules contain multiple IGV's. The IGV's have also been observed within chromaffin granules during assembly in the Golgi. An example of IGV's in granules is shown in Figure 1. In cells stimulated to secrete with acetylcholine the IGV's have been observed in the exocytotic lumens formed during compound exocytosis. Chemical fixation of intact cells destroys IGV's, but they can be detected in chemically fixed isolated granule preparations. The question of IGV contents is being studied now by atomic imaging electron microscopy (3).

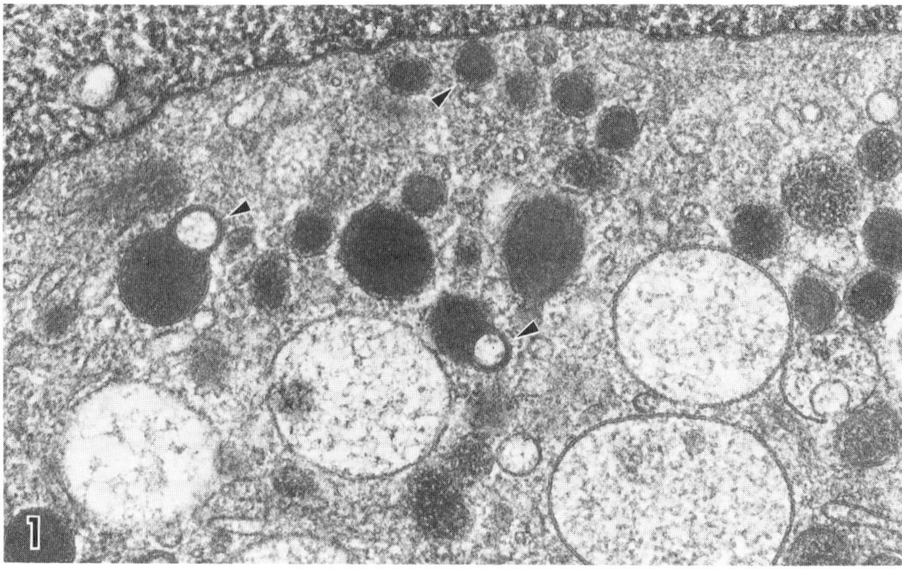

Figure 1. Electron micrograph of chromaffin granules in a rapid frozen, freeze-substituted chromaffin cell. Intragranular vesicles (arrows) are found in 60% of the large granules. Small chromaffin granules (upper arrow) illustrate a subpopulation of granules readily observed in rapid frozen cells. x 100,000.

Calcium in Stimulated Chromaffin Cells

Stimulation of the cell with acetylcholine induces a rapid increase in internal Ca^{++} concentration, detectable by both $^{45}Ca^{++}$ transport and Quin-2 fluorescence studies. In the case of activation by nicotine, the time course of calcium uptake into chromaffin cells, measured either by ^{45}Ca influx or induced fluorescence of Quin-2, is rapid, and terminates in a minute or two. Over the same time course after stimulation, compound exocytotic vacuoles of 1-5 μ in diameter are also rapidly formed, presumably a consequence of compound exocytosis, but are resolved morphologically within 5 minutes. Contact and fusion events can be readily detected and initially seem to occur over a very small region of the granule membrane.

What Does Calcium Do?

The question of how calcium works to promote these changes remains quite a central question in cell biology. While calcium may act directly on the membranes, many recent proposals have focused on possible mediators of calcium action such as cytoskeletal elements, protein kinases, calmodulin, proteases and synexin. In the face of these many possibilities, it is our feeling that in order to evaluate the involvement of specific mediators it is useful if the presumed mediator replicates in some way ultrastructural changes occuring *in vivo* and responds to physiologic calcium signals. To some extent, both of these expectation are born out by interactions of actin (4, 5) and synexin (6) with isolated chromaffin granules.

Cytoskeleton and Secretion

In resting chromaffin cells, cytoskeletal elements, including actin, are closely juxtaposed to chromaffin granules (7). Indeed, mixing F-actin with chromaffin granules under conditions of low calcium concentration ($< 10^{-7}$M) induces an extensive cross-linking of the F-actin filaments and a dramatic increase in the viscosity of the solution. The interaction is trypsin sensitive and heat labile, suggesting a protein component on the granule membrane to be involved in the interaction. Addition of calcium ($K_{1/2}$ = 0.2 μM) induces a dramatic decline in cross-linking, a process not understood at present, but reversible. The fascinating aspect of the interaction is that it could explain how granules, relatively immobilized in the cytoplasm at low calcium concentrations, could become mobilized for further contacts with the plasma membrane upon increases in intracellular Ca^{++} concentration. ATP also promotes the dissociation of granules from F-actin, thus indicating that at least two factors, calcium and ATP, exist in the cytoplasm that could control granule-cytoskeleton interaction.

Synexin and Membrane Fusion

The problem is to define what subsequent steps could lead to contact and fusion between plasma membranes and granule membranes, or indeed between granule membranes, as occurs during compound exocytosis. Electron microscopic data indicate that initial contacts between membranes occur over a limited area as mentioned earlier. Synexin is one example of a Ca^{++} binding protein that can cause such contacts to occur between chromaffin granule membranes (6), and which can support subsequent fusion of juxtaposed membranes in the presence of arachidonic acid (8). Interestingly the structures of the fused granules are quite similar to structures found in stimulated cells. The $K_{1/2}$ for synexin binding to granule membranes is ∿ 5 μM (9), while the $K_{1/2}$ for granule aggregation and fusion is ∿ 200 μM (7). These values are within the ranges of free Ca^{++} concentrations known to occur in stimulated chromaffin cells, and we believe that synexin is thus a viable candidate for the mediator of calcium action leading to membrane fusion and exocytosis.

Synexin Receptors on Membranes

The nature of the synexin receptor on plasma and granule membranes thus becomes of critical interest. Synexin can bind to phosphatidylserine liposomes and cause them to fuse if calcium is present (10). However, we have used a newly devised method to evaluate a wide variety of phospholipids and other lipids as possible receptors, finding that phosphatidylinositol is among the very best of the lipid receptors, while phosphatidylcholine is entirely inactive. Phosphotidylserine is somewhat intermediate between the two. These data have directed our attention to the concept that membrane fusion may proceed by synexin-directed changes in the location of specific phospholipids in juxtaposed membranes.

Calcium and Non-exocytotic Secretion of Ascorbate

While the discussion until this point has emphasized how calcium might direct secretion by exocytosis, it is important to keep in mind that in chromaffin cells, the same calcium signals can induce secretion of substances from the cytosol. One of these substances is ascorbate, a molecule rapidly becoming appreciated as a possible neurotransmitter in the central nervous system, and perhaps now peripherally as well. Chromaffin cells, in response to nicotinic secretagogues, elevated K^+ or veratridine, secrete ascorbate primarily from the cytosol (11). The same calcium channels involved in regulating excytosis also appear to be involved with regulating this non-exocytotically released substance as well. The differences between the two processes can be distinguished at present only pharmacologically. Trifluorerazine has no action on ascorbate secretion. However, trifluoperazine does block catecholamine secretion occurring by true exocytosis and incidently also interferes with synexin activity as well (12).

REFERENCES

1. Pollard, H.B., Creutz, C.E., Fowler, V., Scott, J., and Pazoles, C.J. (1982) Cold Spring Harbor Symp. Quant. Biol. 46: 819-833.
2. Ornberg, R.L. and Reese, T.S. (1981) J. Cell Biology 90: 40-54.
3. Leapman, R.D. and Ornberg, R.L. (1983) Proc. 41st Ann. Meeting of E.M.S.A. ed. G.W. Bailey (San Francisco Press, San Francisco) pp. 390-391.
4. Fowler, V.M. and Pollard, H.B. (1982) Nature 295: 336-338.
5. Fowler, V.M. and Pollard, H.B. (1982) J. Cell Bioch. 18: 295311.
6. Creutz, C.E., Pazoles, C.J. and Pollard, H.B. (1978) J. Biol. Chem. 253: 2858-2866.
7. Kondo, H., Wolosewick, I.J. and Pappas, G.D. (1982) J. Neuroscience 2: 57-65.
8. Creutz, C.E. (1981) J. Cell Biol. 91: 247-256.
9. Creutz, C.E. and Sterner, D.C. (1983) Biochem. Biophys. Res. Comm. 114: 355-364.
10. Hong, K., Dazgunes, N. and Papahadjopoulos, D. (1981) J. Biol. Chem. 3641-3644.
11. Levine, M., Asher, A., Pollard, H.B. and Zinder, O. (1983) J. Biol. Chem. 258: 13111-13115.
12. Pollard, H.B., Scott, J.H. and Creutz, C.E. (1983) Biophys. Biochem. Res. Comm. 113: 908-915.

© 1984 Elsevier Science Publishers B.V.
Endocrinology
F. Labrie, L. Proulx, eds.

PROTEOLYTIC MECHANISMS IN PROHORMONE PROCESSING - CATHEPSIN B-LIKE ENZYMES IN ISLET SECRETION GRANULES

D.F. STEINER, B. SAN SEGUNDO, S.J. CHAN, AND K. DOCHERTY
Department of Biochemistry, University of Chicago, 920 E. 58th Street, Chicago, Illinois 60637

Most small bioactive peptides are derived by fundamentally similar proteolytic processing mechanisms from preprohormones. Since this topic has been reviewed frequently (1-5) our purpose here will be to indicate progress in controversial areas. Earlier, as well as more recent, studies suggest that several kinds of proteolytic enzymes must participate in proteolytic processing. Their biochemical nature and subcellular localization remain important areas of study. Defects in processing of precursors (1,5,6) also are attracting increasing interest as these can be helpful in unravelling both the mechanisms of biosynthesis and cleavage as well as the physiological roles of the product peptide hormones and/or neuropeptides themselves.

Structures of precursors. Most precursor peptides are single chain molecules of variable size, but usually are greater than 8000 daltons (proinsulin and proPP (7) are among the smallest). Bioactive regions may be found almost anywhere along the peptide chains, and they often have a reiterative linear organization with tandemly repeated identical (preproenkephalin) or homologous (preproglucagon) segments (2), suggesting a complex mode of evolution from smaller units. Cleavage sites are almost invariably marked by pairs of basic residues and these are usually quantitatively removed by the action of the proteolytic processing mechanisms (1,8). The frequency of useage of the 4 possible combinations of the basic residues (Lys and Arg) also varies but Lys-Arg and Arg-Arg are the most frequently used (9). As discussed elsewhere in greater detail (1) cleavage at single basic residues, as well as at other special sites including the carboxyl side of Leu, Gln and Tyr also occasionally occurs. Prepeptide processing with its own distinctive features (10,11) should not be considered in the same context as prohormone processing, as it occurs in the rough endoplasmic reticulum during, or immediately after, biosynthesis of the pre(pro)secretory polypeptides (for reviews see 10-12).

Subcellular Localization of Prohormone Processing. Our earlier studies (13) along with those of Howell (14) and Orci et al. (15) demonstrated that movement of newly synthesized proinsulin to the Golgi apparatus via an energy dependent process is necessary for initiation of proteolytic processing. Energy does not appear to be required once this transit step has been completed inasmuch as inhibitors such as antimycin or dinitrophenol no longer inhibit processing if added about 40 minutes after synthesis. Similar findings have been reported for other systems (16,17). We interpret these results to indicate that processing begins in the Golgi area as products are condensed into (pro)secretory granules (1,13). However, conversion in many systems, including the β cells, continues for many hours after granules have already formed, indicating that they contain the full complement of processing enzymes.

The extent of proteolytic processing in the Golgi remains controversial. In the case of proinsulin it seems to be a minor fraction as judged by comparing the topological localization of labeled proinsulin (15) with biochemical data on the progress of conversion towards completion, i.e. in isolated labeled rat islets most of the labeled (pro)insulin has left the Golgi area (or is in condensing vacuoles) within 1 hour after a short pulse-labeling period, but conversion is only about 10% complete at this stage (18). In some other systems proteolysis occurs more rapidly and the products are not stored extensively (19,20), suggesting either that the Golgi or short-lived vesicles derived from it, are involved to a greater extent. In contrast some neurosecretory systems process precursors more slowly with little, if any, processing occuring in the Golgi per se (21). It can be argued that conversion (fragmentation) of precursors should not occur in the Golgi region prior to packaging since this would abbrogate a receptor-mediated mechanism for "sorting" the secretory propeptide into the trans Golgi stack and condensing vacuole, i.e. the many fragments would not be efficiently transferred into granules. However, evidence for such Golgi-associated receptors for proinsulin or any other prohormonal peptides in their cells of origin does not exist at present, nor is it known how such hypothetical receptors would in themselves be sorted or directed into the secretory granule-forming regions of the Golgi apparatus.

The only well-defined Golgi-associated transport receptor is the mannose-6-P receptor (see ref. 22) which has been localized (mainly) to the cis Golgi region in the elegant immunocytochemical studies of Brown and Farquhar (23). Their findings imply that this receptor is strategically poised to detect and divert those proteins destined for lysosomes that bear appropriately phosphorylated mannose-rich carbohydrate side chains. The more or less complete removal from the secretory main-stream into various side paths (e.g. lysosomal, constitutive (24), etc.) of certain products indeed may be largely mediated by specialized receptors, but it seems less likely that the very large amounts of some secreted products (e.g. (pro)insulin in the pancreatic β cells, the numerous distinct pancreatic acinar zymogens and enzymes, provasopressin in the supraoptic nucleus, etc.) require the participation of specific receptors for their intracellular movement. A simpler view would be that these products arrive in the trans Golgi and are concentrated into prosecretory granules by a bulk fluid-flow mechanism analogous to pinocytosis.

It has recently been shown that AtT20 cells derived from a mouse pituitary tumor which normally makes and secretes ACTH via processing and storage of its precursor, proopiomelanocortin (POMC) also can make, correctly process and secrete (pre)proinsulin (25). These findings could be interpreted as supporting the possibility mentioned above that secretory protein movement through the Golgi is accomplished via passive fluid flow. We have recently shown that islet cells of transgenic mice producing rat growth hormone (26) secrete growth hormone in a glucose-regulated fashion (Welsh, M., Brinster,

R. and Steiner, D.F., unpublished data). Since proinsulin is not glycosylated and bears no clear structural resemblance to POMC or to growth hormone it is difficult to believe that these proteins share structural determinants that can be recognized by a "sorting" receptor. It seems even less probable that AtT20 cells or mouse islet cells contitutively produce specific receptors for the transport and sorting of alien proteins such as proinsulin or growth hormone. It might be that some "facilitative" proteins exist in the ER and Golgi apparatus which enhance protein flow along the secretory pathway, perhaps, as suggested by P. Peterson (personal communication), by sensing correct conformation or ordered elements of symmetry in the products.

Proteolytic Cleavage Mechanisms. The nature of the converting proteases and their precise mechanisms of action is yet another area that has been difficult to penetrate experimentally. A bewildering array of proteases has been invoked by various workers to account for the initial endoproteolytic attack at the sites of paired basic residues in different precursors (for reviews see 1-4). At least four quite distinct proteolytic systems are currently being studied in considerable detail by a number of laboratories, each with findings and/or hypotheses that fundamentally disagree, indicating either that there may be several distinct classes of endoproteases accomplishing dibasic cleavage in different tissues or that the correct proteases are escaping identification because of the low levels required. Some of these systems are summarized in Table I.

TABLE I
SOME TENTATIVELY IDENTIFIED PROHORMONE ENDOPROTEASES

Cellular System	Type of Protease	pH Optimum	Cellular Localization	Proposed Mode of Cleavage	Refs.
Ant. Pituitary, Pancreatic Islets	Serine	> 7.0	Secretory Granules	-Lys↓Arg↓	(27,28) (29,47)
Post & Int. Pituitary	Unknown	4.0	Secretory Granules	-Lys↓Arg-	(30)
Pancreatic Islets	Thiol Protease	6.5	Secretory Granules	-Lys-Arg↓	(3,31,32)
Yeast	Unknown	~7.0	Membrane-bound	-Lys-Arg↓	(33)
Yeast	Serine	> 7.0	Soluble	-Lys↓Arg-	(34)

Recent studies in the laboratory of Noe and coworkers (3) as well as our own (26,27) have implicated cathepsin B-like thiol proteases in the processing of proinsulin as well as prosomatostatin and proglucagon (3). Incubation of isolated rat or anglerfish islet secretory granule preparations containing pulse-labeled precursors as substrates, leads to the processing of these precursors by secretory granule proteases that can be inhibited by leupeptin, antipain, pCMBS and alanyl-lysyl-arginyl-chloromethyl ketone (ALACK). However, mature cathepsin B and the other known lysosomal thiol proteases (cathepsins H and L) are unlikely to be converting enzymes because of their inappropriate cleavage specificities which in many instances result in degradation of precursors or their product peptides (1,2). However, cathepsin B is known to readily cleave a number of synthetic substrates having pairs of basic residues, e.g. Cbz-Arg-Arg-AMC and congeners (35). This property suggests that mature cathpsin B (∽30 kd) may cleave such substrates because of conformational changes induced in the protease by the bulky blocking or leaving groups of these compounds. Induction of conformational changes resulting in altered substrate specificity is well known from studies of specialized trypsin-like serine proteases (36). These enzymes usually contain a typical trypsin-like domain to which additional peptide material has been added to narrow the cleavage specificity and/or to confer other properties that render the enzyme more suitable for a special role, e.g. membrane binding, Ca^{++} binding, etc. We have found that insulin secretory granules from islets (31) and from a transplantable rat insulinoma (32) contain a higher molecular weight form of cathepsin B (39 kd) that exhibits a greater selectivity for the dibasic chloromethylketone, ALACK.

Biosynthetic studies with rat islets in our laboratories also indicate that cathepsin B is derived from a precursor which has a molecular weight of 43 kd (2). This precursor form (procathepsin B) appears to be secreted from normal islets in a glucose-dependent manner (Steiner, D.F. and Carroll, R., unpublished) indicating that it can be diverted from lysosomes into secretory pathways. It is of interest that similar larger (latent or active) forms of cathepsin B-like material are secreted in relatively large amounts by a variety of tumors (37,38). Preliminary studies with such tumor enzyme preparations, kindly supplied to us by Dr. John S. Mort (Montreal), indicate that some of these can process proinsulin to insulin (Steiner, D.F. and Mort, J., unpublished). These findings support (but do not prove) the thesis that higher molecular weight forms of cathepsin B may have a more directed protetolytic specificity and may be sorted as converting enzymes into secretory vesicles in the islets (and other tissues). We have recently cloned cDNAs for rat liver cathepsin B in order to study in greater detail the structure of its precursor form, its mechanisms of activation and intracellular transport, its tissue distribution and any closely related forms that can be detected in islet and other endocrine tissues (Chan, S.J., San Segundo, B., and Steiner, D.F., unpublished).

In addition to its potential role as a converting protease, procathepsin B in the secretory granules also may ultimately serve a degradative role (32). Procathepsin B can be activated to its mature form by aspartyl proteases such as pepsin or cathepsin D (37). It is known that turnover of insulin secretory granules occurs (39) but it is unclear whether this is a simple stochastic process or is regulated to occur under special conditions or as granules age within the beta cell. In the latter case it might be proposed that as the granule ages appropriate conditions for the conversion of procathepsin B (perhaps via autoactivation of procathepsin D) to mature enzyme gradually develop. Cathepsin B might then serve to initiate degradation of the C-peptide and insulin accompanied by lysis of the granule in autophagic vesicles (40).

In addition to the trypsin-like endoprotease whose nature remains unsettled there is considerable evidence for the existence of a carboxypeptidase B-like enzyme which removes C-terminal basic residues released by the endoprotease. This enzyme is acidic in pH optimum and soluble, but differs from both lysosomal or pancreatic carboxypeptidases B in several features, including molecular size and its strong stimulation by cobalt ions (41-43). The enzymes from islets (43) and chromaffin granules (41) are closely similar in properties suggesting that the same enzyme or isoenzymes may occur in these tissues.

In addition there is now evidence for an aminodipeptidase activity required for the maturation of both promellitin in honeybee sting glands (44), as well as for maturation of α-mating factor after cleavage at paired basic residues in yeast (45,46). This enzyme is currently being studied in greater detail. Another type of aminopeptidase activity directed toward substrates with N-terminal arginine residues has recently been discovered in posterior pituitary granules and chromaffin granules (30) and may complement processing endoproteases which cleave between basic residues in these tissues (see Table I).

The biochemical nature, evolutionary origin(s) and mechanism(s) for intracellular transport and activation of these proteases during the sorting and packaging of prohormonal peptides continues to provide fascinating and challenging problems for both endocrinologists and cell biologists alike.

ACKNOWLEDGEMENTS

This work was supported by NIH grants AM 13914 and 20595. We thank Cathy Christopherson for her skillful assistance in the preparation of this manuscript.

REFERENCES

1. Docherty K, Steiner DF (1981) Ann Rev Physiol 44:625-638
2. Steiner DF, Docherty K, Carroll R (1984) J Cell Biochem 24:121-130
3. Noe BD, Moran MN (1983) In: Hruby VJ, Rich DH (eds) Peptides: Structure and Function. Pierce Chemical Co., Rockford IL, pp 219-228
4. Chertow BS (1981) Endocrine Rev 2:137-173
5. Robbins DC, Tager HS, Rubenstein AH (1984) New Eng J Med 310:1165-1175
6. Owen MC, Brennan SO, Lewis JH, Carrell RW (1983) New Eng J Med 309:695-698
7. Boel E, Schwartz TW, Norris KE, Fiil NP (1984) EMBO J 3:909-912
8. Yanaihara N, Sakura M, Yanaihara C, Hashimoto T, Rubensteien AH, Steiner DF (1975) Nature 258:365-366
9. Schwartz TW, Wittels B, Tager HS (1983) In: Hruby VJ, Rich DH (eds) Peptides: Structure and Function. Pierce Chemical Co., Rockford IL, pp 229-238
10. Steiner DF, Quinn PS, Patzelt C, Chan SJ, Marsh J, Tager HS (1980) In: Goldsteiner L, Prescott DM (eds) Cell Biology: A Comprehensive Treatise, Vol. IV. Academic Press, New York, pp 175-201
11. Kreil G (1981) Ann Revs Biochem 50:317-348

12. Patzelt C, Steiner DF 1983 In: Randle PJ, Steiner DF, Whelan WJ (eds) Carbohydrate Metabolism and its Disorders, Vol. 3. Academic Press, New York, pp 159-179
13. Steiner DF, Clark JL, Nolan C, Rubenstein AH, Margoliash E, Melani F, Oyer PE (1970) In: Cerasi E, Luft R (eds) On the Pathogenesis of Diabetes Mellitus. Almqvist and Wiksell, Stockholm, pp 57-80
14. Howell SL (1972) Nature New Biology 235:85
15. Orci L, Lambert, AE, Kanazawa Y, Amherdt M, Rouiller C, Renold AE (1971) J Cell Biol 50:565-582
16. Habener JF, Potts JT Jr (1979) Endocrinology 104:265-275
17. Eipper BA, Mains RE (1980) Endocrine Reviews 1:1-27
18. Steiner DF (1967) Trans. N.Y. Acad. Sci. USA, Ser. II 30:60-68
19. Potts JT Jr, Kronenberg HM, Rosenblatt M (1982) Adv Prot Chem 35:323-395
20. Dorling PR, Quinn PS, Judah JD (1975) Biochem J 152:341-348
21. Gainer H, Sarne Y, Brownstein MJ (1977) J Cell Biol 73:366-381
22. Sly WS, Fischer HD (1982) J Cell Biochem 18:67-85
23. Brown WJ, Farquhar MG (1984) Cell 36:295-307
24. Gumbiner B, Kelly RB (1981) Proc Natl Acad Sci USA 78:318-322
25. Moore H-PH, Walker MD, Lee F, Kelly, RB (1983) Cell 35:531-538
26. Palmiter RD, Norstedt G, Gelinas RE, Hammer RE, Brinster RL (1983) Science 222:809-814
27. Powers CA, Nasjletti A (1983) Endocrinology 112:1194-1200
28. Richards RI, Catanzaro DF, Mason AJ, Morris BJ, Baxter JD, Shine J (1982) J Biol Chem 257:2758-2761
29. Pinkus GS, Maier M, ole-MoiYoi O, Austen KF, Spragg J (1983) In: Fritz, Back, Dietze, and Haberland (eds) KININS-III, Pt. A. Plenum Publishing Co., pp 367-376
30. Loh, YP, et al This volume
31. Docherty K, Carroll R, Steiner DF (1983) Proc Natl Acad Sci USA 80:3245-3249
32. Docherty K, Hutton JC, Steiner DF (1984) J Biol Chem 259:6041-6044
33. Julius D, Brake A, Blair L, Kunisawa R, Thorner J (1984) Cell, in press
34. Mizuno K, Matsuo H (1984) Nature 309:558-560
35. Barrett AJ, Kirschke H (1981) Method in Enzymol 80:535-561
36. Neurath H (1984) Science 224:350-357
37. Recklies, AD, Mort JS, Poole AR (1982) Cancer Res 42:1026-1032
38. Mort JS, Leduc MS, Recklies AD (1983) Biochem et Biophys Acta 755:369-375
39. Halban PA, Wollheim CB (1980) J Biol Chem 255:6003-6006
40 Orci L, Ravazzola M, Amherdt M, Yanaihara C, Yanaihara N, Halban P, Renold AE, Perrelet A (1984) J Cell Biol 98:222-228
41. Hook VYH, Eiden LE, Brownstein MJ (1982) Nature 295:341-342
42. Fricker LD, Snyder SH (1982) Proc Natl Acad Sci USA 79:3886-3890
43. Docherty K, Hutton JC (1983) FEBS Letters 162:137-141
44. Kreil G, Mollay C, Hutticher A, Vilas U, Haiml L (1983) In: Sund H, Veeger C (eds) Mobility and Recognition in Cell Biology. Walter de Gruyter, Berlin, pp 471-484
45. Kurjan J, Herskowitz I (1982) Cell 30:933-943
46. Julius D, Blair L, Brake A, Sprague G, Thorner J (1983) Cell 32:839-852
47. Virji MAG, Vassalli J-D, Estensen RD, Reich E (1980) Proc Natl Acad Sci USA 77:875-879

Dr. K. Docherty's present address: The Department of Medicine, University of Birmingham, Queen Elizabeth Hospital, Birmingham, B15 2TH, United Kingdom

Endocrinology
F. Labrie, L. Proulx, eds.

PROTEOLYTIC PROCESSING OF PRO-OPIOMELANOCORTIN BY AN UNIQUE LYS-ARG SPECIFIC CONVERTING ENZYME FROM BOVINE PARS INTERMEDIA SECRETORY VESICLES

Y. PENG LOH, DAVID C. PARISH AND RENU TUTEJA

Section on Cellular Neurobiology, Laboratory of Neurochemistry and Neuroimmunology, National Institute of Child Health and Human Development, National Institutes of Health, Bethesda, Md. 20205, USA

INTRODUCTION

Pro-opiomelanocortin (POMC), also referred to as pro-opiocortin and ACTH/endorphin prohormone is synthesized by the anterior and the intermediate lobe of the pituitary. This prohormone is processed within secretory vesicles (1,2) to form adrenocorticotropin (ACTH), β-lipotropin (β-LPH) and β-endorphin in the anterior and intermediate lobes of the pituitary (3-5). In the intermediate lobe the ACTH appears to be further processed to α-MSH ($AcACTH_{1-13}NH_2$)(3-5). In addition, a 16,000 molecular weight (16K, K=1000) N-terminal glycopeptide (pro-γ-MSH) is cleaved from the prohormone (Fig. 1). Like other prohormones and pro-neuropeptides (7-10), the hormone sequences within POMC which are to be cleaved are flanked by pairs of basic residues, the most common being Lys-Arg pairs. Processing of these hormones to the active hormones involves cleavages at the paired basic residues. In this paper we describe an unique protease from bovine pituitary pars intermedia (intermediate lobe) secretory vesicles, which cleaves the Lys-Arg pairs of POMC.

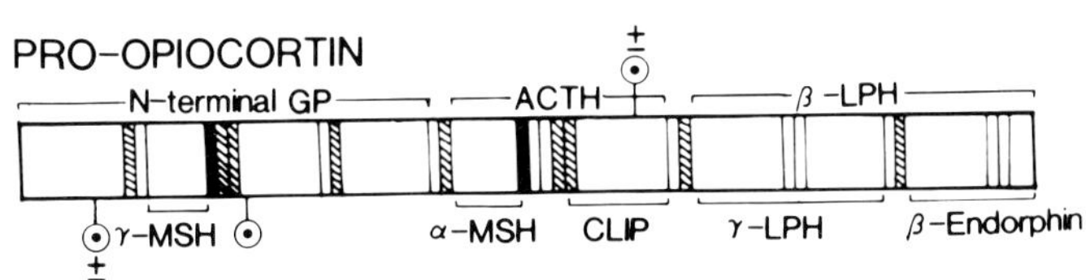

Figure 1. Diagramatic representation of the structure of bovine POMC (6) showing the paired basic amino acid residues(lysine □ , arginine ▨), the glycine residues (■) located at the N-termini of the pairs of basic amino acids, and glycosylation sites ⊙.

MATERIAL AND METHODS

<u>Preparation of bovine pars intermedia secretory vesicles.</u> Bovine pituitaries were collected fresh from the slaughter house and secretory vesicles were prepared from the pars intermedia by differential centrifugation followed by metri-

zamide gradient centrifugation (11). Analysis of the vesicle preparation using different markers for vesicles (radioimmunoassayable α-MSH), mitochondria (monoamine oxidase) and lysosomes (β-glucuronidase) revealed a 94-fold purification of vesicles with respect to lysosomes.

Partial purification of POMC converting enzyme. Secretory vesicles were lysed osmotically and by freezing and thawing. The lysate was centrifuged and the supernatant separated on a G-75 Sephadex column. Fractions (1.6 ml) eluted from the column with 0.1M ammonium formate buffer (pH 7.4) were assayed for PCE activity. Fractions containing PCE activity were pooled and further purified on a concanavalin A (Con A) affinity column. Fractions eluted from the Con A column were assayed for PCE activity. All the activity were found in the Con A bound fractions (Parish et al., in preparation). The Con A affinity purified PCE was used for the studies described in this paper.

Preparation of [^{3}H] amino acid labeled POMC substrate. Radioactive POMC was prepared by incubating mouse neurointermediate lobes in medium (12) containing [^{3}H] phenylalanine, [^{3}H]arginine or [^{3}H]lysine, for 1h at 37° (12). Lobes were homogenized in 0.1N HCl. Labeled POMC was purified from the homogenate by acid-urea gel electrophoresis as previously described (12).

Assay of POMC converting enzyme (PCE). Labeled POMC was incubated with Con A affinity purified PCE from the soluble fraction of bovine intermediate lobe secretory vesicles for 5h at 37°C in a pH 4.0 Na Citrate buffer. The reaction was stopped by the addition of HCl, to a final concentration of 0.1N. The products cleaved by PCE were identified by their immunological properties (immunoprecipitation by specific antisera to the N terminus of ACTH and β-endorphin), molecular weight and co-electrophoresis on acid-urea gels with synthetic peptide markers and products synthesized by the mouse pars intermedia *in situ* (2,13).

RESULTS

Con A affinity purified POMC converting enzyme (PCE) was assayed for activity at various pHs with [^{3}H] labeled mouse POMC as substrate. PCE was more active at acidic pHs (pH 4.0-5.0) than at neutral pH (Loh & Parish, unpublished data). When [^{3}H] phenylalanine labeled mouse POMC was incubated at pH 4.0 in the absence of PCE no processing occurred. However, incubation of [^{3}H]phenylalanine labeled mouse POMC with Con A affinity purified PCE resulted in the formation of several cleavage products: 21-23K ACTH, 13K and 4.5K ACTH, β-LPH, β-endorphin, γ-LPH and 16K glycopeptide (Table I). Since the amino acid sequence of mouse POMC is known, it is possible to determine whether the cpm in the different [^{3}H]phenylanine labeled cleavage products have a stoichiometric relationship consistent with the theoretical one, based on the known number of phenylalanines in the products. Table I shows that the experimentally determined ratios of cpm in 16K GP: (13K + 4.5K ACTH); β-END: γ-LPH and (21-23K + 4.5K + 13K ACTH): (β-END + γ-LPH + β-LPH) are close to that of the theoretical values, further supporting immunological and size identification of the products. The products formed from mouse POMC suggest that cleavages occurred at Lys-Arg pairs of POMC (see Fig. 1). C- and N-terminal analysis of the cleavage products confirmed that the PCE cleaved at the Lys-Arg pairs (Loh & Parish, in preparation).

TABLE I

STOICHIOMETRIC RATIOS OF [^{3}H]PHENYLALANINE CPM IN PRODUCTS CLEAVED FROM [^{3}H] PHENYLALANINE LABELED MOUSE POMC BY PCE.

POMC/Products	cpm in peak	Σcpm in products	No. Phe/ molecule	Theoretical* Ratio	Experimental** Ratio
POMC (t = 0h)	1145		9		
Products formed:					
13K ACTH	54		3		
4.5K ACTH	28		3		
Σ(13K+4.5K ACTH)[a]		82	3	a/b = 1	a/b = 0.98
16K GP[b]	84		3		
21-23K ACTH	617		6		
Σ[(21-23K+13K+ 4.5K)ACTH+16K GP][c]		783	6	c/d = 2	c/d = 2.32
β-END[e]	174		2	e/f = 2	e/f = 2.07
γ-END[f]	84		1		
β-LPH	80		3		
Σ(β-END+γ-LPH+ β-LPH)[d]		338	3		

* Theoretical ratio = ratio of the theoretical number of phenylalanines (phe; determined from the primary sequence) in each part of the POMC molecule indicated.

** Experimental ratio = ratio of the [^{3}H]phenylanine cpm found in different (or sum of) immunologically identified products (denoted by superscript letters) cleaved from POMC by PCE.

DISCUSSION

The results presented show the presence of a prohormone (POMC) converting enzyme in bovine pars intermedia secretory vesicles that cleaves mouse POMC at Lys-Arg pairs to yield the appropriate products seen in the mouse pars intermedia *in situ* (2). PCE is a glycoprotein and has an acidic pH optimum, consistent with the acidic intravesicular pH of these secretory vesicles (11). The subcellular localization in secretory vesicles (the site of prohormone processing), acidic pH optimum and cleavage specificity of the PCE described thus fulfill the minimum criteria (14) for a physiologically relevant prohormone converting enzyme.

A similar activity has also been found in bovine neural lobe secretory vesicles. The neural lobe PCE activity was shown to cleave rat pro-vasopressin to yield neurophysin-glycopeptide and a vasopressin-like peptide (Parish et al, in preparation), consistent with a cleavage of the prohormone at a pair of basic residues. However, the single Arg residue between the neurophysin and the glycopeptide was not cleaved by PCE.

The PCE activities from both the intermediate and neural lobe secretory vesicles have now been purified to apparent homogeneity (Parish et al, in preparation). Protease inhibitor studies suggest that the intermediate lobe and neural lobe PCE are unique enzymes distinct from trypsin or lysosomal cathepsin B.

ACKNOWLEDGMENTS

We thank the National Pituitary Agency, Baltimore, Md., for antiserum to ACTH and Drs. R.E. Mains and B.A. Eipper, Johns Hopkin University, Baltimore, Md. for antiserum to β-endorphin.

REFERENCES

1. Glembotski, C (1981) J Biol Chem 256:7433-7439
2. Loh YP, Gritsch HA (1981) Europ J Cell Biol 26:177-183
3. Eipper BA, Mains RE (1980) Endocrine Rev 1:1 -27
4. Herbert E, Budarf M, Phillips M, Rosa P, Policastro P, Ortes E, Roberts J, Seidah NG, Chretien M (1980) Ann New York Acad Sci 343:79-93
5. Crine P, Seidah NG, Heanotte L, Chretien M (1980) Can J Biochem 58:1318-1322
6. Nakanishi S, Inoue A, Kita T, Nakamura M, Chang ACY, Cohen S, Numa S (1979) Nature 275:423-427
7. Gubler U, Seeburg P, Hoffman BJ, Gage LP, Udenfriend S (1982) Nature 295: 206-208
8. Kakidani H, Furutani Y, Takahashi H, Noda M, Morimoto Y, Hirose T,Asai M, Inayama S, Nakanishi S, Numa S (1982) Nature 298:245-249
9. Land H, Schutz G, Schmale H, Richter D (1982) Nature 295:299-303
10. Chan SJ, Keim P, Steiner DF (1976) Proc Natl Acad Sci 73: 1964-1968
11. Loh YP, Tam WWH, Russell JT (1984) J Biol Chem In press
12. Loh YP, Gainer H (1982) Proc Natl Acad Sci USA 79:108-112
13. Loh YP, Gritsch HA, Chang TL (1982) Peptides 3:397-404
14. Docherty K, Steiner DF (1982) Ann Rev Physiol 44:625-638

19. The Renin-Angiotensin System and Hypertension

Endocrinology
F. Labrie, L. Proulx, eds.

ADVANCES IN THE BIOCHEMISTRY OF THE RENIN ANGIOTENSIN SYSTEM . . . INTRACELLULAR RENIN ANGIOTENSIN SYSTEM IN RAT ADRENAL ZONA GLOMERULOSA CELLS AND RAT TESTICULAR LEYDIG CELLS

TADASHI INAGAMI, KAILASH PANDEY, MITSUAKI NAKAMARU, JAMES C. McKENZIE, KUNIO S. MISONO, KIYOKO NARUSE AND MITSUHIDE NARUSE
Department of Biochemistry and Hypertension Center, Vanderbilt University School of Medicine, Nashville, TN 37232 USA

INTRODUCTION

Renin immunoreactive to anti-renal renin antibodies has been found in many types of tissues (1) often coxisting with angiotensins. To demonstrate that the tissue renin-angiotensin is not due to uptake from or contamination of blood, cloned and cultured cell lines were used to demonstrate the intracellular generation of angiotensin II in renin containing cells (2-5). These cells growing in culture are mostly transformed and may not represent normal conditions. We examined normal Leydig cells and adrenal glomerulosa cells as models of steroidogenic system for the studies of intracellular angiotensin forming system and its regulation.

MATERIALS AND METHODS

Specific renin activity was determined using anti-renin antibody to distinguish it from nonspecfic renin-like activity of protease according to the method described previously (3). Angiotensins were separated by HPLC according to Ganten et al. (6), and determined by radioimmunoassay for angiotensins I and II. Male Sprague-Dawley rats (200 g) were maintained on drinking water containing 3% KCl and 5% glucose for one week or tap water (control) with or without captopril (100 mg/kg/body weight). Plasma samples were collected by decapitation and adrenals were obtained after saline perfusion. Testicular Leydig cells were isolated after collagenase digestion of testis and centrifugation on discontinuous density gradients of metrizamide (7). Renin was detected immunohistochemically in paraffin sections by the avidin-biotin method using anti-rat renin antibodies.

RESULTS

Both adrenal capsules and testicular Leydig cells were found to contain immunosuppressible renin activity and angiotensin II. Zona glomerulosa cells of potassium fed rats, rat on regular chow and Leydig cells were stained positively for renin. Renin in these extrarenal steroidogenic tissues were under acute control of various factors. For example, Leydig cell renin was markedly (30-fold) stimulated by hCG.

Testicular Leydig cells were found to produce high levels of angiotensins which ranged 30-40 pg/10^6 cells for angiotensin II and 150-200 pg/10^6 cells for angiotensin I, respectively. A large portion of angiotensin II was found in culture medium but little, if any, renin was present in the medium. Zona glomerulosa cells were found to contain angiotensin II at 100 pg/10^6 cells.

As shown in Table I adrenal capsular renin was markedly stimulated by potassium feeding which increased the plasma potassium level from 4.5 to 4.7mEq/l. The high potassium loading caused a 10-fold increase in adrenal renin and a 3-fold increase in adrenal aldosterone while causing little change in plasma renin. Captopril reversed the potassium-induced elevation of adrenal aldosterone to the control level, and reduced adrenal angiotensin II to 20-25% of the normal level. Potassium slightly reduced plasma renin.

TABLE I

Effects of Potassium and Captopril on Renin in Rat Adrenal Capsules

Condition	n	Adrenal Renin (ngAI/mg prot/h)	Adrenal Aldosterone (n/mg prot)	Plasma Renin Activity (ngAI/ml/n)
Control	6	2.7 ± 0.2	24.2 ± 1.1	3.0 ± 0.4
Potassium Loaded	6	28.2 ± 1.5**	69.8 ± 8.5**	2.5 ± 0.3*
Captopril	6	6.1 ± 1.0**	21.0 ± 9.6	6.8 ± 0.5**
Potassium + Captopril	5	20.3 ± 2.9**	29.6 ± 2.8*	8.2 ± 1.9**

Values are means ± SEM.
* P 0.05
** P 0.01 vs. control

DISCUSSION

The coexistence of renin and angiotensins in rat Leydig cells and adrenal capsular cells indicates the intracellular production of angiotensin II in those steroidogenic cells. The presence of angiotensin II and absence of renin in the culture medium of Leydig cells (analogous to neuroblastoma cells (2)) indicate that angiotensin II produced in the cell is secreted to perform autocrine or paracrine function whereas renin catalyzes angiotensin production within the cell. The strong effect of hCG on Leydig cell renin, and nephrectomy (8), sodium loading or depletion (9,10,11) and potassium loading (11,12) on adrenal capsular renin indicate metabolically active roles of renin and angiotensins in these tissues.

The mechanism of the control and the function of the adrenal renin has not been clear. Although some correlation has been reported between the increment of adrenal renin and adrenal aldosterone (12), causal relationship has not been known. The present intervention studies using captopril demonstrated that potassium induces increase in adrenal renin and aldosterone but not in plasma renin. This increase of adrenal aldosterone is normalized by captopril under the high potassium load. These observations indicate the potassium stimulation may be mediated by the intracellular angiotensin II produced in the adrenal. The fact that plasma renin remains below a normal level in the potassium fed animals indicates that plasma renin-angiotensin may not play a major role in mediating the potassium stimulated increase in adrenal aldosterone.

Analogous to the examples of Leydig cells and adrenal glomerulosa cells, renin in several extrarenal tissues have been shown to produce angiotensin II. It is intriguing to extraporate the present observations to other tissues and propose that these tissues release angiotensin II rather than renin. The release of a small amount of renin to plasma may not effectively influence the local renin concentration. On the other hand angiotensin II released locally seems to be able to influence cells in the immediate vicinity of the angiotensin generating cells or the angiotensin generating cells themselves.

ACKNOWLEDGMENT

This study was supported by Research and Training Grants HL-14192, HL-22288, HL-24112 and HL-07323 from NIH, Grant-in-Aid 82-1057 from American Heart Association.

REFERENCES

1. Naruse M, Naruse K, Inagaki T, Inagami T (1984) Hypertension 6:275
2. Okamura T, Clemens DL, Inagami T (1981) Proc Natl Acad Sci USA 78:6940
3. Fishman MC, Zimmerman EA, Slater EE (1981) Science 214:921
4. Rightsel WA, Okamura T, Inagami T, Pitcock JA, Takii Y, Brooks B, Brown P, Muirhead EE (1982) Circ Res 50:822
5. Okamura T, Clemens DL, Inagami T (1984) Neurosci Lett in press
6. Ganten D, Hermann K, Bayer C, Unger T, Lang RE (1983) Science 221:4613
7. O'Shaunessy PJ, Wong KL, Payne AH (1981) Endocrinology 109:1061
8. Naruse M, Inagami T (1982) Proc Natl Acad Sci USA 79:3295
9. Aguilera G, Fujita K, Shirar A, Catt KJ (1980) Proceedings of the VI International Congress of Endocrinology, Melbourne, Australia:389

10. Doi Y, Atarashi K, Franco-Saenz R, Mulrow PJ, (1983) Clin Exp Hypertens A5:1119
11. Nakamaru M, Naruse M, Naruse K, Shizume K, Inagami T (1984) Fed Proc 43:1077
12. Doi, Y, Atarashi E, Franco-Saenz R, Mulrow PJ, (1984) Hypertension 6 (suppl I):I-124

© 1984 Elsevier Science Publishers B.V.
Endocrinology
F. Labrie, L. Proulx, eds.

ACTIONS OF ANGIOTENSIN II ON THE BRAIN

IAN A. REID

Department of Physiology, University of California, San Francisco, California 94143, U.S.A.

INTRODUCTION

Angiotensin II acts on the brain to produce a wide variety of cardiovascular, behavioral, endocrine and renal effects. These include elevation of blood pressure, stimulation of drinking and sodium appetite, increased secretion of several pituitary hormones including vasopressin, oxytocin, ACTH and LH, inhibition of renin release by the kidneys, and natriuresis (for reviews see 1-4). The renin-angiotensin system is therefore in a position to exert important effects on blood pressure regulation, fluid and electrolyte intake and excretion, and other functions.

During recent years, there have been significant advances in our understanding of the central actions of angiotensin II. The purpose of this brief review is to summarize the progress.

RELATION OF ANGIOTENSIN II TO THE BRAIN

Angiotensin II is a polar molecule and is therefore excluded from most parts of the brain by the blood-brain barrier. Initially, therefore, it was difficult to understand how blood-borne angiotensin could produce such a variety of central actions. This problem was subsequently resolved with the finding that the receptors for many of the actions of angiotensin are contained in the circumventricular organs, specialized areas of the brain which lack a blood-brain barrier. These include the area postrema (AP), subfornical organ (SFO), organum vasculosum of the lamina terminalis (OVLT) and median eminence (ME) (5).

It has been postulated that angiotensin II is synthesized not only in the circulation by the renal renin-angiotensin system but also in the central nervous system by a brain renin-angiotensin system (6). This proposal originated with the finding that the enzymes and substrates required for the formation of angiotensin II - renin or renin-like enzymes, angiotensinogen and converting enzyme - are present in the brain (6). This concept has proven to be a controversial one and, despite much research effort, definite evidence for the existence of a functional brain renin-angiotensin system is still lacking. The problems have been discussed in detail elsewhere (6-8). One of the major problems is that it has proven extremely difficult to demonstrate the presence of angiotensin II in the brain. Several investigators have found angiotensin-like immunoreactivity in brain extracts, but there are conflicting reports concerning the biochemical nature of this material (9-12).

Another reason for postulating the existence of a brain renin-angiotensin system is that angiotensin II produces such a variety of effects when administered centrally. However, these responses are, in general, the same as those produced by blood-borne angiotensin, and there is evidence that they may be mediated via the same receptors. For example, some of the responses to systemically-administered angiotensin can be blocked by intraventricular injection of saralasin and other angiotensin receptor antagonists (1). Moreover, studies in this laboratory have shown that the binding of systemically-administered radiolabeled angiotensin II to the circumventricular organs can be blocked or reduced by intraventricular injection of saralasin (13). On the basis of these observations, it appears that many of the responses elicited by centrally-administered angiotensin II are mediated via the circumventricular organs, and it is therefore not necessary to postulate the existence of a brain renin-angiotensin system to explain their significance.

In the remainder of this review, current concepts concerning three of the central actions of angiotensin II - elevation of blood pressure and stimulation of vasopressin and ACTH secretion - are summarized.

CENTRAL ACTIONS OF ANGIOTENSIN II

Blood Pressure

Angiotensin II increases blood pressure when injected into the vertebral or carotid arteries, the cerebral ventricles, or specific brain regions (1-3,14-19). In the dog, the blood pressure response to intravertebral angiotensin II is mediated via receptors located in the AP (2,3). With low doses of angiotensin, the increase in blood pressure results from an increase in cardiac output secondary to withdrawal of vagal tone to the heart (15). With higher doses, total peripheral resistance is also increased (2). The blood pressure response to intraventricular angiotensin is not mediated via the AP and recent evidence suggests a role for the OVLT (16). The responses to intraventricular angiotensin result from an increase in sympathetic discharge (3).

In the rat, the AP is not an important central site of action of angiotensin on blood pressure and current evidence indicates that the SFO and OVLT play more important roles (17,18). Depending on the route of administration, centrally-mediated pressor responses to angiotensin in the rat can result from sympathetically-mediated vasoconstriction or from increased release of vasopressin (3,19).

There is evidence that the centrally-mediated pressor action of angiotensin is important in the physiological regulation of arterial pressure as well as in the development and maintenance of some forms of hypertension (2,3,17).

Vasopressin Secretion

Several investigators have reported that angiotensin II stimulates the release of vasopressin when injected into the cerebral ventricles (4). This stimulation has been observed in a number of species including the dog and rat, can be related to the dose of angiotensin, and occurs following acute or chronic administration of the peptide. There have also been reports that angiotensin stimulates vasopressin release when administered systemically in the dog, rat, and human, but there is disagreement concerning the dose of angiotensin required to produce this stimulatory effect (1,4,14). In some studies, systemically-administered angiotensin has failed to stimulate vasopressin secretion (4).

Several factors appear to be responsible for the variability in the vasopressin response to angiotensin II. Species differences are probably important, and it appears that the rat is less sensitive than other species. Another important factor is the use of anesthetics which reduce or abolish the stimulatory effect of angiotensin on vasopressin secretion (4). The state of water balance may also be important because there is evidence that there is an interaction between osmolality and angiotensin in the control of vasopressin secretion (4). A final factor which may influence the vasopressin response to angiotensin II is blood pressure. It is known that elevation of blood pressure suppresses vasopressin secretion, and recent evidence from this laboratory indicates that the increase in blood pressure produced by angiotensin tends to counteract its stimulatory effect on vasopressin secretion (20). It is important to note that in most situations where renin secretion is stimulated and endogenous angiotensin II levels are increased, blood pressure is either normal or low so that the stimulatory effect of angiotensin on vasopressin secretion would be unopposed.

At the present time, it is not clear if the renin-angiotensin system plays a physiological role in the control of vasopressin secretion. However, current evidence indicates that the renin-angiotensin system does not contribute significantly to the stimulation of vasopressin secretion that occurs during hemorrhage, postural changes, caval constriction or water deprivation (1,4).

ACTH Secretion

Angiotensin II has been reported to stimulate the release of ACTH when injected intravenously, into the carotid arteries or into the cerebral ventricles (1,14,21). Angiotensin also increases ACTH release when injected directly into the anterior pituitary (21) or when added to pituitary cells *in vitro* (22). As in the case of vasopressin, there are discrepancies in the literature concerning the dose of angiotensin required to stimulate ACTH secretion. The situation is particularly confusing in the human where angiotensin has variously been reported to increase or inhibit ACTH secretion (23).

Information concerning the site of action of angiotensin II on ACTH secretion is available. As noted above, there is evidence that angiotensin can stimulate ACTH release by direct action on the pituitary (21,22). However, at least a component of the response appears to be mediated by the ME, apparently via the release of CRF (24). Finally, part of the ACTH response to angiotensin may be mediated via vasopressin which has CRF activity and potentiates the ACTH response to CRF (25).

Recent studies in this laboratory have shown that the pressor action of angiotensin tends to counteract its stimulatory effect on ACTH secretion (26). Therefore, the ability of angiotensin to stimulate ACTH release may have been underestimated in the past. Nevertheless, there is currently little evidence that the renin-angiotensin system plays a role in the physiological control of ACTH secretion. On the other hand, evidence has been presented that in high renin forms of human hypertension, the renin-angiotensin system may interact with the pituitary-adrenal axis to stimulate the secretion of cortisol (27).

ACKNOWLEDGMENTS

Research in the author's laboratory was supported by U.S.P.H.S. Grants AM06704 and HL29714.

REFERENCES

1. Ramsay DJ (1982) In: Ganong WF, Martini L (eds) Frontiers in Neuroendocrinology. Raven Press, New York, pp 263-285
2. Ferrario CM, Gildenberg PL, McCubbin JW (1972) Circ Res 30: 257
3. Severs WB, Daniels-Severs AE (1973) Pharmacol Rev 25: 415
4. Share L (1979) Fed Proc 38: 2267
5. Weindl A (1973) In: Ganong WF, Martini L (eds) Frontiers in Neuroendocrinology. Oxford University Press, New York, pp 3-32
6. Ganten D, Printz M, Phillips MI, Scholkens BA (1982) The Renin-Angiotensin System in the Brain. Springer-Verlag, Berlin, Heidelberg
7. Reid IA (1979) Fed Proc 38: 2255
8. Reid IA, Brownfield MS (1982) In: Ganten D, Printz M, Phillips MI, Scholkens BA (eds) The Renin-Angiotensin System in the Brain. Springer-Verlag, Berlin, Heidelberg, pp 284-293
9. Ganten D, Hermann K, Bayer C, Unger Th, Lang RE (1983) Science 221: 869
10. Husain A, Bumpus FM, Smeby RR, Brosnihan KB, Khosla MC, Speth RC, Ferrario CM (1983) Circ Res 52: 460
11. Meyer DK, Phillips MI, Eiden L (1982) J Neurochem 38: 816
12. Semple PF, Macrae WA, Morton JJ (1980) Clin Sci 59: 61s
13. Van Houten M, Mangiapane ML, Reid IA, Ganong WF (1983) Neuroscience 10: 1421
14. Reid IA, Brooks VL, Rudolph CD, Keil LC (1982) Am J Physiol 243: R82
15. Scroop GC, Lowe RD (1969) Clin Sci 37: 605

16. Marson O, Chernicky CL, Barnes KL, Ferrario CM (1983) Neuroscience Abstracts 9: 544

17. Buggy J, Fink GD, Johnson AK, Brody MJ (1977) Circ Res 40 (Supp I): I-110

18. Mangiapane ML, Simpson JB (1980) Am J Physiol 239: R382

19. Lappe RW, Brody MJ (1984) Am J Physiol 246: R56

20. Brooks VL, Keil LC, Reid IA (1983) Physiologist 26: A10

21. Maran JW, Yates FE (1977) Am J Physiol 233: E273

22. Gaillard RC, Grossman A, Gillies G, Rees LH, Besser GM (1981) Clin Endocrinol 15: 573

23. Semple PF, Buckingham JC, Mason PA, Fraser R (1979) Clin Endocrinol 10: 137

24. Rivier C, Vale W (1983) Peptides 7: 253

25. Rivier C, Vale W (1983) Endocrinology 113: 939

26. Brooks VL, Reid IA (1983) Fed Proc 42: 590

27. Atlas SA, Case DB, Sealey, JE, Laragh JH (1981) Clin Sci 61: 265s

© 1984 Elsevier Science Publishers B.V.
Endocrinology
F. Labrie, L. Proulx, eds.

RENIN: A PRESSOR HORMONE

MALCOLM TREE, JEHOIADA J. BROWN, ROBERT FRASER, BRENDA J. LECKIE, ANTHONY F. LEVER, JAMES J. MORTON, J. IAN S. ROBERTSON, PETER F. SEMPLE

MRC Blood Pressure Unit, Western Infirmary, Glasgow, G11 6NT, U.K.

Renin, a blood-borne hormone

In 1898 Tigerstedt and Bergman (1) extracted a potent, heat labile, non-diffusible, pressor material from the renal cortex of the rabbit. On intravenous infusion it raised blood pressure. They named the material 'renin' and speculated that it was formed in the kidney and released into blood where, as a chemical messenger, it produced its effect on blood pressure by constricting blood vessels possibly through a nervous mechanism. Their speculation, the subject of this review, puts them among the founding fathers of endocrinology (Brown-Sequard, Oliver and Schafer).

The enzymic nature of renin was not recognised until 1939 (see ref. 2). It is an aspartyl proteinase formed in the juxtaglomerular apparatus of the renal cortex, mainly in the afferent glomerular arteriole. Immunoperoxidase techniques stain both storage granules and endoplasmic reticulum in the juxtaglomerular cells suggesting that renin is synthesised as well as stored in these cells (3).

Renal renin exists in active and inactive forms. Both have been purified (4,5). Active and inactive renin are released from the kidney into blood. In man active renin cleaves a Leu-Val bond in the N-terminal sequence of a plasma protein substrate to produce the decapeptide, angiotensin I (6). The scissile bond in the corresponding substrates for horse, pig and rat renin is Leu-Leu (7). Angiotensin I is inactive biologically, but undergoes rapid enzymic conversion to the active octapeptide, angiotensin II. All components of this mechanism - renin, renin-substrate, angiotensin I, converting enzyme and angiotensin II circulate in plasma (8).

Control of angiotensin II in blood by renin release: an unusual mechanism for a peptide hormone.

The biological effects of blood-borne peptide hormones are regulated mainly by change in their plasma concentration and plasma peptide concentration is usually regulated by change in the rate of synthesis and release of preformed peptide from the gland. ACTH, TSH, vasopressin, prolactin, gonadotrophic hormone, growth hormone and insulin are all controlled in this way.

Angiotensin II is an interesting exception. Although it derives ultimately from renal renin, it is not released from the kidney as preformed angiotensin II. Indeed, the venoarterial difference for angiotensin II is negative; more angiotensin II enters the kidney in arterial blood than leaves in the renal vein (9). It is the rate of release of renin from the kidney which determines the plasma concentration of renin (10) and thence the plasma concentrations of angiotensin I and angiotensin II. In most physiological and pathological circumstances the plasma concentrations of all three substances change in parallel (8). When plasma renin is inhibited plasma concentrations of angiotensin I and angiotensin II decrease (11). Thus, the activity of blood-borne angiotensin II is regulated by release of the parent enzyme rather than by release of preformed peptide.

There are two possible explanations for this unusual mechanism. Like other chemical messengers, renin may have evolved as a local-tissue hormone acting close to its site of production. Only later in evolution did it enter blood to produce an effect at a distance. In the mammal both actions of renin have been preserved. Renin is likely to be an intrarenal hormone (12) as well as a blood-borne hormone with actions on arterial pressure and corticosteroid secretion (13). Need to maintain this dual role may be the reason why renin, rather than angiotensin II, is released from the kidney. Renin has a relatively long half-life, between 15 and 30 minutes. Because of this, release of renin from the kidney can sustain a plasma concentration of angiotensin II over a wide physiological and pathological range with a renal venoarterial difference for renin as small as +25% (10). Thus, renin can be released into renal blood without generating a large excess of angiotensin II within the kidney. Angiotensin II on the other hand has a short half-life, less than 2 minutes. For release of angiotensin II from the kidney to maintain a peripheral plasma concentration of the peptide in the lower part of the physiological range (say 10pg/ml) would require a secretion rate of 1ng of angiotensin II/kg/min in the conscious sodium-replete dog (derived from infusion data in ref. 14). Allowing a renal plasma flow of 200ml/min for a 20kg dog, this rate of secretion could only be maintained by a renal venoarterial difference for angiotensin II of 1,100%. When arterial angiotensin II is 10pg/ml, renal venous angiotensin II would have to be 110pg/ml. Thus, a normal plasma concentration of angiotensin II in peripheral blood could only be sustained by a supranormal concentration of the peptide in renal blood. It follows that angiotensin II could not influence arterial pressure or corticosteroid secretion as a blood-borne hormone without at the same time producing marked vasoconstriction within the kidney. The need to dissociate renal and extrarenal effects may be the reason why renin rather than angiotensin II is released from the kidney.

A second explanation for release of renin is that the enzyme may be taken up from blood into the vessel wall where it produces angiotensin I and angiotensin II locally with vasoconstrictor effect (15). A mechanism of this sort could not operate by angiotensin II release from the kidney.

Renin and blood pressure

There are several ways in which renin might influence blood pressure: a local action of renin within the kidney may alter sodium excretion and thereby influence blood pressure (12). Angiotensin II entering the kidney in arterial blood may have a similar effect. Best known is the direct vasoconstrictor effect of angiotensin II. In a normal man on a normal dietary intake of sodium, a 5-fold increase in the plasma concentration of angiotensin II produces a small direct pressor effect (13). Interestingly, a 5-fold decrease of plasma angiotensin II concentration has less effect, possibly becasue the dose-response for angiotensin II and arterial pressure is sigmoid in shape and in normal circumstances angiotensin II concentration is at the foot of this curve and thus in a position where an increase will raise blood pressure, but a decrease will have no effect. If this is so, the direct vasoconstrictor effect of plasma angiotensin II is less important in the minute-to-minute regulation of arterial pressure, but more likely to be important in the maintenance of arterial pressure in circumstances such as sodium depletion when blood pressure would otherwise fall. For example, large falls of blood pressure do occur in the sodium-deplete state when inhibitors of renin and angiotensin I converting enzyme are given (Szelke et al. to be published).

The direct effect is not the only action of angiotensin II on blood pressure. A small increase of circulating angiotensin II concentration (4-fold in the rat) can, if sustained for 7 days, produce a large slowly progressive rise of blood pressure (16). Since this action occurs at a much lower level than the direct pressor effect, it could be important in the long-term regulation of arterial pressure. There is evidence from at least one form of hypertension, renin-secreting tumour, that it plays a major role in causing the hypertension (13).

Conclusions

We have dealt here with renin and angiotensin as a blood-borne pressor mechanism. There is a large and interesting literature on the possibility that blood pressure is also influenced by angiotensin generated locally by renin in blood vessels and brain. Neither possibility detracts from the correctness of Tigerstedt and Bergman's original prediction: renin is a blood-borne pressor mechanism; it is released from the kidney into blood; it does control blood pressure and it may as they suggested do so by a nervous mechanism.

References

1. Tigerstedt R, Bergman, P.G. (1898) Skand Arch Physiol **8:**223

2. Pickering GW (1968) High Blood Pressure (2nd ed.) JA Churchill Ltd. London

3. Lindop G, Reid R, Downie T, Corvol P, Menard J, Brown W, Brown JJ, Leckie B, Lever AF, Lucie NP, Robertson JIS (1983) In: Woolf N (ed) Biology and Pathology of the Vessel Wall. Praeger, London, pp 213-228

4. Galen FX, Devaux C, Guyenne TT, Menard J, Corvol P (1979) J Biol Chem **254:**4848-4855

5. McIntyre GH, Pau B, Leckie B, Hallett A, Szelke M (1984) J Hypertension (in press)

6. Tewksbury DA, Dart RA, Travis, J (1981) Biochem Biophys Res Commun **99:**1311-1315

7. Skeggs LT, Kahn JR, Lentz KE, Shumway NP (1957) J Exp Med **106:**439-453

8. Brown JJ, Leckie BJ, Lever AF, McIntyre G, Morton JJ, Semple PF, Robertson JIS (1983) In: Robertson JIS (ed) Handbook of Hypertension. Elsevier, Amsterdam, **1:**pp 278-323,

9. Semple PF, Cumming AMM, Millar JA (1979) Kidney Internat **15:**176-282

10. Hosie KF, Brown JJ, Harper AM, Lever AF, MacAdam RD, MacGregor J, Robertson JIS (1970) Clin Sci **38:**157-176

11. Tree M, Atrash B, Donovan B, Gamble J, Hallett A, Highes M, Jones DM, Leckie B, Lever AF, Morton JJ, Szelke M (1983) J Hypertension **1:**399-403

12. Levens NR, Peach MJ, Carey RM (1981) Circ Res **48:**157-167

13. Brown JJ, Casals-Stenzel J, Cumming AMM, Davies DL, Fraser R, Lever AF, Morton JJ, Semple PF, Tree M, Robertson JIS (1979) Hypertension **1:**159-179

14. Nicholls MG, Tree M, Brown JJ, Douglas BH, Fraser R, Hay GD, Lever AF, Morton JJ, Robertson JIS (1978) Endocrinology **102:**485-493

15. Swales JD (1979) Clin Sci **56:**293-298

16. Brown AJ, Casals-Stenzel J, Gofford S, Lever AF, Morton JJ (1981) Aner J Physiol **241:**H381-388

© 1984 Elsevier Science Publishers B.V.
Endocrinology
F. Labrie, L. Proulx, eds.

RENIN INHIBITORS AND ANGIOTENSIN-CONVERTING ENZYME INHIBITORS: RATIONALE AND COMPARISON OF RESULTS

VICTOR J. DZAU, M.D.

Division of Vascular Medicine and Atherosclerosis, Hypertension Unit, Brigham and Women's Hospital, Harvard Medical School, Boston MA U.S.A.

The renin angiotensin system play a central role in blood pressure regulation (1), Specific inhibition of this system is likely to play an important role in the therapy of hypertension. Since renin and angiotensin-converting enzyme (ACE) are key enzymes in the generation of angiotensin II, pharmacologic inhibition of these enzymes has become a major strategy in the development of anti-hypertensive drugs.

Inhibition of ACE (peptidyl dipeptidase) was first made possible by the discovery of the nonapeptide inhibitor (teprotide) in the snake venom of Barthrops Jararaca (1). Subsequently, an orally active ACE inhibitor, D-3-mercapto-2-methyl propanoyl-L-proline (captopril) was synthesized based on a hypothetical model of ACE extraporlated from the known properties of the active site of carboxypeptidase A (1). Captopril has been approved for clinical use. Recently, a series of substituted N-carboxymethyl-dipeptides have been synthesized (2). One of these compounds, enalapril (MK-421) has been employed for animal and clinical studies. Several other ACE inhibitors are also under active study. ACE inhibition results in a small depressor response in the sodium replete man but significantly lower blood pressure in the sodium deplete subject. ACE inhibitors are effective antihypertensive drugs. The magnitude of its acute depressor effect appears to correlate with pretreatment plasma renin activity (PRA)(1). However, patients with normal or low renin essential hypertension will also exhibit depressor responses but of lesser magnitudes. When combined with a diuretic, ACE inhibitors controlled the blood pressure (BP) of over 80% of patients with essential hypertension. It has been suggested that part of the hypotensive effect of captopril may be mediated by bradykinin, vasodilator prostaglandins or decreasedsympathetic or baroreceptor reflex activity (1). Whether these are universal effects of ACE inhibitors is unclear. Preliminary evidence suggests that prostaglandin accumulation may not occur with enalapril (3).

In addition to its effect on angiotensin I and bradykinin, ACE is also capable of hydrolysing substance P, enkephalins and neurotensin (4). Thus peptidyl dipeptidase is a relatively nonselective enzyme. This multitargeted effect of ACE raises the question of the specificity of the cardiovascular responses to ACE inhibition. More importantly, the concern over unpredicted and undesired side effects with long term·inhibition of this enzyme has been raised. Renin is the first and the rate limiting step in plasma angiotensin production. This enzyme is specific for its substrate, angiotensinogen. To date, no other substrate has been reported. Therefore, renin provides an ideal target for the blockade of this system. The most promising inhibitors of renin include four classes of compounds (Table 1).

TABLE I

RENIN INHIBITORS

1. Renin antibody
2. Modified pepstatin
3. Angiotensinogen analogs
    a. Competitive inhibitor
    b. Statine substitution
    c. Reduced or hydroxy isostere
4. Prosegment peptide

Specific blockade of renin using antibodies raised against purified renin is now possible. Antirenin antisera, purified IgG and Fab have been administered to conscious animals. Complete renin inhibition was accompanied by a hypotensive response in the sodium deplete but not sodium replete animals. Antirenin antibodies normalized the BP of animals with acute renovascular hypertension (5). Recently, monoclonal antibodies to human renal renin have been obtained. These antibodies selectively inhibited human and monkey renin activities. Monoclonal antirenin antibodies lowered BP of sodium deplete monkeys as well as those with renin-dependent hypertension. The overall BP responses to polyclonal or monoclonal antibodies were comparable to those of ACE inhibitors (5-7). This immunological approach provides a highly specific method of renin blockade in vivo but its therapeutic potential is limited by the potential immunogenecity of these foreign proteins and by the lack of activity when orally administered.

Chemical renin inhibitors include peptides from the prosegment of prorenin, general inhibitors of aspartyl proteinases or angiotensinogen analogues: (a) Evin et al (8) synthesized peptide 11-19 of mouse submaxillary gland prorenin and demonstrated its inhibitory activity on the enzyme. More recently, human prosegment peptide has also been synthesized. This peptide has a relatively week inhibitory activity (IC_{50} 10^{-4}M) on human plasma renin (9). However, one may anticipate that further manipulation of the amino acid sequences of these peptides may result in the development of more potent inhibitors of renin in the future. (b) Pepstatin inhibits many aspartyl proteinases. Its application has been limited by its relative insolubility and nonselectivity. The addition of charged amino acids at its carboxyterminus has rendered it more useful (10). (c) The most promising approach in the development of chemical renin inhibitors appears to be the synthesis of angiotensinogen analogues (Table 2).

TABLE 2

SUBSTRATE ANALOGUES AS RENIN INHIBITORS

Compound	Amino Acid Sequence	IC_{50} (M)*
Minimal Substrate	His-Pro-Phe-His-Leu-Leu-Val-Tyr (Val-Ile-His)	
RIP	Pro-His-Pro-Phe-His-Phe-Phe-Val-Tyr-Lys	$7X10^{-6}$
H-77	D His-Pro-Phe-His-Leu$\overset{R}{-}$Leu-Val-Tyr	$1X10^{-6}$
H-142	Pro-His-Pro-Phe-His-Leu$\overset{R}{-}$Val-Ile-His	$1X10^{-8}$
H-261	His-Pro-Phe-His-Leu$\overset{OH}{-}$Val-Ile-His	$6.9X10^{-10}$
SCRIP	His-Pro-Phe-His—Sta— Ile-His	$2X10^{-9}$

R = $-CH_2-NH-$ OH= $-CH(OH)-CH_2-$ *human renin

Analogues of the minimal octapeptide sequence of angiotensinogen have yielded highly specific competitive inhibitors (11). The first modification made in the octapeptide sequences were aimed at producing peptides that bind but not be cleaved by renin. Replacement of either leucyl residues (positions 10 and 11) with D-stereoisomer at the scissile bond resulted in an effective renin inhibitor. Replacement of leucyl residues with phenylalanine yielded an even more potent inhibitor. Addition of a prolyl residue to the aminoterminus and a lysyl residue to the carboxyterminus increased solubility. This renin inhibitory peptide (RIP) has a Ki of 1μM for human renin (11). Recently, several laboratories have synthesized transition-state analogues of renin substrate, based on the theory that enzymes have a greater binding affinity for the transition state than for the ground state of the substrate. These consists of two classes of compounds: (i) those which contain a statine substitution for residues at the scissile bond (e.g. SCRIP)(12) and (ii) those which incorporate transition-state isostere into the octapeptide (13-14). In place of the scissile Leu-Leu peptide bond, the secondary amine-CH_2-NH-(i.e. Leu$\overset{R}{-}$Leu), or the hydroxy-ethylene moiety $-CH(OH)-CH_2-$, (i.e. Leu$\overset{OH}{-}$Leu), were incorporated (Table 2). These transition-state analogues are highly potent inhibitors (IC_{50} 10^{-9} to 10^{-10} M) with increased in vivo stability. However, all these compounds are limited by the relatively short duration of action and susceptibility to digestive enzymes.

In vivo experimental studies employing different renin inhibitors have yielded similar overall results (12-16). All renin inhibitors effectively inhibited plasma renin activities (PRA) in vivo and lowered BP in sodium deplete animals as well as in those with renin-dependent hypertension. The acute depressor responses were comparable to teprotide or captopril in all cases. However, an additional interesting observation was made with the statine-containing renin inhibitor, SCRIP (12). Although a dose-dependent decrease in BP was observed with SCRIP, its effects on BP and PRA appeared to be dissociated. At lower infusion rates (up to 20 μg/kg/min), the slope of inhibition of PRA was steeper than that for the decline of BP. At doses >20μg/kg/min, when PRA was completely suppressed, BP continued to fall in a dose-dependent fashion independent of PRA.

To date, only two clinical trials with renin inhibitors have been reported (17-18). Infusion of H-142 (1 and 2.5 mg/kg/hr) reduced diastolic BP in sodium deplete normal human subjects accompanied by large reductions of circulating angiotensin I and II (17). In a separate study infusion of RIP in doses effective in monkeys (0.2 mg/kg/min) had little effect in sodium deplete or sodium replete man. In higher doses (1 mg/kg/min), RIP resulted in large reduction of systolic and diastolic BP (>40 mmHg) in the supine position. BP was inaudible when the subject was tilted upright. This response was significantly greater than that seen with captopril in the same subject. Similar response were also seen in sodium replete subjects and in a patient with low renin essential hypertension (18).

Although the overall acute PB response to renin inhibitors appeared to be comparable to ACE inhibitors, the responses to RIP in man and SCRIP in animals raises the possibility that the mechanisms of actions of renin and ACE inhibitors may differ to some extent. Are renin inhibitors acting at another site(s) of renin action other than plasma e.g. brain, vascular or intracardiac renin? Is the additional blood pressure response to some of the renin inhibitors due to nonrenin effects? It should be pointed out that all studies with renin inhibitors to date employed short term administration of these compounds. Comparison of chronic effects of renin and ACE inhibitors will provide further information on the differences and similarities of these compounds and their relative therapeutic potentials in hypertension.

ACKNOWLEDGEMENTS

Support by NHLBI grant HL00750, HL 19259 and a grant from RJ Reynold's Inc. Victor J. Dzau is an Established Investigator of American Heart Association.

REFERENCES

1. Dzau VJ (1983) In: Isselbacher et al (eds) Update IV. Harrison's Principles of Internal Medicine, pp 137-146
2. Patchett AA et al (1980) Nature 288:280-283
3. Given BD et al (1984) J Cardiovas Pharma 6:436-441
4. Erdos EG, Skidgel RA (1984) Proceedings of symposium on renin and angiotensin II inhibitors. Institute Scientifique Roussel p 5-6
5. Dzau VJ et al (1983) Clin and Exper Hyper A5 (7&8), 1207-1220
6. Wood JM et al (1984) Proceedings of the Tenth Scientific Meeting of the International Society of Hypertension. Abstract No. 941

7. deClaviere M et al (1984) Proceedings of the Tenth Scientific Meeting of the International Society of Hypertension. Abstract No. 279
8. Evin G et al (1984) Proc Natl Acad Sci USA 81:48-52
9. Evin G et al (1984) Proceedings of Tenth Scientific Meeting of International Society of Hypertension. Abstract No. 44
10. Eid M et al (1981) Biochem J 197:465-471
11. Haber E (1983) Clin and Exper Hyper A5 (7&8): 1193-1205
12. Blain E et al (1984) Hypertension 6 (Suppl I): I-111-I-118
13. Szelke M et al (1983) In: Hruby VJ, Rich DH (eds) Peptides structure and function pp 579-583
14. Szelke M (1984) Proceedings of the symposium on renin and angiotensin inhibition. Institute Scientifique Roussel p 23-24
15. Tree M et al (1983) J Hyper 1:399-403
16. Szelke M et al (1983) Hyper 4:59-69
17. Zusman RM et al (1983) Trans Am Assoc Phys 365-374
18. Webb D et al (1983) Lancet ii, 1486-1487

20. Thermogenesis and Body Weight

Endocrinology
F. Labrie, L. Proulx, eds.

DIET-INDUCED THERMOGENESIS AND BROWN FAT

NANCY J. ROTHWELL AND MICHAEL J. STOCK
Department of Physiology, St.George's Hospital Medical School, London SW17, U.K.

Regulation of energy balance and body composition in mammals now appears to be achieved by controls operating on both food intake and energy expenditure (1). The importance and magnitude of regulatory changes in energy expenditure (diet-induced thermogenesis, DIT) have been assessed only recently, and advances in this area have depended to a large extent on overfeeding studies on laboratory rodents.

OVERFEEDING AND DIT

Most laboratory rodents can be induced to overeat voluntarily simply by presenting them with a choice of varied and highly palatable human food items, often referred to as the 'cafeteria diet'. This feeding regime results in increases in energy intake of up to 80%, but in young animals causes no change in body weight and only small increases in fat and energy content. The hyperphagia of these animals is associated with marked increases in energy expenditure (up to 100%) and reduced levels of energetic efficiency (1,2). Increases in DIT in response to overfeeding have been demonstrated in several species (e.g. mouse, pig, guinea-pig, man) and in many strains of rats including wild ones (3). Some controversy has arisen over the quantitative significance of DIT, so food intakes and body composition of cafeteria-fed rats have now been assessed by two different methods (4), and energy expenditure determined from energy balance and directly from acute and chronic measurements of oxygen consumption (5). These studies confirm the large potential for DIT in young animals, and show that energy equivalent to the entire maintenance requirement can be dissipated as heat via this phenomenon. Only a very small proportion of this increased energy expenditure can be ascribed to the extra energy costs of assimilating nutrients and synthesis of body protein. However, like most physiological systems, the magnitude of the DIT is variable and dependent on many factors, such as the level of hyperphagia, composition of the diet, season, temperature, feeding frequency and the age, sex and genetic background of the animals (6). Thus, modest increases in energy intake (less than 30%) of a high fat diet produce little or no change in energy expenditure, particularly in older animals or those with a genetic predisposition to obesity.

MECHANISMS OF DIT

Increases in energy expenditure resulting from hyperphagia appear to be mediated by the sympathetic nervous system, which causes activation of heat production in brown adipose tissue (BAT). DIT can be inhibited by pharmacological or surgical inhibition of the sympathetic nervous system, mimicked by injection of sympathetic agonists, and is accompanied by increased tissue turnover rates of noradrenaline, particularly in BAT (7). Foster and Frydman (8) have established the quantitative importance of BAT in non-shivering thermogenesis from measurements of in vivo metabolic rate of the tissue. The same techniques have now been applied to hyperphagic cafeteria-fed rats and have shown that the enhanced thermogenic capacity of these animals can be almost entirely ascribed to BAT (9). These very high rates of heat production in brown fat are due to a physiological uncoupling of oxidative phosphorylation involving a proton conductance pathway in the inner mitochondrial membrane (10). The activity of this pathway is enhanced by overfeeding, which also causes hypertrophy and, in young animals, hyperplasia of BAT (11). Conversely, the activity of the sympathetic nervous system and BAT are depressed in animals with reduced levels of DIT such as food-restricted rats (12) or genetically obese rodents (13).

HORMONAL CONTROL OF DIT AND BAT

Noradrenaline appears to be the primary activator of BAT, with other neural systems possibly exerting minor effects on the tissue (e.g. dopaminergic, serotonergic, histaminergic). However, heat production in BAT, and the metabolic rate and energy balance of the whole animal, can be modified by a number of hormonal systems.

Circulating levels of triiodothyronine (T_3) are usually elevated in overfed animals and depressed by food restriction (see 14 for review). Despite the marked thermogenic actions of thyroid hormones, it is generally accepted that their role in non-shivering and diet-induced thermogenesis is largely permissive, and they may be required only to maintain sensitivity to noradrenaline. However, a rise in T_3 levels does appear essential for the delayed thermogenic response to refeeding in fasted animals (15), and the recent report of high levels of the 5'-deiodinase enzyme in BAT (16) could indicate a close relationship between thyroid hormones and DIT.

Insulin has generally been considered as an anabolic hormone which acts mainly to promote fat deposition and a positive energy balance. However, recent evidence has suggested that insulin is required for DIT and may even activate thermogenesis. Experimental diabetes inhibits BAT activity and impairs DIT, while supplementation of animals with insulin can result in lower weight gains and dramatic increases in BAT thermogenesis (1,2,17,18). Furthermore, the acute thermogenic response to a carbohydrate meal is suppressed by inhibition of insulin release with diazoxide (19), or by subdiaphragmatic vagotomy

(P.L.R.Andrews, N.J.Rothwell and M.J.Stock, unpublished data), while responses to fat are unaffected. It is not known whether insulin exerts direct effects on BAT, but a more likely site of action may be the ventromedial hypothalamus, which is known to be insulin-sensitive and appears to be involved in the activation of brown fat thermogenesis (20).

Surgical adrenalectomy can arrest or prevent the development of obesity in genetically obese rodents and older rats fed a cafeteria diet (21,22). This effect is achieved not only by a reduction in food intake, but also by lower levels of energetic efficiency and stimulation of DIT and brown fat activity (22,23). The effects of adrenalectomy can be reversed by treatment with corticosterone or by surgical denervation of brown fat (24), indicating that this steroid inhibits brown fat by suppression of the sympathetic nervous system. However, changes in circulating levels of ACTH may partly be responsible for the effects of adrenalectomy on energy balance (N.J.Rothwell and M.J.Stock, unpublished data).

In addition to the hormones discussed above, many others such as glucagon, melatonin, TSH, endorphins and sex hormones have in some way been implicated in the regulation of energy balance or the control of thermogenesis.

The evolutionary significance of DIT and brown adipose tissue metabolism has been discussed elsewhere, particularly with reference to the advantages of DIT for animals consuming poor quality (e.g. low protein) diets (25). However, sympathetic control of brown fat heat production may also be involved in some of the alterations in energetic efficiency seen in other physiological or pathological conditions such as pregnancy, lactation, fever, injury and cancer cachexia (26).

REFERENCES

1. Rothwell NJ, Stock MJ (1981) Ann Rev Nutr 1:235-256.
2. Rothwell NJ, Stock MJ (1983) In: Girardier L, Stock MJ (eds) Mammalian Thermogenesis. Chapman and Hall, London, pp 208-233.
3. Rothwell NJ, Saville ME, Stock MJ (1982) J Nutr 112:1515-1524.
4. Rothwell NJ, Stock MJ (1982) Br J Nutr 47:461-471.
5. Rothwell NJ, Stock MJ (1982) J Physiol 328:371-377.
6. Rothwell NJ, Stock MJ (1981) In: Cioffi LA, James WPT, Van Itallie TB (eds) The Body Weight Regulatory System: Normal and Disturbed Mechanisms. Raven Press, New York, pp 335-343.
7. Landsberg L, Young JB (1983) In: Girardier L, Stock MJ (eds) Mammalian Thermogenesis. Chapman and Hall, London, pp 99-140.
8. Foster DO, Frydman ML (1978) Can J Physiol Pharmacol 56:110-122.
9. Rothwell NJ, Stock MJ (1981) Pflugers Archiv 389:237-242.

10. Nicholls DG, Locke R (1983) Physiol Rev 6:1.

11. Brooks SL, Rothwell NJ, Stock MJ (1982) Q J Exper Physiol 67:259-268.

12. Rothwell NJ, Stock MJ (1982) Biosci Rep 2:543-549.

13. Trayhurn P, James WPT (1983) In: Girardier L, Stock MJ (eds) Mammalian Thermogenesis. Chapman and Hall, London, pp 234-258.

14. Himms-Hagen J (1983) In: Girardier L, Stock MJ (eds) Mammalian Thermogenesis. Chapman and Hall, London, pp 141-177.

15. Rothwell NJ, Saville ME, Stock MJ (1982) Am J Physiol 243:R339-346.

16. Silva JE, Larsen PR (1983) Nature 305:712.

17. Rothwell NJ, Stock MJ (1981) Metabolism 30:673-678.

18. Seydoux J, Trimble ER, Bouillaud F, Assimacopoulos-Jeannet F, Bas S, Riquer D, Giacobini JP, Girardier L (1984) FEBS Letts 166:141-145.

19. Rothwell NJ, Stock MJ, Warwick BP (1984) Proc Nutr Soc (in press).

20. Perkins MN, Rothwell NJ, Stock MJ, Stone TW (1981) Nature 289:401-402.

21. Yukimura Y, Bray GA (1978) Endocrinol Res Commun 5:189-193.

22. Marchington D, Rothwell NJ, Stock MJ, York DA (1983) J Nutr 113:1395-1402.

23. Rothwell NJ, Stock MJ, York DA (1984) Comp Biochem Physiol (in press).

24. Rothwell NJ, Stock MJ (1984) Comp Biochem Physiol (in press).

25. Rothwell NJ, Stock MJ (1983) In: Draper HH (ed) Advanced Nutrition Research vol 5. Plenum, New York, pp 201-220.

26. Rothwell NJ, Stock MJ (1982) Obesity and Leanness. J Libbey, London.

Endocrinology
F. Labrie, L. Proulx, eds.

BROWN ADIPOSE TISSUE THERMOGENESIS AND OBESITY IN ANIMALS

PAUL TRAYHURN and STEWART W. MERCER
Dunn Nutrition Laboratory, University of Cambridge and Medical Research Council, Downham's Lane, Milton Road, Cambridge CB4 1XJ (United Kingdom)

INTRODUCTION

The mechanisms responsible for the increase in body fat that leads to obesity have been the subject of intensive study over a number of years. The 'pathological' rise in fat stores in obesity must, of course, be differentiated from the 'physiologically programmed' increases in fat occurring at specific periods in an animal's life - e.g. during pregnancy and pre-hibernation - where the deposition of energy relates to a subsequent energy demand. The problem of obesity is in essence one of energy balance; either food intake is higher than normal, or one or more components of energy expenditure is reduced.

Animal models have been extensively used in the study of obesity, and a wide range of such models is available. These include animals where obesity is genetically determined - such as the obese (ob/ob) mouse, the diabetic-obese (db/db) mouse and the Zucker or fatty (fa/fa) rat - and animals in which the condition is experimentally induced. Examples of methods by which obesity can be induced experimentally include the administration of insulin, corticosteroids or gold thioglucose, lesioning of the ventromedial hypothalamus, and the provision of a high fat diet (1).

In several types of animal obesity, notably the genetically inherited forms, it is clear that the condition can develop on a normal energy intake (see 2,3). It is now also apparent that the initiation and early development of obesity in ob/ob and db/db mice, and in the fa/fa rat, occurs before the development of hyperphagia (2,3). Thus a reduction in energy expenditure is the key factor in the aetiology of obesity in these mutants, while hyperphagia is a secondary manifestation of the disorder. This has led to a focus on the routes by which energy expenditure can be reduced, with a particular emphasis on brown adipose tissue.

BROWN ADIPOSE TISSUE

Brown adipose tissue is now recognised as being the principal site of thermoregulatory non-shivering thermogenesis in adult rodents, in addition to being important in the generation of heat in mammalian neonates and during the arousal from hibernation. The central mechanism by which heat is produced in brown adipose tissue is through a proton conductance pathway across the mitochondrial inner membrane, which dissociates respiration from the synthesis of ATP (see 4). The proton conductance pathway can be inhibited by purine nucleotides, such as GDP, which bind to an uncoupling protein of mol. wt. 32,000.

There is now considerable evidence from several experimental approaches, including blood flow measurements and various indices of the activity of the proton conductance pathway, that thermogenesis in brown adipose tissue is decreased in ob/ob and db/db mice and in the fatty rat (see 2,3). The thermogenic activity of the tissue has also been shown to be reduced in several of the experimentally-induced forms of obesity (2,3). Importantly, the decrease in thermogenesis in genetically obese animals has been shown to occur during the suckling period, well before obesity develops. This strongly suggests that the ability of these mutants to become obese on a normal energy intake is related to a low level of energy expenditure on brown adipose tissue thermogenesis.

When hyperphagia develops secondarily in genetically obese mice and rats it does not lead to the same stimulation of thermogenesis in brown adipose tissue as in normal animals (2,3), and this has been interpreted as indicating that the capacity for diet-induced thermogenesis is impaired. An impairment in the dietary stimulus to the tissue is now viewed as a general feature of obese animals, and has been documented in several forms of experimental obesity.

ADRENAL FUNCTION

Obese animals are characterised by a wide range of metabolic and endocrinological abnormalities, including hyperinsulinaemia, hyperlipogenesis and insulin resistance (1). Adrenal function is now emerging as a factor of considerable importance to the overall development of obesity in ob/ob mice and the fatty rat. Adrenalectomy of these animals has wide-ranging and profound effects, including the abolition of hyperphagia and a reduction in the level of hyperinsulinaemia. Although adrenalectomy has little effect on lean animals, the chronic treatment of mice with corticosterone leads to hyperphagia, hyperinsulinaemia and obesity (5).

TABLE 1
EFFECT OF ADRENALECTOMY ON BROWN ADIPOSE TISSUE OF OBESE ob/ob MICE

	Sham		Adrenalectomized	
	Lean	Obese	Lean	Obese
n =	7	6	9	7
Initial body wt. (g)	22.7±1.5	27.6±1.1	21.9±0.7	27.2±1.1
Body wt. gain (g)	1.3±0.3	7.2±0.7	1.3±0.6	4.0±1.1
Brown adipose tissue (interscap. + subscap.) wt. (mg)	126±9	498±29	123±7	320±37
Tissue protein content (mg)	17.6±0.7	16.5±1.3	20.9±1.4	18.3±1.1
Tissue cytochrome oxidase activity (μmol cyto. c oxidized/min)	26.8±2.4	17.1±2.5	31.2±4.2	32.4±2.1
GDP binding (pmol/mg mito. protein)	246±39	149±29	219±18	223±35

Female mice of the 'Aston strain', aged 4-5 weeks and studied 5 days after bilateral adrenalectomy. Methods were as described in Galpin et al. (5).

Adrenalectomy has recently been found to restore the activity of brown adipose tissue in fatty rats to normal, and it also results in a restoration of the response to dietary stimuli, effects which are reversible by the administration of corticosterone (6). Intact corticosterone-treated mice show a reduction in thermogenesis in brown adipose tissue (5), and we have recently found that adrenalectomy of ob/ob mice leads to the same restoration of the activity of the tissue as in the fatty rat (see TABLE 1). This is particularly evident for the proton conductance pathway, as assessed by the GDP binding assay. Lean mice are little affected by adrenalectomy (TABLE 1). Current evidence suggests that the effects of corticosterone may be mediated centrally through the sympathetic nervous system, rather than directly on brown adipose tissue itself (6,7).

GENERAL CONCLUSIONS

The early development of obesity in genetically obese animals takes place on a normal energy intake, and this appears to be due to a reduced level of energy expenditure on thermogenesis in brown adipose tissue; there is no other current explanation. A decrease in brown adipose tissue thermogenesis has also been documented for several forms of experimentally-induced obesity, where the tissue shows little activation in response to overfeeding. Thermogenesis in obese animals may be low primarily because of reduced sympathetic nervous system activity, and in the genetic forms of obesity this may relate to a suppressive effect of corticosteroids.

ACKNOWLEDGEMENTS

SWM was funded by a grant from Unilever plc.

REFERENCES

1. Bray GA, York DA (1979) Physiol Rev 59:719-809
2. Trayhurn P, James WPT (1983) In: Girardier L, Stock MJ (eds) Mammalian Thermogenesis. Chapman and Hall, London and New York, pp 234-258
3. Trayhurn P (1984) Clin Endocrinol Metab 13: in press
4. Nicholls DG, Locke RM (1984) Physiol Rev 64:1-64
5. Galpin KS, Henderson RG, James WPT, Trayhurn P (1983) Biochem J 214:265-268
6. Holt S, York DA, Fitzsimons JTR (1983) Biochem J 214:215-223
7. Vander Tuig JG, Ohshima K, Yoshida T, Romsos DR, Bray GA (1984) Life Sci 34:1423-1432

Endocrinology
F. Labrie, L. Proulx, eds.

THE ROLE OF THE SYMPATHOADRENAL SYSTEM IN THE REGULATION OF DIETARY THERMOGENESIS

LEWIS LANDSBERG, M.D. AND JAMES B. YOUNG, M.D.

Thorndike Laboratory and Dana Research Institute, Department of Medicine, Beth Israel Hospital and Harvard Medical School, 330 Brookline Avenue, Boston, MA 02215

INTRODUCTION: THE SYMPATHETIC NERVOUS SYSTEM (SNS) AND NONSHIVERING THERMOGENESIS (NST)

The SNS plays a major role in the regulation of metabolic heat production in mammalian organisms exposed to cold (NST) (1). The sequence of events between cold exposure and increased heat production has been well delineated in laboratory rodents: i) environmental cold stimulates temperature sensitive neurons in the periphery and within the CNS; afferent impulses from these neurons are integrated in the hypothalamus and result in increased SNS activity in many (but not all) organ systems including brown adipose tissue (BAT) (2); ii) activation of beta-1 adrenergic receptors in BAT markedly increases mitochondrial substrate oxidation via a unique proton conductance pathway (3); iii) BAT blood flow increases many-fold thereby increasing substrate availability and facilitating export of locally produced heat for temperature maintenance. Repeated or continuous exposure to cold results in cold acclimation which is associated with BAT hypertrophy and increased thermogenic respones to the SNS neurotransmitter norepinephrine (NE) (4). In human subjects although i) cold exposure increases sympathetic activity, and ii) catecholamines increase metabolic rate, a role for BAT in the production of sympathetically mediated thermogenesis has been neither proved nor excluded. In recent years, the demonstration that i) diet influences SNS activity (5,6) and that ii) NST resembles in many important respects diet-induced thermogenesis (DIT) (7) has led to the hypothesis that the SNS modulates energy expenditure in relationship to dietary intake.

DIETARY INTAKE AND SNS ACTIVITY

Fasting and caloric restriction

Fasting, or caloric restriction, suppresses the SNS in laboratory rodents (5) and human subjects (8). The available evidence suggests that SNS suppression contributes to the decrease in metabolic rate that accompanies caloric restriction (1,9).

Overfeeding

Caloric excess increases SNS activity in rodents (2) and man (8). Available evidence is consistent with a role for the SNS in the increased metabolic rate associated with overfeeding (10,11).

Diet composition

Various nutrient classes, moreover, appear to exert differential effects on the SNS.

Refined carbohydrates. Sucrose and glucose increase SNS activity in rodents and man (6,12), even when total caloric intake is not increased (13). Although some debate exists, available evidence is consistent with a role for the SNS in the regulation of glucose-induced thermogenesis in humans (11).

Fat. Like refined carbohydrate, fat stimulates the SNS in the rat (13). The effect of fat on SNS activity in man and the relationship between fat intake, thermogenesis, and the SNS requires further study.

Protein. In contrast to the effects of refined carbohydrates and fat, studies in rats indicate that protein does not stimulate the SNS (14). This observation is consistent with the fact that low protein diets are associated with an increase in both SNS activity (15) and thermogenesis (16).

RELATIONSHIP BETWEEN DIETARY INTAKE, THE CENTRAL NERVOUS SYSTEM, AND SNS ACTIVITY

Although much remains to be learned about the relationship between nutritional status and SNS activity a plausible hypothesis relating changes in SNS activity during fasting on the one hand, and carbohydrate feeding on the other, to alterations in insulin-mediated glucose metabolism within the hypothalamus has been advanced (17,18,19,20). The fact that hypoglycemia and 2-deoxyglucose diminish SNS activity (despite adrenal medullary stimulation) implies a role for glucose metabolism in the relationship between dietary intake and SNS activity, while the fact that experimental diabetes (21) diminishes, and insulin infusions (without hypoglycemia) stimulate the SNS is consistent with a role for insulin. Involvement of the ventromedial portion of the hypothalamus is suggested by the fact that gold thioglucose, which ablates insulin-glucose sensitive neurons in this region, disrupts dietary changes in SNS activity by abolishing suppression of the SNS with fasting. Thus, insulin-mediated glucose metabolism within the ventromedial portion of the hypothalamus may be one signal in the relationship between dietary intake and SNS activity; other signals must exist as well since the stimulatory effect of fat on the SNS is not readily explicable in terms of the insulin-glucose model.

PHYSIOLOGICAL SIGNIFICANCE OF DIETARY CHANGES IN SNS ACTIVITY

Fasting and caloric restriction

Suppression of SNS activity during fasting appears to contribute to the diminution in metabolic rate associated with reduced caloric intake by decreasing sympathetically mediated thermogenesis. Such a mechanism, by conserving calories at a time of reduced intake would prolong survival during famine; called into play during therapeutic dieting for weight loss, however, this mechanism would antagonize weight loss and reduce the efficiency of low energy diets. Physiological or pharmacological manipulation of the SNS during therapeutic caloric restriction warrants study as an adjunct to reduced caloric intake in the treatment of obesity.

Overfeeding

Sympathetically mediated thermogenesis in the face of overfeeding provides a mechanism for dissipating excess calories as heat. This capacity would be particularly useful to organisms subsisting on a low protein diet; by increasing metabolic rate these organisms would be able to consume increased quantities of the low protein diet thereby satisfying basic nitrogen requirements for growth and development without storing the excess calories as fat. The fact that low protein feeding increases sympathetic activity, and that protein, unlike carbohydrate and fat, does not stimulate the SNS, supports this hypothesis. Since the capacity to dissipate excess calories defends against the development of obesity, individuals with a reduced capacity for heat dissipation would conserve weight better during periods of caloric restriction but, during periods of freely available foodstuffs, be liable to the development of obesity. SNS function, particularly in response to dietary intake, warrants further study in the obese.

ACKNOWLEDGEMENTS

Supported in part by NIH grants AM 20378, HL 24084, AG 00599.

REFERENCES

1. Landsberg L (1983) In: Girardier L, Stock MJ (eds) Mammalian Thermogenesis. Chapman & Hall, London, pp 99-140

2. Young JB, Saville E, Rothwell NJ, Stock MJ, Landsberg L (1982) J Clin Invest 69:1061-1071

3. Nicholls D, Locke R (1983) In: Girardier L, Stock MJ (eds) Mammalian Thermogenesis. Chapman & Hall, London, pp 8-49

4. Cannon B, Nedergaard J (1983) J Therm Biol 8:85-90

5. Young JB, Landsberg L (1977) Science 196:1473-1475

6. Young JB, Landsberg L (1977) Nature 269:615-617

7. Rothwell NJ, Stock MJ (1983) In: Girardier L, Stock MJ (eds) Mammalian Thermogenesis. Chapman & Hall, London, 208-233

8. O'Dea K, Esler M, Leonard P, Stockigt JR, Nestel P (1982) Metabolism 31:896-899

9. Shetty PS, Jung RT, James WPT (1979) Lancet 1:77-79

10. Jung RT, Shetty PS, James WPT (1980) Europ J Clin Invest 10:179-182

11. Acheson K, Jequier E, Wahren J (1983) J Clin Invest 72:981-986.

12. Welle S, Lilavivathana U, Campbell RG (1980) Metabolism 29:806-809

13. Schwartz JH, Young JB, Landsberg L (1983) J Clin Invest 72: 361-370

14. Kaufman LN, Young JB, Landsberg L (1984) Clin Res 32:478A

15. Young JB, Saville ME, Landsberg L (1983) Clin Res 31:466A

16. Miller DS, Mumford P (1967) J Clin Nutr 20:1212-1222

17. Young JB, Landsberg L (1979) J Clin Invest 64:109-116

18. Young JB, Landsberg L (1980) J Clin Invest 65:1086-1094

19. Rappaport EB, Young JB, Landsberg L (1982) Endocrinology 110:650-656

20. Rowe JW, Young JB, Minaker KL, Stevens AL, Pallotta J, Landsberg L (1981) Diabetes 30:219-225

21. Young JB, Einhorn D, Landsberg L (1983) Diabetes 32(Suppl):26A

Endocrinology
F. Labrie, L. Proulx, eds.

THE MECHANISM OF CHANGES IN ENERGY EXPENDITURE IN RELATION TO CHANGES IN ENERGY INTAKE IN RATS

G.R. HERVEY and G. TOBIN
Department of Physiology, University of Leeds, Leeds LS2 9JT, U.K.

INTRODUCTION

Human energy expenditure varies widely, but in general adults maintain stable body weights. There is abundant evidence that 'voluntary' food intake is physiologically controlled in such a way as to maintain energy balance in the long run. If humans or animals are restricted to an energy intake less than their voluntary intake, they can still maintain stable though reduced body weights. This implies that they can also regulate energy balance by reducing energy expenditure to match a restricted intake. Measurements of metabolic rate confirm this (1).

From the turn of the century onwards impressions of food intake and body weight have suggested that increased energy intake can similarly be compensated by regulatory increase in expenditure: the postulated mechanism was named 'Luxuskonsumption'. Recently the claim has been renewed that such a mechanism exists, widely variable but very effective when fully operative. It has been re-named 'diet-induced thermogenesis', and its site is said to be in brown adipose tissue (2). Whether or not there is adequate experimental evidence for such a mechanism is controversial. The opposing views have been set out in review articles (3 4): anyone wishing to reach an informed judgement must study the evidence critically.

The older impressions that weight can be maintained despite overfeeding may have been misleading because of failure to distinguish intake below voluntary, in which energy expenditure is reduced, from a true free-feeding state, or failure to appreciate that physiological control of food intake was still highly effective.

Nearly all the evidence, old and new, for 'diet-induced thermogenesis' depends on estimates of changes in energy intake and body energy content, not on measurements of energy expenditure. Inferring energy expenditure by difference means that real changes cannot be distinguished from the effects of experimental errors, and regulatory changes cannot be distinguished from other causes of changed expenditure, for example by their time and amplitude relationships. The commonest errors are losses of energy due to such technical difficulties as failure to recover all scattered food and excreta, loss of weight from food due to evaporation, and loss of energy from excreta. Systematic errors cumulate in energy balances, and such errors are inevitably reported as increased expenditure. We believe it is essential to measure all three components of energy balance - intake, expenditure and change in body energy content - independently and with the highest attainable accuracy, and to check end-to-end apparent energy balances against the found changes in body energy content.

OUR EARLIER EXPERIMENTS

Measurements of continuous energy expenditure in rats fed fixed levels of energy intake by stomach-tube confirmed the ability to compensate underfeeding by reduction of energy expenditure (1 5). In rats given 1.0 to 0.7 times their voluntary energy intake energy expenditure fell over the first few days, and then became steady and approximately equal to energy intake. Body weight fell initially and then became steady at a lower level. The fact that a steady weight was maintained after adjustment of energy expenditure suggests that this was a regulatory response. There is no soundly based evidence to identify the tissues in which metabolism is reduced, or the controlling pathway.

In further experiments (1 5) tube-feeding was used to increase energy intake to 1.0 - 1.8 times voluntary intake. In contrast to underfeeding, body weight continued to rise and the rats became progressively fatter, until the experiment ended. Energy expenditure increased over the first few days and then became nearly steady. Metabolizable energy intake in excess of voluntary intake, rate of weight gain and increase in energy expenditure were all found to be proportional. The 95 % confidence limits for the regression of energy expenditure on intake showed that expenditure increased by 36 - 52 kJ for each 100 kJ excess intake.

Rats can be induced to increase their voluntary energy intake by supplementing their normal diet with varied, attractive items ('cafeteria feeding'). When this is done energy intake is not under the experimenter's control, cannot be varied widely, and falls off with time. Body weight rises at first, but eventually ceases to rise, we believe because physiological control of food intake balances the attractiveness of the foods. In an experiment on adult rats we found energy expenditure increased by 33 - 37 kJ per 100 kJ excess intake (95 % confidence limits). Further experiments, which included young growing rats and rats of other strains including that used by Rothwell & Stock (2), gave regressions in the range 20 - 36 kJ / 100 kJ.

The consistency of the increase in energy expenditure as a proportion of excess intake, and the lack of any control of energy balance when regulation of energy intake was by-passed, suggest that the increase in energy expenditure after overfeeding is not a regulatory mechanism. There are at least three evident non-regulatory causes of increased energy costs: the costs of digestion, absorption and early metabolism of extra nutrients; the cost of storing energy as fat; and the costs entailed in supporting a larger body.

There is evidence in the literature and in our own data as to the scale of these costs, which we have discussed (6). Our best estimates, in the context of an experiment with 'cafeteria'-fed adult rats, were: digestion, absorption and early metabolism, 8 kJ / 100 kJ; synthesis of fat, 20 - 25 kJ / 100 kJ; and the cost of being heavier, 4 kJ / 100 kJ. The first of these occurs over a period of 7 hours following a meal, whereas the second takes some days to build up and is then constant throughout the day if intake remains constant. Neither was affected by administration of propranolol, 15 mg/kg i.p., which confirms that they were not brought about by brown adipose tissue. The last component is actually proportional to weight gained, at approx. 0.1 kJ per gram. The total, 32 - 37 kJ / 100 kJ, agrees closely with the observed increase in expenditure of 33 - 37 kJ / 100 kJ. The slightly larger increase in tube-feeding experiments is probably due to greater weight gain. Allowing for errors it seems unlikely that any further component of increased expenditure could exceed 5 kJ / 100 kJ excess intake.

CURRENT EXPERIMENTS

The estimates in the literature of the costs of handling extra energy intake are based on limited data, obtained mainly from agricultural research, and a number of factors must affect these costs. Further study of them has therefore been undertaken. In the first such experiments the rats were fed by stomach-tube and energy intake was increased to 1.0 - 1.5 times voluntary intake, the extra energy being supplied either entirely as carbohydrate or entirely as fat. The base diet, by weight, was 80 % carbohydrate, 15 % protein and 5 % minerals and vitamins. Additional carbohydrate was added as a glucose polymer and some water was omitted, leading to a small increase in volume; fat was added by replacing water by arachis oil, with no change in volume. Energy intake was measured by adiabatic bomb calorimetry of diet and excreta together with scattered food. Energy expenditure was measured in our continuous-running, automated indirect calorimeter, with four rats in each of four cages and a fifth cage serving as blank and recovery check. Carcass energy was determined by analysis of whole bodies less gut contents, followed by bomb calorimetry of fat and fat-free solids. Initial values for carcass energy were found from regressions based on analyses of substantial numbers of comparable rats (6: with improvements to some methods). Each experiment consisted of 10 days of normal voluntary feeding, 10 days of tube-feeding at approximately the same ME intake, and 20 days of feeding three of the groups increased energy intakes.

Table 1 shows energy balances over the entire experiment. The mean discrepancy between apparent energy balance (i.e. the difference between measured ME intake and measured energy expenditure) and the change in energy content of the carcasses was -2.0 % of total intake (n = 8, s.e.m. ±0.5 %).

Table 1. End-to-end energy intakes, energy balances and precision.

Excess nutrient	-	cho	cho	cho	-	fat	fat	fat
Weight added (g/rat/d)	-	2.2	3.8	5.5	-	1.1	1.6	2.1
Total ME intake (kJ)	6692	7364	7754	8504	6266	7044	7562	7616
Total expenditure (kJ)	6362	6668	6718	6936	5916	5839	6254	6120
Apparent balance (kJ)	+330	+696	+1036	+1568	+350	+1205	+1308	+1496
Δ carcass energy (kJ)	+455	+720	+1086	+1637	+652	+1367	+1445	+1744
Discrepancy (% intake)	-1.9	-0.3	-0.6	-0.8	-4.8	-2.3	-1.8	-3.3

Four energy balances, each over five days, for the four cages gave the following regression coefficients (with 95 % confidence limits) for energy expenditure on energy intake: for overfeeding with carbohydrate, 0.28 (±0.03) kJ / kJ; for overfeeding with fat, 0.23 (±0.06) kJ / kJ. The energy cost of supporting a larger body was too small for reliable measurement (ca. 0 - 2 kJ / 100 kJ excess intake).

Thus the energy costs of assimilating and storing excess energy, supplied as carbohydrate or as fat under otherwise similar conditions, at 28 and 23 kJ / 100 kJ respectively differed in the direction to be expected from the more complex metabolism involved in storing energy supplied as carbohydrate, but only to a modest extent; the values are precisely consistent with the previous literature. The experiment provides no basis for expecting substantially different relationships between energy intake, energy expenditure and weight gain when dietary composition is varied. There was again no evidence of unaccounted-for increase in energy expenditure.

REFERENCES

1. Hervey GR, Tobin G (1983) Proc Nutr Soc Aust 8:1-21
2. Rothwell NJ, Stock MJ (1979) Nature (Lond) 281:31-35
3. Hervey GR, Tobin G (1983) Clin Sci 64:7-18
4. Rothwell NJ, Stock MJ (1983) Clin Sci 64:19-23
5. Hervey GR, Tobin G (1982) Proc Nutr Soc 41:137-153
6. Armitage G, Hervey GR, Rolls BJ, Rowe EA, Tobin G (1983) J Physiol 342:229-251

21. Steroids and Cancer

© 1984 Elsevier Science Publishers B.V.
Endocrinology
F. Labrie, L. Proulx, eds.

MECHANISMS OF ESTROGENIC REGULATION OF HUMAN BREAST CANCER CELL GROWTH IN LONG-TERM TISSUE CULTURE

MARC E. LIPPMAN, KAREN K. HUFF, RAIMUND JAKESZ, TOBY HECHT, SUSAN BATES AND ROBERT DICKSON
Medical Breast Cancer Section, Medicine Branch, National Cancer Institute, Bethesda, Maryland (USA)

The mechanisms by which estrogens stimulate the growth of human breast cancer are far from completely understood. Some years ago we demonstrated that clonal lines of human breast cancer cells in long term culture could be stimulated to proliferate more rapidly by physiologic concentrations of estradiol (1-3). Antiestrogens specifically inhibited the growth of these estrogen receptor positive cells and these inhibitory effects could be blocked by simultaneous addition of estradiol and reversed by subsequent administration of estradiol. Despite lack of success by occasional subsequent investigators, many different groups, working with a variety of human breast cancer cell lines have been able to demonstrate such proliferative responses (4-12). These positive findings showing direct effects of estrogens do not rule out contributory effects by other hormones or growth factors which are either endocrine or paracrine in nature (13). To further study these questions we began a systematic survey of the biological activities of factors secreted by breast cancer cells in vitro.

Our studies were initiated in part by the observation that when MCF-7 human breast cancer cells were plated at increasing density there was a proportional increase in initial growth rate - an observation consistent with the elaboration of secreted growth factors. Initial pilot experiments suggested that medium conditioned by MCF-7 cells (at dilutions of 1:2 to 1:16) was able to stimulate the ^{3}Hthymidine incorporation of other MCF-7 cells as well as their proliferation. In order to study this process further, a defined medium system was developed to assist both in the purification of growth promoting activities and in their assay. MCF-7 cells were grown in Improved Minimal Essential Medium (IMEM) supplemented with fibronectin and transferrin with or without estradiol addition (1 nM). Cells were first plated in serum-containing medium, the medium removed, and cells grown in the serum free medium for 2 days. The medium was exchanged for identical fresh medium and harvested at the end of an additional 2 day incubation period. Following sequential removel of fibronectin and transferrin by gelatin sepharose and affinity chromatography, the conditioned medium with or without addition of protease inihibitors (added at the time of media collection) was subjected to different extraction procedures (dialysis and concentration, acid or acid-ethanol extraction) and fractionation by Sephacryl S-200 or Biogel P-60 chromatography.

In previous work we have shown that partial synchrony of MCF-7 cells in culture can be achieved by growth arrest which follows transfer to isoleucine deficient medium for 24 to 30 hours (14). At this time, S fraction determined by flow cytometry, is near zero as is precursor incorporation into DNA although viability remains close to 100% as assessed by trypan blue dye exclusion. If cells are refed with isoleucine deficient medium, DNA synthesis occurs beginning approximately 24 hours later followed by mitosis. If this medium is supplemented with either 1 nM estradiol or concentrated conditioned medium derived from MCF-7 cells, an accelerated and exaggerated growth response occurs beginning at about 16 hours. The effect of conditioned medium - which is superimposable on that seen with addition of 1 nM estradiol to control medium - provides a convenient and assay for growth promoting activity. The proliferative response to conditioned medium is not due to contaminating estradiol by purification criteria, and by radioimmunoassay and radioreceptor assay information.

Specific fractions of column eluates were characterized by six distinct assay methodologies. These are: radioimmunoassay for insulin like growth factor 1 (somatomedin C) IGF-1/SmC; competition in a radioreceptor assay with iodinated EGF (using A431 cells as a source of receptor); transforming activity using normal rat kidney cells in a soft agar cloning assay; monoclonal antibody reactivity (described below) and thymidine incorporation and long term growth promoting activities. These six assay methodologies were applied to conditioned medium derived from MCF-7 cells which had or had not been stimulated with 1 nM estradiol. In addition conditioned media derived from estrogen responsive ZR-75-1 and estrogen unresponsive MDA-MB-231 and HS578T human breast cancers were studied.

MCF-7 cell secrete radioimmunoassayable IGF 1/SmC. Depending upon extraction conditions this material is associated with a higher molecular weight presumptive carrier protein. (IGF-1 activity produced by MCF-7 cells gives a parallel competition curve by radioimmunoassay with authentic IGF-1). Authentic IGF-1 when incubated with MCF-7 conditioned medium shifts to a higher molecular weight form indicative of association with a carrier protein. With acid ethanol extraction, all of the IGF-1 immunoassayable material co-elutes from sephacryl S-200 with authentic IGF-1. Estradiol stimulation has minimal effects (less than 2 fold) on quantities of IGF-1/SmC activity released into the medium.

MCF-7 cells additionally secrete material which competes with ^{125}I-EGF binding to EGF receptor. Multiple peaks of EGF receptor binding activity are obtained on Biogel P-60 columns. Total activity in conditioned medium obtained from estradiol treated cells is enhanced up to 100 fold compared with cells not treated with estradiol. The mechanism of this increased growth factor activity induced by estradiol is not yet completely understood. Possible mechanisms include increased growth factor synthesis and decreased growth factor degradation.

Conditioned medium was also assayed for transforming activity using the cloning of NRK cells in soft agar as an endpoint (15). MCF-7 cells contain potent transforming activity which is also present in high quantities from MCF-7 cells not stimulated by estradiol.

Fractionation of conditioned medium activity using either Sephacryl S-200 or Biogel P-60 columns reveals multiple peaks of autocrine growth promoting activities (that is, when re-applied to other growth arrested MCF-7 cells). These peaks of activity are induced 2 to 8 fold in conditioned medium from estradiol treated MCF-7 cells. Several of these peaks do not correspond to activities identified by the previously described IGF-1/SmC radioimmunoassay or EGF receptor assay.

Concentrated, acid extracted, conditioned medium prepared as described has been used as an immunogen to prepare monoclonal antibodies (MAB). Antibody producing clones were intially screened by ELISA assay for differential reactivity against secreted proteins versus fetal calf serum proteins. Four MABs have been partially characterized. Three react against all breast cancer cell lines tested whether hormone responsive or not. The fourth reacts with antigens produced by MCF-7 and ZR-75-1 cells when stimulated by estradiol but is unreactive against control conditioned medium from these cells grown in the absence of estradiol. This latter MAB reacts with conditioned medium from estrogen unresponsive breast cancer cell lines (MDA-MB-231 and HS578T) in the absence of hormone stimulation. The regulation and function of the antigens identified by these MABs is under investigation.

In summary, human breast cancer cells produce multiple, potent growth regulatory substances at least some of whose activities may be positively and directly regulated in hormone responsive breast cancer cells by addition of physiologic concentrations of estradiol. The possibility that some of these estrogen regulated growth promoting activities are required for in vivo growth is being characterized in a nude mouse assay system in which estradiol supplementation is an absolute requirement for tumor formation.

REFERENCES

1. Lippman ME, Bolan G, Huff K (1976) Cancer Research 36:4595

2. Allegra JC, Lippman ME (1978) Cancer Research 38: 3823
3. Aitken SC, Lippman ME (1982) Cancer Research 42: 1727
4. Leung BS, Qureshi S, Leung JS (1982) Cancer Research 42:5060-5066
5. Darbre P, Yates J, Curtis S, King RJB (1983) Cancer Research 43:349-354
6. Chalbos D, Vignon F, Keydar I, Rochefort H (1982) J Clin Endocrinol Metab 55(2): 276-287
7. Page M, Field J, Everett N, Green C (1983) Cancer Research 43:1244-1250
8. Katzenellenbogen B, Norman MJ, Eckert RL, Peltz SW, Mangel WF (1984) Cancer Research 44:112-119
9. Natoli C, Sica G, Natoli V, Serra A, Iacobelli S (1983) Breast Cancer Res Treat 3:23-32
10. Huseby RA, Maloney TM, McGrath CM (1984) Cancer Research 44:2654-2659
11. Barnes D, Sato G (1979) Nature 281:388-389
12. Weichselbaum RW, Hellman S, Piro A, Nove J, Little JB (1978) Cancer Research 38:2339-2342
13. Ikeda T, Sirbasku DA (1984) J Biol Chem 259(7): 4049-4064
14. Jakesz R, Smith CA, Aitken S, Huff K, Schuette W, Shackney S, Lippman M (1984) Cancer Research 44:619-625
15. Delarco JW, Todaro GJ (1978) Proc Natl Acad Sci USA 75:4001-4005

Endocrinology
F. Labrie, L. Proulx, eds.

THE 52 K ESTROGEN REGULATED PROTEIN SECRETED BY HUMAN MAMMARY CANCER

H. ROCHEFORT, F. CAPONY, M. GARCIA, O. MASSOT, F. MAY, F. VEITH, F. VIGNON and B. WESTLEY

Unité d'Endocrinologie Cellulaire et Moléculaire, U 148 INSERM, 60 rue de Navacelles, 34100 Montpellier (France)

Estrogens promote the development of breast cancer and stimulate the growth *in vitro* of some breast cancer cell lines (1), however the mechanism of their cancerogenic and mitogenic action is unknown. We have used the hormone-responsive MCF7 breast cancer cell line to analyse the mechanism by which estrogens regulate both the biosynthesis of specific proteins and cell proliferation. Estrogen regulated proteins have been recently shown in several metastatic breast cancer cell lines by ^{35}S-methionine labelling of protein followed by their SDS polyacrylamide electrophoresis. Of particular interest is a protein of 52,000 mol wt (52 K) whose production in the culture medium by estrogen receptor positive metastatic breast cancer cell lines is specifically increased by estrogens and inhibited by antiestrogens (2). The 52 K protein is a glycoprotein produced by the estrogen treated MCF7 cells in low amount (≃15 ng/ml of medium) accounting for 20 to 40 % of total released proteins in the culture medium and representing (with the related cellular protein) approx. 0.3 % of total protein synthesis. On the basis of its high hormonal specificity (3), this protein can be used as a simple *in vitro* test to evaluate the estrogenic and antiestrogenic activity of a drug. This protein is more closely related to the control of cell proliferation by estrogen than the progesterone receptor, but is not a marker of action of any mitogen, since it is not stimulated by prolactin, insulin, epithelial growth factor and charcoal-treated fetal calf serum (3).

We will report on three series of results recently obtained by our laboratory concerning : 1. The development and use of monoclonal antibodies to the 52 K protein. 2. The distribution of this protein in estrogen responsive human tissues and its potential use as a marker of breast cancer. 3. Its possible role in mediating the mitogenic activity of estrogen on breast cancer cells.

MONOCLONAL ANTIBODIES

In order to study the structure, function and distribution of this protein, it is necessary to purify it and to detect it in a complex medium or tissue using specific probes. We have developed monoclonal antibodies (MAbs) to the 52 K protein using partially purified antigen isolated from 25 l of medium conditioned by MCF7 cells. In collaboration with CLIN-MIDY Research Laboratory, MAbs were raised, cloned and purified after fusion of lymphocytes from immunised high responder Biozzi's selected mice with the murine myeloma P3-X63-Ag8-653 (4). The 7 MAbs that were cloned and purified were all of the IgG1 isotype and their KD ranged from 0.35 to 2.3 nM. The antibodies specifically recognized the secreted and a cellular 52 K protein as evidenced by double immunoprecipitation and by immunoblotting after electrophoretic separation and transfer. In MCF7 cell extracts, smaller forms (processed or proteolysed ?) of 48,000 and 34,000 mol wt were also immunoreactive but forms heavier than 52 K (precursors ?) have been detected. Double determinant immunoradiometric assay indicated that the 7 MAbs recognized three distinct regions of the Mr 52,000 protein and allowed the 52 K protein to be assayed in biological fluids. These antibodies did not react with the external plasma membrane of MCF7 cells, as shown by immunofluorescence analysis. By contrast, the cytoplasm of MCF7 cells (but not that of the human T47D cell line) was stained by the peroxidase anti-peroxidase complex after plasma membrane permeation, indicating that the protein is secreted by exocytosis rather than shedded from plasma membrane (4).

DISTRIBUTION OF THE 52 K PROTEIN IN ESTROGEN RESPONSIVE TISSUE AND POTENTIAL USE AS A MARKER

Since the 52 K protein is secreted from epithelial cancer cells, it is potentially interesting as a circulating and/or cellular marker of estrogen-responsiveness. Available MAbs allowed us to investigate this possibility and to first study the distribution of the 52 K protein in human tissues directly collected from patients. The estrogen regulated 52 K protein had been shown to be secreted by metastatic breast cancers cells in primary cultures (5). We then examined frozen sections of several human tissues by the peroxidase-anti-peroxidase technique (6). Negative control were routinely performed with an excess of antigen, or with irrelevant IgG antibodies showing the staining specificity. In 20 out of 25 primary breast cancer, specific immunoperoxidase staining was observed in the cytoplasm of epithelial cells. The 5 samples that were not stained contained no detectable estrogen receptor. No staining was observed in normal human mammary glands collected during reduction mammoplasties and in normal uteri whether tissues were collected at the follicular or luteal phase. Two endometrial cancers were also negative. Tentative conclusions from these first results are : a) The 52 K protein is not a general marker of estrogen responsiveness as is the progesterone receptor or the 28 K protein (7), but has some specificity for mammary tissue. b) the 52 K protein does not seem to be a differentiation marker of mammary cells since it was not found in normal epithelial mammary cells. c) the 52 K protein appears to be related to estrogen regulated tumoral mammary cells.

More extensive clinical studies based on the immunostaining of several breast disease (malignant, pre-malignant or benign) are necessary before to propose its clinical use as a marker.

THE 52 K PROTEIN AND THE AUTOCRINE CONTROL OF CELL PROLIFERATION BY ESTROGEN

The identity and biological functions of the 52 K protein are presently unknown. The 52 K protein is not a major milk protein such as human casein or -lactalbumin, which have different molecular weights. The relation of the 52 K protein with other estrogen-regulated proteins : (28 K protein (7)), several virus-related proteins (gp52) or a 54 K membrane protein (8), which have been described in human breast cancer cells has been excluded in collaboration with several investigators who have provided their specific antibodies. The identification of the 52 K protein to a plasminogen activator was recently excluded after purification (9). The 52 K protein therefore does not seem to correspond to a kwown mammary protein. We have raised the hypothesis (10) that this protein could be an estrogen regulated growth-transforming factor acting in an autocrine manner to stimulate the growth of breast cancer cells (11). Vignon et al (12) have recently shown that in a chemically defined culture medium (13), estradiol stimulates both the growth of MCF7 cells and the production of the secreted 52 K protein thus excluding a sole permissive effect of estrogen on growth. This result confirmed that these two effects of estradiol do not require the presence of unidentified serum factors. Several indirect lines of evidence suggest that estrogen-induced secreted proteins mediate the mitogenic effect of estrogen (2,3,10). In fact, proteins from serum free media conditioned by estrogen stimulated MCF7 cells increase the growth of resting MCF7 cells, and the mitogenic activity is retained by Con A Sepharose chromatography and eluted with the glycoprotein fraction (14). By contrast, the conditioned media from estrogen withdrawn MCF7 cells are inactive. Moreover, in the antiestrogen resistant cell lines R27, and RTx6, tamoxifen remains, as in the wild type MCF7 cells unable to stimulate the production of the estrogen regulated 160 K secreted protein and of the pS2 mRNA (15) but became able, as an estrogen, to increase the production of the 52 K protein (16). These results also suggest that tamoxifen might decrease the production of estrogen induced growth factor in antiestrogen sensitive cells and increase that production in some antiestrogen resistant cells.

Several lines of evidence suggest that this protein might play a role in human mammary cancerogenesis : 1. Its production is increased by estrogen, a mitogen of epithelial mammary cells. 2. It is present in estrogen receptor positive breast cancer cells but not in normal mammary gland or normal uterus. 3. It is closely related to the effect of estrogen and antiestrogen on cell proliferation. It is therefore tempting to propose as a working hypothesis that the 52 K protein is an estrogen regulated growth factor, coded by one as yet uncharacterized mammary oncogene and expressed at a higher level in transformed cells. Several growth factors have recently been related to oncogenes (17) and it is conceivable that some of them are regulated by steroids. The availability of several monoclonal antibodies, the purification of the protein and the cloning of its cDNA and gene might provide evidence for or against this hypothesis.

ACKNOWLEDGEMENTS

This work was mostly supported by the "Institut National de la Santé et de la Recherche Médicale", and by contracts from the "Caisse Nationale d'Assurance Maladie des Travailleurs Salariés", SANOFI-CLIN-MIDY (n°81039) and the "Association pour le Développement de la Recherche sur le Cancer".

REFERENCES

1. Banbury Report I (1981) "Hormones and Breast Cancer", Pike MC, Siiteri PK, Welsch CW (eds). Cold Spring Harbor Laboratory.
2. Westley B, Rochefort H (1980) Cell 20:353-362.
3. Rochefort H, Chalbos D, Capony F, Garcia M, Veith F, Vignon F, Westley B (1984) In: Gurpide E, Calandra R, Levy C, Soto RJ (eds) Hormones and Cancer. Alan R. Liss, Inc., New York, Vol. 142, pp 37-51.
4. Garcia M, Derocq D, Simon D, Pau B, Rochefort H. Submitted for publication.
5. Veith FO, Capony F, Garcia M, Chantelard J, Pujol H, Veith F, Zajdela A, Rochefort H (1983) Cancer Res 43:1861-1868.
6. Garcia M, Salazar-Retana G, Richer G, Domergue J, Capony F, Pujol H, Laffargue F, Pau B, Rochefort H (1984) J Clin Endocrin Met, in press.
7. Edwards DP, Adams DJ, Savage N, McGuire WL (1980) Biochem Biophys Res Commun 93:804-812.
8. Brabon AC, Williams JF, Cardiff RD (1984) Cancer Res 44:2704-2710.
9. Massot O, Capony F, Garcia M, Rochefort H (1984) Mol Cell Endocrinol 35:167-175.
10. Rochefort H, Coezy E, Joly E, Westley B, Vignon F (1980) In: Iacobelli S, King RJB, Lindner HR, Lippman ME (eds) Progress in Cancer Research and Therapy, Hormones and Cancer. Raven Press, New York, Vol 14, pp 21-29.
11. DeLarco JE, Todaro GJ (1978) Proc Natl Acad Sci (USA) 75:4001-4005.
12. Vignon F. Effects of estrogens in human breast cancer cells growing in serum-free media, in preparation.
13. Barnes D, Sato G (1980) An Biochem 102:255-270.
14. Vignon F, Derocq D, Chambon M, Rochefort H (1983) C R Acad Sci (Paris) 296:151-156.
15. Masiakowski P, Breathnach R, Bloch J, Gannon F, Krust A, Chambon P (1982) Nucl Acids Res 10:7895-7903.
16. Westley B, May FEB, Brown AMC, Krust A, Chambon P, Lippman ME, Rochefort H (1984) J Biol Chem, in press.
17. Heldin CH, Westermark B (1984) Cell 37:9-20.

Endocrinology
F. Labrie, L. Proulx, eds.

EPIDEMIOLOGY OF STEROID DEPENDENT CANCER

R.D. BULBROOK
Imperial Cancer Research Fund, P.O. Box 123, London WC2A 3PX (Gt. Britain)

CLASSICAL EPIDEMIOLOGY

Cancers of the breast, endometrium and ovary have a number of determinants of risk in common. The international incidence rates for the three cancers are highly correlated (1) and in 9 surveyed areas of America the same high correlation was also found (2). A woman who develops one of these cancers has an increased risk of developing either of the remaining two (1). Exogenous estrogens certainly increase the risk of endometrial cancer (3) and probably have the same effect for breast (4) and ovarian cancer (5). Geographical variation in the incidence of the cancers is correlated with Gross National Product and with fat intake (6).

Some aspects of reproductive function are also shared. High risk is associated with nulliparity, low fertility, and a late age at first child: multiparity is protective (7). Obesity is certainly related to a high risk of endometrial cancer but its association with breast and ovarian cancer is less clear.

The inference from these results is that one of the prime determinants of risk is an excessive exposure to estrogens and this view is supported by a considerable amount of evidence from studies on experimental animals.

ANALYTICAL EPIDEMIOLOGY

From 1955 onwards a great deal of work was done in an attempt to replace inferences with actual measurements of endocrine function in patients with cancer of the breast and endometrium and in appropriate controls. As far as breast cancer is concerned, assays of urinary estrogen metabolites led to inconclusive results and the expectation that measurements of blood levels of estradiol would lead to a decisive demonstration of hyperestrogenism has not been fulfilled (8). The balance of the evidence for increased blood and urinary levels of estrogens in endometrial cancer indicates that this does occur but interpretation of the results is complicated because of over-matching the cases by using obese controls (9). Sex-hormone-binding globulin (SHBG) levels in obese women are particulary low so that in addition to an augmented estrogenic stimulus due to increased peripheral aromatisation of androgens there is an additional effect due to lack of protein binding.

There arose, therefore, a paradoxical situation where the clear leads given by classical epidemiologic research could not be substantiated by analytical work. This gave rise to a number of alternative hypotheses such as estriol as a protective agent; altered estrogen metabolism; tissue sensitivity; a major role for prolactin or the androgens; and, above all, to the luteal phase dysfunction hypothesis in which a controlling or modulating effect for progesterone was postulated.

BIOLOGICAL AVAILABILITY OF ESTRADIOL

The resolution of some of the problems described above may result from new work on the biological availability of estradiol. The main point is that estradiol bound to SHBG is not available for biological action and assays of total estradiol in blood may not be the appropriate measurement.

There are now three case-control studies which show that the levels of non-protein-bound estradiol are significantly higher in women with breast cancer than in controls (8,10,11). In a comparison between normal British and Japanese women (i.e., a high and a low risk population) it was found that the former had marginally higher levels of free estradiol in their blood, significantly higher levels of albumin-bound estradiol and a striking diminution of the amount bound to SHBG--30% compared to 53% (12).

Perhaps the most convincing evidence comes from a recent prospective study in which blood samples were collected from 5000 normal British women. In 11 of 13 women whose blood was obtained before breast cancer was diagnosed, free estradiol levels were at or above the 80th percentile of the normal population range (13).

The importance of measuring biologically available estradiol in endometrial cancer is shown by the finding that in obese patients total estradiol was increased two-fold compared with slender patients, but bioavailable estradiol was increased four-fold (14).

No comparable data exists for ovarian cancer.

Since the metabolic clearance rates of many steroids are related to protein binding (9) patients with breast and endometrial cancer should have high clearance rates. The available data indicate that this is so for estrone in breast cancer cases (15).

CONCLUSIONS

There is a certain plausibility about the concept that the biological availability of estradiol is of cardinal importance in the genesis of breast, endometrial and possibly ovarian cancer. Abnormalities in protein binding do not appear to be confined only to these cancers. In osteoporotic women, where there is evidence that the condition stems from hypoestrogenism, measurements of total blood estradiol have not been informative whereas available estradiol levels are raised (16). Logically, it should follow that bone densities should be high in patients with these cancers: there is one report to this effect (17).

There are, however, a number of irritating inconsistencies in the data, mainly concerned with the levels or capacity of SHBG. At equal levels of SHBG, patients with breast cancer and controls have different amounts of estradiol bound to the protein suggesting displacement by another blood component, possibly of dietary origin. The double risk due to obesity in endometrial cancer has been mentioned. It should follow that over-weight would be a powerful determinant of risk in breast cancer. But this is not so: excess weight is a weak factor, not found in all surveys. Nutrition rather than weight may be the important variable. SHBG capacity is extremely sensitive to thyroid function but the thyroid seems to have little or no effect on the incidence of breast cancer.

The biological role of protein binding of estradiol is still poorly understood but if future work substantiates the findings described above, it might eventually be possible to explore preventive measures based on the manipulation of the amounts of estradiol that are biologically available.

REFERENCES

1. Berg JW (1975) Cancer Res 35:3345
2. Winkelstein W, Sacks ST, Ernster VL, Selvin S (1977) Amer J Epidemiol 105: 407
3. Henderson BE, Casagrande JT, Pike MC, Mack T, Rosario I, Duke A (1983) Br J Cancer 47:749
4. Hoover R, Gray LA, Cole P, MacMahon B (1976) New Engl J Med 295:401
5. Hoover R, Gray LA, Fraumeni JF (1977) Lancet 2:533
6. Armstrong B, Doll R (1975) Int J Cancer 15:617
7. Joly DJ, Lilienfeld AM, Diamond EL, Bross ID (1974) Amer J Epidemiol 99:190
8. Reed MJ, Cheng RW, Noel CT, Dudley HAF, James VHT (1983) Cancer Res 43:3940
9. Siiteri PK, Murai JT, Hammond GL, Nisker JA, Raymoure WJ, Kuhn RW (1982) Recent Prog Horm Res 38:457
10. Siiteri PK, Hammond GL, Nisker JA (1981) In: Pike MC, Siiteri PK, Welsch CW (eds) Banbury Report No. 8; Hormones and Cancer. Cold Spring Harbor Laboratory, pp 87-101
11. Moore JW, Clark GMG, Bulbrook RD, Hayward JL, Murai JT, Hammond GL, Siiteri PK (1982) Int J Cancer 29:17
12. Moore JW, Clark GMG, Takatani O, Wakabayashi Y, Hayward JL, Bulbrook RD (1983) J Natl Cancer Inst 71:749
13. Bulbrook RD, Moore JW, Wang DY, Clark GMG (1984) To be published
14. Gambone JC, Pardridge WM, Lagasse LD, Judd HL (1982) Obstet Gynecol 59:416
15. Kirschner MA, Cohen FB, Ryan C (1978) Cancer Res 38:4029
16. Davidson BJ, Ross RK, Paganini-Hill A, Hammond GD, Siiteri PK, Judd HL (1982) J Clin Endocrinol Metab 54:115
17. Kantin AV, Rokhlin GD (1975) Vopr Onkol 21:34

Endocrinology
F. Labrie, L. Proulx, eds.

SPECTACULAR RESPONSE TO COMBINED ANTIHORMONAL TREATMENT IN ADVANCED PROSTATE CANCER

FERNAND LABRIE, ANDRE DUPONT, ALAIN BELANGER, AND MEMBERS OF LAVAL UNIVERSITY PROSTATE CANCER PROGRAM *

Departments of Medicine and Molecular Endocrinology, Laval University Medical Center, Quebec G1V 4G2, Canada

Cancer of the prostate is a frequent disease which is the second cause of death due to cancer in man. The probability of diagnosis of prostate cancer in white and black men in the US is 5.2 and 9.6% respectively, thus indicating that approximately 1 out of 20 white males and 1 out of 10 black males will be victims of this disease during their lifetime. Moreover, in more than 50% of patients, the cancer can only be detected at a late stage when it has already spread to distant tissues, especially the bones. Moreover, it should be mentioned that 50% of the cases of prostate cancer are diagnosed between the ages of 45 and 67, at a time when most men have their highest level of social responsabilities.

REPLACEMENT OF SURGICAL CASTRATION AND ESTROGENS BY LHRH AGONISTS, A NEW CLASS OF DRUGS FREE OF SECONDARY EFFECTS

Since surgical castration presents serious psychological limitations in a large proportion of patients, while estrogens have serious and often lethal cardiovascular complications, there was the obvious need for a more acceptable means of neutralizing the secretion of androgens by the testes (1). Following our observation in experimental animals that chronic treatment with synthetic analogs of the hypothalamic hormone luteinizing hormone-releasing hormone (LHRH) blocks testicular androgen secretion with secondary atrophy of the prostate (2), the hope was immediately raised that such treatment could be used for the treatment of prostate cancer. We could show fairly quickly that the same chemical castration can be easily achieved in man (3-5).

NOT ONLY THE TESTES BUT ALSO THE ADRENALS PRODUCE MALE HORMONES ACTING ON THE PROSTATE CANCER

While, in any other animal species, the testes are the almost exclusive source of male hormones, this is not the case in man. It is of major importance to realize that the normal human prostate as well as the prostate cancer cells receive close to 50% of their stimulation by male hormones originating from the adrenal glands. Surgical or medical castration is thus no more than a partial treatment

---

*C. Bossé, R. Delisle, J.G. Girard, J.G. Houle, J.P. Emond, G. Monfette, J.P. Paquet and A. Vallières.

for prostate cancer. The dramatic consequence of this fact that only 50 to 60% of the male hormones acting on the cancer have been removed by orchiectomy or medical castration (achieved by estrogens or LHRH agonists alone), is that the prostate cancer remains under the influence of an important amount of male hormones originating from the adrenals following such incomplete treatment. With this knowledge, we felt that a major step forward in the treatment of prostate cancer would be the neutralization of the so-far unrecognized role of the adrenal male hormones in the growth of prostate cancer.

THE MALE HORMONES OF ADRENAL ORIGIN ARE BLOCKED BY AN ANTIANDROGEN

Although the male hormone precursors are only by-products of the adrenal glands, it is not possible to block their formation without interfering at the same time with the formation of cortisol, the stress hormone essential for life. We have thus chosen to avoid this problem by blocking the action rather than the formation of these precursors of male hormones using a pure antiandrogen.

Flutamide and Anandron are called pure antiandrogens since they have no activity by themselves but act exclusively by blocking the action of male hormones in the prostate cancer tissue.

ALL PROSTATE CANCERS PREVIOUSLY UNTREATED SHOW A POSITIVE AND OBJECTIVE RESPONSE TO THE NEW TREATMENT AS COMPARED TO ONLY 60 TO 80% BY PREVIOUS TREATMENTS

The new combined antihormonal treatment has now been administered for 2½ years. Two hundred patients have received the treatment for periods of time sufficient to permit an objective evaluation of the results obtained. Objective assessment of the effect of treatment is made using all the techniques and assays available: bone scanning, X-Ray, intravenous pyelography, level of serum prostatic acid phosphatase, urinary flow, ultrasonography of the prostate and CAT scan. The main clinical parameters used are pain, urinary symptoms, appetite, body weight, well-being and performance.

The most dramatic finding is that all patients who received this new treatment as their first treatment showed, with no exception so far, a positive and objective response. The improvement in the signs and symptoms of prostate cancer is extremely rapid. In fact, pain disappeared in all patients within days. All patients returned to normal life activities with no secondary side-effects, thus enjoying an excellent quality of life.

It should be mentioned that previous endocrine treatments such as surgical castration and estrogens caused a positive response in only 60 to 80% of patients, while the present treatment has so far induced a positive response in 100% of patients.

SURVIVAL IS IMPROVED AT LEAST 10-FOLD AT 2 YEARS BY THE NEW TREATMENT

Since all patients not treated previously experience a remission of their disease with the combined treatment, the next question is the duration of this positive response and the effect on the duration of life or survival. While all previous studies have shown that the death rate after 1½ year of treatment varies from 24 to 37%, this value is now reduced to 3.3% by the new treatment, thus representing a 7 to 11-fold improvement in survival (Fig. 1). It should be mentioned that the only patient who died in our study started treatment when he was at the terminal phase of his disease with a life expectancy of only 2 to 3 weeks. He could live for 9 months with a good quality of life.

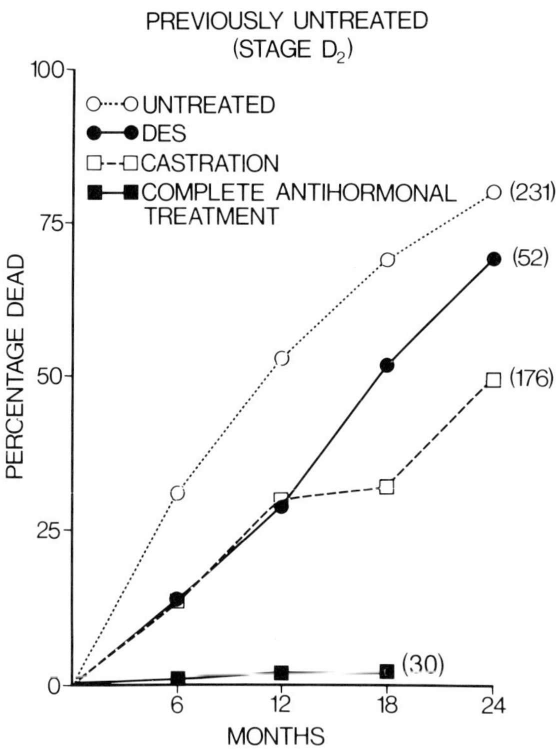

Fig. 1. Comparison of the objective positive response following the new combined treatment (LHRH agonist or orchiectomy in association with a pure antiandrogen) and partial androgen neutralization (DES or castration) (6) in previously untreated stage D2 prostate cancer patients.

CONCLUSION

The most important conclusion from this study is that prostate cancer previously untreated is exquisitely sensitive to male hormones. When, in the past, only part of the male hormones, namely those of testicular origin, were neutralized by surgical castration or estrogens, a positive response was obtained in 60% to 80% of cases. When the combined antihormonal treatment is applied, thus resulting in more complete neutralization of male hormones of both testicular and adrenal origin, a positive response has been seen in all patients with no exception so far.

Not only a much larger proportion (100 versus 60-80%) of patients respond to the new treatment but the effect of treatment on the duration of life is at least increased by 10-fold at 2 years. It is extremely important to recall that exposure of patients to estrogens, surgical castration or LHRH agonists alone induces the formation of cancers insensitive to male hormones. Moreover, the new combined antihormonal treatment has no secondary effect. It thus appears logical to propose that the combined antihormonal treatment should be started immediately after diagnosis of prostate cancer in order to obtain remission in a greater proportion of patients, to increase survival and to minimize the appearance of androgen-resistant cell clones. Consequently, orchiectomy, estrogens or LHRH agonists alone should not be further used for the treatment of prostate cancer without concomitant administration of a pure antiandrogen.

The availability of such a treatment that has no secondary effect, markedly increases survival and permits a return to normal activity with an excellent quality of life is of major importance. In fact, it is estimated that 75,000,000 men presently living in the world have or will have clinical prostate cancer during their lifetime. A 5-year increase in survival corresponds to 275,000,000 man-years or more than the total activity of the total population of the U.S. during a full year. In addition to the dramatic advantages already observed in prostate cancer, it is expected that the same principles of complete blockade of all hormonal influences on the cancer will apply to other hormone-sensitive diseases, especially breast cancer, where complete blockade of estrogenic influences has never been achieved at the start of treatment.

REFERENCES

1. Huggins C, Stevens RE, Hodges CW (1941) Arch Surg 43:209

2. Labrie F, Auclair C, Cusan L, Kelly PA, Pelletier G, Ferland L (1978) In Hansson V (ed), Endocrine Approach to Male Contraception, Int J Androl (Suppl 2), pp 303-308

3. Labrie F, Bélanger A, Cusan L, Séguin C, Pelletier G, Kelly PA, Lefebvre FA, Lemay A, Raynaud JP (1980) Androl 1:209

4. Labrie F, Dupont A, Bélanger A, Cusan L, Lacoursière Y, Monfette G, Laberge JG, Emond JP, Fazekas ATA, Raynaud JP, Husson JM (1982) J Clin Invest Med 5: 267

5. Labrie F, Dupont A, Bélanger A, Lacoursière Y, Raynaud JP, Husson JM, Gareau J, Fazekas ATA, Sandow J, Monfette G, Girard JG, Emond J, Houle JG (1983) The Prostate 4: 579

6. Jordan WP Jr, Blackard CE, Byar DP (1977) South Med J 70:1411

22. Autoimmune Thyroiditis

© 1984 Elsevier Science Publishers B.V.
Endocrinology
F. Labrie, L. Proulx, eds.

ABERRANT MAJOR HISTOCOMPATIBILITY CLASS II (HLA-DR) EXPRESSION AS A NEW FACTOR IN ENDOCRINE AUTOIMMUNE DISORDERS

MARCO LONDEI, RICARDO PUJOL-BORRELL, GIANFRANCO BOTTAZZO

Department of Immunology, Arthur Stanley House, Middlesex Hospital Medical School, 40-50 Tottenham Street, London W1P 9PG. Correspondence to Dr G F Bottazzo MD MRCP MRCPath at the above address

INTRODUCTION

The recent demonstration of HLA-DR expression on monolayers of stimulated normal thyrocytes in vitro and, the presence of these molecules in vivo on thyroid glands from Graves' and Hashimoto patients but not on 'healthy' glands has offered a new insight into the understanding of the pathogenesis of organ-specific autoimmune diseases (1-2).

Since MHC Class II molecules are normally confined to cells actively involved in immune reactions (B lymphocytes, activated T-lymphocytes; macrophages and dendritic cells collectively referred to as 'antigen-presenting cells' or APCs) and since these molecules play a crucial role in initiating the immune response to any antigen, a new role could be indicated for thyroid epithelial cells in organ-specific autoimmunity. These findings led us to a new hypothesis to try to explain the phenomena leading to autoimmunity in the thyroid gland and more broadly, in organ-specific autoimmune disease (3).

THE EVIDENCE

Aberrant HLA-DR expression in thyroditis and other autoimmune disorders

HLA-DR molecules, contrary to the HLA-A,B,C antigens (Class I MHC) have a restricted distribution. Apart from immunocytes of various kinds these antigens have been found in other tissues such as the vascular endothelium and some epithelia under physiological and pathological conditions. However, they are normally not present on epithelial cells of the endocrine glands. We demonstrated by indirect immunofluorescence that normal human thyroid follicular cells could be induced in vitro to express HLA-DR antigens when cultured with mitogenic lectins (1).

Soon we found that expression of DR molecules was a common feature in glands of Graves and Hashimoto patients indicating that the phenomenon already observed *in vitro* was present *in vivo* only in glands of 'autoimmmune' patients (2). A similar aberrant expression was also found in diabetic insulitis, primary biliary cirrhosis and autoimmune enteropathy suggesting wider implications for the original finding.

Interferon-(IFN)-Gamma induces aberrant expression of HLA-DR

It is difficult to envisage lectins as 'switching on' DR synthesis in vivo, as they did under experimental conditions. Therefore we looked for more acceptable physiological mediators for this induction.

The most widely studied modulator of DR expression is Interferon-gamma, a factor produced by T-lymphocytes. For this reason we tested the capacity of IFN-gamma to induce MHC Class II molecules in cultures of normal DR negative thyrocytes. IFN-gamma in concentrations as low as 1 U/ml gave positive results when incubated with monolayers of thyrocytes, whereas IFN-alpha, IFN-beta and Interleukin (Il)-2 were unable to induce DR activation (4).

These results indicate that environmental factors which are known to stimulate IFN-gamma, can eventually lead to the triggering of thyrocytes to become antigen presenters of their own surface autoantigens.

One of the critical tests in our hypothesis was to prove that the MHC Class II molecules expressed on thyrocytes had the same physiological role in presenting antigens as do regular antigen-presenting cells (APCs).

We demonstrated that thyrocytes spontaneoulsy positive for DR were able to present a 20 amino acid peptide of the hemagglutinin of influenza strain A virus, but not the intact virus, to a T-cell clone that selectively proliferated in the presence of the same antigen presented by HLA-matched APCs. An irrelevant peptide introduced as a control was inactive. Moreover, as with other proliferative responses, a monoclonal antibody against the DR 'backbone' or invariant region could block the response to the influenza antigen (5).

Our results indicate that DR^+ thyrocytes acquire only some of the properties of APCs but are unable to process or 'digest' large proteins as do macrophages. We believe that they could present surface autoantigens to immunocompetent cells mainly because these are already processed in specialized endocrine cells before being inserted as a final product on the plasma membrane.

A new strategy to dissect the autoimmune response

Cloned T-lymphocytes from glands of patients with Graves' disease gave us the opportunity to validate such a hypothesis by a new approach. Lymphocytes already activated in vivo were extracted from autoimmune glands and expanded in the presence of mitogen-free IL-2, to allow their growth. Some of the clones showed a proliferative response only in the presence of autologous thyrocytes but not when cultured with autologous peripheral blood mononuclear cells or HLA mismatched thyrocytes.

This proliferative response could be inhibited by monoclonal antibodies to the MHC Class II molecules; furthermore we could visually observe a direct binding between the thyrocytes and the cloned T-lymphocytes (6).

CONCLUSION

The model that we suggest is shown in the Fig.

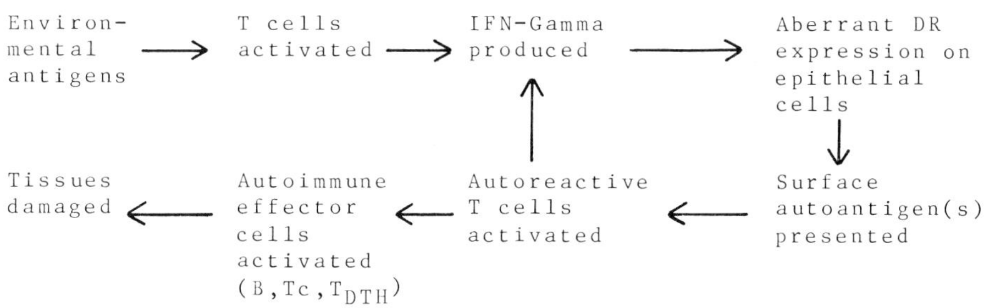

Fig Sequence of events leading to organ specific autoimmune disease as proposed in our hypothesis.

An initial, probably non-specific antigenic challenge triggers the activation of T-lymphocytes in a genetically predisposed individual. The resulting production of factors, particularly INF-Gamma could lead to the aberrant expression of DR antigen on endocrine and other epithelial cells. This will allow certain MHC Class II molecules with the right configuration, for example various polypeptide chains related to DR-3, DR-4, DR-5, etc, to associate themselves closely with a surface autoantigen. This molecular complex will then attract specialized organ-specific T-helper lymphocytes. More interferon-gamma will be secreted and this will maintain the aberrant DR expression on the endocrine cells. Specifically sensitized lymphocytes will send signals to the other cells of the immune system, allowing them to make autoantibodies and the process will culminate in the expansion of cytotoxic T-cell clones.

We envisage that organ-specific T-suppressor lymphocytes will gradually lose their capacity to overcome this abnormal autoantigen presentation in patients with a suitable genetic make-up and this could lead to the presence of the organ-specific antibodies in the patient's serum and to the known slow destructive process observed in the autoimmune atrophy of the endocrine glands.

REFERENCES

1. Pujol-Borrell R., Hanafusa T., Chiovato L., Bottazzo G.F. Lectin-induced expression of DR antigen on human cultured follicular thyroid cells. Nature (London) 303:71-73 (1983).

2. Hanafusa T., Pujol-Borrell R., Chiovato L., Russell R.C.G., Doniach D., Bottazzo G.F. Aberrant expression of HLA-DR antigen on thyrocytes in Graves' Disease: relevance for autoimmunity. Lancet ii:1111-1115 (1983).

3. Bottazzo G.F., Pujol-Borrell R., Hanafusa T., Feldmann M. Role of aberrant HLA-DR expression and antigen presentation in induction of endocrine autoimmunity. Lancet ii:1115-1119 (1983).

4. Todd I., Pujol-Borrell R., Hammond L.J., Bottazzo G.F., Feldmann M. Interferon gamma induces HLA-DR expression by thyroid epithelium. Submitted for publication.

5. Londei M., Lamb J.R., Bottazzo G.F., Feldmann H. Epithelial cells expressing aberrant MHC class II determinants can present antigen to cloned human T lymphocytes. Submitted for publication.

6. Londei M., Bottazzo G.F., Feldmann M. T cell clones recognising autologous thyroid cells from Graves' disease patients. Submitted for publication.

Endocrinology
F. Labrie, L. Proulx, eds.

MECHANISM OF POSTPARTUM THYROID DISEASE

NOBUYUKI AMINO, YOSHINORI IWATANI, HARUO TAMAKI, HIDEMITSU MORI, KIYOSHI MIYAI and OSAMU TANIZAWA

Department of Laboratory Medicine, Osaka University Medical School, Osaka 553, Japan

INTRODUCTION

Pregnancy markedly influences the clinical course of Hashimoto's disease and Graves' disease (1-3). Both diseases are ameliorated during pregnancy. However diseases are aggravated after delivery and transient thyrotoxicosis and/or hypothyroidism are frequently observed (3-5). Subclinical autoimmune thyroiditis is also aggravated after delivery and thyroid dysfunction was found in 5.5 per cent of postpartum women in general population (6). We examined the mechanisms of occurrence of postpartum thyroid dysfunction.

MATERIAL AND METHODS

Fifteen patients with Hashimoto's disease were observed during and after delivery. For cross-sectional analyses, 20 non-pregnant normal subjects and 77 females with Hashimoto's disease were studied. To examine the postpartum relapse of Graves' thyrotoxicosis, we observed 41 pregnancies in 35 patients with Graves' disease who were considered to be in a state of clinical remission. Anti-thyroid microsomal antibodies (MCHA) were measured by tranned red cell hemagglutination assay. TSH-binding inhibitory immunoglobulins (TBII) were measured by the method of Shewring & Smith (7). Peripheral T, B, Tγ and K lymphocytes were determined by E, EAC, EA rosette formation and ADCC plaque formation, respectively. Large granular lymphocytes (LGL) were enumerated by inspection of cell smear. Peripheral T lymphocyte subsets were determined with monoclonal antibodies using FACS analysis.

RESULTS

In Hashimoto's disease, titers of MCHA and complement dependent cytotoxic antibody, peripheral lymphocyte counts and goiter size decreased during pregnancy but increased after delivery. At the time of postpartum aggravation percentages of B and K lymphocytes were significantly higher than normal nonpregnant females (Table 1). The percentages of LGL also increased transiently after delivery. The percentages of Leu 1 (total T), Leu 2a (suppressor) and Leu 3a (helper) T cells were decreased but helper T/suppressor T cells ratio was normal even at postpartum aggravation. These data suggest that both humoral and cellular immune reactions are important in the postpartum aggravation. Postpartum development of hypothyroidism recurred in all 8 patients with Hashimoto's disease who had previous history of postpartum transient hypothyroidism. To predict the postpartum development of hypothyroidism, various parameters in early pregnancy were analyzed and MCHA titers were found to be useful. All patients, who had MCHA titers of 2^{11}x10 or more, in early pregnancy, developed postpartum hypothyroidism (Fig. 1).

In Graves' disease 18 of 41 cases showed transient increase of free T_4 index at 10-15 weeks of pregnancy but became euthyroid in later half of pregnancy. After delivery 10 cases relapsed Graves' thyrotoxicosis. At the time of relapse, activities of TBII were not detectable even by sensitive radioreceptor assay, although significant increase of peripheral B lymphocytes and decrease of Tγ lymphocytes were observed (Fig. 2). However significant increase of TBII activity was observed 1-2 months later in all patients who relapsed Graves' thyrotoxicosis. Data suggest that cellular immunity may be more important than

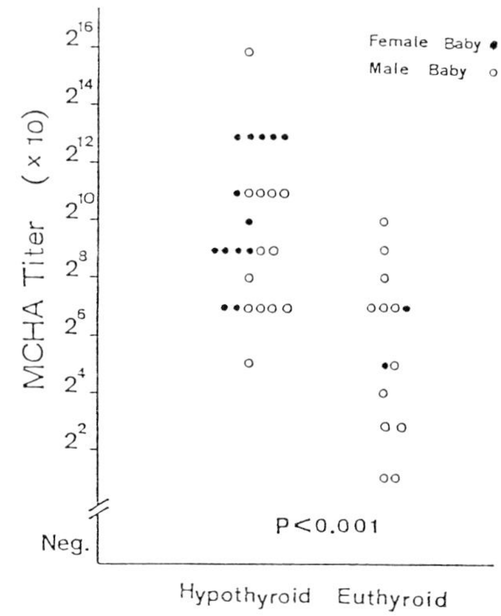

Fig. 1. Comparison of titers of anti-thyroid microsomal antibody in early pregnancy in Hashimoto's patients who developed postpartum hypothyroidism and those did not develop hypothyroidism.

TABLE 1.

Peripheral T, B, and K lymphocytes in healthy subjects and patients with Hashimoto's disease

	No. Examined	Total Lymphocyte (Count/mm^3)	Percentage		
			T cells	B cells	K cells
Nonpregnant controls	20	1768±465	75.9±5.5	21.8±5.1	4.6±1.6
Hashimoto					
Nonpregnant	25	1899±468	76.5±7.8	19.0±7.5	5.4±2.4
Pregnant	16	1555±297	73.8±11.6	25.3±12.9	3.1±1.2†
Postpartum[a]	36	2339±429§	68.9±9.1†	27.6±8.9†	6.2±2.4*

Values are means±SD. a: Values at the time of postpartum aggravation of Hashimoto's disease. Difference from healthy controls at P<0.05 (*), P<0.01 (†), and P<0.001 (§).

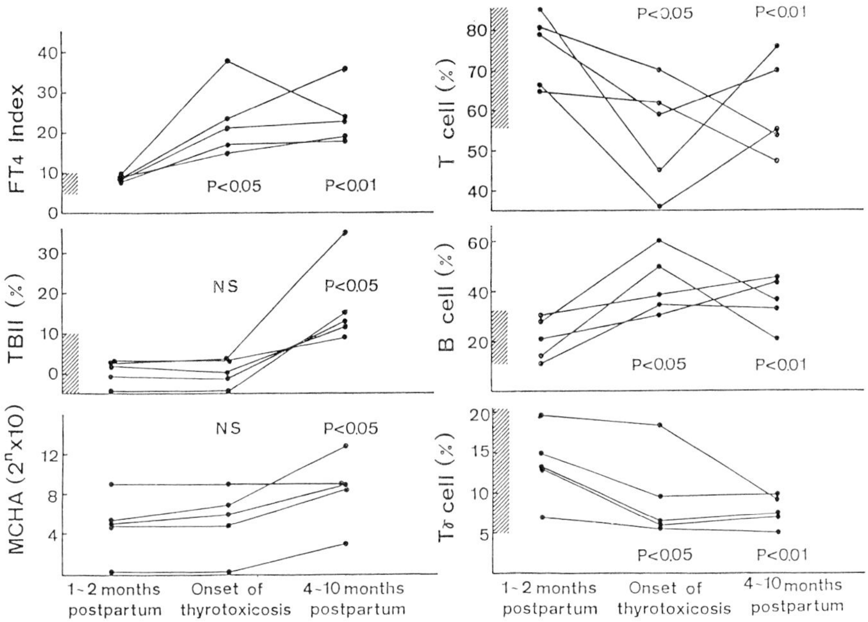

Fig. 2. Changes of circulating thyroid hormone, antibodies and lymphocyte subsets at postpartum relapse of Graves' thyrotoxicosis.

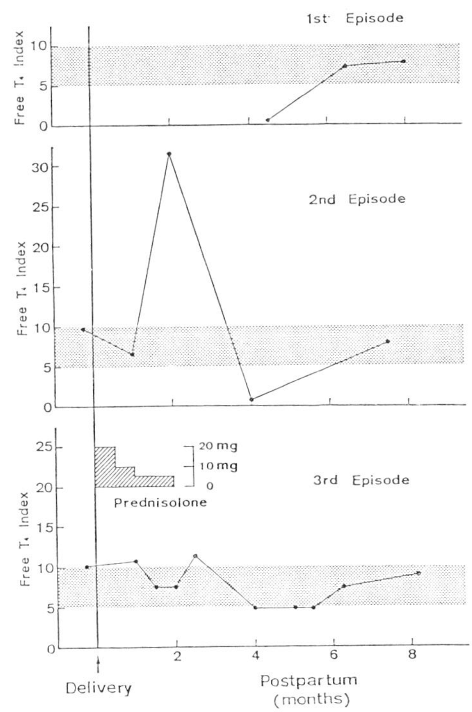

Fig. 3. Prevention of postpartum development of hypothyroidism by short-term prednisolone therapy.

humoral immunity in the initiation of Graves' thyrotoxicosis, or that local immune reactions may be different form immunological abnormalities detected in peripheral blood. Postpartum relapse of Graves' thyrotoxicosis could be predicted by increase of free T_4 index at both 10-15 and 30-32 weeks of pregnancy.

Prevention of postpartum development of hypothyroidism in Hashimoto's disease was tried by short-term prednisolone therapy. As shown in Fig. 3 development of hypothyroidism could be prevented in the third postpartum period. Short-term prednisolone therapy delayed postpartum recurrence of Graves' thyrotoxicosis.

Other autoimmune disease often ameliorate during pregnancy and are aggravated more frequently after delivery. "Immune rebound hypothesis" (Fig. 4) is proposed as the mechanism of postpartum development of thyroid dysfunction.

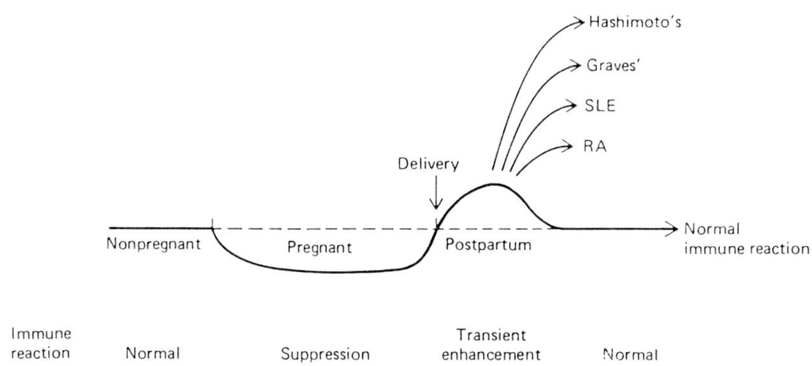

Fig. 4 Immune rebound hypothesis regarding the postpartum onset of autoimmune diseases. Possible immunosuppression in pregnancy may disappear at delivery. "Transient enhancement" of the immune reactions may occur after delivery.

REFERENCES

1. Amino N et al. (1976) J Clin Endocrinol Metab 42: 296
2. Amino N et al. (1977) J Clin Endocrinol Metab 44: 130
3. Amino N et al. (1977) Ann Intern Med 87: 155
4. Amino N et al. (1982) J Clin Endocrinol Metab 55: 108
5. Amino N, Miyai K (1983) In: Davies TF (ed) Autoimmune Endocrine Disease. John Wiley & Sons, New York, pp 247-272
6. Amino N et al. (1982) New Engl J Med 306: 849
7. Shewring G, Smith BR (1982) Clin Endocrinol 17: 409

© 1984 Elsevier Science Publishers B.V.
Endocrinology
F. Labrie, L. Proulx, eds.

MODULATION OF LYMPHOCYTE FUNCTION IN AUTOIMMUNE THYROID DISEASE

A.M. McGREGOR, A.P. WEETMAN, ROSEMARY HASSMAN, D.P. RENNIE, MARIAN LUDGATE, CATHERINE GUNN, SUVINA RATANACHAIYAVONG, and R. HALL
Department of Medicine, Welsh National School of Medicine, Heath Park, Cardiff, CF4 4XN, Wales, U.K.

INTRODUCTION

Autoimmune thyroid disease (AITD) arises in genetically predisposed individuals and though the aetiology remains uncertain the pathogenic mechanisms inducing the disease are increasingly well understood (1). Since AITD is due to immune-mediated events, the most effective means of controlling the disease will ultimately depend on modulating the aberrant autoimmune response. For this to be feasible a clear understanding of the immune response made to an autoantigen is necessary. Developments in cellular immunology and immunoassay techniques have permitted studies *in vivo* and *in vitro* in man and in rat models of AITD. Using such technology it has become possible to i) investigate the autoimmune response, ii) examine the individual constituents of the response, iii) locate the site within the immune system where the process is occurring and iv) study the potential for influencing the autoimmune response by physiological, pharmacological and immunological manipulation of the processes involved. This paper seeks to highlight our work in this field.

INVESTIGATION OF THE AUTOIMMUNE RESPONSE

Peripheral blood mononuclear cells (PBM) obtained from patients with AITD and cultured *in vitro* in the presence of a non-specific mitogen (pokeweed mitogen) will synthesise and secrete detectable amounts of antithyroid autoantibodies (2). In such systems, a number of limitations exist; i) measurement of autoantibody by haemagglutination is tedious and imprecise, ii) interpretation of results achieved in long-term cultures in terms of their relevance to the *in vivo* situation is uncertain and finally iii) the use of mitogens as opposed to specific antigens to generate an autoimmune response is again of questionable relevance. To try to circumvent these limitations a number of modifications have been made. Development of enzyme-linked immunosorbent assays (ELISA) for the detection of thyroid autoantibodies (1,3,4) has significantly improved our ability to detect autoantibodies, in serum or secreted *in vitro*, to thyroglobulin and the thyroid microsome. Likewise establishment of culture and assay systems permitting investigation of spontaneous as opposed to mitogen-driven autoantibody secretion have allowed analysis of lymphocyte function which reflects more closely the *in vivo* situation (5). The ability to demonstrate antigen- as opposed to mitogen-driven autoantibody synthesis by PBM from some patients with AITD at critical low doses of autoantigen (6) and the subsequent enhancement of this response by direct presentation of auto-antigen to purified antigen-presenting cells (monocytes) within the PBM population (7) have further increased the means for investigating the autoimmune response. Finally, establishment of animal models of experimental AITD in rats by either antigen/adjuvant innoculation (8) or neonatal thymectomy and sublethal whole-body irradiation (9) has provided access to all the constituents of the immune system without the ethical constraints inherent in investigating AITD in man.

DISSECTION OF THE AUTOIMMUNE RESPONSE

Great caution is required in interpreting data obtained in ELISA assay systems using crude antigen preparations to coat the plate and seeking with such material to detect autoantibodies to pure antigens presumed to be present within the crude preparation (McGregor et al, submitted for publication). Likewise the significance of obtaining cell-mediated responses to crude antigen preparations in migration-inhibition assay systems when no such responses are attainable to purified thyroid antigens questions the validity of such techniques (Ludgate et al, submitted for publication). Using monoclonal antibodies to purified human thyroid antigens it is clear that both poly- and monoclonal autoantibodies are recognising discrete antigens (Weetman et al, submitted for publication) and most likely epitopes within these antigens (1) so that assay and culture systems which investigate the autoimmune response should rely on the use of highly purified rather than crude antigens if they are to have any relevance. Using pure antigens it has been possible to characterise the central role of the antigen-presenting cell both *in vivo* (10) and *in vitro* (7) in generating the autoimmune response. Furthermore access to tissue from varying sites within the immune system both in rats (11) and in man (12) has clarified the important role the bone marrow and lymph nodes draining the site of the active autoimmune process may have, in addition to the thyroid, in the production of autoantibodies in AITD. Development of monoclonal antibodies to human thyroid autoantigens in particular to the thyroid microsome, besides helping to elucidate the structure of the antigen and its localisation, have permitted characterisation of the role antibodies to the microsome play in binding to and killing thyroid cells (Weetman et al, submitted for publication).

REGULATION OF THE AUTOIMMUNE RESPONSE

Whilst enumeration of total numbers of "suppressor" T cells in both man (13) and rats (9) with AITD suggests differences which relate to disease activity, the significance of these changes and their relevance to the disease remain questionable. They are much more likely to represent a non-specific, secondary event. In contrast functional alterations in antigen-specific suppressor T cells could be of considerable importance. Such defects have been reported in patients with AITD (14) but we have been unable to confirm these observations (Ludgate et al, submitted for publication) using a similar system. A role for thyroid hormones themselves in regulating the immune system has attracted considerable interest (14). Neither in rats with AITD nor in man, *in vivo* or *in vitro* have we succeeded in demonstrating any immune-modulating effect of thyroid hormones (15, 16, Hassman et al, submitted for publication).

CONTROL OF THE AUTOIMMUNE RESPONSE

Demonstration of an immunosuppressive effect of methimazole (MMI) on autoantibody synthesis in man (17) and rats (8) has been followed by localisation of the site of action. MMI is taken up by antigen-presenting cells (Weetman et al, submitted for publication), and inhibits antigen presentation to these cells (7) probably by interfering with the generation of oxygen radicals (18). Not surprisingly perchlorate, like MMI, also has immunosuppressive properties (19). The ability of irradiation *in vivo* (20) and *in vitro* (21) to influence the autoimmune process further highlights the importance of considering the influence of therapeutic agents on the immune system and the relevance of such effects for disease control. Furthermore the recognition that agents such as iodine (22) and lithium (Hassman et al, submitted for publication) may have potential for immune regulatory effects further emphasises the need to examine immune system-directed therapeutic manoeuvres to control AITD. In this context the potent immunosuppressive cyclosporin A, acting primarily to interfere with T cell-mediated processes may have a role to play where such phenomena are implicated (9). Similarly development of conjugates between lethal toxins, such as ricin, and antigens or anti-idiotypic antibodies directed at B lymphocytes making autoantibodies may provide a means,in deleting these clones of cells secreting autoantibody (23),for disease control.

CONCLUSIONS

Systems for the investigation of AITD both *in vivo* and *in vitro* have been developed. Using such techniques we have further defined the constituents involved in the autoimmune response and the sites in the immune system where such events occur has been established. Regulation within the immune system itself in AITD in response to physiologic stimuli such as thyroid hormones has been examined. Recognition of the influence of conventional antithyroid therapy on the immune response in AITD besides leading to characterisation of their site action has highlighted the need to focus therapy for AITD on the immune system. In this context preliminary data with powerful immunosuppressive agents and with ricin toxin conjugates suggest potential means for more effective disease control in the future.

ACKNOWLEDGEMENTS

The support of the Wellcome Trust and the Medical Research Council (U.K) is gratefully acknowledged, as is the secretarial assistance of Miss Annette Berry.

REFERENCES

1. Weetman AP, McGregor AM (1984) Endocrine Reviews 5 (no 2):309
2. McGregor AM, McLachlan SM, Clark F et al (1979) Immunology 36: 81
3. McGregor AM, Borst GC, Wistar R et al (1981) Clin Research 29:296
4. Weetman AP, Rennie DP, Hassman R et al (1984) Clin Chim Acta 138:237
5. Weetman AP, McGregor AM, Hall R (1982) J Immunol Meth 54:47
6. McGregor AM, Borst GC, Wistar R et al (1981) Annal Clin Endocrinol. 11th Meeting ETA Abstract 71
7. Weetman AP, McGregor AM, Hall R (1983) Clin Immunol Immunopathol 28:39
8. Rennie DP, McGregor AM, Keast D et al (1983) Endocrinology 112:326
9. McGregor AM, Rennie DP, Weetman AP et al (1983) Life Sciences 32:97
10. Weetman AP, McGregor AM, Hall R (1983) Immunology 50:315
11. Weetman AP, McGregor AM, Rennie DP et al (1982) Immunology 46:465
12. Weetman AP, McGregor AM, Wheeler MH (1984) Clin Exptl Immunol 56:330
13. Ludgate ME, McGregor AM, Weetman AP (1984) Brit Med J 288:526
14. Strakosch CR, Wenzel BE, Row VV et al (1982) N Engl J Med 307:1499
15. Weetman AP, McGregor AM, Rennie DP et al (1982) Clin Exptl Immunol 50:51
16. Weetman AP, McGregor AM, Ludgate M et al (1984) J Endocrinol 101:81
17. McGregor AM, Petersen MM, McLachlan SM et al (1980) N Engl J Med 303:302
18. Weetman AP, Holt ME, Campbell AK et al (1984) Brit Med J 288:518
19. Weetman AP, Gunn C, Hall R et al (1984) Lancet 1:906
20. McGregor AM, Petersen MM, Capiferri R et al (1979) Clin Endocrinol 11:437
21. McGregor AM, McLachlan SM, Rees Smith B et al (1979) Lancet 2:469
22. Weetman AP, McGregor AM, Campbell H et al (1983) Acta Endocrinol 103:210
23. Rennie DP, McGregor AM, Wright J et al (1983) Lancet 2:1338

Endocrinology
F. Labrie, L. Proulx, eds.

MEMBRANE ANTIGENS IN THYROID AUTOIMMUNE DISEASES

ALDO PINCHERA, GIANFRANCO FENZI, STEFANO MARIOTTI, PAOLO VITTI, ENRICO MACCHIA, LUCA CHIOVATO, CLAUDIO MARCOCCI, LUIGI BARTALENA
Cattedra di Endocrinologia and Patologia Medica 2, University of Pisa, Pisa, Italy

INTRODUCTION

Several antigen-antibody systems have been identified in thyroid autoimmune disorders, involving different constituents of the thyroid gland (1). In the classical view thyroglobulin (Tg) is considered the main soluble antigen of the colloid, while the microsomal antigen (M) was regarded as typically intracytoplasmic and associated with the smooth endoplasmic reticulum membranes (2). More recently, evidence was obtained in our labóratory that antigenic determinants of Tg are also associated with membrane structures (3,4). Furthermore, M is expressed on the surface of thyroid cells and cannot be readily separated from the TSH receptor complex (3-5). Recent investigations on the various thyroid cell membrane associated antigens will be discussed in the present report.

THYROGLOBULIN IS ASSOCIATED TO THYROID CELL MEMBRANE

Human Tg autoantibody purified by affinity chromatography (TgAb) was used to assess the presence of Tg on the surface of intact thyroid cells and on thyroid plasma membrane. ^{125}I-labeled TgAb was shown to bind human thyrocytes in primary culture but not to human fibroblasts (3). The binding to thyrocytes could be inhibited by addition of unlabeled TgAb or Tg, whereas microsomal autoantibody (MAb) was not effective. These data indicate that Tg antigenic determinants are present on the thyroid cell surface. To assess whether the presence of Tg on thyroid cell surface could merely be due to simple adherence, further experiments were performed on human thyroid plasma membrane purified by sucrose gradient centrifugation. The membrane preparation was extensively washed to remove weakly associated proteins. After labeling with ^{125}I, lithium diiodosalycilate solubilized material was incubated with purified TgAb, and the resulting precipitate was applied to PAGE. Evidence of Tg antigenic determinants was obtained by autoradiography (6). These data clearly demonstrate that Tg is strictly associated with the thyroid plasma membrane. The question of whether colloid and membrane Tg are antigenically heterogeneous remains to be studied. In preliminary experiments carried out with a panel of Tg monoclonal antibodies we have so far detected no antigenic difference.

RELATIONSHIP BETWEEN THE MICROSOMAL (M) AND CELL SURFACE ANTIGENS

The nature of M antigen is still not fully characterized. It is believed to be a lipoprotein membrane component of exocytotic vesicles transporting newly syn-

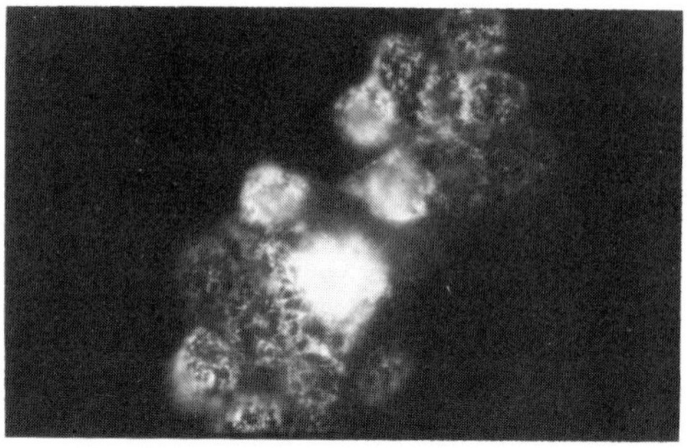

Fig. 1. Indirect immunofluorescence stain on FRT_L cells cultured in the presence of TSH with MAb and fluorescinated anti-human gammaglobulin conjugate.

thesized Tg from the Golgi apparatus to the colloid (1). The notion that these vesicular structures are in continous dynamic exchange with thyroid cell membrane (7) suggested the possibility that M antigen is not only intracellular, but is also expressed on the cell surface. Support to this concept was provided by the demonstration that ^{125}I-MAb was able to bind to intact human thyroid cells in primary culture (8). A dose-dependent inhibition of the binding was elicited by unlabeled MAb preparations, but not by TgAb. A highly significant positive correlation between the inhibitory activity of ^{125}I-MAb binding and the MAb titer was found in a large series of sera from patients with thyroid autoimmune disorders (8). Other authors reached the same conclusions using an indirect immunofluorescence technique on viable human thyroid cells (5). These data provide clear evidence that M antigen is present on thyroid cell surface. In more recent experiments, we have studied the relationship between functional status of the thyroid and the expression of M antigen on the cell surface using continuously cultured rat thyroid cells, which require TSH for growth (9,10). In these cells we were able to show the presence of M antigen on the cell surface (Fig. 1). Withdrawal of TSH from the culture medium impaired the functional status of the cells, blocked the cell growth, and interestingly also elicited a time-dependent decrease of the surface M antigen. Readdition of TSH to the culture medium produced the reappearance of M antigen on the cell surface after 24 hours. Thus, evidence has been obtained that the expression of the M antigen is strictly dependent on the functional status of thyroid cells.

RELATIONSHIP BETWEEN TSH RECEPTOR AND M ANTIGEN

TSH receptor antibodies (TRAb) present in sera of patients with Graves' disease are known to stimulate thyroid adenylate cyclase and to inhibit TSH binding to its receptor, but no strict correlation between these two activities has been found (11,12). A possible explanation for this discrepancy is the multicomponent structure of the TSH receptor (13). Using monoclonal antibodies prepared fusing murine myeloma cells with peripheral lymphocytes from patients with Graves' disease, evi

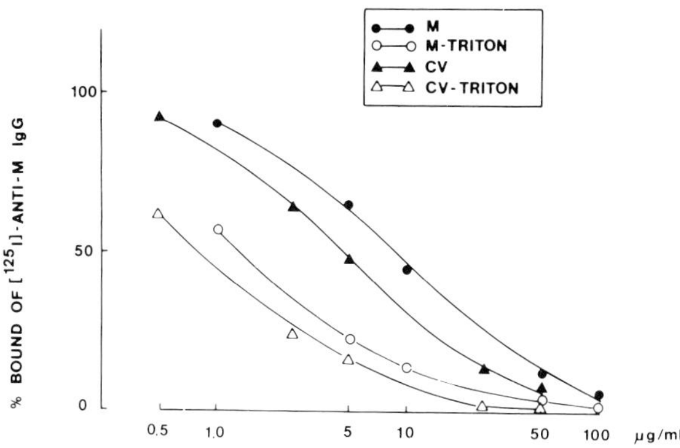

Fig. 2. Inhibition of ^{125}I-MAb binding to human thyroid microsomes coated on plastic wells by addition of graded amounts of particulate (M) or solubilized (M-Triton) microsomal fractions and by particulate (CV) or solubilized (CV-Triton) human thyroid coated vescicles.

dence was obtained supporting the concept that the TSH receptor is a complex structure in which at least a binding and a stimulation site can be antigenically distinguished (14). The coexistence of TSH receptor and M antigen on the thyroid cell surface raises the question of the relationship between these antigenic determinants.

Coated vesicles are recently identified cell structures containing a high density of polypeptide hormone receptors (15,16). Coated vesicles were prepared from human thyroid and identified by elecron microscopy. Particulate and solubilized preparations of thyroid coated vesicles were shown to produce a dose-dependent inhibition of MAb binding to thyroid microsomes (Fig. 2), indicating that these structures contain high concentration of M antigen. Further studies are required to elucidate the significance of this finding.

In other experiments radiolabeled solubulized human thyroid plasma membrane has been used in the attempt to separate M antigen and TSH receptor by immunoprecipitation. The immunoprecipitates obtained by incubation of the radiolabeled solubilized membrane material with TSH or MAb were submitted to PAGE and analyzed by autoradiography. Only a single polypeptide band with an apparent MW of 63 K was found to react with TSH. Among others, the same band was precipitated by MAb, suggesting that TSH receptor comprised common determinants with the M antigen from which cannot be separated.

CONCLUSIONS

Several antigens are expressed on thyroid cell membrane and are recognized by autoantibodies present in patients with thyroid autoimmune disorders. Tg is not only a soluble antigen of the colloid, but is also strictly associated with the cytoplasmic membranes and the thyroid cell surface. M antigen, once reported to be intracellular, has been demonstrated on thyroid cell surface and in thyroid coated vesicles, where also TSH receptor, the putative antigen of TSAb, is represented. These two entities are stricly associated and cannot be readily separated after immunoprecipitation and PAGE. It is conceivable that antigenic determinants expressed on thyroid cell surface are in continuous dynamic exchange with intracellular antigens and can be modulated by the functional status of the cell.

REFERENCES

1. Pinchera A, Fenzi GF, Bartalena L, Chiovato L, Marcocci C, Baschieri L (1980) In: Pinchera A, Doniach D, Fenzi GF, Baschieri L (eds) Autoimmune Aspects of Endocrine Disorders. Academic Press, Amsterdam, pp 57-74
2. Volpè R (1982) Autoimmunity in the Endocrine System. Springer Verlag, Berlin
3. Fenzi GF, Bartalena L, Chiovato L, Marcocci C, Rotella CM, Zonefrati R, Toccafondi R, Pinchera A (1982) Clin Exp Immunol 47: 336-344
4. Fenzi GF, Pinchera A, Bartalena L, Monzani F, Macchia E, Baschieri L (1980) In: Stockigt JR, Nagataki S (eds) Thyroid Research VIII. Australian Academy of Sciences, Canberra pp 703-706
5. Khoury E, Hammond L, Bottazzo GF, Doniach D (1981) Clin Exp Immunol 45: 316-328
6. Monzani F, Fenzi GF, Lippi F, Bartalena L, Macchia E, Pinchera A, Baschieri L (1982) Ann Endocrinol (Paris) 43: 55
7. Ekholm R, Engström LE, Ericson LE, Melander A (1975) Endocrinology 97: 337-344
8. Pinchera A, Fenzi GF, Bartalena L, Chiovato L, Marcocci C, Toccafondi R, Rotella CM, Zonefrati R (1980) In: Stockigt JR, Nagataki S (eds) Thyroid Research VIII. Australian Academy of Sciences, Canberra,pp 707-710
9. Ambesi-Impiombato FS, Parks LAM, Coon HG (1980) Proc Natl Acad Sci USA 77: 3475-3479
10. Valente WA, Vitti P, Kohn LD, Brandi ML, Rotella CM, Toccafondi R, Tramontano D, Aloy SM, Ambesi-Impiombato FS (1983) Endocrinology 112: 71-79
11. Fenzi GF, Mariotti S, Bartalena L, De Groot LJ (1981) In: Coen MP, Foà PP (eds) Special Topics in Endocrinology and Metabolism, vol 2. Alan Liss, New York, pp 43-84
12. Macchia E, Fenzi GF, Monzani F, Lippi F, Vitti P, Grasso L, Bartalena L, Baschieri L, Pinchera A (1981) Clin Endocrinol (Oxf) 15: 175-182
13. Kohn LD, Valente WA, Laccetti P, Cohen JL, Aloj SM, Grollman EF (1983) Life Science 32: 15-30
14. Valente WA, Vitti P, Yavin Z, Yavin E, Rotella CM, Grollman EF, Toccafondi R, Kohn LD (1982) Proc Natl Acad Sci Usa 79: 6680-6685
15. Goldstein JL, Anderson RGW, Brown MS (1979) Nature 279: 679-684
16. Posner BI, Kahn MN, Bergeron JM (1982) Endocr Rev 3:280-298

23. IGF and Related Growth Factors

© 1984 Elsevier Science Publishers B.V.
Endocrinology
F. Labrie, L. Proulx, eds.

IGF I AND II: IN VITRO AND IN VIVO EFFECTS

E.RUDOLF FROESCH, CHRISTOPH SCHMID, EUGEN SCHOENLE, AND JUERGEN ZAPF

Metabolic Unit, Department of Medicine, University of Zurich, 8091 Zurich (Switzerland)

IGF I and II homologues of insulin

The structures of IGF I/SM C and of IGF II have been elucidated by Rinderknecht and Humbel (1,2). They are structurally closely related to insulin and stem from a common precursor. IGF I and II analogues appear to be present in all mammals so far studied.

Differences between insulin and the IGFs

It appears that the synthesis and the processing of insulin and of IGF are very different. Rat IGF is synthesized and secreted by the perfused rat liver and it is likely that IGF I originates mostly from the human liver. The synthesis of IGF I is followed by rapid secretion of the molecule without storage. The processes of IGF synthesis and secretion appear to be very similar to those of albumin. The carrier proteins of IGF are also synthesized and secreted by the rat liver probably independently of IGF. IGF secretion is minimal in livers of hypophysectomized rats whereas binding protein release is decreased only by about 30 % (3).

The actions of small molecular IGF are threefold: The IGFs mimic the effects of insulin on adipose tissue, striated muscle and on the perfused rat heart (4). The relative effectiveness on these tissues in vitro is 1 : 100 in favour of insulin in the case of adipose tissue, 1 : 10 in the case of striated muscle, and 1 : 5 in the case of the rat heart muscle. In all likelihood the IGFs act on adipose tissue via the insulin receptor and on the rat heart via the IGF receptor. Recent results from our laboratory tend to indicate that the positive inotropic effect on contractility of the rat heart occurs at approximately 50 % of total insulin receptor occupancy by insulin as well as by IGF. No qualitative differencies between the effects of insulin and IGF on these tissues have as yet been demonstrated.

Furthermore, there is evidence that IGFs support differentiation and clonal colony formation of fetal and adult human chondrocytes.

In all these test systems, cells in primary culture tend to differentiate in a defined medium containing as the only growth promoting factor IGF I or IGF II. When similar experiments with calvaria cells are carried out with crude platelet-derived growth factor, the cell number increases more markedly and alkaline phosphatase as a marker of osteoblasts decreases when expressed per dish and even more markedly per cell (8).

Insulin-like and growth promoting effects of IGF in vivo

Bolus injections of IGF I and IGF II lead to hypoglycemia and to an increased turnover of glucose (10). If ^{14}C-glucose is injected together with a bolus of IGF I or II, glucose incorporation into striated muscle is markedly enhanced. Lipogenesis of adipose tissue is stimulated to a smaller extent in agreement with the in vitro findings according to which IGF has a smaller affinity to adipose tissue than to muscle. These results can be interpreted to mean that the large amount of rapidly injected IGF overrides the capacity of the binding protein and rapidly diffuses as free molecule into the interstitial space where it interacts with insulin- and IGF-receptors. In such experiments growth promoting effects of IGFs cannot be demonstrated. For the latter, small amounts of IGF were infused subcutaneously to hypophysectomized rats by Alzetosmotic minipumps. The rats gained weight, their tibial epiphyseal width increased, the costal cartilage of the rats incorporated more ^{3}H-thymidine and all these effects were dose-dependent (11). IGF I was clearly more effective than IGF II and endogenous rat IGF induced by the infusion of growth hormone appears to be more effective than IGF I. Thus, IGF I alone induces growth in vivo in the absence of other pituitary and pituitary-dependent hormones. Some differences between the effects of growth hormone and those of IGF treatment were observed. Growth hormone led to the reappearance of the large molecular 150'000 dalton binding peak of serum, IGF did not. The large molecular binding peak is responsible for the long half-life (4 h) of IGF in the rat. Therefore, growth hormone has a major effect on the circulatory form of IGF I and probably also on its distribution and presentation to the target organs (12).

The IGFs are potent growth stimulating factors on cultured cells. Mitogenic effects on DNA synthesis and cell replication have been demonstrated on fibroblasts of different animal species, on chondrocytes of various species, on rat calvaria cells and on many different cell lines mostly of mesodermal origin (5,6). Stimulation by IGF of colony formation of erythroid precursor cells (9) and of differentiation of muscle and bone cells have been demonstrated in our and in other laboratories (7,8).

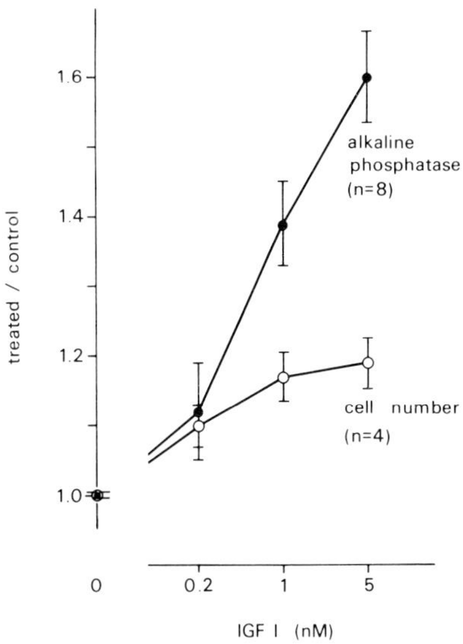

<u>Fig. 1</u>
<u>Cell number and alkaline phosphatase activity in primary cultures of rat calvaria cells grown for six days in the presence of IGF I (mean + SEM, 2 experiments)</u>
Rat calvaria cells were grown in culture without and with IGF I in a defined medium containing no serum or other growth factors. Alkaline phosphatase activity rose out of proportion to the cell number, indicating that IGF is a mitogen that supports differentiation (from Schmid et al. 1984).

The hypothesis of Salmon and Daughaday (13) according to which the growth promoting effects of growth hormone are mostly mediated by the somatomedins has been proven to be true despite opposing views of Isaksson et al. (14). Some experiments of nature, two of which have been studied in detail, support this hypothesis. The pygmies in Central Africa are of small stature and have low levels of IGF I and normal levels of growth hormone (15). They do not respond to growth hormone with an increase of IGF I levels and do not retain nitrogen. The pymies appear to be small because of an IGF I deficit. Eigenmann et al. (16) have made similar observations in 3 different size poodles (standard, miniature and toy). Growth hormone secretion is similar but IGF I levels differ in the same direction as body size.

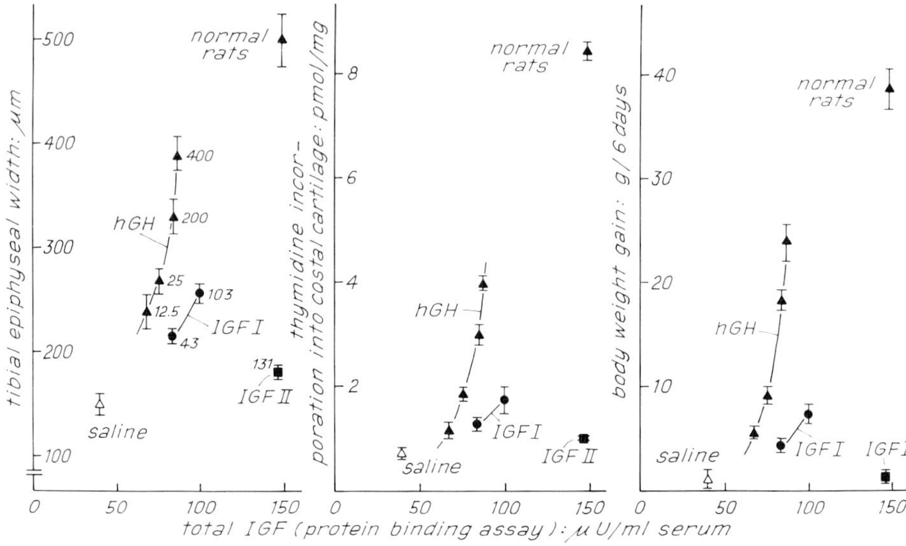

Figure 2
Comparison of growth effects of directly administered IGF I or IGF II with endogenous rat IGF induced by GH administration. Hormones were administered during 6 days to hypox rats in the following dosages: IGF I: 43 ug/day, 103 ug/day; IGF II 131 ug/day; GH 0, 12.5, 25, 200, 400 mU/day. Each point represents the mean of values obtained from four rats. (from Schoenle et al.).

Many problems will be answered when enough IGF will become available to allow experiments like those in the hypophysectomized rats to delineate which hormones contribute to growth and differentiation of tissues and to what extent.

ACKNOWLEDGEMENT

These studies have been supported by the Swiss National Science Foundation (grants 3.380-0.78, 3.167-0.81).

REFERENCES

1. Rinderknecht E, Humbel RE (1978) J Biol Chem 253:2769-2776
2. Rinderknecht E, Humbel RE (1978) FEBS Lett 89:283-286
3. Schwander J, Hauri C, Zapf J, Froesch ER (1983) Endocrinology 113:297-305
4. Zapf J, Schoenle E, Froesch ER (1978) Eur J Biochem 87:285-296
5. Froesch ER, Zapf J, Audhya,TK, Ben-Porath E, Segen BJ, Gibson KD (1976) Proc Natl Acad Sci USA 73:2904-2908

6. Zapf J, Froesch ER, Humbel RE (1981) Current Topics in Cellular Regulation 19:257-309

7. Schmid Ch, Steiner Th, Froesch ER (1983) FEBS-Letters 161:117-121

8. Schmid C, Steiner Th, Froesch ER (1984) FEBS-Letters, in press

9. Kurtz A, Jelkmann W, Bauer Ch (1982) FEBS-Letters 149:105-108

10. Oelz O, Jakob A, Froesch ER (1970) Eur J clin Invest 1:48-53

11. Schoenle E, Zapf J, Humbel RE, Froesch ER (1982) Nature 296: 252-253

12. Schoenle E, Hauri Ch, Steiner Th, Zapf J, Froesch ER (Submitted for publication)

13. Salmon WD, Jr, Daughaday WH (1957) J Lab Clin Med 49:825-836

14. Isaksson OGP, Jansson J-V, Gause IAM (1982) Science 216:1237-1238

15. Merimee TJ, Zapf J, Froesch ER (1981) New Eng J Med. 305:965-968

16. Eigenmann JE, Patterson, DF, Froesch ER (1984) Acta Endocrinol (Kbh), in press.

Endocrinology
F. Labrie, L. Proulx, eds.

PHYSIOLOGY OF SOMATOMEDIN-C/INSULIN-LIKE GROWTH FACTOR I

LOUIS E. UNDERWOOD, JUDSON J. VAN WYK, A. JOSEPH D'ERCOLE, DAVID R. CLEMMONS, and MARJORIE SVOBODA

Department of Pediatrics and Medicine, University of North Carolina, Chapel Hill, NC, USA

Concentrations of somatomedin-C(Sm-C)/insulin-like growth factor I(IGF-I) are modulated in humans by several factors, the most important being growth hormone (GH) and nutritional status. In addition to considering the feedback regulation of Sm-C/IGF-I on growth hormone secretion, and the role of nutrients in the regulation of Sm-C/IGF-I, this presentation will focus on current understanding of somatomedin production and the possible importance of the multiple sites of somatomedin synthesis.

SITES OF SOMATOMEDIN SYNTHESIS: EVIDENCE FOR AUTOCRINE/PARACRINE ACTIONS

The liver was originally believed to be the sole site of somatomedin production. Although recent findings have not diminished the importance of liver, they have shown that somatomedins are synthesized by a variety of tissues. D'Ercole *et al.* (1) first proposed that the somatomedins are synthesized at multiple sites when they reported that immunoreactive somatomedin-like peptides were secreted into the culture medium by explants of a variety of fetal mouse tissues. Subsequently it was shown that a somatomedin-like peptide could also be measured in media in which human fibroblasts were cultured (2,3), and that GH and platelet derived growth factor could stimulate release of this peptide. We have also reported that Sm-C/IGF-I can be extracted directly from rat tissues (4). In the latter studies we observed that most tissues from hypophysectomized rats contained far less activity than tissues from normal animals. Furthermore, after oGH is administered, tissue Sm-C/IGF-I concentrations are raised earlier than serum values. In tissues, peak values occur 8-12 hours after GH, 6-10 hours before maximal serum concentrations are attained (Figure 1).

Because its production is widespread, we and others have proposed that Sm-C/IGF-I acts locally at its site of origin, and that its transport in blood (endocrine model of hormone action) may not be necessary for it to stimulate growth of most tissues (1). Instead, Sm-C/IGF-I may act directly on the cells that produce it (autocrine action) or on neighboring cells (paracrine action). Regardless of whether it stimulates growth entirely by local actions, plasma Sm-C/IGF-I concentrations seem to reflect tissue production. Measurements of plasma concentrations, therefore, are useful in determining variables that influence tissue production.

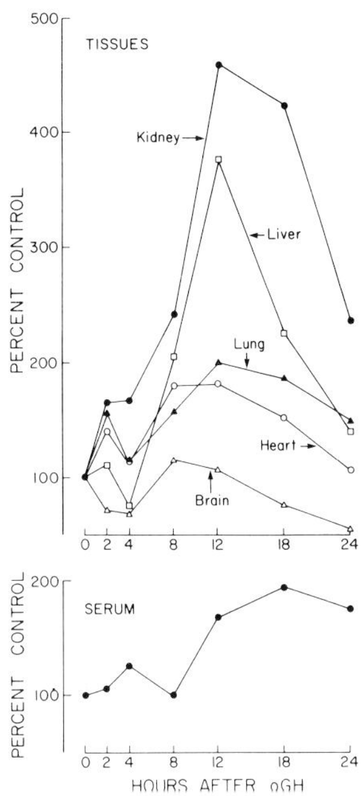

Fig. 1. Tissue and serum Sm-C/IGF-I responses to intraperitoneal injection of 1 mg of ovine GH into hypophysectomized rats. Measurements were made by RIA and are expressed as percent of the control (before oGH) value. Note that the rise and fall in tissue concentrations precede similar changes in serum concentrations. From D'Ercole et al (1984) Proc Natl Acad Sci (USA) 81:935-939.

FEEDBACK REGULATION: INHIBITION OF GH SECRETION BY SM-C/IGF-I

The suggestion that somatomedin might exert feedback inhibition of GH secretion first came from observations on patients with Laron-type dwarfism. These patients, who are unable to synthesize Sm-C/IGF-I, have markedly elevated serum GH concentrations. Support for the possibility that these high GH levels reflect loss of feedback inhibition by Sm-C/IGF-I comes from several recent studies. Specifically, Sm-C/IGF-I has been shown to stimulate production of somatostatin by *in vitro* explants of hypothalamic tissue and to inhibit GH secretion by pituitary *in vitro* (5). Sm-C/IGF-I also blocks the stimulation of GRF-induced growth hormone release by cultured pituitary cells (6). Finally, intracerebroventricular injections of Sm-C/IGF-I (500 ng) (7) and another purified IGF preparation (8) have been shown to obliterate endogenous spikes of GH in the plasma of rats. Abe *et al.* (7), showed that, in addition to Sm-C/IGF-I, intracerebroventricular installation of GH also suppressed plasma GH for the 6 hours of study. This suppression occurs despite the fact that there was no rise in Sm-C/IGF-I in peripheral blood. This GH effect raises the possibility that Sm-C/IGF-I is synthesized in the pituitary and/or hypothalamus, and exerts its effect at or near its site of production. This conforms to our observation that more somatomedin is extractable from human and rat pituitaries than from other tissues (unpublished).

ROLE OF NUTRITION IN THE REGULATION OF SM-C/IGF-I

The importance of nutritional status in the regulation of plasma somatomedin concentrations was recognized from bioassay studies that showed that somatomedins are reduced in children with protein-calorie malnutrition (9-10). Using the more specific RIA for Sm-C/IGF-I, which avoids problems of bioassay inhibitors, we have extended these studies and have shown that moderately obese human volunteers who are fasted for 10 days have a marked decline in Sm-C/IGF-I (11) to values that are approximately 20-30% of basal values. This fall of plasma Sm-C/IGF-I correlates with changes in nitrogen balance (r=0.74).

In a follow-up study, normal adult volunteers were fasted for 5 days on 3 occasions (12). After each fast, they were refed one of 3 diets. During fasting the serum Sm-C/IGF-I fell from a mean prefast value of 1.85±0.39 (SD) to 0.67±0.16 units/ml. Refeeding a normal diet (1.35 g protein and 35.3 kcal/kg) for 5 days caused the Sm-C/IGF-I to rise to 1.26±0.20 U/ml (68% of prefast). Refeeding an isocaloric diet that was protein deficient (32% of control) returned the Sm-C/IGF-I to only 0.90±0.24 U/ml (normal vs. protein deficient diet, $p<0.05$). Refeeding a diet deficient in both protein and energy (10.8 kcal/kg) led to a further fall in Sm-C/IGF-I (mean after 5 days of refeeding, 0.31±0.06 U/ml). The changes in Sm-C/IGF-I during each fasting and refeeding period correlated with changes in mean daily nitrogen balance (r=0.90, $p<0.001$). From this study we conclude that intake of both energy and protein are regulators of serum Sm-C/IGF-I and that the serum concentrations of this peptide are good indicators of acute directional changes in nitrogen balance.

In a third study we fasted normal volunteers for 5 days, then refed diets of variable energy-adequate protein or variable protein-adequate energy (13). This study confirmed that both energy and protein are important determinants of Sm-C/IGF-I concentrations. Energy, however, is probably more important because there is a threshhold energy requirement below which protein has no effect on Sm-C/IGF-I. Additionally, the rate of restoration of Sm-C/IGF-I to normal is better facilitated by ingestion of a full complement of energy (13).

The results of a series of studies in nutritionally deprived rats suggest a possible mechanism for the dietary modulation of Sm-C/IGF-I in humans (14,15). These experiments, performed on fasted-refed adult rats and nutrient deprived neonatal rats, show that fluctuations in serum Sm-C/IGF-I are closely paralleled by changes in binding of GH to somatogenic receptors in liver. Nutrient deprivation leads to a reduction in GH binding. This mechanism is supported by studies of Merimee et al (16) who showed that Sm-C/IGF-I failed to increase in fasted subjects in response to GH injection.

The measurement of plasma levels of Sm-C/IGF-I may be useful in assessing changes in nutritional status in patients undergoing nutritional repletion. In a recently completed study on 6 malnourished hospitalized patients with bowel disease who were undergoing hyperalimentation, we observed that the plasma concentration of Sm-C/IGF-I began to rise within 2 days of the initiation of adequate nutritional replacement, and reached values more than 2.5-fold higher than basal by 10 days. Concurrently, no significant changes occurred in serum prealbumin, transferrin or retinol-binding protein. We believe, therefore, that measurement of this peptide may be useful as a means of monitoring the adequacy of nutritional replacement therapy in hospitalized patients.

ACKNOWLEDGMENTS

This work was supported by National Institutes of Health research grants AM01022, HD08299 and HL26309, and NIH training grant AM07129. The Clinical Research Unit of the North Carolina Memorial Hospital is supported by grant RR00046 of the General Clinical Research Centers Program of the Division of Research Resources, NIH. Judson Van Wyk is a recipient of a Career Research Award 5 K06 AM14115 and A. Joseph D'Ercole is a recipient of Research Career Development Award HD00435 from the N.I.H.

REFERENCES

1. D'Ercole AJ, Applewhite GT, Underwood LE (1980) Develop Biol 75:315-328
2. Clemmons DR, Underwood LE, Van Wyk JJ (1981) J Clin Invest 67:10-19
3. Atkison PR, Weidman ER, Bhaumick B, Bala RM (1980) Endocrinology 106:2006-2012
4. D'Ercole AJ, Stiles AD, Underwood LE (1984) Proc Natl Acad Sci (USA) 81:935-939
5. Berelowitz M, Szabo M, Frohman LA, Firestone S, Chu L, Hintz RL (1981) Science 212:1279
6. Brazeau P, Guillemin R, Ling N, Van Wyk J, Humbel R (1982) C.R. Seance Acad Sci Paris (III)295:651-654
7. Abe H, Molitch ME, Van Wyk JJ, Underwood LE (1983) Endocrinology 113:1319-1324
8. Tannenbaum GS, Guyda HJ, Posner BI (1983) Science 220:77
9. Grant DB, Hambley J, Becker D, Pimstone BL (1973) Arch Dis Child 48:596-600
10. Hintz RL, Susskind R, Amatayakul K, Thanangkul O, Olson R (1978) J Pediatr 92:153-156
11. Clemmons DR, Klibanski A, Underwood LE, MacArthur JW, Ridgway EC, Beitins IZ, Van Wyk JJ (1981) J Clin Endocrinol Metab 53:1247-1250
12. Isley WL, Underwood LE, Clemmons DR (1983) J Clin Invest 71:175-182
13. Isley WL, Underwood LE, Clemmons DR (1984) JPEN (in press)
14. Maes M, Underwood LE, Ketelslegers J-M (1983) J Endocrinol 97:243-252
15. Maes M, Underwood LE, Gerard G, Ketelslegers J-M (1984) Endocrinology (in press)
16. Merimee TJ, Zapf J, Froesch ER (1982) J Clin Endocrinol Metab 55:999-1002

© 1984 Elsevier Science Publishers B.V.
Endocrinology
F. Labrie, L. Proulx, eds.

IGF RECEPTORS: THE HUMAN PLACENTA CONTAINS TWO SPECIES OF IGF-I RECEPTORS

HELEN A. JONAS AND LEN C. HARRISON
Department of Diabetes and Endocrinology, University of Melbourne, Department of Medicine, Royal Melbourne Hospital, 3050, Victoria, Australia

Insulin-like growth factors (human IGF-I and IGF-II), multiplication-stimulating activity (rat MSA) and insulin are structurally related hormones with overlapping biological activities (1,2). Distinct binding sites for IGF-I, IGF-II, MSA and insulin exist in a number of tissues. The insulin receptor has a low affinity for IGF-I, IGF-II and MSA; the type I IGF receptor has a higher affinity for IGF-I than IGF-II and MSA and a low affinity for insulin; and the type II IGF receptor has a higher affinity for IGF-II and MSA than IGF-I and no affinity for insulin (3-5).

Like insulin receptors, IGF-I receptors can be down-regulated by either IGFs or insulin (see (3)), are recognized by antibodies to the insulin receptor (8-10) and consist of similarly sized oligomers (Mr > 300K) composed of disulphide-linked 130K and 95K subunits (4-8). The 130K subunits contain the hormone binding sites (4-7) while the 95K subunits have hormone-stimulated tyrosine kinase activities (11). The identification of similarly sized biosynthetic precursors (Mr = 180K) (12) and concordant receptor defects in some patients with severe insulin resistance (3,13) suggest that both receptors are encoded by the same or closely related genes.

Type II IGF-I receptors are antigenically distinct (10) and consist of a single polypeptide (Mr = 260K) (4). They are not subject to down-regulation (3) but rather to "up-regulation" by insulin (14-17).

In most tissues, IGFs and MSA promote growth more readily than does insulin, and in tissues containing no type I IGF receptors (e.g. adipocytes (1,4) 100 fold higher concentrations of IGFs are required to elicit insulin's metabolic actions (1-3). Thus, it has generally been considered that insulin and IGF receptors mediate, respectively, the metabolic and mitogenic functions of these hormones. On the other hand, in some cells and tissues containing Type I IGF receptors (e.g. soleus/cardiac muscle, BC_3H-1 mouse myocytes and human skin fibroblasts (3)) low concentrations of IGFs and MSA can stimulate glucose and amino acid transport. Recent evidence suggests that these metabolic effects are mediated via type I rather than type II IGF receptors (18). It is not known whether the metabolic and mitogenic effects of IGF-I are mediated via IGF-I binding to the same site or to separate sites on its own (type I) or type II receptors.

Our studies indicate that the human placenta contains two types of IGF-I receptors which can be delineated on the basis of their reactivity with autoantibodies to the insulin receptor.

Reactivity of human placental IGF-I receptors with auto-antibodies to the insulin receptor. ^{125}I-IGF-I labelled receptors from Triton solubilized human placental membranes could be immunoprecipitated by autoantisera B-2, B-5 and B-8, but not by sera B-6 and B-10 (9). Further studies with serum B-2 revealed a finite population of IGF-I receptors (usually 50-80% of original binding activity) which could not be immunoprecipitated with serum dilutions < 1/250.

Binding characteristics of immunoprecipitable and non-immunoprecipitable IGF-I receptors. Curvilinear Scatchard plots were obtained when IGF-I binding to solubilized membranes was assayed by polyethlene glycol (PEG) precipitation. However, precipitation of ^{125}I-IGF-I binding sites by serum B-2 and S.aureus yielded a linear plot, consistent with a single class of lower affinity sites (Kd = 7.1×10^{-10}M, Ro = 0.13×10^{-12}mol/mg protein). In contrast, after immunodepletion of solubilized receptors by B-2 IgG pre-bound to S.aureus, residual IGF-I binding assayed by PEG precipitation yielded a single class of higher affinity binding sites (Kd = 2.1×10^{-10}M, Ro = 0.077×10^{-12}mol/mg) (Fig. 1). Porcine insulin was 120 fold less potent than IGF-I in

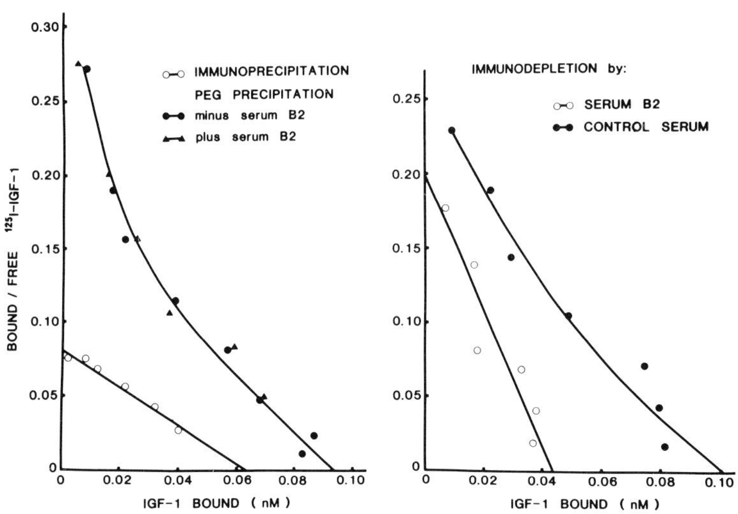

Fig. 1. Scatchard plots of IGF-I binding to the B-2 immunoprecipitable lower affinity receptors (left hand figure, open circles) and to the B-2 non-reactive, higher affinity receptors (right hand figure, open circles).
The closed symbols represent IGF-I binding to the total IGF-I receptor population.

competing with ^{125}I-IGF-I for its low affinity (B-2 reactive) site and 1100 fold less potent in competing for the high affinity (B-2 non reactive) site. The relative potency of IGF-I compared to MSA was 25 for both IGF-I receptors.

After pretreatment of placental membranes with dithiothreitol (DTT), barely detectable levels of the low affinity, B-2 immunoprecipitable receptors remained. However, the average binding affinity of the PEG-precipitable receptors (i.e. the total receptor population) increased, consistent with the loss of the low affinity receptors, but not the high affinity receptors (Fig. 2).

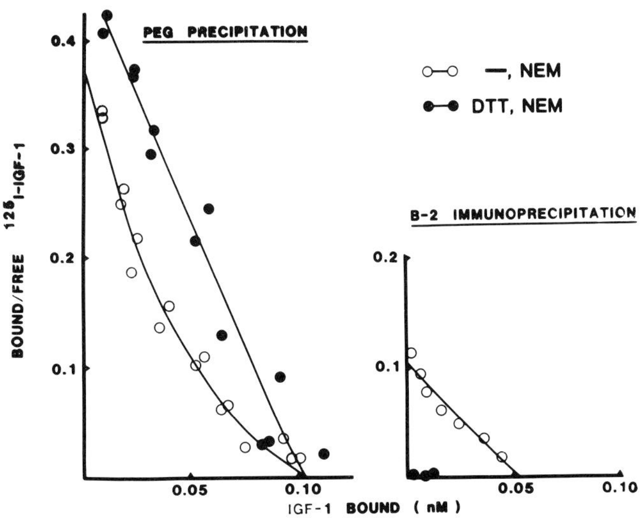

Fig. 2. Effect of reduction on the binding properties of placental IGF-I receptor subtypes. Placental membranes (5 mg/ml) were pretreated with or without 20 mM DTT (20 min at 22°C) followed by 50 mM N-ethylmaleinimide (NEM), washed, solubilized and subjected to IGF-I binding analyses. Total receptors were precipitated by PEG, and B-2 reactive receptors, by serum B-2 and S. aureus

Immunoprecipitation of ^{125}I-labelled receptors from human placental membranes. Analysis by SDS-polyacrylamide gel electrophoresis and autoradiography of ^{125}I-labelled receptors precipitated by autoantiserum B-10 (which recognizes only insulin receptors (9)) or autoantiserum B-2 revealed, in both cases, specific reduced bands of Mr = 130K and 90K; the same subunits were also seen after sequential precipitation with B-10 and B-2 antisera to enrich the proportion of IGF-I receptors recovered.

CONCLUSIONS

We conclude that the IGF-I receptor recognized by B-2 antibodies is more closely related to the insulin receptor than is the non-immunoreactive IGF-I receptor, in terms of its antigenicity, cross-reactivity with insulin, and susceptibility to dithiothreitol (19), and appears to have an identical subunit composition to the insulin receptor. Neither receptor can be defined as a classical IGF-II receptor, because of its high affinity for IGF-I, moderate affinity for MSA, and low affinity for insulin. The finding of two distinct species of IGF-I receptor raises the possibility that cell or tissue-specific isotypes of the IGF-I receptor could mediate the different biological actions of IGF-I.

ACKNOWLEDGEMENTS

This work was supported by the National Health and Medical Research Council of Australia. ^{125}I-IGF-I, IGF-I and MSA were kindly provided by Drs. R. Baxter (Sydney), R. Humbel (Zurich) and M. Czech (Worcester).

REFERENCES

1. Zapf J, Rinderknecht E, Humbel RE, Froesch ER (1978) Metabolism 27: 1803-1827
2. King GL, Kahn CR, Rechler MM, Nissley SP (1980) J Clin Invest 66: 130-140
3. Rechler MM, Kasuga M, Sasaki N, de Vroede MA, Romanus JA, Nissley SP (1983) In: Spencer EM (ed) Insulin-Like Growth Factors/Somatomedins. Walter de Gruyter & Co, Berlin, pp 459-490
4. Massague J, Czech MP (1982) J Biol Chem 257: 5038-5045
5. Kasuga M, Van Obberghen E, Nissley SP, Rechler MM (1982) Proc Natl Acad Sci USA 79: 1864-1868
6. Chernausek SD, Jacobs S, Van Wyk JJ (1981) Biochemistry 20: 7345-7350
7. Baumick B, Bala RM, Hollenberg MD (1981) Proc Natl Acad Sci USA 78: 4279-4283
8. Kull FC Jr, Jacobs S, Su Y-F, Svoboda ME, Van Wyk JJ, Cuatrecasas P (1983) J Biol Chem 258: 6561-6566
9. Jonas HA, Baxter RC, Harrison LC (1982) Biochem Biophys Res Commun 109: 463-470
10. Kasuga M, Sasaki N, Kahn CR, Nissley SP, Rechler MM (1983) J Clin Invest 72: 1459-1469
11. Jacobs S, Kull FC Jr, Earp HS, Svoboda ME, Van Wyk JJ, Cuatrecasas P (1983) J Biol Chem 258: 9581-9584
12. Jacobs S, Kull FC Jr, Cuatrecasas P (1983) Proc Natl Acad Sci USA 80: 1228-1231
13. Massague J, Freidenberg GF, Olefsky JM, Czech MP (1983) Diabetes 32: 541-544
14. Zapf J, Schoenle E, Froesch ER (1978) Eur J Biochem 87: 285-296
15. King GL, Rechler MM, Kahn CR (1982) J Biol Chem 257: 10001-10006
16. Massague J, Blinderman LA, Czech MP (1982) J Biol Chem 257: 13958-13963
17. Oppenheimer CL, Pessin JE, Massague J, Gitomer W, Czech MP (1983) J Biol Chem 258: 4824-4830
18. Yu K-T, Czech MP (1984) J Biol Chem 259: 3090-3095
19. Massague J, Czech MP (1982) J Biol Chem 257: 6729-6738

Endocrinology
F. Labrie, L. Proulx, eds.

MECHANISM OF ACTION OF CARTILAGE-DERIVED FACTOR (CDF) AND MULTIPLICATION-STIMULATING ACTIVITY (MSA)

FUJIO SUZUKI, YUJI HIRAKI, HIROYUKI INOUE AND YUKIO KATO
Department of Biochemistry and Calcified-Tissue Metabolism, Faculty of Dentistry, Osaka University, 1-8, Yamadaoka, Suita, Osaka 565 (Japan)

INTRODUCTION

Salmon and Daughaday proposed that stimulation of growth by growth hormone is mediated by a systemic somatomedin (1). However, the effect of somatomedin is smaller than that of growth hormone itself on linear growth of the skeleton in hypophysectomized rats (2). In addition, somatomedins are not so effective in stimulating growth of animal cells in culture as serum or non-somatomedin growth factors, such as epidermal growth factor (EGF), fibroblast growth factor (FGF) or certain tumor-derived growth factors (3). Therefore, it is not clear whether somatomedin mediates the whole action of growth hormone on bone growth.

Recently, we found that fetal bovine cartilage contains somatomedin-like growth factors (4-7). This cartilage-derived factor (CDF) stimulates proteoglycan synthesis, RNA synthesis and DNA synthesis in rabbit chondrocytes in culture (4-6). In the present study, the actions of CDF and MSA (multiplication-stimulating activity, a family of fetal somatomedins) in rabbit costal chondrocytes in culture, were compared. In addition, the growth promoting effects of CDF and MSA in the presence of various non-somatomedin growth factors.

MATERIALS AND METHODS

Materials.

MSA was purified from serum-free medium that had been conditioned by a cloned line of Buffalo rat liver cells. CDF was purified from fetal bovine cartilage as described previously (6). EGF and FGF were purchased from Collaborative Research, Inc., USA.

Cell culture.

Chondrocytes were dispersed from rib cartilage of young rabbits weighing 300-600 g and growth-cartilage cells were cultured in 6-mm microwells or 60-mm dishes, as described previously (8,9).

Assays.

$[^3H]$Thymidine incorporation. Confluent cultures of chondrocytes were pre-incubated for 24 h in Dulbecco's modified Eagle's medium (DMEM) containing 0.3 % fetal calf serum (FCS). Then the cells were incubated in DMEM containing test samples and 0.3 % FCS. At the indicated times, 5 μl of [^{3}H]thymidine solution (260 μCi/ml) was added, and the cells were incubated for 3 h more. The cell layers were then washed three times with cold phosphate-buffered saline and precipitated with 5 % trichloroacetic acid and with ethanol-ethylether (3:1, V/V). The residues in the wells were solubilized with 0.3 N NaOH. The solution was neutralized and radioactivity was measured.

[^{35}S]Sulfate incorporation. Confluent cultures of chondrocytes were pre-incubated for 24 h in DMEM containing 0.3 % FCS. The cells were then exposed for 24 h to 0.5 μCi of $H_2{}^{35}SO_4$ in DMEM containing test samples and 0.3 % FCS. Proteoglycan synthesis was monitored by measuring incorporation of $^{35}SO_4{}^{2-}$ into materials precipitated with cetylpyridinium chloride after treatment with pronase E, as described previously (4).

RESULTS

The role of CDF on skeletal growth was evaluated by comparing its effect on cultured chondrocytes with those of MSA, a somatomedin purified from conditioned medium of Buffalo rat liver cells, and other non-somatomedin growth factors. In cultures of rabbit costal chondrocytes exposed to medium containing CDF began to increase [^{3}H]thymidine incorporation into DNA after 14-16 h, reached a maximum at 24 to 28 h, after CDF addition, and then decreased. The time-course of MSA-induced DNA synthesis was similar to that of CDF-induced DNA synthesis. The incorporation of [^{3}H]uridine into RNA was also increased within 1-2 h in the cells incubated with the peptides. These stimulations of nucleic acid synthesis were followed by cell division in serum-free medium. On the other hand, CDF and MSA enhanced the synthesis of sulfated proteoglycans, as measured in terms of increased incorporation of [^{35}S]sulfate, [^{3}H]glucosamine or [^{3}H]serine into material precipitated with cetylpyridinium chloride, was consistently higher than the extent of CDF and MSA stimulation of total protein synthesis.

EGF and FGF also stimulated DNA synthesis, RNA synthesis and cell division of chondrocytes in culture, but did not stimulate nor inhibit proteoglycan synthesis. MSA and EGF or FGF had synergistic effects on the growth of chondrocytes (TABLE I). CDF mimicked these effects of MSA: CDF and MSA had similar stimulatory effects on DNA synthesis in chondrocytes even in the presence of EGF, FGF or both. On the contrary, EGF and FGF had additive effects on DNA synthesis and cell division of chondrocytes. On the other hand, EGF and FGF had little effect on the incorporation of $^{35}SO_4{}^{2-}$ per DNA basis, although they increased the incorporation of the label per dish (TABLE I). Addition of MSA or CDF with EGF resulted in increase in $^{35}SO_4{}^{2-}$

TABLE I

STIMULATION OF GROWTH AND PROTEOGLYCAN SYNTHESIS BY ADDITION OF EGF WITH MSA, CDF OR FGF

Addition	DNA/dish		$^{35}SO_4^{2-}$ uptake	
			per dish	per DNA mass
	μg	% increase	dis. min^{-1}	dis.min^{-1} μg^{-1}
None (before incubation)	3.1 ± 0.3	0		
None (after incubation)	7.4 ± 0.3	138	3675 ± 535	487 ± 45
MSA	9.2 ± 0.6	197	6617 ± 866	719 ± 49
CDF	10.2 ± 1.7	229	6394 ± 779	684 ± 51
FGF	12.9 ± 0.3	316	5911 ± 918	465 ± 22
EGF	13.1 ± 0.3	323	5978 ± 240	457 ± 11
EGF + MSA	18.4 ± 3.0	594	6985 ± 600	387 ± 31
EGF + CDF	17.5 ± 1.6	565	6719 ± 203	364 ± 34
EGF + FGF	21.7 ± 1.2	700	5016 ± 426	250 ± 14

All cultures were started in DMEM containing EGF (1 ng/ml), FGF (0.3 μg/ml), MSA (0.5 μg/ml) or CDF (2 μg/ml) in the presence of 0.3 % FCS. After incubation for 2 days, the medium was replaced by appropriate medium with 2 μCi of $H_2{}^{35}SO_4$. After further incubation for 24 h, DNA and ^{35}S-labeled proteoglycans were analyzed.

incorporation per dish but caused a slight decrease in incorporation on a DNA basis (TABLE I). TABLE I also shows that addition of FGF with EGF also increased the incorporation of $^{35}SO_4^{2-}$ per dish but caused a marked decrease in its incorporation on a DNA basis. These findings suggest that the actions of somatomedins on chondrocytes are quite different from those of EGF and FGF and that somatomedin-like growth factors and non-somatomedin mitogens have complementary effects on chondrocytes.

DNA synthesis in cells treated with CDF for only the initial 5 h also increased 23 h after removal of CDF (Fig. 1). Therefore, initial 5 h exposure of chondrocytes to CDF is sufficient for full stimulation of DNA synthesis. MSA also gave similar results. On the contrary, EGF must be continuously present in medium for stimulation of DNA synthesis. FGF also required a continuous exposure to cells for full stimulation of DNA synthesis. Moreover, an early removal (5 h) of CDF or MSA from the medium did not affect the interaction of CDF or MSA with EGF or FGF for their synergistic stimulation of DNA synthesis in chondrocytes. Thus, a transient exposure to CDF or MSA with EGF or FGF followed by a continuous exposure to EGF or FGF resulted in $G_1 \rightarrow$ S transition. These findings suggest that somatomedin-related factors affect an early distinct state in G_1 phase in the cell cycle in chondrocytes and trigger some signals for entry into the DNA synthetic phase.

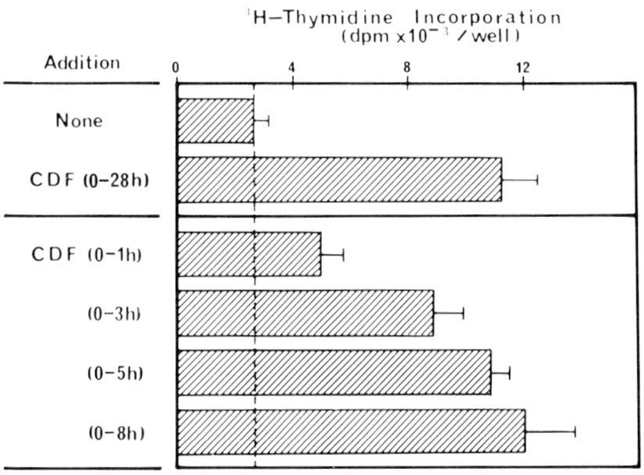

Fig. 1. Effects of limited exposures of chondrocytes to CDF on their DNA synthesis. Chondrocytes were grown to confluency in 6-mm microwells. The cells were preincubated for 24 h in 0.1 ml of DMEM containing 0.3 % FCS, and then the medium was replaced by 0.1 ml of DMEM supplemented with CDF (2 μg/ml). After incubation for the indicated periods, the cultures were rinsed three times with DMEM and washed free of CDF. Then incubation was continued with DMEM and the cultures were pulsed with [^{3}H]thymidine for the last 3 h from 25 to 28 h after the addition of CDF.

REFERENCES

1. Salmon WD Jr, Daughaday WH (1957) J Lab Clin Med 49:825-836
2. Schoenle E, Zapf J, Humbel RE, Froesch ER (1982) Nature 296:252-253
3. Kato Y, Watanabe R, Hiraki Y, Suzuki F, Canalis E, Raisz LG, Nishikawa K, Adachi K (1982) Biochim Biophys Acta 716:232-239
4. Kato Y, Nomura Y, Daikuhara Y, Nasu N, Tsuji M, Asada A, Suzuki F (1980) Exp Cell Res 130:73-81
5. Kato Y, Nomura Y, Tsuji M, Ohmae H, Kinoshita M, Hamamoto S, Suzuki F (1981) Exp Cell Res 132:339-347
6. Kato Y, Nomura Y, Tsuji M, Ohmae H, Nakazawa T, Suzuki F (1981) J Biochem 90:1377-1386
7. Kato Y, Nomura Y, Tsuji M, Kinoshita M, Ohmae H, Suzuki F (1981) Proc Natl Acad Sci USA 78:6831-6835
8. Suzuki F, Yoneda T, Shimomura Y (1976) FEBS Lett 70:155-158
9. Kato Y, Hiraki Y, Inoue H, Kinoshita M, Yutani Y, Suzuki F (1983) Eur J Biochem 129:685-690

24. Control of Pituitary Cell Activity

Endocrinology
F. Labrie, L. Proulx, eds.

PARACRINE INTERACTION IN RAT ANTERIOR PITUITARY

CARL DENEF

Laboratory of Cell Pharmacology, University of Leuven, School of Medicine, Campus Gasthuisberg, B-3000 Leuven, Belgium

GONADOTROPH-MEDIATED STIMULATION OF BASAL AND DOPAMINE-INHIBITED PRL RELEASE

We recently presented evidence for the existence of a specific intercellular communication between gonadotrophs and lactotrophs in anterior pituitary reaggregate cell cultures studied in a superfusion system (1,2). In cultures consisting of an enriched lactotroph population to which gonadotrophs from a highly-enriched population obtained by unit gravity sedimentation of pituitary cells from 14-day-old female rats were added, LHRH (10^{-11}-10^{-8} M) was capable of stimulating basal as well as dopamine inhibited PRL release. The magnitude of stimulation was in proportion to the number of gonadotrophs in the coculture. Medium conditioned by purified gonadotrophs also stimulated PRL release, suggesting that gonadotrophs might activate the secretory activity of the lactotrophs by the release of a paracrine factor. Although the nature of this factor remains unknown, it was shown not to be LHRH itself, LH, FSH or PRL. The factor was ultrafiltrable and its M.W. was estimated to be smaller than 10,000.

The gonadotroph-lactotroph interaction is characterized by a high degree of specificity. In reaggregates containing gonadotrophs, lactotrophs, thyrotrophs and somatotrophs in about equal proportions (obtained from 14-day-old male rat pituitary), only PRL release was stimulated by physiological concentrations of LHRH. At higher concentrations of LHRH (10^{-8} M) there was no effect on TSH release but there was some stimulation of GH release (3). Corticotrophin-releasing factor (CRF) (10^{-8} M) failed to influence PRL, GH, LH and TSH release. Human pancreatic growth hormone releasing factor [hpGHRF(1-44)] (10^{-12}-10^{-9} M) stimulated GH release but not LH, TSH or PRL release. Vasoactive intestinal peptide (10^{-9}-10^{-7} M) and angiotensin II (AII) (10^{-10}-10^{-8} M) stimulated PRL release (4,5) but not TSH or LH release (unpublished observations). In reaggregates consisting mainly of gonadotrophs and thyrotrophs (obtained by unit gravity sedimentation) TRH (10^{-8} M) stimulated TSH release but failed to affect LH release (2). In lactotroph-gonadotroph cocultures TRH also failed to stimulate LH release (2).

MODULATION OF STIMULATED PRL AND GH RELEASE BY ENDOCRINE "HELPER" AND "SUPPRESSOR" CELLS

Stimulated PRL release

AII stimulates PRL release in reaggregates of the total pituitary cell population (4,5) as well as in reaggregates prepared from enriched lactotroph populations from adult male or 14-day-old female rats (unpublished). However, the potency and the maximal effect of AII was considerably weaker in lactotroph-enriched populations in which gonadotrophs were virtually absent than in populations containing both lactotrophs and gonadotrophs. In the latter populations the dynamics of secretion as a function of time was also different from that in the former. When the lactotroph population with the weakest response was supplemented for 5 percent with cells from a highly enriched population of large gonadotrophs from 14-day-old females (70 % gonadotrophs), the PRL response to AII was enhanced when the peptide was superfused at a concentration of 1 nM. When the proportional number of these large gonadotrophs in the coculture was increased to 15 percent or when AII was used at a concentration of 10 or 100 nM the PRL response became weaker than in the gonadotroph-poor lactotroph population (6). In contrast, there was no correlation between the presence of gonadotrophs and the PRL response to TRH. We interpret these findings by advancing the hypothesis that large gonadotrophs can potentiate the response of the lactotrophs to AII but that they may also engage in inhibitory interactions. Up to a certain number of these cells stimulation would prevail but when present in higher number stimulation would gradually be overruled by inhibition. If this hypothesis is correct, a higher concentration of AII would be expected also to favor the inhibitory interaction and this was indeed found. On the other hand, lactotroph populations containing small gonadotrophs were highly sensitive to AII on their own and the magnitude of the response did not decline at high concentrations of AII. When large gonadotrophs were added to the latter population the PRL response did not diminish either at high concentrations of AII. Taken together these data support the hypothesis that large gonadotrophs are capable to function as "helper" as well as as "suppressor" cells of the lactotrophs' responsiveness to AII whereas small gonadotrophs are mainly "helper" cells.

Stimulated GH release

When reaggregates from the total pituitary cell population (adult or immature rats) were cultured in serum-free defined medium (for constituents see ref. 7), dexamethasone (80 nM) allowed a 10-20 fold stimulation of GH release by VIP and PHI (0.1-10 nM) but not by TRH (10 nM). In a somatotroph-rich population (60-70 % somatotrophs) the GH response to VIP was weak but it could be reinduced by coculturing the somatotrophs with a lactotroph-enriched population (35 % lactotrophs). In contrast, the GH response to 0.1 nM hpGHRF(1-44) was depressed in the latter coculture situation (unpublished). The GH response to VIP (1-10 nM) could also be depressed by adding large gonadotrophs from 14-day-old females to the coculture.

These data again suggest that gonadotrophs seem to produce agent(s) inhibiting the response of other cell types to their secretagogues. In addition, helper and suppressor activity may also be displayed by lactotrophs under certain experimental conditions. Since the lactotroph-enriched population was also enriched with 8 % corticotrophs, the latter cell type may also be involved.

MODULATION OF INTERCELLULAR COMMUNICATION BY STEROID AND THYROID HORMONES

Addition of testosterone (0.1-100 nM), estradiol (0.01-10 nM) or 5 α-dihydrotestosterone (1-100 nM) to the culture medium (serum-supplemented or serum-free) for 10 days inhibited the PRL response to LHRH, the order of potency being testosterone > estradiol > 5 α-dihydrotestosterone (3). The response was slightly inhibited by adding T_3 (0.5-5 nM) or dexamethasone (10 nM) to serum-free defined medium (unpublished). On the other hand, as already mentioned, the GH response to VIP required the presence of a glucocorticoid. T_3 (0.05-1 nM) dose-dependently changed the secretory pattern of PRL release in response to 10 nM AII but not to 0.1 nM AII.

CONCLUSION

The present data show that multiple and complex interactions may occur between different anterior pituitary cell types and that these interactions are not random. The underlying mechanism may be the release of paracrine factors. A key peptide possibly involved in some of the cellular interactions may be AII. Angiotensin-like immunoreactivity has been shown in the gonadotrophs and lactotrophs (8), and we have consistently found pg amounts of AI immunoreactivity in acid extracts of reaggregate cell cultures from a highly enriched population of gonadotrophs using a highly selective AI antiserum (unpublished observations). If this material is released by appropriate stimuli in the close vicinity of lactotrophs there may be an effective response even with minute amounts of the peptide as AI is rapidly converted to AII in pituitary cell reaggregate cell cultures (5). Thus, the present findings are consistent with the hypothesis that angiotensin may have a local regulatory role in the pituitary.

Moreover, AII is capable of amplifying as well as blunting its own action presumably through a gonadotroph-lactotroph cell-to-cell communication mechanism. In preliminary experiments we have found evidence that the "helper" and "suppressor" activity of these cells is mediated by the release of humoral factor(s). When AII is superfused in medium previously conditioned for 1 h with the gonadotroph-rich aggregates, the PRL response enhances severalfold. If these data can be confirmed, there is good evidence to propose that AII may not only be involved in paracrine actions on its own but also in controlling the release of other presumptive autocrine or paracrine agents.

ACKNOWLEDGEMENTS

The excellent technical assistance of R. Dewals, A. De Wolf and M.J. Vanderheyden and secretarial work of M. Bareau is gratefully acknowledged. The authors are grateful to the U.S. National Hormone and Pituitary Program and the National Institute of Arthritis, Diabetes and Digestive and Kidney Diseases and Dr. A.F. Parlow for providing rat PRL, GH, LH, FSH and TSH RIA kits.

This work was supported by grants from "Geconcerteerde Onderzoeksakties", F.G.W.O. and Queen Elisabeth Medical Foundation.

REFERENCES

1. Vanderschueren B, Denef C, Cassiman JJ (1982) Endocrinology 110:513
2. Denef C, Andries M (1983) Endocrinology 112:813
3. Denef C (1984) In : Proceedings of the 3rd European Workshop on Pituitary Adenomas. Blackwell Scientific, London, in press
4. Schramme C, Denef C (1983) Neuroendocrinology 36:483
5. Schramme C, Denef C (1984) Life Sci 34:1651
6. Denef C (1984) Hormone Res : in press
7. Denef C, Baes M, Schramme C (1984) Endocrinology 114:1371
8. Steele MK, Brownfield MS, Ganong WF (1982) Neuroendocrinology 35:155

Endocrinology
F. Labrie, L. Proulx, eds.

STUDIES OF HORMONE STORAGE AND SECRETION IN THE MULTIPOTENTIAL GONADOTROPE

GWEN V. CHILDS
Department of Anatomy, The University of Texas Medical Branch, Galveston, Tx 77550

INTRODUCTION

Studies of gonadotropin storage have shown that, in most species, luteinizing hormone (LH) and follicle stimulating hormone (FSH) are stored in the same cells (reviewed in ref. 1). These studies have relied on serial sections stained for LH or FSH, or double stains applied to the same field or section. Many of the studies have also demonstrated the presence of gonadotropes that contain only one of the hormones. Questions about the significance of this subtype arise. Are the monohormonal gonadotropes a special class of cell, or are they in fact multipotential and thus capable of synthesizing both hormones when stimulated?

Currently there is a controversy about gonadotropin storage that is focused on the relative percentages of monohormonal and multihormonal gonadotropes (reviewed in ref. 1). Most of the studies rely on serial sections and the thickness of the section can artifactually shift the relative proportions of each type (1). Similarly, the relative proportions are dependent on the type and specificity of the antisera and the ease with which one can localize both gonadotropins in fixed-embedded tissue sections.

In this study, we tested various combinations of fixatives and embedding media for their effect on stains for gonadotropin alpha and beta chain subunits. This report correlates evidence from multiple approaches that together both validate and confirm the percentages of each subtype. We also show how the specificity of the stain is affected by the fixation protocol. Finally, evidence for the dissociation of storage sites of alpha and beta chains will be presented along with a description of the effect of GnRH on subunit storage in multihormonal cells.

MATERIALS AND METHODS

Several fixation-embedding protocols were applied to pituitaries from male or cycling female rats. Protocol 1 included fixation in glutaraldehyde or p-formaldehyde, dehydration in ethanol, infiltration in propylene oxide, and polymerization at 60°C in Araldite 6005. Protocol 2 included blocks exposed to freeze fixation, followed by freeze drying and embedding in Araldite 6005 at 60°C. Sections were etched in sodium methoxide or hydrogen peroxide prior to staining.

Protocol 3 involved the use of aldehyde fixation followed by dehydration in a water soluble embedding plastic (glycol methacrylate) and embedding in the same at 4°C. This protocol excluded all organic solvents, etching agents, and heat polymerization steps. Protocol 4 involved the use of whole monolayer cells fixed in 1% glutaraldehyde that were stained before exposure to dehydrating agents and plastic (preembedding stains).

The pituitary tissues were prepared in the above protocols as described in references 1-3. Serial sections of embedded tissues, or whole cell monolayers were then stained in preembedding or postembedding stains with the avidin-biotin peroxidase complex.

The stained cells were then counted and expressed as a percentage of the total cell population. Serial fields were matched to learn if the cells contained all three subunits. Third, the monolayer cells were stained with dual stains for alpha chains and one of the beta chains, or both beta chains (1). Parallel fields were stimulated with 10^{-10}M [D-Lys^6] GnRH to learn if this affected storage sites of the subunits (1,4).

RESULTS

We began by testing various fixatives and embedding protocols for their effect on the immunoreactivity of gonadotropins. The measure employed was the efficiency of the reaction as determined by the optimal working dilution of the primary antisera. This was defined as the dilution on the steepest part of the titration curve that gave a dense, low background stain.

Optimal staining following protocol 1 was achieved with a 1:5000-1:10,000 dilution of anti-bLHβ, or a 1:2000-1:5000 dilution of anti-hFSHβ. However, no staining was seen for alpha subunits with any of the antisera tested to date. This suggests that the greatest specificity of staining for beta subunits will occur following the use of Protocol 1. Protocols 2 and 3 allowed a 3-5 fold dilution of both beta chain antisera for optimal staining and, alpha chain reactivity was preserved. This may reflect the deleterious effect of the organic solvents and aldehyde fixation, used in Protocol 1, on the antigens, especially the alpha subunits.

Protocol 4 eliminated dehydration and embedding altogether. This and the fact that it is applied to whole cells, allowed a striking 30 fold increase in staining efficiency, particularly for FSH beta chains and alpha chains. Dual stains with this protocol allowed one to view the different storage sites of the subunits in whole multipotential cells. Figure 1 shows 2 cells stained for alpha chains in the first stain (gray-black) and LH-beta in the second stain (orange). Cell a stains only for alpha chains; therefore, it may be a thyrotroph, or a monohormonal FSH cell. Cell b stains for both LH-alpha (center of cell) and for LH-beta. These orange staining regions for LH-beta may be filled with rough endoplasmic reticulum. The staining pattern thus demonstrates that alpha and beta chains can be sequestered in separate regions in the gonadotrope during a phase of the secretory cycle.

The quantitative studies have also demonstrated that the percentages of gonadotropes in the overall cell population do not vary with the fixative or embedding protocols. There are 10% LH cells, 12% FSH cells, 22% alpha chain reactive cells and 6% thyrotropes. The dual beta chain stains show that there are 16-17% total gonadotropes. Therefore, the percentage of alpha chain cells appears to be the sum of gonadotropes and thyrotropes. In female rats (mixed cycles), there are 50% multihormonal gonadotropes (LH-FSH) and 20-25% monohormonal gonadotropes in tissues or dissociated cells irrespective of the protocol employed (1,2). These findings validate one another and confirm the data first obtained in ultrathin serial plastic sections (3).

Hormone storage in stimulated gonadotropes. The above studies showed that the fixation and embedding protocol affected the efficiency of the immunocytochemical reaction, but it did not affect the overall counts of the different types of gonadotropes. The proportions of different subtypes can be altered, however, following castration, ovariectomy, or GnRH stimulation. There is clearly a shift to a higher percentage of multihormonal (LH-FSH) gonadotropes (from 70% to 91% in the male and from 50% to 75% in the female) following the surgeries with a corresponding drop in the proportion of monohormonal gonadotropes. In dissociated gonadotropes, there is a similar shift after stimulation with 10^{-10}M [D-Lys^6] GnRH (from 50% to 75% in the female-4 h after exposure). These data suggest that the monohormonal gonadotropes may in fact be multipotential, especially since the overall percentages of gonadotropes do not increase.

The multipotential gonadotrope is affected dramatically by the GnRH stimulation. Figure 2 shows that cell processes form within 10 min after stimulation. Sometimes these contain different amounts of each beta chain immunoreactivity. Often the site of binding of GnRH can be correlated with the extension of microvilli and cellular processes that become filled with stain for LH or FSH, as if the movement of the stores are directed to the region of the stimulation. Figure 3 shows that the processes persist for up to 4 h after stimulation. The black stain indicates GnRH binding (4)and the red stain shows FSH storage. Figure 4 is an electron micrograph of a process labeled for biotinylated GnRH (4).

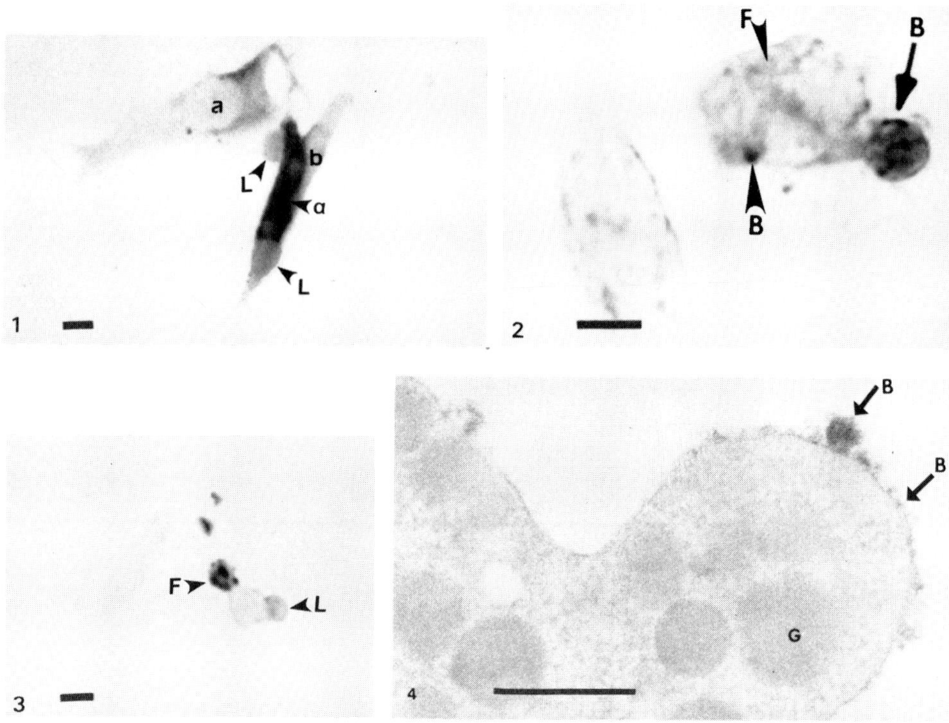

Figures #1-3 show dual stains for alpha chains and LH-β(#1); LHβ and FSHβ (#2) and Biotinylated GnRH and FSHβ (#3). Stimulated gonadotropes dissociate their stores of subunits (#1 and 2), often in processes that bind GnRH (#3 and 4). Arrows indicate site of each stain: a=alpha, L=LHβ F=FSHβ and B=biotinylated GnRH. Bar - #1-3 = 10 μm; #4 = 0.5 μm, G = secretory granules.

Conclusions. These studies have validated past work that showed the gonadotrope population to be heterogeneous. In addition, we show that multihormonal gonadotropes may store their subunits in separate regions, perhaps partly to effect non-parallel release of the two hormones. Furthermore, our data show that GnRH stimulation may mediate release by directing the stores to one specific site. One could postulate that the site(s) could be further modified by steroids or inhibin to allow only the release of one of the gonadotropins. Thus, non-parallel release could stem both from monohormonal gonadotropes, and from specific regions on multihormonal cells.

REFERENCES

1. Childs, GV (1983) Stain Technology, 58:281
2. Childs, GV, Hyde C, Naor, Z, and Catt, K. (1980) Endocrinology, 113:2120
3. Childs, GV, Ellison, DG and Garner, L, (1980) Am J. Anat 158:397
4. Childs, GV, Naor, Z, Hazum, E, Tibolt, R, Westlund, KN, and Hancock, MB, (1983) Peptides 4:549

Endocrinology
F. Labrie, L. Proulx, eds.

MONOAMINE-PEPTIDE INTERACTIONS IN THE REGULATION OF PITUITARY CELL FUNCTION

ANDRES NEGRO-VILAR, EDUARDO SPINEDI, AND CRAIG JOHNSTON
Reproductive Neuroendocrinology Section, Laboratory of Reproductive and Developmental Toxicology, National Institute of Environmental Health Sciences, NIH, Research Triangle Park, NC 27709 (United States)

Peptidergic and aminergic neurotransmitters interact at different integrative levels to modulate endocrine function and these interactions involve complex and diverse cellular mechanisms with distinct peculiarities for each individual hormonal system.

Neuroendocrine mechanisms regulating ACTH and β-endorphin release represent one of the more complex regulatory system(s). Indeed, several hypothalamic peptides have been identified and determined to have clear-cut stimulatory effects on the release of ACTH from the anterior pituitary (AP). Corticotropin releasing factor (CRF), arginine vasopressin (AVP), oxytocin (OT) and angiotensin II (AII) are among the most conspicuous neural peptides involved in the release of the proopiomelanocortin-derived (POMC) peptides from the AP. The recently isolated CRF is by far the most potent releaser of ACTH, both *in vivo* and *in vitro* (1-3). The following order of potency of corticotropin releasing activity (CRA) was determined (3) *in vitro*: CRF>AVP>OT>AII. Rat CRF is slightly more potent than ovine CRF in this *in vitro* system. The actions of several of the above peptides are mediated by specific membrane receptors. AII receptors in AP cell membranes have been characterized with K_D values which agree with the doses required to elicit ACTH release. Saralasin, a specific AII receptor blocker, binds to the AII membrane receptor with high affinity (4) and abolishes the release of ACTH induced by AII (3). CRF receptors in rat AP membranes (7,8) have affinity and specificity that agree with the biological activity of the peptide *in vitro*. We described (9) the presence of AVP receptors using an AP dispersed cell system, and correlated the binding characteristics of the peptide with its ACTH releasing potency. The K_D of the receptor (1.63 nM at 37°C) agrees with the dose of AVP required to significantly increase ACTH release *in vitro* (1 nM) and with the levels of AVP (9) reported in hypophyseal portal blood ($\sim$ 1 ng/ml). Two additional reports have confirmed the presence of AVP receptors in AP cell membranes (10,11). Binding affinities of different AVP analogs and of OT correlate well with the ACTH-releasing activities of those compounds. CRF and AII did not displace AVP binding even at concentrations exceeding by several orders of magnitude the amounts required to enhance ACTH release *in vitro*.

Therefore, the action of at least three of the major peptides involved in ACTH release is expressed via specific membrane receptors. Moreover, post-receptor activation of hormone release may involve different metabolic pathways, since CRF enhances cAMP production prior to releasing ACTH (12), whereas AVP does not (11). This raises the interesting possiblity that other intracellular messenger system(s) may mediate the effects of AVP. The potentiation of the CRA of CRF by AVP, however, is mediated by cAMP (13). Little is known about the intracellular messenger system(s) mediating the action of AII at the pituitary level.

Central aminergic systems are known to be involved in the regulation of AP release of ACTH and β-endorphin (14), primarily by modulating the release of hypothalamic peptide hormones with intrinsic CRA. Attention has focused on direct AP effects of some aminergic neurotransmitters. Epinephrine (EPI; 15,16) and serotonin (5-HT; 17) enhance release of ACTH *in vitro* in a concentration-dependent fashion. The effects of EPI involve both α-adrenergic (15) and β-adrenergic receptors (18). Alpha- (19) and β-adrenergic (20) receptors in AP cell membranes have been characterized. The effects of 5-HT on ACTH release can be blocked by metergoline, a specific 5-HT receptor blocker, in a concentration-dependent manner. Although 5-HT receptors in the AP have not yet been characterized, a high affinity uptake system for 5-HT in AP cells has been described (21). How these amines are delivered to the corticotrophs is an important question. To determine whether the vascular connection between the hypothalamus and the AP might supply the amines to that organ, we analyzed the levels of these monoamines in hypophyseal portal plasma and compared them with those found in peripheral plasma. The results showed that, in addition to the expected high levels of dopamine (DA), higher levels of EPI, but not 5-HT, were found in portal versus peripheral plasma (22). Moreover, studies in adrenalectomized rats indicated that a significant portion of the EPI found in portal plasma was derived from a central source. These results, suggest a physiological role for central EPI in the direct regulation of ACTH and β-endorphin release from the AP (22). The intriguing observation was also made that 5-hydroxyindole-3-acetic acid (5-HIAA) was 2-4 fold more concentrated in portal than in peripheral plasma (21). The lack of higher concentrations of 5-HT in the portal circulation suggests alternative sources of 5-HT supply to the AP. Another possible source is the recently described 5-HT innervation in the rat adenohypophysis (23). However, transplantation of the AP under the kidney capsule for 5 days did not change 5-HT content in the gland (24). Furthermore, the AP lacks any significant L-aromatic aminoacid decarboxylase activity and is therefore unable to directly synthesize 5-HT from 5-hydroxytryptophan. These results suggest that the AP must receive 5-HT from other sources. Another likely explanation is that 5-HT in blood is taken up by the high affinity system present in certain AP cells (21). Since 5-HT seems to be preferentially taken up by gonadotrophs (25) and does not seem to affect the release of LH *in vitro* (Spinedi and Negro-Vilar, unpublished), the intriguing possibility that the amine may be taken up by one cell type and subsequently released to modify the activity (or response) of neighboring cells must be considered. A similar type of interaction has been suggested for AII, which is found in gonadotrophs (26) but primarily stimulates ACTH (3) and PRL (26-29) secretion from the AP.

The action of 5-HT to directly enhance ACTH release may also involve an amine-peptide interaction mechanism. Addition of 5-HT to the cell culture medium greatly potentiates the release of ACTH induced by AVP (17). This 5-HT-peptide interaction is specific (it can be nullified by 5-HT receptor blockers) and selective, since it was not observed to occur with CRF or AII. In addition, blockade of 5-HT receptor with metergoline *in vitro* blunted ACTH release in response to median eminence (ME) extracts (17) from intact rats but not from ME extracts obtained from vasopressin-deficient Brattleboro rats, suggesting that in the absence of endogenous AVP, the 5-HT/AVP interaction was absent (Spinedi and Negro-Vilar, unpublished). Dispersed AP cells from animals pretreated 72 hours prior to the experiment with p-chlorophenylalanine (PCPA), an inhibitor of 5-HT synthesis, demonstrated a diminished ACTH response to two different doses of AVP suggesting that depletion of endogenous stores of 5-HT decreased responsiveness of corticotrophs to the peptide. These results, taken together, indicate that the 5-HT/AVP interaction may play a physiologically relevant role in the regulation of ACTH/β-endorphin release.

Several testable models may explain the intriguing peptide-amine interaction uncovered by our studies. A simple model system is one in which the amine and peptide interact with specific membrane receptors eliciting ACTH release through independent mechanisms. Another model would have the same intracellular messenger (IM) stimulated by both factors, with a potentiation resulting from an enhanced response of the IM system. The amine-peptide interaction may also occur at the membrane receptor level if both receptors for AVP and 5-HT are part of an integrated receptor complex. Finally, the possibility of a true paracrine effect where the amine is taken up by a cell adjacent to the corticotroph and later released to act on the corticotroph in conjunction with the peptide must be considered. It can be predicted that as more such interactions between factors regulating AP hormone secretion are uncovered, our understanding of the complex mechanisms regulating hormone release at the pituitary level should vastly improve.

References

1. Vale W, Vaughn J, Smith M, Yamamoto G, Rivier J, Rivier C (1983) Endocrinology 113:1121
2. Vale W, Spiess J, Rivier C, Rivier J (1981) Science 213:1394
3. Spinedi E, Negro-Vilar A (1983) Neuroendocrinology 37:446
4. Mukherjee A, Kulkarni P, McCann SM, Negro-Vilar A (1982) Endocrinology 110: 665
5. Hauger RL, Aguilera G, Baukal A, Catt KJ (1982) Mol Cell Endocrinol 25:203
6. Capponi AM, Favrod-Coune CA, Gaillard RC, Muller AF (1982) Endocrinology 110: 1043
7. Wynn PC, Aguilera G, Morell J, Catt KJ (1983) Biochem Biophys Res Comm 110: 602
8. Koch B, Lutz-Bucher B (1983) Neuroendocrinol Lett 5:227
9. Gibbs D, Vale W (1983) Brain Res 280:176
10. Lutz-Bucher B, Koch B (1983) Biochem Biophys Res Comm 115:492
11. Gaillard RC, Schoenenberg P, Favrod-Coune CA, Muller AF, Bockaert J, Jard S (1984) Proc Nat Acad Sci 81:2907
12. Giguere V, Labrie F, Cote J, Coy DH, Sueiras-Diaz J, Schally AV (1982) Proc Nat Acad Sci 79:3466
13. Giguere V, Labrie F (1982) Endocrinology 111:1752
14. Negro-Vilar A, Ojeda SR (1981) In: McCann SM (ed) International Review of Physiology. University Park Press, Baltimore, pp. 97-156
15. Giguere V, Cote J, Labrie F (1981) Endocrinology 109:757
16. Vale W, Rivier C, Lang L, Minick S, Guillemin R (1978) Endocrinology 103:1910
17. Spinedi E, Negro-Vilar A (1983) Endocrinology 112:1217
18. Mezey E, Reisine TD, Palkovits M, Brownstein MJ, Axelrod J (1983) Proc Nat Acad Sci 80:6728
19. Peters JR, Foord SM, Dieguez C, Scanlon MF, Hall R (1983) Endocrinology 113: 133
20. Petrovic SL, McDonald JK, Snyder GD, McCann SM (1983) Brain Res 261:249
21. Johns MA, Azmitia EC, Krieger DT (1982) Endocrinology 111:754
22. Johnston CA, Gibbs DM, Negro-Vilar A (1983) Endocrinology 113:819
23. Westlund KN, Childs GV (1982) Endocrinology 111:1761
24. Johnston CA, Spinedi E, Negro-Vilar A (1984) Neuroendocrinology, in press.
25. Nunez EA, Gershon MD, Silverman AJ (1981) J Histochem Cytochem 29:1336
26. Steele MK, Brownfield MS, Ganong WF (1982) Neuroendocrinology 35:155
27. Steele MK, Negro-Vilar A, McCann SM (1981) Endocrinology 109:893
28. Aguilera G, Hyde CL, Catt KJ (1982) Endocrinology 111:1045
29. Schramme C, Denef C (1983) Neuroendocrinology 36:483

© 1984 Elsevier Science Publishers B.V.
Endocrinology
F. Labrie, L. Proulx, eds.

DISCUSSION OF THE EVIDENCE FOR AND POSSIBLE CONSEQUENCES OF DISSIMILAR CONCENTRATIONS OF DOPAMINE IN BLOOD OF VARIOUS HYPOPHYSIAL PORTAL VESSELS

JOHN C. PORTER and MARIANNE J. REYMOND*
Cecil H. and Ida Green Center for Reproductive Biology Sciences, Departments of Obstetrics and Gynecology and Physiology, The University of Texas Health Science Center at Dallas, Southwestern Medical School, Dallas, Texas 75235, U.S.A.

INTRODUCTION

The hypophysial portal vessels have characteristics of end-arteries, and this fact raises the possibility that neurohypophysiotropic control of the secretion of hormones by cells of the pars distalis is not equally manifested throughout this gland. If there exists a lack of homogeneity in the concentrations of a hypophysiotropic hormone in blood of the various portal vessels, the adenohypophysial cells in the field vascularized by one portal vessel may be under a different level of hypothalamic control than are cells in the field vascularized by another portal vessel. The consequences of such disparity, if it were to exist, could be pronounced for cells that secrete prolactin since such cells are known to be tonically inhibited by a prolactin release-inhibiting hormone from the hypothalamus. The hormone that inhibits the release of prolactin is now believed to be dopamine (1), a neurohormone released into hypophysial portal blood (2).

MATERIAL AND METHODS

Adult female rats (Long-Evans strain) undergoing regular four 4-day estrous cycles were used on the second diestrous day. Each animal was anesthetized with urethane, and a single hypophysial portal vessel was cannulated and blood collected from the vessel, as described previously (3, 4). Blood was collected from a medial portal vessel or from a lateral portal vessel. Simultaneously with the collection of hypophysial portal blood, blood was collected at 7 µl/min from a femoral artery. Plasma from portal or aterial blood was analyzed for dopamine, norepinephrine, and epinephrine using a radioenzymatic assay (5). In order to evaluate the rate of biosynthesis of L-dihydroxyphenylalanine (DOPA) in the

---

*Present address: Divison of Endocrinology, Department of Internal Medicine, CHUV, Lausanne, Switzerland

lateral or medial median eminence, female rats were treated with 3-hydroxybenzlhydrazine (NSD1015) to inhibit the activity of aromatic L-amino acid decarboxylase (6, 7). After 60 min, the brains were removed, and segments of the median eminence were excised with a tubular punch as described by Selmanoff (8). The tissue segments were analyzed for DOPA as described by Zürcher and Da Prada (9).

RESULTS AND DISCUSSION

The rates of collection of plasma from medial portal vessels and lateral portal vessels were 66 ± 8 µl/h (mean ± SE, N=17) and 48 ± 5 µl/h (N=20), respectively. Despite a greater mean blood flow in medial portal vessels than in lateral portal vessel, the concentration of dopamine in the medial portal vessels was significantly greater ($P<0.005$) than that in the lateral portal vessels, being 3.12 ± 0.48 ng/ml and 1.59 ± 0.23 ng/ml, respectively. The concentration of dopamine in plasma from the lateral portal vessels on the right side of the pituitary stalk was 1.56 ± 0.30 ng/ml and on the left side of the stalk was 1.62 ± 0.36 ng/ml. Inasmuch as the concentration of dopamine in portal plasma was 20 to 40 times greater than that in portal plasma of the same animals, it is evident that dopamine in portal plasma is due to the release of hypothalamic dopamine. On the basis of these findings, we calculate that the rate of release of dopamine into the medial portal vessels was 2.5 times that released into the lateral portal vessels.

In contrast to that of dopamine, the plasma concentrations of norepinephrine and epinephrine in lateral portal vessels were not different from the plasma concentrations of norepinephrine and epinephrine in the medial portal vessels. Moreover, the concentrations of norepinephrine and epinephrine in portal plasma were equal to or less than those in arterial plasma of the same animals, indicating that there is no net secretion of these two catecholamines into portal blood by neurons of the hypothalamus.

If dopamine that enters a lateral portal vessel is derived from dopamine released by neurons terminating in the lateral median eminence and if dopamine that enters a medial portal vessel is derived from dopamine released by neurons terminating in the medial median eminence, it is reasonable to ask whether less dopamine is released in the lateral median eminence than in the lateral median eminence. At present, it is not possible to quantify the rate of release of dopamine from hypothalamic neurons apart from the rate of secretion of dopamine into hypophysial portal blood. However, it has been found that dopamine released into portal blood is derived form newly synthesized dopamine, and inhibition of decarboxylation of DOPA by means of an inhibitor of aromatic

L-amino acid decarboxylase activity leads to prompt reduction in the release of dopamine into portal blood. Therefore, it is reasonable to believe that the rate of synthesis of DOPA in the axonal endings of dopaminergic neurons innervating a segment of the median eminence is an accurate reflection of the synthesis and release of dopamine in the same segment.

Thus, rats were treated with NSD 1015. Sixty min later each animal was decapitated, and the lateral median eminences and median eminence were excised. When these tissues were analyzed for DOPA, it was found that the rate of accumulation of DOPA in the lateral median eminence was not different from that in the medial median eminence. This finding is difficult to reconcile with the observation that the rate of release of dopamine into portal blood into the lateral portal vessels is appreciably less than that into the medial portal vessels. Either the assumption that the rate of synthesis of DOPA is an accurate reflection of dopamine release is incorrect or that dopamine released into the lateral median eminence has a different fate than that released into the medial median eminence.

It is interesting to speculate on the consequences of the difference in the concentrations of dopamine in plasma of the lateral and medial portal vessels. It is possible that the concentration of dopamine in portal blood perfusing one group of lactotropes of the pars distalis is sufficient to inhibit the release of prolactin, whereas the concentration of dopamine in portal blood simultaneously perfusing another group of lactotropes is not sufficient to inhibit the release of prolactin, resulting in hypersecretion of prolactin by the uninhibited cells. In view of the effect of dopaminergic agonists and antagonists on growth and hypertrophy of lactotropes (10-16), it is reasonable to suspect that a low concentration of dopamine in blood perfusing lactotropes may be associated with an anomalous growth of these cells and the formation of tumor-like collections of prolactin-secreting cells in the pars distalis. If such speculation has validity, a higher incidence of prolactin-secreting adenomas would be expected to occur in the lateral zones of the pars distalis than in the medial zone. Moreover, the incidence of prolactin-secreting tumors of the pars distalis of the rat would be expected to increase with aging since aging is associated with a reduction in the release of dopamine into hypophysial portal blood.

ACKNOWLEDGEMENT

The assistance of Kay Stanley in the preparation of this manuscript is greatly appreciated.

REFERENCES

1. MacLeod RM (1976) In: Martini L, Ganong WF (eds) Frontiers in Neuroendocrinology. Raven Press, New York, vol 4:169-194
2. Ben-Jonathan N, Oliver C, Weiner HJ, Mical RS, Porter JC (1977) Endocrinology 100:452-458
3. Porter JC, Mical RS, Kamberi IA, Grazia YR (1970) Endocrinology 87:197-201
4. Porter JC (1975) Methods Enzymol 39:166-183
5. Ben-Jonathan N, Porter JC (1976) Endocrinology 98:1497-1507
6. Demarest KT, Alper RH, Moore KE (1979) J Neural Transm 46:183-193
7. Demarest KT, Moore KE (1980) Endocrinology 106:463-468
8. Selmanoff M (1981) Endocrinology 108:1716-1722
9. Zürcher G, Da Prada M (1979) J Neurochem 33:631-639
10. Quadri SK, Lu KH, Meites J (1972) Science 176:417-418
11. MacLeod RM, Lehmeyer JE (1973) Cancer Res 33:849-855
12. Lloyd HM, Meares JD, Jacobi J (1975) Nature 255:497-498
13. Kalbermann LE, Machiavelli GA, De Nicola AF, Weissenberg LS, Burdman JA (1980) J Endocrinol 87:221-224
14. Thorner MO, Martin WH, Rogol AD, Morris JL, Perryman RL, Conway BP, Howards SS, Wolfman MG, MacLeod RM (1980) J Clin Endocrinol Metab 51:438-445
15. Sobrinho LG, Nunes MC, Calhaz-Jorge C, Mauricio JC, Santos MA (1981) Acta Endocrinol (Copenh) 96:24-29
16. Prysor-Jones RA, Jenkins JS (1981) J Endocrinol 88:463-469

25. Relaxin

Endocrinology
F. Labrie, L. Proulx, eds.

RELAXIN : STRUCTURE FUNCTION RELATIONS

GEOFFREY W. TREGEAR AND HUGH D. NIALL
Howard Florey Institute of Experimental Physiology and Medicine, University of Melbourne, Parkville, Victoria, Australia, 3052

The ovarian peptide relaxin is characterized by its action in remodelling the reproductive tract before parturition, thus facilitating the birth process. Although predominantly a hormone of pregnancy, relaxin has also been detected in the non-pregnant female as well as in the male (see ref. 1-3 for review).

The amino acid sequences of relaxin from pig, rat, tiger shark, dogfish shark and human have now been established. The hormone consists of two peptide chains (A & B) joined by disulfide bonds with an intra-chain disulfide loop in the A chain in a manner exactly analogous to that of insulin. A surprising difference between relaxin and most other peptide hormones is the considerable structural variation between species. For example, pig and rat relaxins differ in over 50% of amino acid positions whereas pig and rat insulins differ in only 8%. These differences explain the poor immunological cross-reactivity between relaxins of different species and also a number of the observed differences in their specific biological activity.

The application of recombinant DNA technology has led to the isolation and characterization of the genes coding for rat(4), pig(5) and human relaxins(6,7). Analysis of the nucleotide sequence from cDNA and genomic clones, and a comparison of the deduced amino acid sequences reveals a common structural organization for the relaxin precursor protein. There is a signal peptide of 25 residues, followed by a B-chain of about 30 amino acids, a C-peptide of about 105 amino acids, and an A-chain of 22 to 24 amino acids. In the human, pig and rat genomic clones, an intron interrupts the coding region of the C-peptide. The physiological role of the C-peptide which is considerably longer than the related insulin peptides, and the nature of the enzymes responsible for its removal from the ends of the A and B chain are important unresolved issues.

In the case of human relaxin two separate gene sequences have been identified(6,7). Only one of these genes (G2) is expressed in the ovary during pregnancy, and it is unclear whether the other gene is expressed at another tissue site, or whether it represents a pseudo-gene. The two human relaxin genes show considerable nucleotide and amino acid homology to each other, particularly in the B and C peptide. However, there are some notable regions of sequence divergence, particularly in the amino terminal region of both A and B chains (see Fig.1). The fact that G2 relaxin is synthesized and expressed in the ovary suggests that this is the sequence which is involved in the physiology of pregnancy.

Human relaxin and human insulin genes contain an intron at a similar position in the C-peptide, suggesting that these hormones arose by gene duplication. Recent studies (8) on the chromosomal position of the relaxin genes using mouse/human cell hybrids have established that the human insulin and human relaxin genes are in fact positioned on different chromosomes. Both human relaxin genes are located on the short arm region of chromosome 9, whereas the insulin gene is located on chromosome 11.

Fig.1 compares the known amino acid sequences of relaxins from different species. In addition to the 6 cysteine residues and flanking glycine residues, only the isoleucine at position 7 in the B chain, the arginine at positions 12 and 16, and the leucine at position 32 have been conserved. The cysteine residues are clearly essential to maintaining the overall disulfide bond configuration, and most of the other residues have been predicted to be on the surface of the molecule (9). The variation in amino acid sequence at most positions in the relaxin molecule is remarkable, and is in marked contrast to the situation with virtually all other peptide hormone families. Another feature of the relaxin structures is the variation in length seen at the amino and carboxyl terminal regions of the B-chain, and to a lesser extent at the amino terminus of the A-chain.

The chemical synthesis of relaxin has been particularly difficult largely as a result of the unusual solubility and structural characteristics of the isolated B-chain(10). Despite these difficulties, preliminary studies have provided valuable information regarding the structural features important for biological activity(10). The synthesis of pig relaxin, and more recently the two forms of human relaxin has been successfully achieved. An interesting finding was that the synthetic peptides representing the two forms of human relaxin were of equal potency as assessed in the standard uterine contraction bioassay. The synthetic relaxins and their structural analogue have confirmed that the full length of the A and B chains is not required for biological activity. Up to 6 amino acids may be

RELAXIN A-CHAINS

	-2		1				5					10					15					20		22
HUMAN-1	Arg	Pro	Tyr	Val	Ala	Leu	Phe	Glu	Lys	Cys	Cys	Leu	Ile	Gly	Cys	Thr	Lys	Arg	Ser	Leu	Ala	Lys	Tyr	Cys
HUMAN-2	Gln	Leu	Tyr	Ser	Ala	Leu	Ala	Asn	Lys	Cys	Cys	His	Val	Gly	Cys	Thr	Lys	Arg	Ser	Leu	Ala	Arg	Phe	Cys
PIG			Arg	Met	Thr	Leu	Ser	Glu	Lys	Cys	Cys	Gln	Val	Gly	Cys	Ile	Arg	Lys	Asp	Ile	Ala	Arg	Leu	Cys
RAT	Gln	Ser	Gly	Ala	Leu	Leu	Ser	Glu	Gln	Cys	Cys	His	Ile	Gly	Cys	Thr	Arg	Arg	Ser	Ile	Ala	Lys	Leu	Cys
SHARK	Ala	Thr	Ser	Pro	Ala	Met	Ser	Ile	Lys	Cys	Cys	Ile	Tyr	Gly	Cys	Thr	Lys	Lys	Asp	Ile	Ser	Val	Leu	Cys
DOGFISH	Glu	Gly	Ser	Pro	Gly	Met	Ser	Ser	Lys	Cys	Cys	Thr	Tyr	Gly	Cys	Thr	Arg	Lys	Asp	Ile	Ser	Ile	Leu	Cys

RELAXIN B-CHAINS

	-4				1				5					10					15					20					25					30		32
HUMAN-1					Lys	Trp	Lys	Asp	Asp	Val	Ile	Lys	Leu	Cys	Gly	Arg	Glu	Leu	Val	Arg	Ala	Gln	Ile	Ala	Ile	Cys	Gly	Met	Ser	Thr	Trp	Ser	Lys	Arg	Ser	Leu
HUMAN-2				Asp	Ser	Trp	Met	Glu	Glu	Val	Ile	Lys	Leu	Cys	Gly	Arg	Glu	Leu	Val	Arg	Ala	Gln	Ile	Ala	Ile	Cys	Gly	Met	Ser	Thr	Trp	Ser	Lys	Arg	Ser	Leu
PIG					Gln	Ser	Thr	Asn	Asp	Phe	Ile	Lys	Ala	Cys	Gly	Arg	Glu	Leu	Val	Arg	Leu	Trp	Val	Glu	Ile	Cys	Gly	Ser	Val	Ser	Trp	Gly	Arg	Thr	Ala	Leu
RAT	Arg	Val	Ser	Glu	Glu	Trp	Met	Asp	Gln	Val	Ile	Gln	Val	Cys	Gly	Arg	Gly	Tyr	Ala	Arg	Ala	Trp	Ile	Glu	Val	Cys	Gly	Ala		Ser	Val	Gly	Arg	Leu	Ala	Leu
SHARK		Gln	Ser	Leu	Ser	Asn	Ala	Gly	Ser	Gly	Ile	Lys	Leu	Cys	Gly	Arg	Gly	Phe	Ile	Arg	Ala	Ile	Ile	Phe	Ala	Cys	Gly	Gly	Ser	Arg						
DOGFISH					Gln	Asn	Ala	Glu	Pro	Gly	Ile	Lys	Leu	Cys	Gly	Arg	Glu	Phe	Ile	Arg	Ala	Val	Ile	Tyr	Ser	Cys	Gly									

Fig.1. Comparison of the amino acid sequences of the A and B chains of the human relaxins with other members of the relaxin family. The boxed areas highlight residues which are conserved.

removed from the C-terminus of the B-chain without affecting activity. Similarly, up to 3 amino acids may be removed from the amino terminus of the A-chain before activity is lost, and many of the individual amino acids may be substituted with only minor activity changes. These synthetic studies and those provided by expression of chemically synthesized genes for relaxin in bacterial and yeast systems should provide sufficient human relaxin to permit detailed physiological studies of the hormone, and will aid in the design of structural analogues for possible therapeutic use.

ACKNOWLEDGEMENTS

In this review we have attempted to summarize the published work of others as well as presenting some recent data from our own laboratory concerning the molecular biology of relaxin. The many contributors to this work have been listed in the references to papers published or submitted and are acknowledged below. This work was supported by grants from the National Health & Medical Research Council of Australia, and by NIH grant HD11980.

REFERENCES

1. Bryant-Greenwood GD (1982) Endocrine Reviews 3:62-90

2. Weiss G (1984) Ann Rev Physiol 46: 43-52

3. Schwabe C (1983) In : Bigazzi M, Greenwood FC, Gasparri F (eds) Biology of Relaxin and its Role in the Human. Excerpta Medica, Amsterdam, pp 22-31

4. Hudson P,Haley H, Cronk M, Shine J, Niall H (1981) Nature 291 : 127-131

5. Haley J, Hudson P, Scanlon D, John M, Cronk M, Shine J, Tregear G, Niall H (1982) DNA 1: 155-162

6. Hudson P, Haley J, John M, Cronk M, Crawford R, Haralambidis J, Tregear G, Shine J, Niall H (1984) Nature 301: 628-631

7. Hudson P, John M, Crawford R, Haralambidis J,Scanlon D,Gorman J, Tregear G, Shine J, Niall H (1984) Submitted for publication

8. Crawford RJ, Hudson P, Shine J, Niall HD, Eddie RL, Shows TB (1984) Submitted for publication

9. Blundell T, Gowan LK, Schwabe C (1983) In : Bigazzi M, Greenwood FC, Gasparri F (eds) Biology of Relaxin and its Role in the Human. Excerpta Medica, Amsterdam, pp 14-21

10. Tregear GW, Du YC, Wang KZ, Southwell C, Jones P, John M, Gorman J, Kemp B, Niall HD (1983) In : Bigazzi M, Greenwood FC, Gasparri F (eds) Biology of Relaxin and its Role in the Human. Excerpta Medica, Amsterdam, pp 42-55

© 1984 Elsevier Science Publishers B.V.
Endocrinology
F. Labrie, L. Proulx, eds.

EXTRALUTEAL SOURCES OF RELAXIN

MARIO BIGAZZI and GILLIAN D. BRYANT-GREENWOOD

Poggiosecco Hospital, INRCA, Florence, Italy; Dpt of Anatomy and Reproductive Biology, Univ. of Hawaii, Honolulu, USA.

Relaxin (RLX) has been measured in human blood only during pregnancy, its secretory granules have been identified in cells of the porcine gestational corpus luteum and its extraction and purification achieved from ovaries of several species of pregnant animals. Therefore RLX has been considered for long time, an hormone exclusively of the pregnant female and solely secreted from the corpus luteum [1]. More recent studies demonstrated its presence in other tissues of the pregnant or cyclic female and also in the male and yielded evidence that the major source of RLX may vary in different species [2,3] (Table 1). Generally extraluteal sources contains RLX in low levels, perhaps because of a continous release of the hormone.

This makes more difficult the isolation/identification and the direct proof of active synthesis of RLX. A second problem comes from the species variability of the sources, the structure and even the effects of RLX, which do not allow a

TABLE 1

SOURCES OF RELAXIN

FEMALE		MALE	
OVARY		EPIDYDYMUS	
		PROSTATE GLAND	seminal fluid
CORPUS LUTEUM	peritoneal fluid	SEMINAL VESCICLES	
(****) cycle	blood	(****)	
pregnancy	urine		
puerperium?	milk		
FOLLICLE	follicular fluid	HUMAN DISEASE	
(**)		OVARIAN CYST	cyst fluid
		(***)	
UTERUS		FIBROCYSTIC DISEASE	cyst fluid
ENDOMETRIUM	uterine fluid?	OF MAMMARY GLAND	
(**)		(*)	
		PROSTATE ADENOMATA	seminal fluid
DECIDUA		(***)	
PLACENTA	amniotic fluid?		
BASAL PLATE			
(****)			

(*) RIA, Bioassay
(**) Ria, Bioassay, Immunohist.
(***) RIA, Bioassay, Isolation
(****) RIA, Bioassay, Immunohist., Isolation

direct comparison among studies on different animals. Finally we may expect that RLX produced by most of the extraluteal sources does not enter the general circulation but rather acts locally.

We will focus on the secretion of RLX from the ovarian follicle and the decidua, because recent studies point to some local effects of the hormone, which seem related to ovulation and parturition.

Bryant-Greenwood and colleagues demonstrated, in pig, that RLX is present in periovulatory follicular fluid and is produced by the follicle wall _in vitro_ [4]. Also human follicular fluid contains RLX, which apparently increases as ovulation approaches [5]. In pig the principal site of production seems to be the theca [6] with some contribution of the granulosa cells [7], while in human Balboni and colleagues [8] showed that cells which stain specifically by immunofluorescence and peroxidase methods are more numerous in the granulosa, and appear in the theca only near ovulation. Colloidal gold stain showed that in the follicular cell RLX is packaged in granules as in the corpus luteum.

Relaxin synthesised by theca/granulosa coula act perhaps directly on to affect the contractility and collagen metabolism of the follicle wall. It is also targets the granulosa cells to produce plasminogen activator, collagenase and proteoglycanase which enter the follicular fluid and presumably act on the follicle wall, as inferred from _in vitro_ experiments [9].

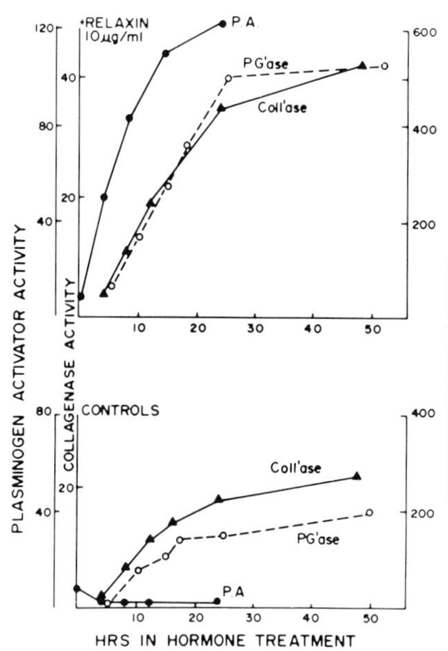

Fig. 1 Effect of RLX on collagenolytic enzymes released from PMSG primed rat granulosa cells _in vitro_.

In presenting the decidual secretion of RLX, we refer mainly to studies in the human, because according to the type of placentation, the decidual reaction and probably decidual function may vary greatly. In fact, the human species has an hemochorial type of placentation, characterized by remarked development of the decidua. Many studies have shown that human decidua must be considered an endocrine organ which produces many bioactive substances and which shows specific endocrine functions, specific hormone regulation and a secretoty polarity towards the amniotic compartment [10].

The presence of RLX in decidua, whole placenta and placenta basal plate of pregnant women at term has been demonstrated by isolation, bioassay and radioimmunoassay [11,12,13]. The actual concentrations reported varied over a wide range depending on the assay used for the RLX measurement, the RIA values were much lower than the biopotency refered to porcine relaxin. The low levels of RLX contained in decidua and the sensitivity of the RIA method currently available, make difficult any dynamic studies to demonstrate an active synthesis in such tissue. A de novo synthesis of RLX in human decidua is supported by results of in vitro studies. Decidua cultured in medium containing labelled amino acids, released a substance which was precipitated by excess anti-pRLX antibody, furthermore the radioactivity of the immunocomplex decreased progressively with inhibition of the protein synthesis (Fig. 2).

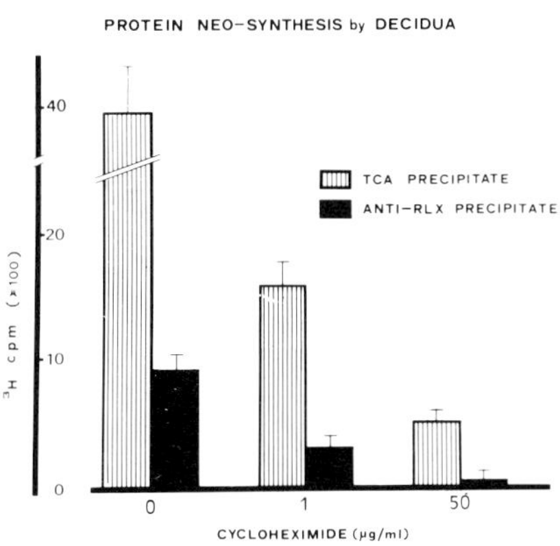

Fig. 2. Radioactivity found in the precipitation after TCA or anti+RLX antibody exposure of medium of in vitro cultures of human decidua incubated with labelled aminoacids.

A further proof of active secretion of RLX in decidua has been given by immunofluorescence stu- dies which showed specific reac- tion with anti-RLX antibodies in the cytoplasm of some decidual cells [14]. These results have been recently confirmed by biotin avidin immunoperoxidase. Such cells, observed at EM do not show evidence of granules, confirming that RLX is continu- ously secreted by decidua, by analogy with decidual PRL [10], and in accordance with the hypothesis that RLX in decidua may be considered a maintenance hormone, acting locally [15]. It has been claimed that the local effect of decidual RLX may be elicited by the contiguous muscle and collagen of the uterus. Recent studies indicate that RLX also acts on amnion/chorion cells, inducing a release of proteolytic enzymes into the amniotic fluid. Plasminogen activator (Fig. 3) and collagenase are released from amnion/chorion cells in vitro in the presence of RLX in the culture medium. These findings have permitted speculation on a role for decidual RLX, together with decidual PRL and PGF, 2 , in the event of parturition[16]. The roles played by RLX as a local hormone which just now are beginning to be recognized, seem to overshadow the effects attributed to systemic RLX.

Recent experiments in rats also suggest that RLX released locally may produce systemic effects indirectly through other systems. The peritoneal administration

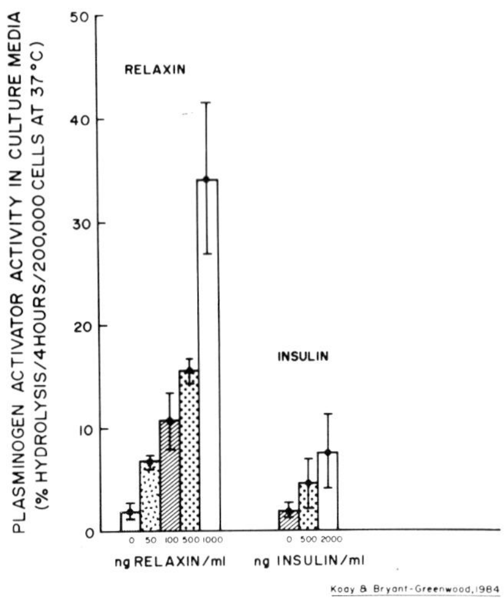

Fig. 3. Physiological dose-response effect of relaxin on plasminogen activator secretion by amnion/chorion cells in vitro after 32 hours incubation with hormone.

of porcine RLX (NIH-RXN P1) to male rats is followed by a striking reduction of the blood clotting time (Fig. 4). This effect can be attributed to the massive degranulation observed in the peritoneal mast cells after RLX administration [18].

This RLX-mediated effect also could explain the finding of changes in the microcirculation [19] and on the volume of the spleen [20] found under similar experimental conditions, and perhaps explains the therapeutic effect of RLX observed many years ago on vascular diseases [21].

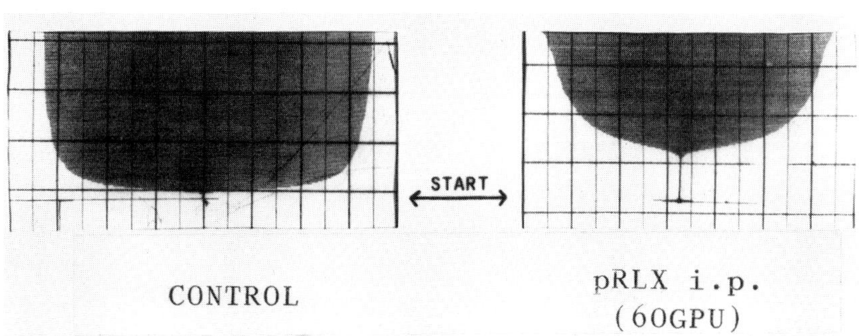

Fig. 4. Changes in blood coagulation following I.P. administration of RLX to male rat

REFERENCES

1) Schwabe C, Steinetz Bl, Weiss G, Segaloff A, Mc Donald J, O'Byrne E, Hochman J, Carrier B and Goldsmith L, (1978) Rec Prog Horm Res 24: 123 - 211

2) Bryant-Greenwood GD, (1982) Endocr Rev 3: 62 - 90

3) In: Bigazzi M, Greenwood FC, and Gasparri F. (eds) Biology of Relaxin and its role in the human (1983). Excerpta Medica, Amsterdam, International Congress Serie N. 610

4) Bryant-Greenwood GD, Jeffery R, Ralph MM and Seamark RF (1980) Biol Reprod 23: 792 -798

5) Noci I, Nardi E, Scarselli G, Petrucci F, Chelo E, La Malfa A, Tantini C, Bruni V, and Bigazzi M. In: Bigazzi M, Greenwood F.C. and Gasparri F. (eds) Biology of Relaxin and its role in the human, Excerpta Medica, Amsterdam, p.p. 270 - 272

6) Evans G, Wathes DC, King GJ, Armstrong DT, Porter DG (1983) J. Reprod Fert 69: 677 - 683

7) Loecken MR, D'Eletto R, Weiss G (1981) 63 Annual Meeting of the Endocrine Society, Cincinnati, OH (Abs 1056)

8) Balboni GC, Bigazzi M, Scarselli G, Vannelli G (1984) 7th International Congress of Endocrinology, Quebec, Canada (Abs 184)

9) Too CK, Bryant-Greenwood GD, and Greenwood FC. (1984) Endocrinology In press

10) Bigazzi M. (1983) Seminars in Reproductive biology 1: 4, 343 - 356

11) Bigazzi M, Nardi E, Bruni P, Petrucci F (1980) J Clin endocrinol Metab 51: 939 - 941

12) Fields PA, Larkin LH (1981) J Clin Endocrinol Metab 52: 79 - 85

13) Yamamoto S, Kwok SCM, Greenwood FC, Bryant-Greenwood GD (1981) J Clin Endocr Metab 52: 601 - 604

14) Bigazzi M, Bruni P, Nardi E, Petrucci F, Pollicino G, Franchini M, Scarselli G, and Farnararo M. (1982) Ann NY Acad Sci, 380: 87 - 99

15) Bryant Greenwood GD, (1982) Endocrine Rev 3: 62-90

16) Koay ESC, Greenwood FC and Bryant Greenwood GD (1984) in Physiology of Pregnancy and Periportal period Revew Press (in press)

17) Bigazzi M, Bettoni M, Petrucci F, Del Mese A, Baui G (1984), in preparation

18) Baui G, Bigazzi M, Bianchi S, Petruci F (1984) in preparation

19) Del Mese A, Casali R, Novelli GP, Petrucci F and Bigazzi M (1984) 7th International Congress of Endocrinology Quebec City, Canada (Abs 949)

20) Petrucci F, Baui G, Bettoni M, Del Mese A, Bianchi S and Bigazzi M (1984) in preparation

21) Casten GG, Gilmore MD, Houghton FE and Samuels SS (1960) Angiology 11: 408-419

© 1984 Elsevier Science Publishers B.V.
Endocrinology
F. Labrie, L. Proulx, eds.

RELAXIN: A MULTIPURPOSE HORMONE

D.G. PORTER
Pre-Clinical Veterinary Studies, Department of Anatomy, The Medical School, Bristol, U.K.

Relaxin was discovered in the mid-1920s by Hisaw[1] and promptly over-shadowed by the discovery of progesterone. Only sporadic attention was given to the hormone until an inopportune flurry of clinical interest in the 1950s relegated the hormone to the category of a dangerous myth[2]. Recent elegant work on purification and sequencing however have restored at least chemical respectability to Hisaw's hormone but the constant reporting of novel actions of relaxin may strain the credulity of even the polypeptide's most ardent devotees. It may be necessary therefore for us to recognize that relaxin may be a multipurpose hormone, having actions at least within the reproductive system, which are as fundamental and as diverse as are those of the corticosteroids for the physiology of the body in general.

The classic actions of relaxin are threefold[2]: (1) upon the collagenous structures of the cervix (2) and the 'pubic' symphysis, and (3) upon the smooth muscle of the uterus. Reports have existed in the literature for many years however that pointed to wider responsibilities for relaxin. Its presence in an elasmobranch, in birds, and in male animals, and claims that it modified milk secretion, all encouraged the view that the concept of relaxin as merely a pre-partum hormone was too restrictive. Table 1 underscores the wide range of processes in which relaxin has been implicated. In my own laboratory we have been involved recently with three non-classical aspects of the physiology of relaxin.

The report that relaxin is present in the *ovarian follicle*[3] was of great interest since it cast doubt even on the long-held view that as far as the female mammal was concerned the polypeptide was primarily a hormone of pregnancy. In a collaborative study[4] we were able to identify the theca as the principal site of relaxin production by the porcine follicle rather than the granulosa layer as had been reported earlier[5]. Moreover, we showed that relaxin output by the theca increased as ovulation approached, although our study did not ascertain whether or not this trend continued up to the moment of ovulation. No experimental work appears to have been done on the possibility that relaxin may play a part in folliculogenesis or ovulation or both. The classic actions of the peptide prompt speculation that relaxin may promote the changes in collagen which occur as the follicle expands and its wall ruptures. Another possibility is that relaxin may modulate smooth muscle

Reported actions and sources (or putative sources) of relaxin

Actions (stimulatory unless otherwise indicated)		Sources (and putative sources)	
Pelvic ligaments	Soften	Corpus luteum	Prostate
Cervix	Soften	Follicle wall: theca	Non mammals
Uterus	Growth	Decidua	Tetrahymena
	Water imbibition	(Endometrium: glands)	Elasmobranch ovaries: 2 species
	Collagen rearrangement		
a. Myometrium	Inhibition		
	Co-ordination		
	Glycogen deposition		
b. Endometrium	Arteriolar endothelial proliferation	(Syncytio-trophoblast)	Avian testes
	Granulocyte aggregation		
Mammary gland			
a. Myoepithelium	Blocks oxytocin stimulation		
b. Alveolar epithelium	Growth		
c. Ducts	Growth		
d. Fibroblasts	Mitosis		
	Protein synthesis		
Vagina	Opening		
	Oestrogen-induced cornification		
Brain	Inhibits oxytocin release		
Fat cells (mature, female)	Insulin binding		
Spermatozoa	Motility		

Table 1

activity in the follicle. Although the subject is controversial, recent studies provide persuasive evidence that smooth muscle may be involved in the process of ovulation[6]. On whether relaxin might act as an inhibitor, or would improve co-ordination of the muscle as ovulation approaches it is only possible to speculate. Relaxin could have a role unrelated to the three classical actions. Interestingly it has been reported that relaxin stimulates follicular production of plasminogen activator[7], a substance implicated in the inflammatory changes which precede follicular wall breakdown, but this has not gone unchallenged[8].

It is probable that relaxin plays a part in the pre-partum inhibition of myometrial activity. However oxytocin and $PGF_{2\alpha}$ can override myometrial inhibition produced by relaxin, which may be important in permitting labour to occur 'on time' but it would seem potentially hazardous as inappropriate oxytocin release which can occur in women[9] might prejudice the fetus. It would seem logical therefore if relaxin *inhibited the central release of oxytocin*. Because of the difficulties of measuring release of oxytocin per se we monitored intramammary pressure in the anaesthetized, suckling rat[10] as a specific indicator of oxytocin release. Our experiments demonstrated[11] a dual action of relaxin, namely on the mammary gland, where it reduced the sensitivity of the myoepithelium to exogenous oxytocin and also centrally, where it inhibited oxytocin release. We confirmed the latter action by intracerebroventricular injections of purified porcine relaxin in amounts (40ng) small enough to exert no action peripherally on the mammary gland, but which interrupted significantly the pattern of milk ejection in spontaneously ejecting rats. Although we do not know yet the precise site or mechanism of action of relaxin centrally this is the first demonstration of the action of the hormone on yet another target, namely nervous tissue. The physiological significance of this needs further study. It may mean that relaxin restrains myometrial activity pre-partum by a double mechanism, but whether it has relevance for lactation is not known. It has been reported that relaxin is secreted from a non-ovarian source during suckling in the sow[12,13], but this has been disputed. Evidence of secretion of relaxin during lactation in other species is not available but there are reports of actions of relaxin, although not always consistent on milk secretion in several species[2].

Relaxin is secreted in increasing amounts as term approaches in several, but not the human[14], species. In the rat high affinity binding of relaxin to the myometrium increases to a peak in late gestation (day 17) and falls abruptly pre-partum[15]. This is difficult to reconcile with paradoxical findings that relaxin is unable to inhibit rat (or mouse[16]) myometrial activity *in vitro* when strips are taken from animals after ∿ day 15 of pregnancy. Further we have found that the ability of relaxin to provoke cAMP generation in the uterus is likewise lost *in vitro* after day 15[17]. We do not know whether this represents another *in vivo* vs *in vitro* discrepancy[18] or is physiologically significant, because in the pregnant pig relaxin appears to inhibit contractions Fig.1([19]) . Also intra-arterial infusion of relaxin to ovariectomized pregnant sows, permitted to deliver by withdrawal of progestational replacement therapy, arrested early labour contractions, but despite continuous infusion of the hormone the inhibitory effect of the polypeptide was evenutally 'overriden'[19].

The crucial experiments of eliminating relaxin and observing the effects on reproductive processes are difficult to conduct so that it remains impossible to say that relaxin is absolutely essential for any specific reproductive mechanism. The best evidence is that that ovariectomized sows maintained on progesterone can deliver with normal livebirth rates if relaxin is provided when progestational replacement therapy is withdrawn, whereas without relaxin the stillbirth rate is high[20]. Our work in progress in intact sows also points to a close relationship of the evolution of mechanical and electrical activity in the myometrium with the decline in relaxin titres, whereas PGFM titres increase before the development of significant uterine activity[19].

These studies provide information on only a limited number of facets of the

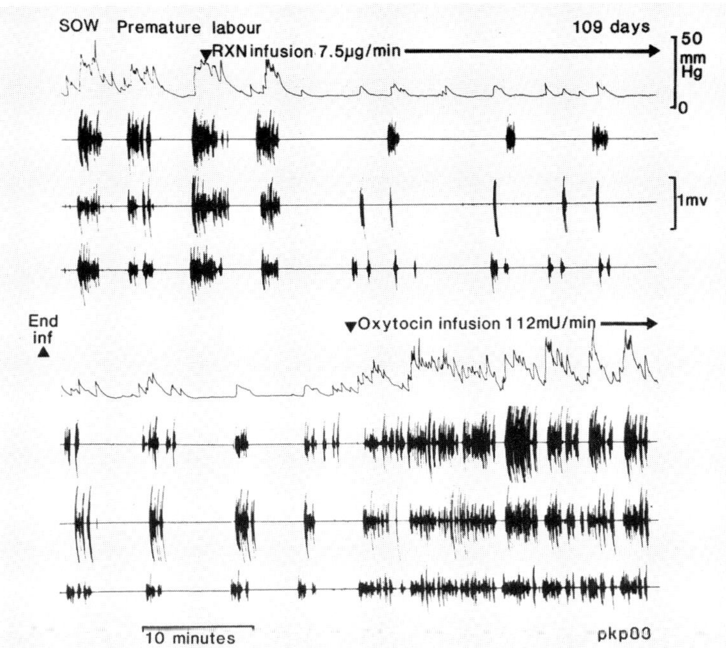

Fig. 1. Intrauterine pressure and electromyographic records from three stainless steel electrodes in the myometrium (10cms apart) from a sow in premature labour on day 109 of pregnancy. Upper traces show effect of an infusion of pure porcine relaxin on labour contractions. The infusion was ended after 60 minutes, shortly before lower traces were recorded. The inhibited uterus was sensitive to an infusion of oxytocin which induced delivery of three dead piglets.

spectrum of actions of relaxin at present under investigation in different laboratories. However not only do they corroborate the view that relaxin has clear actions at a number of sites in the reproductive system, but they also extend the range of these actions. The effects are often subtle, and as happened in the early research on corticosteroids[21] our yardsticks may be too crude to dissect out the numerous threads that this ancient hormone contributes to the weave of reproductive processes. The recent clear demonstration that relaxin exists in several forms in rat plasma[22], the ratios of which change with time during pregnancy is consistent with the concept of multiple responsibilities. But actions on the diverse tissues shown in Table 1 suggests that the relaxin family of polypeptides may have protean responsibilities ranging from permissive to essential.

REFERENCES

1. Hisaw FL (1926) Proc Soc exp Biol Med 23: 661-663
2. Porter DG (1979) In: Finn CA (ed) Oxford Reviews of Reproductive Biology Vol.1 Clarendon Press, Oxford, pp 1-57
3. Bryant-Greenwood GD, Jeffrey R, Ralph MM, Seamark RF (1980) Biol Reprod 23: 792
4. Evans G, Wathes DC, King GJ, Armstrong DT, Porter DG (1983) J Reprod Fert 69: 677-683
5. Loeken MR, Channing CP, D'Eletto R, Weiss G (1983) Endocrinology 112: 769-771
6. Martin GG, Talbot P (1981) J Exper Zool 216: 469
7. Too CKL, Weiss TJ, Bryant-Greenwood GD (1982) Endocrinology 112: 1424-1426
8. Martinat N, Combarnous Y (1983) Endocrinology 113: 433-435
9. Viegas OAC, Arulkumaran S (1984) The Lancet, I (8384) 1015
10. Lincoln DW, Hill A, Wakerley JB (1973) J Endocr 57: 459-476
11. Summerlee AJS, O'Byrne KT, Paisley AC, Breeze MF, Porter DG (1984) Nature 309: 372-374
12. Afele S, Bryant-Greenwood GD, Chamley WA, Dax EM (1979) J Reprod Fert 56: 451
13. Sherwood OD, Nara BS, Welk FA, First NL, Rutherford JE (1981) Biol Reprod 25: 65
14. O'Byrne EM, Flitcraft JF, Sawyer WI, Hochman J, Weiss G, Steinetz BG (1978) Endocrinology 102: 1641
15. Mercado-Simmen RC, Bryant-Greenwood GD, Greenwood FC (1982) Endocrinology 110; 220
16. Wiqvist N (1959) Acta endocr Copenh 32: Suppl.46 15-32
17. Breeze MF, Gilling JAG, Creek J, Porter DG (Unpublished data)
18. Finn CA, Porter DG (1975) The Uterus. Handbook of Reproductive Biology. Paul Elek Ltd, London. pp 178-179.
19. Porter DG, Watts A, Jones R (Unpublished data)
20. Nara BS, Welk FA, Rutherford JE, Sherwood OD, First NL (1982) J Reprod Fert 66: 359-365
21. Munroe NA, O'Hare MJ (1982) The Human Adrenal Cortex. Springer-Verlag, Berlin
22. Sherwood OD, Key RH, Tarbell MK, Downing SJ (1984) Endocrinology 114: 806-813

ACKNOWLEDGEMENTS

I am indebted to my colleagues, Drs. M.F.Breeze, W.A.Kelly, A.J.S.Summerlee and D.C.Wathes and Messrs. K.T.O'Byrne and A.Watts for most of the experimental work reported here. I thank Miss Anne Moffatt, Mr. R.Jones, Miss J.Creek and Miss A.Hockey for their technical assistance, Mrs.S.Somers for typing the manuscript and the M.R.C. and A.F.R.C. for financial support.

Endocrinology
F. Labrie, L. Proulx, eds.

CLINICAL STUDIES ON RELAXIN

GERSON WEISS
Department of Obstetrics and Gynecology, New York University School of Medicine, New York, N.Y. 10016 (U.S.A.)

INTRODUCTION

Studies on the physiology of relaxin in women were hampered for over 50 years by an inability to measure circulating relaxin due to insensitive bioassays. In 1976, O'Byrne and Steinetz described an RIA utilizing antiserum R6, raised in a rabbit against purified porcine relaxin, which cross-reacted with a substance in human pregnancy serum (1). Utilizing this RIA, immunoreactive relaxin was detected during term pregnancy in the ovarian vein draining the corpus luteum in higher concentrations than in either peripheral blood or the contralateral ovarian vein (2). Corpora lutea of pregnant women contain relaxin which has both biological and immunological activity. The biological activity parallels the immunoactivity of relaxin. The ratio of biologic to immunologic activity ranges from 1.3-4.4:1, suggesting that most human relaxin is detected by this antiserum (3). This antiserum was used to measure human relaxin in the studies reported herein.

RELAXIN SECRETION

Relaxin is detectable in human serum throughout pregnancy from the time of the missed menses, two weeks after conception. Levels rapidly rise and are highest in the first trimester. By the end of the first trimester, serum concentrations have fallen by approximately 20 per cent. Concentrations then remain stable throughout pregnancy. Early detection and first trimester predominance are secretion characteristics shared with hCG. Relaxin concentrations in the first trimester of pregnancy are higher in HMG-hCG induced ovulations which result in multiple gestations rather than singleton gestations from HMG-hCG induced ovulations. This suggests that the level of hCG in the mother regulates the amount of circulating relaxin. Luteectomy during pregnancy results in a prompt fall in circulating relaxin levels. There are no significant differences between antepartum and intrapartum relaxin concentations. There is no prelabor elevation in serum relaxin concentrations in women as there are in pigs and rats (4). Relaxin is occasionally found in the sera of nonpregnant luteal phase women. It is also found in the corpora lutea of nonpregnant women at 1 to 2 orders of magnitude lower concentration than in the corpora lutea of pregnancy.

Serum relaxin concentrations were determined in several pathological pregnancy categories. Relaxin levels in third trimester women with toxemia of pregnancy are similar to levels in normal women. In contrast, the levels in women beyond the forty-third week of pregnancy are significantly lower than third trimester levels. In women in premature labor between 29 and 36 weeks, relaxin was significantly lower than in normal age-matched pregnancies.

After delivery, circulating relaxin levels gradually fall to below assay detectability in approximately three days. There is no difference in the serum relaxin concentrations in nursing and non-nursing women, suggesting that prolactin in nursing postpartum women is not luteotrophic (4).

The stimulus for relaxin secretion appears to be a signal from the developing blastocyst. Relaxin secretion can be induced by hCG when given to women on day 8-10 of the luteal phase. This treatment produces an abrupt rise in progesterone but relaxin does not become detectable for 2 to 6 days. The timing of the hCG stimulus is critical. When hCG injections are given on day 2 or 3 of the luteal phase, no relaxin was detectable. There was no significant change in progesterone response either. These data suggest that luteal responsiveness varies as the corpus luteum matures.

ACTIONS OF RELAXIN DURING PREGNANCY

Human relaxin from the corpus luteum of pregnancy can decrease the amplitude of spontaneous contractions of human myometrium in vitro. In contrast, progesterone has little activity alone in this system. However, progesterone synergizes with relaxin in this inhibitory action. Doses of relaxin and progesterone, which independently are ineffective, together inhibit myometrial contraction amplitude. Since relaxin and progesterone are both luteal products, and the corpus luteum is necessary for the maintenance of early pregnancy, it is likely that these hormones act in concert physiologically in the maintenance of human pregnancy. In fact, the secretion pattern of relaxin, its human myometrial action, and the necessity of the corpus luteum in the maintenance of early human pregnancy suggest that the major actions of circulating relaxin in women are at the beginning of pregnancy (4).

There is no evidence to suggest that the fetus makes relaxin. Relaxin is generally undetectable in fetal blood. It was found in only 10 percent of approximately 40 amniotic fluid samples in low concentrations. Relaxin is detectable in human decidual tissue and placenta at term in concentrations several orders of magnitude below that contained in the corpora lutea of term pregnancy. Immunoactive relaxin has also been detected in myometrium, fat and skin in low concentrations. It is of great interest to know whether relaxin is made locally in these tissues or sequestered from blood relaxin derived from other tissue sources.

We have shown that the baboon is a good model for human relaxin secretion since both species have similar secretion patterns and control mechanisms (5). Relaxin is detectable in several different types of tissues of the pregnant baboon months after removal of the corpus luteum bearing ovary when peripheral levels are undetectable, suggesting local production as well as luteal production. The concentrations of relaxin in decidua in these animals is higher than the concentrations of relaxin in decidua of intact animals. Human pregnancy can proceed uneventfully in the absence of the corpus luteum after the mid-first trimester. However, local decidual production of relaxin may contribute to the maintenance of uterine quiescence and cervical ripening during late pregnancy.

RELAXIN IN THE MALE

Relaxin is present in human seminal plasma in concentrations one to two orders of magnitude greater than that contained in pregnancy serum. The presence of relaxin in the ejaculate of men with congenital absence of the vas deferens and seminal vesicles suggest a prostatic source. Antisera to relaxin promptly immobilizes human sperm whereas antisera to insulin, also present in seminal plasma, has no effect on motility. The immobilization of sperm by relaxin antisera can be prevented by pretreatment with excess quantities of relaxin (6). Relaxin augments the penetration of sperm into cervical mucus. Treating washed sperm with physiologic concentrations of relaxin results in significantly increased sperm penetration into cervical mucus as compared with treatment with albumin or buffer. The improvement of motility of sperm in cervical mucus is much greater than the improvement of motility of sperm in buffer, suggesting that there are co-factors present in cervical mucus which maximize the effect of relaxin. The act of centrifuging and washing human sperm decreases its motility in cervical mucus. Replacement of the seminal plasma results in improvement of motility. A similar level of improvement of motility of sperm can be obtained by addition of physiologic concentations of relaxin into buffer(7). This implies that relaxin is the factor in seminal plasma which augments sperm motility. The addition of relaxin to whole semen improves motility of sperm in aged (5 hours after ejaculation) semen or poorly motile sperm. These data suggest that relaxin plays a major role in sperm motility. Human relaxin has potential clinical usefulness in fertility regulation. Relaxin secretion in seminal plasma by the male represents a novel physiological mechanism for hormone delivery. This exocrine male secretion is delivered to the female during coitus where it seems to facilitate sperm penetration through the female reproductive system.

ACKNOWLEDGMENTS

Supported by NIH grant HD-12395 and a grant from the Mellon Foundation.

REFERENCES

1. O'Byrne, EM, Steinetz, BG (1976) Proc. Soc. Exp. Biol. Med. 152:272-276

2. Weiss, G, O'Byrne EM, Steinetz BG (1976) Science 194:948-949

3. O'Byrne EM, Flitcraft JF, Sawyer WI et al. (1978) Endocrinology 102:1641-1644

4. Weiss G (1983) Clinics in Perinatology 10:641-651

5. Castracane VD, D'Eletto R, Weiss G (1983) In: Greenwald S. Terranova PF (eds) Factors Regulating Ovarian Function. Raven Press, 415-419

6. Sarosi P, Schoenfeld C, Berman J et al. (1983) Endocrinology 112:1860-61.

7. Brenner SH, Lessing JB, Schoenfeld C, et al (1984) Fertil. Steril.,in press

26. Steroid Receptors

Endocrinology
F. Labrie, L. Proulx, eds.

PROBES FOR STEROID RECEPTORS

JEAN-PIERRE RAYNAUD, TIIU OJASOO, ALAIN JOUQUEY, MARTINE MOGUILEWSKY AND GEORGES TEUTSCH
Roussel-Uclaf, Paris, France

INTRODUCTION

By demonstrating in 1959 selective accumulation of ^{3}H-labeled hexestrol in the reproductive organs of immature female goats and sheep, Glascock and Hoekstra (4) initiated research into the mechanism of action of steroid hormones by the use of radioactive probes. However, the development of synthetic steroids for the detection and assay of steroid receptors only really took off with the ability to measure bound radioactivity in high-speed supernatant (cytosol) from target organ homogenates. This chapter describes the radioligands developed by Roussel Uclaf.

CRITERIA FOR THE SELECTION OF STEROID PROBES

A probe must meet several requirements : (a) it should bind to a functional receptor, (b) it should bind to one receptor only, (c) it should form a stable complex with this receptor, (d) it should bind as little as possible to plasma proteins, (e) it should not be degraded on in vitro incubation, (f) it should be labeled with high specific activity.

Because the natural hormones do not fulfil all these criteria (21), the following synthetic probes were developed at Roussel-Uclaf : ^{3}H-moxestrol (R 2858) for the estrogen receptor (ER) (17), ^{3}H-promegestone (R 5020) or its 21S-hydroxy metabolite (RU 27987) for the progestin receptor (PR) (8,9), ^{3}H-metribolone (R 1881) for the androgen receptor (AR) (2,23), and ^{3}H-RU 26988 or ^{3}H-RU 28362 for the glucocorticoid receptor (GR) (11,14,22).

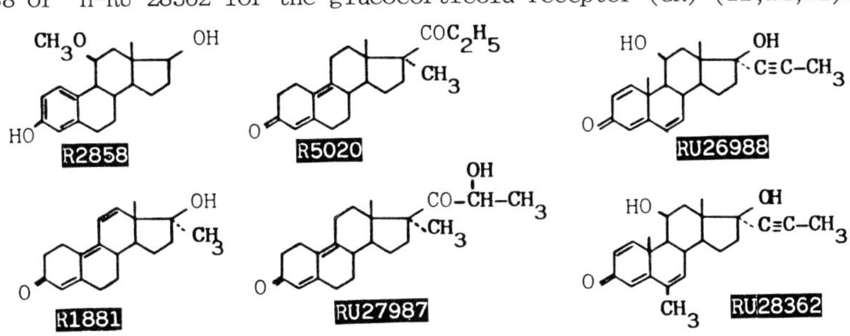

a) Biological activity. Steroid probes must have demonstrated biological potency indicating that they recognize a functional receptor. Moxestrol, promegestone, RU 27987 and metribolone are amongst the most potent available synthetic hormones (12,15,16,18). The glucocorticoid potency of RU 28362 (24) is greater than that of RU 26988 (5) but less than that of dexamethasone.

b) Receptor binding specificity. Moxestrol binds with high affinity uniquely to ER. The search for highly specific ligands for the other receptors is hampered by the overlap in the binding specificity of 3-keto-$\Delta 4$ steroids (20). RU 26988 and RU 28362 can be considered the most "pure" since they bind virtually exclusively to GR under standard screening conditions (19) ; both promegestone and RU 27987 exhibit less GR and AR binding than progesterone (22) ; metribolone binds equally effectively to AR and PR and slightly to the mineralocorticoid receptor (MR) and, consequently, to assay AR, triamcinolone acetonide, which has a complementary specificity profile, is added in excess to the incubation medium (1,25). No specific synthetic probe has yet been developed for the measurement of MR but the GR binding of ^{3}H-aldosterone can be prevented by an excess of either RU 26988 or RU 28362.

c) Binding affinity. Moxestrol associates at nearly the same rate as estradiol with cytosol ER but the complex formed dissociates 2 to 10 times more slowly (3).This indicates that the moxestrol complex is sufficiently stable to perform exchange assays. Similarly, promegestone and RU 27987 dissociate more slowly than progesterone from PR (8,16) and metribolone more slowly than testosterone from AR (13). The association rate of ^{3}H-RU 28362 to cytosol GR of rat thymus is higher than that of dexamethasone (DXM) (k_{+1}=1.5 and 0.8 x$10^6 M^{-1} min^{-1}$ respectively at 0°C) ; the dissociation rate is only a little faster for the RU 28362 than DXM complex (k_{-1}= 7 and 9 x$10^{-4} min^{-1}$ respectively at 0°C ; 37 and 48 x$10^{-4} min^{-1}$ at 15°C)(unpublished data). However, ^{3}H-RU 26988 dissociates considerably more rapidly than DXM or ^{3}H-RU 28362 and is therefore a less suitable probe (10).

d) Specific and non-specific binding in plasma. The majority of assay techniques rely on methods for separating firmly-bound hormone from weakly-bound or free hormone. Thus, even in the presence of low binding to specific plasma proteins such as sex-steroid binding protein (SBP) or corticosteroid binding globulin (CBG), a suitable assay technique will measure only high-affinity binding. Moxestrol does not bind to either semi-purified human SBP or CBG and shows very low non-specific binding in human plasma (12). The binding of RU 27987 to CBG is similar to that of promegestone (about 1% of that of progesterone) ; since its binding to human serum albumin is weaker, it is a more suitable ligand for nuclear PR exchange assays and for PR assay in plasma-contaminated samples (9). Metribolone binding to SBP (6) is so weak that it is dissociated by dextran-coated charcoal (DCC) adsorption. When ^{3}H-RU 28362 is incubated at 0°C with 1/50 diluted human plasma, no specific binding is measured either by equilibrium dialysis or the DCC technique whereas RU 26988 competes slightly for ^{3}H-corticosterone binding in rat plasma (unpublished data).

e) Degradation upon incubation. During incubation with cytosol, unstable radioligands may undergo enzymatic transformation into degradation products (21). Dihydrotestosterone, in particular, is readily converted into androstanediols whereas metribolone is relatively resistant to degradation because of its triene structure. Under our experimental conditions, no metabolic conversion of moxestrol, promegestone, RU 27987, nor RU 28362 has been detected.

f) Specific activity. In general, high specific activity (s.a.) engenders the risk of increased non-specific binding emphasizing the importance of the position and number of tritium atoms introduced into the steroid structure. Roussel-Uclaf's policy has been to tritiate steroids in positions C-6,7 resulting in radioligands of a s.a. of ca. 50 Ci/mmol except for 2^3H-RU 26988 (15 Ci/mmol) and 6^3H-RU 28362 (37 Ci/mmol). New England Nuclear (Boston, Mass) who markets several Roussel-Uclaf radioligands under licence has chosen to label the compounds with higher s.a. (70-90 Ci/mmol) as follows : 11-methoxy-^{3}H-moxestrol, 17α-methyl-^{3}H-promegestone and 17α-methyl-^{3}H-metribolone.

CONCLUSION

Because of their long-standing experience in steroid synthesis, Roussel-Uclaf have been able to develop several probes which have now become standard laboratory reagents for the assay of steroid hormone receptors in normal and pathological tissues. Over a thousand steroids have been tested in a routine screening system to find improved ligands, to detect potentially active drugs, and to map receptor binding sites (19). Studies are in progress on labels other than tritium, e.g. iodine for imaging, metals such as boron for spectrometric detection, fluorescent markers for fluocytometry. High-affinity ligands with conjugated double bonds can be used for affinity labeling or, if naturally fluorescent, can be detected directly by observation with high-performance photomultipliers (7). The final aim in all these studies is quantification and visualisation of receptor in the absence and presence of ligand. The new techniques will have to relate the kinetics and subcellular distribution of the ligand to the availability of the receptor and will have to be compatible with developments in, for example, scanning electron microscopy.

REFERENCES

1. Asselin J, Melançon R, Gourdeau Y, Labrie F, Bonne C, Raynaud JP (1979) J steroid Biochem 10:483-486

2. Bonne C, Raynaud JP (1976) Steroids 27:497-507

3. Bouton MM, Raynaud JP (1978) J steroid Biochem 9:9-15

4. Glascock RF, Hoekstra WG (1959) Biochem J 72:673

5. Gomez-Sanchez EP, Gomez-Sanchez CE, Ferris MW (1983) J steroid Biochem 9:1819-1822

6. Karr JP, Kirdani RY, Murphy GP, Sandberg AA (1978) Arch Andro 1:123-129

7. Martin PM, Magdelenat HP, Benhyahia B, Rigaud O, Katzenellenbogen JA (1983) Cancer Res 43 4956-4965

8. McGuire WL, Raynaud JP, Baulieu EE (eds) (1977) Progesterone Receptors in Normal and Neoplastic Tissues, Prog Cancer Res Ther Vol 4, Raven Press, NY

9. Moguilewsky M, Philibert D, Bouton MM, Raynaud JP (1983) J steroid Biochem Suppl 19:126S,n°378

10. Moguilewsky M, Raynaud JP (1980) J steroid Biochem 12:309-314

11. Nichols NR, Olsson CA, Funder JW (1983) Endocrinology 113:1096-1101

12. Ojasoo T, Raynaud JP (1978) Cancer Res 38:4186-4198

13. Ojasoo T, Raynaud JP (1983) In : Jasonni VM, Nenci I, Flamigni C (eds) Steroids in Endometrial Cancer, Prog Cancer Res Ther Vol 25, Raven Press, NY, pp 11-28

14. Philibert D, Moguilewsky M (1983) In : Abstracts, 65th Annual Meeting of the Endocrine Society, n°1018

15. Raynaud JP (1973) Steroids 2:249-258

16. Raynaud JP, Brown N, Coussedière D, Pottier J, Delettré J, Mornon JP (1980) In : Beato M (ed) Steroid-induced Uterine Proteins, Elsevier-North Holland Biomedical Press, Amsterdam

17. Raynaud JP, Martin P, Bouton MM, Ojasoo T (1978) Cancer Res 38:3044-3050

18. Raynaud JP, Ojasoo T (1983) J Gyn Obst Biol Repr 12:697-710

19. Raynaud JP, Ojasoo T (1983) In : Eriksson H, Gustafsson JÅ (eds) Steroid Hormone Receptors : Structure and Function, Amsterdam, pp 141-170

20. Raynaud JP, Ojasoo, Bouton MM, Philibert D (1979) In : Ariëns EJ (ed) Drug Design vol VIII, Academic Press, NY, pp 169-214

21. Raynaud JP, Ojasoo T, Vaché V (1979) In : Thompson EB, Lippman ME (eds) Steroid Receptors and the Management of Cancer. CRC Press Inc, Boca Raton, pp 215-232

22. Raynaud JP, Ojasoo T, Vaché V (1981) In : McKerns KW (ed) Reproductive Processes and Contraception, Plenum Press, NY, pp 163-179

23. Shain SA, Boesel RW (1978) Invest Urol 16:169-174

24. Teutsch G, Costerousse G, Deraedt R, Benzoni J, Fortin M, Philibert D (1981) Steroids 38:651-665

25. Zava DT, Landrum B, Horwitz KB, McGuire WL (1979) Endocrinology 104: 1007-1012

Endocrinology
F. Labrie, L. Proulx, eds.

ANTIESTROGEN BINDING PROTEINS

BENITA S. KATZENELLENBOGEN, MARGARET A. MILLER, ALAKA MULLICK, AND YHUN YHONG SHEEN
Department of Physiology and Biophysics, University of Illinois and University of Illinois College of Medicine, Urbana, Illinois 61801 U.S.A.

INTRODUCTION

Antiestrogens are non-steroidal compounds that are capable of antagonizing many of the actions of estrogens (1,2). They are of particular interest because of their successful employment in the treatment of hormone dependent breast cancer due to their ability to control the growth of these cells. Antiestrogens bind with high affinity to the estrogen receptor (ER) present in target cells and, in addition, they bind to an antiestrogen binding site (AEBS) that is estrogen-noncompetable (1-5). In this paper, we present some of our recent studies on the interactions of antiestrogens with ER and AEBS.

MATERIAL AND METHODS

MCF-7 cells were obtained from the Michigan Cancer Foundation (Detroit, MI). The T47D, MDA-MB-231, and ZR-75 cells were obtained from the EG and G Mason Research Institute (Worcester, MA). Cells were grown as described previously (5). Sources for antiestrogens are given in references 4-6.

RESULTS

Interaction of High Affinity Antiestrogens With the Estrogen Receptor (ER)

Antiestrogens compete with estrogen for binding to ER and the antiestrogen-occupied complex localizes in the cell nucleus (1,2). Studies with high affinity radiolabeled antiestrogens (CI628M, H1285, trans-4-hydroxytamoxifen) in MCF-7 and in ZR-75 human breast cancer cells indicate that antiestrogens all favor maintenance of a 5.5 S form of the nuclear ER complex that may be an important aspect of the nuclear interaction of these compounds in these breast cancer cells. Hence, when cells were incubated with tritiated estradiol or tritiated antiestrogen and nuclear salt extracts were analyzed on high salt sucrose gradients, the sedimentation profiles of the nuclear receptor complexes with antiestrogen and with estradiol were found to be different (6,7). While the sedimentation profile of the nuclear receptor complex with estradiol varied with the buffer composition of the sucrose gradients, being 4.1 S in phosphate-thioglycerol-glycerol and predominantly 5.5 S in Tris-EDTA buffered gradients, the antiestrogen receptor complex showed the same sedimentation (5.5 S) regardless of the buffer composition. To examine the nature of the nuclear receptor further, we have used the affinity labeling antiestrogen, tamoxifen aziridine (8), and chemical crosslinking and density shift experiments (9-11). The observation that several different antiestrogens all favor maintenance of a 5.5 S form (Mr $\sim$ 130,000) of the nuclear ER complex suggests that this may be an important aspect of the nuclear interaction of these compounds. The basis for this difference in stability of the 5 S nuclear receptor with antiestrogen versus estrogen remains under intensive investigation. Whether this represents differences in sensitivity to proteolysis, differences in phosphorylation, or other ligand-induced differences remains under analysis.

Interaction of Antiestrogens With Antiestrogen Binding Sites (AEBS) Distinct From The Estrogen Receptor

In contrast to the restriction of ER to estrogen target cells such as those of the uterus and mammary gland, the AEBS are present in a wide variety of estrogen target and non-target tissues and in ER -positive and -negative human breast cancer cell lines (MCF-7, T47D, MDA-MB-231) that differ markedly in their sensitivity to antiestrogens (3-5). Differential centrifugation studies with enzyme markers (4-5) indicated that AEBS were associated with the microsomal fraction. In further fractionation studies, we have used the method of Adelman et al., (12) to study in detail the microsomal association of AEBS (Table 1). Using rat liver, the richest source of AEBS, we find that more than half of the microsomal binding sites are associated with the rough endoplasmic reticulum, smaller amounts are present in the smooth endoplasmic reticulum fraction (which is contaminated to some extent with rough endoplasmic reticulum) with very little of these bindings sites being present in the ribosome. Hence, the majority of the microsomal AEBS are associated with the membrane component of the rough endoplasmic reticulum, a finding in agreement with a recent study (13), using a slightly different microsomal fractionation procedure. Hence, our findings and those of Watts and Sutherland (13) suggest that almost all of the AEBS in cells are associated with microsomes, whereas the ER is largely nuclear after hormone interaction, and we find little if any AEBS associated with purified nuclei. The AEBS are destroyed by proteases (3-5) and their membrane association is observed by their rapid sedimentation on sucrose gradients.

In order to gain greater insight into the role of these AEBS in the actions of antiestrogens, we and others have examined the biopotency of different antiestrogens and tried to correlate their effectiveness as antiestrogens with their affinity for ER and/or AEBS (3-5). The order of affinities of different antiestrogens for AEBS is CI628 > trans-tamoxifen > trans-hydroxytamoxifen > CI628M > H1285 > LY117018. As seen in Table 2, this order of affinities does not parallel the affinity of these compounds for the ER nor the potency of these

TABLE 1

MICROSOMAL ANTIESTROGEN BINDING SITES

Fraction*	% Distribution (Mean ± Range)
Rough Endoplasmic Reticulum	55 ± 4
"Smooth Endoplasmic Reticulum"	32 ± 21
Ribosomes	13 ± 11

*Microsomes from female (day 22) rat liver were prepared and fractionated by the method of Adelman et al. (12). Values are the mean ± range from two separate experiments.

TABLE 2

AFFINITY OF COMPOUNDS FOR ESTROGEN RECEPTOR AND ANTIESTROGEN BINDING SITES AND THEIR POTENCIES IN GROWTH INHIBITION

	BINDING AFFINITY			GROWTH INHIBITION
	ER*	AEBS**	ER/AEBS	Potency***
LY117018	160	5	32	+5
H1285	120	13	9.2	+5
CI628M	90	18	5.0	+5
Trans-OH-Tam	185	38	4.9	+5
Tamoxifen	2	100	0.02	+3
CI628	3	156	0.02	+3
BPEA	0	4	0	0

*Affinity for estrogen receptor (ER) where the affinity of estradiol is set at 100. Values are from references 4,5,6,14 and unpublished data.
**Affinity for estrogen-noncompetable antiestrogen binding sites (AEBS) where the affinity of tamoxifen is set at 100. Values are from references 4,5 and unpublished data.
***Potency in inhibiting the growth of MCF-7 cells _in vitro_. Values are from reference 14 and unpublished data.

compounds as antiestrogens. In addition, we have synthesized and studied the properties of t-butylphenoxyethyldiethylamine (BPEA) that was designed to incorporate the features important in antiestrogen binding to AEBS but lacking the features required for binding to the ER. Hence, as shown in Table 2, BPEA has an affinity for AEBS 4% that of tamoxifen, but has no affinity for ER. We find that this compound has no effect, either stimulatory or inhibitory, on proliferation of MCF-7 cells over a wide range of concentrations (from 10^{-11} M to 10^{-5} M). At these high concentrations, we would expect this compound to fully occupy the AEBS. In addition, this compound exhibits no uterotrophic activity and no antiuterotrophic activity when assayed in immature female rats. Hence, we conclude that occupancy exclusively of the AEBS does not result in growth suppression. In sum then, our findings suggest that affinity for the ER most closely corresponds with the potency of these compounds as antiestrogens. Studies with BPEA, which binds exclusively to the AEBS and not at all to the ER, should be particularly instructive in determining the influence of AEBS on the distribution of antiestrogens and their biopotency.

ACKNOWLEDGEMENTS

This work was supported by National Institutes of Health Grants CA18119 and CA31870.

REFERENCES

1. Horwitz KB, McGuire, WL (1978) In: McGuire WL (ed) Breast Cancer: Advances in Research and Treatment. Plenum, New York, vol 2, pp 155-204

2. Katzenellenbogen BS, Bhakoo HS, Ferguson ER, Lan NC, Tatee T, Tsai TL, Katzenellenbogen JA (1979) Recent Prog Hormone Res 35: 259-300

3. Sutherland RL, Murphy LC, Foo MS, Greene MD, Waybourne AM, Krozowski ZS (1980) Nature 288: 273-275

4. Sudo K, Monsma FJJr, Katzenellenbogen BS (1983) Endocrinology 112:425-434

5. Miller MA, Katzenellenbogen BS (1983) Cancer Res 43: 3094-3100

6. Eckert RL, Katzenellenbogen BS (1982) J Biol Chem 257: 8840-8846

7. Miller MA, Greene GL, Katzenellenbogen BS (1984) Endocrinology 114: 296-298

8. Katzenellenbogen JA, Carlson KE, Heiman DF, Robertson DW, Wei LL, Katzenellenbogen BS (1983) J Biol Chem 258: 3487-3495

9. Monsma FJJr, Katzenellenbogen BS, Miller MA, Ziegler YS, Katzenellenbogen JA (1984) Endocrinology 115: in press

10. Eckert RL, Mullick A, Rorke EA, Katzenellenbogen BS (1984) Endocrinology 114: 629-637

11. Miller MA, Mullick A, Katzenellenbogen BS (1984) Proceedings 7th International Congress of Endocrinology, in press

12. Adelman MR, Blobel G, Sabatini DD (1974) Methods Enzymol 31: 201-215

13. Watts CKW, Sutherland RL (1984) Biochem Biophys Res Commun 120: 109-115

14. Katzenellenbogen BS, Norman MJ, Eckert RL, Peltz SW, Mangel WF (1984) Cancer Res 44: 112-119

Endocrinology
F. Labrie, L. Proulx, eds.

MONOCLONAL ANTIBODIES AS PROBES FOR ESTROGEN RECEPTOR

GEOFFREY L. GREENE, WILLIAM J. KING AND MICHAEL F. PRESS

The Ben May Laboratory for Cancer Research and Department of Pathology, The University of Chicago, Chicago, Illinois 60637 U.S.A.

Monoclonal rat antibodies to MCF-7 human breast cancer estrogen receptor have been used to study the structure and cellular location of receptor in reproductive tissues and cancers as well as to develop assays for receptor that do not depend on the binding of hormone to the receptor protein. Fusion of splenic lymphocytes from Lewis rats, immunized with affinity-purified estrogen receptor from MCF-7 cell cytosol, with two different mouse myeloma lines [1,2], provided 13 cloned hybridoma cell lines; each of these (with one possible exception) secretes a unique idiotype of antibody that recognizes a distinct region of the receptor molecule (Table 1).

TABLE 1

CROSS REACTIVITY OF MONOCLONAL ANTIBODIES TO HUMAN ESTROPHILIN

	Receptor Source						
	Breast Cancer		Uterus				Oviduct
Antibody[a]	MCF-7	Human	Human	Monkey	Calf	Rat	Hen
Rat serum	+	+	+	+	+	+	+
D58P3μ	+	+	+	+	+	+	−
D75P3γ	+	+	+	+	−	−	−
D547Spγ	+	+	+	+	+	+	−
F88Spγ	+	+	+		+	+	+
F344Spμ	+		+		+	+	+
G5Spγ	+	+	+		+		−
G13Spγ	+						
H23Spγ	+	+	+	+		+	+
H142Spγ	+	+	+	+		+	+
H165Spγ	+	+	+	+		+	+
H221Spγ	+	+	+	+	+	+	+
H222Spγ	+	+	+	+	+	+	+
H226Spγ	+	+	+	+	+	+	+

[a]IgM antibodies indicated by μ and IgG by γ. P3 and Sp indicate hyrbidomas derived from P3-X63-Ag8 and Sp2/0-Ag14 mouse myeloma cells, respectively. Reproduced from [3].

These antibodies have high affinity (K_d=10^{-9}-10^{-10}M) for both steroid-occupied and unoccupied estrogen receptor and recognize nuclear as well as cytosol forms of the receptor molecule. Although they vary in their cross reactivity with estrogen receptors from various animal species, each antibody appears to be completely specific for the 65,000-dalton steroid-binding subunit of the estrogen receptor complex, as judged by extensive sucrose gradient and immunoblot analyses of cytosol and nuclear extracts from a variety of tissues and cell lines. Cross reactivity patterns (Table 1) indicate both sequence homology and heterogeneity among mammalian and nonmammalian estrophilins. Some determinants (eg. H222 and H226) are common to all tested estrogen receptors, including those from hen oviduct, whereas others (eg. D547 and D58) are present only in mammalian receptors and one (D75) appears to be restricted to primate estrophilin.

Three monoclonal antibodies (D547, D75, H222) have been used to devise simple immunoradiometric (IRMA) [4] and immunocolorimetric (ICMA) [5] sandwich assays for receptor in reproductive tissues and tumors. Polystyrene beads coated with D547 adsorb either occupied (ER) or unoccupied (R) receptor present in a tissue or tumor extract. Radiolabeled (IRMA) or peroxidase-conjugated (ICMA) D75 or H222 is then used to measure the amount of receptor bound to the bead. When tumor cytosols from 18 human breast cancers were analyzed for receptor content by the IRMA method (^{125}I-D75)and the results were compared with estrophilin content determined by specific [^{3}H]estradiol binding to receptor on sucrose density gradients, a linear correlation (m=0.94, r=0.98) was obtained. This sandwich assay has since been modified to an immunocolorimetric assay at Abbott Laboratories and tested against an additional 64 breast cancer cytosols with equally good results. The sensitivity of the D547/D75 combination is about 17 fmol of receptor per milliliter of cytosol (1.7 fmol/mg protein). A newer version of the ICMA assay (D547/H222) has a sensitivity of about 2 fmol of ER per milliliter of cytosol (0.2 fmol/mg protein). A commercial diagnostic kit that is simple, rapid, and does not depend on the binding of estradiol to receptor should be available in the near future.

As part of our ongoing effort to elucidate the distribution and dynamics of the estrogen receptor protein in target tissues in the presence and absence of estrogens and antiestrogens, we have developed an immunocytochemical assay (ER-ICA) for visualizing receptor directly in tissues and cells. Five monoclonal antibodies (D547, D58, D75, H222, H226) have been used individually to localize estrophilin by an indirect immunoperoxidase technique in frozen, fixed sections of human breast tumors, human uterus, rabbit uterus, and in other mammalian reproductive tissues, as well as in fixed MCF-7 cell cultures [6-8]. Specific immunoperoxidase staining for receptor in estrogen-sensitive tissues is confined to the nucleus of all stained cells, regardless of hormone status. Staining is absent in nontarget tissues, such as colon epithelium, and in receptor-negative breast cancers; in addition, it can be abolished by the addition of highly purified receptor to primary antibody. Heterogeneous staining has been observed in MCF-7 cells as well as in receptor-poor and receptor-rich breast cancers, possibly reflecting either variations in cell cycle or the presence of estrogen-sensitive and insensitive cells. Little or no cytoplasmic staining for estrophilin has been observed in any of the tissues or tumor cells examined thus far, including those deprived of exogenous estrogens. In a study of 117 human breast cancers by the ER-ICA method, the presence or absence of nuclear staining was significantly associated with the concentration of cytosolic estrogen receptor determined by steroid-binding assay. Staining intensity, epithelial cellularity and the proportion of tumor cells stained also correlated significantly with receptor concentration.

In view of the exclusively nuclear localization of specific immunoperoxidase staining for receptor in all estrogen-sensitive tissues and cells studied thus far, it appears that both cytosol and nuclear forms of the receptor may reside in the nuclear compartment in the presence and absence of steroid. We have seen little or no increase in nuclear staining intensity in MCF-7 cells and in uteri from immature rabbits or from postmenopausal women following short-term exposure of cells or tissue to estradiol. A notable exception is the increase in nuclear staining intensity observed by McClellan et al. [9] in monkey endometrium following in vitro exposure to 100nm estradiol. These observations are consistent with the hypothesis that unoccupied estrophilin recovered in the low salt cytosol fraction of a tissue homogenate represents receptor that is loosely associated with nuclear components and that binding of estradiol to receptor leads to a tighter association, a phenomenon previously interpreted as indicating translocation of the receptor from the cytoplasm to the nucleus. We are currently using the ER-immunocytochemical assay in combination with electron microscopy to determine the intranuclear localization of receptor as a function of hormone manipulation in MCF-7 cells and in human uterus.

ACKNOWLEDGEMENTS

These studies were supported by Abbott Laboratories, the American Cancer Society (BC-86), the NCI (CA-02897) and by the Women's Board of the University of Chicago Cancer Research Foundation.

REFERENCES

1. G.L. Greene, C. Nolan, J.P. Engler and E.V. Jensen: Monoclonal antibodies to human estrogen receptor. Proc. Natl. Acad. Sci. USA 77, 5115-5119 (1980).

2. L.S. Miller, I.I.E. Tribby, M.R. Miles, J.T. Tomita, and C. Nolan: Hybridomas producing monoclonal antibodies to human estrogen receptor. Fedn. Proc. 41, 520 (1982).

3. G.L. Greene, N.B. Sobel, W.J. King and E.V. Jensen: Immunochemical studies of estrogen receptors. J. Steroid Biochem. 20, 51-56 (1984).

4. G.L. Greene and E.V. Jensen: Monoclonal antibodies as probes for estrogen receptor detection characterization. J. Steroid Biochem. 16, 353-359 (1982).

5. C. Nolan, L.W. Przywara, L.S. Miller, V. Suduikis, J.T. Tomita. A sensitive solid-phase enzyme immunoassay for human estrogen receptor. Current Controversies in Breast Cancer. F.C. Ames, G.R. Blumensheim, and E.D. Montague, eds., Univ. of Texas Press, Austin, 1984. pp. 433-441.

6. W.J. King and G.L. Greene: Monoclonal antibodies to estrogen receptor localize receptor in the nucleus of target cells. Nature 307, 745-747 (1984).

7. M.F. Press and G.L. Greene: An immunocytochemical method for demonstrating estrogen receptor in human uterus using monoclonal antibodies to human estrophilin. Lab. Invest., 50, 480-486 (1984).

8. W.J. King and G.L. Greene: A comparison of immunocytochemical and steroid-binding assays for estrogen receptor in human breast tumors. Cancer Research, 1984, in press.

9. M.C. McClellan, N.B. West, D.E. Tacha, G.L. Greene and R.M. Brenner: Immunocytochemical localization of estrogen receptors in the Macaque reproductive tract with monoclonal antiestrophilins. Endocrinology, 1984, in press.

Endocrinology
F. Labrie, L. Proulx, eds.

GLUCOCORTICOID RECEPTORS AND THE PHYSIOLOGICAL ROLES OF GLUCOCORTICOID HORMONES

JOHN W. FUNDER
Medical Research Centre, Prince Henry's Hospital, Melbourne 3004, Australia

For over 40 years glucocorticoid hormones have been a physiological enigma, involved in an array of 'pleiotypic' and/or permissive effects, and in an ill-defined stress response. The term glucocorticoid derives from a classic bioassay, that of mouse liver glycogen deposition. In most species, including man, cortisol (hydrocortisone, compound F) is the predominant glucocorticoid; in the rat and mouse it is corticosterone (compound B).

These physiological gucocorticoids (in contrast with synthetic glucocorticoids) circulate >90% protein bound, largely to a high-affinity globulin (transcortin or corticosteroid binding globulin - CBG). Their specificity is not absolute; high therapeutic doses of hydrocortisone, for example, overlap into the mineralocorticoid (aldosterone) domain of action, and result in fluid and electrolyte retention.

Glucocorticoids are secreted on demand by the adrenal cortex, under the immediate control of pituitary ACTH, and probably of other congeners of ACTH in the longer term. ACTH has two patterns of secretion - circadian, with a major peak around waking, minor meal-related peaks, and troughs of very low levels; and episodic, in response to stress (e.g. fever, hypoglycaemia).

In addition to two modes of secretion (diurnal, episodic) there appears to be increasing evidence that glucocorticoids act via two distinct types of receptors - Type I, with very high affinity for the naturally-occurring glucocorticoids, and moderate affinity for dexamethasone; and Type II, 'classical' glucocorticoid receptors, with moderate affinity for dexamethasone, and lower affinity for cortisol and corticosterone.

Classical (Type II) glucocorticoid receptors have been described over the past 15 years using ^{3}H-dexamethasone (^{3}HDM), or less frequently ^{3}H-triamcinolone acetonide, as a probe for binding studies. These synthetic fluorinated steroids have two advantages for such studies - that of high affinity for Type II sites, and of minimal binding to CBG which often contaminates cytosol preparations. The affinity of steroids for Type II receptors parallels their anti-inflammatory potency; it is moderate for dexamethasone (K_d 3-10 nM), and even lower for B and F. Type II receptors appear widely distributed, having been described in all mammalian tissues examined.

Over the past decade, intracellular binding sites with higher affinity for corticosterone than dexamethasone have also been described in a variety of tissues in the rat. McEwen and his associates, for example, reported that the hippocampus and septum of adrenalectomized rats showed much higher levels of nuclear-bound ^{3}HB than ^{3}HDM after in vivo isotope injection (1); they designated these hippocampal 'corticosterone-preferring' sites, and subsequently suggested a receptor role on the basis of the restoration of protein I (synapsin, a M_r 80K phosphoprotein) levels in adrenalectomized rat hippocampus by B but not by equal doses of DM (2).

Similar sites (affinity B > DM) have been reported in a variety of other tissues in the rat; in these reports more extensive specificity studies, involving a range of other steroids, have perhaps paradoxically led to difficulties of interpretation in terms of potential physiological roles. Central to this dilemma has been the finding of equivalent affinity of these sites for aldosterone and corticosterone for example, in cultured rat aortic fibroblasts and smooth muscle cells (3), and rat pituitary tumor (GH) cells in culture (4).

Since these sites had similar affinity for corticosterone and aldosterone, they were cautiously designed 'corticoid receptors I' (3) or 'mineralocorticoid receptor-like' sites (4). In other studies, in which affinity of the sites for corticosterone was not reported, hippocampal sites binding aldosterone with higher affinity than DM were termed 'mineralocorticoid' receptors (5). Renal mineralocorticoid receptors, in contrast with the 'corticoid I receptors' or 'mineralocorticoid-like' receptors, have an apparent affinity for aldosterone $\sim$10x that for B, in both tissue-slice (6) and broken-cell studies (7).

Recent studies comparing the binding of ^{3}H-aldosterone and ^{3}H-B in hippocampal and renal cytosols (7) strongly suggest the identity of renal mineralocorticoid receptors and hippocampal 'B-preferring' sites, and by extension the aldosterone-binding sites in rat cultured cells (3,4), brain (5,8), gut (9), pituitary (10), lung (11) and mammary gland (12). Though such sites are widespread, they do not appear ubiquitous; in the thymus gland, for example, they are either absent or below detection limits (7).

Classically, renal mineralocorticoid receptors were termed Type I, to distinguish them from dexamethasone-binding glucocorticoid receptors (6). Even in hemoglobin-free cytosols prepared from carefully perfused kidneys, aldosterone appears to have a $\sim$10x higher affinity than B for such sites, when tracer is confined to Type I sites by concurrent excess of the Type II-specific ligand RU26988. If, however, renal cytosols are preadsorbed onto hydroxylapatite, and washed free of any possibly contaminating CBG, the specificity profile alters dramatically, with B and aldosterone showing equivalent high affinity for Type I sites. Conversely, if hippocampal cytosols, which are essentially CBG-free, are made 1% with adrenalectomized rat plasma, the resultant specificity profile (aldosterone $\sim$10x higher affinity than corticosterone) is identical to that seen in untreated renal cytosols. Plasma in which CBG is destroyed (56° for 30′) is ineffective in parallel, control studies.

These (7) and subsequent studies (13,14) have been interpreted as evidence for a role for extravascular CBG, in vivo and in vitro, in conferring mineralocorticoid specificity (i.e., aldosterone-selectivity) on sites which would otherwise be preferentially occupied by B, reflecting its higher plasma free levels. A countercurrent model, based on recurrent vascular loops, has been proposed as the mechanism whereby extravascular CBG can act as a renewable, non-saturable sink for the sequestration of B in the renal inner medulla-papilla (13).

In tissues such as the hippocampus, however, where there are negligible levels of extravascular CBG, the predominant occupant of such Type I sites in the rat will be corticosterone rather than aldosterone. These sites have very high affinity for corticosterone; accordingly they will be essentially saturated at the peak of diurnal secretion, and considerably less saturated at the troughs. This is in marked contrast with Type II receptors, which have a much lower affinity for physiological glucocorticoids, and for saturation require levels found following stress.

We would therforee propose that at the receptor level glucocorticoids operate in two modes, reflecting the bimodal pattern of their secretion in response to ACTH (diurnal, episodic stress). High affinity, Type I receptors are filled (and, relatively, empty) over the diurnal range of ACTH secretion and plasma glucocorticoid levels; in terms of their affinity, they are ideally suited to act as daily zeitgeber, to mediate glucocorticoid effects on such functions as mood, appetite and sleep/wake patterns (hippocampus) or fluid and electrolyte transport (gut and renal cortical epithelia).

Type II glucocorticoid receptors, in contrast, have a much lower affinity for the naturally-occurring glucocorticoids (but not, it should be noted, for dexamethasone). Consequently, these sites are only substantially occupied in response to stressed levels of ACTH and glucocorticoids; in terms of their affinity and ubiquity, they are ideally suited to integrate whole-body responses to metabolic challenge. Physiologically, we respond to hypoglycemia or pyrexia by an elevated cortisol; these stimuli probably reflect the primordial metabolic domain of glucocorticoid action.

In addition, glucocorticoids appear to have been recruited into a wide range of developmental functions (from glutamine synthetase in the retina, to surfactant, to the transition from hemoglobin F to hemoglobin A, to the appearance of gut enzymes). In this developmental context, therefore, glucocorticoids can also be appropriately seen as stress hormones, though unlike the adventitious stresses of hypoglycemia or pyrexia such stress is programmed. Given the spectacular differences between intra- and extra-uterine life (for example, in oxygenation/alimentation/heat conservation), birth must thus surely rank as <u>the</u> outstanding stress-event, in a physiological sense.

In summary, then, glucocorticoids are secreted in two modes, diurnal and in response to stress, which may be episodic or programmed. Over the diurnal range of glucocorticoid levels, high affinity (Type I) receptors will be more, or less, occupied: they may thus serve as receptors for glucocorticoids acting as zeitgebers, integrating in a time dimension a variety of neural, secretory and perhaps other processes. When glucocorticoid levels rise above the diurnal baseline in response to stress, lower affinity, Type II ^{3}H-dexamethasone-binding receptors will be filled; they may thus serve as receptors for glucocorticoids acting as the endocrine equivalent of the sympathetic nervous sytem, integrating in a space dimension a whole-body response to stress.

ACKNOWLEDGEMENT

These studies were supported by the National Health and Medical Research Council of Australia.

REFERENCES

1. McEwen BS, De Kloet R, Wallach G (1976) Brain Res 105:129-136.

2. Nestler EJ, Rainbow TC, McEwen BS, Greengard P (1981) Science 212:1162-1164.

3. Meyer WJ, Nichols NR (1981) J Steroid Biochem 14:1157-1168.

5. Moguilewsky M, Raynaud JP (1980) J Steroid Biochem 12:309-314.

6. Funder JW, Feldman D, Edelman IS (1972) J Steroid Biochem 3:209-218.

7. Krozowski ZS, Funder JW (1983) Proc Natl Acad Sci USA 80:6056-6060.

8. Beaumont K, Fanestil DD (1983) Endocrinology 113:2043-2051.

9. Suthers MB, Pressley LA, Funder JW (1976) Endocrinology 99:260-269.

10. Krozowski ZS, Funder JW (1981) Endocrinology 109:1221-1224.

11. Krozowski ZS, Funder JW (1981) Endocrinology 109:1811-1813.

12. Quirk SJ, Gannell JE, Funder JW (1983) Endocrinology 113:1812-1817.

13. Stephenson G, Krozowski ZS, Funder JW (1984) Amer J Physiol 15:F227-F233.

14. Stephenson G, Hammet M, Hadaway G, Funder JW (1984) Amer J Physiol (in press).

27. Pathogenesis of Graves' Disease

© 1984 Elsevier Science Publishers B.V.
Endocrinology
F. Labrie, L. Proulx, eds.

THE ROLE OF NONTHYROID RECEPTORS IN STUDIES OF THE PATHOGENESIS OF GRAVES' DISEASE

SIDNEY H. INGBAR

Thorndike Laboratory, Beth Israel Hospital, Boston, Mass., U.S.A.

Although their biological significance is unknown, it is clear that receptors or binding sites for TSH exist outside of the thyroid gland, in biological materials as disparate as mammalian adipose tissue and bacterial membranes (1,2). This discussion will consider briefly how fat cell membranes have contributed to studies of the pathogenesis of Graves' disease and how they might prove useful in this respect in the future.

PURIFICATION OF GRAVES'-SPECIFIC IMMUNOGLOBULINS

Fat cell membranes (FCM) have served as a vehicle for the first substantial purification of Graves'-specific immunoglobulins (GSIG)(1). Graves' serum contains GSIG, IgG found in the blood of healthy normals, and classical antithyroid antibodies common to other autoimmune diseases. At present, receptor-purification, exploiting the interaction of GSIG with the TSH receptor is the only feasible means of separating them from other IgG. Human thyroid membranes proved unsatisfactory for this purpose, however, since the IgG they yielded were little enriched in biological activity and were contaminated with other thyroid-directed antibodies copurified in the process (3). Because of the known lipolytic effects of TSH and Graves'-IgG (4), as well as the likelihood that adipose tissue does not contain antigens with which other thyroid-directed IgG would interact, we examined FCM as a vehicle for the receptor purification of GSIG. Among various species studied, guinea pig FCM resembled human thyroid membranes most closely in their TSH-binding properties, including binding affinity. FCM did not bind antithyroid microsomal antibodies, but did bind GSIG with TSH-binding inhibitory (TBI) activity. From these findings, a method for the preparation of receptor-purified GSIG (RP-GSIG) was developed.

RP-GSIG obtained in this manner are free of measurable antimicrosomal antibodies, have been enriched in TBI specific activity by as much as 250-fold, and have shown parallel increases in adenylate cyclase stimulating activity.

Preparations such as this are currently being used to develop monoclonal antibodies against GSIG. In addition to their potential use as reagents in clinically-applicable tests for GSIG, such monoclonal antibodies might very well be useful probes of the heterogeneity of epitopes in GSIG, both in individual patients and among different patients with Graves' disease.

INTERACTIONS OF GSIG WITH HUMAN THYROID MEMBRANES

Methods for radioiodinating RP-GSIG that left their TBI activity intact made possible the first direct examination of the interaction of GSIG and the human thyroid membrane (5). ^{125}I-labeled RP-GISG (GISG*) displayed time- and temperature-dependent binding to human thyroid membranes. Binding of GSIG* was saturable, since it was progressively inhibited by increasing concentrations of unlabeled Graves'-IgG. More importantly, binding of GSIG prepared with FCM was disease specific, since it was essentially unaffected by even higher concentrations of normal IgG or Hashimoto's-IgG. Thus, with respect to their ability to interact with pathogenic factors in the circulation of patients with Graves' disease, guinea pig FCM are more disease-specific than human thyroid membranes are.

Maximum binding was achieved more slowly with GSIG* than with TSH, perhaps explaining why the maximum stimulatory response of adenylate cyclase to Graves'-IgG occurs later than that to TSH. In general, however, properties of the binding interaction of the two, including the effects of temperature, pH, and various cations, were quite similar. These findings provided evidence of a commonality between the binding site for TSH and that for GSIG, a possibility discussed in more detail later.

FAT CELL-BINDING IMMUNOGLOBULINS

Since FCM exhibit greater disease specificity with respect to their interaction with GSIG than human thyroid membranes do, they have been employed in a method for detecting and quantitating GSIG in preparations of IgG or in serum. The method assesses the extent of interaction between components in ^{125}I-labeled solubilized FCM and IgG in the test specimen (fat cell-binding IgG, FBI). To date, the FBI method seems to afford a greater degree of sensitivity and specificity than other methods for detecting GSIG. This may be due to the greater Graves' disease-specificity of FCM than of human thyroid membranes, to the fact that the test measures all binding interactions between the test IgG and components of the FCM, or both. As discussed below, the test probably detects, therefore, GSIG that bind to some components in the FCM other than the principal binding site for TSH.

HETEROGENEITY OF GRAVES'-SPECIFIC IgG

Abundant evidence exists that IgG with biological activities characteristics of GSIG are polyclonal in origin, though of restricted heterogeneity (6). Similarly, there is ample evidence of functional heterogeneity of IgG that interact with the TSH receptor. This derives from studies of patients with hypothyroidism due to so-called "blocking" or "inhibitory" antibodies against the TSH receptor, as well as studies of monoclonal antibodies either raised against the TSH receptor or derived from fusion of Graves' disease lymphocytes and mouse myeloma cells. (See discussions by L. Kohn and J. Konishi immediately following.) Among such IgG, some block the binding of TSH and inhibit the response thereto; some stimulate thyroid adenylate cyclase, but do not block TSH-binding; some both inhibit TSH-binding and stimulate cyclase; and still others inhibit the cyclase response to TSH but do not inhibit its binding. The general concept that has been developed is that there are two domains of the TSH receptor, one concerned with TSH-binding, but not directly with adenylate cyclase activation, and the other mainly concerned with and necessary for activation. In this light, whether or not GSIG inhibit the binding of TSH, and whether they activate or inhibit adenylate cyclase, depends upon how they interact with these domains of the TSH receptor.

Our studies with FCM (1,5,7), and with preparations of GSIG purified with their use, provide strong support for the existence of functionally heterogeneous species of GSIG, both within and among patients with Graves' disease. Thus, the ability of preparations of unlabeled IgG from the serum of patients with Graves' disease to inhibit the binding of GSIG* to human thyroid membranes was closely correlated with their TBI activity (r=0.98). This is best explained if certain of the GSIG* share a common binding site with TSH in the human thyroid membrane, and if the GSIG in different patients with Graves' disease are capable of inhibiting the binding of both to the extent that they themselves bind at the same site. This conclusion is consonant with the general concept that GSIG are antibodies against the TSH receptor.

A greater complexity was indicated, however, in studies of the converse relationship, the ability of TSH to inhibit the binding of GSIG*. Although some inhibition of binding occurred, complete inhibition was not produced by even high and increasing concentrations of TSH. Further, when GSIG* from different patients were studied, the ability of TSH to inhibit their binding varied widely. These findings suggest that there is heterogeneity among the GSIG of the individual patient, some interacting with the TSH-binding site, per se, whereas the remainder interact with other components of the TSH receptor.

Further evidence to the same point was obtained in studies with the FBI technique. In studies of a large number of sera from patients with Graves' disease, there was no correlation between their FBI values and their TBI activity; many sera displayed elevated FBI values but had little or no TBI activity. In addition, standard concentrations of TSH decreased elevated FBI values in patients whose TBI activity was strong, but had little or no effect on the elevated FBI values of patients with negligible TBI activity. This suggests that there are two generic types of GSIG that bind to the FCM, one that binds to the same site as TSH and whose binding is inhibited by TSH, and another that binds to a different component of the TSH receptor.

If, as studies with monoclonal antibodies would suggest, IgG that block the binding of TSH are largely inhibitory, and those that bind to the receptor but do not have TBI activity are largely stimulatory, then studies of FBI values and of the ability of TSH to decrease them may be a quite simple means of quantitating stimulatory and inhibitory GSIG in the individual patient with Graves' disease.

REFERENCES

1. Endo K, Amir SM, Ingbar SH (1981) J Clin Endocrinol Metab 52:1113-1123
2. Weiss M, Ingbar SH, Winblad S, Kasper DL (1983) Science 219:1131-1133
3. Ochi Y, Hosoda S, Hachiga T, Yoshimura M, Miyazaki T, Kajita Y (1979) Acta Endocrinol (Copenh) 91:89-98
4. Hart IR, McKenzie JM (1971) Endocrinology 88:26-30
5. Endo K, Borges M, Amir S, Ingbar SH (1982) J Clin Endocrinol Metab 55:566-576
6. Zakarija M (1980) Horm Res 13:1-15
7. Shinozawa T, Ingbar SH (1983) Program of the 65th Annual Meeting of the Endocrine Society, San Antonio, June 8-10, p86 (abstract)

Endocrinology
F. Labrie, L. Proulx, eds.

MONOCLONAL ANTIBODIES, THE THYROTROPIN RECEPTOR AND AUTOIMMUNE THYROID DISEASE

LEONARD D. KOHN
National Institute of Health, Bethesda, Maryland 20814 USA

A membrane ganglioside and glycoprotein are components of the cell surface receptor for TSH (1-4). TSH binding to the glycoprotein is the initial high affinity recognition event on the cell surface. The ganglioside acts as an emulsifying agent to allow the hormone to interact with other membrane components within the hydrophobic environment of the lipid bilayer, i.e., components of the adenylate cyclase complex. Clinical data has led to a belief that antibodies to thyroid membranes exist in the sera of Graves' patients and are important in the pathogenesis of the hyperthyroid state. Unclear is whether these antibodies are directed against the TSH receptor or if there are multiple antibodies to the receptor, one for adenylate cyclase activation, one for goiter production (growth), and one even for connective tissue complications.

A monoclonal antibody approach has been used to resolve questions concerning the structure of the TSH receptor and its relation to autoantibodies in Graves' disease (1-4). The first step of this approach involved the injection of crude solubilized thyroid membrane preparations into mice followed by spleen cell fusion with non-IgG producing mouse myeloma cells. The second step involved fusion of lymphocytes from patients with active Graves' disease with a non-IgG secreting mouse myeloma cell line. Anti-TSH receptor producing clones were identified as monoclonal antibodies to the TSH receptor by the following criteria. (i) The antibody had to inhibit TSH binding to thyroid membranes or, conversely, be itself prevented from binding to thyroid membranes by TSH. (ii) Inhibition had to be reasonably specific and had to be competitive as opposed to noncompetitive or uncompetitive. (iii) The antibody had to competitively inhibit TSH-stimulated thyroid functions i.e., adenylate cyclase activity, iodide uptake, or thyroid hormone release or, conversely, had to mimic TSH activity and exhibit properties of competitive agonism.

After identification of over 30 antibodies satisfying the criteria above, all can be broadly grouped into three classes. "Inhibitor" antibodies resemble autoantibodies in Graves' sera which inhibit TSH binding. They competitively inhibit ^{125}I-TSH binding, TSH-stimulated adenylate cyclase activity, and TSH-stimulable thyroidal iodine release or uptake. They do not stimulate thyroid adenylate cyclase activity, T_3/T_4 release, or iodide uptake. No "inhibitor" is reactive with TSH, i.e., they are not TSH antibodies. They do not inhibit TSAb function.

"Stimulators" mimic the activity of thyroid stimulating TSABs in Graves' patients. They exhibit direct, TSH-like, stimulatory action with respect to adenylate cyclase activity, iodide uptake and T_3/T_4 release. They are competitive agonists when included with low concentrations of TSH in assays measuring adenylate cyclase activity. Despite significantly weaker inhibition of ^{125}I-TSH binding than the first group, they exhibit equally potent competitive inhibition of TSH-stimulable adenylate cyclase activity. They exhibit the species specificity of TSAbs.

The antibodies in the "inhibitory" group are uniformly directed against the glycoprotein component of the TSH receptor. In contrast, the stimulating antibodies interact with ganglioside preparations of thyroid membranes. Mixing experiments confirm that inhibitor and stimulator monoclonal antibodies are directed at distinct biochemical determinants of the membrane; differences in effects of inhibiting antibodies on TSH as opposed to TSAbs were not the result of a difference in binding constants.

The third group of "mixed" monoclonal antibodies are potent inhibitors of TSH binding as well as potent stimulators of adenylate cyclase activity. These antibodies react with both the glycoprotein receptor component and the ganglioside yet, like "stimulators", are relatively insensitive to "inhibitors" in mixing experiments. These results suggest that "mixed" antibodies are directed against a unique set of receptor determinants different from "stimulators" and "inhibitors" yet common to both. The best explanation is that there are common carbohydrate determinants on the glycoprotein and ganglioside or that the true "physiologic TSH receptor" exists as a functional complex of ganglioside and glycoprotein.

In sum, the monoclonal data would appear to confirm the two component receptor model envisaged from *in vitro* binding experiments and to show that the autoantibodies in Graves' sera are related to different components of the TSH receptor. An important clinical implication for a Graves' patient who has both an "inhibiting" and stimulating antibody present in his or her serum: the phenotypic expression will be a hyperthyroid state. This is evident since the inhibitor antibody will not inhibit TSAb activity, only TSH activity.

Immunoprecipitation data (2) indicate that the glycoprotein component of the TSH receptor is composed of two subunits of ~25K and ~50 to 60K. Crosslinking studies suggest that the receptor exists as a complex of the two subunits with a ~molecular weight of 80 to 90K or as a tetrameric structure of ~160 to 180K. The ~25K subunit appears to be related to the ~15K fragment of the TSH receptor purified after tryptic digestion of solubilized membrane preparations. There is a Con A binding site on the glycoprotein component but the Con A site is not involved in the TSH binding site. The glycoprotein receptor component also contains a site which recognizes immunoglobulin-reactive agents; thus, protein A, can precipitate solubilized receptor and can inhibit TSH binding. Finally, there is an phosphatidylinositol attachment site on the glycoprotein receptor component which can prevent reconstitution of TSH receptor into liposomes (i) by decreasing its incorporation into the lipid matrix and (ii) by inhibiting the binding activity of that fraction of which is incorporated.

The ganglioside (4) of the TSH receptor is thyroid-specific disialoganglioside which is less than 0.1% of the total thyroidal ganglioside pool as evaluated by solid phase assays or direct autoradiography. The disialoganglioside appears to have one neuraminidase sensitive and one insensitive sialic moiety. It can be presumed from previous inhibition studies that the sialic residues may have a G_{D1b} configuration.

The receptor structure defined above also signals TSH induced growth activity, maximal growth expression requiring both receptor components. Thus antibodies from all groups, i.e., "stimulator" "mixed" or "inhibitor" can cause growth of the cells to a greater or lesser degree. Indomethacin partially inhibits the "mixed" antibodies; has, however, no affect on "stimulator" antibodies; yet completely inhibits "inhibitor" antibody growth activity. In short, it would appear that the TSH receptor modulated growth activity of the thyroid cell involves phospholipid modulation as well as cAMP signals; phospholipid signalling is linked more to the glycoprotein receptor component, adenylate cyclase action to the ganglioside component.

Non thyroidal TSH "receptors" have been argued to be important in the pathogenesis of exophthalmos and the connective tissue complications of Graves' disease as a result of studies of experimental exophthalmos (1). The monoclonal approach has been used to evaluate this thesis (1). Monoclonal antibodies derived from the lymphocytes of patients with

Graves' disease and exophthalmos were compared to those from Graves' patients without exophthalmos. One stimulating antibody (307H6) derived from the exophthalmos group was found to stimulate thymidine uptake in fibroblasts as well or better than in thyroid cells and to also stimulate collagen biosynthesis in these fibroblasts. This antibody had all the characteristics of a stimulator antibody to the TSH receptor defined above; its existence as only one of over a dozen TSAb monoclonals and as originating from a patient with exophthalmos clearly established that a unique stimulator TSAb could exist which also stimulated fibroblasts.

Of further interest in this regard were observations evolved during the testing of a range of monoclonal antibodies to the TSH receptor which were in the "inhibitory" group. None of the antibodies had growth activity with respect to fibroblasts even if they exhibited growth activity with respect to thyroid cells. None stimulated cAMP activity in fibroblasts. Surprisingly, however, several had potent activities as stimulators of collagen biosynthesis in fibroblasts. In studies using the same collagen biosynthesis assay (involving measurement of [^{3}H]proline incorporation into fibroblasts), IgG preparations from 17 of 20 patients with Graves' ophthalmopathy were shown to stimulate collagen synthesis. This activity correlated with the severity of the ophthalmopathy; was not associated with TSAb activity in a thyroid cell cAMP assay in 50% of cases; disappeared in remission; and was not evident in IgGs from 12 normals of 7 of 8 Graves' with no exophthalmos, 4 Hashimoto's, 7 nontoxic goiters, or 4 thyroid atrophy patients. The activity of the "exophthalmogenic" IgGs were comparable to the positive monoclonals above. These observations provide strong support for expression of a TSH receptor on a nonthyroidal tissue as a causative factor in human as well as experimental exophthalmos.

REFERENCES

1. Kohn LD (1984) In "The Thyroid" (S. Werner, S. Ingbar, and L. Braverman, eds.), 5th Edition, in press, Harper and Row, Hagerstown, Md.

2. Kohn LD, Valente WA, Laccetti P, Cohen JL, Aloj SM, and Grollman EF (1983) Life Sciences 32, 15-30.

3. Kohn LD, Yavin E, Yavin Z, Laccetti P, Vitti P, Grollman EF, and Valente WA (1983). In "Monoclonal Antibodies: Probes for Study of Autoimmunity and Immunodeficiency" (G. Eisenbarth and R. Haynes, eds.), pp. 221-258. Academic Press, New York.

4. Laccetti P, Tombaccini D, Aloj SM, Grollman EF., and Kohn LD (1984). In "Ganglioside Structure Function and Biomedical Potential" (R. Ledeen, R. Yu, M. Rapport, and K. Suzuki, eds.) 365-367 Plenum Press, New York.

Endocrinology
F. Labrie, L. Proulx, eds.

THYROTROPIN-RECEPTOR BLOCKING ANTIBODIES

JUNJI KONISHI, YASUHIRO IIDA, KANJI KASAGI, KEIGO ENDO, TAKASHI MISAKI and KANJI TORIZUKA

Department of Nuclear Medicine, Kyoto University School of Medicine, Sakyo-ku, Kyoto, 606 (Japan)

INTRODUCTION

It is now well established that the serum from patients with Graves' disease contains immunoglobulins which inhibit the binding of TSH to its receptor (1) and elicit the thyroid stimulating activity (2). However, the correlation between these two activities is generally poor (3). The most striking finding which indicated the presence of heterogeneity in TSH receptor antibodies with respect to TSH receptor binding and intrinsic thyroid stimulating activity was the detection of TSH-binding inhibitor immunoglobulins (TBII) in hypothyroid patients (4-8). This paper is concerned with TBII observed in patients with primary hypothyroidism and in particular: a) Incidence and biological activities of TBII b) Clinical and laboratory findings in TBII-positive patients and c) Role of the antibodies in thyroid diseases.

INCIDENCE OF TBII IN HYPOTHYROID PATIENTS

TBII were assay by a radioreceptor assayed of TSH using Triton-solubilized human thyroid membranes as the receptor (9). As shown in Fig. 1, seven out of 43 patients with goitrous Hashimoto's disease (16%) showed a significant inhibition of TSH binding in comparison to 16 normal controls. On the other hand, TBII were detected in 9 patients out of 43 consecutive patients with primary myxedema (21%).

Five patients (12%) showed especially potent TBII activity resulting in more than 50% inhibition of ^{125}I-TSH binding in the assay. In the same figure, 6 patients with primary myxedema who had been known to have potent TBII before this study were also plotted as triangles. Among hypothyroid patients all cases having potent TBII belonged to the nongoitrous group.

CLINICAL FETAURES OF TBII-POSITIVE PATIENTS

In comparison to 34 patients with primary myxedema having no detectable TBII, the sex ratio (female/male) was higher in cases with potent TBII (10/1

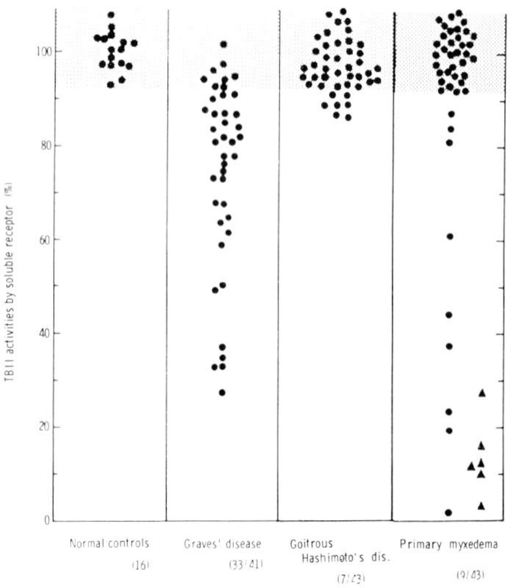

Fig.1.Detection of TBII in various thyroid diseases. Cases previously known to have potent TBII were plotted as triangles in the same figure.

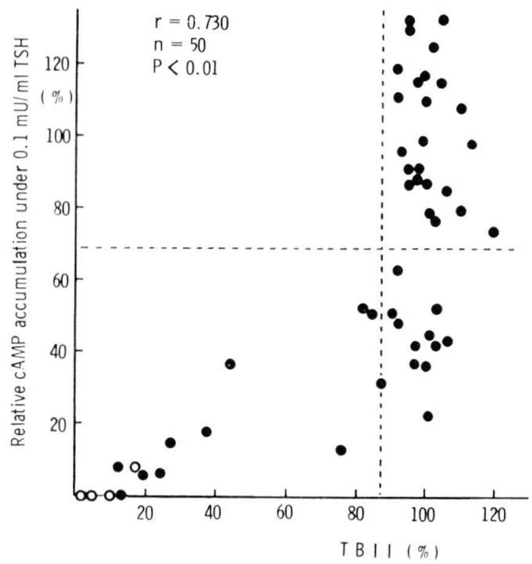

Fig.2. Correlation of TBII and thyroid-stimulation blocking activity in patients with primary myxedema. Open circles represent patients who gave birth to infants with transient hypothyroidism.

versus 23/11). Their ages at onset ranged from 15 to 49 years, while those of TBII-negative patients distributed from 1 to 84 with increasing incidence in the elderly. One of the most characteristic features was the ocurrence of transient hypothyroidism in newborn babies from these patients. Since the first case reported in 1980 (5), three cases has been found to have TBII because of this clinical complication in infants. In addition, another patient who had been found to have TBII before marriage delivered a baby with transient hypothyroidism as anticipated. Thus, this unique complication was so far observed in all infants born to mothers having potent TBII. These cases were represented by open circles in Fig. 2.

LABORATORY FINDINGS IN TBII-POSITIVE PATIENTS

No significant difference was observed in serum TSH levels between TBII-positive and negative groups of patients. Although thyroid uptake was generally low in these patients, both 30 min ^{99m}Tc-pertechnetate uptake and 24 hr radioiodine uptake in TBII-positive patients were significantly lower than those in TBII-negative patients. Antithyroid antibodies were positive in all except one case of TBII-positive patients. However, there was no significant difference in the titers of antithyroid antibodies between these 2 groups.

BIOLOGICAL ACTIVITIES OF TBII IN HYPOTHYROID PATIENTS

None of IgG preparations from hypothyroid patients caused any significant increase of cAMP in cultured human thyroid cells (10).

When 3mg each of IgG preperations from 43 patients with primary myxedema were added together with 0.1 mU/ml bTSH to cultured thyroid cells, 20 preparations (47%) caused significant inhibition of cAMP increase in comparison to 14 normal control IgGs, while 4 out of 18 preparations (22%) from patients with goitrous Hashimoto's disease were inhibitory. These IgGs were also inhibitory against cAMP increase induced by thyroid stimulating antibodies from Graves' patients, but not against that induced by prostaglandin E_1. All of the IgGs with TBII activity were potent inhibitor of the TSH-induced cAMP increase. Further, about a third of TBII-negative IgGs from patients with primary myxedema was also inhibitory. TSH-binding inhibitory activity of the patients' IgGs was significantly correlated with their thyroid-stimulation blocking activity (Fig2).

Analysis of both TSH-binding and thyroid-stimulation by TSH under the presence of these IgGs by double reciprocal plots indicated the competitive nature of the inhibition by these IgGs. Papain digestion of one IgG preparation resulted in the complete preservation of both activities in Fab fragment. The most potent TBII among these reacted only with anti-K antibody and the reaction resulted in loss of thyroid-stimulation blocking activity as well as loss of TBII. The direct binding of the TBII to human thyroid membranes was observed after purification of the ^{125}I-labeled IgG by receptor adsorption using guinea pig fat cell membranes. The binding was significantly inhibited by TSH as well as the unlabeled TBII (11). The TBII blocked not only the thyroid stimulation induced by TBII-positive Graves' IgGs but also that induced by TBII-negative Graves' IgGs, suggesting the close proximity of the binding sites of both stimulators to TSH receptors.

TSH-RECEPTOR BLOCKING ANTIBODIES IN GRAVES'DISEASE

The blocking nature of the TBII in hypothyroid patients is in marked contrast to the thyroid stimulating activity of TBII usually observed in Graves' dosease. However, blocking type of antibodies have also been reported in Graves' patients after radioiodine treatment (12), suggesting the heterogeneity in receptor antibodies in this condition. We have recently experienced a case of Graves' disease who developed hypothyroidism after 3 years of antithyroid drug treatment, concomitant with the switching of the nature of TBII from stimulating to blocking type.

CONCLUSION

Analysis of the IgG from patients with primary myxedema indicated that TBII in these patients were blocking antibodies against TSH receptors. Clinical and laboratory findings in TBII-positive patients, being compatible with the nature of TBII, supported the pathogenic role of the antibodies. Further, the detection of such antibodies in few patients with Graves' disease indicated the importance of the analysis of TSH receptor antibodies for the understanding of the pathogenesis of both hyper- and hypo-thyroid autoimmune disorders.

ACKNOWLEDGMENT

This study was supported by the Research Grant for the Intractable Diseases from the Ministry of Health and Welfare of Japan. We are indebted to Drs. N.Matsuura, M.Ninomiya, T. Mori and T. Ishihara for giving us sera with high TBII activities and corresponding clinical information. We are most grateful to Dr. K. Kuma, Kobe, for supplying human thyroid tissues and to Dr. J. G. Pierce, UCLA, for providing the purified bTSH. Miss K. Aoki provided excellent secretarial assistance.

REFERENCES

1. Smith BR, Hall R (1974) Lancet 2: 427-31
2. McKenzie JM, Zakarija M, Sato A (1978) Clinics in Endocrinol Metab 7: 31-45
3. Volpe R (1981) In: Auto-immunity in the Endocrine System. Springer-Verlag, Berlin, pp33-40
4. Endo K, Kasagi K, Konishi J et al. (1978) J Clin Endocrinol Metab 46:734-9
5. Matsuura N, Yamada Y, Nohara Y et al.(1980) N Engl J Med 303: 738-41
6. Ninomiya M, Goji K, Takahashi T et al. (1983) Acta Paediat Japon 87: 939-44 (Japanese)
7. Konishi J, Iida Y, Endo K et al. (1983) J Clin Endocrinol Metab 57: 544-9
8. Iseki M, Shimizu M, Oikawa T et al. (1983) J Clin Endocrinol Metab 57: 384-7
9. Iida Y, Konishi J, Kasagi K et al. (1982) Endocrinol Jpn 29:227-31
10. Kasagi K, Konishi J, Iida Y etal. (1982) J Clin Endocrinol Metab 54: 108-14
11. Konishi J, Iida Y, Endo K et al. (1982) In: Imura H, Kuzuya H (eds) Hormone Receptors and Receptor Diseases (ICS No 603) Excerpta Medica, Amsterdam, pp79-86
12. Beck K, Bliddal H, Siersbaek-Nielsen K, Friis T (1982) Clin Endocrinol (Oxf) 17:395-402

Endocrinology
F. Labrie, L. Proulx, eds.

IMMUNOGENETICS OF GRAVES' AND HASHIMOTO'S DISEASES

H. Tamai, H. Uno, Y. Hirota, S. Matsubayashi, K. Kuma, H. Matsumoto, L.F. Kumagai, T. Sasazuki and S. Nagataki

Department of Psychosomatic Medicine, Faculty of Medicine, Kyushu University (H.T., Y.H., S.M.), Fukuoka; Department of Human Genetics Medical Research Institute, Tokyo Medical and Dental University (H.U., T.S.), Tokyo; Kuma Hospital (K.K.), Kobe; Department of Legal Medicine, Osaka Medical School (H.M.), Takatsuki; Department of Internal Medicine, School of Meidcine, University of California Davis (L.F.K.); and First Department of Internal Medicine, School of Medicine, Nagasaki University (S.N.) Nagasaki; Japan

The etiology of Graves' and Hashimoto's diseases is unknown, but it is evident that Graves' disease occurs frequently within one genealogical family. Consanguineous occurrence of Graves' disease has led to the possibility that hereditary factors may be important in its pathogenesis (1). It has been reported from many laboratories that the susceptibility to autoimmune thyroid diseases is real linkage to certain immunogenetic factors (2). An increased frequency of certain HLA antigens has been found in patients with Graves' disease (3-4) and those with Hashimoto's disease (5). The present study was undertaken to investigate immunogenetic factors in Graves' and Hashimoto's diseases and to elucidate the relationships if any, of genetic determinants in Graves' disease and Hashimoto's disease.

MATERIALS AND METHODS

Families:

The studies were performed on 243 members of 37 families in which two or more first degree relatives were affected with Graves' disease. In 27 families, 173 members were studied and 70 (40%) had Graves' disease and none had Hashimoto's disease. In the remaining 10 families consisting 70 members, 26 (37%) had Graves' disease and 14 (20%) had Hashimoto's disease among first degree relatives.

Examinations:

Physical examinations, measurements of thyroid function consisting of determinations of serum concentrations of T4, T3 and TSH, values for T3 uptake, and titers of thyroid autoantibodies as well as TRH tests were performed on all subjects. Needle biopsies to confirm the diagnosis of Hashimoto's disease were performed in subjects who had high titers of thyroid autoantibodies or who were suspected of having Hashimoto's disease by clinical examination.

HLA typing and Immunoglobulin allotypes:

Our approach to the inheritance problem was to study immunogenetics in many families with multiple cases of Graves' and Hashimoto's diseases. This was done by determining HLA-A, B and C antigens and the immunoglobulin allotype, Gm, in all 243 members of 37 families.

Identification of disease-associated haplotypes:

Initially a complete analysis of HLA and Gm haplotypes was performed in all members in each family. Subsequently the particular HLA and Gm haplotypes that were found to be concordant in two members with Graves' disease in each family were defined as being the disease-associated haplotypes for that specific family. The data in the remaining members of the family were then examined to determine those in whom one or both of the disease-associated haplotypes was present or lacking, and this was correlated with the presence or absence of thyroid disease.

RESULTS AND DISCUSSION

Fig. 1 shows a family affected with Graves' disease. Haplotypes of HLA a, b, c,

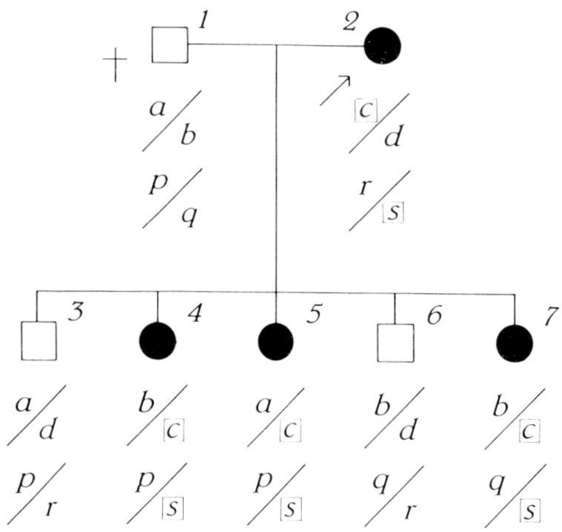

● Graves'disease, *a* : HLA-A-,B15,Cw-, *b* : HLA-A-,B40,Cw-, *c* : HLA-Aw24,B-,Cw-, *d* : HLA-Aw24,Bw51,Cw3, *p* : Gm(1,21,17,26), *q* : Gm(1,11,13,10,15,16,17), *r* : Gm(1,2,21,17,26), *s* : Gm(1,21,17,26).

Fig. 1 A family affected with Graves' disease.

d, and haplotypes of Gm p, q, r, s were determined by analysis of HLA-A, B and C antigens and Gm phenotypes of all members of the family. As stated earlier, the disease-associated haplotypes were defined as being those concordant in two members with Graves' disease. In this family, the disease-associated haplotypes of HLA (c) and Gm (s) were identified from patients No. 2 and No. 4. Among additional subjects, two (No. 5 and 7) had disease-associated haplotypes of both HLA and Gm were also affected with Graves' disease. The other two siblings (No. 3 and 6) had neither of the disease-associated haplotypes and were not affected with Graves' disease.

Fig. 2 shows a family affected with Graves' and Hashimoto's diseases. In this family, the disease-associated haplotypes of HLA and Gm were identified from patients with Graves' disease, No. 2 and No. 6 (c and r). Among the other three siblings, one (No. 3) was affected with Hashimoto's disease and she had the disease-associated haplotypes of HLA and Gm. One other sibling (No. 5) had the disease-associated haplotype of Gm only and was not affected with thyroid disease. Another sibling (No. 4) did not have either of the disease-associated haplotypes and was not affected with Graves' or Hashimoto's disease.

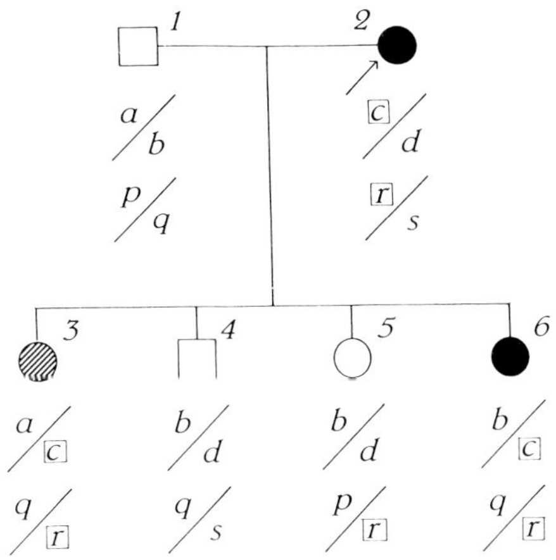

● Graves' disease, Hashimoto's disease, a : HLA-A2,B40,Cw3, b : HLA-A9,Bw51,Cw-, c : HLA-A26,B40,Cw-, d : HLA-A-,B7,Cw-, p : Gm(1,3,5,13,23), q : Gm(1,13,15,16,17), r : Gm(1,2,21,17,26), s : Gm(1,17,21)

Fig. 2 A family affected with Graves' and Hashimoto's diseases.

The results of 37 families in which two or more first degree relatives were affected with Graves' disease are shown in Table 1. Among 96 patients with Graves' disease, 74 patients, i.e., two members in 37 families, served as the basis for identification of disease-associated haplotypes. Among the remaining 22 patients with Graves' disease, 21 had disease-associated haplotypes of both HLA and Gm, and one had only the Gm haplotype. All of the 14 patients with Hashimoto's disease had the same haplotypes of HLA and Gm of Graves' disease for their respective families. This patient with Graves' disease who did not have the disease-associated haplotype of HLA may be explained by a recombination between HLA and the HLA-linked susceptibility gene for Graves' disease. In this study, all 96 patients with Graves' disease except for one and all 14 patients with Hashimoto's disease had the same disease-associated haplotypes of both HLA and Gm as deter-

Table 1.

Association among Graves' and Hashimoto's diseases, HLA and Gm haplotypes in 37 families (243 subjects) in which two or more first degree relatives were affected with Graves' disease.

	concordance of disease-associated haplotypes of				
	both HLA and Gm	only HLA	only Gm	neither HLA nor Gm	Total
Graves' disease	95 (74 + 21)	0	1	0	96 (74 + 22)
Hashimoto's disease	14	0	0	0	14
Others	37	16	38	42	133
Total	146	16	39	42	243

mined from the members with Graves' disease in their families. In each family, the results strongly support the hypothesis that in Graves' and Hashimoto's diseases, two genes linked to HLA and Gm control the susceptibility to both diseases, and that common immunogenetic factors are involved in the pathogenesis of both disorders. Furthermore, among 146 subjects who also had the disease-associated haplotypes of both HLA and Gm, 37 (25.5%) were euthyroid. Additional genetic or environmental factors must play important roles in the development of Graves' or Hashimoto's disease. It should be emphasized, however, that from results in the present study, those family members who do not have immunogenetic factors for their particular family are very unlikely to develop Graves' or Hashimoto's disease.

CONCLUSION

1) Hereditary immunogenetic factors play important roles in the development of both Graves' and Hashimoto's diseases. 2) The results in our study indicate that 2 genes linked to HLA and Gm control the susceptibility for Graves' and Hashimoto's diseases. 3) Common immunogenetic determinants are involved in the pathogenesis of both diseases. 4) Since it was evident that a large number of family members with disease-associated haplotypes may remain euthyroid for years, other factors, as yet undefined, must be involved in the onset of Graves' and Hashimoto's diseases. 5) In the absence of disease-associated haplotypes, the development of Graves' or Hashimoto's disease is highly unlikely.

REFERENCES

1) Tamai, H., Ohsako, N., Takeno, K., Fukino, O., Takahashi, H., Kuma, K., Kumagai, L.F. and Nagataki, S., J Clin Endocrinol Metab. 51: 1123, 1980.

2) Uno, H., Sasazuki, T., Tamai, H., and Matsumoto, H., Nature 292: 768, 1981.

3) Grumet, F.C., Payne, R.O., Konishi, J., and Kriss J.P., J Clin Endocrinol Metab. 39: 1115, 1974.

4) Farid, N.R., Barnard, J.M., and Marshall, W.H., Tissue Antigen 8: 181, 1976.

5) Moens, H., and Farid, N.R., New Engl J Med 299: 133, 1978.

28. Growth Factors other than IGF

Endocrinology
F. Labrie, L. Proulx, eds.

THE FUNCTIONAL DOMAINS OF THE EGF-RECEPTOR, THEIR STRUCTURE AND MECHANISM OF ACTIVATION

J. SCHLESSINGER, R. KRIS, I. LAX, T.A. LIBERMANN AND Y. YARDEN
Department of Chemical Immunology, The Weizmann Institute of Science, Rehovot 76100, Israel

INTRODUCTION

Epidermal growth factor (EGF) mediates its mitogenic effect through binding to a specific membrane receptor (1,2).

The membrane receptor of EGF is a 170,000 dalton glycoprotein which possesses an intrinsic tyrosine specific kinase activity. The EGF receptor kinase activity is similar to the tyrosine specific kinase activity associated with the transforming proteins encoded by oncogenes belonging to the src gene family (3-5).

Partial amino acid sequence analysis of six peptides derived from human EGF receptor very closely matched a part of the deduced sequence of the V-erb-B transforming protein of avian erythroblastosis virus (AEV) (6). It was proposed that the virus acquired part of the cellular gene sequence of EGF-receptor. This truncated receptor lacked the external binding domain but retained the transmembrane and cytoplasmic domain involved in stimulation of cell proliferation (6). Ullrich et al. recently described the complete amino acid sequence of EGF receptor deduced from human cDNA clones (7).

It appears that EGF-receptor can be divided into three functional domains. An external domain of 621 amino acids which contains the EGF binding site and at least 11 asparagine linked glycosylation sites; a single 23 amino acid hydrophobic transmembrane domain and the cytoplasmic domain of 542 amino acids possessing the kinase activity and the autophosphorylation site(s) (7).

As previously proposed the V-erb-B protein appears to be a truncated EGF receptor. It lost most of the N-terminal extracellular domain thus losing the EGF binding domain (7). The C-terminal region of V-erb-B protein is shorther than EGF-receptor by 32 amino acids. However, a tetra peptide from the viral env gene is expressed as part of the C-terminal region of the V-erb-B protein (7,8).

An interesting conclusion from the sequence of EGF receptor is that the EGF-binding domain is connected to the cytoplasmic kinase domain by a single strech of 23 amino acids. Hence, these two domains are separated by the plasma membrane. It is well established that the binding of EGF to the external domain activates the cytoplasmic tyrosine kinase, even with highly purified EGF-receptors (9).

Hence the question remains what is the mechanism which leads to the signal transduction between these domains leading to the activation of the cytoplasmic portion? This and other questions of mechanism will be addressed in this paper.

The orientation of EGF receptor within the plasma membrane of A-431 cells. We have prepared antibodies against a synthetic peptide from the C-terminal region of EGF-receptor and the V-erb-B protein (10). This antibody recognizes various forms of the V-erb-B protein and the EGF receptor from various tissues and species (10). Immunofluorescence analysis indicates that this antibody labels only permeabilized A-431 cells (Fig. 1a). It does not labele intact A-431 cells. Thus, indicating that it recognizes cytoplasmic determinates of the EGF-receptor.

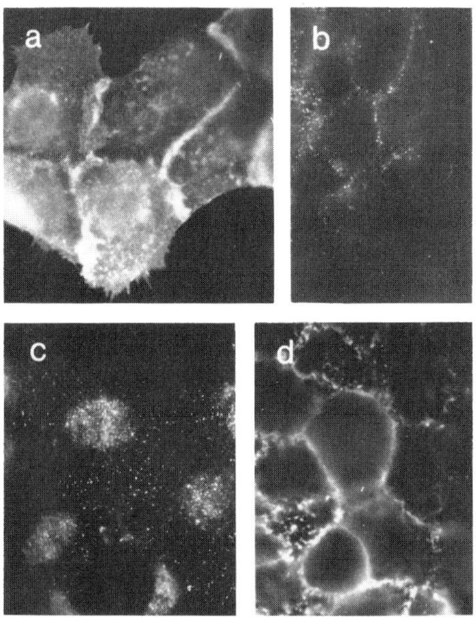

Fig.1. Fluorescence labeling of A-431 cells. A) Permeabilized A-431 cells were labeled with an antibody against a synthetic peptide from the C-terminal region of EGF-receptor (10) washed and then labeled with fluorescein conjugated goat anti-rabbit antibodies. B) Same labeling procedure of intact cells. C) Preimmune antibodies and D) Labeling of intact A-431 cells with antibody recognizing external determinants of EGF-receptors (11). Magnification X 400.

This result provides an experimental confirmation to the proposal that the C-terminal region of EGF receptor is the cytoplasmic domain (5-7).

EGF receptor as an allosteric dimer. We have previously shown that EGF induces the aggregation of EGF-receptors (2) and that cross-linking of the receptor molecules with antibody can mimic the effects of EGF (2,11).

Hence, on the basis of these results and on the basis of the structural domains of EGF receptor as revealed by its primary structure we propose the following model for the activation of the kinase activity of the receptor molecule by EGF.

We propose that an individual 170,000 dalton EGF receptor (E) appears in equilibrium with an aggregated dimeric (E_2) state (Fig. 2). The equilibrium constant for aggregation is defined as K_D. It is proposed that the affinity of the aggregated receptor (E_2) to EGF (X) is larger than the affinity of the monomeric receptor (E) to the growth factor ($K_2 > K_1$). To simplify the model we assume that the sites on the dimer are identical and that they do not interact with each other. It is postulated that EGF drives the clustering of the extracellular domains, consequently bringing together the cytoplasmic domains to a close proximity which leads to the activation of the kinase domain.

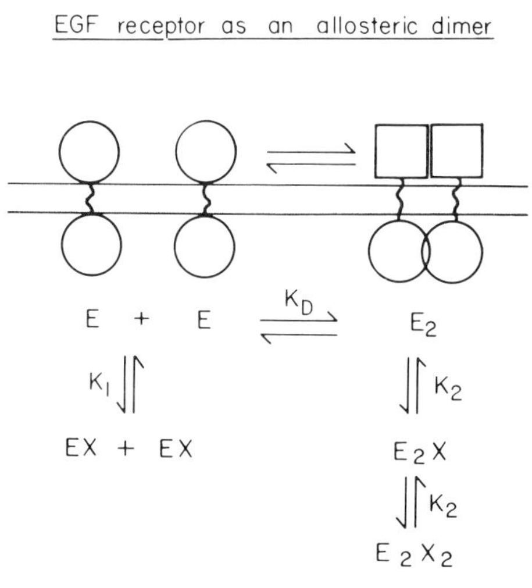

Fig. 2. An aggregation model for the activation of the kinase activity of the receptor molecule by EGF.

Several recent results are consistent with this aggregation model.

We have recently shown that monoclonal antibodies which bind to sugar residues of EGF receptor activate the EGF sensitive kinase (12). Moreover, the EGF-induced phosphorylation reaction is dependent on the concentration of the EGF-receptor suggesting that on aggregation step is involved in the activation of this enzyme (12).

These and other studies which are currently in progress will clarify the initial steps involved in the transmembrane signaling of the EGF-receptor system.

ACKNOWLEDGEMENTS

This work was supported by grants from NIH (CA 25820) and from U.S.-Israel Binational Science Foundation.

REFERENCES

1. Carpenter G, Cohen S (1979) Ann. Rev. Biochem 48:193-216
2. Schlessinger J, Schreiber AB, Levi A, Lax I, Libermann TA, Yarden Y (1983) Critical Rev. Biochem CRC 14:93-111
3. Cohen S, Carpenter G, King L Jr (1980) J Biol Chem 255:4834-4842
4. Ushiro H, Cohen S (1980) J Biol Chem 255:8363-8365
5. Lax I, Bar-Eli M, Yarden Y, Libermann TA, Schlessinger J (1984) Proc. Natl Acad USA (in press)
6. Downward J, Yarden Y, Mayes E, Scrace G, Totty N, Stockwell P, Ullrich A, Schlessinger J, Waterfield M (1984) Nature 307:521-527
7. Ullrich A, Coussens L, Hayflick JS, Dull TJ, Gray A, Tam AW, Lee J, Yarden Y, Libermann TA, Schlessinger J, Downward J, Mayes ELV, Whittle N, Waterfield MD, Seeberg PH (1984) Nature 309:418-425
8. Yamamoto Y, Nishida T, Miyajima N, Kawai S, Ooi K and Toyoshima K (1983) Cell 35:71-78
9. Yarden Y, Harari I, Schlessinger J (1984) J Biol Chem (submitted)
10. Kris R, Lax I, Gullick B, Waterfield M, Ullrich A, Schlessinger J (1984) (in preparation)
11. Schreiber AB, Libermann TA, Lax I, Yarden Y, Schlessinger J (1983) J Biol Chem 258:846-853
12. Yarden Y, Schlessinger J (unpublished results)

© 1984 Elsevier Science Publishers B.V.
Endocrinology
F. Labrie, L. Proulx, eds.

IN VIVO CARDIOVASCULAR, RENAL AND ENDOCRINE EFFECTS OF EPIDERMAL GROWTH FACTOR IN SHEEP

BRUCE A. SCOGGINS, ALDONNA BUTKUS, JOHN P. COGHLAN, DAVID T.W. FEI, JOHN G. McDOUGALL, HUGH D. NIALL, JOHN R. WALSH AND XIAOMING WANG

Howard Florey Institute of Experimental Physiology and Medicine, Parkville, 3052, (Australia)

INTRODUCTION

Since the first demonstration of an epidermal growth factor in extracts of mouse submandibular glands by Cohen in 1962 (1) there have been many studies examining its effects and mechanism of action in in-vitro cell and tissue preparations (2,3). Few experiments have reported the physiological effects of the peptide in conscious animals.

The in-vivo effects of mouse epidermal growth factor (mEGF) in sheep have been concerned with three aspects of the physiology of the peptide.

a) the role of EGF in fetal development (4).
b) the inhibition of wool growth following mEGF administration (5).
c) the effects of mEGF on thyroid, pituitary, pancreatic and adrenal function (6).

This report describes in detail the cardiovascular, renal and effects on ACTH release of mEGF in conscious animals for the first time.

MATERIALS AND METHODS

Experimental

Sheep. Adult cross bred merino ewes (35-45 kg) were used. All animals had carotid arterial loops and were housed in individual metabolism cages. Sheep with an autotransplanted adrenal gland (7) or a cervical renal transplant (8) or bilateral adrenalectomy were also used. For intracerebroventricular infusion (IVT) sheep had a lateral ventricular guide tube implanted. All surgical procedures were carried out at least 3 months prior to experimentation. Each day all animals received 800 g of a lucerne-oaten chaff diet containing 50-100 mmol/kg Na and 150-250 mmol/Kg K.

Preparation of mEGF. EGF was preapred from mouse submandibular glands by homogenisation and extraction followed by gel permeation and ion exchange chromatography.

Hormone assays. ACTH, AVP, and plasma renin concentration (PRC) were measured by radioimmunoassay. Cortisol and aldosterone in adrenal venous blood were measured by a double isotope dilution derivative assay.

RESULTS

Effects of 24 hours intravenous infusions

mEGF (125 μg/h) for 24 hours in 5 sheep produced a 50% fall in food intake, a rise in heart rate from 58 ± 3 to 129 ± 7 b/min and a fall in plasma [K] from 4.3 ± 01. to 3.6 ± 0.2 mmol/l. There was no change in MAP, Na or K excretion, plasma [glucose], urine output or water intake. Within 7-14 days all sheep started to shed their fleece. In adrenalectomised sheep (n=3) on a basal intravenous cortisol and aldosterone replacement regime mEGF infusion for 24 hours resulted in death either during the infusion or soon after.

Cardiovascular effects of mEGF

mEGF (125 μg/h for 5 hours) in 5 sheep produced large effects on cardiac output (CO); heart rate (HR) and total peripheral resistance (TPR) (Table 1). After 3.5 h a fall in MAP was also observed. PRC was increased and AVP unchanged. Administration of captopril (20 mg iv) reduced MAP by 15 mmHg. In adrenalectomised sheep on basla steroid replacement large falls in MAP (15-20 mmHg) were seen within 2-3 hours. Increased PRC and AVP were found in these animals after 3 hours. Plasma [ACTH] responses were similar in intact and adrenalectomised sheep. At 62.5 μg/h for 3 hours mEGF had little or no effect on HR or MAP in intact sheep.

TABLE 1
HEMODYNAMIC EFFECTS OF mEGF (125 μg/h) IN INTACT SHEEP (n=5)

CO (l/min)	5.4 ± 0.1	6.0 ± 0.1*	7.6 ± 0.2*	8.2 ± 0.2*
HR (b/min)	70 ± 9	78 ± 9	115 ± 11*	128 ± 7*
MAP (mmHg)	73 ± 2	73 ± 4	70 ± 4	67 ± 3*
TPR (units)	13.4 ± 0.5	12.3 ± 0.7	9.2 ± 0.5*	8.2 ± 0.4*
SV (ml/b)	78 ± 10	77 ± 9	66 ± 7*	64 ± 4*

* p <0.01 cf pre-infusion value.

Renal effects of mEGF

Within 30 min of starting the iv mEGF (125 μg/h for 6 hours) in 5 sheep there was an increase in urine flow (8 ± 1 to 42 ± 9 ml/min), urinary Na (0.05 ± 0.01 to 0.1 ± 0.03 mmol/min) and K excretion (0.07 ± 0.01 to 0.14 ± 0.01 mmol/min). The effect on urine flow persisted but urinary Na and K excretion returned to normal within 1-2 hours. Both GFR (^{51}CR EDTA clearance) and renal plasma flow (^{125}I-pAH clearance) fell gradually over the period of infusion.

Infusion of mEGF directly into the renal artery at 0.125 - 125 μg/h for

60 min produced an increase in urine flow at 12.5 μg/h. K excretion increased at 12.5 μg/h but there was no increase in Na excretion at any rate of infusion.

Effects of mEGF on plasma [ACTH]

Intravenous mEGF (125 μg/h) increased plasma [ACTH] from 33.2 ± 21 to 1715 ± 305 pg/ml (n=5) within 60 min. After 5 hours plasma [ACTH] was 933 ± 284 pg/ml. In another series of sheep (n=3) which received mEGF (125 μg/h) for 24 hours plasma [ACTH] started to fall back towards control levels after 8 hours. At 24 hours plasma [ACTH] was not significantly elevated. The threshold for the effect of mEGF on [ACTH] was 37.5 μg/hour and an increase in plasma [ACTH] was seen within 30 min.

Effects of mEGF on aldosterone and cortisol secretion

Infusion of mEGF at 0.8 - 80 μg/h directly into the adrenal arterial supply of Na replete (n=3) or Na depleted (n=3) sheep with an autotransplanted adrenal gland had no significant effects on aldosterone or cortisol secretion rates.

Effects of IVT mEGF infusion

Infusion of mEGF at 12.5 μg/h for 24 hours in 4 sheep produced a small increase in MAP (74 ± 2 to 87 ± 1 mmHg). There were only small effects on plasma [ACTH], heart rate, urine volume, Na and K excretion, water intake and food intake.

DISCUSSION

EGF produces large effects on the cardiovascular system. Within 30 min there was a fall in peripheral resistance probably in vascular beds such as the skin and gut - both tissues in which EGF receptors and effects of the peptide have been identified. Cardiac output increased due to an increased heart rate. Blood pressure was maintained close to the normal range due to stimulation of the renin-angiotensin system. In the adrenalectomised sheep on basal steroid replacement EGF produced large falls in blood pressure. Although both AVP and PRC are elevated in the absence of the adrenal medulla the circulation is compromised in these animals and death occurred following 24 hour infusions.

Recent identification of EGF gene expression in the mouse kidney (Coghlan et al, personal communication) and the observed effects of mEGF on urine flow and Na excretion in sheep are of interest. However the effects of mEGF on renal electrolyte excretion were relatively small and transient.

Although Waters (9) has demonstrated in-vitro that the effects of EGF on plasma cortisol levels may be due to a direct effect on cholesterol precursor synthesis the present in-vivo sutdies showed little effect of EGF on cortisol (and also aldosterone) secretion. The marked increase in plasma ACTH levels observed in sheep suggests that in-vivo ACTH probably plays a major role in stimulating cortisol secretion in response to EGF infusion. The effects of mEGF on plasma [ACTH] are much greater than those found with infusions of CRF (100 μg/h) into the same sheep (n=4) (pre CRF 15 ± 10 pg/ml: 108 ± 14 pg/ml after 30 min of CRF infusion).

In conclusion: mEGF produces a wide spectrum of endocrine, renal and cardiovascular effects in sheep. Very few peptides of biological origin produce the range of effects found with EGF. Although a number of the changes are transient, lasting only a few hours, other effects persist for at least 24 hours. Many of the actions of the peptide observed in in-vivo experiments in sheep are clearly not related to the mitogenic activity of EGF. The physiological significance of these effects remains to be determined.

ACKNOWLEDGEMENTS

These studies were supported by an Institute grant from the National Health and Medical Research Council of Australia.

REFERENCES

1. Cohen S (1982) J Biol Chem 237; 1555
2. Carpenter G (1980) Birth Defects XVI: 61
3. Cohen S (1983) Cancer 51: 1787
4. Thorburn GD, Water MJ, Young IR, Dolling M, Buntine D, Hopkins PS (1981) Ciba Foundation Symposium 86: 172
5. Moore GPM, Panaratto BA, Robertson D (1981) Search 12: 128
6. Waters MJ, Corcoran J, Tennison MM, Jorgenson G, Eastman RC, Bourke JR, Thorburn GD (1982) Proceedings Endocrine Society of Australia 25: 34
7. McDonald IR, Goding JR, Wright RD (1958) Aust J Exp Biol Med 36: 83
8. Wright RD, Hardy KJ, Potocnik SJ, McDougall JG (1982) Kidney Intern 22: 309
9. Singh-Asa P, Waters MJ, Risbridger G (1982) Proceedings Endocrine Society of Australia 25: 9

29. Hormones and Bone Metabolism

Endocrinology
F. Labrie, L. Proulx, eds.

THE DESIGN AND BIOLOGICAL EVALUATION OF A PARATHYROID HORMONE ANTAGONIST EFFECTIVE *IN VIVO*

MICHAEL ROSENBLATT, GEORGE A. TYLER, SAMUEL H. DOPPELT, NOBORU HORIUCHI, ROBERT M. NEER, AND JOHN T. POTTS, JR

Endocrine Unit, Massachusetts General Hospital and Department of Medicine, Harvard Medical School, Boston, MA 02114

INTRODUCTION

Parathyroid hormone (PTH) plays a critical role in calcium homeostasis through its direct action on kidney and bone and indirect effects on gut to prevent hypocalcemia. Through its rapid effects on target tissue, PTH is responsible for regulation of calcium levels within the narrow physiological range essential for the normal activity of muscle, nerve, enzymes, blood clotting factors and other hormones.

For the last decade, efforts have been made in our laboratory to elucidate the nature of the PTH-receptor interaction leading to expression of hormonal activity. Extensive structure-activity studies in multiple bioassay systems[1] have been performed and the structural elements within the PTH molecule necessary for receptor-binding and for expression of hormone action have been identified as well-delinated and separable domains. From these studies, directions were established leading to the design and synthesis of a PTH antagonist which can inhibit the major parameters of PTH action in kidney and bone *in vivo*.[2,3]

<u>Design of a PTH Antagonist Effect *In Vivo*</u>

PTH is an 84-amino acid single-chain polypeptide. All of the structural determinants necessary for full biological activity of PTH reside within the N-terminal one-third (residues 1--34) of the native hormone.[1,4] Within the molecule, there is a domain responsible for receptor binding, the region 3--34, and a small but critical region (positions 1 and 2) necessary for hormone action. Based on these findings, potent *in vitro* antagonists were prepared. An analog of the 3--34 region, [Nle-8,Nle-18,Tyr-34]bPTH-(3--34)amide, proved to be the most potent *in vitro* antagonist yet designed. *In Vitro*, this compound is a competitive inhibitor which has avidity for PTH receptors comparable to PTH and is devoid of PTH-like angonist activity.[1,5,6] However, in two *in vivo* studies,[7,8] the analog failed to display inhibitory properties; in other *in vivo* investigations, it demonstrated weak, but definite, PTH-like agonist properties in the dog,[9] the rat[10] and in a canine isolated perfused bone system.[11] Taken together, these studies revealed the 3--34 analog to be a weak agonist for several parameters of PTH action, including stimulation of hypercalcemia, urinary phosphate and cAMP excretion, and production of 1α,25-dihydroxyvitamin D_3.

Our approach to generating an *in vivo* PTH inhibitor was to modify the N-terminus through further truncation to eliminate the last traces of agonist activity from the 3--34 sequence without losing completely avidity for PTH receptors.

A series of fragments of PTH containing N-terminal deletions were synthesized and evaluated in a renal radioreceptor assay for PTH.[12] Stepwise deletions at the N-terminus produce a progressive decline in receptor avidity, and identify the region 25--34 as the principal binding domain of the hormone.[13] The intermediate sequence 7--34 binds well to PTH receptors, although avidity was diminished to 1/10-1/100th of the 3--34 sequence. In addition, substitution of norleucine for methionine is poorly tolerated *in vivo*.[14]

Using these directions established *in vitro* and *in vivo*, we selected for synthesis the analog [Tyr-34]bPTH-(7--34)-amide. The peptide was prepared by the solid-phase method of Merrifield[15,16] and purified by gel-filtration followed by semi-preparative high pressure liquid chromatography.[17]

In Vivo Evaluation of a PTH Antagonist

The biological properties of this analog *in vivo* were evaluated for effects on PTH-stimulated urinary phosphate and cAMP excretion. Highly purified native bPTH-(1--84) (kindly provided by Dr. Henry T. Keutmann) or the antagonist, or a combination of both peptides was infused intravenously into vitamin D-deficient thyroparathyroidectomized rats and urine volume, phosphate, and cAMP levels determined every 30 min for 2.5-3.5 h. When inhibitor was administered, its infusion began 1h prior to beginning PTH infusion. The inhibitor was infused at a molar dose-rate 200-fold greater than native PTH. Figure 1 depicts a compilation of data obtained from 40 test animals. The analog displayed no PTH-like agonist properties and completely inhibited the PTH-stimulated phosphaturic response.

Further studies have been undertaken to assess effects of the 7--34 analog on the PTH-mediated calcemic response. A newly developed *in vivo* assay, based on the serum calcium-elevating response to PTH which occurs in acutely thyroparathyroidectomized rats, was used.[3] Given in intravenous boluses before, simultaneous with, and after a single bolus of PTH (antagonist:agonist=30:1 for each bolus), the antagonist completely blocked the calcemic response to PTH (Figure 2).

Hence, structure-activity studies have led to the design and synthesis of the first inhibitory analog of PTH active *in vivo*. This antagonist exerts its effects through competing with PTH for occupancy of receptor sites. When administered in sufficiently high dosage, this analog inhibits completely the principal actions of PTH *in vivo*, namely stimulation of phosphaturia and urinary cAMP excretion and elevation of serum calcium levels. These studies establish feasibility and future directions for design of PTH inhibitors.[2] Attempts are

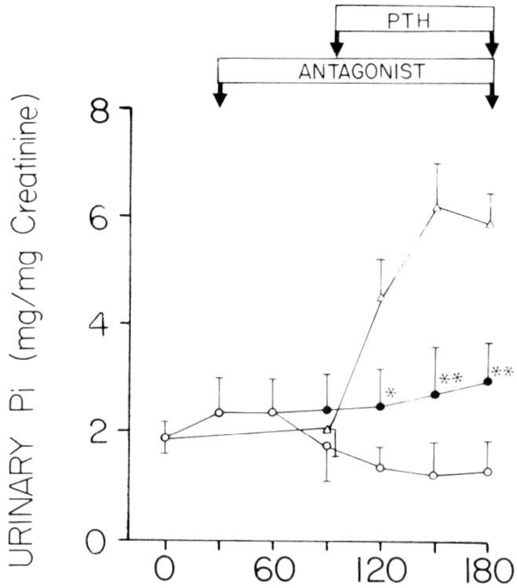

Fig 3. Evaluation of the effects of [Tyr-34]bPTH-(7--34)amide on urinary phosphate excretion *in vivo* in rats. Data shown are compiled from a total of 40 animals. Fifteen rats (Δ) comprised the control group and received native bPTH-(1--84) alone intravenously at a molar dose rate of 0.27 nmol/h. Twenty-one rats received the inhibitor at a dose rate of 54 nmol/h and PTH (0.27 nmol/h) (●). Analog infusion was begun one hour prior to beginning the PTH infusion. Four animals (O) received antagonist alone. Determinations in animals receiving antagonist and PTH differ significantly from animals receiving PTH alone, *p< 0.025 and **p<0.01 by Student's t-test. (Reprinted with permission.)

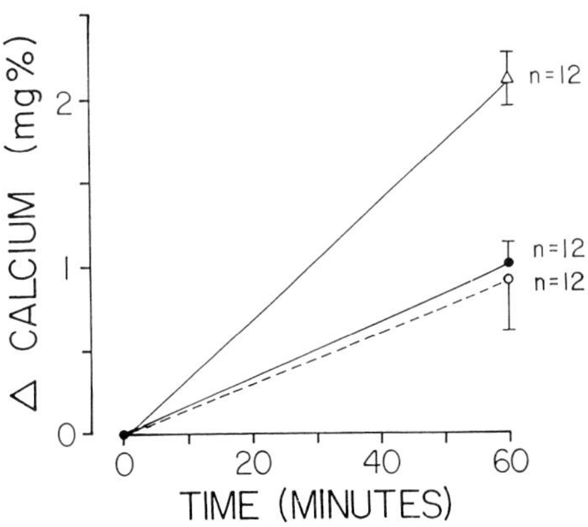

Fig 2. Inhibition of PTH-stimulated calcemic response in acutely thyroparathyroidectomized rats. Data shown are for animals receiving 5 M.R.C. Units hPTH-(1--34) (Δ), [Tyr-34]-bPTH-(7--34)amide + hPTH-(1--34), (●), and controls (no peptide) (O). (Reprinted with permission.)

now underway to design more potent antagonists. Finally, recent evidence from several laboratories indicates that the hypercalcemia of malignancy may be mediated by tumor-secreted factors, which are not PTH but which interact with PTH receptors. Therefore, the potential utility of a PTH antagonist in treating hypercalcemia of several etiologies warrants further investigation.

ACKNOWLEDGEMENTS

This work was supported in part by Grant No. AM11794 from the N.I.A.D.D.K.

REFERENCES

1. Potts JT Jr, Kronenberg HM, Rosenblatt M (1982) Adv Protein Chem 35:323-396
2. Horiuchi N, Holick MF, Potts JT Jr, Rosenblatt M (1983) Science 220:1053-1055
3. Doppelt S, Federico P, Tyler GA, Rosenblatt M, Neer RM (1983) Calcif Tissue Int A45 (in press)
4. Tregear GW, van Reitschoten J, Greene E, Keutmann HT, Niall HD, Reit B, Parsons JA, Potts JT Jr (1973) Endocrinology 93:1349-1353
5. Rosenblatt M, Callahan EN, Mahaffey JE, Pont A, Potts JT Jr (1977) J Biol Chem 252:5847-5851
6. Goldring SR, Dayer JM, Rosenblatt M (1981) J Clin Endocrinol Metab 33:375-380
7. Gray DA, Parsons JA, Potts JT Jr, Rosenblatt M, Stevenson RW (1982) Br J Pharm 76:259-263
8. McGowan JA, Chen TC, Fragola J, Puschett JB, Rosenblatt M (1982) Science 219:67-69
9. Segre GV, Tully GL III, Rosenblatt M, Laugharn JA, Reit B, Potts JT Jr (1979) Calcif Tissue Int [Abstr] 28:171
10. Horiuchi N, Holick MF, Rosenblatt M, Keutmann HT, Potts JT Jr (1983) Am J Physiol 244 (Endocrinol Metab 7):E589-95
11. Martin KJ, Bellorin-Font E, Freitag J, Rosenblatt M, Slatopolsky E (1981) Endocrinology 109:956-959
12. Rosenblatt M, Segre GV, Tyler GA, Shepard GL, Nussbaum SR, Potts JT Jr (1980) Endocrinology 106:545-550
13. Nussbaum SR, Rosenblatt M, Potts JT Jr (1980) J Biol Chem 225:10183-10187
14. Rosenblatt M, Coltrera MD, Shepard GL, Gray DA, Parsons JA, Potts JT Jr (1981) Biochemistry 20:7246-7250
15. Tyler GA, Rosenblatt M (1983) J Chromatogr 266:313-318

© 1984 Elsevier Science Publishers B.V.
Endocrinology
F. Labrie, L. Proulx, eds.

THE EFFECT OF PARATHYROID HORMONE ON BONE CELLS

G.A. RODAN, S.B. RODAN, R.J. MAJESKA, J.J. EGAN AND G. GRONOWICZ

Department of Oral Biology, Univ. of Connecticut Health Center, School of Dental Medicine, Farmington, CT 06032 (USA)

The major physiological and pathological effect of parathyroid hormone (PTH) on bone is stimulation of bone resorption, a cellular process carried out by osteoclasts. The mechanism for PTH activation of osteoclasts is not known and so far, there is no convincing evidence for the presence of PTH receptors in these cells. PTH receptors have been demonstrated in osteoblasts by autoradiographic and functional criteria (1,2,3,4) and considerable information is now available on the effect of PTH on these cells. The osteoblastic PTH receptor (K_D 0.6 nM) (5) is coupled to adenylate cyclase (AC) and interaction with the hormone leads to rapid cellular accumulation of cAMP. PTH activation of AC in cell membranes requires GTP and Mg^{2+} (4) and hormone stimulation of AC is associated with an increase in the affinity of the enzyme for Mg^{2+}. In whole cells, hormone dependent cAMP accumulation peaks around 5 min even in the presence of phosphodiesterase inhibitors. The short duration for AC activation is probably due to desensitization, a general phenomenon characteristic of biological signal transduction. The immediate refractoriness to hormone stimulation appears to be due to alterations in receptor AC coupling and may involve changes in the guanine nucleotide binding subunit of the AC system. This is reflected in a reduction in the Mg^{2+} affinity of the guanine nucleotide stimulated AC. In addition, the receptors are internalized and reduce in number (down regulation). As a result of desensitization each cell presumably sees a single pulse of cAMP following hormone exposure, which should initiate the hormonal changes in the target cell. Cyclic cAMP acts via protein kinase (PK) and PTH was indeed shown to activate cAMP PK in osteoblastic cells within 1 min. Significantly lower concentrations of PTH are needed to produce 50% PK activation than those required to produce 50% AC stimulation, effective hormone concentrations thus approaching the physiologically relevant range. The role and location of PTH receptors which are activated at higher concentrations is not known. Both PK I and PK II are activated by PTH in osteoblasts, but the specific proteins phosphorylated as a result of PK activation have not been characterized (6).

One of the earliest PTH effects is a shape change characterized by retraction of cellular processes. These morphological changes parallel changes in the distribution of microfilaments, visualized by rhodamine conjugated phalloidin (7). Biochemically, these changes are associated with myosin and actin depolymerization, which peak at 5 min and are accompanied by a reduction in myosin light chain phosphorylation. These effects show a PTH dose dependence and are inhibited by the antagonist [Nle^{8}, Nle^{18}, Tyr^{34}] bPTH (3-34)amide. Similar changes are produced by cAMP elevating agents or by a reduction in intracellular calcium through chelation to Quin 2. It is not known if these are alternate pathways or if cAMP causes calcium reduction, for example via a cAMP PK stimulated calcium pump. The role of osteoblastic shape change in the mechanism of action of PTH in these cells is not known. It was proposed that in osteoblast derived lining cells, shape changes may increase the accessibility of osteoclasts to bone matrix (8). In matrix forming cells, PTH reduces collagen synthesis (9) by reducing the level of mRNA (10). PTH also reduces alkaline phosphatase by a cAMP mediated process (11) probably by inhibition of *de novo* synthesis. The sensitivity to PTH is increased by glucocorticoids which, at physiological concentrations stimulate osteoblastic expression in osteosarcoma cells and augment PTH activation of AC (12). Glucocorticoids increase *de novo* synthesis of alkaline phosphatase in these cells and at the same time potentiate the inhibitory effects of PTH on this process. Along with the inhibition of osteoblastic features PTH stimulates the proliferation of osteoblastic cells (13). These effects are consistent with the reported stimulation of bone formation by low concentrations of PTH *in vivo* (14, 15).

At the cellular level the following effects could account for all the effects of PTH on bone: Increased osteoclastic bone resorption, which may be mediated by other cells including osteoblasts, inhibition of osteoblastic (differentiated) functions, and possibly stimulation of proliferation in precursor cells, resulting later in accelerated bone formation. Many of these effects involve regulation of gene expression. The mechanism of action of PTH at this level is not known. Progress is being made in the elucidation of the molecular pathway for the conveyance of the PTH message from the surface of the cell to the genome. There is clear evidence that cAMP is a second messenger for PTH without excluding the potential participation of calcium in PTH action. One of the more recent observations involves effects on the cytoskeleton, which has been implicated in the regulation of gene expression.

ACKNOWLEDGEMENTS

This work was supported by an NIH Grant AM-17848.

REFERENCES

1. Silve CM, Hradek GT, Jones AL, Arnaud CD (1982) J Cell Biol 94: 379.
2. Wong GL, Cohn DV (1975) Proc Natl Acad Sci USA 72: 3167
3. Peck WA, Burks JK, Wilkins J, Rodan SB, Rodan GA (1977) Endocrinology 100: 1357
4. Rodan SB, Rodan GA (1981) Biochim Biophys Acta 673: 55
5. Pliam NB, Nyiredy KO, Arnaud CD (1982) Proc Natl Acad Sci USA 79: 2061
6. Livesey SA, Kemp BE, Re CA, Partridge NC, Martin TJ (1982) J Biol Chem 257: 14983
7. Gronowicz G, Egan JJ, Rodan GA (1984) Calcif Tissue Int In Press
8. Rodan GA, Martin TJ (1981) Calcif Tissue Int 33: 349
9. Wong GL, Luben RA, Cohn DV (1977) Science 197: 663
10. Kream BE, Rowe DW, Gworek SC, Raisz LG (1980) Proc Natl Acad Sci USA 77: 5654
11. Majeska RJ, Rodan GA (1982) Calcif Tissue Int 34: 59
12. Rodan SB, Rischer MK, Egan JJ, Epstein PM, Rodan GA (1984) Endocrinology In Press
13. Majeska RJ, Rodan GA (1981) Calcif Tissue Int 33: 36A
14. Parsons JA, Reit B (1974) Nature 250: 254
15. Tam CS, Heersche JN, Murray TM, Parson, JA (1982) Endocrinology 110: 506.

Endocrinology
F. Labrie, L. Proulx, eds.

OSTEOCLAST ACTIVATING FACTOR

GREGORY R MUNDY, DONALD R BERTOLINI
University of Texas Health Science Center, Department of Medicine/Endocrinology, 7703 Floyd Curl Drive, San Antonio, Texas 78284

In 1972, bone resorbing activity was identified in the supernatant media harvested from cultures of peripheral blood leukocytes activated by the mitogen phytohemagglutinin and by dental plaque [1]. Because its effects on bone were to stimulate osteoclastic bone resorption, the activity was called osteoclast activating factor or OAF. Since that time, many studies have revealed that this bone resorbing activity in fact represents a family of bone resorbing factors whose biological effect is the same, namely an increase in osteoclastic bone resorption, but whose structural relationships and cellular origins remain unclear.

Most of the studies on OAF to date have been performed on the unseparated bone resorbing activity present in culture media harvested from activated peripheral blood leukocytes. Thus, all of these studies must be considered in light of the recent findings that this activity probably represents a number of distinct factors whose cellular source of origin, structure and regulation of production may vary under different circumstances. Nevertheless, some general statements can be made about the generic or total bone resorbing activity present in activated leukocyte culture supernatants. This activity is produced only when the leukocytes are exposed to an antigen to which they have been previously exposed or to a non-specific mitogen such as phytohemagglutinin [2-4]. The bone resorbing activity has similar biological effects to those of parathyroid hormone (PTH). It has a steep dose response curve, produces a prolonged effect after short exposure, stimulates osteoclast activity including increasing the size of the osteoclast ruffled border, and its effects are inhibited by cortisol, calcitonin and phosphate [3]. It is probably a local rather than a systemic factor, since when it is injected systemically it fails to cause hypercalcemia, unlike PTH [3]. Like other bone resorbing factors such as PTH and prostaglandins of the E series, its effects on bone collagen synthesis in vitro are inhibitory [3]. The biological activity in culture supernatants is clearly heterogeneous and comprises smaller and larger forms [5]. Production of OAF appears to depend on prostaglandin synthesis, since leukocytes cultured in the presence of indomethacin or other structurally unrelated inhibitors of prostaglandin synthesis fail to produce bone resorbing activity [6-8]. Bone resorbing activity is restored when prostaglandins of the E series are added to the leukocyte cultures.

In recent years, it has become apparent that osteoclast activating factor represents a family of bone resorbing factors with the same biological effect. For purposes of convenience, we classify this family of OAFs into three sub-groups according to their cell of origin - T cell OAFs, B cell OAFs and monocyte OAFs.

T Cell OAFs

Evidence that the T lymphocyte produces an osteoclast activating factor was first suggested by experiments in which OAF was present in leukocyte cultures after exposure to phytohemagglutinin or conconavalin A. These agents are relatively specific for T cells. In early cell separation experiments, Horton et al [9] and later Chen et al [10] separated T lymphocytes by their capacity to rosette with sheep red blood cells. Enriched T cell populations were found to produce an osteoclast activating factor when cultured with an appropriate mitogen. In later experiments using mouse T cells, Horowitz et al [11] were able to specifically deplete non T cells from leukocyte cultures and found that the cell source of origin of OAF from mouse cells was an activated T cell. Recent studies with the T cell malignancy associated with the unique type C retrovirus which causes adult T cell lymphoma have shown that both lymphoma cells and cord blood lymphocytes which carry the virus produce an OAF constitutively [12]. These T cells have the surface characteristics of helper-inducer cells. Since almost all patients with this type of lymphoma develop hypercalcemia or destructive bone lesions, this OAF is clearly a bone resorbing factor of important biological as well as pathologic significance.

B Cell OAFs

Horton et al[9] and later Chen et al [10] found that lymphocytes which were partially adherent and did not rosette with sheep red blood cells also produce an OAF, but unlike T cells they could produce it without exposure to a mitogen. They concluded that these B cells released an OAF constitutively. Because of the relationship of lymphoid malignancies of the B cell with bone destruction and hypercalcemia, these observations led to studies on established lymphoid cell lines derived from patients with myeloma and Burkitt's lymphoma [13]. Bone resorbing activity was found both in media harvested from lymphoid cell lines from both types of B cell malignancy. Later studies showed that cultured freshly aspirated myeloma cells from patients with myeloma also produced a similar bone resorbing factor [14]. This factor was a macromolecular protein similar to the macromolecular protein present in activated leukocytes culture supernatants. Burkitt's lymphoma is frequently associated with localized osteoclastic bone resorption and myeloma is almost always associated with discrete or diffuse bone resorption, as well as hypercalcemia in more than 20% of patients. Histomorphometric examination of the skeleton in myeloma reveals that the myeloma cells occur adjacent to increases in osteoclast number and activity [14-15]. The relationship of this B cell OAF to the OAF present in patients with T cell malignancies remains unknown.

Monocyte OAFs

Cultures of peripheral blood monocytes produce at least two distinct types of bone resorbing activity.

a. Prostaglandins of the E series

When monocytes are cultured with fetal rat long bones, the monocytes release prostaglandins of the E series which in turn resorb bone [16]. This release of bone resorbing activity by the monocytes can be inhibited by co-culture with indomethacin and other structurally unrelated inhibitors of prostaglandin synthesis. Monocytes are important sources of prostaglandins and the production of prostaglandins by monocytes may stimulate osteoclasts directly in addition to being a requirement for lymphocyte OAF production (see above).

b. Interleukin I like activity

Recently it has been found that interleukin I, the protein which stimulates thymocyte activation and probably is responsible for a series of other biological effects such as fibroblast proliferation, release of bacterial pyrogen, and release of prostaglandins and collagenase from synovial cells and gingival fibroblasts, is capable of resorbing bone [17]. It is not clear whether the bone resorbing activity resides in the interleukin I molecule or is a closely related protein which co-purifies with interleukin I. The effects can be observed both in mouse calvarial cultures as well as in fetal rat long bone cultures. The effects are neither dependent on prostaglandin synthesis nor is the production of this factor related to prostaglandin synthesis.

Occasionally patients with malignancies of cells of the monocyte-macrophage series develop bone destruction and hypercalcemia [18]. The pathogenesis of this increased bone resorption is unknown but may be due to osteoclast activating factors released by these malignant cells.

Thus, the osteoclast activating factors represent a family of bone resorbing factors present in supernatant medias harvested from cultured peripheral blood leukocytes. The relationship of these factors to each other is unknown at the present time. However, one or more of these factors acting in concert may be responsible for regulation of normal bone turnover and formation of the bone marrow cavity by activation of endosteal osteoclasts. These factors may be important in the lymphoid malignancies associated with bone destruction and hypercalcemia such as adult T cell lymphoma and the B cell malignancies such as myeloma and Burkitt's lymphoma, as well as in the less frequent monocyte malignancies associated with hypercalcemia. They may also be important in the localized bone destruction which occurs around accumulations of chronic inflammatory cells in conditions such as periodontal disease, rheumatoid arthritis and in cholesteatoma. Understanding the relationship of these factors to each other and the control of their production and their effects should prove of major importance in understanding the process of normal bone turnover and bone remodeling.

ACKNOWLEDGEMENTS

This work was supported by grants AM-28149 and CA29537 and RR-134 from the National Institutes of Health.

REFERENCES

1. Horton JE, Raisz LG, Simmons HA, Oppenheim JJ, Mergenhagen SE (1972) Science 177:793-795

2. Luben RA, Mundy GR, Trummel CL, Raisz LG (1974) J Clin Invest 53:1473-1480

3. Raisz LG, Luben RA, Mundy GR, Dietrich JW, Horton JE, Trummel CL (1975) J Clin Invest 56:408-413

4. Trummel CL, Mundy GR, Raisz LG (1975) J Lab Clin Med 85:1001-1007.

5. Mundy GR, Raisz LG (1977) J Clin Invest 60:122-128

6. Yoneda T, Mundy GR (1979a) J Exp Med 149:279-283

7. Yoneda T, Mundy GR (1979b) J Exp Med 150:338-350

8. Bockman R, Repo MA (1981) J Exp Med 154:529-534

9. Horton JE, Oppenheim JJ, Mergenhagen SE, Raisz LG (1974) J Immunol 113:1278-1287

10. Chen P, Trummel C, Horton J, Baker JJ, Oppenheim JJ (1976) Eur J Immunol 6:732-736

11. Horowitz M, Vignery A, Gershon RK, Baron R (1984) Proc Natl Acad Sci (in press)

12. Bertolini DR, Sarin P, Mundy GR (1984) Calcif Tiss Int (abstract) in press

13. Mundy GR, Luben RA, Rasiz LG, Oppenheim JJ, Buell DN (1974) New Engl J Med 290:867-871

14. Mundy GR, Raisz LG, Cooper RA, Schechter GP, Salmon SE (1974) New Engl J Med 291:1041-1046

15. Valentin-Opran A, Charhon SA, Meunier PJ, Edouard CM, Arlot ME (1982) Brit J Haematology 52:601-610

16. Dominguez JH, Mundy GR (1980) Calcif Tiss Int 30:127-133

17. Gowen M, Wood DD, Ihrie EJ, McGuire MKB, Russell RGG (1983) Nature 306:378-380

18. Koeffler HP, Mundy GR, Golde DW, Cline MJ (1978) Cancer 41:2438-2443

Endocrinology
F. Labrie, L. Proulx, eds.

MALIGNANCY-ASSOCIATED HYPERCALCEMIA

A.E. BROADUS, K.L. INSOGNA, E.C. WEIR, A.M.C. VIGNERY, W.J. BURTIS, J.W. GODSALL, and A.F. STEWART

Department of Internal Medicine, Yale University, New Haven, Connecticut, 06510, USA

Two general mechanisms appear to be responsible for malignancy-associated hypercalcemia (MAHC): a) local osteolytic hypercalcemia, which results from bone resorption mediated by malignant cells occurring primarily in or metastatic to bone (e.g., myeloma, breast carcinoma) and b) humoral hypercalcemia of malignancy, which results from bone resorption mediated by a circulating factor(s) produced by neoplasms remote from bone (e.g., squamous cell, renal, bladder, and ovarian carcinomas). Interest in humoral hypercalcemia of malignancy (HHM), the primary focus of this brief review, has increased markedly in the past several years. This increased interest reflects 1) the reported frequency of the syndrome as well as the precision with which it has been characterized biochemically *in vivo* (1-3), 2) the increased availability of animal models which closely mimic the human syndrome (4-8), 3) the increasingly powerful tools which have been developed for detection and isolation of the putative mediators *in vitro* (4-10), and 4) the recognition that the active principal is rarely, if ever, related to the gene product for parathyroid hormone (PTH) and therefore likely represents a novel peptide of great potential biological significance (4-10).

The two most active hypotheses at present are that the mediator in question is "growth factor-like" (8) or "PTH-like" (1-7,9,10). These two hypotheses are clearly not mutually exclusive. In addition, other mechanisms may apply in certain unusual examples of HHM (see below). Our own work has been largely concerned with the "PTH-like" hypothesis and has proceeded in the four interrelated phases described below.

The first phase was the descriptive phase *in vivo*. In essence, we employed a biochemical rather than a clinical classification scheme, viewing an increase in nephrogenous cyclic AMP (NcAMP) excretion as evidence for a systemic mediator and regarding such patients as examples of HHM. Based on this classification, a humoral mechanism applies in some 80% of unselected, untreated patients with MAHC. In contrast to patients with primary hyperparathyroidism, the prototype of humoral hypercalcemia, patients with HHM display: 1) a marked mean increase in fractional calcium excretion, 2) a profound mean reduction in circulating 1,25-$(OH)_2D$, 3) normal or reduced serum immunoreactive PTH in a variety of region-specific assays, 4) circulating cytochemical bioactivity which elutes ahead of PTH on gel filtration and which is largely uninhibited by preincubation with anti-PTH antisera (2), and

5) intense osteoclastic bone resorption and near-complete uncoupling of bone turnover on histomorphometric analysis (1-3). These findings portray HHM as a syndrome of purely resorptive hypercalcemia and indicate that the mediator in question is "PTH-like" in only a very limited sense. Our experience has more than doubled since the publication of the original clinical series (1) and indicates that 95% of patients with MAHC can be reliably classified biochemically (only 8 of 125 consecutive patients were regarded as unclassifiable). Four patients appeared to have a humoral syndrome but had suppressed NcAMP; these included 3 patients with a lymphoma and apparent 1,25-$(OH)_2D$-mediated hypercalcemia and 1 patient with an ovarian carcinoma and suppressed values for all parameters. We have studied the H500 Leydig cell tumor in the Fisher rat and a novel carcinogen-induced squamous cell carcinoma in the mouse in like fashion; both animal models are remarkably similar to the human syndrome, the sole exception being that circulating 1,25-$(OH)_2D$ has been increased in the animal models (4,5).

The second phase of our work involved developing techniques for pursuing the mediator(s) _in vitro_. Our strategy was to assume that the mediator in question would display the same actions _in vitro_ that it displays _in vivo_. Correspondingly, the detection systems we have employed include a canine renal cortical adenylate cyclase system, a conventional bone-resorbing system, the cytochemical bioassay for PTH (in collaboration with D. Goltzman), and an adenylate cyclase assay in cultured rat osteosarcoma cells (kindly supplied by G. Rodan). The sources of material have included human tumors, the rat and mouse models, and cultured cells from several of these systems. We have observed an essentially 100% correspondence between _in vivo_ evidence of HHM and the presence of activity in a combination of these detection systems in both tumor extracts and conditioned medium from cultured tumor cells, whereas activity has been absent in tumor extracts from patients with local osteolytic hypercalcemia and absent or negligible in control tumors. In 3 of the detection systems, activity in tumor extracts and media is completely inhibited by the synthetic PTH analog, $[Nle^8,Nle^{18},Tyr^{34}]bPTH\text{-}(3\text{-}34)NH_2$, but the adenylate cyclase-stimulating activity is completely untouched by preincubation with PTH antisera, including a panel of 4 amino-terminal antisera (courtesy of G. Segre). We interpret these data as indicating that the factor(s) is specifically interacting with PTH receptors, at least in certain tissues, but is clearly distinct from native PTH.

The third phase has been concerned with protein purification. Work to date has largely been performed with a human squamous cell tumor (selected on the basis of marked activity in crude extracts) and the rat Leydig cell tumor. A combination of solvent-precipitation, gel filtration, and reverse-phase high performance liquid chromatography has generated material from the human tumor which is some 30,000-

fold purified and which maintains maximal activity in the cyclase and bone-resortion assays (11). The protein appears to be quite basic and has an estimated molecular weight of approximately 25,000 daltons. Material from tumors and conditioned medium from the Leydig cell model has been similarly purified and also has an estimated molecular weight of approximately 25,000 daltons (12). Work with both systems has advanced to preparative scale, and an immunization program using highly purified material has been initiated.

The fourth phase has involved the focusing of molecular techniques on the problem, in collaboration with A. Webb, D. Goltzman, and H. Kronenberg. Messenger RNA was prepared from several human tumors and both animal model tumors and also from 2 control tumors (a mouse myeloma and a human lymphoma). This mRNA was microinjected into _Xenopus_ oocytes, with assay of the medium in the cytochemical bioassay (CBA) for PTH. CBA activity has been observed in each of the media from experimental mRNA-injected oocytes, parallels that of the PTH standard in the assay, and is completely inhibited by the PTH_{3-34} analog. No such activity has been observed in the media of oocytes injected with control mRNA. Using these techniques, mRNA from the rat system has been enriched some 20-fold by preparative acrylamide gel electrophoresis.

Humoral hypercalcemia of malignancy is a common paraneoplastic syndrome which results from the elaboration by tumors of a systemic factor(s) which is clearly distinct from native parathyroid hormone. The factor in question appears to be a basic protein of 25,000 daltons.

REFERENCES

1. Stewart AF, Horst L, Deftos LJ, Cadman EC, Lang R, Broadus AE (1980) N Engl J Med 303:1377
2. Goltzman D, Stewart AF, Broadus AE (1981) J Clin Endocrinol Metab 53,899
3. Stewart AF, Vignery A, Silvergate A, Ravin ND, Livolsi V, Broadus AE, Baron R (1982) J Clin Endocrinol Metab 55:219
4. Insogna KL, Stewart AF, Vignery AMC, Weir EC, Namnum PA, Baron RE, Kirkwood JM, Deftos LJ, Broadus AE (1984) Endocrinology 114:888
5. Hayes T, Gkonos P, Charney E, Jacoby R, Baron R, McGuire J, Stewart A (1983) Clin Res 31:387A
6. Rodan SB, Insogna KL, Vignery AMC, Stewart AF, Broadus AE, D'Souza SM, Bertolini DR, Mundy GR, Rodan GA (1983) J Clin Invest 72:1511
7. Strewler GJ, Williams RD, Nissenson RA (1983) J Clin Invest 71:769
8. Ibbotson K, D'Souza SM, Osborne CK, Niall M, Martin TJ, Mundy GR (1983) Science 221:1292
9. Stewart AF, Insogna KL, Goltzman D, Broadus AE (1983) Proc Natl Acad Sci 80:1454
10. Simpson EL, Mundy GR, D'Souza SM, Ibbotson KJ, Bockman R, Jacobs RJ (1983) N Engl J Med 309:325

11. Stewart AF, Vignery A, Burtis WJ (1984) Clin Res 32:410A
12. Insogna K, Weir E, Stewart A, Godsall W, Broadus A (1984) Am Soc Bone Min Res A54
13. Broadus A, Goltzman D, Webb, A, Kronenberg H (1984) Clin Res 32:518A

30. Central Nervous System Peptides and Homeostasis

Endocrinology
F. Labrie, L. Proulx, eds.

CRF: INTEGRATION OF THE NEUROENDOCRINE AND AUTONOMIC NERVOUS SYSTEM RESPONSES TO STRESS

MARVIN R. BROWN and LAUREL A. FISHER

Peptide Biology Laboratory, The Salk Institute, 10010 North Torrey Pines Road, La Jolla, California 92037

Corticotropin releasing factor (CRF) is released into hypophyseal portal blood following stress, and is thought to be the principle physiologic stimulator of ACTH release (12,16). This notion is based on the observations that ACTH secretion can be prevented by systemic administration of either antisera directed against CRF or a CRF receptor antagonist (13,14). The hypothesis that CRF might be involved in the regulation of the autonomic nervous system and visceral organ physiology is supported by the neuroanatomic distribution of this peptide (15). In addition, we have previously noted that several of the hypophysiotropic peptides are capable of eliciting neurobiological actions that complement their pituitary actions (2). Thus, it is conceivable that a brain peptide involved in stimulating ACTH secretion following stress might also participate in generating other stress-induced changes of animal physiology, such as those in the autonomic nervous system.

CNS Effects of CRF on the Sympathetic Nervous System and Adrenal Medulla

CRF given intracerebroventricularly (icv) to the rat or dog elicits dose-related elevations of plasma epinephrine and norepinephrine concentrations (1,4). Since no significant increases of plasma CRF levels are detected following icv administration of CRF (10), it is unlikely that this peptide leaks from the central nervous system (CNS) to modify plasma catecholamine concentrations through a peripheral site of action. Further evidence that the elevation of plasma catecholamine levels following icv administration of CRF results from a CNS action of this peptide is provided by experiments in which animals were given intravenous (iv) injections of CRF antisera and icv injections of CRF. This antisera given iv prevents the changes in plasma catecholamine levels following iv injection of CRF but not following icv injection of CRF. Thus, these results support the contention that CRF given icv acts within the CNS to increase plasma concentrations of catecholamines.

CRF-induced Hyperglycemia

CRF given icv produces an increase in plasma glucose concentrations that is not prevented by hypophysectomy or adrenalectomy but is prevented by ganglionic blockade with chlorisondamine or by systemic administration of somatostatin (4). CRF-induced hyperglycemia is accompanied by an elevation of plasma glucagon concentrations and a relative lowering of plasma insulin concentrations. We conclude that CRF-induced hyperglycemia is mediated by catecholamine-evoked elevations of plasma glucagon levels and suppression of insulin secretion with a resultant increase of hepatic glucose production.

CNS Effects of CRF on the Cardiovascular System

CRF injected icv increases mean arterial pressure and heart rate in the dog and rat (1,9). In contrast, intravenous administration of CRF lowers mean arterial pressure (5,8). Recent studies in the rat demonstrate that CRF given icv produces an increase in cardiac output and stroke volume, and a decrease in peripheral vascular resistance (Brown and Fisher, unpublished data). Thus, in spite of high plasma catecholamine concentrations, CRF-induced cardiovascular changes represent those of increased flow and decreased resistance favoring maximum tissue perfusion. CRF-induced tachycardia may be mediated by increased cardiac sympathetic nervous stimulation and/or decreased cardiac parasympathetic nervous innervation. To further explore the CNS effects of CRF on heart rate, experiments were carried out in animals receiving the α-adrenergic agonist, phenylephrine. Phenylephrine given intravenously produces an increase of mean arterial pressure accompanied by a baroreceptor reflex-mediated slowing of heart rate. Icv administration of CRF blunts the reflex bradycardia in response to phenylephrine-induced elevations of mean arterial pressure, suggesting that CRF interferes with baroreceptor reflex-induced changes in heart rate.

CRF-induced elevations of mean arterial pressure and heart rate are not prevented by hypophysectomy or adrenalectomy, or by administration of a vasopressin receptor antagonist or the angiotensin converting enzyme inhibitor, captopril (8). CRF-induced elevations of mean arterial pressure and heart rate are prevented by administration of the ganglionic blocker, chlorisondamine (8,9). We conclude that CRF influences sympathetic and parasympathetic nervous efferents so as to increase venous return and elevate heart rate thereby resulting in an increase in cardiac output. CRF-induced increases in mean arterial pressure are secondary to an increase in cardiac output rather than an increase in peripheral vascular resistance.

Is CRF Involved in the Physiologic Regulation of the Autonomic Nervous System?

Three methods have been used to assess the role of endogenous brain CRF in the physiologic regulation of the autonomic nervous system. The first technique consisted of passive immunization with icv injections of CRF antisera. No consistent effect of the CRF antisera was observed on stress-induced elevations of plasma catecholamines levels.

The second approach used to assess the role of endogenous brain CRF in the regulation of the autonomic nervous system involved glucocorticoid treatment (6). The rationale for these experiments was based on the observations that dexamethasone inhibits stress-induced release of CRF into the hypophyseal portal system (12) and that adrenalectomy leads to an increase of brain and spinal cord concentrations of CRF as assessed by immunocytochemistry (11). Thus, it seemed reasonable to speculate that glucocorticoids may be used as a tool to inhibit brain CRF release. Indeed, dexamethasone treatment suppressed ether-vapor-induced elevations of plasma epinephrine and norepinephrine concentrations (6). Similarly, corticosterone, administered at a dose that produces 50% inhibition of ACTH secretion, also suppressed ether-vapor-induced elevations of plasma epinephrine and norepinephrine concentrations. Consistent with these results, removal of endogenous glucocorticoids by acute bilateral adrenalectomy (24 hours prior to the experiment) produced an accentuated elevation of plasma norepinephrine levels in response to ether-vapor exposure and this effect was prevented by administration of dexamethasone (6). Dexamethasone treatment does not cause a generalized impairment of sympathetic nervous system function since neither CRF- nor CGRP-induced elevations of plasma catecholamine levels are prevented by glucocorticoid administration (6). These studies support the idea that endogenous brain CRF may participate in the regulation of the sympathetic nervous system and adrenal medulla.

The third method used to study the role of endogenous brain CRF in the regulation of the sympathetic nervous system utilizes the newly developed CRF receptor antagonists. α-helical-CRF(9-41) given intracisternally suppresses insulin- and ether-vapor-induced elevations of plasma epinephrine levels but not those of norepinephrine (7). The question of why the CRF antagonists inhibit stress-induced elevations of plasma epinephrine levels but not norepinephrine levels is not resolved at this time. Since exogenous CRF administration elevates both epinephrine and norepinephrine concentrations in plasma, several possibilities exist that may explain this finding. First, the CRF receptor antagonists could possess different binding affinities to brain CRF receptors involved in the regulation of adrenal epinephrine release versus noradrenergic nerve release of norepinephrine. Second, the CRF antagonist may not gain access to the site of action of endogenous CRF that is involved in the regulation of norepinephrine release. Third, endogenous CRF may not participate in the regulation of peripheral norepinephrine release. Fourth, endogenous CRF may participate in the regulation of norepinephrine release, but if CRF receptors are blocked, other redundant pathways may co-opt this function. These results do suggest, as previously reported, that adrenal medullary epinephrine secretion and peripheral noradrenergic activity are regulated independently (2,3).

In conclusion, CRF, in addition to the regulation of pituitary ACTH secretion, may be involved in the physiologic regulation of the autonomic nervous system. CRF acts within the CNS to modify sympathetic, parasympathetic and adrenomedullary efferent pathways that in turn result in metabolic and cardiovascular changes. These neuroendocrine-induced changes in metabolic substrate availability and cardiovascular function may represent a generalized adaptive response to various types of stress that is coordinated by a single peptide, CRF.

ACKNOWLEDGEMENTS

Research supported by NIH grant AM26741. This research conducted in part by the Clayton Foundation for Research - California Division. MRB is a Clayton Foundation Investigator. The authors thank D. Weigand and S. Logan for manuscript preparation.

REFERENCES

1. Brown MR, Fisher LA (1983) Brain Res 280:75
2. Brown MR, Fisher LA (1984) J Amer Med Assn 251:1310
3. Brown MR, Fisher LA (1984) Am J Physiol 247:E41
4. Brown MR, Fisher LA, Spiess J, Rivier C, Rivier J, Vale W (1982) Endocrinology 111:928
5. Brown MR, Fisher LA, Spiess J, Rivier J, Rivier C, Vale W (1982) Regul Pept 4:107
6. Brown MR, Fisher LA, Vale WW (1983) Soc Neurosci Abstr 9:391
7. Brown MR, Fisher LA, Vale WW, Rivier JE (1984) Soc Neuro Abstr in press
8. Fisher LA, Jessen G, Brown MR (1983) Regul Pept 5:153-161
9. Fisher LA, Rivier J, Rivier C, Spiess J, Vale W, Brown MR (1982) Endocrinology 110:2222
10. Lenz HJ, Fisher LA, Rivier J, Vale W, Brown MR (1982) Gastroenterology 84:1228
11. Merchenthaler I, Hynes MA, Vigh S, Schally AV, Petrusz P (1983) Brain Res 275:373
12. Plotsky PM, Vale W (1984) Endocrinology 114:164
13. Rivier C, Rivier J, Vale W (1982) Science 218:377
14. Rivier J, Rivier C, Vale W (1984) Science 224:889
15. Swanson LW, Sawchenko PE, Rivier J, Vale WW (1983) Neuroendocrinology 36:165
16. Vale W, Spiess J, Rivier C, Rivier J (1981) Science 213:1394

Endocrinology
F. Labrie, L. Proulx, eds.

THE ROLE OF PEPTIDES IN THE CONTROL OF FOOD INTAKE

STEPHEN C. WOODS and DANIEL PORTE, JR

Depts. of Psychology and of Medicine, and the Regional Primate Research Center, Univ. of Washington, and the Veterans Administration Research Center, Seattle, WA, U.S.A.

INTRODUCTION

Interest has recently focused upon the possibility that naturally occurring hormones may be important modulators of appetite. The control of food intake by endogenous compounds has obvious appeal over the use of exogenous drugs, and this research area has mushroomed over the decade since synthetic peptides have been widely available and applied to behavioral research.

Peptides probably function at many levels and areas of the brain in the control of food intake, but this short review will be limited to the role of peptides as within-meal satiety factors and as signals related to adiposity.

ADIPOSITY IS REGULATED

The amount of fat in the body is precisely regulated (1,2). The easiest demonstration of this is that adipose mass is rigorously defended. Adipose mass can be reduced via food restriction or dieting. However, once the regimen is relaxed, overeating occurs until the original level of adiposity is regained. This is the sad conclusion of most instances of weight loss in obese humans (3). Analogously, forced overfeeding results in increased body fat; and when the procedure is finished, hypophagia and weight loss occur (4). These and other types of experiments which make the same point are summarized elsewhere (1,2,5); the important concept is that information related to adipose mass is integrated into the overall control over food intake.

EVIDENCE THAT INSULIN PROVIDES AN ADIPOSITY-RELATED SIGNAL TO THE BRAIN

We believe that insulin provides a signal to the brain which is directly related to adipose mass. When we initially proposed this hypothesis in 1976 (6), there was little evidence that insulin could cross the blood brain barrier, and it was thought that insulin had no effect upon brain cells since they could utilize glucose in its absence. Since then, considerable evidence has been provided supporting the concept that insulin is an important signal to the brain.

Insulin is secreted into the blood in direct proportion to adipose mass (7). This is especially true of basal insulin which is highly correlated with adiposity both among and within individuals (1,7). However, insulin secretion is responsive to the fluxes and needs of fuels (especially glucose) in the body; it rises after meals and it wanes during exercise and stress (8). Only if one integrates total insulin secretion over large intervals, or else prevents eating, stress and exercise (i.e., attains "basal" conditions), can adiposity be inferred from plasma insulin. We therefore consider plasma insulin to be an unlikely herald of adiposity to the brain. However, we (9) and others (10) have found that insulin penetrates into the cerebrospinal fluid (CSF) from the blood and that CSF insulin levels are an integral over time of plasma values (9). CSF insulin, like plasma insulin, is elevated in obese animals (11). CSF insulin, therefore, may approximate total insulin secretion over time and be better correlated with adiposity than moment-to-moment plasma values.

Our group, like others, has found immunoreactive insulin to be present in the brain in small quantities and to be relatively concentrated in specific sites, including the hypothalamus (12). Although controversy exists as to the source of brain insulin, with some believing that a significant amount is synthesized within the brain itself (13), we have shown that when insulin is administered into the plasma, it gains access to the CSF (9), and others have shown that when insulin is administered into the plasma, it binds to specific brain insulin receptors (14). When insulin is administered into the CSF, it penetrates into the brain and attaches to specific binding sites (15). At least some of the insulin present within the brain therefore probably originates within the plasma.

In a direct test of our hypothesis that insulin provides a functional adiposity signal to the brain, we administered insulin into the CSF of baboons and observed a dose-related decrease of food intake and body weight (16). Similar results have more recently been found for rats (17), and the administration of insulin antibodies into the hypothalamus of rats causes increased eating (18).

PEPTIDES AND SATIETY

Gibbs et al. initially reported that the administration of either extracted cholecystokinin or its synthetic C-terminal octapeptide (CCK-8) causes a dose-dependent reduction of meal size, and this basic finding has been replicated in many species including humans (see 19, 20). Since then, numerous other gut peptides have been reported to reduce meal size when administered just prior to the initiation of eating (20,21). The hypothesis is that these peptides are secreted in response to food in the gut, and that they build up during a meal until a sufficient signal is generated to turn off eating (see 19). The mechanism by which these satiety peptides influence eating is not clear.

OPIOID PEPTIDES INCREASE MEAL SIZE

Most of the known opioid peptides, including enkephalins, beta-endorphin, and dynorphine, increase meal size (21,22). Because these peptides are intimately involved with hedonic and motivated behaviors, it is possible that they act by increasing the positive aspects of food (see 21). It is not clear whether these compounds are secreted during meals in a way analogous to the gut peptides. It is more likely that these opioid peptides are central neuromodulators of the reinforcing and gustatory aspects of food.

INTERACTION OF SATIETY PEPTIDES WITH CENTRAL INSULIN

At some level, the myriad signals related to adiposity, the contents of the meal being consumed, and the social setting, must all become integrated to determine meal offset. We are testing the hypothesis that insulin acting at the brain interacts with satiety peptides to create a feeling of satiety (23). Baboons were initially given CCK-8 intravenously until the largest dose which did not reduce meal size was determined (the "probe" dose). Insulin was then infused directly into the CSF at a dose which had no effect on food intake. When the probe dose of CCK-8 was then given intravenously, meal size was reduced by around 90%. Insulin within the CSF therefore appears to change the sensitivity to the satiating effect of CCK-8. When an animal eats excess food, it gets fatter and secretes more insulin. Some of this insulin enters the CSF, gains access to critical brain areas, and increases the gain of the CCK satiating response. The animal eats smaller meals until its former weight is attained. Analogously, when one diets and loses weight, insulin secretion is reduced and less insulin penetrates into the CSF and brain. More CCK (and presumably other satiety peptides as well) is required to stop eating, so larger meals are consumed until weight is returned to normal.

ACKNOWLEDGMENTS

This research was supported by NIH Grants AM17844, AM12829, AM17047, and RR00166.

REFERENCES

1. Bray G (1976) The Obese Patient. Saunders, Philadelphia
2. Keesey RE (1980) In: Stunkard AJ (ed) Obesity. Saunders, Philadelphia, pp 144-165
3. Johnson D, Drenick EJ (1977) Arch Intern Med 137: 1381-1382
4. Sims EAH, Goldman RJ, Gluck CM, Horton ES, Keleher DC, Rowe DW (1968) Trans Assoc Am Physicians 81: 153-170
5. Woods SC, Porte,Jr D (1983) Adv Met Dis 10: 457-468
6. Woods SC, Porte,Jr D (1976) In: Novin D, Bray GA, Wyrwichka W (eds) Hunger Basic Mechanisms and Clinical Impressions. Raven Press, New York, pp 273-280

7. Woods SC, Decke E, Vasselli JR (1974) Psych Rev 81: 26-43

8. Porte,Jr D, Woods SC (1983) In: Ellenberg M, Rifkin H (eds) Diabetes Mellitus. Theory and Practice (3rd Ed). Med Exam Publ, New Hyde Park, NY, pp 267-294

9. Woods SC, Porte,Jr D (1977) Am J Physiol 233: E331-E334

10. Margolis RU, Altszuler N (1967) Nature (London) 215: 1375-1376

11. Stein LJ, Dorsa DM, Baskin DG, Figlewicz DP, Ikeda H, Frankmann SP, Greenwood MRC, Porte,Jr D, Woods SC (1983) Endocrinology 113:2299-2301

12. Baskin DG, Porte,Jr D, Guest K, Dorsa DM (1983) Endocrinology 112:898

13. Havrankova J, Brownstein M, Roth J (1981) Diabetologia 20(Suppl):268-273

14. Van Houten M, Posner BI (181) Diabetologia 20(Suppl):255-267

15. Baskin DB, Woods SC, West DB, Van Houten M, Posner BI, Dorsa DM, Porte, Jr D (1983) Endocrinology 113:1818-1825

16. Woods SC, Lotter EC, McKay LD, Porte,Jr D (1979) Nature 282:503-505

17. Brief DJ, Davis JD (1981) Soc Neurosci Abstr 7:655

18. Strubbe JH, Mein CG (1977) Physiol Behav 19: 309-313

19. Smith GP, Gibbs J (1979) Prog Psychobiol Physiol Psychol 8:179-242

20. Woods SC, West DB, Stein LJ, McKay LD, Kenney NJ, Porte SG, Lotter EC, Porte,Jr D (1981) Diabetologia 20:305-313

21. Morley JE, Levine AS (1982) In: Hoebel BG, Novin D (eds) The Neural Basis of Feeding and Reward. Haer Institute, Brunswick, Maine, pp 499-506

22. McKay LD, Kenney NJ, Williams RH, Woods SC (1981) Life Sciences 29:1429-1434

23. Woods SC, Ikeda H, Stein LJ, Figlewicz DP, West DB, Porte,Jr D (1983) Appetite 4:233

Endocrinology
F. Labrie, L. Proulx, eds.

BRAIN PEPTIDES AND CARDIOVASCULAR CONTROL

DETLEV GANTEN, THOMAS UNGER, RUDOLF E. LANG

German Institute for High Blood Pressure Research and Department of Pharmacology, University of Heidelberg, Im Neuenheimer Feld 366, D-6900 Heidelberg, FRG

Using immunohistochemical and biochemical methods, an ever increasing number of peptides have been found in the brain. Evidence favouring a role of angiotensin, opioid peptides, substance P, vasopressin, kinins, corticotropin releasing factor and other peptides such as bombesin and somatostatin in central blood pressure regulation arises from neuroanatomical observations as well as from pharmacological and biochemical studies:

1) These peptides have been localized in brain areas known to be important in cardiovascular control. 2) Specific peptide receptors with high affinity have been discovered in the brain. 3) Upon central administration the peptides produce blood pressure effects which can be prevented by competitive antagonists. 4) They interact with other blood pressure-controlling neuroregulators, e.g. catecholamines or GABA. 5) Central inhibition of brain peptide synthesis or interaction with brain peptide receptors results in marked cardiovascular effects. 6) Peptide levels and the activity of synthesizing enzymes is altered in hypertensive states. 7) Supersensitivity to the pressor action of some brain peptides in experimental models of hypertension has been described (for review see 1).

Angiotensin circulates as a hormone in the blood and is also present in the brain (2,3). Angiotensin II (ANG II) induces salt appetite and drinking behavior by an action on the brain and it reduces salt excretion by the kidney; the latter is brought about by a direct action of hormonal plasma ANG II on the kidney tubules and by releasing the mineralocorticoid hormone aldosterone from the adrenal gland which in turn promotes water and salt reabsorption. Further, ANG II increases the secretion of AVP from the posterior lobe of the pituitary. AVP then causes the reabsorption of water from the urine. In addition to its peripheral salt and volume preserving actions, ANG II increases blood pressure by an action within the central nervous system and by direct vasoconstriction of the peripheral arterioles. As a circulating hormone in the blood and as a neuropeptide in the central nervous system ANG II thus acts in a coordinated way to prevent water and salt loss. In the case of pathophysiological disturbances, overactivity of hormonal and neuronal angiotensin results in the development of high blood pressure. Inhibitors of the renin angiotensin system are clinically used as antihypertensive agents.

The opioid peptides provide a further example of an integrating function of neuropeptides. Enkephalins, endorphins and other opioid peptides occur in the central nervous system and in peripheral nerves as neuropeptides. In addition, they are released as hormes from the pituitary gland into the blood and they are also secreted (together with the catecholamines) from the adrenal gland. Cardiovascular effects have been described at all locations, probably mediated via different receptors (4,5).

Substance P is not only involved in the transmission of afferent sensory input to the brain but appears to generate a complex behavioral pattern known as the "arousal" or "defense" reaction. It induces motor activation, increase in blood pressure, selective release of stress hormones from the pituitary gland and generalized stimulation of the sympatho-adrenal system (6,7).

Corticotropin releasing factor (CRF) may also participate in the integration of cardiovascular and humoral responses to different kinds of stress. CRF has been localized in a number of hypothalamic and extrahypothalamic nuclei including the limbic system and cardiovascular centers in the medulla oblongata. Apart from releasing ACTH and ß-endorphin from the pituitary, it also increases blood pressure by stimulation of sympathetic tone. Humoral and neuronal pathways are thus activated to achieve a concerted cardiovascular response to stress (8).

Vasopressin is instrumental in fluid and volume homeostasis and like angiotensin seems to exert its effects centrally and peripherally. However, its central actions may be even more complex than those of ANG II. The pressor effects on one hand and the pressor inhibiting action on the other, evoked by its central application, suggest that this peptide can activate blood pressure increasing and blood pressure lowering pathways. This may be explained by the fact that AVP can be stimulated by isoosmotic hypovolaemia as well as by normo- or hypervolaemic hyperosmolality. In the first case (e.g. following haemorrhage) an antidiuretic and pressor action of AVP would be logical to regain volume homeostasis and to improve the haemodynamic situation. In the case of stimulation of AVP by hyperosmolality a depressor action together with renal water reabsorption might be the more adequate response, since there is no volume deficit and blood pressure may be normal or already increased (4).

Mode of action: No meaningful generalisation about the mode of action can probably be made for so large a group of molecules which represent the neuropeptides, but there are some special features which merit to be pointed out in this context. Neuropeptides frequently coexist with each other or with monoamine transmitters, thereby greatly increasing the number of different chemical signals that a neuron can release and use in communicating with other cells. It is possible that the "synaptic cocktail" consisting of peptides, monoamines and amino acids is being released simultaneously if these are packaged together in one vesicle of a given nerve ending. They may, however, also be released separately. Peptide actions in general take place over a slower time course and over longer distances ("neuro-hormonal" action) than is the case for rapid synaptic transmission. A fundamental difference between biogenic amines, amino acids and peptides is their mode of synthesis and metabolism. Peptides are not as rapidly degraded as classic transmitters and they are probably not recycled. The different speed of synthesis, transport and replenishment opens up interesting possibilities, e.g. that the same repeated stimulus will in a graded way elicit different postsynaptic patterns in peptidergic and non-peptidergic neurons. The relevance of this for cardiovascular control remains to be investigated; the functional subdivision of the autonomic nervous system according to the colocalization of peptides has, however, opened new vistas for the understanding and possible treatment of hypertensive desease.

REFERENCES

1. Ganten D, Pfaff D (eds) (1983) In: Central Cardiovascular Control; Current Topics in Neuroendocrinology, Vol. 3. Springer-Verlag Berlin, Heidelberg, New York.

2. Printz M, Ganten D, Unger Th, Phillips MI (1982) Minireview: The brain renin angiotensin system 1982. In: Exp Brain Res (Suppl 4) The renin angiotensin system in the brain, eds Ganten D, Printz M, Phillips MI, Schölkens BA, Berlin, Heidelberg, New York, Springer, pp 2-52

3. Ganten D, Hermann K, Bayer C, Unger Th, Lang RE (1983) Angiotensin synthesis in the brain and increased turnover in hypertensive rats. Science 221,4613:869-871

4. Lang RE, Gaida W, Ganten D, Hermann K, Kraft K, Unger Th (1983) Neuropeptides and central blood pressure regulation. In: Current Topics in Neuroendocrinology (Vol 3): Central cardiovascular control - basic and clinical aspects, eds Ganten D, Pfaff D, Springer Berlin, Heidelberg, New York, Tokyo, pp 103-123

5. Holaday JW (1983) Cardiovascular effects of endogenous opiate systems. Ann Rev Pharmacol Toxicol 23: 541-594

6. Unger Th, Rascher W, Schuster C, Pavlovic R, Schömig A, Dietz R, Ganten D (1981) Central blood pressure effects of substance P and angiotensin II: Role of the sympathetic nervous system and vasopressin. Europ J Pharmacol 71: 33-42

7. Pernow B (1983) Substance P. Pharmacol Rev 35: 85-141

8. Brown MR, Fischer LA, Spiess J, Rivier I, Rivier C, Vale W (1982) Corticotropin releasing factor (CRF): effects on the sympathetic nervous system (SNS), vasopressin release and cardiovascular regulation. Endocrinology (Suppl) 110:225.

© 1984 Elsevier Science Publishers B.V.
Endocrinology
F. Labrie, L. Proulx, eds.

RECEPTORS AND ACTIONS OF ANGIOTENSIN II (AII) AND CORTICOTROPIN-RELEASING FACTOR (CRF) IN SPECIFIC REGIONS OF THE CENTRAL NERVOUS SYSTEM

G. AGUILERA, P.C. WYNN, R.L. HAUGER, M.C. HOLMES, M.A. MILLAN, F.A.O. MENDELSOHN, C. GREWE, AND K.J. CATT

Endocrinology Reproduction Research Branch, National Institute of Child Health and Human Development, National Institutes of Health, Bethesda, MD 20205

The individual functions of the endocrine and nervous systems have been extensively studied, but little is known about the integration of the two systems during homeostatic adaptations to stress. Both AII and CRF are present in the brain, and mimic several behavioral, visceral and endocrine stress responses on intraventricular injection (1,2), suggesting that they may act in the central coordination of endocrine and neural mechanisms involved in homeostasis. Since such actions must be expressed through specific binding sites in the central nervous system (CNS), we have characterized brain receptors for AII and CRF, and compared their anatomical distributions with the central actions of both peptides.

ANGIOTENSIN II RECEPTORS IN THE BRAIN.

The well-established CNS effects of AII include stimulation of drinking, increased sodium appetite and blood pressure, and modulation of pituitary hormone release. These effects, and the presence of AII receptors and all components of the renin-angiotensin system in the CNS, suggest that AII may act as a neuropeptide. Specific AII receptors were found in homogenates of several brain regions, with highest concentrations in the SFO, OVLT and AP (3). To determine whether the central effects of AII are accompanied by relevant changes in receptor concentration, AII receptors were analyzed in the circumventricular organs of control and 48-hr water deprived rats (3). In 10 experiments, AII

Abbreviations: AA anterior amygdoloid area; ACg anterior cingulate cortex; Acb nucleus accumbens; AC amygdala complex; AP area postrema; Arc arcuate nucleus; BST bed nucleus stria terminalis; Cl claustrum; CPu caudate putamen; DM dorsomedial hypothalamic nucleus; EPI external plexiform layer, olfactory bulb; Fr prefrontal cortex; FrPaM fronto-parietal cortex, motor; FrPaS fronto-parietal cortex, sensory; Hi hippocampus; IP interpeduncular nucleus; LC locus coeruleus; ME median eminence; MPA medial preoptic area; MPN median preoptic nucleus; NTS nucleus tractus solitarius; OA anterior olfactory nucleus; OVLT organum vasculosum lamina terminalis; PCg posterior cingulate cortex; PeV periventricular nucleus; PVA paraventricular thalamic nucleus, anterior; PVN paraventricular nucleus; Pn pontine nucleus; RSpl retrosplenial cortex; Sbc subiculum; Sch suprachiasmatic nucleus; SFO subfornical organ; SuC superior colliculus; Str striate cortex; TS triangular septum.

binding sites in the SFO were increased by 50% ($p<0.005$), with no change in other areas. This increase could represent positive regulation of SFO receptors by the plasma AII levels during dehydration, with consequent enhancement of the drinking response.

Analysis of ^{125}I-[Sar]AII binding in rat brain sections by _in vitro_ autoradiography revealed a characteristic pattern of AII receptors, predominately localized at known sites of action of the peptide (4). Structures involved in the drinking response to AII, including the SFO, OVLT, medial preoptic area, and median preoptic nucleus, all contained moderate to high densities of AII receptors (Fig. 1-A), suggesting that the neural connections between these nuclei are angiotensinergic. The absence of AII receptors in the SON, which is connected to the latter pathway and is involved in drinking and vasopressin secretion, is consistent with reports that injection of AII into the SON does not affect drinking or vasopressin release. The effects of AII on vasopressin release are probably exerted at the level of the PVN, in view of the presence of abundant AII receptors (Fig 1-B) and immunoreactive AII in this area.

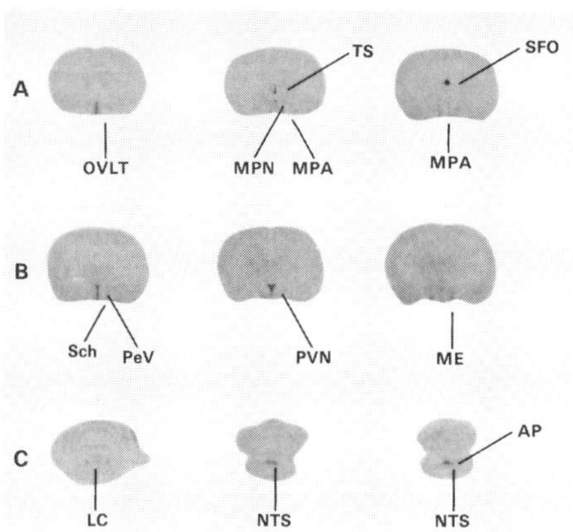

Fig 1. Autoradiographic mapping of AII receptors in rat brain.

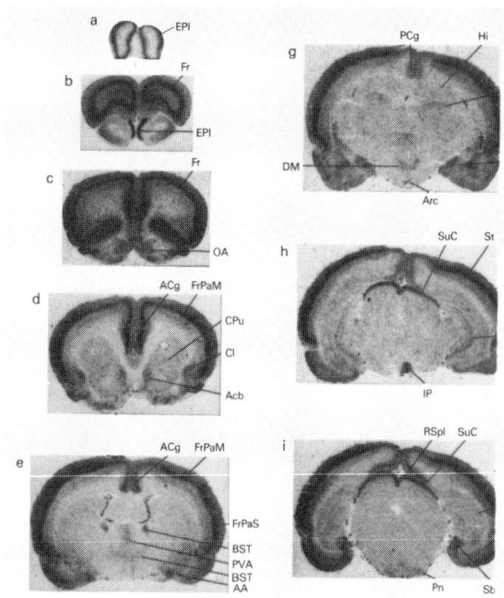

Fig 2. Autoradiographic mapping of CRF receptors in rat brain.

AII receptors were also present in the NTS, locus coeruleus, median preoptic nucleus, and area postrema (Fig. 1-A, C), areas relevant to the known central actions of AII on blood pressure. The central actions of AII are probably exerted through modulation of sympathetic activity, and several of the structures that contain AII receptors, including the NTS, locus coeruleus, and peri- and paraventricular hypothalamic nuclei, are associated with the central adrenergic system. AII is known to act on peripheral noradrenergic neurones to stimulate norephinephrine release (4), and may also be involved in the central regulation of norepinephrine and dopamine release in the brain regions. AII receptors also occur in a number of areas related to the limbic system (olfactory tract, superior colliculus, olivary nucleus and spinal trigeminal tract) indicating additional actions for AII in the control of hypothalamic and autonomic nervous system functions.

CRF RECEPTORS IN THE BRAIN

Receptors for CRF with similar properties to those described in the anterior pituitary (Ka 3.9±1.2 x 10^8) were identified in membrane-rich preparations from olfactory bulb, amygdala and cortex (5). As in the anterior pituitary, CRF stimulated adenylate cyclase activity (by 40%) in vesicular preparations from frontal cortex and amygdala, but had no effect in areas lacking CRF receptors. Autoradiographic analysis of ^{125}I-Tyr-CRF binding to frozen brain sections showed CRF receptors mainly in 2 functionally distinct systems, the neocortex and the limbic system (Fig. 2). CRF receptors were abundant throughout the cerebral cortex, with relatively high densities in the anterior cingulate cortex, frontoparietal and temporal cortex. They were most dense in the outer cortical layers, with the highest concentration in cortical layer IV followed by layers I to III. Cells containing immunoreactive CRF are scattered in all parts of the cortex within layers I and IV, suggesting that the peptide may act as an intracortical neurotransmitter (1). The claustrum, which is closely related to sensory areas of the neocortex, has efferent projections ending mainly in the cortical layer IV, which contains most of the cortical CRF receptors. Variable concentrations of CRF receptors were found in a number of structures related to the limbic system and the control of the autonomic nervous system (Fig 2). Correspondingly, cell bodies and fibers containing immunoreactive CRF are present in most of the areas in which CRF receptors are found (1). Also, intracerebral injections of CRF are known to cause many of the behavorial and viceral responses observed during stress and electrical stimulation of the limbic system (1). These findings support the view that the peptide acts as a neurotransmitter within the CNS, mediating responses to stress via CRF receptors in the limbic system. Incubation of rat hippocampus slices with nanomolar concentrations of CRF increases spontaneous discharge frequency in pyramidal neurones (1). This effect, and the local neuronal activation observed after microinjection on CRF in the locus coeruleus (6), is probably mediated by the receptors observed in these areas. The CRF receptors in the arcuate nucleus may be related to the inhibitory effect of CRF on sexual behavior when injected into the arcuate-ventromedial area of the hypothalamus (7).

Whereas both immunoreactive CRF and receptors are present in the cerebral cortex and limbic system, no CRF receptors were found in the median eminence or the PVN and periventricular nucleus of the hypothalamus. These regions possess the highest content of immunoreactive CRF in the brain, and are the source of CRF released into the portal circulation (1). These areas also contain AII (2) and high concentrations of AII receptors (Fig 1-B), suggesting that this peptide could be a regulator of CRF release. In this regard, blockade of endogenous AII formation in the brain by intraventricular injection of the converting enzyme inhibitor, Captopril, markedly reduces the plasma ACTH response to ether stress. In adult male rats, plasma ACTH levels rose from 33±4 to 262±24 pg/ml after 30 sec exposure to ether vapor. Following central converting enzyme inhibition, the rise in plasma ACTH levels was reduced by 55%, indicating that AII is necessary for the full response to stress. That AII stimulates CRF release is also suggested by the report that stimulation of ACTH secretion by intraventricular AII is blocked by anti-CRF serum (8). AII receptors and immunoreactive AII are also found in areas with projections to the PVN, including the locus coeruleus and dorsal vagal complex, important centers of autonomic nervous control, and in the suprachiasmatic nuclei, major regulatory centers of circadian rhythms (4). It is also possible that AII acts directly at the pituitary level (5), and by stimulating the release of other corticotropic factors such as vasopressin and norepinephrine (2).

High concentrations of CRF receptors were also found in the cerebellar cortex, mainly the granular layer. These receptors could mediate a modulatory role of the cerebellum on visceral function, as suggested by the existence of hypothalamic-cerebellar connections (9). The presence of functional CRF receptors in relevant areas of the brain supports the view that CRF has an important role as a neuropeptide in coordinating the integrated response to stress.

REFERENCES

1. Vale W, Rivier C, Brown MR, Spiess J, Koob G, Swanson L, Bilezikjian F, Bloom F, Rivier J (1983) Recent Prog in Hormone Res 39, 245
2. Phillips MI (1978) Neuroendocrinology 25:354-77
3. Catt KJ, Mendelsohn FAO, Millan MA, Aguilera G (1984) J Cardiovasc Res, in press
4. Zimmerman B (1972) Fed Proc 31:1344-50
5. Aguilera G, Wynn PC, Harwood JP, Hauger RL, Millan MA, Grewe C, Catt KJ (1984) Fed Proc, in press
6. Valentino RJ, Foote SL, Aston-Jones G, (1983) Brain Research 270:363
7. Sirinathsinghji DJS, Rees LH, Rivier J, Vale W (1983) Nature 305:232
8. Rivier C, Vale W (1983) Regulatory Peptides 7:253
9. Dietricks E (1984) Science 223:591

31. Regulation of Testicular Function

Endocrinology
F. Labrie, L. Proulx, eds.

HORMONAL CONTROL OF SERTOLI CELL FUNCTION

J.P. MATHER, P.L. MORRIS, V. PEREZ-INFANTE, Y.A. SALOMON, A. NAKHLA, G.L. GUNSALUS and C.W. BARDIN

The Population Council, 1230 York Avenue, New York, NY 10021

The Sertoli cell of the seminiferous tubule of the testis is a hormone-responsive cell which plays a crucial role in spermatogenesis. Early work on the hormonal regulation of Sertoli cell function focused on the effects of follicle stimulating hormone (FSH) and testosterone (T), both of which are required for full testicular function (1,2). More recently, insulin (3,4) and retinoids (5,6) have also been shown to stimulate Sertoli cell secretory activity.

The complex nature of the regulation of growth of the Sertoli-derived TM_4 cell line in serum free hormone-supplemented medium led us to believe that Sertoli cell function was under the control of a number of factors other than those mentioned above. We have used four measurements to identify the hormones, vitamins, transport proteins, and growth factors which affect Sertoli cell function *in vitro* by defining those elements which influence: 1) growth of the TM_4 cell line; 2) secretion of androgen binding protein (rABP) and/or transferrin (rTF) in primary Sertoli cell-enriched cultures derived from immature rat testis; 3) adenylate cyclase activity in TM_4 cells or primary Sertoli cell cultures; and 4) steroid or epidermal growth factor binding to specific receptors.

This approach was considered useful for determining which factors should be studied as possible regulators of specific Sertoli cell functions which may be characterized in future years. Detailed comparative studies of rTF and rABP secretion have shown that these two proteins are differentially regulated *in vitro* (6). The cyclical nature of Sertoli cell protein secretion in synchrony with the cycle of the seminiferous epithelium but with various proteins showing peak secretion at different stages of the cycle suggests that many proteins secreted by this cell are not coordinately regulated and may respond to different subsets of hormonal stimuli and groups of germ cells (7). The advantage of using Sertoli cell-enriched primary cultures and the TM_4 cell line is that only direct hormonal effects on Sertoli cells are measured.

We will summarize the results of these several studies below. Table 1 lists nineteen hormones, growth factors, transport proteins, and vitamins which elicit responses in Sertoli cells. Also shown are the receptor levels, in or on these cells, for some of these factors. The presence of specific receptors for steroids (8), epidermal growth factor (EGF) (9), and retinol (10,11) correlates well with Sertoli cell responsiveness to these factors.

Table 1: Sertoli cell responsiveness to and receptors for hormones, growth factors, vitamins and transport proteins in vitro.

Factor or Hormone	TM_4 cells: Receptor[1] Levels	TM_4 cells: Response AdCy[3]	TM_4 cells: Response Growth[2]	1° Sertoli cells: Receptor[1] Levels	1° Sertoli cells: Response AdCy[3]	1° Sertoli cells: Response Protein Secretion[4]
Insulin	ND	ND	+	ND	ND	A,T
Testosterone	68 ± 7	ND	+	85 ± 5	0	A,T
Estradiol	34 ± 4	ND	-	50 ± 6	0	A
Hydrocortisone	ND	ND	+	ND	0	A
Progesterone	10.0	ND	+	ND	0	A
Prostaglandin E_1	ND	S	0	ND	S	A
Iosproterenol	ND	S	0	ND	S	A
Calcitonin	ND	S	0	ND	S	A
αMSH	ND	S	ND	ND	S	ND
ACTH	ND	S	+	ND	S	A
FSH	ND	S	+	ND	S	A
EGF	35	ND	+	6	M	A,T
Somatomedin C	ND	ND	+	ND	ND	A,T
Ceruloplasmin	ND	ND	+	ND	M	A,T
Transferrin	ND	ND	+	ND	ND	A
HDL	ND	ND	+	ND	ND	ND
Vitamin E	ND	0	+	ND	M	A
Retinoic acid	ND	0	+	ND	M	T
Retinol	yes[5]	0	+	yes[6]	M	T

ND, not determined. 1) steroid receptors are expressed as fmoles/mg protein, EGF receptors as fmoles/10^6 cells. 2) +, growth stimulatory; -, growth inhibitory; 0, no effect. 3) S, stimulatory; M, modulates acute response to FSH, isoproterenol and/forskolin. 4) stimulates rABP (A) or rTF (T) secretion. 5) Reference 10. 6) Reference 11.

The Sertoli cell adenylate cyclase (AdCy) system can be stimulated by a number of hormones including, FSH, isoproterenol, ACTH, αMSH, prostaglandins E_1 and E_2, and calcitonin as well as the non-hormonal stimulators, forskolin and cholera toxin (12). There is a good correlation between the ability of these hormones to stimulate AdCy and their ability to increase rABP secretion in primary Sertoli cell cultures. A number of other factors, including ceruloplasmin, EGF, and vitamins E and A, which do not have a direct effect on AdCy, can modulate the acute response of this enzyme to FSH, isoproterenol, and/or forskolin (12).

Insulin and somatomedin C both stimulate the growth of TM_4 cells (13) and the survival of primary Sertoli cells *in vitro* (4). In addition, they stimulate both rABP and rTF secretion (4,6). Since the stimulation of rABP secretion is additive at optimal concentrations it seems likely that insulin and somatomedin C act via independent pathways.

Epidermal growth factor receptors are present on both TM_4 and primary Sertoli cells in culture. EGF is a major growth stimulator for the TM_4 cell line and stimulates both rTF and rABP secretion in primary Sertoli cell cultures. Receptors for testosterone, estradiol, and progesterone are present in Sertoli cells and these steroids, as well as hydrocortisone, all stimulate rABP secretion (4,6). Of these steroids only testosterone stimulates rTF secretion.

The transport proteins TF, ceruloplasmin, and high density lipoprotein all stimulate the growth of TM_4 cells (14,15). TF will stimulate rABP secretion under conditions where endogenous rTF secretion is low. Ceruloplasmin has given variable results as a stimulator of rTF and rABP secretion.

Finally, vitamins A and E, both known through animal studies to be required for male fertility, increase the growth of TM_4 cells and modulate the AdCy response to FSH. Retinol and retinoic acid are the major stimulators of rTF secretion *in vitro*.

The number of responses described above indicates that the humoral control of Sertoli cell function is much more complex than previously thought. It is also apparent that each functional activity is influenced by a different subset of hormones, growth factors, vitamins, and transport proteins. It is not known currently whether the specific responses studied reflect the major effects elicited by a specific hormone. Conversely, the occurrence of a measurable hormonal response *in vitro* does not tell us when in development or in which stages of the seminiferous cycle the Sertoli cell responds to these factors, if at all. An *in vitro* response to a hormone or the presence of receptors does tell us that the Sertoli cell is capable of responding to these factors but implies their role in testicular physiology should be further explored. Finally, the functional activity of Sertoli cells has been shown to be controlled not only by soluble factors but also by Sertoli-germ cell (16) and Sertoli-peritubular myoid cell interactions (17,18) and by insoluble extracellular matrix components (19). The critical role of this cell in spermatogenesis and the complex nature of the regulation of its functional activities makes Sertoli cell culture a fruitful and challenging system for further study.

REFERENCES

1. Fritz IB (1978) In: G Litwack (eds) Biochemical Action of Hormones. vol. V Academic Press, Inc., New York, p 249

2. Means AR, Dedman JR, Tash JS, Tindall DJ, Sickle M, and Welsh MJ (1980) Ann Rev Physiol 42:59-70

3. Karl A and Griswold MD (1980) Biochem J 186:1001-1003

4. Rich KA, Bardin CW, Gunsalus GL, and Mather JP (1983) Endocrinology 113:2284-2293

5. Skinner MK and Griswold MD (1982) Biol Reprod 27:211-221

6. Perez-Infante V, Bardin CW, Gunsalus GL, Musto N, Rich KA, and Mather JP (1984) Endocrinology (submitted)

7. Wright WW, Parvinen M, Musto NA, Gunsalus GL, Phillips DM, Mather JP, and Bardin CW (1983) Biol Reprod 29:257-270

8. Nakhla AM, Mather JP, and Bardin CW (1984) J Clin Endocrinol (in press)

9. Chen C-L, Mather JP, Morris PL, and Bardin CW (1984) Proc Natl Acad Sci USA (submitted)

10. Carson DD, Rosenberg LI, Blaner WS, Kato M, and Lannarz WJ (1984) J Biol Chem 259:3117-3123

11. Huggenvik J and Griswold MD (1981) J Reprod Fertil 61:403-408

12. Salomon Y, Bardin CW, Gunsalus GL, Byer AL, and Mather JP (1984) Molec Cell Endocrinol (submitted)

13. Mather JP and Furlanetto R (1983) In: EM Spencer (eds) Insulin-like Growth Factors/Somatomedins: Basic Chemistry, Biology and Clinical Importance. Walter de Gruyter & Co., New York, p 451-458

14. Perez-Infante V and Mather JP (1982) Ann NY Acad Sci 383:488-490

15. Mather JP (1982) In Vitro 18:990-996

16. Parvinen M (1982) Endocrinol Rev 3:404-417

17. Tung PS and Fritz IB (1980) Biol Reprod 23:227-242

18. Mather JP and Phillips DM (1984) J Ultrastruct Res (in press)

19. Mather JP, Wolpe SD, Gunsalus GL, Bardin CW, and Phillips DM (1984) Ann NY Acad Sci (in press)

© 1984 Elsevier Science Publishers B.V.
Endocrinology
F. Labrie, L. Proulx, eds.

THE INTERACTIONS OF SERTOLI CELL GLYCOPROTEINS WITH GERMINAL CELLS IN THE TESTIS

MICHAEL D. GRISWOLD, JODI HUGGENVIK, MICHAEL K. SKINNER, S. R. SYLVESTER
Program in Biochemistry/Biophysics, Washington State University, Pullman, WA 99164-4660 (USA)

INTRODUCTION

Because of their unique morphological arrangement in the testis, the Sertoli cells have traditionally been regarded as "nurse" cells whose function is to provide an appropriate biochemical milieu in which germinal cell development can proceed (1). Even though it is clear that Sertoli cells secrete several glycoproteins and metabolites, evidence for the direct *in vivo* interaction between these products and germinal cells has been lacking. It has been and remains the goal of our research to identify, characterize and localize in the testis the major glycoprotein secretion products of Sertoli cells. In addition, we have examined the synthesis of these glycoproteins in an effort to determine the regulation of Sertoli cell functions both in cell culture and *in vivo*.

METHODS AND MATERIALS

The methods used in these studies have been described in detail elsewhere.

Cell culture - Sertoli cells from 20 day old rats were prepared and maintained in culture in Ham's F-12 medium (2).

Immunofluorescence - Paraffin embedded sections of Bouin's fixed adult rat testes were deparaffinized and rehydrated. Sections were preincubated in buffer containing 1% calf serum for 10 min prior to staining. Rabbit antisera to rat transferrin or to rat DAG-protein were diluted 50 to 100 fold and incubated on the tissue overnight. The slides were washed with buffer, and incubated with 1:100 dilution of biotinylated goat anti-rabbit IgG for 2 hr. The slides were further washed and incubated with FITC-avidin, re-washed and viewed with a Nikon Model-Ke microscope equipped for epifluorescence illumination and photomicroscopy (3).

Results and Discussion - When Sertoli cells from 20 day old rats are placed in cell culture, they continue to synthesize and secrete glycoproteins (4). If these secretion products are labeled with ^{35}S-methionine and analyzed by 2-dimensional polyacrylamide gel electrophoresis and fluorography several major polypeptides are detected (Fig. 1). Many of these polypeptides exhibit charge heterogeneity characteristic of sialated glycoproteins. Several of the major polypeptides on this electrophoretogram have been purified and identified. Polypeptides numbered 1 and 2 have been shown to be testicular

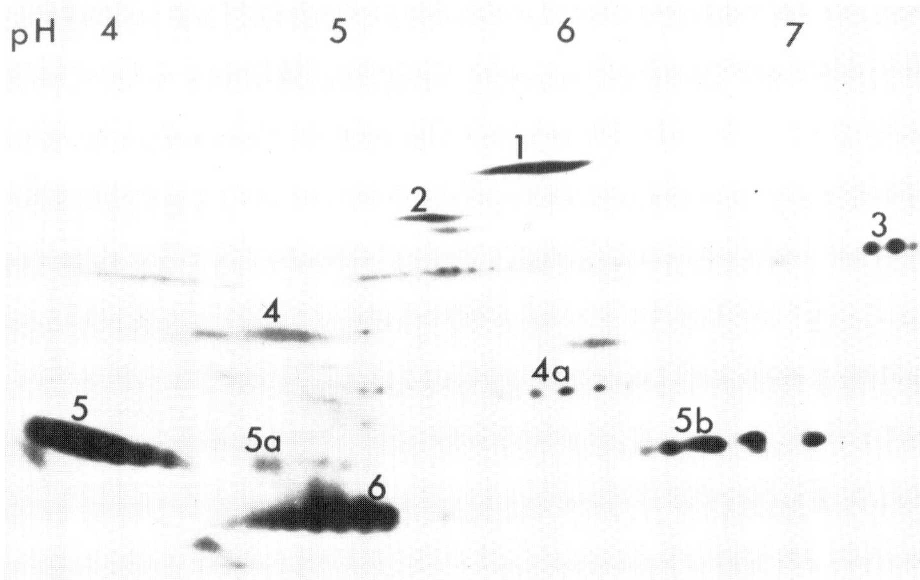

Fig. 1. Fluorogram of 2-dimensional polyacrylamide gel electrophoresis analysis of ^{35}S-methionine labeled proteins secreted by cultured Sertoli cells. The molecular weight of the polypeptides are 1-130 Kdal; 2-115 Kdal; 3-75 Kdal; 5-41 Kdal; 6-29 Kdal.

ceruloplasmin and a proteolytic fragment of testicular ceruloplasmin, respectively (5). Number 4a has been shown to be secreted by peritubular myoid cells which are present in low numbers in Sertoli cell cultures (4). Number 3 has been identified as testicular transferrin (6) and numbers 5 and 6 are monomers of a disulfide linked acidic glycoprotein (DAG-protein) (4). By a number of different analytical procedures, it was estimated that transferrin accounts for 7-15% and DAG-protein for 30-50% of the total mass of the secreted proteins. Most of our further studies have focused on the biochemistry and localization of transferrin and the DAG-protein.

Testicular transferrin was purified from spent Sertoli cell culture medium by a combination of hydrophobic chromatography and immuno-affinity chromatography. The polypeptide portion of rat testicular transferrin is identical to that of rat hepatic transferrin (7). The synthesis of transferrin by cultured Sertoli cells was examined by radioimmunoassay and by hybridization

TABLE I

SECRETION OF TRANSFERRIN AND ACCUMULATION OF TRANSFERRIN mRNA BY CULTURED SERTOLI CELLS

The transferrin was measured by a radioimmunoassay of spent medium from cultured Sertoli cells accumulated over a 2 day period on days 4-6 of cultures. The mRNA was measured in similar cultures on day 4 by hybridization of poly A^+ RNA to nick translated DNA for transferrin.

Hormone treatment	mg Transferrin/ 10^5 cells/48hr (avg. of 9 determinations)	cpm ^{32}P DNA hybridized/ ng cellular DNA (avg. of 12 determinations)
control	25 $\pm$ 5	90,960$\pm$18,800
FSH, Insulin, Retinol, Testosterone	164 $\pm$ 22	209,190$\pm$68,000

of mRNA to a nick translated cloned cDNA probe constructed from purified transferrin mRNA. (8, 9) Using these analyses, it was shown that the secretion of transferrin and the presence of transferrin mRNA were maximal and were stimulated when the cells were cultured in the presence of FSH, insulin, retinol and testosterone. (Table I) Antisera to transferrin was used to localize the protein on fixed paraffin embedded sections of testis (3). The transferrin was localized in the interstitium as hepatic or serum transferrin and in the acrosome region of developing spermatids, presumably as testicular transferrin (Fig. 2, left).

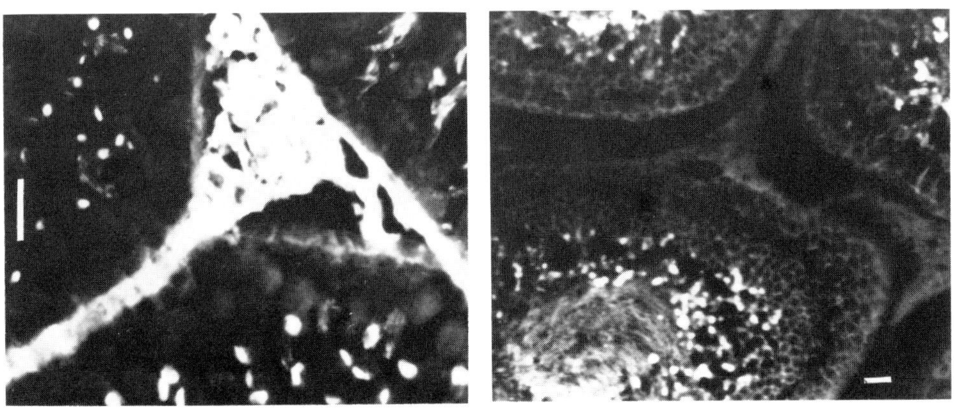

Fig. 2. Localization by immunofluorescence, in paraffin sections of testis, of transferrin (left) and DAG-protein (right). Bar = 25 microns.

DAG-protein was purified by column chromatography and by high performance liquid chromatography. Biochemical studies have shown that DAG-protein is a heavily glycosylated, sulfated, hydrophobic protein (10). Antisera to DAG-protein has been used to localize the protein in tissue sections in a procedure similar to the studies with transferrin. A unique pattern of localization showed DAG-protein present on released testicular spermatozoa, in the tubular milieu, and in the epididymal lumen (Fig. 2, right). Further studies have shown that DAG-protein is actively synthesized and secreted by the caput epididymus. The DAG-protein becomes localized on the sperm membrane over the anterior acrosome, the neck region and the distal tail (10).

Thus, two of the major secretion products of the Sertoli cells can be shown to interact with specific but separate stages of germinal cells during spermiogenesis. The function of the transferrin is presumably to supply Fe^{+3} to developing spermatids - a "nurse" cell activity of the Sertoli cells. The function of the DAG-protein is unknown but apparently is confined to interactions with spermatozoa.

ACKNOWLEDGMENTS

These studies were supported by a grant from the National Institute of Child Health and Human Development (no. HD 10808).

REFERENCES

1. Fawcett SW (1975) In: Hamilton D W, Grup R D (eds.) Handbook of Physiology, vol. 5, American Physiological Society, Bethesda, MD, pp 21-56
2. Wilson RM, Griswold MD (1979) Exp. Cell Res. 123:127-135
3. Sylvester SR, Griswold MD (1984) Biol. of Reprod. in press
4. Kissinger C, Skinner MK, Griswold MD (1982) Biol. of Reprod. 27:233-240
5. Skinner MK, Griswold MD (1983) Biol. of Reprod. 28:1225-1229
6. Skinner MK, Griswold MD (1980) J. Biol. Chem. 225:1923-1925
7. Skinner MK, Cosand WL, Griswold MD (1984) Biochem. J. 218:313-320
8. Skinner MK, Griswold MD (1982) Biol. of Reprod. 27:211-221
9. Huggenvik J, Sylvester SR, Griswold MD (1984) Annals of N.Y. Acad. Sci. in press
10. Sylvester SR, Skinner MK, Griswold MD (1984) submitted

Endocrinology
F. Labrie, L. Proulx, eds.

SERTOLI CELL-GERM CELL INTERACTIONS AND THE HORMONAL CONTROL OF SPERMATOGENESIS

J. ANTON GROOTEGOED, RIA B. OONK, RUUD JANSEN and
HENK J. VAN DER MOLEN

Department of Biochemistry (Division of Chemical Endocrinology),
Medical Faculty, Erasmus University Rotterdam, The Netherlands

Incubation conditions which support the differentiation *in vitro* of isolated spermatogenic cells from mammalian species, have not yet been defined. Isolated mid-pachytene spermatocytes from rats, for example, do not develop into spermatids, but degenerate within a few days after isolation. One could speculate therefore, that specific metabolic pathways do not occur in the spermatogenic cells, so that exogenous compounds are required which may be produced by Sertoli cells. This could result in hormonal control of spermatogenesis, through hormonal regulation of the production of these compounds by Sertoli cells, which are target cells for follitropin, testosterone and other hormones.

In experiments designed to trace compounds which could be important for developing germ cells, we have used isolated rat Sertoli cells, pachytene spermatocytes and round spermatids. In addition, spermatogenic epithelium was obtained from immature rats, after removal of the interstitial tissue and the cells from the tubular wall by collagenase treatment of decapsulated testes. This spermatogenic epithelium contains spermatocytes and spermatids, which remain in contact with Sertoli cells during incubation (1).

LACTATE PRODUCTION BY SERTOLI CELLS

Isolated rat spermatogenic cells cannot produce ATP at a high rate using glucose or many other energy yielding substrates. The ATP content of spermatocytes and spermatids, however, is maintained during short-term incubation in the presence of pyruvate or lactate (2,3). Observations on pyruvate and lactate oxidation by spermatogenic cells indicate, that a high concentration of lactate (3-6 mM) may be essential to support ATP production via the mitochondrial metabolism of endogenous pyruvate (3). In the spermatogenic microenvironment, lactate could come from Sertoli cells. Isolated Sertoli cells metabolize glucose via glycolysis at a high rate, which results in net production of lactate (1,4).

INTERCELLULAR PATHWAY OF LEUCINE CATABOLISM

A number of enzyme activities are abundant in Sertoli cells, but virtually absent in spermatogenic cells. Branched-chain amino acid aminotransferase is one of these enzymes (5). Via this enzyme activity, Sertoli cells convert leucine to α-ketoisocaproate (Table I). This pathway occurs in many tissues. However, in rat spermatogenic epithelium *in vitro*, α-ketoisocaproate is reduced to α-hydroxyisocaproate (Table I). This reduction occurs in spermatocytes and spermatids, but not in Sertoli cells, and is catalyzed most likely by the male germ cell-specific lactate dehydrogenase isoenzyme LDH-C_4 (6,7). Hence, in rat spermatogenic epithelium, there is a unique intercellular pathway for leucine catabolism which involves both Sertoli cells and spermatogenic cells.

The NAD-dependent reduction of exogenous α-ketoisocaproate was observed during incubation of isolated spermatogenic cells in the presence of 3-6 mM sodium L-lactate, but not in the presence of pyruvate (7). This can be explained, because exogenous pyruvate is converted to lactate (3), which may result in a highly oxidized NAD^+/NADH system (9). Hence, the present results indicate that spermatogenic cells *in situ* in the spermatogenic epithelium, are exposed to a relatively high concentration of lactate, and reduce α-ketoisocaproate concomitantly with the conversion of exogenous lactate to pyruvate.

TRANSPORT OF FLUOROCITRATE FROM SERTOLI CELLS INTO GERM CELLS

Fluoroacetate, which has been used as a rat poison, inhibits spermatogenesis *in vivo* at a sublethal dose (10). Fluoroacetate is activated to fluoroacetyl CoA which then condenses with oxaloacetate to give fluorocitrate. Fluorocitrate is a potent inhibitor of aconitase, one of the enzymes which catalyze the citric acid cycle. In isolated germ cells, however, exogenous acetate does not support ATP production (not shown), indicating that acetate is not activated to acetyl CoA. Hence, one may wonder why fluoroacetate is lethal to the germ cells *in vivo*. In spermatogenic epithelium from 5-week-old rats *in vitro*, the rate of conversion of $[2\text{-}^{14}C]$pyruvate to $^{14}CO_2$ via the citric acid cycle was strongly inhibited by fluoroacetate during a 20 h incubation period (5.5 ± 0.6 and 0.3 ± 0.1 nmol/mg protein per h, in the absence or presence of 0.5 mM fluoroacetate respectively; means ± S.D.). However, pyruvate oxidation (not shown) and ATP production by isolated spermatocytes and spermatids was inhibited by fluorocitrate, but not by fluoroacetate (Table II). These observations indicate, that fluorocitrate is produced from fluoroacetate by Sertoli cells and transported subsequently into the germ cells. This transport of fluorocitrate illustrates that Sertoli cells and germ cells *in situ* may communicate via the cell-to-cell transport of intermediates of metabolism other than lactate.

HORMONAL CONTROL OF SPERMATOGENESIS

Our results show that metabolic intermediates from Sertoli cells are utilized by spermatogenic cells. It remains to be shown, however, that the supply of one or more compound(s) limits the number of developing germ cells. Lactate could be a good candidate, because the concentration which may be required (3-6 mM) exceeds the concentration of lactate in rat blood (1 mM). Furthermore, the net production of lactate by Sertoli cells *in vitro* is stimulated by follitropin. This stimulation was observed for Sertoli cells from immature 3-6 week-old rats (11), which is during the period of development that follitropin probably is involved in the differentiation of Sertoli cells and the initiation of spermatogenesis.

Stimulation (approximately 3-fold) of lactate production by Sertoli cells was obtained within 3 hours after addition of follitropin (NIH-FSH-S13; ED_{50}=10 ng/ml), but also by insulin (ED_{50}=50 ng/ml), following a 3-day incubation period in the absence of hormones (12). This rapid stimulation was not dependent on *de novo* protein synthesis (12). Within 24 hours after addition of follitropin, however, the cells became refractory to the hormone, whereas the cells could be stimulated still by insulin; and *vice versa* (not shown). Hence, it is important to define incubation conditions and the combination of hormone additions which might result in long-term stimulation of glucose metabolism by Sertoli cells.

REFERENCES

1. Jutte NHPM, Jansen R, Grootegoed JA, Rommerts FFG, Clausen OPF, van der Molen HJ (1982) J Reprod Fert 65:431-438
2. Jutte NHPM, Grootegoed JA, Rommerts FFG, van der Molen HJ (1981) J Reprod Fert 62:399-405
3. Grootegoed JA, Jansen R, van der Molen HJ (1984) Biochim Biophys Acta, in the press
4. Robinson R, Fritz IB (1981) Biol Reprod 24:1032-1041
5. Grootegoed JA, Jutte NHPM, Jansen R, van der Molen HJ (1983) In: Dumont JE, Nunez J, Denton RM (eds) Hormones and Cell Regulation Vol. 7. Elsevier, Amsterdam, pp 299-316

6. Blanco A, Burgos C, Gerez de Burgos NM, Montamat EE (1976) Biochem J 153:165-172

7. Grootegoed JA, Jansen R, van der Molen HJ (1984) Ann N Y Acad Sci , in the press

8. Tanaka K, Hine DG, West-Dull A, Lynn TB (1980) Clin Chem 26: 1839-1846

9. Brooks DE, Mann T (1972) Biochem J 129:1023-1034

10. Sullivan JL, Smith FA, Garman RH (1979) J Reprod Fert 56:201-207

11. Jutte NHPM, Jansen R, Grootegoed JA, Rommerts FFG, van der Molen HJ (1983) J Reprod Fert 68:219-226

12. Oonk RB, Grootegoed JA, Reuvers PJ, van der Molen HJ (1984) Proceedings of the Third European Testis Workshop, Lyon, in the press

TABLE I
RATES OF NET PRODUCTION OF α-KETOISOCAPROATE AND α-HYDROXYISOCAPROATE BY SERTOLI CELLS AND SPERMATOGENIC EPITHELIUM
Sertoli cells and spermatogenic epithelium were isolated from 3-week-old sterile or intact rats respectively, as described elsewhere (1) and incubated for 20 h in Eagle's minimum essential medium which contained 2 mM L-leucine. The quantitative data were obtained by gas-liquid chromatography of the spent incubation medium, essentially as described by Tanaka (8) (means ± S.D.).

	α-ketoisocaproate	α-hydroxyisocaproate
	(nmol/mg protein per 20 h)	
Sertoli cells	205 ± 22	non-detectable
Spermatogenic epithelium	26 ± 5	124 ± 17

TABLE II
ATP CONTENT OF SPERMATOCYTES AND SPERMATIDS AFTER 20 h OF INCUBATION IN THE ABSENCE OR PRESENCE OF FLUOROACETATE OR DL-FLUOROCITRATE
The germ cells were isolated and incubated, and ATP was estimated, as described elsewhere (3) (means ± S.D.).

	Spermatocytes	Spermatids
	(nmol ATP/10^6 cells)	
Control	13.5 ± 1.5	6.1 ± 0.7
Fluoroacetate (0.5 mM)	12.6 ± 1.5	5.2 ± 0.1
DL-Fluorocitrate (0.02 mM)	2.0 ± 0.1	0.4 ± 0.1

© 1984 Elsevier Science Publishers B.V.
Endocrinology
F. Labrie, L. Proulx, eds.

HORMONAL REGULATION OF SPERMATOGENESIS IN PRIMATES

GARY R. MARSHALL, EBERHARD NIESCHLAG

Max Planck Clinical Research Unit for Reproductive Medicine, and Department for Experimental Endocrinology, University Womens' Hospital, Steinfurter Str. 107, D-4400 Münster, F.R. Germany

INTRODUCTION

Spermatogenesis is the process by which many highly differentiated spermatozoa are produced from only a few undifferentiated spermatogonia. Through mitosis, spermatogonia proliferate and finally produce spermatocytes. These cells, then, through meiosis, produce spermatids which develop during spermiogenesis. The germ cells and the Sertoli cells compose the seminiferous epithelium.

It has been known for half a century that pituitary hormones, primarily LH and FSH, regulate spermatogenesis (1). LH stimulates Leydig cells to produce testosterone which has direct effects on the seminiferous epithelium. FSH also exerts its effects directly on the epithelium. FSH and testosterone most likely act on the Sertoli cells which, in turn, provide the proper local conditions for spermatogenesis (2). The precise role of each of these hormones in regulation of spermatogenesis is controversial.

The major conclusion which has been derived from experiments done primarily in rats is that testosterone can maintain or restore spermatogenesis in hypophysectomized rats but FSH is also needed for stimulating the first wave of spermatogenesis, that is, initiating the process. In these experiments spermatogenesis is not stimulated fully because fewer germ cells than normal are produced, i.e., spermatogenesis is qualitatively but not quantitatively maintained. There are, however, few experimental studies in primates and some clinical observation suggest that the above conclusion may not be entirely applicable to primates. Therefore we did experiments to develop a similar concept for primates.

ROLE OF TESTOSTERONE IN SPERMATOGENESIS

Maintenance of spermatogenesis.

After hypophysectomy, the testicular volumes of monkeys decline to 30% of their former values and the seminiferous epithelium comprises only Sertoli cells and spermatogonia. When monkeys are implanted immediately following pituitary extirpation with testosterone filled Silastic capsules sufficient to raise serum testosterone levels 8 to 10 fold above normal, testicular volumes decline to only 60% of the normal value (3). The numbers of all germ cells more advanced than Ad and Ap spermatogonia decline but in relative terms the proliferation of more advanced spermatogonia is reduced and this results in a reduced number of all other germ cells. Testosterone can maintain spermatogenesis but not quantitatively. All of the events of spermatogenesis are maintained but spermatogonial proliferation is much impaired.

Restoration of spermatogenesis.

Testosterone can, when administered in amounts which elevate circulating testosterone 10 to 25 fold over normal adult levels, also stimulate spermatogenesis in the regressed testes of hypophysectomized and pituitary stalk-sectioned monkeys (4). The testicular volumes increase from the regressed size of 30% of presurgical volume to 60%. Complete but quantitatively reduced spermatogenesis occurs as judged by fewer sperm in ejaculates and histological appearance of the testes.

Clearly testosterone can maintain as well as restore spermatogenesis in adult monkeys but it is unable to stimulate testicular volumes and germ cell numbers to fully normal levels. These results suggest that another factor, almost certainly FSH, is necessary for fully normal spermatogenesis.

ROLE OF FSH IN SPERMATOGENESIS

Immunization of adult rhesus monkeys against FSH results in a decline in the testicular volume as well as a reduction in the thickness of the seminiferous epithelium (5). Furthermore pulsatile administration of GnRH at 1 µg/min for 6 min every 1.5 hr to a stalk-sectioned monkey resulted in complete restoration of testicular volume after 10 weeks of treatment. GnRH is the hypothalamic factor, normally released in a regular episodic fashion, which stimulates the pituitary gland to release LH and FSH. The circulating testosterone and LH levels were elevated about 4 to 5 fold 45 min after a GnRH pulse began. In similar animals, exogenously administered testosterone which yields even higher circulating levels only restored testicular volumes to 60% of presurgical values. The immunization studies and the results of the pulsatile GnRH treatment, although preliminary, strongly suggest that both gonadotropins are needed for quantitatively normal spermatogenesis in adult primates.

INITIATION OF SPERMATOGENESIS

Both LH and FSH are necessary for the initiation of spermatogenesis in immature rats, but prepubertal boys bearing testosterone secreting testicular tumors may have complete spermatogenesis in the region of the tumor (6). To investigate this issue further we did the following study.

Four one-year old, i.e. immature, monkeys were administered testosterone which elevated serum levels 10 fold over normal adult concentrations (7). The testicular testosterone concentrations were 4 times greater than those of untreated immature monkeys but 80% of normal adult levels. The testicular volumes were 5 times larger than those of similarly aged animals but only 10% of those of adults. Spermatozoa, even motile ones, were found in some of the ejaculates and complete spermatogenesis occurred in the testes of three monkeys. Spermatogenesis had advanced to maturation phase in the fourth. In comparison, only immature Sertoli cells and spermatogonia were found in the testes of untreated immature animals. In contrast to immature rats, complete spermatogenesis can be stimulated in immature primates.

CONCLUSION

Spermatogenesis can be maintained in mature and stimulated in immature nonhuman primates by testosterone alone, but the stimulation is not complete in quantitative terms in so far as fewer germ cells are produced. The reduced number of germ cells is due primarily to the fewer advanced spermatogonia being produced. It may be speculated from these results and the complete stimulation of the testes by pulsatile administration of GnRH that FSH acts primarily to increase the efficiency of spermatogonial proliferation.

REFERENCES

1. Hodgson Y, Robertson DM, de Kretser DM (1983) In: Greep RO (ed) International Review of Physiology. University Park Press, Baltimore, pp 275 - 327

2. Parvinen M (1982) Endocrine Rev 3: 404

3. Marshall GR, Jockenhövel F, Lüdecke DK, Nieschlag E (1984) 7th International Congress of Endocrinology, Abstract

4. Marshall GR, Wickings EJ, Lüdecke DK, Nieschlag E (1983) J Clin Endocrinol Metab 57: 152

5. Wickings EJ, Usadel KH, Dathe G, Nieschlag E (1980) Acta endocrinol 95: 117

6. Chemes HE, Pasqualini T, Rivarola MA, Bergada C (1982) Int J Andrology 5: 229

7. Marshall GR, Wickings EJ, Nieschlag E (1984) Endocrinology in press

32. Opioid Peptides in the Brain and Endocrine Tissue

Endocrinology
F. Labrie, L. Proulx, eds.

ENDORPHIN AND ENDOPSYCHOSIN: MU/DELTA AND SIGMA OPIATE LIGANDS OF THE PITUITARY GLAND AND BRAIN

WILLIAM R. MILLINGTON [1,2], PATRICIA C. CONTRERAS [1,3], MICHAEL D. HIRSCH [1] AND THOMAS L. O'DONOHUE [1]

1. Experimental Therapeutics Branch, National Institute of Neurological and Communicative Disorders and Stroke, Bethesda, MD 20205

2. Department of Physiology, Uniformed Services University of the Health Science, Bethesda, MD 20014

3. Department of Medicine, Howard University School of Medicine, Washington, DC 20059

Four different types of opiate receptors have been proposed to be responsible for the spectrum of pharmacological actions of opiates. Mu receptors are thought to mediate analgesia; delta receptors may be involved in the mediation of reward processes and seizure; kappa receptors may mediate analgesia and sedation; and sigma receptors mediate the psychotomimetic actions of opiates (1). Neurons and endocrine cells secrete peptides are derived from at least three common prohormones which interact with opiate receptors (2). Neurons in the brain and periphery and endocrine cells in the adrenal medulla synthesize and secrete peptides derived from pro-enkephalin which are thought to preferentially interact with delta receptors. Neurons in the brain and spinal cord synthesize peptides derived from pro-dynorphin which preferentially interact with the kappa subtype of receptor. Neurons and endocrine cells of the pituitary gland as well as a number of other organs synthesize and secrete the opiate and non-opiate peptides derived from pro-opiomelanocortin (POMC): β-lipotropin, β-endorphin, ACTH and α-MSH; β-endorphin is thought to interact primarily with the mu and delta subtypes of receptors.

In this paper, we will briefly review recent results of studies of presynaptic regulatory processes and their post-synaptic significance in the POMC system and describe data indicating that there is also an endogenous peptide which interacts with the sigma opiate receptor.

The discovery of the potent analgetic property of β-endorphin (β-END) initially suggested that β-END releasing neurons might be coupled to a specific postsynaptic receptor which selectively mediates analgesia. The subsequent characterization of opiate receptor subtypes clearly demonstrated, however, that β-END is not a selective ligand for mu receptors which are thought to mediate the analgetic response to opiates. Recent findings indicate, however, that receptor specificity may not be the sole determinant of the response to β-END but that presynaptic modifications of the β-END molecule may be equally as important in determining the transynaptic response to the peptide. Indeed the recognition that β-END is synthesized as part of a larger precursor molecule, POMC, which contains the sequences of multiple bioactive peptides has led to the discomforting realization that the complexities of chemical transmission by such multisecretory neurons may not be adequately predicted by the traditional "one neuron-one transmitter-one receptor" paradigms developed from the study of unisecretory monoaminergic neurons. Here we will highlight several recent studies which show that differential post-transitional processing of POMC-derived peptides profoundly alters their bioactivities and imparts regional specificity to the opiomelanotropinergic (OMT) neuronal system.

β-END and α-MSH are the predominant peptides expressed by the POMC processing pathway of neuronal tissue (3). C-terminal cleavage products of β-END ($β\text{-END}_{1-27}$; $β\text{-END}_{1-26}$) have also been identified in the brain and both α-MSH and β-END peptides occur in N-terminally acetylated and non-acetylated forms (4,5). β-END and α-MSH peptides coexist within the processes of an extensive fiber distribution which emanates from perikarya localized in the medial basal hypothalamus and projects to subcortical structures throughout the forebrain (3). This OMT neuronal system appears to be heterogenous with respect to POMC processing in that OMT neuronal processes contain and presumably release different relative amounts of β-END and α-MSH in different terminal projection fields. Indeed, the relative concentrations of α-MSH and β-END vary across brain regions by more than a six-fold range (6). In addition, the observations of regional differences in the extent of acetylation of β-END and α-MSH peptides further indicates that the POMC neuronal system possesses regionally heterogeneous processing mechanisms (4,5). These observations suggest that there are either separate neuronal populations which process POMC differently, or else the ratios of OMT peptides are varied across different axon collaterals of individual neurons. In either case, the existence of a regional heterogeneity for OMT peptide ratios suggests that the expression of OMT peptides may be regionally selective. In this manner, processing might impart functional specificity to seperate neuronal pathways within the OMT neuronal system. The processing of β-END and α-MSH is similar in the brain and the intermediate lobe of the pituitary gland (IL) but one difference is that in the IL, peptides are almost totally N-acetylated (3), whereas in brain there is a lower ratio of N-acetylated forms (7,8). Recent studies have demonstrated the existence of an enzyme which can acetylate both α-MSH and β-END (9-13). Further studies indicate that this enzyme can be induced by stimuli which induce POMC biosynthesis (14).

The post-translational processing of β-END and α-MSH dramatically alters the bioactivities of both peptides. Although α-MSH is considerably more potent than its des-acetyl derivative in a variety of behavioral paradigms (7) the opiate activity of β-END is reduced by a factor of 1,000 following N-terminal acetylation (8). C-terminal cleavage of β-END_{1-31} to β-END_{1-27} also dramatically reduces its agonistic opiate activity and, moreover, transforms the peptide into an endogenous opiate antagonist with a potency that is four-fold greater than that of naloxone (9). The post-translational processing of β-END and α-MSH also affects the behavioral outputs resulting from the postsynaptic interaction of the two co-released peptides. Thus, the stretch-yawn-syndrome (SYS), a characteristic response to icv injected α-MSH, is inhibited by the co-administration of β-END_{1-31} and the acetylation of β-END reduces its ability to inhibit the α-MSH-induced SYS (10). Surprisingly, C-terminal cleavage of β-END_{1-31} to β-END_{1-27} results in a peptide which can produce SYS instead of inhibiting α-MSH induced SYS. These data demonstrate that post-translational modifications of β-END can profoundly affect both the relative potency of the peptide, as well as the qualitative nature of the biological response that it produces, presumably via interaction with mu, delta, and possibly other postsynaptic receptors.

Another subtype of receptors that interact with opioids are sigma receptors, which are believed to mediate the psychotominetic effects of opioids. It is generally believed that phencyclidine (PCP) receptors are sigma receptors because PCP generalizes to a SKF 10,047 stimulus (17) and SKF 10,047 generalizes to a PCP stimulus (18). Furthermore, only opioids with psychotomimetic properties displace ^{3}H-PCP binding (19).

A possible endogenous peptide ligand for sigma receptors is β-endopsychosin, which has been isolated from porcine brains (20,21). Like PCP, β-endopsychosin inhibits ^{3}H-PCP binding, depresses spontaneous neuronal electrical activity in the hippocampus and cerebral cortex, and produces contralateral rotation in the rat after unilateral intranigral administration. Furthermore, the distribution of β-endopsychosin parallels the regional distribution of PCP receptors. For example, there is a high concentration of β-endopsychosin in the hippocampus and cerebral cortex, which may be relevant to the psychotomimetic properties of some opioids and PCP. Studies in progress involve the determination of the structure and synthesis of β-endopsychosin.

All of the opiate peptides derived from pro-enkephalin, pro-dynorphin, and POMC commonly share an the enkephalin sequence of amino acids. However, post-translational processing may produce the important structural differences which produce mu, kappa or delta receptor subtype selectively. It will be interesting to see if the endogenous ligand for the sigma receptor also has structural similarities to the other opiate peptides.

REFERENCES

1. Martin WR (1984) Pharmacological Reviews 35:283-323.
2. Hollt V (1983) Trends in Neurosciences 6:24-26.
3. O'Donohue TL, Dorsa DM (1982) Peptides 3:353-395.
4. Dennis M, Seidah NG, Chretien M (1983) Life Sci. 33:49-52.
5. Zakarian S, Smyth DG (1982) Nature 296:250-252.
6. Millington, WR, Mueller GP, O'Donohue TL (in press) Peptides.
7. O'Donohue TL, Handelmann GE, Miller RL, Jacobowitz DM (1982) Science 215:1125-1127.
8. Deakin JFW, Dostrovsky JO, Smyth DG (1980) Biochem. J. 189:501-506.
9. O'Donohue TL, Chappel MC (1982) Peptides 3:69-75.
10. Chappel MC, Loh YP, O'Donohue TL (1982) Peptides 3:405-410.
11. O'Donohue TL (1982) J. Biol. Chem. 258:2163-2167.
12. Woodford TA, Dixon JE (1979) J. Biol Chem. 254:4993-4999.
13. Glembotski CC (1982) J. Biol. Chem. 257:10501-10509.
14. Chappel MC, Millington WR, Mueller GP, O'Donohue TL (1984) submitted.
15. Hammond RG, Nicolas P and Li CH (1984) Proc. Natl. Acad. Sci. 81:1389-1390.
16. Hirsch MD, O'Donohue TL (1984) Soc. Neurosci. Abstr.
17. Shannon HE (1981) J. Pharmacol Exp. Ther. 216:543-551.
18. Shannon HE (1983) J. Pharmacol Exp. Ther. 225:144-152.
19. Quirion R, Hammer RP Jr, Herkenham M, Pert CB (1981) Proc. Natl. Acad. Sci. USA 78:5881-5885.
20. O'Donohue TL, Pert CB, French ED, Pert A, DiMaggio DA, Everist H, Quirion R (1983) In: Hruby VJ, Rich EH (eds) Peptides Structure and Function. Pierce Chemical Co., pp 433-436.
21. Quirion R, DiMaggio DA, French ED, Contreras P, Shiloach J, Pert CB, Everst H, Pert A, O'Donohue TL (1984) Peptides.

Endocrinology
F. Labrie, L. Proulx, eds.

NEO-ENDORPHINS AND DYNORPHINS PROCESSED OUT OF PROENKEPHALIN B

HISAYUKI MATSUO

Department of Biochemistry, Miyazaki Medical College, Kiyotake, Miyazaki 889-16, Japan

Since 1975 when enkephalins were first identified in mammalian brain, a variety of endogenous opioid peptides containing N-terminal enkephalin unit have been isolated in neural tissues. All the peptides have been known to be derived from either of three distinct precursors; proopiomelanocortin, proenkephalin A and proenkephalin B. The recent development of DNA analysis provides precise knowledge of structures of the precursors. However, our knowledge of the processing event intervening from the precursor to the mature peptides has been still very limited. In this review, I have chosen neo-endorphin-dynorphin system involved in proenkephalin B for discussing about processing mechanism.

Initial identification of α-neo-endorphin(α-NE), immediately followed by dynorphin(Dyn A), induced successive isolation of several "big" Leu-enkephalin(Leu-enk), such as PH-8P(Dyn[1-8]), β-neo-endorphin(β-NE), rimorphin(Dyn B) and Dyn-32 (Fig. 1). In addition, immunoreactive Leu-morphin(Dyn B-29) has been reported to exist in pituitary. At the time when α-NE and Dyn A were identified in 1980, these "big" Leu-enkephalins were thought to be putative intermediates to Leu-enkephalin, since they contain in common an N-terminal Leu-enk, followed by paired basic residues, such as R-K or R-R. However, All the "big" Leu-enk identified were found to elicit an opioid activity more potent than Leu-enk itself and are distributed in neural system in their own fashion. Yet the cells producing NE and Dyn do not contain detectable amounts of Leu-enk. These facts indicate a possibility that they may not only serve as biosynthetic intermediate of Leu-enk, but also play a physiological function of their own, even though there still remain many questions to be answered.

α-neo-endorphin:Tyr-Gly-Gly-Phe-Leu-**Arg-Lys**-Tyr-Pro-Lys
β-neo-endorphin:Tyr-Gly-Gly-Phe-Leu-**Arg-Lys**-Tyr-Pro
dynorphin-32 :Tyr-Gly-Gly-Phe-Leu-**Arg-Arg**-Ile-Arg-Pro-Lys-Leu-Lys-Trp-Asp-Asn-Gln-Lys-Arg-Tyr-Gly-Gly-Phe-Leu-**Arg-Arg**-Gln-Phe-Lys-Val-Val-Thr
dynorphin A :Tyr-Gly-Gly-Phe-Leu-**Arg-Arg**-Ile-Arg-Pro-Lys-Leu-Lys-Trp-Asp-Asn-Gln
PH-8P(Dyn[1-8]):Tyr-Gly-Gly-Phe-Leu-**Arg-Arg**-Ile
dynorphin B-29 :Tyr-Gly-Gly-Phe-Leu-**Arg-Arg**-Gln-Phe-Lys-Val-Val-Thr-Arg-Ser-Gln-Glu-Asp-Pro-Asn-Ala-Tyr-Tyr-Glu-Leu-Phe-Asp-Val
dynorphin B :Tyr-Gly-Gly-Phe-Leu-**Arg-Arg**-Gln-Phe-Lys-Val-Val-Thr

Fig.1. Structures of neo-endorphins and dynorphins

It is now well known that neo-endorphins and dynorphins share a common parent molecule, named proenkephalin B. As schematized in Fig. 2, proenkephalin B contains three units of Leu-enk and seven pairs of consecutive basic amino acid residues (4 sets of K-R, 2 R-R and 1 R-K).

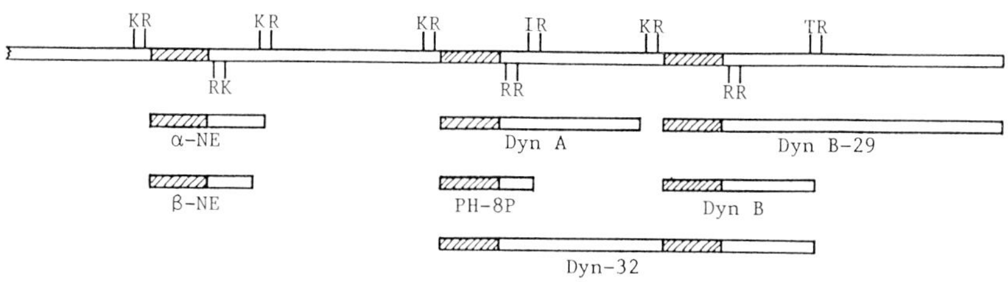

Fig. 2. Schematic processing-pattern of proenkephalin B.

When the structure of proenkephalin B is compared with those of their products so far identified, three distinct patterns are revealed to exist in the processing mechanism:

1) Cleavage at K-R pair giving rise to β-NE, Dyn A and Dyn B-29: Dyn-32 may be the case. Many of the known proteolytic cleavages of precursors occur at pairs of basic amino acid residues, which are known to be typical processing signals. In this context, we have demonstrated the presence of a unique proenkephalin-converting enzyme(1). The enzyme purified from bovine adrenal chromaffin

granules converts proenkephalin to enkephalins by cleaving specifically at the site of consecutive basic residues. However, formation of [Arg^6]-enk was not observed during the enzymatic reaction. Furthermore, [Arg^6]-enks were not converted to enkephalins.by the enzyme. Accordingly, the enzyme was proved to be a unique converting enzyme distinct from either trypsin-like or carboxypeptidase B-like proteases. Participation of the enzyme in the enkephalin processing is conceivable. Note that R-K and R-R pairs remain uncleaved in neo-endorphins and dynorphins. Preferential cleavage at the site of K-R implies that R-R or R-K may not be an obligatory processing signal in the processing of proenkephalin B.

2) Cleavage between the K-R signal leading to α-neo-endorphin: When a cleavage occurs at the consecutive basic residues, both basic residues are usually absent from the resultant products. However, there is important exceptions in which one basic resiude remains within the product peptide, as seen in the case of α-neo-endorphin. A basic residue, K remains at the C-terminus of α-NE but is removed from β-NE which terminates in Pro. The presence of proline before the K-R signal may alter susceptibility of K-R signal to the enzyme. However, the ratio of α-NE to β-NE is much greater than unity in most brain regions, indicating that the cells producing α-NE may contain another enzyme specificaly cleaving between K-R signal. In respect with these, we have very recently reported the isolation of a novel protease which specifically recognizes paired basic residues but cleaves the peptide bond between consecutive basic residues(2). The enzyme was isolated from yeast, but the presence of a similar enzyme system may be possible in mammals.

3) Cleavage before a single arginine: Natural occurence of PH-8P and Dyn B(rimorphin), whose C-terminal residues are not followed by a basic pair signal, but by a single Arg in the molecule of proenkephalin B. indicates that another type of processing may take place at the site before a special Arg residue. It has been evidenced that a similar processing of peptide E portion in proenkephalin A results in the formation of "adrenorphin (methorphamide)", which is the first C-terminally amidated opioid peptide identified in mammals(3, 4). As seen in Fig. 3, adrenorphin would be processed out of the precursor before the linkage of Arg-Pro, followed by C-terminal amidation. Recently, it has been

reported that putative processing enzymes with unusual specificity toward the single arginine residue are present in rat brain(5) and Aplysia(6).

Proenkephalin B

------Lys-Arg↓-Tyr(210)-Gly-Gly-Phe-Leu-Arg-Arg(215)-Ile↓-Arg-Pro-------

PH-8P   Tyr-Gly-Gly-Phe-Leu-Arg-Arg-Ile

Proenkephalin A

------Lys-Arg↓-Tyr(210)-Gly-Gly-Phe-Met-Arg(215)-Arg-Val-[Gly]↓-Arg(220)-Pro----

Adrenorphin   Tyr-Gly-Gly-Phe-Met-Arg-Arg-Val-NH_2

Fig. 3. Location of adrenorphin and PH-8P in their precursors.

ACKNOWLEDGEMENTS

This work was supported in part by research grant from the Ministry of Education, Science and Culture of Japan.

REFERENCES

1. Mizuno, K., Miyata, A., Kangawa, K., Matsuo, H. (1982) Biochem Biophys Res Commun 108:1235-1242
2. Mizuno, K., Matsuo, H. (1984) Nature in press
3. Matsuo, H., Miyata, A., Mizuno, K. (1983) Nature 305:721-723
4. Weber, E.,et al. (1983) Proc Natl Acad Sci USA 80: 7362-7366
5. Devi, L., Goldstein, A. (1984) Proc Natl Acad Sci USA 81: 1892-1896
6. Wallace, E.F., Weber, E., Barchas, J.D., Evans, C.J. (1984) Biochem Biophys Res Commun 119: 415-422

Endocrinology
F. Labrie, L. Proulx, eds.

"ENKEPHALINASE" AND METABOLISM OF ENKEPHALINS

JEAN-CHARLES SCHWARTZ, BRUNO GIROS, CLAUDE GROS, MARION LEBOYER, CATHERINE LLORENS, BERNARD MALFROY, ISABELLE PACHOT, HELENE POLLARD

Unité 109 de Neurobiologie, Centre Paul Broca de l'INSERM - 2 ter rue d'Alésia - 75014 PARIS (FRANCE)

JEAN-CLAUDE MAZIE
Institut Pasteur, 25 rue du Docteur Roux - 75015 PARIS (FRANCE)

INTRODUCTION

The enkephalins can be cleaved by a variety of peptidases but it progressively appears that two enzyme activities are mainly if not solely involved in their physiological inactivation (reviewed by Schwartz, 1983). The first, responsible for the cleavage of the Gly^3-Phe^4 amide bond, is generally termed "enkephalinase". It is primarily associated with synaptic membranes and is potently and selectively inhibited by Thiorphan. Its inhibition allows an increased recovery of enkephalins released from striatal slices and, in vivo, a diminished responsiveness to various nociceptive stimuli. In addition an aminopeptidase activity sensitive to bestatin, an inhibitor of microbial origin seems to be physiologically involved in the hydrolysis of endogenous enkephalins as shown by the strong potentiation of the effects of Thiorphan as regard both protection of the peptide and antinociceptive effect (De la Baume et al., 1983).

LOCALISATION OF "ENKEPHALINASE" USING MONOCLONAL ANTIBODIES

The enzyme is present not only in brain but also in a variety of peripheral tissues among which the kidney is the richest. Purification of the enzyme allowed to establish its identity with a previously known "neutral proteinase from rabbit kidney brush border" (EC 3.4.24.11) whose presence in CNS and function anywhere had remained unknown . Starting from the rat renal enzyme purified close to homogeneity (Malfroy and Schwartz, 1982) we have recently developped monoclonal antibodies (Buttin et al., 1978). Using the PAP method a strong "enkephalinase"-IR was localised not only, as expected on brush borders from renal tubuli and intestine but also on the ependymal cells lining the whole ventricular system and on tanycytes (Fig. 1). Enkephalins, as well as a variety of other bioactive peptides cleavable by "enkephalinase" are known to be present in CSF, suggesting that their turnover therein should be rather rapid. In addition the observation does not support the largely debated hypothesis that tanycytes are physiologically involved in the transport of peptide messengers between CSF and pituitary.

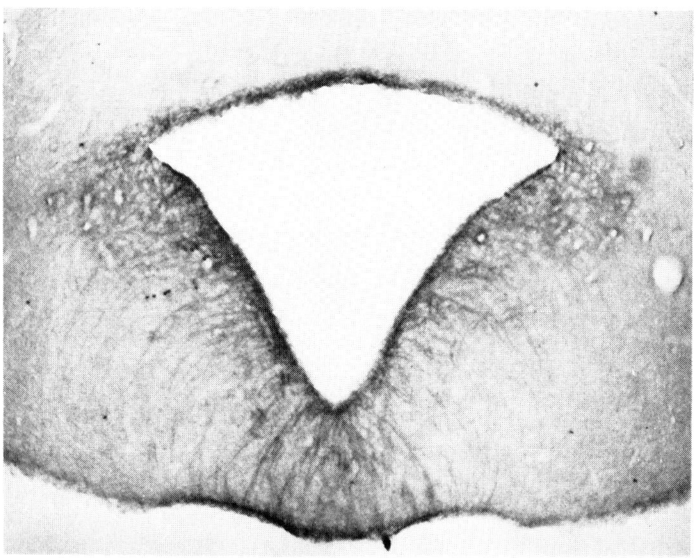

Fig. 1. Immunohistochemical localisation of "enkephalinase" on as frontal section of rat diencephalon

EFFECT OF PEPTIDASE INHIBITORS ON THE METABOLISM OF ENDOGENOUS ENKEPHALIN

When the metabolism of "classical" i.e. non-peptide neurotransmitters is inhibited a rise in their steady state level is observed at a rate which may be indicative of their synthesis rate. With the development of inhibitors of the two enzyme activities implicated in the metabolism of enkephalins it became feasible to test whether this is the case for neuropeptides. Thiorphan or Bestatin alone did not elicit, after 1 h, any significant change in striatal (Met^5)enkephalin level (Table 1). However with the two peptidase inhibitors together, enkephalin level rose by about 75 % in 1 h, confirming the involvement of the two pathways, and suggesting that they have to be inhibited together before the steady state is altered. Also, they suggest a much more rapid turnover of enkephalins than is generally thought.

TABLE 1

EFFECTS OF THIORPHAN AND BESTATIN ON (MET^5)ENKEPHALIN LEVELS IN MOUSE STRIATUM

Groups of 5 to 17 mice received either saline or the peptidase inhibitors (50 µg, i.c.v.) 1h before sacrifice. The peptide was isolated by polystyrene bead column chromatography and radioimmunoassayed.

	(MET^5)ENKEPHALIN LEVELS (pmol/mg protein)
Controls	18.9 ± 2.2
Thiorphan	17.3 ± 1.7$^{N.S.}$
Bestatin	16.8 ± 1.7$^{N.S.}$
Thiorphan + Bestatin	33.1 ± 4.1* (+ 75 %)

N.S. non significant ; * $p < 0.002$

In addition, we have recently developped a sensitive RIA against Tyr-Gly-Gly, the characteristic product of the action of "enkephalinase" on enkephalins. The levels of this metabolite in mouse brain regions approximately represent 30 % of those of (Met^5)enkephalin. In animals treated with Thiorphan, striatal levels are strongly reduced in 60 min (Table 2). This indicates that a major fraction of Tyr-Gly-Gly emanates from the hydrolysis of the opioid pentapeptides by "enkephalinase" (neither dynorphin nor β-endorphin are good substrates). The observation also confirms the rapid turnover of enkephalins and suggests that the level of endogenous Tyr-Gly-Gly might represent a useful index of enkephalinergic neuron activity.

TABLE 2

TYR-GLY-GLY LEVELS IN MOUSE STRIATUM AFTER I.C.V. INJECTION OF THIORPHAN

Mice received either saline or Thiorphan (100 µg) i.c.v. 1 h before sacrifice. The peptide was isolated on SEP-PAK columns and radioimmunoassayed.

	TYR-GLY-GLY LEVELS (pmol/mg protein)
Controls (9)	6.6 ± 0.5
Thiorphan (5)	1.9 ± 0.3* (- 71 %)

* P < 0.01

REFERENCES

1. Schwartz JC (1983) Trends Neurosci. 6 : 15-18.

2. De la Baume S, Yi CC, Schwartz JC, Chaillet P, Marcais-Collado H, Costentin J (1983) Neuroscience 8 : 143-151.

3. Malfroy B, Schwartz JC (1982) Biochem. Biophys. Res. Commun. 106 : 276-285.

4. Buttin G, Le Guern C, Phalente L, Lin ECC, Medrano L, Cazenave P.A. (1978) In : Potter F.M., Warner N (eds) Current topics in Microbiology and Immunology. Springer Verlag, Bale, pp 1301-1309.

Endocrinology
F. Labrie, L. Proulx, eds.

CHARACTERIZATION OF ENKEPHALIN CONVERTASE, AN ENKEPHALIN SYNTHESIZING CARBOXYPEPTIDASE

KAREN M. BRAAS, DAVID R. LYNCH, STEPHEN M. STRITTMATTER AND SOLOMON H. SNYDER

Departments of Neuroscience, Pharmacology and Experimental Therapeutics, and Psychiatry and Behavioral Sciences, The Johns Hopkins University School of Medicine, 725 North Wolfe Street, Baltimore, Maryland 21205, U.S.A.

INTRODUCTION

Peptidergic hormones and neurotransmitters are generally derived from large mw precursors (1). The enkephalins are synthesized from proenkephalin A and B in which the active peptides are flanked by pairs of basic amino acids. Cleavage by trypsin-like enzymes yields peptides with basic amino acid carboxyl terminal extensions which are cleaved by carboxypeptidase B-like enzymes to the active opioid peptides. Numerous carboxypeptidase B-like enzymes are distributed in lysosomes and other subcellular organelles throughout brain and peripheral tissues (2-4). Enkephalin convertase (EC), a novel carboxypeptidase B-like enzyme, which appears to be associated with enkephalin biosynthesis, has been characterized in brain, pituitary, and adrenal (5). In the adrenal, EC is selectively localized to adrenal chromaffin granules (6), where enkephalins are stored, and the regional distribution of EC activity in the brain resembles that of the enkephalins. EC has been purified to apparent homogeneity, characterized, and shown to be distinct from other known carboxypeptidases (5). The active-site-directed inhibitor guanidinoethylmercaptosuccinic acid (GEMSA) has nanomolar affinity for EC, but displays micromolar potency for other carboxypeptidases (7). [^{3}H]GEMSA binds selectively to EC in crude homogenates of brain, pituitary, and adrenal (8). The high specificity of [^{3}H]GEMSA labeling has permitted us to visualize EC in brain sections using autoradiography. We have also localized EC in brain and enkephalin-containing neuroblastoma cell lines by immunocytochemical techniques using specific antisera against purified EC.

METHODS

Whole Brain Studies. [^{3}H]GEMSA (30 Ci/mmol) was obtained from Dr. S. Hurt of New England Nuclear (Boston, MA). Male Sprague-Dawley rats were anesthesized, perfused and the brains rapidly frozen (9,10). Cryostat sections (8 μM) were incubated with 4 nM [^{3}H]GEMSA in the presence or absence of inhibitors. Autoradiograms were generated by exposing the slides to LKB Ultrofilm or emulsion coated coverslips. Nonspecific binding was determined in the presence of 10 μM GEMSA. For immunocytochemistry, rats were anesthesized and perfused with 2.5°/∘ glutaraldehyde. Cryostat sections (8 μm) were stained with antisera against purified EC (1:10,000 - 1:20,000) using the avidin-biotin complex immunocytochemical technique (11).

Cell Culture Studies. NG108-15 (108CC15) cells were cultured as previously described (12). To induce differentiation, cultures were treated with 1.0 mM dibutyryl cAMP or 2.0 mM sodium butyrate for 5-7 days. The cells were fixed with 2.5°/∘ glutaraldehyde and stained with antiserum against EC (1:200,000), or the enkephalins (1:10,000 - 1:15,000) using the peroxidase anti-peroxidase (PAP) complex immunocytochemical technique (12-14).

RESULTS AND DISCUSSION

Whole Brain Studies. [^{3}H]GEMSA binding to rat brain sections and homogenates was saturable and specific with a K_D of 3-5 nM (10). [^{3}H]GEMSA binding was highest in the median eminence. Additional regions with high levels of binding included the lateral septum, bed nucleus of the stria terminalis, hippocampus, dentate gyrus, central nucleus of the amygdala, pre-optic and magnocellular nuclei of the hypothalamus, interpeduncular nucleus, dorsal parabrachial nucleus, locus coeruleus, nucleus of the solitary tract, and the substantia gelatinosa of the spinal trigeminal tract (see Fig. 1).

Immunocytochemical staining of fixed brain sections using specific antisera primarily localized EC-like immunoreactivity to perikarya. Regions exhibiting highest staining included the caudate putamen, bed nucleus of the stria terminalis, central nucleus of the amygdala, and the hippocampus.

The [^{3}H]GEMSA binding and EC-like immunoreactivity distributions corresponded to a number of enkephalin-containing regions of the brain. The brain regions which exhibited binding or immunoreactivity have also previously been shown to contain either proenkephalin A or proenkephalin B as well as Met- and/or Leu-enkephalin-like immunoreactivity (15-17). Radioreceptor and autoradiographic methods have demonstrated regional opiate receptor distributions throughout the nervous system that are similar to those observed for the endogenous opioid peptides. Regional distributions of EC activity, [^{3}H]GEMSA binding, and EC-like immunoreactivity appeared to parallel both the receptor and peptide localizations.

Cell Culture Studies. Regulation of the cellular content of EC and the endogenous opioid peptides Met- and Leu-enkephalin was investigated in the neuroblastoma x glioma hybrid cells NG108-15. Untreated cells and cells induced to differentiate were stained using antisera to EC or the enkephalins. In untreated NG108-15 cells, EC-like and enkephalin-like immunoreactivities were found in cell bodies and short processes of a select population of cells. When cells were induced to differentiate with dibutyryl cAMP or sodium butyrate for 5-7 days, staining was found throughout the cytoplasm of perikarya and the extensive processes which were expressed. The volume fraction of stained cells and the cellular content of EC paralleled that observed for the enkephalins in both untreated cells and cells induced to differentiate. These neuronal cell lines may prove useful in investigations of enkephalin biosynthesis and post-translational processing. These studies demonstrate that EC is selectively associated with the biosynthesis of enkephalins in both intact brain and neuronal cell lines.

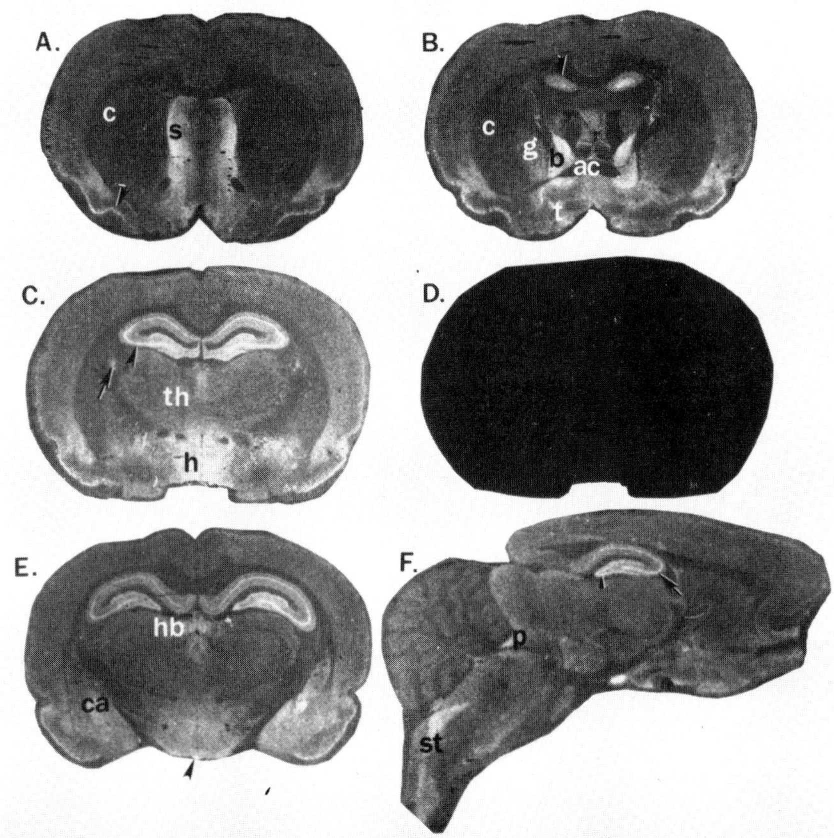

Fig. 1. Autoradiographic Localization of [^{3}H]GEMSA in Rat Brain.
(A) Binding in a coronal section of the rostral forebrain. The highest densities of labeling are the lateral septum (s) and the pyriform cortex (➤). The caudate putamen (c) and the frontal cortex have lower densities.
(B) Densely labeled areas include the bed nucleus of the stria terminalis (b), olfactory tubercle (t), and the rostral hippocampus (➤). The globus pallidus (g) is moderately labeled, while the caudate putamen (c) is weakly labeled, and the anterior commissure (ac) is unlabeled. (C) Labeling is dense in the dentate gyrus, hippocampal CA3-4 pyramidal cell region (➤), and the

stria terminalis (→). The preoptic hypothalamus (h) contains higher labeling than the thalamus (th), where the periventricular nucleus is labeled. (D) [^{3}H]GEMSA binding in the presence of 10 μM GEMSA. (E) Binding in the caudal forebrain. The area with the highest binding is the median eminence (➤). Within the amygdaloid nuclear complex, the central nucleus (ca) has the highest density of labeling. Also labeled is the habenula (hb). (F) Binding in a sagittal section of the brain. Distinct binding is present in the dorsal parabrachial nucleus (p) and the nucleus of the solitary tract (st). The dentate gyrus (➤) and hippocampus are also densely labeled.

ACKNOWLEDGEMENTS

Supported by USPHS grants DA-00266, NS-16375, RSA DA-00074 to S.H.S., training grant GM-07309 to D.R.L. and S.M.S., UPSPHS postdoctoral fellowship NS-07073 to K.M.B., and a grant from the McKnight Foundation. We thank Drs. L.D. Fricker and T.R. Plummer for enzymes and carboxypeptidase inhibitors, Drs. J.F. Wilber and R.J. Miller for antisera, and Drs. M. Nirenberg and B. Hamprecht for cultured cells.

REFERENCES

1. Docherty K, Steiner DF (1982) Ann Rev Physiol 44:625-638
2. Hook VYH, Eiden LE, Brownstein MJ (1982) Nature 295:341-342
3. Barrett AJ (1977) Proteinases in mammalian cells and tissues. Elsevier/North-Holland
4. Ninjoor V, Taylor SL, Tappel AL (1974) Biochem Biophys Acta 370:308
5. Fricker LD, Snyder SH (1983) J Biol Chem 258:10950-10955
6. Fricker LD, Snyder SH (1982) Proc Natl Acad Sci USA 79:3886-3890
7. Fricker LD, Plummer TH, Snyder SH (1983) Biochem Biophys Res Commun 111:994-1000
8. Strittmatter SM, Lynch DR, Snyder SH (submitted)
9. Young WS III, Kuhar MJ (1979) Brain Res 179:255-270
10. Strittmatter SM, Lo MMS, Javitch JA, Snyder SH (1984) Proc Natl Acad Sci USA 81:1599-1603
11. Childs G, Unabia G (1982) J Histochem Cytochem 30:713-716
12. Braas KM, Childers SR, U'Prichard DC (1983) J Neurosci 3:1713-1727
13. Sternberger, LA, Hardy PH, Cuculis JJ, Meyer HG (1970) J Histochem Cytochem 18:315-333
14. Moriarty GC, Halmi NS (1972) J Histochem Cytochem 20:590-603
15. Petrusz P, Merchenthaler J, Maderdrut JL (1984) In: Bjorklund A, Hokfelt T (eds) Handbook of Chemical Neuroanatomy, Elsevier, Amsterdam (in press)
16. Watson SJ, Khachaturian H, Akil H, Coy DH, Goldstein A (1982) Science 218:1134-1136
17. Weber E, Barchas JD (1983) Proc Natl Acad Sci USA 80:1125-1129

33. Biosynthesis and Processing of Peptide Hormones II

© 1984 Elsevier Science Publishers B.V.
Endocrinology
F. Labrie, L. Proulx, eds.

PROCESSING OF PROSOMATOSTATIN EXPRESSED BY A METALLOTHIONEIN-SOMATOSTATIN FUSION GENE IN TRANSGENIC MICE AND CULTURED FIBROBLASTS

M.J. LOW, R. PALMITER, R.E. HAMMER, R. BRINSTER, R.H. GOODMAN, AND J.F. HABENER
Laboratory of Molecular Endocrinology and Howard Hughes Medical Institute, Massachusetts General Hospital; Department of Medicine, New England Medical Center, Boston, Massachusetts; Department of Biochemistry, University of Washington, Seattle, Washington; School of Veterinary Medicine, University of Pennsylvania, Philadelphia, Pennsylvania

INTRODUCTION

Somatostatin is a ubiquitous neuropeptide of 14 (SS-14) or 28 (SS-28) amino acids that is expressed in multiple tissues and that regulates secretory activities. Both SS-14 and SS-28 arise by post-translational cleavages from prosomatostatin, a precursor of the somatostatins. To investigate the cellular mechanisms involved in the processing of prosomatostatin we have analyzed the products of the expression of a metallothionein-somatostatin fusion gene after introduction into fibroblasts and into the germ line of mice. We ligated a DNA fragment containing the entire coding sequence for rat pre prosomatostatin into a plasmid containing the metallothionein promoter and the 3' end of the human growth hormone gene.

MATERIAL AND METHODS

To test the integrity of this recombinant DNA we introduced it by endocytosis into a hamster kidney fibroblast cell line. The fibroblasts synthesized and exported nanogram amounts of immunoreactive somatostatin and zinc induced tenfold increases in the amounts of somatostatin synthesized indicating that the metallothionein promoter was active. We next introduced the recombinant DNA into the germ line of mice by micro-injection into fertilized mouse zygotes and transplantation of the zygotes into pseudopregnant mice.

RESULTS

Eleven offspring born from these surrogate mothers contained rat somatostatin DNA sequences determined by DNA tail blots. Blood levels of immunoreactive somatostatin in four of the animals were 50 to 100 times above normal. The growth characteristics, however, of the transgenic mice expressing the rat somatostatin gene were no different from those of the control siblings without fusion genes. Extracts of 15 different organs of the transgenic mice contained elevated levels of somatostatin. 31 of 45 second generation mice resulting from transgenic probands contained fusion genes indicating multiple insertional loci of the genes which segregated independently. By gel filtration immunoreactive somatostatin in extracts of the cultured fibroblasts and in livers and kidneys of transgenic mice co-chromotographed in positions corresponding to prosomatostatin, SS-28, SS-14, and a 7K intermediate form of prosomatostatin.

DISCUSSION

The successful introduction of an actively expressed somatostatin gene into the germ line of mice and into a stable cell line will facilitate further studies by site-specific mutagenesis of the structural elements in preprosomatostatin that are involved in the post-translational processing of SS-14 and SS-28. In addition analyses of the organ-specific expression of the somatostatin gene in the transgenic mice may provide insights into specific organs that are, or are not, effective in specifically processing a prohormone to its bioactive products.

Endocrinology
F. Labrie, L. Proulx, eds.

PRECURSORS AND PRODUCTS IN THE FORMATION OF NEUROHYPOPHYSIAL HORMONES*

B.T. PICKERING, R.W. SWANN, S.D. BIRKETT, P. O'SHAUGHNESSY, D.C. WATHES & D.G. PORTER

M.R.C. Neuronal Peptides Research Group, Department of Anatomy, University of Bristol, Bristol BS8 1TD, U.K.

Just 30 years after du Vigneaud and his colleagues (1) elucidated the structure of oxytocin, the sequence of the primary biosynthetic precursor of the hormone was deduced by Land et al. (2), using cDNA and gene-splicing techniques. Similarly this group (3) had also deduced the sequence of the precursor for vasopressin (Figure 1).

signal-VASOPRESSIN-Gly.Lys.Arg-neurophysin-Arg-GLYCOPEPTIDE

signal-OXYTOCIN-Gly.Lys.Arg-neurophysin-His

Fig. 1. Bovine preprovasopressin (upper) and prepro-oxytocin (refs 2 & 3).

The hormones share common precursors with their associated neurophysins, as predicted by Sachs and his colleagues in the 1960s (4), supported by indications of parallel biosynthesis (5) and substantiated by the isolation of such molecules (6). The successful translation of hypothalamic mRNA (7) led to the deduction of the precursor sequences and of the structure of the vasopressin gene (8). We (9) have evidence for two vasopressin precursors in the rat but do not yet know the difference between them. Thus the first chapter in the story of the synthesis of the hormones is complete and leads into new questions about processing of the precursors and the biological functions of the constituent peptides.

Functions of precursor constituents

Neurophysin is still without a physiological function and, although we have recent evidence for a trophic action on glial cells in the hypothalamus (10), all functions previously ascribed to neurophysins have subsequently been shown to be due to contaminants (11). It seems unlikely, however, that the great conservation of structure, seen in neurophysin molecules, is related solely to the molecule's role in the hormone precursor or, indeed, in the granule. The vasopressin precursor contains an additional component : the vasopressin-glycopeptide (3,6). This had been isolated from pituitary glands and sequenced (12,13), and is free in the granules of the neurohypophysis (5). The only role

*Supported by grants from M.R.C., The Wellcome Trust and Roche Products Ltd.

postulated for this molecule is intracellular. Prevention of glycosylation during synthesis, by injecting rats with tunicamycin, leads to an accumulation of product in the endoplasmic reticulum (14) i.e. to a failure of the packaging mechanism. This is compatible with a role for carbohydrate side-chains as signals for intracellular trafficking, directing the precursor from the RER to the Golgi (15). However, postulating such a function for the vasopressin-glycopeptide raises the problem of how oxytocin is handled.

Precursor processing

Early evidence suggested that precursor processing occurs inside the secretory granule during its journey along the axon (5). Granule movement through the cell is not essential for processing which continues normally even when granules are arrested with colchicine (16). Cleavage of the hormonal peptide from its neurophysin (Fig. 1) involves the usual (17) pair of basic residues, and neurohypophysial granules contain an enzyme system to process such linkages (18). In addition, the cleavage sequence contains a glycine which could act as a nitrogen donor for the amidation of the hormones (19). There is no basic pair separating the vasopressin-glycopeptide sequence from neurophysin; just a single arginine (Fig. 1). Only conformation of the precursor can distinguish this arginyl bond from the others in the molecule and it is not surprising that this cleavage appears to proceed more slowly than the hormone-neurophysin one, leading to significant amounts of what North refers to as proneurophysin (neurophysin linked to vasopressin-glycopeptide) in the glands of cattle (20) and guinea-pigs (21). A molecule similar to proneurophysin is present in the pituitary of the turtle, although we cannot be sure whether it represents an incompletely processed precursor, as in mammals, or is the end-product in reptiles (22).

Extrahypothalamic systems

Investigation of the control of processing would be facilitated by systems amenable to studies *in vitro*. It has long been known that small cell carcinomas of the lung may synthesise vasopressin and oxytocin and such tumours synthesise vasopressin by way of a precursor much like that in the hypothalamus (23). Interestingly, these tumours secrete significant amounts of apparently unprocessed precursor into the medium. Our discovery that corpus luteum contains a peptide which is indistinguishable from oxytocin (24) offered an alternative system to study.

Radioactive oxytocin has been characterised in extracts of luteal cells after incubation with (^{35}S)cysteine (25). Because of the avidity with which (^{35}S) cysteine binds to peptides non-specifically or by disulphide interchange, great care must be taken to ensure that the label has been truly incorporated. In Fig. 2a dispersed ovine luteal cells, incubated with (^{35}S)cysteine for 2h or 7h, have been extracted and the radioactive peptides which bound to an affinity column of neurophysin coupled to Sepharose have been separated by h.p.l.c. (9). Peak 2 which has the retention time of oxytocin was collected, oxidised with performic acid and rechromatographed on h.p.l.c. The oxidised material showed a shorter retention time (less hydrophobic) than peak 2 and, indeed, co-eluted with the performic acid-oxidised product of authentic oxytocin.

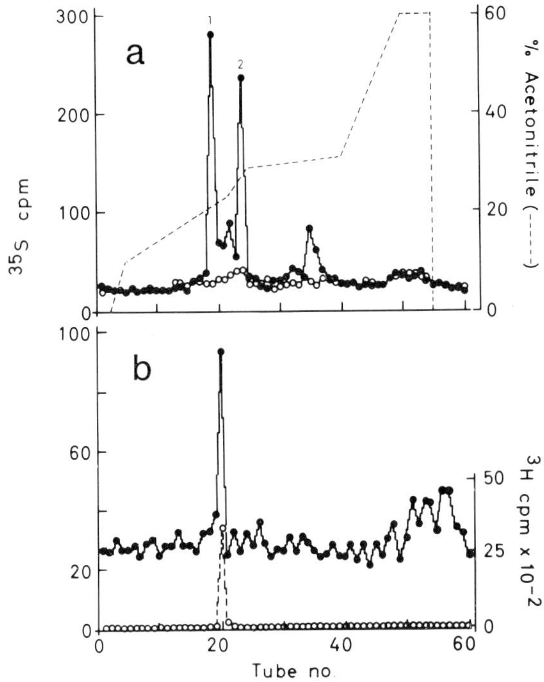

Fig. 2. H.p.l.c. of: a) peptides which bind to neurophysin, from ovine luteal cells incubated with (^{35}S)cysteine for 2h (o——o) or 7h (●——●); b) performic acid-oxidised peptides recovered from peak 2 (●——●) and performic acid-oxidised authentic (^{3}H)oxytocin (o -- o).

Immunoprecipitation of luteal cell extracts with antisera to either neurophysin or oxytocin precipitated a component with similar electrophoretic mobility to the hypothalamic precursor for oxytocin (Fig. 3). While free radioactive oxytocin could be detected only in the cells incubated with label for 7h (Fig. 2), the putative precursor was present in those incubated for 2h as well. Incorporation was prevented by cycloheximide (2.8 μg/ml). Like the lung tumour, luteal cells released significant amounts of unprocessed precursor into the medium.

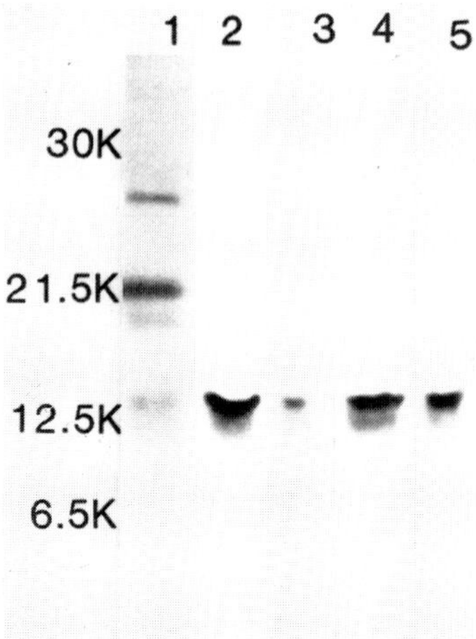

Fig. 3. Autoradiograms of SDS gels of immunoprecipitates from ovine luteal cell extracts prepared with: antineurophysin (lanes 2 & 4) or anti-oxytocin (lanes 3 & 5). Luteal cells incubated with (^{35}S)cysteine for 2h (lanes 2 & 3) or 7h (lanes 4 & 5). Lane 1: peptides precipitated with acetone from an extract of rat SON 1h after (^{35}S)cysteine had been injected *in vivo*.

Thus the corpus luteum synthesises oxytocin and does so by a mechanism resembling that in the hypothalamus. A similar conclusion has been reached by Ivell & Richter (26) using cDNA probes. While the component present in Peak 1 of Fig. 2 has the elution properties of arginine vasopressin, and immunoreactive vasopressin is associated with this peak, we do not believe that the radioactivity is associated with authentic vasopressin.

The gonadal production of 'neurohypophysial' hormones promises to be a fruitful system. Peptides resembling oxytocin, vasopressin and neurophysins have been detected in ovaries and testes from several species (27-30) and, although definitive evidence for local synthesis in the testis is still lacking, immunocytochemical studies suggest that the oxytocin is in Leydig cells (31). There are suggestions of roles for locally synthesised oxytocin in corpus luteum (27) but its function in testis is completely unknown. It may be related to steroidogenesis (32) but there is an intriguing relationship between the appearance of oxytocin in the testes of young rats and the onset of spontaneous contractility in their seminiferous tubules (33).

REFERENCES

1. Du Vigneaud V, Ressler C, Trippett S (1953) J Biol Chem 205:949-957
2. Land H, Grez M, Ruppert S, Schmale H, Rehbein M, Richter D, Schutz G (1983) Nature 302:342-344
3. Land H, Schutz G, Schmale H, Richter D (1982) Nature 295:299-303
4. Sachs H, Fawcett CP, Takabatake Y, Portanova R (1969) Recent Prog Hormone Res 25:447-491

5. Pickering BT, Jones CW, Burford GD, McPherson M, Swann RW, Heap PF, Morris JF (1975) Ann NY Acad Sci 248:15-35

6. Russell JT, Brownstein MJ, Gainer H (1980) Endocrinology 107:1880-1891

7. Schmale H, Richter D (1980) FEBS Lett 121:358-362

8. Schmale H, Heinsohn S, Richter D (1983) EMBO J 2:763-767

9. Swann RW, González CB, Birkett SD, Pickering BT (1982) Biochem J 208:339-349

10. Worley RTS, Pickering BT (1984) Cell Tissue Res (In Press)

11. Pickering BT, Jones CW (1978) In: Li CH (ed) Hormonal Proteins and Peptides, Vol 5. Academic Press, New York, pp 103-158

12. Smyth DG, Massey DE (1979) Biochem Biophys Res Commun 87:1006-1010

13. Seidah NG, Benjannet S, Chrétien M (1981) Biochem Biophys Res Commun 100: 901-907

14. González CB, Swann RW, Pickering BT (1981) Cell Tissue Res 217:199-210

15. Olden K, Bernard BA, White SL, Parent JB (1982) J Cell Biochem 18:313-335

16. Birkett SD, Swann RW, González CB, Pickering BT (1983) Arch Biochem Biophys 225:430-435

17. Steiner DF, Quinn PS, Chan SJ, Marsh J, Tager HS (1980) Ann NY Acad Sci 343: 1-16

18. Chang T-L, Gainer H, Russell JT, Loh YP (1982) Endocrinology 111:1607-1614

19. Bradbury AF, Finnie MDA, Smyth DG (1982) Nature 298:686-688

20. North WG, Mitchell TI, North GM (1983) FEBS Lett 152:29-34

21. Robinson ICAF, Jones PM (1983) Neuroscience Lett 39:273-278

22. Licht P, Pickering BT, Papkoff H, Pearson A, Bona-Gallo A (1984) J Endocr (In Press)

23. Yamaji T, Ishibashi M, Katayama S, Itabashi A, Ohsawa N, Kondo Y, Mizumoto Y, Kosaka K (1981) J Clin Invest 68:1441-1449

24. Wathes DC, Swann RW (1982) Nature 297:225-227

25. Swann RW, O'Shaughnessy PJ, Birkett SD, Wathes DC, Porter DG, Pickering BT (1984) FEBS Lett submitted

26. Ivell R, Richter D (1984) EMBO J (In Press)

27. Wathes DC, Swann RW, Birkett SD, Porter DG, Pickering BT (1983) Endocrinology 113:693-698

28. Wathes DC, Swann RW, Hull MGR, Drife JO, Porter DG, Pickering BT (1983) Progr Brain Res 60:513-519

29. Fields PA, Eldridge RK, Fuchs A-R, Roberts RF, Fields MJ (1983) Endocrinology 112:1544-1546

30. Nicholson HD, Swann RW, Burford GD, Wathes DC, Porter DG, Pickering BT (1984) Regul Pept 8:141-146

31. Guldenaar SEF, Pickering BT (1984) J Anat (In Press)

32. Adashi EY, Hsueh AJW (1981) Nature 293:650-652

33. Worley RTS, Nicholson HD, Pickering BT (1984) Proc 3rd Workshop Eur Study Grp. Molecular and Cellular Endocrinology of the Testis. Saez JM (ed). I.N.S.E.R.M.:Paris (In Press)

Endocrinology
F. Labrie, L. Proulx, eds.

BIOSYNTHESIS AND PROCESSING OF OPIOID PEPTIDE PRECURSORS

D. L. KILPATRICK

Roche Institute of Molecular Biology, Roche Research Center, Nutley, New Jersey 07110

INTRODUCTION

The adrenal medulla is a relatively rich source of the opioid peptides [Met]enkephalin and [Leu]enkephalin and has served as a convenient system for the elucidation of their biosynthetic pathway (1). The pentapeptides are derived from a multi-enkephalin precursor, proenkephalin. While much is known about the structure of proenkephalin and the EC peptides derived from it, little is known about the mechanisms which regulate its biosynthesis and processing. Previous studies have shown that denervation of the rat adrenal gland leads to a marked increase in the number of enkephalin-immunoreactive chromaffin cells (2) and the content of adrenal enkephalin-containing (EC) peptides (3,4). This suggests that proenkephalin biosynthesis in the rat adrenal gland may be under neural regulation. Here it is shown that following splanchnicectomy there is a several-fold increase in the rat adrenal content of proenkephalin mRNA thus demonstrating that denervation stimulates proenkephalin biosynthesis by a pre-translational mechanism.

MATERIALS AND METHODS

Analysis of Rat Adrenal Poly(A)$^+$RNA

Adrenal glands were obtained from male Sprague-Dawley rats (150-200 gm) (Taconic Farms; Germantown, NY) which had been unilaterally denervated for various lengths of time. Poly(A)$^+$RNA from innervated and denervated glands was purified by the guanidinium thiocyanate/CsCl gradient method (5) followed by oligo-dT column chromatography (6). Northern analysis of poly(A)$^+$RNA was carried out according to Thomas (7). Proenkephalin mRNA was quantitated by RNA blots (8) using rat brain poly(A)$^+$RNA as a standard. Autoradiogram densities were converted to pg of hybridized human proenkephalin cDNA by scintillation counting of rat brain standard dots.

Preparation of ^{32}P-Labelled DNA Probes

A synthetic 30 nucleotide long oligodeoxynucleotide complementary to a portion of human and bovine proenkephalin mRNAs was labelled using polynucleotide kinase and γ-^{32}P-ATP. Human proenkephalin cDNA was labelled by nick-translation to a specific activity of 2-5 x 10^8 cpm/µg.

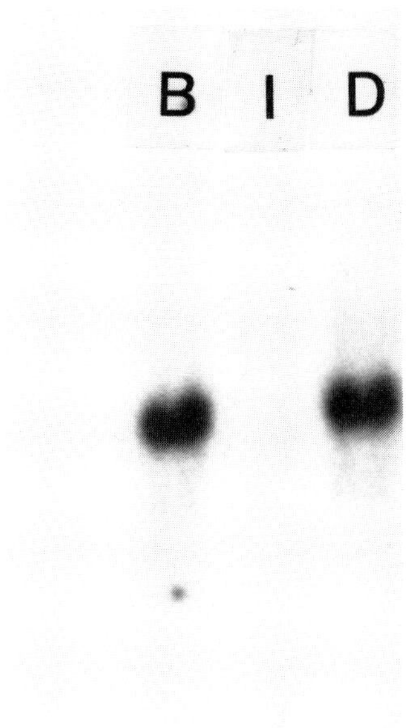

Fig. 1. Effect of splanchnicectomy on rat adrenal proenkephalin mRNA. Innervated (I) and denervated (D) adrenal glands (0.3-0.4 gm) were obtained from 13 rats which had been unilaterally denervated for 24 hr. Poly(A)$^+$RNA was prepared from each group of glands, electrophoresed on 1% agarose gels containing 10 mM methyl mercury, and hybridized with ^{32}P-labelled probe after transfer onto nitrocellulose. Six µg of rat brain poly(A)$^+$RNA (B) was included as a standard. (Figure taken from ref. 9).

RESULTS

Adrenal poly(A)$^+$RNA fractions from rats which had been unilaterally denervated for 24 hr were submitted to Northern analysis and hybridized with a synthetic ^{32}P-labelled proenkephalin DNA probe (Fig. 1). In the sample from innervated adrenal glands, the amount of proenkephalin mRNA was below the limit of detection. Substantial quantities of proenkephalin mRNA were clearly evident in the poly(A)$^+$ fraction from denervated adrenal glands, however.

Using RNA blots, the changes in proenkephalin mRNA were determined at various time points following splanchnicectomy (data not shown). An increase in rat adrenal proenkephalin mRNA is evident within 12 hr following unilateral denervation. Maximal levels of proenkephalin mRNA in the denervated samples were reached between 24 and 48 hr and thereafter the levels declined. This time course is in agreement with the previously observed increase in adrenal EC peptides (4).

The increase in proenkephalin mRNA following splanchnicectomy is not due to an increase in the total population of rat adrenal poly(A)$^+$RNA. Denervation in fact causes a 200-400% decrease in total RNA and poly(A)$^+$RNA of rat adrenal glands (9). Thus, the increase in proenkephalin mRNA in denervated adrenals is even greater when expressed per μg poly(A)$^+$RNA than when expressed per adrenal gland. The DNA content of denervated adrenals did not change relative to innervated glands, indicating no net loss of cells in these experiments.

DISCUSSION

Both the increase in rat adrenal proenkephalin mRNA and total EC peptides following splanchnic nerve sectioning are of similar magnitude (approximately 10-fold)(4,9). The increase in proenkephalin-derived EC peptides can therefore be completely accounted for by an increase in the steady state levels of proenkephalin mRNA. The marked decreases in rat adrenal RNA content following denervation suggest that splanchnic innervation exerts a strong trophic influence on rat adrenal gene expression. The observed increase in proenkephalin mRNA may therefore reflect innervation-dependent repression of adrenal proenkephalin gene expression in the rat which is reversed upon denervation. The expression of the skeletal muscle proteins tropomyosin and troponin (10) appear to be regulated in such a manner.

An alternative to this derepression model is the possibility that denervation causes an induction of proenkephalin gene expression, similar to that observed for the catecholamine biosynthetic enzymes (11). However, it has been shown that catecholamines do not increase concomittantly with EC peptides following rat adrenal denervation (4). Whatever the mechanism, these studies demonstrate that innervation has a profound effect on proenkephalin gene expression in the rat adrenal gland. It is also clear that although EC peptides and catecholamines are co-stored and co-released from adrenal chromaffin granules, their biosynthesis is not coordinately regulated in response to denervation.

ACKNOWLEDGEMENTS

Drs. Gideon Fleminger, Richard Howells, Hans-Werner Lahm and Sidney Udenfriend each made major contributions to this work.

REFERENCES

1. Udenfriend, S, Kilpatrick DL (1983) Arch Biochem Biophys 221:309-232
2. Schultzberg M, Lundberg JM, Hokfelt T, Brandt J, Elda, RP, Goldstein M (1978) Neuroscience 3:1169-1189
3. Lewis RV, Stern AS, Kilpatrick DL, Gerber LD, Rossier J, Stein S, Udenfriend S (1981) J. Neuroscience 1:80-82
4. Fleminger, G, Lahm H-W, Udenfriend S (1984) Proc Natl Acad Sci USA 81:3587-3590
5. Chirgwin JM, Przybyla AE, MacDonald RJ, Rutter WJ (1979) Biochemistry 18:5294-5299
6. Norgard MV, Tocci MJ, Monahan JJ (1980) J Biol Chem 225:7665-7672
7. Thomas PS (1980) Proc Natl Acad Sci USA 77:5201-5205
8. White BA, Bancroft FC (1982) J Biol Chem 257:8569-8572
9. Kilpatrick DL, Howells RD, Fleminger G, Udenfriend S (1984) (in preparation)
10. Matsuda R, Spector D, Strokman RC (1984) Proc Natl Acad Sci USA 81:1122-1125
11. Guidotti A, Costa E (1977) Biochem Pharmacol 26:817-823

© 1984 Elsevier Science Publishers B.V.
Endocrinology
F. Labrie, L. Proulx, eds.

BIOSYNTHESIS AND PROCESSING OF HUMAN VIP/PHM-27 PRECURSOR

HIROSHI OKAMOTO*, NOBORU YANAIHARA†, YUMIKO HAYAKAWA, NOBUYUKI ITOH AND KEN-ICHI OBATA

Department of Biochemistry, Toyama Medical and Pharmaceutical University School of Medicine, Toyama 930-01, Japan, and †Laboratory of Bioorganic Chemistry, Shizuoka College of Pharmacy, Shizuoka 422, Japan

INTRODUCTION

Vasoactive intestinal polypeptide (VIP), a 28-amino acid peptide, was originally isolated from porcine duodenum (1). VIP is present not only in gastrointestinal tissues but also neural tissues possibly as a neurotransmitter, and exhibits a wide range of biological actions (2). However, the biosynthetic mechanism of VIP remains to be elucidated. Recently, we reported that VIP was synthesized from a precursor (pro-VIP) in human neuroblastoma cells and that the synthesis of pro-VIP was stimulated by Bt_2cAMP (3). More recently, we have cloned the DNA sequence complementary to the mRNA coding for human VIP and analyzed the nucleotide sequence (4). As shown in Fig. 1, the entire amino acid sequence of the precursor, deduced from the nucleotide sequence, indicates that the precursor protein contains not only VIP but also a novel peptide of 27 amino acids, PHM-27 (5), which differs by only 2 amino acids from porcine PHI-27 (6).

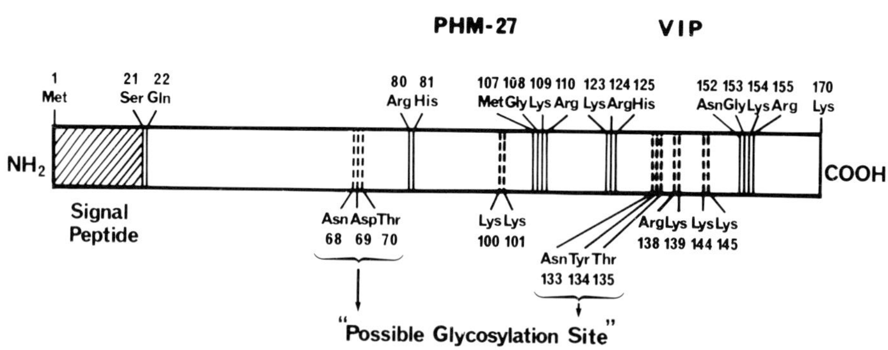

Fig. 1. Structure of Human Prepro-VIP/PHM-27

*All correspondence should be addressed to Prof. Hiroshi Okamoto, Department of Biochemistry, Toyama Medical and Pharmaceutical University School of Medicine, Toyama 930-01, Japan.

In order to clarify the mechanism of the induction of pro-VIP/PHM-27 synthesis by Bt_2cAMP, we have now used a prepro-VIP/PHM-27 cDNA hybridization method to determine the amount of the specific mRNA in neuroblastoma cells and the transcriptional activity of nuclei isolated from neuroblastoma cells (7).

EXPERIMENTAL PROCEDURES

Cell Culture. A human neuroblastoma cell line (NB-1) was originally established by Miyake *et al.* (8). The cells were cultured in RPMI 1640 (Nissui Seiyaku Co., Ltd. Tokyo) supplemented by 10% fetal bovine serum and 0.05% kanamycin in 75-cm^2 Corning tissue culture flasks (7). Cells were stimulated at 37°C for 48h with 1 mM Bt_2cAMP.

Nuclear RNA Synthesis In Vitro. Nuclei were isolated from neuroblastoma cells, and the nuclear pellet was suspended in 20 mM Tris-Cl, pH 8.0, 5 mM $MgCl_2$, 0.1 mM EDTA, 2 mM DTT, and 40% glycerol. For transcription, 50 μl of the nuclear suspension were incubated in a 150 μl reaction mixture containing 15% glycerol, 20 mM Tris-Cl, pH 8.0, 5 mM $MgCl_2$, 150 mM KCl, 2 mM DTT, 0.4 mM of ATP, GTP and CTP and 125 μCi of [α-^{32}P]UTP at 26°C for 30 min (7). The proteinase K-digested sample was combined with 2.0 ml of guanidinium thiocyanate solution and incubated at 60°C for several minutes until the chromatin dissolved. The sample was layered over 1.5 ml of 5.7 M CsCl, 0.1 M EDTA, pH 7.0, and centrifuged at 35,000 rpm at 20°C for 16h in a Beckman SW 60Ti rotor. The RNA pellet was then dissolved in sterile water and precipitated by addition of 0.1 volume of 3 M sodium acetate pH 7.0 and 2.5 volumes of ethanol (7).

Filter Hybridization. PstI-digested plasmid pVIP-1 was coupled to DPT paper (15 μg of plasmid/cm^2 filter), and hybridization mixtures of 120 μl contained 0.5 M NaCl, 20 mM Hepes, pH 7.4, 33% deionized formamide, 0.4% SDS, 2 mM EDTA, 100 μg/ml yeast tRNA, 1000 cpm of prepro-VIP/PHM-27 [^{3}H]cRNA, and two filters containing immobilized pBR322 DNA and pVIP-1 DNA (7). Hybridizations were carried out for 3 days at 45°C.

RESULTS

Induction of Pro-VIP/PHM-27 Synthesis by Bt_2cAMP. After treatment of neuroblastoma cells with 1 mM Bt_2cAMP for 48h, the synthesis of pro-VIP/PHM-27 was markedly induced and the mRNA hybridized to prepro-VIP/PHM-27 cDNA was also increased (TABLE I). However total protein synthesis and the amount of total RNA were only increased by a very small amount.

TABLE I

EFFECT OF Bt_2cAMP ON PRO-VIP/PHM-27 SYNTHESIS AND PREPRO-VIP/PHM-27 mRNA LEVEL IN HUMAN NEUROBLASTOMA CELLS

Total protein synthesis was determined by radioactivity of TCA-insoluble materials of aliquots of cell extracts from neuroblastoma cells incubated at 37°C for 2h with [^{35}S]methionine in the presence or absence of 1 mM Bt_2cAMP (7). The band corresponding to pro-VIP/PHM-27 was excised from the gels to determine the radioactivity of pro-VIP/PHM-27. The amount of prepro-VIP/PHM-27 mRNA was determined by measuring the radioactivity of the band corresponding to prepro-VIP/PHM-27 mRNA. The numbers in parentheses were related to that uninduced by Bt_2cAMP.

Treatment	Protein		RNA	
	Total	Pro-VIP/PHM-27 synthesis	Total	Prepro-VIP/PHM-27 mRNA
	cpm/4×10^{5} cells		μg/2×10^{6} cells	cpm/2×10^{6} cells
None	3.4×10^{6} (1.0)	440 (1.0)	18 (1.0)	105 (1.0)
1 mM Bt_2cAMP	6.2×10^{6} (1.8)	4,810 (10.9)	27 (1.5)	1,210 (11.5)

TABLE II

TRANSCRIPTION OF PREPRO-VIP/PHM-27 mRNA IN ISOLATED NUCLEI

Nuclei were isolated from 1 mM Bt_2cAMP-induced cells and from uninduced cells. Isolated nuclei were allowed to incorporate [^{32}P]UTP. The [^{32}P]RNA was isolated, purified, and hybridized to DPT filters carrying immobilized pVIP-1 DNA or pBR322 DNA. Hybridized radioactivity was eluted from the filters and determined by liquid scintillation counting. The efficiency (27-29%) of hybridization was assessed by determination of the recovery of added [^{3}H]cRNA standard. Nonspecific hybridization to pBR322 filters has been substracted from cpm hybridized to pVIP-1 filters.

Cell treatment	Input of [^{32}P] RNA	[^{32}P]RNA hybridized to		Prepro-VIP/PHM-27 mRNA synthesis
		pVIP-1	pBR322	
	cpm	cpm	cpm	%
Experiment 1				
Control	1.02×10^{7}	56	53	0.0000
Bt_2cAMP	1.05×10^{7}	232	112	0.0042
Experiment 2				
Control	1.32×10^{7}	58	60	0.0000
Bt_2cAMP	1.49×10^{7}	240	80	0.0037

Effect of Bt_2cAMP on VIP/PHM-27 gene expression. Nuclei isolated from induced and uninduced cells were transcribed *in vitro*, and the relative rates of prepro-VIP/PHM-27 mRNA synthesis were determined by hybridization of the nuclear RNA products to immobilized pVIP-1.

The results are shown in Table II. Although the transcriptional activity was not detectable in nuclei isolated from uninduced cells, transcription of prepro-VIP/PHM-27 mRNA was actually observed in isolated nuclei from induced cells.

An RNA species corresponding to mature prepro-VIP/PHM-27 mRNA was detected in nuclear RNA isolated from induced cells and a possible prepro-VIP/PHM-27 mRNA precursor was faintly found at the position of about 4-kb (7).

DISCUSSION

From the present experiments, it may be concluded that cAMP exerts its effect on the transcription rate of VIP/PHM-27 gene in human neuroblastoma cells. The intracellular cAMP level may be increased by some hormones or neurotransmitters via the receptor-adenylate cyclase system. If such transmitters are demonstrated not only *in vitro* but also *in vivo*, then they may be the natural regulator of VIP/PHM-27 synthesis. Furthermore, the control mechanism of the processing step of VIP/PHM-27 precursor is of great importance in understanding the biosynthesis of VIP and PHM-27. Although VIP is preceded by a pair of basic amino acids, Lys-Arg, in the precursor protein, PHM-27 is preceded by only one basic amino acid, Arg (Fig. 1). Furthermore, both VIP and PHM-27 contain a pair of internal basic amino acid residues, such as Lys-Lys and Arg-Lys. These could reflect a differential tissue-specific processing pathway, yielding either VIP or PHM-27, or both. In addition, possible glycosylation sites are found in prepro-VIP/PHM-27. This suggests that the VIP/PHM-27 precursor may be a glycoprotein.

REFERENCES

1. Mutt V, Said SI (1974) Eur J Biochem 42:581-589
2. In: Said SI (ed) Vasoactive Intestinal Peptide, Advances in Peptide Hormone Research Series. (1982) Raven Press, New York
3. Obata K, Itoh N, Okamoto H, Yanaihara C, Yanaihara N, Suzuki T (1981) FEBS Lett 136:123-126
4. Okamoto H, Itoh N, Obata K (1983) Regulatory Peptides 6:320
5. Itoh N, Obata K, Yanaihara N, Okamoto H (1983) Nature 304:547-549
6. Tatemoto K, Mutt V (1981) Proc Natl Acad Sci USA 78:6603-6607
7. Hayakawa Y, Obata K, Itoh N, Yanaihara N, Okamoto H (1984) J Biol Chem, in press
8. Miyake S, Shimo T, Kitamura Y, Nojyo T, Nakamura S, Imashuku S, Abe T (1973) Autonomic Nervous System 10:115-120 (in Japanese)

34. Hormonal Control of Electrolyte Balance

Endocrinology
F. Labrie, L. Proulx, eds.

HORMONAL REGULATION OF GLOMERULAR ULTRAFILTRATION

KARL L. SKORECKI, BARBARA J. BALLERMANN, BARRY M. BRENNER

Laboratory of Kidney and Electrolyte Physiology, Brigham and Women's Hospital and Harvard Medical School, Boston, MA 02115

INTRODUCTION

A large volume of plasma normally courses through the microvascular network comprising the mammalian renal glomerulus. The excess transcapillary hydraulic over the opposing oncotic pressure difference results in the separation of a nearly ideal ultrafiltrate. In recent years it has become evident that this ultrafiltration process is regulated by a variety of circulating and intrarenal hormones. By combining physiologic studies using direct micropuncture of glomeruli in vivo with biochemical studies using isolated glomeruli and cultured glomerular cells in vitro, new insights have been gleaned into the mechanisms whereby hormones influence glomerular filtration at the single nephron level. This paper will focus on the role of angiotensin II (AII).

PHYSIOLOGIC STUDIES

Advances in micropuncture methodology have made possible a precise description of the forces governing glomerular ultrafiltration (1). As described in detail elsewhere (2), the mean net force favoring ultrafiltration, P_{UF}, is given by the difference between the mean glomerular transcapillary hydraulic pressure gradient (ΔP) and the corresponding mean transcapillary gradient of colloid osmotic pressure ($\Delta\pi$) The rate of ultrafiltration for a single glomerulus (SNGFR) is equal to the product of the mean net driving pressure (P_{UF}) and the ultrafiltration coefficient (K_f). K_f, in turn, is the product of the local effective hydraulic conductivity of the capillary wall (k) and the total surface area available for filtration (S). Accordingly, changes in SNGFR may be evoked by alterations in K_f or P_{UF}, the latter ultimately determined by the value of ΔP, the oncotic pressure at the afferent end of the glomerular capillary network (π_A) and the initial glomerular capillary plasma flow rate (Q_A). Therefore, all vasoactive substances that affect the whole kidney glomerular filtration rate (GFR) must do so by influencing one or more of these determinants of SNGFR.

The action of AII on the glomerular microcirculation of the rat was first studied by Myers et al. (3). In that study, infusion of pressor doses of AII resulted, on average, in relative stability of SNGFR, despite a significant decline in Q_A. This fall in Q_A was associated with increases in afferent arteriolar resistance (R_A) and efferent resistance (R_E). The mean value of ΔP increased with AII infusion, due primarily to a marked increase in P_{GC}. The average value of the efferent arteriolar oncotic pressure (π_E) rose concomitantly with ΔP so that filtration pressure equilibrium was preserved. Given persistence of filtration pressure equilibrium, SNGFR is determined solely by Q_A, ΔP and π_A. Since, on average, π_A was unchanged by AII infusion, the observed near constancy of SNGFR resulted from offsetting effects of a reduction in Q_A and elevation of ΔP. Of interest is the extent to which the rise in ΔP observed with AII is dependent on the simultaneous rise in renal perfusion pressure that regularly occurs with the dose of AII employed in these studies. To examine this question, Myers et al. (3) carried out experiments with an identical dose of AII in a separate group of Munich-Wistar rats in which partial constriction of the aorta prevented the rise in renal perfusion pressure. When the aorta was constricted during infusion of AII, the increase in R_A was strikingly attenuated. Average changes in R_E, SNGFR, Q_A, ΔP and π_E, however, were similar to those seen when the rise in arterial pressure was permitted. These observations suggest that the increase in R_A that occurs when arterial pressure increases, is secondary to the rise in renal perfusion pressure - perhaps the consequence of a myogenic reflex. This possibility received further support from a series of experiments by Ichikawa et al. (4). Thus, in response to a subpressor dose of AII administered via the renal artery, the changes in the mean values of R_E, Q_A, SNGFR, ΔP and π_E were similar to those seen with systemic infusion of pressor doses of AII, whereas, on average, R_A and renal arterial pressure again failed to increase appreciably. These studies suggest that the predominant microcirculatory action of AII is confined to the efferent arteriole, a conclusion subsequently confirmed by others (5).

In order to study the effect of AII infusion on the glomerular capillary ultrafiltration coefficient, K_f, Blantz et al. (6) examined the effects of varying doses of AII on plasma-loaded rats. Under circumstances of plasma loading, filtration pressure disequilibrium obtained, thus enabling the determination of unique values for K_f with AII infusion. Significant reductions in the mean value of K_f to $\sim$ 50% of control were noted. It has also been noted that the AII-induced glomerular hemodynamic changes could be reversed by the infusion of verapamil or manganese; known inhibitors of excitation-contraction coupling in smooth muscle cells that act by interfering with transmembrane calcium transport (4,7).

Vasopressin also has been shown to modulate SNGFR. Ichikawa and Brenner (8) systematically investigated the glomerular actions of various antidiuretic peptides in the chronically water-diuretic Munich-Wistar rat. During infusion of arginine vasopressin, the average value of ΔP rose significantly despite near constancy of P_{GC}, due to a marked fall in tubule pressure following transition from water diuresis to ADH-induced antidiuresis. Despite this increase in ΔP, SNGFR, on average, failed to change due to an ADH-induced reduction in the mean value of K_f that served to offset the increase in ΔP. The same response was observed with other antidiuretic peptides (Pitressin and DDAVP).

The effect of a number of other hormones on glomerular hemodynamics has been shown to be mediated ultimately by the action of AII. These included parathyroid hormone, prostaglandin E_2 and prostaglandin I_2 (9-12). These hormones, all of which activate adenylate cyclase, as well as dibutyryl cAMP itself, when infused in vivo cause a reduction in K_f which can be mitigated by angiotensin blockade (8-12). This suggests that these substances act via local cAMP mediated renin release and AII generation to bring about the observed reduction in K_f (11-16). Indeed, a number of studies have demonstrated the presence of all the biochemical requirements for the local glomerular elaboration of AII (16-19). In addition to the hormones noted above, more recently Blantz and coworkers (20) have demonstrated that the glomerular hemodynamic effects of β-adrenergic stimulation are also mediated in part through the action of AII (presumably also as a result of local renin release) as indicated by the effect of AII inhibition. In contrast, the effects of vasopressin on glomerular hemodynamics do not require the intermediacy of AII. The dramatic fall in K_f and rise in glomerular capillary resistances elicted by vasopressin infusion, are not reversed by angiotensin blockade (8).

BIOCHEMICAL STUDIES

Insights into the cellular mechanisms of action of AII have come from studies in isolated glomeruli and cultured glomerular cells. Ligand binding studies in isolated rat renal glomeruli using ^{125}I-AII have demonstrated a single class of high affinity receptors with an equilibrium dissociation constant of approximately 0.4 nM (21). From this value and the known circulating levels of AII, it was determined that occupancy of only a small fraction of total receptors was sufficient to elicit a physiologic response.

Autoradiographic studies using ^{125}I-AII in vitro (21) and using ^{3}H-AII in vivo (22) localized these receptors to the surface of glomerular mesangial cells. The potency order for displacement of tracer AII by analogues of AII was shown to differ from the potency order described for rat mesenteric smooth muscle, indicating heterogeneity of AII receptor subtypes, in agreement with the heterogeneous physiologic response to AII analogues reported by Taub et al. (23) in the peripheral and renal circulations. Regulation of AII receptor density by alterations in circulating levels of AII in response to changes in salt intake were also demonstrated (21). High salt intake was associated with upregulation and low salt intake with downregulation of receptor density, without any change in receptor affinity. In addition, the administration of captopril to suppress circulating AII levels in animals fed a low salt diet resulted in upregulation of receptor number implying that receptor density is regulated by circulating AII concentrations per se.

As was noted above, the capacity for local glomerular production of AII has been demonstrated in a number of studies (16-19). It thus appears, that the capacity for regulation of glomerular hemodynamics resides locally within the glomerulus, both in terms of synthetic source and target for the vasoactive peptide. An understanding of the potential mechanisms whereby alterations in glomerular hemodynamics are brought about by occupancy of AII receptors in the glomerulus has emanated from studies in cultured glomerular cells. Radioligand binding studies have demonstrated high affinity binding sites for AII on glomerular mesangial cells in primary culture (24-25), confirming the autoradiographic localization studies in whole glomeruli (21). Furthermore, incubation of cultured mesangial cells with AII is associated with a calcium-dependent contractile response whose kinetic parameters parallel the kinetics of hormone binding (24-26).

Glomerular mesangial cells contain abundant bundles of myofilaments, dense surface patches and dense bodies, similar to vascular smooth muscle cells (25-26). In addition, human mesangial cells have been shown by immunofluorescence to contain actomyosin in situ (26,27). In a variety of other AII-responsive systems, it has been shown that after binding to its receptor, AII is thought to stimulate hydrolysis of membrane polyphosphoinositides which results in enhanced cytosolic calcium availability (28,29). In vascular smooth muscle, the latter signal is associated with stimulation of myosin light chain kinase, leading to the contractile response (30).

Based on the combined physiologic and biochemical evidence cited above, it has been proposed that the K_f-lowering effects of AII in the glomerulus may be brought about by contraction of mesangial cells, which are anatomically ideally located to act as modulators of glomerular capillary patency and, thereby, filtration surface area.

In addition to effects of mesangial cell contraction, AII-associated phospholipase activation with enhanced prostaglandin E_2 release has been demonstated in cultured glomerular mesangial cells (31-33). In this same study, a similar response to vasopressin, with specificity for the pressor receptor subtype was also noted. Release of prostaglandins locally may serve to modulate the hemodynamic consequences of AII on the glomerular microcirculation (33-34). This may be of particular physiologic relevance under those circumstances in which it is desirable to dissociate the systemic hemodynamic effects of high circulating levels of AII from its renal hemodynamic consequences.

DISEASE MODELS

The role of altered AII action in the glomerulus in the pathogenesis of a number of disease states has been explored using a variety of approaches in experimental disease models. A reduction in K_f has been observed in several experimental models of renal injury including gentamicin nephrotoxicity (35,36), uranyl-nitrate induced ARF (20,37), puromycin aminonucleoside-induced nephrotic syndrome (38), and partial ureteral obstruction (39) in rats. In each of these cases the reduction in K_f could be mitigated at least in part by inhibition or blockade of angiotensin. This suggests a functional AII-mediated component as part of the lesion in these experimental models. Such an AII effect may be mediated by perturbations in local intrarenal AII production or binding or altered interactions with other vasoactive hormones.

Most recently a number of studies have explored the physiologic and biochemical basis for the glomerular hemodynamic abnormalities of experimental streptozotocin-induced diabetes mellitus in rats. Reduced renal vascular sensitivity to AII has been demonstrated in early experimental diabetes mellitus (40). At the single nephron level, augmented single nephron glomerular plasma flow rates and glomerular hyperfiltration have been demonstrated and thought to contribute to the eventual development of diabetic glomerulopathy (41,42). In order to determine the biochemical basis for this hemodynamic disturbance, Ballermann et al. (43) compared AII binding parameters in glomeruli isolated from normal rats, and from insulin treated and non-insulin treated rats with streptozotocin-induced diabetes mellitus 3 to 4 weeks after induction of disease. With low, intermediate and high salt intakes, AII receptor density varied inversely with the plasma renin concentration in all three groups. However, despite lower plasma renin concentrations in untreated diabetic rats, AII receptor density was reduced at all levels of salt intake when compared to control and insulin-treated diabetic rats. AII receptor affinity was not different among the groups studied. Normalization of blood sugars was not achieved in the insulin treated diabetic group so that the reduction in AII-receptor density could not be explained on the basis of hyperglycemia per se. Administration of captopril to control and untreated diabetic rats on a low salt diet resulted in upregulation of receptor density in both groups indicating that regulation of receptor density in response to circulating AII levels was preserved although reset in untreated diabetic rats. It has been demonstrated that for systems in which there is a substantial receptor reserve, responsiveness to hormone is a nearly linear function of receptor number at low hormone occupancy (44). This circumstance applies to the glomerular receptor for AII (21), such that the 30-35% lowering of glomerular AII receptor density for any given plasma renin concentration in untreated diabetic rats could account for the observed diminished glomerular vasoreactivity.

CONCLUSION

A number of circulating and intrarenal hormones modulate glomerular hemodynamic parameters at the single nephron level. Among these, AII plays a central role, by binding to specific receptors located on glomerular mesangial cells where a contractile response is elicited. This response modulates the single nephron glomerular ultrafiltration coefficient. This latter parameter varies therefore with circulating and local intrarenal levels of AII and with mesangial AII receptor characteristics. Local glomerular renin release and production of AII may serve as a common pathway for the action of a number of other vasoactive hormones on the glomerulus. Alterations in AII production or receptor characteristics underlie abnormalities of glomerular function in a number of experimental models of disease including diabetes mellitus.

ACKNOWLEDGEMENT

We gratefully acknowledge the expert secretarial and editorial assistance provided by Ms. Michelle Hardiman.

Support for studies performed by the authors was provided by USPHS grants AM19467 and AM30410

REFERENCES

1. Baylis C, Brenner BM (1978) Rev Physiol Biochem Pharmacol 80:1-46, 1978
2. Brenner BM, Ichikawa I, Deen WM (1981) In: Brenner BM, Rector FC (eds) The Kidney. Saunders, Philadelphia, pp. 289-327
3. Myers BD, Deen WM, Brenner BM (1975) Circ Res 37:101-110
4. Ichikawa I, Miele JF, Brenner BM (1979) Kidney Int 16:137-147
5. Edwards RM (1983) Am J Physiol 244:F526-F534
6. Blantz RC, Konnen KS, Tucker BJ (1976) J Clin Invest 57:419-434
7. Langer GA, Serena SD, Nudd LM (1975) Am J Physiol 229:1003-1007
8. Ichikawa I, Brenner BM (1977) Am J Physiol 233:F102-F117
9. Ichikawa I, Humes HD, Dousa TP, Brenner BM (1978) Am J Physiol 234:F393-F401
10. Schor NI, Ichikawa I, Brenner BM (1981) Kidney Int 20:442-451
11. Dworkin LD, Ichikawa I, Brenner BM (1983) Am J Physiol 244:F95-F104
12. Torres VE, Northrup TE, Edwards RM, Shah SV, Dousa TP (1978) J Clin Invest 62:1334-1343
13. Sraer J, Ardaillou R, Loreau M, Sraer JD (1974) Endocrinol 1:285-294
14. Schlondorff D, Yoo P, Alpert BE (1978) Am J Physiol 235:458-464

15. Dousa TP, Barnes LD, Ong SH, Steiner AL (1977) Proc Natl Acad Sci USA 74:3569-3573
16. Hofbauer KG, Konrads A, Schwartz K, Werner U (1978) Klin Wschr 50:51-59
17. Celio M, Inagami T (1981) Proc Natl Acad Sci USA 78:3897-3800
18. Frega MS, Davalos M, Leaf A (1980) Kidney Int 18:323-327
19. Levens NR, Peach MJ, Carey RM (1981) Circ Res 48:157-167
20. Blantz RC, Pelayo JC (1983) Federation Proc 42:3071-3074
21. Skorecki KL, Ballermann BJ, Rennke HG, Brenner BM (1983) Federation Proc 42:3064-3070
22. Osborne MJ, Droz B, Meyer P, Morel F (1975) Kidney Int 8:245-254
23. Taub KJ, Caldicott WJH, Hollenberg NK (1977) Kidney Int 59:528-535
24. Foidart JJ, Sraer F, Delarue P, Maheiu P, Ardaillou R (1980) FEBS Lett 121:333-339
25. Ausiello DA, Kreisberg JJ, Roy C, Karnovsky MJ (1980) 65:754-760
26. Kreisberg J (1983) Federation Proc 42:3053-3057
27. Scheinman JI, Fish AJ (1978) Am J Path 92:125-146
28. Farese RV, Larson RE, Sabir MA, Gomez-Sanchez C (1981) J Biol Chem 256:11093-11097
29. Elliot ME, Alexander RC, Goodfriend TL (1982) Hypertension 4:II-52-II-58
30. Anderson JM, Gimbrone MA, Alexander RW (1981) J Biol Chem 256:4693-4696
31. Kreisberg JI, Karnovsky MJ, Levine L (1982) Kidney Int 22:355-359
32. Scharschmidt LA, Dunn MJ (1983) J Clin Invest 71:1756-1764, 1983.
33. Scharschmidt LA, Lianos E, Dunn MJ (1983) Federation Proc 42:3058-3063
34. Baylis C, Brenner BM (1978) Circ Res 43:889-898
35. Baylis C, Rennke HG, Brenner BM (1977) Kidney Int 12:344-353
36. Schor N, Ichikawa I, Brenner BM (1981) Kidney Int 19:288-296
37. Blantz R, Gushwa L (1982) Kidney Int 21:215(abstract)
38. Ichikawa I, Rennke HG, Hoyer JR, Badr KF, Schor N, Troy JL, Lechene CP, Brenner BM (1983) J Clin Invest 71:91-103
39. Ichikawa I, Brenner BM (1979) Am J Physiol 236:F131-F140
40. Reineck HJ, Kreisberg JI (1983) Kidney Int 23:247 (abstract)
41. Hostetter TH, Troy JL, Brenner BM (1981) Kidney Int 19:410-415
42. Hostetter TH, Rennke HG, Brenner BM (1982) Am J Med 72:375-380
43. Ballermann BJ, Skorecki KL, Brenner BM Am J Physiol (In Press)
44. Levitzki A (1980) In: Schulster D, Levitzki A (eds) Cellular Receptors for Hormones and Neurotransmitters, John Wiley and Sons Ltd, pp. 9-28

Endocrinology
F. Labrie, L. Proulx, eds.

CONTROL OF TRANSEPITHELIAL SODIUM TRANSPORT AND Na,K-ATPase SYNTHESIS BY OXYTOCIN AND ALDOSTERONE IN THE TOAD URINARY BLADDER OF BUFO MARINUS*

BERNARD C. ROSSIER
Institut de Pharmacologie de l'Université, rue du Bugnon 21, CH-1011-Lausanne, Switzerland

INTRODUCTION

The urinary bladder of the toad *Bufo marinus* is a useful experimental model for studying the mechanism of action of hormones that control transepithelial sodium transport. Aldosterone and neuropituitary hormones (vasopressin, vasotocin, oxytocin) are probably the most important factors involved (1). In amphibia aldosterone and vasotocin (the natural agonists) increase sodium rabsorption by distinct mechanisms: aldosterone by the induction of proteins (i.e.aldosterone-induced protein) and vasotocin by a cAMP mediated process (2,3). We have previously reported that aldosterone induces *de novo* synthesis of Na,K-ATPase in the toad bladder (see review in ref 4). The induction was mineralocorticoid specific (e.g. related to the occupancy of Type I binding sites (10) and inhibited by Actinomycin D (4) or sodium butyrate (5). These latter observations suggest that the induction is a transcriptional mediated event. The induction of Na,K-ATPase occured late in the action of aldosterone on sodium transport, suggesting that it might be physiologically related to the late mineralocorticoid response (4,5). In this study, we have reexamined the synergistic action of aldosterone and oxytocin on sodium transport. We have studied whether oxytocin could also control the synthesis of Na,K-ATPase alone or in combination with aldosterone.

METHODS

Sodium transport response was measured by the short circuit current method as previously described (6). Oxytocin (Syntocinon, Sandoz) was added to the serosal compartment at a supramaximal concentration (50 mU/ml).

Na,K-ATPase biosynthesis was studied in homologous and paired pools of tissue incubated in presence of ^{35}S methionine (30 min pulse) as previously described (7). The alpha subunit of Na,K-ATPase was selectively immunoprecipitated and the relative rate of synthesis (over control) determined by scan densitometry (7).

*Supported by Swiss National Science Foundation
Grant no 3.646.80.

RESULTS AND DISCUSSION

Effects of oxytocin on sodium transport and Na,K-ATPase biosynthesis.

Upon addition of a supramaximal dose of oxytocin, we observed a rapid increase (Within 2 to 5 minutes) of sodium transport which peaked 3- to 4-fold above control values after 15 minutes. In agreement with others (8), the sodium transport then decreased progressively for the next two hours, but from then on (up to 20 hours of incubation) remained significantly (2-fold) higher than the control base-line. As shown in Table 1 and Figure 1, the rate of synthesis of the alpha subunit of Na,K-ATPase was significantly (1.9-fold) increased over control values at steady state (e.g. 20 hours after oxytocin addition).

TABLE 1

EFFECTS OF OXYTOCIN AND ALDOSTERONE ON THE RELATIVE RATE OF SYNTHESIS OF THE ALPHA SUBUNIT OF Na,K-ATPase

Experiment Number	Control	Relative change (Test/Control) Oxytocin (50mU/ml)	Aldosterone (80nM)	Aldosterone + Oxytocin
1	1.0	1.8	3.4	4.5
2	1.0	1.6	2.3	2.9
3	1.0	2.3	4.5	4.5
Mean $\pm$ SEM	1.0	1.9 $\pm$ 0.2	3.4 $\pm$ 0.6	4.0 $\pm$ 0.5

Homologous pools of urinary bladder tissue were incubated for 20 h in presence or abscence of hormones. Tissue labeling and immunoprecipitation of the alpha subunit and its resolution on SDS-PAGE were as described (7). The relative changes represent changes in peak heights of the immunoprecipitated products in densitometric scans of autoradiograms.

As shown in Figure 1, this effect was also mimicked by cAMP (2mM). In addition, both the cAMP- and oxytocin-dependent increase of alpha subunit synthesis rate were inhibited by pretreatment with Actinomycin D (2μg/ml). This inhibitor of transcription completely abolished the aldosterone-dependent sodium transport, but it abolished only the sustained (after 5-6 h) oxytocin-dependent sodium transport.

Effects of aldosterone on sodium transport and Na,K-ATPase biosynthesis

Upon addition of a supramaximal dose of aldosterone (final concn. 80nM), the increase in sodium transport was characterized by three distinct phases :

i) a *latent period* of about 45 minutes during which neither sodium transport nor transepithelial electrical resistance were significantly modified, ii) an *early response* (2 to 3 h)

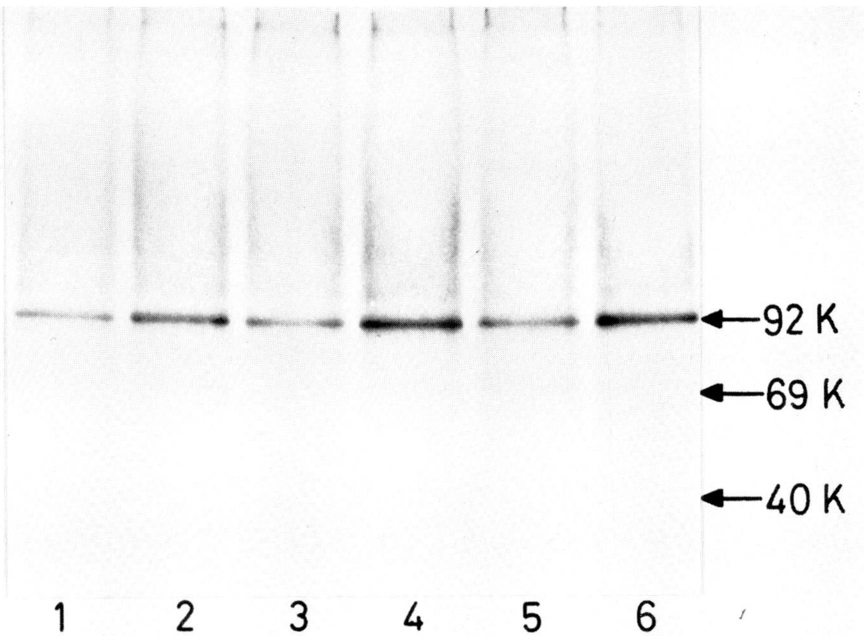

FIGURE 1. *Effects of oxytocin, aldosterone and cAMP on the rate of biosynthesis of the alpha subunit of Na,K-ATPase. Toad bladder tissues were incubated for 20 h either without hormone (lane 1), with aldosterone (80nM) (lane 2), with oxytocin (50mU/ml) (lane 3), with aldosterone (80nM) + oxytocin (50mU/ml) (lane 4), with cAMP (2mM, serosal side) (lane 5) or with cAMP (2mM) + aldosterone (80nM) (lane6). Immunprecipitation was performed on total cell extracts containing the same amount of radioactivity (see Methods).*

during which sodium transport increased rapidly and resistance fell concomitantly, iii) a *late response* during which sodium transport still increased substantially but without any further change in resistance. A steady state was reached 6 to 8 hours after the addition of aldosterone. From then on, the response was either maintained or slowly decreased to lower values even in continued presence of the hormone. After 20 hours of incubation, sodium transport of aldosterone-treated tissue remained, however, always significantly higher than base-line values. As shown in Table 1 and Figure 1 and as previously reported (7), the rate of synthesis of the alpha subunit of Na,K-ATPase was significantly increased (3.4-fold) over control values at steady state (e.g. 20 hours after aldosterone addition).

Synergistic effects of oxytocin (or cAMP) and aldosterone on sodium transport and Na,K-ATPase biosynthesis.

When aldosterone and oxytocin were added simultaneously (at their respective supramaximal concentrations) the sodium transport response (after 90 min) was always significantly higher than that observed when each hormone was given alone (synergism of potentiation). Cyclic AMP (2mM) was as effective as oxytocin in potentiating the effect of aldosterone. Cyclic AMP alone, however, was able to mimic the oxytocin response for only 2 hours and was much less effective in maintaining the sodium transport higher than base-line values. As shown in Table 1 and Figure 1, the effects of oxytocin and aldosterone on the rate of synthesis of the alpha subunit of Na,K-ATPase were synergistic but the observed potentiation was not statistically significant. The same appeared to be true for the interaction between cAMP and aldosterone (Figure 1).

CONCLUSIONS

Our results indicate that sodium transport and Na,K-ATPase synthesis are controlled by oxytocin (or cAMP) and aldosterone in a synergistic manner. The induction of Na,K,-ATPase was apparently mediated by a transcriptional step as suggested by the Actinomycin D sensitivity of the two hormonal responses. The discrepancy between the magnitude of the observed potentiation (sodium transport vs Na,K-ATPase synthesis) suggests that other important determinants of sodium transport (e.g. sodium channels) could also be involved in this synergism (11). Finally this hormonal interaction could be interpreted in the context of modulation of the cAMP-dependent protein kinases by aldosterone (9).

REFERENCES

1. Rossier BC, Geering K, Kraehenbühl JP (1979) Colloques Inserm 85:185-194
2. Fanestil DD, Park CS (1981) Annu Rev Physiol 43:637-649
3. Handler JS, Preston AS, Orloff J (1969) J Clin Invest 48:823-833
4. Rossier BC (1984) Curr Top Membr Transp 20:125-145
5. Truscello A, Geering K, Gäggeler HP, Rossier BC(1983)J Biol Chem 258:3388-3395
6. Rossier BC,Geering K,Gäggeler HP,Claire M,Corvol P (1980)Am J Phys 239:F433-439
7. Geering K, Girardet M, Bron C, Krähenbühl JP, Rossier BC (1982) J Biol Chem 257:10338-10343
8. Finn AL, Krug EF (1973) Am J Phys 224:1018-1023
9. Liu AYC (1984) Trends Pharmacol Sci 5:106-108
10. Geering K,Claire M,Gäggeler HP,Rossier BC(1984)Am J Phys(Cell Phys)(accepted)
11. Garty H, Edelman IS (1983) J Gen Physiol 81:785-803

Endocrinology
F. Labrie, L. Proulx, eds.

RENAL MINERALOCORTICOID TARGET CELLS

DIANA MARVER
University of Texas Health Science Center, Southwestern Medical School, Departments of Internal Medicine and Biochemistry, Dallas, Texas

The loss of adrenal function is associated with renal salt wasting, hyperkalemia, metabolic acidosis, a reduction in glomerular filtration rate, a decrease in urinary concentrating capacity, and an impairment in the capacity to excrete a water load (1). Both mineralocorticoids and glucocorticoids participate in the correction of these defects. Those responses attributable to mineralocorticoids include correction of salt wasting, hyperkalemia, and acidosis. Glucocorticoids also directly or indirectly influence K^+ and H^+ excretion by either enhancing the glomerular filtration rate (K^+) or proximal tubule ammoniagenesis, Na/H exchange capacity and phosphate turnover (H^+) (2,3). Furthermore, following adrenalectomy, there is a modest fall in renal cortical NaK ATPase with a 30-50% fall in outer medullary enzyme activity. The cortical steroid-dependent enzyme is localized to the collecting tubule (CCT) while that of the outer medulla is attributable to the medullary thick ascending limb of Henle (mTALH). Mineralocorticoids correct the cortical enzyme levels, and glucocorticoids the medullary enzyme levels if administered following adrenalectomy (4-8). While the effect of aldosterone on CCT NaK ATPase enhances the Na reabsorptive and K secretive capacity of the distal nephron, the influence of glucocorticoids on mTALH NaK ATPase activity would be expected to help correct the incapacity to excrete a water load since free water is generated at this segment. It has also been suggested that plasma ADH levels, elevated secondary to a reduction in ECF also diminish the ability to excrete a water load normally, and this state is corrected by mineralocorticoids (9).

A permissive action of picomolar concentrations [well below those concentrations of steroid required to occupy either the renal Type I (mineralocorticoid) or Type II (glucocorticoid) receptors (10)] on distal nephron ADH-mediated water flow has also been documented (11). This action of corticosteroids explains the final defect in adrenal insufficiency, namely the inability to maximally concentrate urine, since the ADH-sensitive collecting duct system is responsible for free water reabsorption. A glucocorticoid effect on the hypertonicity of the medulla, generated at the level of the thick ascending limb would also be expected to play some role in establishing the osmotic gradient for free water reabsorption in the presence of ADH and permissive levels of corticosteroids.

Two sites of aldosterone action along the nephron have been studied in some detail. They include the cortical and outer medullary collecting duct. While the former is responsible for steroid-dependent Na reabsorption and K secretion, the medullary collecting duct elaborates aldosterone-dependent H^+ secretion. Adrenalectomy markedly depresses the ability of the latter segment to secrete acid, and acute aldosterone, but not dexamethasone added to in vitro microperfused inner stripe medullary collecting duct tubules returns this secretory capacity to normal values within several hours post-addition (12). Increases in acid secretion are preceded by increases in the mineralocorticoid marker enzyme, citrate synthase (13).

In comparison, acute actions of aldosterone on the cortical collecting tubule include an increase in lumen to bath Na^+ transport, as determined in in vitro microperfusion experiments (14) and an elevation of citrate synthase and NaK ATPase activities (5,15). In this segment, marked increases in citrate synthase can be demonstrated as early as 1.5 hours after hormone administration while those in NaK ATPase are significantly elevated after some 2-3 hours post hormone administration. Neither are acutely increased if equivalent doses of dexamethasone rather than aldosterone are given, suggesting that they are mineralocorticoid-specific. This is supported by the studies of Mujais et al (6) who found that chronic replacement of circulating levels of aldosterone but not corticosterone by implantation of minipumps in adrenalectomized rats increased NaK ATPase in cortical collecting tubules. Thus, under steady-state conditions, this segment appears to have a transepithelial potential difference and a net Na and K flux which varies as a function of changes in plasma aldosterone concentrations within the physiological range (16).

Less clear is the action of aldosterone at other distal nephron sites including the thick ascending limb of Henle (TALH), the distal convoluted tubule and the connecting segment. For instance, modest doses of aldosterone have been shown to bind to apparent Type I mineralocorticoid receptors in the connecting segment using autoradiographic analyses (17), while acute doses of aldosterone increase citrate synthase levels in the medullary TALH (13). When Farman and Bonvalet elevated ambient ^3H aldosterone concentrations for autoradiographic analyses of nuclear-bound steroid complexes, they also found enhanced labeling of structures such as the distal convoluted tubule in addition to the TALH. Whether these constitute aldosterone-specific sites or crossover binding to other classes of receptors remains to be seen. Certainly chronic high dose steroid therapy using deoxycorticosterone acetate brings about both enhanced NaK ATPase activities and increases in the basolateral membrane surface area in all distal nephron cortical segments (18,19). Again, whether this is mediated via a particular receptor, the direct physiological consequences of binding to some combination of Type I, II, and III sites, or whether the hypertrophy is linked to volume expansion and enhanced Na load to the distal nephron is unclear, but has been discussed in some depth in a recent publication (20).

ACKNOWLEDGEMENTS

The author wishes to acknowledge the support of NIH-NIAMD grant number AM 25176 for some of the studies outlined above.

REFERENCES

1. Marver D (1981) IN: Munson P (ed) Vitamins and Hormones, Vol 38. Academic Press, New York, pp 55-117
2. Welbourne TC, Phenix P, Thornley-Brown C, Welbourne CJ (1976) Proc Soc Exp Biol Med 153:539-542
3. Freiberg JM, Kinsella J, Sactor B (1982) Proc Natl Acad Sci USA 79:4932-4936
4. Marver D, Schwartz MJ, Petty K, Lombard WE (1980) In: Licardus B, Schrier RW, Ponec J (eds) Hormonal Regulation of Sodium Excretion. Elsevier/ North- Holland Biomedical Press, Amsterdam, pp 229-236
5. Petty KJ, Kokko JP, Marver D (1981) J Clin Invest 68:1514-1521
6. Mujais SK, Chekal MA, Jones WJ, Hayslett JP, Katz AI (1984) J Clin Invest 73:13-19
7. Charney AN, Silva P, Besarab A, Epstein FH (1974) Am J Physiol 227:345-350
8. Rayson BM, Lowther SO (1984) Am J Physiol 246:F656-F662
9. Schrier RW, Bichet DG (1981) J Lab Clin Med 98:1-15
10. Marver D (1980) Endocrinology 106:611-618
11. Schwartz MJ, Kokko JP (1980) J Clin Invest 66:234-242
12. Stone DK, Kokko JP, Jacobson HR (1983) J Clin Invest 72:77-83
13. Marver D, Lombard WE (1981) Kidney Int 19:248
14. Wingo CS, Kokko JP, Jacobson HR (1984) Kidney Int 26: in press
15. Marver D, Schwartz MJ (1980) Proc Natl Acad Sci USA 77:3672-3676
16. Schwartz GJ, Burg MJ (1978) Am J Physiol 235:F576-F585
17. Farman N, Vandewalle A, Bonvalet JP (1982) Am J Physiol 242:F69-F77
18. Kaissling B, LeHir M (1982) Cell Tissue Res 224:469-492
19. LeHir M, Kaissling B, Dubach UC (1982) Cell Tissue Res 224:493-503
20. Marver D (1984) Am J Physiol 246:F111-F123

© 1984 Elsevier Science Publishers B.V.
Endocrinology
F. Labrie, L. Proulx, eds.

THE HEART IS AN ENDOCRINE GLAND

MARC CANTIN, JOLANTA GUTKOWSKA, GAETAN THIBAULT, RAUL GARCIA, MADHU ANAND-SRIVASTAVA, PAVEL HAMET, ERNESTO SCHIFFRIN, JACQUES GENEST

Clinical Research Institute of Montreal, 110 Pine Ave West, Montreal, Quebec Canada, H2W 1R7

INTRODUCTION

Since the discovery of "granules" in guinea pig atrial cardiocytes by Kisch in 1956 (1), it has been well established that the atria of mammals (2) and the atria and ventricles of non mammalian vertebrates (3) contain a large Golgi complex and secretory-like granules. These granules were shown by ultrastructural cytochemistry to be made up of proteins (4) and to contain glycoproteins (5) and, by ultrastructural radioautography, to incorporate both ^{3}H-leucine (6) and ^{3}H-fucose (7) in a pattern identical to that of other peptide-secreting endocrine cells. We have established that atrial granules isolated by ultracentrifugation produce a rapid onset and short-lived (20 min), diuresis and natriuresis (8). ANF in the rat is a long molecule of 152 amino acids, the cDNA of which has now been cloned (9), following the sequencing of various fragments with extension in the N-terminus: first the 1-33AA (2-33, 3-33 and 8-33AA) (10), then the 1-73AA (11) and the 1-106AA (12). A short form (1-16AA) synthetized by P. Schiller (Clinical Research Institute of Montreal) was found to possess no biological activity (13). A longer version (8-33AA) synthetized by R. Nutt (Merck Sharp & Dohme Research Laboratories) is as active as the native form (3-33AA) in inducing diuresis and natriuresis (10), vasodilatation and inhibition of the arterial contraction produced either by catecholamines or by angiotensin II (14). We have used this synthetic peptide for all further work.

Localization of receptors

Binding sites. Receptors for the ligand have been found in the zona glomerulosa and zona fasciculata of the beef adrenal cortex (15,16) as well as in anterior and posterior pituitary homogenates.

Radioimmunoassay

Rat atria. A direct radioimmunoassay for ANF has been developed (17). A significantly higher ANF content has been found in the right (2.5 fold) than in the left atrium thus confirming previous morphometric studies at the ultrastructural level (18) and previous immunohistochemical findings of higher granularity in right atrial cardiocytes (19).

Rat plasma. A direct radioimmunoassay to measure immunoreactive ANF in rat plasma has been developed. The results indicate that immunoreactive ANF is indeed present in rat plasma in measurable concentration.

Effects on the adrenals. The effect of 8-33 ANF on adrenal steroidogenesis has been studied in primary cultures of bovine adrenal cells. The polypeptide produces a potent 40-70% inhibition of angiotensin II, ACTH, PGE_1, and forskolin-stimulated secretion of aldosterone production from zona glomerulosa cells with an ED_{50} of 120 pM (15). An equipotent inhibitory effect of ANF on cortisol production was also observed in zona fasciculata cells (15). Analogous results have been obtained with dispersed zona glomerulosa cells of the rat: ANF inhibits hypersecretion of aldosterone induced by angiotensin II, ACTH or potassium. In vivo, the aldosterone response to AII or ACTH is also inhibited in the unanesthetized rat.

Effect on arteries. The infusion of ANF into a high resistance isolated perfused rat kidney produced a rapid decrease (33 ± 5 mmHg) in perfusion pressure which lasted for 18 ± 3 min. ANF produces a potent, dose-dependent relaxant effect on rabbit and rat arterial strips previously made to contract by application of either norepinephrine or angiotensin II. After the application of ANF, the vascular strips were refractory to subsequent stimulation by either Ne or AII. These effects of ANF on vascular smooth muscles, which suppose the presence of receptors, are not mediated by prostaglandins, adrenergic or muscarinic receptors or by an impairment of Ca^{++} influx but are mimicked by sodium nitroprusside (20).

Physiopathology

Hypertension. The intravenous injection of an ED_{50} natriuretic dose (1 μg) of the synthetic peptide induced a fall in blood pressure of 61 ± 6 mmHg in two-kidney, one-clip and of 45 ± 6 mmHg in one-kidney, one-clip hypertensive rats. This decrease in blood pressure lasted more than 40 min in the former group of rats and 34 ± 2 min in the latter. The absence of a positive correlation between natriuresis or diuresis and the fall of blood pressure after ANF administration and the lack of change in hematocrit suggest that the effect of ANF on blood pressure is mainly due to vasodilatation and not to a fall in circulatory volume.

Expansion of blood volume. The relationship observed since several decades between expansion of blood volume and the ensuing diuresis and natriuresis had remained unexplained. We have found that the natriuresis and diuresis which follow blood volume expansion in 240 g female Sprague-Dawley rats (intrajugular infusion of 0.33 ml/min of 0.9% NaCl) are significantly diminished by intravenous injection of 0.5 ml of antiserum from rabbits injected with 8-33 ANF whereas pre immune rabbit serum has no such effect. These results suggest that blood volume expansion induces increased release of ANF from atria and preliminary radioimmu noassay results indicate that it is so.

Adenylate cyclase

Arteries. ANF 8-33 inhibits adenylate cyclase activity in aortic washed particles, mesenteric arteries and renal artery homogenates in a concentration dependent manner with an apparent Ki between 0.1 to 1 nM (21). ANF is also able to inhibit the stimulatory effect of hormones (isoproterenol, epinephrine, norepine phrine, dopamine, glucagon) and of certain agents such as sodium fluoride and forskolin which inhibit adenylate cyclase by receptor-independent mechanisms. In addition, ANF showed an additive effect with the inhibitory response of angio tensin II on adenylate cyclase from rat aorta. In contrast ANF showed no effect on adenylate cyclase activity of such tissues as spleen, squeletal muscle, adre nal medulla and testis which do not harbour target cells for ANF.

Anterior and posterior pituitary

8-33 ANF was also found to inhibit adenylate cyclase activity in rat anterior and posterior pituitary homogenates in a concentration dependent manner. The maximum inhibitions observed were 42% in anterior pituitary with an apparent Ki of 10^{-10}M and 25% with an apparent Ki of 10^{-11}M in posterior pituitary. CRF, VIP, prostaglandins stimulated adenylate cyclase to various degrees in anterior pituitary homogenates and ANF inhibits the stimulatory effect of all these agents. Here again, ANF was also able to inhibit the stimulation exerted by NaF and forskolin. Similarly, the stimulatory effect of N-Ethylcarboxamide adenosine (NECA), sodium fluoride and forskolin on adenylate cyclase in posterior pituitary homogenates were also inhibited by ANF (22). Preliminary data indicate that ANF inhibits the release of ACTH from rat anterior pituitary cell cultures only at very high concentrations (10^{-6}M) but stimulates ADH secretion from rat isolated posterior pituitary lobes at physiological range (10^{12} to 1^{10}M).

c-GMP

An ED_{50} dose of 8-33 ANF increases the plasma level (3.8 fold) as well as the renal excretion (10 fold) of cGMP. The relatively lesser (2 fold) increase of renal clearance indicates that the increase in urinary excretion is by and large due to the increase in tubular secretion (23). The effect of 8-33 ANF was also evaluated on a highly enriched population of proximal convoluted tubular cells from rat renal cortex (24): a 5-fold increase of cGMP was observed after 30 sec of incubation and the effect lasted 2 min (23).

SUMMARY

The evidence presented here indicates that atrial cardiocytes, apart from their contractile function, are bona fide endocrine cells which synthetize a peptide of known composition (152AA) through identified pathways (25,26). Part of the peptide is released into the circulation where it can be measured by RIA. A synthetic fragment (8-33AA) of the peptide is endowed with potent and variagated effects on several target tissues: massive diuresis and natriuresis of rapid onset and short duration, inhibition of the secretion of aldosterone from beef and rat zona glomerulosa and, to a lesser extent, of cortisol from beef zona fasciculata, vasodilatation and inhibition of the arterial contraction induced by catecholamines or angiotensin II. This peptide is a potent antihypertensive agent. The presence of receptors in the anterior and posterior pituitary as well as the significant decrease of adenylate cyclase activity observed in both portion of the gland indicate that the hormone may act at these levels as well. Thus the heart is raised from the status of a pump to that of a putative endocrine integrator of cardiovascular homeostasis.

REFERENCES

1. Kisch B (1956) Exp Med Surg 14:99-112
2. Jamieson JD, Palade GE (1964) J Cell Biol 23:151-172
3. Yunge L, Ballak M, Beuzeron J, Lacasse J, Cantin M (1980) Can J Physiol Pharmacol 58:1463-1476
4. Huet M, Cantin M (1974) Lab Invest 30:525-532
5. Huet M, Cantin M (1974) Lab Invest 30:514-524
6. Yunge L, Benchimol S, Cantin M (1980) Cell Tiss Res 207:1-11
7. Yunge L, Benchimol S, Cantin M (1979) J Mol Cell Cardiol 11:375-388
8. Garcia R, Cantin M, Thibault G, Genest J (1982) Experientia 38:1071-1073
9. Zivin RA, Condra JH, Dixon RAF, Seidah NG, Chrétien M, Nemer M, Chamberland M, Drouin J Proc Natl Acad Sci (USA) submitted
10. Seidah NG, Lazure C, Chrétien M, Thibault G, Garcia R, Cantin M, Genest J, Nutt RF, Brady SF, Lyle TA, Peleveda WJ, Colton CD, Ciccerone TM, Veber DF (1984) Proc Natl Acad Sci (USA) 81:2640-2644
11. Thibault G, Garcia R, Cantin M, Genest J, Lazure C, Seidah G, Chrétien M (1984) FEBS Lett 167:352-356
12. Lazure C, Seidah NG, Chrétien M, Thibault G, Garcia R, Cantin M, Genest J Biochem Biophys Res Commun (in press)
13. Nguyen TMD, Schiller PW In: De Léan et al. Endocrinology (in press)
14. Garcia R, Thibault G, Nutt RF, Cantin M, Genest J (1984) Biochem Biophys Res Commun 119:685-687
15. De Léan A, Racz K, Gutkowska J, Nguyen TT, Cantin M, Genest J Endocrinology (in press)

16. De Léan A, Gutkowska J, McNicoll N, Schiller PW, Cantin M, Genest J Life Science (submitted)

17. Gutkowska J, Thibault G, Januszewicz P, Cantin M, Genest J Biochem Biophys Res Commun (in press)

18. Cantin M, Timm-Kennedy M, El-Khatib F, Huet M, Yunge L (1979) Anat Rec 193:55-76

19. Cantin M, Gutkowska J, Thibault G, Milne RW, Ledoux S, MinLi S, Chapeau C, Garcia R, Genest J (1984) Histochemistry 80:113-127

20. Garcia R, Thibault G, Cantin M, Genest J (1984) Am J Physiol (Reg Integr Comp Physiol (in press)

21. Anand-Srivastava MB, Franks DJ, Cantin M, Genest J Biochem Biophys Res Commun (in press)

22. Anand-Srivastava MB,Cantin M, Genest J Endocrinology (submitted)

23. Hamet P, Garcia R, Pang SC, Thibault G, Tremblay J, Gutkowska J, Cantin M, Genest J (submitted)

24. Vinay P, Gougoux A, Lemieux G (1981) Am J Physiol 241:F403

25. Yunge L, Benchimol S, Cantin M (1979) J Mol Cell Cardiol 11:375-388

26. Yunge L, Benchimol S, Cantin M (1980) Cell Tiss Res 207:1-11.

35. Developmental Endocrinology

Endocrinology
F. Labrie, L. Proulx, eds.

ONTOGENESIS OF PITUITARY HORMONES

PAUL M. DUBOIS[a], MARTINE BEGEOT[a], MICHEL L. AUBERT[b], FIONA J. HEMMING[a], GERARD MOREL[a]

a) C.N.R.S.-ERA 981, University of Lyon-Sud, B.P. 12, 69600 Oullins (France) ; b) Dept. of Pediatrics, University of Geneva, Geneva (Switzerland)

INTRODUCTION

For fourty years, numerous reviews have shown the rapid increase in our knowledge of the ontogeny of pituitary hormones in man (1-3) as well as in animals (4). These reviews insist on the appearance of pituitary hormones as early as the second month of gestation in man. Several reports also give some information about the early appearance of hypothalamic hypophysiotropic hormones. However, the participation of hypothalamic hormones in the differentiation of the pituitary hormones has still not been demonstrated.

Little information exists concerning the initial differentiation of the cells secreting the pituitary hormones. Increased knowledge of factors which could act on the pituitary anlage between the first stage in the formation of Rathke's pouch and the appearance of hormones offers possible insight into the differentiation of the pituitary cells. Indeed, many questions arise : what is the nature of these factors? What is their origin? How do they act? When do they act? Are they the same in the embryo as in the adult? Can the hypothalamic regulating factors of pituitary hormones participate in the differentiation of pituitary hormones? Do growth factors act? Do they act alone? Do they act with other factor(s)? Does every cell type differentiate according to its own model or are they all the same? To try to answer these questions, the methods used have included the study of congenital malformations in man or those induced either in experimental animals by ablation of fetal endocrine glands (5), or by administration of drugs, grafts of fetal pituitary gland or pituitary primordia (6), and culture of fetal pituitary gland or pituitary anlage with enriched serum medium (7-10). It was then suggested than in early fetal life the pituitary cells have a capacity for self-differentiation and that the beginning of the secretion of pituitary hormones is relatively autonomous and unrestrained. This was probably due to the use of grafts in a host where the endocrine environment is not well known and also to use of culture medium enriched with either fetal calf or horse serum of uncertain composition.

However, at present, culture of pituitary primordia in a synthetic medium, immunocytochemistry to detect the differentiated cells and radioimmunoassay to measure the quantities of secreted hormones, seem to be more suitable methods for elucidating the nature, origin and time of action of the factors inducing the differentiation of pituitary cell types. We summarize here our observations concerning 3 cell types (somatotrophs, gonadotrophs and lactotrophs) : the model of the schedule of differentiation is different for each cell type.

FIRST EXAMPLE : SOMATOTROPH DIFFERENTIATION (11)

Immunoreactive somatotropes could be detected, by light and electron microscopy, in cultured primordia explanted on day 14 of gestation or later. The size and numbers of immunoreactive somatotrophs depended on culture medium composition. Culture medium (Parker's 199) enriched with insulin (1 nM/ml) and either cortisol or corticosterone (280 nM) was suitable for development of this cell type. Culture medium enriched with insulin (1 nM/ml) alone was not suitable for development of somatotrophs. Addition of growth hormone-releasing factor (GHRH) to the medium, enriched with insulin (1 nM/ml), during the first culture day did not accelerate the first appearance of somatotrophs. Increased insulin concentration (500 nM/ml) reduced somatotroph numbers. So, the appearance of somatotrophs depends on insulin and glucocorticoid concentration, not on GHRH presence. It is noteworthy that insulin and glucocorticoid exist in man, as well as in rat, at an early stage of development while GHRH, on the contrary, appears much later, after the appearance of the first immunoreactive somatotrophs.

SECOND EXAMPLE : GONADOTROPH DIFFERENTIATION (12, 13)

Immunoreactive gonadotrophs could be detected in the primordia explanted at 11 or 12 days of gestation and cultured in medium (Parker's 199) enriched with insulin (500 nM) and gonadoliberin (GnRH). Synthetic GnRH (10^{-9}M or 10^{-12}M) was added to the culture medium during the first day of culture only. No immunoreactive cells were observed when GnRH was added to the synthetic medium deprived of insulin. These data suggest that GnRH can stimulate the differentiation of gonadotrophs in early fetal life in synergy with insulin. This is supported by the intracellular presence of immunoreactive GnRH which is probably of fetal origin since it has been detected in fetal rat hypothalamus at 12 days of gestation (13). Moreover, no immunoreactive GnRH was detected in rat placenta during gestation and, in early fetal life, transfer of GnRH from mother to fetus is very unlikely since only very small amounts of radioactivity were detected in 11-day-old fetuses after injection of (^{125}I)-GnRH into pregnant rats (12). GnRH receptors can be found in the pituitary gland from 12-day-old fetuses and they increase from 20 days of gestation (13).

THIRD EXAMPLE : LACTOTROPH DIFFERENTIATION

In vitro, immunoreactive lactotrophs were detected in primordia explanted at 13 days and cultured in medium enriched with whole or dialyzed fetal calf serum (14). So, estradiol was not involved in lactotroph differentiation. Addition of GnRH (10^{-9}M) to synthetic medium (Parker's 199 enriched with insulin) induced differentiation of immunoreactive lactotrophs (15). However, the effect of GnRH on lactotroph differentiation is mediated by gonadotrophs since the GnRH-induced lactotroph differentiation was inhibited when an anti-rat LH serum (recognizing native LH and its α-subunit) was added to the culture medium, but it was not inhibited when an anti-LHβ serum (recognizing both native LH and its β-subunit) was used. Further addition of highly purified LH-α subunit (10^{-7} or 10^{-9}M) to culture medium induced lactotrope differentiation. In man, LH-α subunit exist in the gonadotrophs (16, 17) in normal as well as in anencephalic fetuses. Moreover, in the latter, lactotrophs are more numerous and larger than in normal fetuses (18). These data suggest than the α-subunit of LH could be involved in the lactotroph differentiation.

So, the differentiated cells could be committed very early by the effective factors, programming the beginning of hormone synthesis. Thus, only some of the factors which regulate the secretion of pituitary hormones in adult seem to be involved in the initial differentiation of these cell types. It seems that the differentiation processes follow different patterns according to the cell type. Moreover, there is evidence that the undifferentiated cells of the pituitary anlage are not capable of self-differentiation.

ACKNOWLEDGEMENTS

The authors thank Pr R. Guillemin, The Salk Institute, for his generous gift of GRF, Dr M.P. Dubois for his gift of antiserum, Dr Y. Combarnous, I.N.R.A., for his gift of LH and of α-subunit of LH. The authors thank also Mrs M. Tschora for patient secretarial assistance. This work was supported by grant from C.N.R.S. (ERA 981 and ATP n°8206), from I.N.S.E.R.M. (PRC n°135009 and CRE n°834001).

REFERENCES

1. Kaplan SL, Grumbach MM, Aubert ML (1976) Rec Prog Horm Res 32:161-243
2. Gluckman PD, Grumbach MM, Kaplan SL (1980) In: Tulchinsky D, Ryan KJ (eds) Maternal-fetal Endocrinology. Saunders Co, Philadelphia, pp 196-232
3. Winter JSD (1983) In: Saez JM, Bertrand J, Ducharme JR, Collu R (eds) Ontogenesis of the endocrine system. INSERM, Paris, pp 117-134
4. Gluckman PD, Grumbach MM, Kaplan SL (1981) Endocrine Rev 2:363-395
5. Jost A (1953) Rec Prog Horm Res 8:379-418
6. Gash DM, Roos TB, Chambers WF (1975) Neuroendocrinology 19:214-226
7. Franchimont P, Pasteels JL (1972) C R Acad Sc (Paris) 1799-1802
8. Groom GV, Boyns AR (1973) J Endocrinol 59:511-522
9. Siler-Khodr TM, Morgenstern LL, Greenwood FC (1974) J clin Endocrinol Metab 39:891-905
10. Goodyer CG, Hall CSG, Guyda H, Robert F, Giroud CJP (1977) J clin Endocrinol Metab 45:73-85
11. Hemming FJ, Bégeot M, Dubois MP, Dubois P (1984) Endocrinology 114:2107-2112
12. Bégeot M, Morel G, Rivest RW, Aubert ML, Dubois MP, Dubois PM (1984) Neuroendocrinology 38:217-225
13. Aubert M, Bégeot M, Winiger BP, Morel G, Sizonenko P, Dubois PM (1984) Endocrinology:in press
14. Bégeot M, Dubois MP, Dubois PM (1984) C R hebd Acad Sc (Paris) 288:in press
15. Bégeot M, Hemming FJ, Martinat N, Dubois MP, Dubois PM (1983) Endocrinology 112:2224-2226
16. Dubois PM, Dubois MP (1974) In: Forest MG, Bertrand J (eds) Endocrinologie Sexuelle de la Période Périnatale. INSERM, Paris, pp 34-61
17. Hagen C, McNeilly AS (1975) J Endocrinol 67:49-57
18. Bégeot M, Dubois MP, Dubois PM (1984) J clin Endocrinol Metab 58:726-730

Endocrinology
F. Labrie, L. Proulx, eds.

MATURATION OF NEUROENDOCRINE CONTROL OF PITUITARY HORMONE SECRETION - STUDIES IN THE OVINE FETUS

PETER D GLUCKMAN
Department of Paediatrics, University of Auckland, Auckland, New Zealand

The establishment of hypothalamic control over adenohypophysial secretion is a gradual process. In vitro studies suggest that the differentiation of Rathkes pouch and the onset of adenohypophysial secretion is not necessarily dependent on hypothalamic influences. However in vitro and immunohistochemical studies suggest that hypothalamic stimulating factors influence adenohypophysial secretion by the time that the primitive portal vascular system appears (see 1 for review). The chronically catheterised fetal sheep offers an experimental approach to the study of the maturation of the neuroendocrine axis at stages subsequent to this (60 days to term (147 days)). The sheep is a neurally precocial species whose brain growth spurt occurs prenatally; this must be contrasted to altricial species such as the rat whose neural maturation occurs after birth.

Numerous studies of isolated fetal blood samples from many non-altricial species have demonstrated that fetal growth hormone (GH) concentrations are markedly elevated compared to postnatal concentrations (see 1). In general these studies have been noteable for the large scatter in fetal GH values observed. Recently we reexamined the pattern of GH secretion in the sheep fetus using frequent sampling. The basic characteristic of fetal GH release from at least 70 days of gestation is a markedly exaggerated pulsatility. The amplitude of the fetal pulses is greater than that seen in infant lambs (table 1). The interpulse nadir, which presumably reflects basal secretion by the pituitary, is also higher in the fetus than in the infant lamb. The available data suggests a rapid change in the pattern of GH secretion in the few days prior to parturition with GH secretion decreasing (1).

Using recently developed techniques for fetal stereotaxic neurosurgery (2) we examined GH secretion following lesions of the median eminence (ME) or of the arcuate - ventromedial (A-VM) region of the hypothalamus. Lesions of the ME lead to a loss of pulsatility and basal GH concentrations in these fetuses are similar to in the neonatal lamb (table 2). Thus the fetal pituitary is dependent on hypothalamic stimulation both for the high basal GH secretion and for the exaggerated pulsatile release. These observations rule out both pituitary autonomy as an explanation of high fetal GH concentrations and the possibility of direct extrahypothalamic stimulation. Lesions of the A-VM region also markedly reduce pulsatility. As exogenous growth hormone releasing factor (GRF) stimulates GH release in the sheep from at least 70 days of gestation (3,4) and as cell bodies for GRF are located in the medial-basal hypothalamus, these observations suggest that pulsatile GRF release drives fetal GH secretion. The basis for the generation of the pulses has not yet been resolved - the pulses are not synchronous with pulses of TSH or LH release suggesting specificity of the GH pulse generator. Despite an increase in pituitary GH content during this period, the magnitude of the GH response to exogenous GRF in utero decreases with advancing maturation and is less after birth than prenatally (3,4).

TABLE 1

THE ONTOGENY OF PULSATILE HORMONE RELEASE IN THE SHEEP FETUS

	Growth hormone (ng/ml)		Thyrotropin (uU/ml)*		
	Pulse height	Interpulse nadir	Pulse height	Interpulse nadir	
Fetus	92 ± 20	102 ± 15 (18)	7.4 ± 9.6	2.1 ± 3.8	(19)
Infant lamb	23.7 ± 6.5**	5.8 ± 0.5** (7)	2.1 ± 1.1**	< 0.1**	(10)
Ewe	5.8 ± 2.2**	6.3 ± 0.4** (7)	1.5 ± 0.4**	< 0.1**	(6)

* mean ± S.E.
** $p < 0.01$ compared to fetuses

We postulate that a major feature of fetal GH release is a deficiency of somatostatin (SRIF) secretion. Current models of the interactions between SRIF and GRF suggest that SRIF is a non competitive antagonist of GRF (5) and that in addition SRIF may tonically influence somatotropic activity. Thus the pattern of GH secretion in utero may reflect the secretion of GRF not counteracted by SRIF release. Such a hypothesis could explain both the high basal levels of GH and the exaggerated pulsatility observed in the fetal sheep in late gestation. While exogenous SRIF inhibits fetal GH release (see 1) and SRIF is present in the fetal hypothalamus, there is no experimental evidence of SRIF release by the hypothalamus in utero. Lesions of the preoptic region of the fetal hypothalamus (n = 2), the site of SRIF cell bodies, are not associated with an increase in GH secretion.

A paradox of GH secretion in utero is that despite this hypersecretory state, GH does not exert a major effect on fetal growth and neither fetal IGF-1 nor IGF-II concentrations are affected either by decapitation in midgestation (n = 3) or by ME lesions at 110 days of gestation (n = 5). Binding studies fail to demonstrate somatotropic receptors in the ovine liver until 3 - 6 days postnatally (6). As recent evidence suggests that GH secretion is regulated in part by a negative feedback loop functioning through GH (7) and/or IGF-I stimulated SRIF release, a similar receptor immaturity within the neuroendocrine unit could be a possible basis for the high fetal GH release. Whether the differentiation of the GH receptor is in some way linked to the events of parturition or whether it is a maturationally dependent event is not clear.

TABLE 2

EFFECT OF LESIONS OF THE FETAL MEDIAN EMINENCE ON PULSATILE HORMONE RELEASE

	Growth hormone (ng/ml)		Thyrotropin (uU/ml)
	Pulse height	Interpulse nadir	Pulse height
Shams	259 ± 38	65 ± 7	10.2 ± 2.4
Lesions	13 ± 3**	9 ± 2**	2.0 ± 1.0*

* $p < 0.05$
** < 0.01 - compared to shams

The hypothesis that the maturation of GH control commences with a phase of pulsatile GRF release associated with an immaturity of the feedback loop has parallels in studies of both fetal TSH and LH secretion. We have observed markedly pulsatile TSH release in the sheep fetus. Both the pulse height and amplitude are markedly greater than in the infant lamb or adult ewe where there is little evidence of pulsatile TSH release (table 1). Further the interpulse nadir in the fetus <120 days was less than in older fetuses and was <0.1 uU/ml in all postnatal studies (table 1). The pulsatility is reduced by lesions of the ME (table 2).

The exaggerated pulsatility in the fetus may reflect either or both of two mechanisms. Triiodothyronine (T_3) levels in the fetal circulation are low as a consequence of placental inner ring deiodinase converting secreted thyroxine to reverse T_3 (8); following placental separation at birth, T_3 levels rise. This would explain the pronounced fall in pulse amplitude in association with birth. However there is a fall in basal TSH secretion in the fetus after 120 days and this suggests maturational changes in the pituitary - thyroidal axis before birth. Previous studies have suggested immaturity of negative feedback by thyroid hormones in the fetus (see 9).

While studies in the neonatal rat have suggested a lack of hypothalamic influence on fetal TSH release (10), the observation that TSH release is modified by fetal ME lesions demonstrates hypothalamic influences on TSH release are present in utero in a more precocial species. The major influence on TSH release at birth is hypothermia and we recently demonstrated that a reduction in amniotic fluid temperature stimulates fetal TSH release from at least 106 days of gestation (11). This further suggests that hypothalamic thermoregulatory mechanisms have differentiated by this stage of gestation.

Studies of fetal gonadotropin release have shown that in the midgestation fetus, gonadotropin release is pulsatile, with the pulse amplitude equivalent to that seen during puberty (12). The decrease in LH secretion late in gestation correlates with the development of an inhibitory effect on LH of exogenous estradiol (13). Studies in the rodent suggest that this depends upon the development of extrogen receptors in the hypothalamic-pituitary unit (see 16).

In each of these axes pulsatile hormone release is apparent in midgestation, with markedly exaggerated pulse heights. In each case immaturity of the negative feedback loop is postulated to play a role. Little is known of the regulation of receptor differentiation which may be central to interpreting developmental changes in the neuroendocrine axis.

ACKNOWLEDGEMENTS

These studies were supported by the Medical Research Council of New Zealand.

REFERENCES

1. Gluckman PD, Grumbach MM & Kaplan SL (1981) Endocr Rev 2:363-395
2. Gluckman PD & Parsons Y (1983) J Devel Physiol 5:101-128
3. Ohmura E, Jansen A, Chernick V, Winter J, Friesen HG, Rivier J & Vale W (1984) Endocrinol 114:299-301
4. Gluckman PD (1984) J Devel Physiol (in press)
5. Vale W, Vaughan J, Yamamoto G, Spiess J & Rivier J (1983) Endocrinol 112:1553-1555
6. Gluckman PD, Butler JH & Elliott TB (1983) Endocrinol 112:1607-1612
7. Berelowitz M, Firestone SL & Frohman LA (1981) Endocrinol 109:714-719
8. Roti E, Gnudi A & Braverman LE Endocr Revs 4:131-149
9. Fisher PA, Dussault JH, Sack J, Chopra IJ (1977) Rec Prog Horm Res 33:59-107
10. Strbak V & Greer MA (1979) Endocrinol 105:488-492
11. Fraser M, Gunn T, Butler J & Gluckman P (1983) Proc Endo Soc Aust 26 (Supple 2) 32
12. Clark SJ, Ellis N, Styne DM, Gluckman PD, Kaplan SL & Grumbach MM (1984 Endocrinol (in press)
13. Gluckman PD, Marti-Henneberg C, Kaplan SL & Grumbach MM (1983) Endocrinol 112:1618-1623

Endocrinology
F. Labrie, L. Proulx, eds.

PRENATAL DEVELOPMENT OF A FUNCTIONAL CIRCADIAN CLOCK

STEVEN M. REPPERT and WILLIAM J. SCHWARTZ

Children's and Neurology Services, Massachusetts General Hospital and Harvard Medical School, Boston, MA, USA

In mammals, the suprachiasmatic nuclei (SCN) of the anterior hypothalamus function as a circadian pacemaker generating numerous hormonal and behavioral rhythms (1,2). This endogenous clock is normally entrained to the 24-hr day by environmental lighting which acts via a monosynaptic retinohypothalamic pathway to the SCN.

Developmental studies in both humans and rats indicate that circadian rhythms are not overtly manifested until well into the postnatal period (3). Indirect studies in rats have suggested that the circadian pacemaker underlying the rhythms is functional prior to this time and that the developing circadian clock might be functional and entrainable by the mother during fetal life (4). Such indirect studies do not eliminate the possibility, however, that some aspect of the birth process itself starts and sets the timing of the developing clock*.

We set out to determine whether a circadian clock actually is functioning in the SCN before birth by using the ^{14}C-labeled deoxyglucose (dG) technique to directly monitor the functional activity of the nuclei in fetal rats. The dG method, which provides an in vivo determination of the rates of glucose utilization (and therefore energy metabolism) of individual brain structures (7), was chosen for our developmental studies because it provides an effective assay for oscillatory activity of the SCN in adult rats (8,9).

For the experiments, timed pregnant Sprague-Dawley rats were exposed to various environmental lighting regimens, outfitted with intra-atrial catheters on gestational day 10, and injected iv with dG at specified gestational ages and clock times. At 45 min after injection, the animals were sacrificed, fetal brains were removed and frozen, and serial 20-μm coronal sections were cut and processed for autoradiography. The optical density of each SCN was measured, and changes of the optical density of the SCN between animals were compared by using the optical density of the adjacent hypothalamus as an internal reference standard for each fetal brain.

In a series of three experiments, we proved that a circadian clock oscillates in the SCN during fetal development and that the maternal circadian system entrains the timing of the fetal clock to ambient lighting (10). First, dams were exposed to diurnal lighting (12 hrs light per day) during pregnancy until day 19 of

---

*Time of day of birth in the rat is coupled to the photoperiod by a circadian mechanism (5,6).

gestation when they were placed and thereafter maintained in constant darkness. The pregnant animals were then injected with dG either during the subjective night (12-hr period when the lights would have been off) on gestational day 20 or during the subjective day (12-hr period when the lights would have been on) on gestational day 21. The resultant autoradiographs showed that the maternal and all fetal SCN are metabolically active during the subjective day and relatively inactive during the subjective night. Thus, the fetal SCN manifest a clear day-night variation of glucose utilization and the fetal rhythm is synchronous with that in the mother. In the second experiment, a 12-hr phase shift in the lighting cycle during pregnancy, which shifts the maternal circadian system by 12 hrs, results in a corresponding phase shift in the rhythm of fetal SCN metabolic activity. In the third experiment, blind dams were used to show that environmental lighting acts through the maternal circadian system to entrain the rhythm of fetal SCN metabolic activity; the fetal rhythm is synchronous with the circadian time of the blind mothers and not affected directly by ambient lighting. We have subsequently shown that a daily rhythm of metabolic activity in the fetal SCN is detectable by the dG method from the 19th through the 21st days of gestation; no daily rhythm was found on gestational day 18 (11). Evolution of the fetal rhythm from the 19th day of gestation occurs by increasing daytime metabolic activity, with nighttime activity remaining low. Although the appearance of the fetal metabolic rhythm coincides with the start of SCN synaptogenesis (12), the rich neuropil characteristic of the adult SCN is clearly not essential for expression of the daily rhythm of metabolic activity in the fetus.

Since the maternal circadian system entrains the timing of the fetal clock, the first step towards elucidating the specific mechanism of maternal entrainment was to examine the effects of maternal SCN ablation (13). For these studies, either a complete SCN lesion (bilateral electrolytic) or a sham procedure was performed on dams on gestational day 7; they were injected with dG either during subjective night on gestational day 20 or during subjective day on gestational day 21. In contrast to fetuses from intact and sham-operated dams, there is no daily rhythm of SCN metabolic activity in fetuses from dams with bilateral SCN ablation; fetal SCN metabolic activity within each of these litters (8-10 fetuses/litter) is scattered over the inactive to active range. Hence, maternal SCN ablation abolishes maternal entrainment of the fetal circadian clock. The resulting scatter of fetal SCN metabolic activity within each litter suggests that the individual fetal clocks are still oscillating but that relative to one another each is at a different phase of its daily oscillation. In support of this interpretation, we have shown that rats born to mothers with SCN lesions and reared in constant conditions all exhibit different phases of rhythmic drinking behavior as monitored from day 25 postnatally (Reppert and Schwartz, unpublished data). It therefore appears that the mother entrains an endogenous clock in the fetal SCN similar to the way environmental lighting entrains the clock in the adult nuclei. The maternal output signal(s) used to entrain the fetal clock has not yet been elucidated.

In summary, our results show that at a time in development well before the maturation of the neural mechanisms necessary for both the photic entrainment* and overt expression of circadian rhythms, the mother acts as a transducer between the environment and the fetal brain, coordinating the phase of the developing biological clock to her own clock time which, in turn, is entrained by ambient lighting (Fig. 1). One function of this unique form of communication from mother to fetus may be to better prepare the developing mammal for entry into the external environment. Recent dG studies with pregnant squirrel monkeys suggest that the SCN are also functional during late fetal life in the primate and that, as in the rat, the maternal circadian system coordinates the timing of the fetal primate clock to ambient lighting (15). The existence of this form of maternal to fetal communication in such diverse species as the rat and monkey suggests that the phenomenon is generalized among mammals and may even be present in humans.

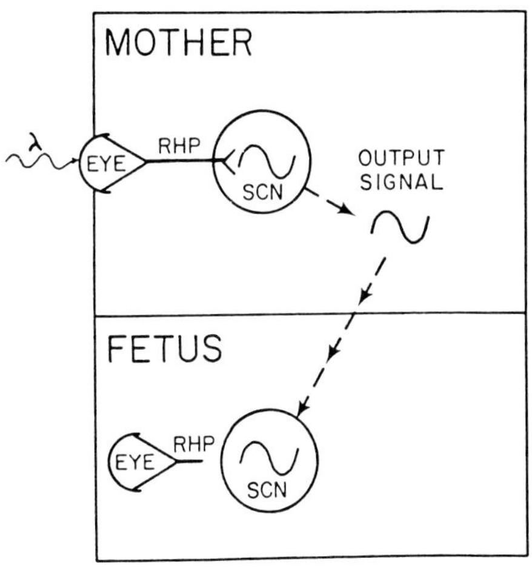

Fig. 1. Conceptual model of maternal-fetal coordination. RHP, retinohypothalamic pathway; SCN, suprachiasmatic nucleus.

---

*The retinohypothalamic pathway does not innervate the rat SCN until postnatal day 3 to 4 (14).

ACKNOWLEDGEMENTS

Supported by March of Dimes Basil O'Connor Starter Research Grant 5-335 and PHS Grant HD 14427 to SMR. WJS is supported by Teacher-Investigator Award NS 00672.

REFERENCES

1. Rusak B, Zucker I (1979) Physiol Rev 59:449-526
2. Moore RY (1981) In: Martin JB, Reichlin S, Bick K (eds) Neurosecretion and Brain Peptides. Raven Press, New York, pp 449-458
3. Davis FC (1981) In: Aschoff J (ed) Handbook of Behavioral Neurobiology, vol 4, Biological Rhythms. Plenum, New York, pp 257-274
4. Deguchi T (1975) Proc Natl Acad Sci USA 72:2914-2920
5. Lincoln DW, Porter DG (1976) Nature (London) 260:780-781
6. Reppert SM (1983) Pediatr Res 17:154A
7. Sokoloff L, Reivich M, Kennedy C, Des Rosiers MH, Patlak CS, Pettigrew KD, Sakurada O, Shinohara M (1977) J Neurochem 28:897-916
8. Schwartz WJ, Gainer H (1977) Science 197:1089-1091
9. Schwartz WJ, Davidson LC, Smith CB (1980) J Comp Neurol 189:157-167
10. Reppert SM, Schwartz WJ (1983) Science 220:969-971
11. Reppert SM, Schwartz WJ (1984) J Neurosci in press
12. Koritsanszky S (1981) Acta Morphol Acad Sci Hung 29:227-239
13. Reppert SM, Schwartz WJ (1984) Pediatr Res 18:144A
14. Stanfield B, Cowan WM (1976) Brain Res 104:129-133
15. Reppert SM, Schwartz WJ (1984) Neurosci Lett in press

Endocrinology
F. Labrie, L. Proulx, eds.

ONTOGENESIS OF FETAL CATECHOLAMINE BIOSYNTHESIS

GLADYS TEITELMAN, LORAINNE IACOVITTI, TONG H. JOH AND DONALD J. REIS

Laboratory of Neurobiology, Cornell University Medical College, 1300 York Avenue, New York, NY 10021 (U.S.A.)

The neural crest is a transient structure that appears on the dorsal surface of the neural tube of vertebrate embryos. Soon after it forms, cells from the neural crest migrate widely_ and subsequently differentiate into a variety of cell types including the neurons of the sympathetic and parasympathetic ganglia and the chromaffin cells of the adrenal medulla. Since in adults these cells synthesize catecholamines (CA) or acetylcholine (ACh) as neurotransmitters, the question arises as to whether the expression by neural crest cells of a neurotransmitter phenotype is predetermined or is regulated by environmental cues.

To examine this issue, we first determined when, in embryogenesis, the CA cells which populate the sympathetic nervous system first differentiate biochemically to express their CA phenotype. Our criteria of differentiation has been the immunocytochemical detection of the CA biosynthetic enzymes tyrosine hydroxylase (TH) and dopamine-B-hydroxylase (DBH) which specifically subserve the biosynthesis of norepinephrine (NE), and phenylethanolamine N-methyltransferase (PNMT), which converts NE into epinephrine (E). Cells containing TH and DBH are first observed in the sympathetic ganglia of 11 day old rat embryos (E11) (Fig. 1).[1] After differentiation the cells initially migrate to the

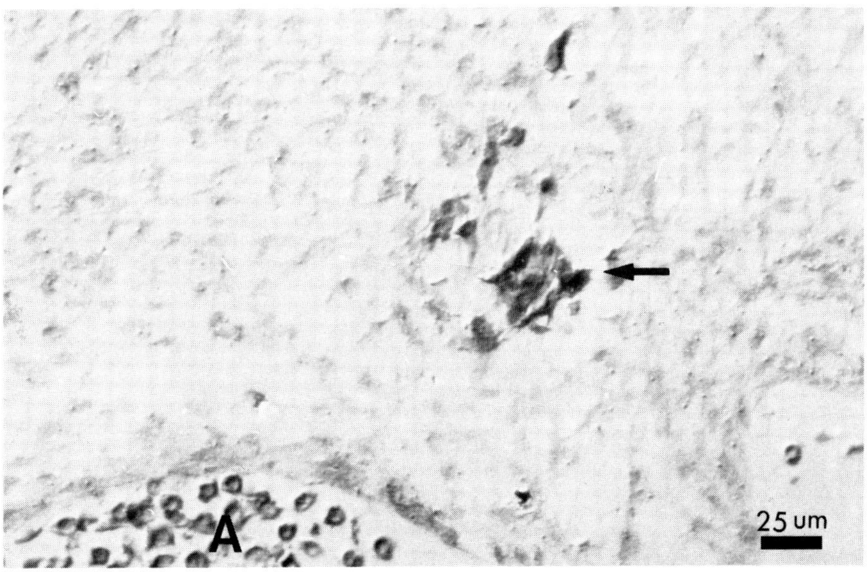

Fig. 1. Immunocytochemical localization of TH in cells (arrow) of the rat sympathetic ganglia at day 11 of development. A = aorta.

paraaortic ganglia and, at E 16, are seen in the adrenal gland. By E18, the adrenal medullary cells containing TH and DBH first express PNMT(1). The delay in the appearance of PNMT and its restriction to adrenal medullary cells seems to support the suggestion raised by others(2) that the initial expression of this enzyme may be elicited by factors released by the adrenal cortex. However, we have recently discovered that sympathetic neurons of chick, in contrast to rat, contain PNMT(3). This observation raises anew the question as to the nature of the signals which initiate PNMT synthesis and whether the same signal is produced by all sympathetic organs that are populated by PNMT cells.

Next we examined whether the ability to express CA enzymes is restricted to sympathetic cells or is also elicited in other neural crest derivatives by appropriate environmental signals. Our experimental model for this study has been the ciliary ganglion (CG) of chick embryos, which is a cholinergic parasympathetic ganglion which originates in the mesencephalic neural crest. We have examined the neurotransmitter plasticity of CG neurons by testing whether they will express CA enzymes when maintained in vitro. As shown in Fig. 2, ciliary neurons in culture contain TH immunoreactivity (Fig. 2). In vitro, these cells also express amino acid decarboxylase

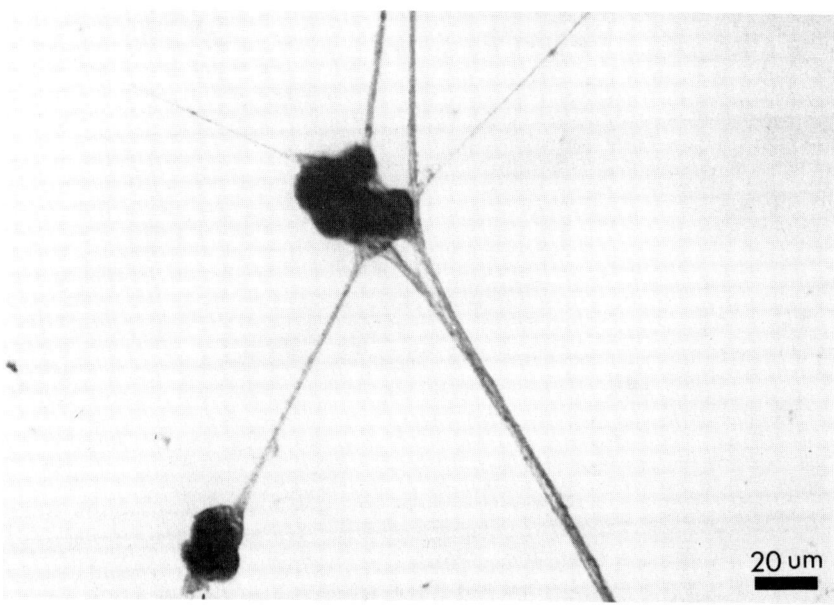

Fig. 2. Immunocytochemical localization of TH in chick ciliary neurons maintained for 5 days in culture.

(AADC) and PNMT (4), two other CA biosynthetic enzymes. This observation indicates that not only sympathetic but also parasympathetic derivatives of neural crest have the ability to synthesize CA enzymes. However, environmental cues determine whether any or all of these enzymes are expressed.

Thirdly, we sought to determine whether the stability of a CA phenotype is also determined by the environment. We have recently discovered a population of cells containing TH in several organs of the rat and mouse embryo which in the adult do not harbor CA cells(5). In these cells, the CA phenotype disappears after midgestation. Thus, they have been named transient catecholaminergic cells (TC cells) as a means of indicating that either the cells and/or their capacity to express the CA biosynthetic enzymes is evanescent. The finding of TC cells in the pancreas of mouse embryos prior to and during the time when glucagon and insulin first appear has raised the possiblity that, in this organ, TC cells might transmute into those containing peptide hormones. We therefore have attempted to determine, by use of an immunocytochemical technique for localizing two antigens within the same cell, whether TC cells of the mouse embryonic pancreas also contain pancreatic hormones. We have found that on the 12th day of development, the mouse embryonic pancreas contains cells which stain for only TH, only glucagon and those which are phenotypic hybrids and contain both antigens (Fig. 3). At

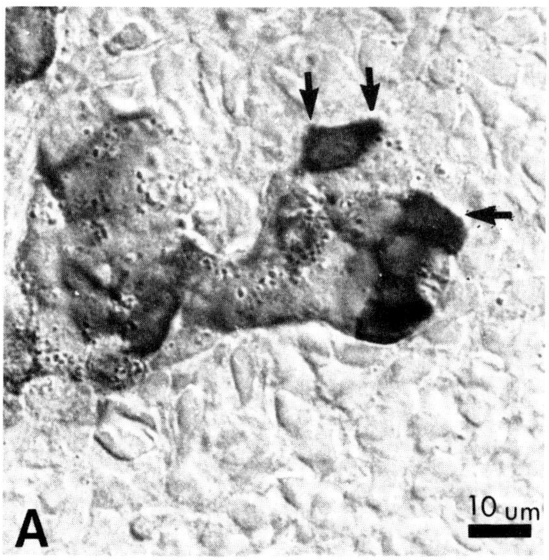

Fig. 3. Immunocytochemical localization of glucagon (A) and TH (B) in the same section of pancreas of 12 day old mouse embryo. Note the presence of some cells containing only glucagon (single arrow in A), only TH (single arrow in B) and TH-glucagon (double arrow).

E14.5, when insulin is first detected, approximately 10% of all cells containing TH also stain for insulin. Since the cells containing TH disappear by E15.5, prior to the appearance of somatostatin, no double label experiments have been carried out using this peptide. These observations indicate that from days 11 to 15 a population of cells which continuously express TH differentiate into peptide-containing pancreatic cells. During this time the cells begin to synthesize pancreatic hormones while the biosynthesis of TH gradually disappears and the TH-containing cells are gradually transformed into endocrine cells. Moreover, these findings suggest that the initial metabolic committment of TC cells is mutable since it can be modified in response to the changing environment provided by the developing pancreas. In summary, our studies provide support for the contention that the appearance of a CA phenotype is regulated by environmental signals which also determine whether the cells retain their initial expression or whether they interconvert and express other phenotypes.

REFERENCES

1. Teitelman G, Baker H, Joh TH, Reis DJ (1979) Proc Natl Acad Sci US 76:509-513
2. Wurtman RJ, Pohorecky LA and Balega BS (1972) Pharmacol Rev 24:411-426
3. Teitelman G, Skaper S, Baker H, Park DH, Joh TH, Adler R (1984) Dev Brain Res 13:283-291
4. Iacovitti L, Teitelman G, Grayson L, Joh TH, Reis DJ (1983) Soc Neurosci Abstr 9:304
5. Teitelman G, Gershon MD, Rothman TP, Joh TH, Reis DJ (1981) Dev Biol 86:348-355
6. Teitelman G, Joh TH, Reis, DJ (1981) Proc Natl Acad Sci USA 78:5225-5229

36. Calcium and Calmodulin in Hormone Action

Endocrinology
F. Labrie, L. Proulx, eds.

CALCIUM AND GLUCOCORTICOID ACTION IN HEPATOCYTES

GUY G. ROUSSEAU and LOUIS HUE

International Institute of Cellular and Molecular Pathology, and University of Louvain Medical School, 75 avenue Hippocrate, B-1200 Brussels (Belgium)

INTRODUCTION

Steroid hormones regulate cell function by binding to receptors that interact with nuclear chromatin and control gene expression. In cytosol from rat (HTC) and human (IM-9) cell lines, Ca^{2+} modulates the affinity of glucocorticoid agonists and antagonists for the receptor (1). This phenomenon can be demonstrated *in vitro* at free Ca^{2+} concentrations (0.1-1 μM) known to occur within intact cells. A similar effect of Ca^{2+} was also found with the mineralocorticoid receptor from rat kidney, but not with the androgen receptor from rat prostate, nor the estrogen or the progesterone receptor from rat uterus. This prompted us to study whether glucocorticoid binding and action could be modulated in intact cells by manipulating the Ca^{2+} environment. We have investigated this question using suspensions of hepatocytes freshly isolated from rat liver, a target tissue for glucocorticoid hormones.

MATERIAL AND METHODS

Binding studies

Hepatocytes were isolated from male Wistar rats (2) and incubated for 30 min at 37° C in Krebs-Ringer's bicarbonate buffer containing 0.1 % (w/v) bovine serum albumin (BSA) and 10 mM glucose (10^7 cells/ml). The cells were collected by centrifugation for further incubation at 37° C or for preparation of cytosol.

For binding studies, the hepatocytes were incubated in the same buffer containing 1 mM EGTA or 2.5 mM $CaCl_2$ for 20 min. ^{3}H-Dexamethasone (Radiochemical Centre, Amersham, UK) was then added, with or without 100-fold excess of nonradioactive dexamethasone. At the times indicated, samples were taken for preparation of a nuclear fraction (3). Specific binding was calculated, from the radioactivity in the pellets, by difference between the two sets of incubations. Nonspecific binding was a linear function of free steroid concentration and, depending on the latter, ranged from 10 % to 30 % of total binding.

For cell-free binding studies, cytosol was obtained as described previously (1). Cytosol aliquots were incubated for 16 h at 0° C with 0.5-15 nM ^{3}H-dexamethasone, with or without excess of nonradioactive dexamethasone, and the concentration of receptor-bound steroid was determined by a charcoal adsorption assay (1).

Enzyme induction studies

Hepatocytes were washed in serum-free Swim's S-77 medium (GIBCO) containing 2 % (w/v) BSA, penicillin-streptomycin (50 U/ml), and either 1 mM EGTA or 2.5 mM $CaCl_2$. After centrifugation, they were incubated at 37° C in the same medium under sterile conditions (2 x 10^6 cells/ml), with or without dexamethasone. At the times indicated, aliquots were taken for determination of lactate dehydrogenase (LDH) (4) and tyrosine aminotransferase (TAT) (5) activity.

RESULTS

A Scatchard plot of the binding data obtained with cytosol showed a single linear slope, consistent with a homogeneous population of receptor sites. Extrapolation yielded about 15,000 sites/cell, which is within the range of values found for other cell types. The effect of Ca^{2+} on dexamethasone binding to cytosol was then studied. Fig. 1 shows that Ca^{2+} *decreased* the affinity for dexamethasone three-fold, without effect on receptor site concentration. These findings are identical to those in HTC and IM-9 cells (1). Thus, isolated hepatocytes appeared to be a suitable model for the *in vivo* studies.

When target cells are exposed to a glucocorticoid agonist at 37° C, the steroid becomes associated with the nucleus within a few minutes, presumably as a result of an interaction of the receptor-steroid complex with chromatin. We therefore examined the effect of Ca^{2+} on the specific binding of dexamethasone to the nuclear fraction in intact hepatocytes. Fig. 2 shows that Ca^{2+} *increased*

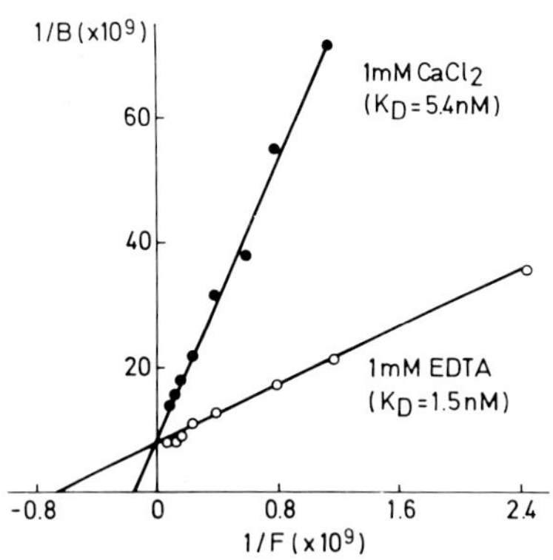

Fig. 1. Double-reciprocal plot of the cell-free binding of dexamethasone to the glucocorticoid receptor, with Ca^{2+} or EDTA, in hepatocyte cytosol at equilibrium (0° C, 16 h)

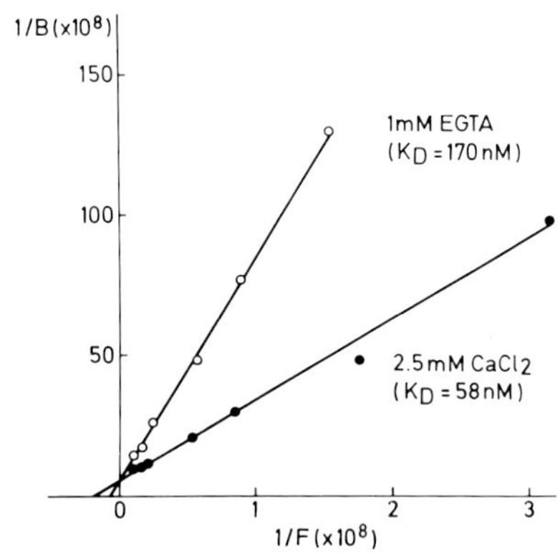

Fig. 2. Effect of Ca^{2+} or EGTA on dexamethasone binding to the glucocorticoid receptor in intact hepatocytes at 37° C. Double-reciprocal plot of specific binding to the nuclear fraction at equilibrium (30 min).

the affinity of the apparently homogeneous class of receptor sites for dexamethasone. As expected (1) the affinity was lower at 37° C than at 0° C. In the presence of Ca^{2+} the apparent affinity constant (K_D) was around 50 nM, which is close to the concentration of free glucocorticoids in plasma. Removal of Ca^{2+} from the incubation medium led to a three-fold decrease in affinity. Receptor site concentration (about 25,000/cell) was identical under both conditions. Nonspecific binding was identical with Ca^{2+} and with EGTA, indicating that steroid uptake was not affected by these ions. Addition of 1 mM EGTA to an incubation containing 3.5 mM $CaCl_2$ did not affect dexamethasone binding, ruling out a nonspecific effect of EGTA on receptor affinity.

These data suggested that receptor occupancy at glucocorticoid concentrations within the physiological range is controlled by Ca^{2+}, which might therefore influence enzyme induction by dexamethasone in hepatocytes. Primary suspension cultures of hepatocytes were exposed to 100 nM dexamethasone in the presence of 2.5 mM $CaCl_2$ or 1 mM EGTA. At least 80 % of the cells survived the 8 h incubation period, based on leakage of LDH activity. After a lag-period of about 2 h TAT activity increased in the steroid-treated cells as compared to control cells. The increase in activity after 8 h was 1.9-fold (range 1.8-2.1 in 3 expts) in the presence of EGTA. With Ca^{2+}, the lag-period was unchanged but the increase was greater at all time-points reaching 4.4-fold (range 3.5-6 in 3 expts) after 8 h. A representative experiment in shown in Fig. 3.

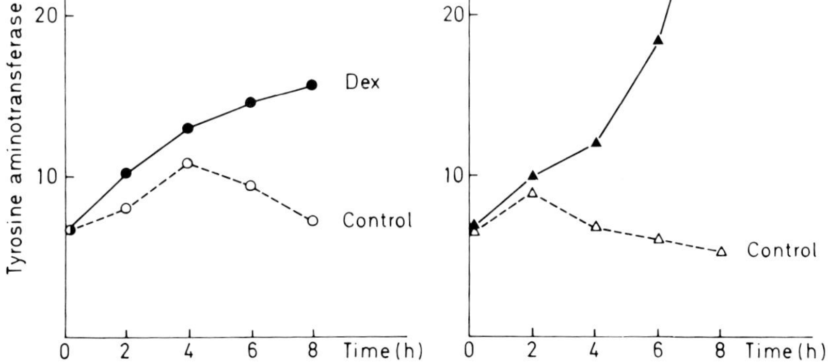

Fig. 3. Effect of Ca^{2+} on tyrosine aminotransferase induction by dexamethasone (100 nM) in intact hepatocytes.

DISCUSSION

These results suggest that Ca^{2+} modulates the glucocorticoid response of normal hepatocytes. It is tempting to speculate that the stimulatory effect of Ca^{2+} on enzyme induction by dexamethasone is related to the increased receptor occupancy by the steroid seen in the nuclei of cells incubated with Ca^{2+}. The latter observation must be reconciled with the fact that, in all the systems studied so far, including hepatocytes, Ca^{2+} actually decreases the affinity of the cytosolic receptor for dexamethasone. One possibility is that the consequences of the putative conformational changes induced by calcium (1) differ whether the receptor assumes the nuclear binding (i.e. dephosphorylated) form or the cytosolic 'untransformed' (i.e. phosphorylated, see ref. 6) form. Alternatively, calcium might stimulate a step beyond the formation of the nuclear receptor-steroid complex.

We have been unable to find conditions under which the nuclear binding of dexamethasone was modified by catecholamines, angiotensin, or vasopressin. The calcium movements induced by these hormones could be too short-lived or occurred outside the nuclear compartment.

ACKNOWLEDGEMENTS

The help of M.A. Gueuning is gratefully appreciated. We thank Dr. M. Rider for a gift of purified albumin. This work was supported by the FRSM (Belgium). L. Hue is Maître de Recherches of the FNRS.

REFERENCES

1. Van Bohemen CG, Eliard PH, Rousseau GG (1983) Molec Physiol 4: 95-110
2. Hue L, Feliu JE, Hers HG (1978) Biochem J 176: 791-717
3. Kaufmann SH, Quddus FF, Shaper JH (1982) Endocrinology 110: 708-716
4. Vassault A (1983) In: Bermeyer HU (ed) Methods of Enzymatic Analysis. Verlag Chemie, Weinheim, 3: 118-126
5. Rousseau GG, Amar-Costesec A, Verhaegen M, Granner DK (1980) Proc Nat Acad Sci USA 77: 1005-1009
6. Schmidt TJ, Litwack G (1982) Physiol Rev 62: 1131-1192

© 1984 Elsevier Science Publishers B.V.
Endocrinology
F. Labrie, L. Proulx, eds.

THE CALCIUM MESSENGER SYSTEM AND SUSTAINED CELLULAR RESPONSE

HOWARD RASMUSSEN, WALTER ZAWALICH, KUMIKO KOJIMA and ITARU KOJIMA

Departments of Internal Medicine and Cell Biology, Yale University School of Medicine, 333 Cedar Street, New Haven, CT 06510 USA

INTRODUCTION

It has become increasingly clear that Ca^{2+} is an intracellular messenger in the action of a variety of hormones and extracellular messengers (1). Our concept of how this calcium messenger system functions was based largely on analogy with how it appeared to operate in excitable systems (2). In these systems, its operation appeared simple and straightforward: an increase in intracellular free $[Ca^{2+}]$ led to the activation of calcium-dependent systems by binding to a specific calcium receptor protein such as troponin C or calmodulin, and this Ca^{2+}-protein interaction triggered cellular response. Hence, amplitude and duration of response was a function of the amplitude and duration of the calcium message.

Ca^{2+} AND cAMP AS INTERRELATED MESSENGERS

However, as this concept was extended to systems that display sustained rather than brief cellular responses, its inadequacies became evident. First, in nearly all such systems not only Ca^{2+} but cAMP serves a messenger function. At least five patterns of this synarchic regulation by Ca^{2+} and cAMP have been recognized: 1) coordinate; 2) hierarchical; 3) redundant; 4) antagonistic; and 5) sequential (1). Out of this newer formulation developed the concept that intracellular messengers can alter cellular responses by a process of <u>sensitivity modulation</u> as well as by amplitude modulation (1). By definition, sensitivity modulation in the calcium messenger system is the activation of a Ca^{2+}-sensitive enzyme or process by a change in the sensitivity of the system to activation by Ca^{2+} without a change in $[Ca^{2+}]$. It is apparent that a rise in [cAMP] and the subsequent phosphorylation of a component of the Ca^{2+}-sensitive response element is a common means by which sensitivity modulation occurs.

CALCIUM MESSENGER TRANSIENTS AND SUSTAINED CELLULAR RESPONSE

A second discovery pointed up the inadequacy of our original notion as to how the calcium messenger system operates. The rise in the calcium ion concentration in the cell cytosol, $[Ca^{2+}]_c$, is transient even though the response is sustained (3,4) in a variety of hormonally responsive cells. The question rises as to how a cell displays a sustained response to a transient message. This question has three possible answers: 1) calmodulin-dependent reactions display hysteresis so that once activated they will remain activated at a $[Ca^{2+}]_c$ lower than that necessary to put them in the activated state; 2) a simultaneous or subsequent increase in $[cAMP]_c$ by the process of positive sensitivity modulation increases the sensitivity of response elements in the calcium messenger system sufficiently so that they remain active at low $[Ca^{2+}]_c$; and 3) the calcium messenger system is more complex than previously thought and sustained response is dependent on the operation of a second non-calmodulin branch in this system. Although several Ca^{2+}-calmodulin regulated response elements have been shown to display hysteresis, it is evident that this behavior does not account for sustained cellular response. It is clear that if $[cAMP]_c$ as well as $[Ca^{2+}]_c$ rises, as occurs in systems displaying coordinate or hierarchical synarchic regulation, then sustained response can be achieved via a cAMP-dependent positive sensitivity modulation of response elements in the calcium messenger system. However, it is equally clear that this can not account for the sustained phase of cellular response in a variety of Ca^{2+} regulated systems.

Dual Pathways of Information Flow in the Calcium Messenger System

In order to consider the third alternative, it is first necessary to consider two other topics: 1) the early events following hormone-receptor interactions in the calcium messenger system; and 2) the properties of a unique enzyme, the calcium-activated, phospholipid-dependent protein kinase (C-kinase). It has been known for 30 years that there a relationship exists between phosphatidylinositol (PtdIns) turnover and the early events in the calcium messenger system. Recent improvements in methodology have led to a more detailed analysis of the turnover of PtdIns's, and a tentative consensus is developing: following hormone-receptor interaction, the initial event is the hydrolysis of phosphatidylinositol 4,5-bisphosphate ($PtdIns4,5P_2$) and possibly PtdIns4P (5). The hydrolysis of $PtdIns4,5P_2$ leads to the production of two products: inositol triphosphate ($InsP_3$) and diacylglycerol (DG) rich in unsaturated fatty acid. Shortly thereafter, the $[Ca^{2+}]_c$ rises transiently due both to the $InsP_3$-induced release of Ca^{2+} from an intracellular (presumably microsomal) pool (6), and an increased entry of Ca^{2+} into the cell. The increase in DG content is thought to have a messenger function. To discuss this, it is necessary to consider the C-kinase. This enzyme is a Ca^{2+}-activated protein kinase which does not employ calmodulin as a Ca^{2+}-receptor subunit, but undergoes a positive sensitivity modulation in the presence of DG and a mixture of phospholipids, particularly phosphatidylserine (7). In their presence, the V_{max} of the enzyme increases 5-fold, and the sensitivity to activation by Ca^{2+} is dramatically increased. Particular phorbol esters, e.g., 12-O-tetradecanoyl-phorbol-13-acetate (TPA), can replace DG as a positive sensitivity modulator of the enzyme (8).

Based on the observations that C-kinase and Ca^{2+} act synergistically in the platelet release reaction (9), we tested the hypothesis that the C-kinase pathway has a specific function in cells displaying a sustained response. We did so by testing the separate and combined effects of a calcium ionophore, A23187, and a phorbol ester, TPA, on cellular response in isolated adrenal glomerulosa cells (10), and in isolated rat pancreatic islets (11).

The peptide hormone angiotensin II (AII) induces an hydrolysis of $PtdIns4,5P_2$ and $PtdIns_4P$, and the production of $InsP_3$ and DG within 10-15 seconds after its addition to isolated adrenal glomerulosa cells. These changes are followed by an efflux of Ca^{2+} from a dantrolene-sensitive pool, and an increase in Ca^{2+} uptake across the plasma membrane. Shortly thereafter, the rate of aldosterone secretion increases monotonically to a sustained rate 4-5 times greater than the basal rate. Addition of A23187 causes no $PtdIns4,5P_2$ hydrolysis but increases both Ca^{2+} influx and intracellular Ca^{2+} release, and causes an initial increase in aldosterone secretory rate. However, this does not reach the value seen after AII action, nor is it sustained. Conversely, TPA addition causes no initial increase in secretory rate, but does induce a very slow rise to values only 20-25 percent of those induced by AII. Combined A23187 and TPA induce a change in aldosterone secretory response qualitatively and quantitatively similar to that induced by AII.

The use of A23187 and TPA in isolated perifused rat islets gives even more dramatic results. Islets perifused with 10 mM glucose (after a period of exposure to 2.75 mM glucose) display a biphasic pattern of insulin secretion: an initial sharp rise, followed by a sharp fall (phase 1) and then a more gradual rise to a sustained plateau (phase 2). Perifusion with either A23187 or tolbutamide leads to a normal or supranormal phase 1 but no phase 2 response. Conversely, TPA does not induce a phase 1 response, only a submaximal phase 2 response. Combined A23187 and TPA, or tolbutamide and TPA induce a biphasic insulin secretory response similar to that seen after glucose addition. If tolbutamide and TPA are added to the perifusate simultaneously with forskolin, an activator of adenylate cyclase, then the insulin secretory response is nearly identical to that seen after perifusion of islets with 10.7 mM glucose.

We interpret these data in terms of a model in which the flow of information from cell surface to cell interior in the calcium messenger system follows two branches: a calmodulin branch which displays amplitude modulation, is activated by the transient rise in $[Ca^{2+}]_c$, and is responsible for the initial phase of cellular response; and a C-kinase branch which displays sensitivity modulation, is activated both by the rise in the DG content of the plasma membrane and the transient rise in $[Ca^{2+}]_c$, and is largely responsible for the sustained phase of cellular response.

It is already clear that this model is applicable to a variety of other cell types that display sustained responses to the sustained presence of an extracellular messengers. It is also evident that changes in $[cAMP]_C$ influence events in the C-kinase as well as calmodulin branch of the calcium messenger system.

ACKNOWLEDGEMENTS

This work was supported by a grant (AM19813) from the National Institutes of Health.

REFERENCES

1. Rasmussen H (1981) Calcium and cAMP As Synarchic Messengers. John Wiley and Sons, New York
2. Weber A, Murray JM (1973) Physiol Rev 53:612-673
3. Morgan JP, Morgan KG (1983) Pflügers Arch 395:75-77
4. Snowdowne KW, Borle AB (1984) Am J Physiol 246 (Endocrinol Metab 9):E198-E201
5. Downes P, Michell RH (1982) Cell Calcium 3:467-502
6. Streb H, Irvine RE, Berridge MJ, Schultz I (1983) Nature 306:67-69
7. Takai Y, Kishimoto A, Kawahara Y, Minakuchi R, Sano K, Kikkawa U, Mori T, Yu B, Kaibuchi K, Nishiguka Y (1981) Adv Cyclic Nucleotide Res 14:301-313
8. Castanga M, Takai Y, Kaibuchi K, Sano K, Kikkawa U, Nishizuka Y (1982) J Biol Chem 257:7847-7851
9. Kaibuchi K, Takai Y, Sawamura M, Hoshyima M, Fujikura T, Nishizuka Y. (19) J Biol Chem 258:6701-6704
10. Kojima I, Lippes H, Kojima K, Rasmussen H (1983) Biochem Biophys Res Commun 116:555-562
11. Zawalich W, Brown C, Rasmussen H. (1983) Biochem Biophys Res Commun 117:448-455

© 1984 Elsevier Science Publishers B.V.
Endocrinology
F. Labrie, L. Proulx, eds.

RECENT STUDIES ON CALMODULIN-REGULATED CALCINEURIN AND CYCLIC NUCLEOTIDE PHOSPHODIESTERASE

CATHERINE J. PALLEN, RAJENDRA K. SHARMA, AND JERRY H. WANG
Department of Medical Biochemistry, Faculty of Medicine, University of Calgary, Calgary, Alberta, Canada T2N 1N4

INTRODUCTION

Many well characterized cascade regulatory systems are themselves regulated through the action of calmodulin (CaM). The mechanism of interaction of CaM with its target proteins is a multistep process involving the binding of Ca^{2+} to CaM followed by a series of conformational changes of CaM (1). The activated CaM can then associate with certain regulatory proteins to modulate their activities. While mediating the activity of various protein kinases and of adenylate cyclase, CaM also regulates the activity of a phosphatase, calcineurin (CaN), and cyclic nucleotide phosphodiesterase (PDE), thus acting at both the initiating and terminating ends of certain regulatory cascades. The following focuses upon certain aspects of our work on calcineurin and cyclic nucleotide phosphodiesterase which may lead to a better understanding of the regulatory actions of these enzymes.

MATERIALS AND METHODS

CaM, CaN, and PDE were purified from bovine brain as previously described (2). Assays of calcineurin-phosphatase activity are as described elsewhere (3,4) or are included in manuscripts which are in preparation. The isozyme forms of PDE were separated and investigated as described elsewhere (5).

RESULTS AND DISCUSSION

Calcineurin-phosphatase

Calcineurin was discovered as an inhibitor of CaM-stimulated cyclic nucleotide PDE (6). It was first shown to possess phosphoprotein phosphatase activity towards phosphorylase kinase and inhibitor-1 (7), and subsequently towards several brain phosphoproteins including synapsin-1, the regulatory subunit of cAMP-dependent protein kinase, myelin basic protein, and phosphocasein and phosphohistone (8-11). In addition to these phosphoprotein substrates, calcineurin also dephosphorylates several non-protein substrates such as p-nitrophenyl phosphate and free phosphotyrosine (3), and phosphoenol pyruvate (12). The finding that CaN can dephosphorylate free phosphotyrosine led us to investigate whether CaN possesses phosphotyrosyl-protein phosphatase activity. We find that CaN has activity towards epidermal growth factor (EGF) receptor of human placental membranes (13), a substrate phosphorylated on tyrosine residues following EGF stimulation.

Chernoff and Li (14) have found that CaN can dephosphorylate EGF receptor from A431 human carcinoma cells and phosphotyrosyl-casein.

In addition to exhibiting an extremely wide substrate specificity, CaN also has an absolute requirement for a metal ion activator and its activity towards all substrates is further stimulated by CaM. We have found that the phosphatase activity towards the non-protein substrates is best stimulated by Ni^{2+}, followed by Mn^{2+} and then Ca^{2+}, in either the presence or absence of CaM (4,12), while Ni^{2+}- or Mn^{2+}-stimulated CaN have similar activities towards phosphocasein (unpublished results). King and Huang (10) find that Ni^{2+} is the most efficient stimulator of CaN activity towards the protein substrates histone H1, G-substrate, and phosphorylase _a_, however the efficiency of Ni^{2+}-stimulated over Ca^{2+}-stimulated phosphatase activity depends upon the substrate used. In contrast, Gupta et al. (11) have reported that Ni^{2+} inhibits CaN activity towards ^{32}P-myelin basic protein. These results may be due to differential properties of calcineurin-phosphatase towards different substrates.

The mechanism of activation of CaN by Ni^{2+} is a multistep process with the rate-limiting step being a conformational change in the enzyme following Ni^{2+} binding (4). Although we have not investigated the mechanism of Mn^{2+} activation, studies in which Ni^{2+}-activation of CaN precluded subsequent Mn^{2+}-activation while simultaneous addition of the two metals resulted in an intermediate level of enzyme activity suggest that the two metal ions compete for binding. The interconversion of the Mn^{2+}- and Ni^{2+}-activated forms of CaN can be facilitated by incubation of either activated enzyme with Ca^{2+}/CaM (4). During the initial stages of such an incubation, CaN activity is stimulated by Ca^{2+}/CaM, however, over a period of hours, the enzyme reaches a Ca^{2+}/CaM-inactivated state from which it can be reactivated by the addition of Ni^{2+} or Mn^{2+} regardless of which of these metal ions had been originally used to activate the enzyme (Scheme 1). Thus, pretreatment of calcineurin with either Ni^{2+} or Mn^{2+} enhances the activation of CaN by Ca^{2+}/CaM, and may be a physiological mechanism by which CaN activity is regulated by Ca^{2+}/CaM supposing that the enzyme _in vivo_ has available Ni^{2+} or Mn^{2+}. During these studies we observed that Ni^{2+} will support CaM stimulation of CaN but not of PDE, suggesting that the activation of these two enzymes by CaM have different metal ion requirements. The requirements for different metal-induced CaM conformations for the activation of different enzymes may be a manifestation of the stepwise conformational changes of CaM induced by Ca^{2+}.

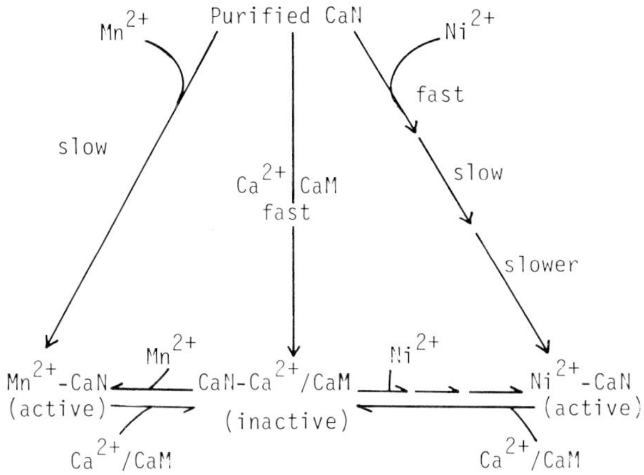

SCHEME 1

Isozymes of the CaM-regulated brain cyclic nucleotide phosphodiesterase

The calmodulin-regulated cyclic nucleotide phosphodiesterase is one of the key enzymes in the interaction between Ca^{2+}/CaM and cyclic AMP regulatory systems. The enzyme has been purified from both bovine brain (15,16) and bovine heart (17) and shown to be a dimeric protein. In an early study, we reported the purification of bovine brain CaM-regulated PDE to apparent homogeneity. The purified sample exhibited a single polypeptide band when analyzed by gel electrophoresis in the presence of SDS according to the procedure of Weber and Osborne. (18) More recently, we found that the purified enzyme could be resolved into two polypeptides of MW 63,000 and 60,000 by using the gel electrophoresis procedure of Laemmli (19).

We have investigated the nature of the two polypeptides in the purified PDE by using specific monoclonal antibodies as probes. Several monoclonal antibodies to PDE have been prepared in our laboratory. Immunoblotting experiments have shown that some of these antibodies show cross-reactivity toward both 60K and 63K polypeptides whereas the others are specific for the 60K polypeptides. When purified PDE was incubated with an excess amount of a cross-reacting antibody, A_6, and then subjected to sucrose-density ultracentrifugation, two poorly resolved peaks of PDE activity could be observed. These activity peaks represent enzyme-antibody complexes as judged by their sedimentation rates (Fig. 1B). Gel electrophoretic analysis of the protein samples in the active fractions showed that both 60K and 63K dalton polypeptides were present. In contrast, when a similar experiment was carried out using a 60K-specific monoclonal antibody, A_2, three PDE activity peaks were resolved by ultracentrifugation. Peak I which sedimented at the rate of the free enzyme contained 63K polypeptides, peak III contained

60K polypeptides and peak II contained both polypeptides of approximately equal intensity (Fig. 1A). These results suggest that there are three isozymes of CaM-regulated PDE in the purified brain enzyme samples: two homodimeric enzymes containing 60K or 63 subunits and a heterodimeric form. The existence of isozymes of brain CaM-regulated PDE have been confirmed by other studies which are described elsewhere in detail (5).

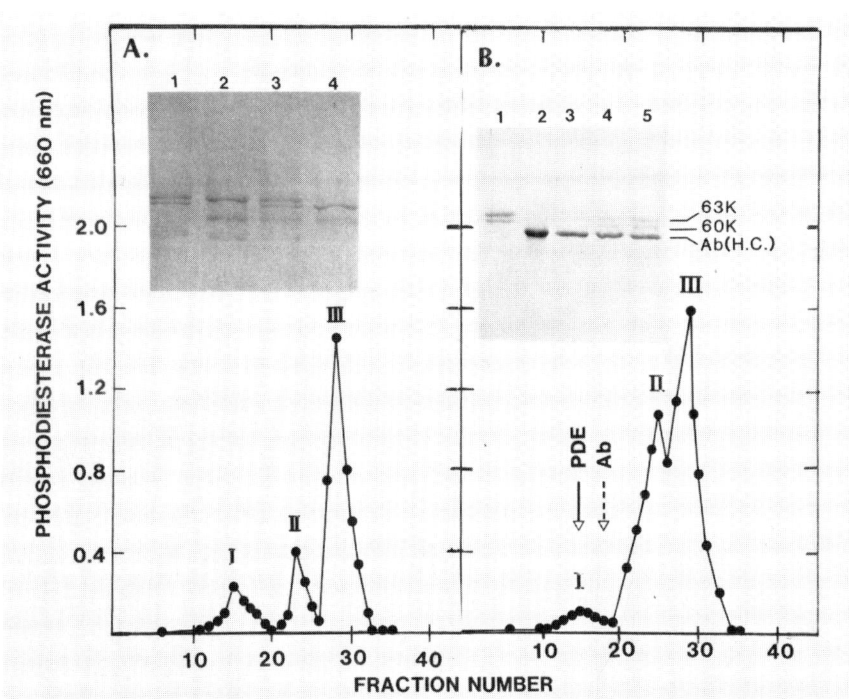

Concluding remarks

Hormonal, neuronal, and many other regulatory effects depend on highly complex interactions between various second messenger systems. The two CaM-regulated enzymes discussed here play important roles in coordinating Ca^{2+} and cAMP systems. Although the physiological significance of the existence of CaM-dependent PDE isozymes in mammalian brain is unknown, our results suggest that the regulation of cellular cAMP concentration by CaM is more complex than previously recognized. In addition, CaN appears to be a multifunctional phosphatase with a complex requirement for an response to certain metal ions. Whether any of the in vitro phosphatase substrates represent physiological substrates is unknown, however the fact that CaN is a phosphatase implies a role for CaM in controlling the regulatory aspects of certain dephosphorylations, with a possible involvement in tyrosyl-protein phosphorylation/dephosphorylation.

REFERENCES

1. Wang, J.H., Sharma, R.K., Huang, C.Y., Chau, V., and Chock, P.B. (1980). Ann. N.Y. Acad. Sci. 356:190-204.
2. Sharma, R.K., Taylor, W.A. and Wang, J.H. (1983). Methods Enzymol. 102:210-219.
3. Pallen, C.J., and Wang, J.H. (1983). J. Biol. Chem. 258:8550-8553.
4. Pallen, C.J., and Wang, J.H. (1984). J. Biol. Chem., in press.
5. Sharma, R.K., Adachi, A.-M., Adachi, K., and Wang, J.H. (1984). J. Biol. Chem., in press.
6. Wang, J.H., and Desai, R. (1976). Biochem. Biophys. Res. Commun. 72: 926-937.
7. Stewart, A.A., Ingebritsen, T.S., Manalan, A., Klee, C.B., and Cohen, P. (1982). FEBS Lett. 137: 80-84.
8. Yang, S.-D., Tallant, E.A., and Cheung, W.Y. (1982). Biochem.Biophys. Res. Commun. 106:1419-1425.
9. Blumenthal, D.K., and Kreb, E.G. (1983). Biophys. J. 41:409a.
10. King, M.M. and Huang, C.Y. (1984). Biochem. Biophys. Res. Commun. 114:955-961.
11. Gupta, R.C., Khandelwal, R.L., and Sulakhe, P.V. (1984). FEBS Lett. 169: 251-255.
12. Wang, J.H., Pallen, C.J., Brown, M.L., and Mitchell, K.J. (1984). Fed. Proc. 43:1897.
13. Pallen, C.J., Valentine, K.A., Wang, J.H., and Hollenberg, M.D. (1984). Fed. Proc. 43:1896.
14. Chernoff, J., and Li, H.-C. (1984). Fed. Proc. 43:766.
15. Morrill, M.E., Thompson, S.T. and Stellwagen, E. (1979), J. Biol. Chem. 254, 4371-4374.
16. Sharma, R.K., Wang, T.H., Wirch, E. and Wang, J.H. (1980) J. Biol. Chem. 255, 5916-5923.
17. LaPorte, D.C., Toscano, W.A. and Storm, D.R. (1979) Biochemistry 18, 2820-2825.
18. Weber, K. and Osborne, M. (1969) J. Biol. Chem. 244, 44-6-4412.
19. Laemmli, U.K. (1970) Nature (London) 227, 680-685.

ACKNOWLEDGEMENTS

This work was supported by grants from the Medical Research Council of Canada, The Alberta Heritage Foundation for Medical Research, and the Alberta Cancer Foundation.

37. Thyroid and the Brain

Endocrinology
F. Labrie, L. Proulx, eds.

THYROID HORMONE METABOLISM IN THE BRAIN

P. REED LARSEN, J. ENRIQUE SILVA, MICHAEL M. KAPLAN, JACK L. LEONARD AND T. J. VISSER

Howard Hughes Medical Institute Laboratory and Thyroid Diagnostic Center, Brigham and Women's Hospital, Harvard Medical School, Boston, MA 02115

INTRODUCTION

In recent years, it has become apparent that most of the T3 in the cerebral cortex is derived from local T4 to T3 conversion (1-3). In this presentation, we discuss the enzymology of the brain deiodinases, their regulation, and speculate on the physiological consequences of such a system. In early studies of thyroid hormone regulation of TSH release in the rat, we identified a propylthiouracil (PTU)-insensitive deiodinase which efficiently converted T4 to T3 in the anterior pituitary (4,5). Subsequently, we found that the brain rapidly converted T4 to T3 by a similar process which was blocked by iopanoic acid (6,7). Equilibrium studies performed with ^{125}I-T_4 and ^{131}I-T_3 in rats demonstrated that in the cerebral cortex between 70% and 80% of the T3 specifically bound to the nucleus was derived from local production of T3 within the central nervous system. As a consequence, nuclear T3 receptors in the brain were virtually saturated with T3. These results suggested that local iodothyronine deiodination would be very critical in determining brain T3 concentrations.

Kaplan and Yaskoski first studied the enzymology of T4 and T3 metabolism in homogenates of rat cerebral cortex, cerebellum and hypothalamus (8). They found that in hypothyroidism the T4 5'-deiodinase was markedly increased while T3 5-deiodinase activity was reduced. In the developing rat, there was a peak of T4 5'-deiodinase activity between 2-6 weeks of age in all three tissues. The pattern of T3 5-deiodination was quite different, being extremely high in the newborn rat, falling to levels typical of the adult by about 4 weeks. Enzymatic T3 5-deiodinase activity was highest in the hypothalamus.

In early studies, it appeared that, as in the case of the liver, the enzyme converting T4 to T3 would accept either T4 or reverse-T3 (rT3) as the substrate for 5'-deiodination. However, there were several problems with the concept that reverse-T3 and T4 deiodination were occurring by the same pathway since PTU partially inhibited 5'-deiodination of rT3 but not T4. Drs. Visser, Kaplan and Leonard subsequently determined that 5'-deiodination of rT3 could occur by two processes in cerebrocortical microsomes. One pathway was sensitive and the other insensitive to 1 mM PTU (10). T4 to T3 conversion occurred only via the PTU-insensitive enzyme. Using PTU as a tool, the deiodinases are tentatively classified as in Table 1.

TABLE 1.
IODOTHYRONINE DEIODINASES IN THE CENTRAL NERVOUS SYSTEM

	TYPE I(5')	TYPE II(5')	TYPE III(5)
REACTION	rT3 → 3,3'T2 ?T4 → T3	T4 → T3 rT3 → 3,3'T2	T3 → 3,3'T2 T4 → rT3
"Km" (nM)	30(rT3)	2(T4 or rT3)	5(T3); 40(T4)
PTU SENSITIVITY	COMPLETE	NONE	PARTIAL
HYPOTHYROIDISM	NO CHANGE	INCREASE	DECREASE
HYPERTHYROIDISM	NO CHANGE	DECREASE	INCREASE

The Type II 5'-deiodinase and Type III 5-deiodinase are the enzymes initially described by Kaplan and Yaskoski (8,9). Of interest is the contrast between Type I and Type II activities with respect to alterations in thyroid status and to Km. The Type III deiodinase prefers T3 as substrate but is also the enzyme responsible for reverse-T3 production from T4 in the CNS (11).

Subsequently, the time course of the response of the Type II enzyme to hypothyroidism was studied (12). Within 24 hours of thyroidectomy, there were 4 to 6-fold increases in Type II activity in cerebral cortex, whereas no change was found in liver Type I activity or CNS Type III activity during this period. Thus, this deiodinase responds rapidly to T4 deprivation. It was also noted that T3 caused a rapid normalization of enzyme activity within a period of four hours. In later studies comparing the effectiveness of T3 and its analogs, we found that the enzyme activity could be reduced 50% by 0.2 μg T4/100g bw, whereas the ED_{50} for T3 was 5μg/100g bw. This suggested that this was not a transcriptionally-mediated event, an impression further enhanced by finding that the ED_{50} for reverse-T3 was approximately 2μg/100g bw (13).

We also evaluated the effect of cycloheximide on the suppression of enzyme activity produced by T3 (14). Either cycloheximide or T3 caused a 25-40% inhibition of enzyme activity within 4 hours. The combination of the two caused greater than a 90% decrease in enzyme activity, indicating that induction of protein synthesis was not required for the T3 effect. The enzyme production rate in hypothyroid rats was reduced, the increased enzyme activity in the hypothyroid brain being a consequence of an approximately 15-fold lower turnover rate. Our current speculation is that T4 and rT3 (or T3) might somehow regulate enzyme activities by influencing the degradation or inactivation of this enzyme.

The three deiodinase activities are found in mixed nerve-cell cultures(15). In these cultures, T3 degradation is extremely rapid with the T3 half-life on the order of 60 minutes. Preliminary data obtained by exposing such cultures to cytosine-arabinoside suggests that the T4 5'-deiodinase activity is contained in nondividing, presumably neuronal, cells.

The increase in Type II and decrease in Type III deiodinase in hypothyroid rats suggested a mechanism for the brain to defend itself against the effects of hypothyroidism (16). Silva and Larsen found that in the newborn rat with graded hypothyroidism, thyroid hormone-dependent enzymes remain normal until serum T4 reaches very low levels (16). Furthermore, injection of minute quantities of T4 (about 60 ng) caused a 3-fold greater increase in cerebrocortical T3 than did a similar injection in euthyroid two-week old pups. Injection of 200-300 ng T4/100g bw caused significant increases in aspartic transaminase in hypothyroid central nervous system tissue 24 hours later, with no effect on hepatic mitochondrial α-glycerophosphate dehydrogenase (α-GPD). While Dratman, et al, (18) suggested that these increases in T3 production in hypothyroidism were largely a reflection of increased Type II activity, Silva and Matthews (19) recent results point to an equally important role of the reduced T3 degradation by the Type III enzyme in this state.

If we extrapolate from these results to the clinical situation, it would appear that maintenance of optimal intracellular T3 concentrations in the central nervous system requires some T4, and that T3 given in replacement quantities could be detrimental to the developing brain by depriving it of this substrate.

REFERENCES

1. Crantz FR, Silva JE, Larsen PR (1982) Endocrinology 110:367-375.
2. van Doorn J, Roelfsema F, van der Heide D (1982) Acta Endocrinol 101:386-396.
3. van Doorn J, van der Heide D, Roelfsema F (1983) J Clin Invest 72:1778-1792.
4. Silva JE, Larsen PR (1978) J Clin Invest 61:1247-1259.
5. Silva JE, Kaplan MM, Cheron RG, Dick TE, Larsen PR (1978) Metabolism 27: 1601-1607.
6. Crantz FR, Larsen PR (1980) J Clin Invest 65:935-938.
7. Silva JE, Leonard JL, Crantz FR, Larsen PR (1982) J Clin Invest 69:1176-1184.
8. Kaplan MM, Yaskoski KA (1980) J Clin Invest 66:551-562.
9. Kaplan MM, Yaskoski KA (1981) J Clin Invest 67:1204-1214.
10. Visser TJ, Leonard JL, Kaplan MM, Larsen PR (1982) Proc Nat Acad Sci (USA) 79:5080-5084.
11. Kaplan MM, Visser TJ, Yaskoski KA, Leonard JL (1983) Endocrinology 112:35.
12. Leonard JL, Kaplan MM, Visser TJ, Silva JE, Larsen PR (1981) Science 214: 571.
13. Silva JE, Leonard JL, Larsen PR (1983) Program of the 65th Annual Meeting of The Endocrine Society (San Antonio), Abstract 487, p. 202.
14. Leonard JL, Silva JE, Kaplan MM, Mellen SA, Visser TJ, Larsen PR (1984) Endocrinology 114:998-1004.

15. Leonard JL, Larsen PR (1984) Brain Research (in press).

16. Larsen PR, Silva JE, Kaplan MM (1981) Endocrine Reviews 2:87-102.

17. Silva JE, Larsen PR (1982) J Clin Invest 70:1110-1123.

18. Dratman MB, Crutchfield FL, Gordon JT, Jennings AS (1983) Am J Physiol 245 (Endocrinol Metab 8): E185-E193.

19. Silva JE, Matthews PS (1984) (submitted for publication).

BRAIN DEVELOPMENT IN THE IODINE DEFICIENT OVINE FETUS

B.S. HETZEL, B.J. POTTER, M. MANO, B. BELLING, G. McINTOSH and B. CRAGG
CSIRO Division of Human Nutrition, Kintore Avenue, Adelaide, South Australia. 5000, and Department of Physiology, Monash University, Clayton, Victoria. 3168

The relationship between brain development and iodine deficiency in man has been established by clinical and epidemiological studies of the syndrome of endemic cretinism (1). Final proof of the causal relationship of iodine deficiency to retarded brain development required demonstration in an animal model. This has now been achieved in the sheep and more recently in the marmoset (monkey). The establishment of the sheep model has led to studies of the mechanisms involved, particularly the role of maternal and fetal hypothyroidism and the possibility of a direct effect of iodine deficiency itself suggested by clinical and epidemiological evidence (2).

(1) EFFECT OF SEVERE IODINE DEFICIENCY (Table 1)

Severe iodine deficiency has been produced in sheep (3) with a low-iodine diet of crushed maize and pelleted pea pollard (8-15μg iodine/kg), which provided 5-8μg iodine/d. After a period of 5 months, although body weights were maintained, iodine deficiency was evident with the appearance of goiter, low plasma T_4 and T_3 values, elevated TSH levels, and low daily urinary excretion of iodine. Control animals received the same diet, but were supplemented with 2 mg sodium iodide administered by subcutaneous injections each week. The ewes were mated with normal fertile rams, the dates of conception established, and fetuses delivered at 56, 70, 98 and 140 d gestation by hysterotomy while the ewes were under sedation and epidural anaesthesia.

Goitre was evident from 70 d in the iodine-deficient fetuses; thyroid histology revealed evidence of hyperplasia from 56 d gestation.

The iodine-deficient fetuses at 140 d were grossly different in physical appearance from the control fetuses. Absence of wool growth, goitre, varying degrees of subluxation of the lower leg joints, deformation of the skull, and retrognathia were frequently present in the deficient animals. Definite evidence of hypothyroidism was shown also by the delayed bone maturation observed in the fetuses at term.

The lowered brain weight and brain DNA as early as 70 d (Table 1) indicate a reduction in cell number due to slowed neuroblast multiplication, which normally occurs from 40 to 80 d in the sheep. Although brain protein was reduced in the deficient fetuses, the ratio of protein : DNA remained unchanged, indicating no significant change in the size of the brain cells. After 80 d, neuroglial development also appears to be slowed since both the DNA and protein content were reduced to less than normal in the 98 d and 140 d fetal brains (3).

Retardation of fetal brain development was revealed also by histological studies at 140 d gestation. Delayed maturation of the cerebellum was shown by reduced migration of cells from the external granular layer to the internal granular layer and increased density of Purkinje cells. In the cerebral hemispheres the cells were more densely packed in the motor and visual areas and the pyramidal neurons in the hippocampus were denser in the CA1 and CA4 regions indicating severe retardation in neuropil growth in both subfields (3).

(2) EFFECT OF FETAL THYROIDECTOMY

Fetal thyroidectomy has been carried out at 56-60 d and at 98 d gestation. At 140 d similar but less severe changes in fetal development were produced, compared to those observed following iodine deficiency. There were more severe changes following the earlier fetal thyroidectomy (4,5).

(3) EFFECT OF MATERNAL THYROIDECTOMY

A study of the effect of maternal thyroidectomy carried out 6 weeks before pregnancy has revealed a transient effect on brain weight and DNA in mid-gestation which had disappeared by the end of gestation (6).

(4) EFFECT OF THE COMBINATION OF MATERNAL THYROIDECTOMY AND FETAL THYROIDECTOMY (Table 2).

Maternal thyroidectomy, carried out 6 weeks before conception, was followed by fetal thyroidectomy at 98 d gestation.

In this case the 140 d old fetuses were more severely affected than those following iodine deficiency (7). There was a more severe reduction of both maternal and fetal thyroid hormones following the surgical procedures than following iodine deficiency (Table 2).

(5) EFFECT OF IODISED OIL IN THE IODINE DEFICIENT SHEEP

The injection of iodised oil (1 ml Neohydriol = 400 mg iodine) at 100 d gestation produced a remarkable reversal of the effects of severe iodine deficiency by 140 d. There was increase in body weight, restoration of wool growth, great improvement in skeletal retardation and significant increase in brain weight and DNA, and restoration of the histological changes(5,6). There was also restoration of maternal and fetal plasma T_4 to the levels in the control animals which were given the same dose of iodised oil before pregnancy.

(6) EFFECT OF THYROXINE IN THE IODINE DEFICIENT SHEEP

Thyroxine (0.5 mg subcutaneously on alternate days) was followed by similar improvement in the growth and development of the iodine deficient fetus although less than that following iodised oil injection. In view of the extensive evidence of failure of passage of maternal thyroxine in the sheep during the latter half of pregnancy (8) these effects must be attributed to iodine transfer across the placental barrier following metabolism of thyroxine in the mother [5].

TABLE 1

EFFECT OF IODINE DEFICIENCY ON MATERNAL AND FETAL THYROID FUNCTION AND FETAL BRAIN DEVELOPMENT IN THE SHEEP.

		Gestational Age[a] (d)			
		56(d)	70(d)	98(d)	140(d)
Maternal Plasma T_4 (nmol/L)	ID[+]	(5)37[b]	(6)17[b]	(5)15[b]	(7)19[b]
	C	(3)126	(4)134	(5)141	(3)137
Fetal Plasma T_4 (nmol/L)	ID	3[c]	4[b]	4[b]	6[b]
	C	10	25	125	216
Brain weight (g)	ID	(5)1.79	(7)4.20[d]	(5)19.0	(7)46.4[c]
	C	(3)1.68	(4)5.01	(5)22.1	(3)53.8
Brain Cell number (mg DNA)	ID	8.86	14.2[d]	27.8[c]	62.6[b]
	C	8.37	16.2	32.5	74.5

a No. observations shown in parentheses.
b $P<0.001$ c $P<0.01$ d $P<0.05$ (two tailed T test)
ID Iodine Deficiency C Control

TABLE 2

EFFECT OF A COMBINATION OF MATERNAL THYROIDECTOMY BEFORE PREGNANCY AND FETAL THYROIDECTOMY (98 d) ON FETAL BRAIN DEVELOPMENT IN SHEEP AT 140 d GESTATION (mean ± SEM).

			Plasma T_4 (nmol/L)		Total Brain	
		Body Weight (kg)	Maternal	Fetal	Weight (g)	Cell No. (mg DNA)
MFTX	(6)[a]	2.45±0.09	<3	<8	42.95[b]±5.23	55.22[b]±5.41
MFSO	(6)	3.84±0.28	70±5	189±11	55.64 ±1.89	74.24 ±2.91

MFTX Superimposed maternal and fetal thyroidectomised group
MFSO Superimposed maternal and fetal sham-operated control group
a No. of animals in parentheses
b $P<0.05$ as for Table 1.

(7) EFFECT OF 3.5-dimethyl-3' isopropyl-L-thyronine (DIMIT) IN THE IODINE DEFICIENT FETUS.

DIMIT (2mg) subcutaneously on alternate days) at 100 d gestation produced no significant effect in the iodine deficient fetus. Failure to cross the placenta was suggested by lowered maternal but not fetal TSH.

DISCUSSION

The findings indicate severe brain retardation associated with a gross reduction of maternal and fetal thyroxine following the iodine deficient diet. Reduced brain weight and brain DNA were first observed at 70 d gestation before the fetal thyroid is fully functional (8). The histological findings at 140 d indicate significant retardation of cell migration in both cerebellum and cerebral hemispheres and reduced neuropil due to reduced arborization (3,5).

The findings following maternal, fetal and combined thyroidectomy suggest that the effect of iodine deficiency on fetal brain development is mediated by the combination of reduced maternal and fetal thyroid secretion and not by a direct effect of iodine. The effect of reduced maternal secretion occurs in the first half of pregnancy and the effect of reduced fetal secretion in the latter half of pregnancy. The conclusion is consistent with recent evidence in the rat of the passage of maternal thyroxine across the placental barrier early in pregnancy (9).

Further support is provided by more recent observations in Papua New Guinea where a correlation between maternal thyroxine levels during pregnancy and subsequent motor performance in 10-12 year old children subjected to severe iodine deficiency in pregnancy has been observed (10).

REFERENCES

(1) Hetzel, B.S. (1983). Lancet 2, 1126-1129.

(2) Pharoah, P.O.D., Buttfield, I.H., Hetzel, B.S. (1971). Lancet 1, 308-310.

(3) Potter, B.J., Mano, M.T., Belling, G.B., McIntosh, G.H., Hua, C., Cragg, B.G., Marshall, J., Wellby, M.L., Hetzel, B.S. (1983). Neuropathology and Applied Neurobiology 8, 303-313.

(4) McIntosh, G.H., Potter, B.J., Hetzel, B.S., Hua, C., Cragg, B.G. (1982). J. Comp. Path. 92, 599-607.

(5) Hetzel, B.S., Potter, B.J. (1983). In: Dreosti, I.E., Smith, R.M. Eds. Neurobiology of Trace Elements, Chapter 3, p. 83-133.

(6) Potter, B.J., McIntosh, G.H., Hetzel, B.S. (1981). In: B.S. Hetzel, R.M. Smith Eds. Fetal Brain Disorders - Recent Approaches to the Problem of Mental Deficiency. Elsevier/N.Holland, Amsterdam pp. 119-148.

(7) McIntosh, G.H., Potter, B.J., Mano, M.T., Hua, C., Cragg, B.G., Hetzel, B.S. (1983). Neuropathology and Appl. Neurobiology 9, 215-223.

(8) Fisher, D.A., Dussault, J.H., Sack, J., Chopra, I.J. (1977). Recent Progr. Hormone Res. 33, 59-116.

(9) Obregon, M.J., Mallol, J., Pastor, R., Morreale de Escobar, G., Escobar del Rey, F. (1984). Endocrinology 114, 305-307.

(10) Pharoah, P.O.D., Connolly, K., Hetzel, B.S., Ekins, R. (1981). Devel. Med. Child, Neurolog, 23, 76-82.

© 1984 Elsevier Science Publishers B.V.
Endocrinology
F. Labrie, L. Proulx, eds.

THYROID HORMONES AND MICROTUBULES DURING BRAIN DEVELOPMENT

JACQUES NUNEZ
CNRS-INSERM U 35 Hôpital Henri Mondor 94010 Créteil (France)

INTRODUCTION

The most significant effects of thyroid hormones take place during the critical period of brain development i.e. when the neurones begin to differentiate. Although each mature neurone seems unique in its function all neurones undergo a common major morphological transformation during this period i.e. the extension of cell process which will produce the axons and the dendrites. Such a fundamental change in cell shape is regulated both *in vivo* (1,2) and *in vitro* (3,4) by thyroid hormones. Hypothyroidism, when established before the critical period of brain development, produces several defects; however, the most dramatic one is an impaired neurite outgrowth. This might lead to the observed reduction in the number of contacts between neurones, and therefore to the decreased electric activity of the brain.

The modifications in cell shape occurring during neurite outgrowth are probably caused by profound changes in the organization of the cytoskeleton. Since the formation of nerve cell processes requires massive neurotubulin assembly (5,6) this parameter has been chosen as a marker of the action of thyroid hormones on neurite outgrowth.

RESULTS AND DISCUSSION

Preliminary informations (7) were obtained by following the kinetics of microtubule assembly with normal brain preparations. Fig.1 shows that the rates of microtubule polymerisation increase with age whatever the animal species. Maximal rates were always obtained during the critical period of brain development. At a fetal stage and just after birth, when most nerve cells are still undifferentiated in the rat and mouse brain, microtubules assembled very poorly. In the guinea pig, a species which has a mature brain at birth, such a situation was seen only at fetal stages.

Hypothyroidism, when established in the rat before the onset of thyroid function (∿ 16 days of gestation), slows this evolution although normal values were observed at adulthood (8). This correlates well with the morphological data: thyroid hormone deficiency reduces the length and the branching of the dendrites of the neurons in the cortex (1) and of the dendritic tree of the Purkinje cells in the cerebellum (2); the length of the parallel fiber, the axon of the grain cells in the cerebellum, is also reduced (9). Both the morphological defects and the decrease in microtubule assembly can be corrected after thyroid hormone administration but such a reversibility is in relation with the age at which therapy is begun.

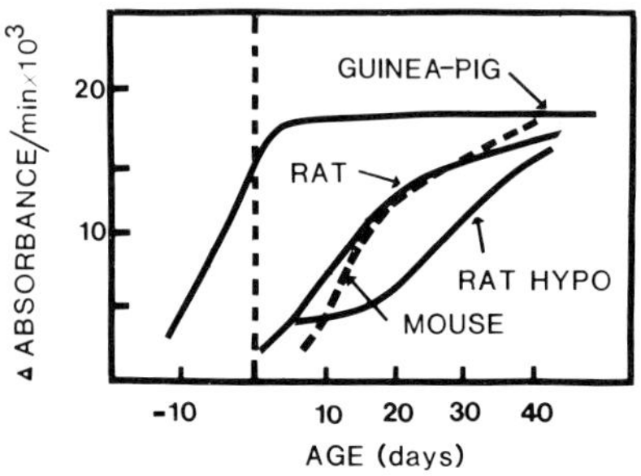

Fig.1. Initial rates of assembly during brain development (1mg tubulin/ml) in different species and in hypothyroid rats.

Tubulin assembly includes a rate limiting initiation step, with the formation of "seeds" or "nuclei", and then an elongation step which allows the formation of the microtubules (see 10). Several parameters related to the initiation step are modified during brain development and in hypothyroidism. Adding microtubule fragments, obtained by sonication, to increase the number of seeds, restored normal rates of assembly both with immature and with hypothyroid preparations. Similarly both MAP_2 and TAU, the two major microtubule-associated proteins (MAPs) which have been shown to act as promotors of tubulin polymerisation, restored normal rates of assembly. These results suggested that the composition or concentration of MAPs (i.e. their activity) varies during brain development and is under thyroid hormone control.

A clear difference in the composition of MAPs during brain development was seen (11) by mono and two dimensional polyacrylamide gel electrophoresis (12). At the level of the TAU fraction (60-68 K) four closely spaced bands are separated in the adult preparation whereas only two (50-63 K) are present at young stages of development. Two dimensional analysis reveals that this group of MAPs is composed with at least 25 different entities. In hypothyroidism the composition of the TAU fraction changes more slowly than in the control of the same age with TAU_3 being almost absent at day 15 after birth (Fig.2). At least 1/3 of the iso-TAU entities are absent as shown by two dimensional analysis.

The different "young" and "adult" TAUs are probably coded by different genes as shown both by peptide mapping analysis (11) and after isolation of their m-RNA (13). Similar conclusion might be true also for "young" and "adult" MAP_2.

Several other MAPs are present in the "young", "adult" and hypothyroid preparations; differences in the gel profile were also noted at the level of these minor entities during normal brain development and in hypothyroid preparations. One of these minor MAP with a molecular weight of $\sim$ 200 K might be ankyrin (14).

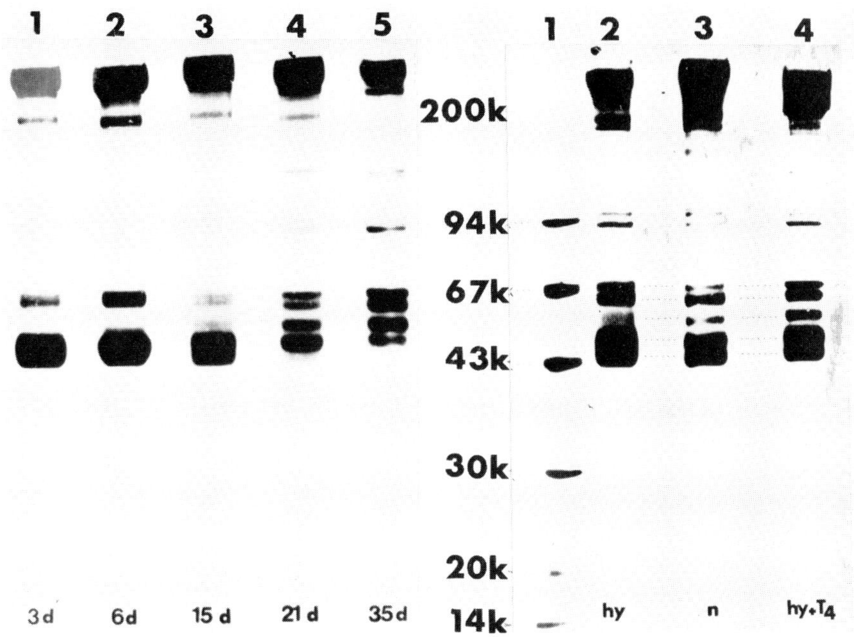

Fig.2. Polyacrylamide gel electrophoresis of the microtubule-associated proteins. Left panel, lanes 1 to 5 from 3,6,15,21 and 35 days old rat brain. Right panel: lane 1 molecular weight markers; lane 2 from hypothyroid rat (hy); lane 3 from normal rat (n); lane 4 from hypothyroid rat receiving thyroid hormone (hy + T_4) at birth.

"Young" and "adult" microtubule preparations also differ in several other respects: 1) "young" MAP_2 and "young" TAU are both less active in promoting microtubule assembly than the corresponding adult entities (11). 2) The pattern of cyclic AMP-dependent phosphorylation on polyacrylamide gels of "young" and "adult" ^{32}P-labeled TAUs is different (11). 3) The sensitivity to calcium ions and to the calmodulin-Ca^2 complex is greater with "young" microtubules than with the adult preparations (15). 4) "Young" microtubules are very unstable and differ in size from the adult ones when analyzed by ultramicroscopic and ultracentrifugation techniques (12).

These and other data showing that the various MAPs are differently located depending on the brain region and the type of neuronal process (16) suggest that each one of these proteins might specify different developmental and (or) cellular events during brain differentiation. Thyroid hormone would act during this process as an epigenic factor i.e. to synchronize the program of construction of the neuronal network by regulating sequentially and geographically microtubule assembly and therefore neurite outgrowth.

REFERENCES

1. Eayrs JT (1960) Brit Med Bull 16:122-127
2. Legrand J (1967) Arch Anat Microsc Morphol Exp 56:205-244
3. Puymerat J, Loudes C, Faivre-Bauman A and Tixier-Vidal A (1982) Cold Spring Harb Conf on Cell Prolif 9:1033-1051
4. Romijn AM, Habets MC, Raaka BM and Stanley F (1982) Dev Sci 2:583-589
5. Yamada KM, Spooner BS and Wessels MK (1970) Proc Natl Acad Sci 66:1206-1212
6. Seed NW, Gilman AG, Amano T and Niremberg MN (1970) Proc Acad Sci 66: 160-167
7. Lennon AM, Francon J, Fellous A and Nunez (1980) J Neurochem 35:804-813
8. Fellous A, Lennon AM, Francon J and Nunez J (1979) Europ J Biochem 101: 365-376
9. Lauder JM (1977) in Thyroid Hormones and Brain development Ed Grave GD Raven Press New York pp 235-252
10. Scheele R and Borisy G in "Microtubules". Roberts K and Hyams JS Eds (1979) Academic Press pp 175-254
11. Francon J, Lennon AM, Fellous A, Mareck A, Pierre M and Nunez J (1982) Europ J Biochem 129:465-471
12. Passareiro H and Nunez J Unpublished results
13. Ginzburg I, Scherson T, Giveon D, Behar L and Littauer UZ (1982) Proc Nat Acad Sci 79:4892-4896
14. Bennett V and Davis J in Organisation of the cytoplasm. Cold Spring Harbor Symposia (1982) Vol XLVI pp 647-657
15. Erneux C, Passareiro H and Nunez J (1984) FebsLetters. In press.
16. Matus A, Bernhardt R and Hugh-Jones T (1981) Proc Nat Acad Sci 78:3010-3040

Endocrinology
F. Labrie, L. Proulx, eds.

EFFECT OF EARLY THYROID TREATMENT ON BRAIN DEVELOPMENT

JEAN H. DUSSAULT

Dept. Endocrinology and Metabolism, Thyroid Research Unit, Centre Hospitalier de l'Université Laval, Ste-Foy, Quebec, Canada G1V 4G2

Thyroid hormones play an important role in the development of the central nervous system. The most striking effects are observed during its maturation where absence of thyroid hormones produces multiple morphological and biochemical alterations and in man finally leads to irreversible mental retardation (1). Since the brain is a very heterogenous organ, a first step to elucidate the mechanism of action of thyroid hormones in this organ is to identify the primary targets of the hormones. The rat will serve as a model for this purpose.

The demonstration of local conversion of T_4 to T_3 in the brain with highly saturated T_3 receptors by Crantz, Larsen and collaborators (2) suggest that T_3 is particularly important in the brain. Saturation experiments reveal the presence of a single class of binding sites not evenly distributed in the adult cortex and concentrated in the neuronal population with a mean Ka of 0.53 0.04 x 10^{10} M^{-1} (M SEM). On the other hand, there is considerable heterogeneity in the nuclear T_3 binding capacity of the structures studied. The highest concentrations of nuclear T_3 receptors were found in the amygdala, the hypocampus and the cortex while the lowest were in the brain stem and the cerebellum with a 9 fold difference between the lowest and the highest capacities measured (3).

The maturation of connectivity of the cortical neurons namely pyramidal cells can be quantitated by measuring the number and distribution of dendritic spines along their shaft (4). At 5 days after birth, pyramidal cells are quite immature and only a few spines are found occasionally along the shaft. The number of spines then increases up to 30 days of age as well as their distance from teh cell. Thyroidectomy at 10 days of age will reduce significantly the number of spines/apical shaft of pyramidal cells of the rat visual cortex at 20 days of age. Early replacement therapy will restored the ratio at 40 days of age but not if treatment is started at a later age (30 days).

In the cerebellum an organ that matures predominantly postnataly, the Purkinge cells are the only efferent neurons of the cortex and are formed just before birth. The mitotic activity in the external germinal layer is manifested by an increase in width of this layer up to 8 days of age and stop by 21 days. During this period the granule cells migrate toward the internal granular layer differentiating in the process. Their dendrites establish contact with the affarent fibers, their axons splits into aT shape and establish contact with the Purkinge cells establishing the wiring pattern of the adult cerebellum. In the hypothyroid rat the external layer is still present at 21 days, death occurs in the cells of the internal layer and the immature wiring pattern persist. Thus the neuronal circuit is quantitatively and quantitatively different from the normal circuit (5).

In the developing auditory system, perinatal hypothyroidism induce irreversible damage to the auditory function as determined by brainstem response audiometry (BSRA). This susceptibility to thyroid hormones deficiency occurs prior to 10 days postnatally (and perhaps as early as 5 days), before the onset of cochlear activity normally seen at 12 days of age, and is prevented by early replacement therapy (6). Some recent anatomical data suggest that the changes induced in auditory cortex pyramids by perinatal hypothyroidism are either very sensitive to a minor degree of hypothyroidism or have a shorter critical period during which treatment may reverse the damage (7). Thus this two complementary studies have the same conclusions on the presence of a critical period in the development of the auditory system where minor degree of hypothyroidism produces irreversible damage.

Biochemically hypothyroidism induces a decrease of nucleic acid synthesis and of enzymes associated with synaptosomes (glutamate and succinate dehydrogenase). In 'vivo' the cerebellar ornithine decarboxyalse (ODC) is regulated by thyroid hormones in the first week of life. Hypothyroidism decreases significantly the activity of the enzyme, activity which is restored by T_3 replacement therapy (8). In 'vitro' (immature astrocytes) the activity of glutamyltransferase is also regulated by thyroid hormones. After 7, 14 and 21 days the activity of this enzyme involved in the astrocytic differentiation is markedly increased 24 hours after the addition of physiological concentration of T_3. The characteristics of the response change with the age of the culture indication that the effect of thyroid hormones depend on the degree of the maturation of the cells. In the same cell type, T_3 added after 2 weeks of culture will regulate specific soluble proteins phosphorylation: a rapid and transient increase of 34 K dalton protein and a progressive decrease in the phosphorylation of two proteins (20 K and 21 K) (9). As for the effect of thyroid hormones on neurotransmitters there is an increase in substance P and dopamine in various anatomical regions of the brain in 60 days old rat rendered hypothyroid at birth (10).

In human untreated congenital hypothyroidism leads to permanent mental retardation. 85% of the infants have an abnormal I.Q. if treated after age 3 months. Prospective studies on the impact of screening programs for congenital hypothyroidism have shown that early therapy will permit a normal mental development at age 7 years in the great majorities of children (90%) (11).

In summary thyroid hormones are essential for the normal development of the central nervous systems, their effect being related to specific time period in the maturation of diverse regions of the SNC.

REFERENCES

1. Raiti S, Newns GH (1971) Arch Dis Child 46:692.
2. Crantz FR, Larsen PR (1980) J Clin Invest 65:935-938.
3. Ruel J, Faure R, Dussault JH (1982) Abstract, American Thyroid Association, Quebec.
4. Morreale de Escobar G, Escobar del Rey F, Ruiz-Marcos A (1983) In: Dussault JH, Walker P (eds) Congenital Hypothyroidism. Marcel Dekker, Inc, New York, pp 85-126.
5. Legrand J (1977) In: Berenberg SR (ed) Brain, Fetal and Infant. Martinus Nijhoff Medical Division, The Hague, pp 137-164.
6. Hébert R, Dussault JH (1984) Dev Brain Res (accepted for publication).
7. Ruiz-Marcos A, Salas J, Sanchez-Toscano F, Escobar del Rey F, Morreale de Escobar G (1983) Dev Brain Res 9:205-213.
8. Ruel J, Chénard C, Coulombe P, Dussault JH (1984) Can J Physiol Pharmacol (accepted for publication).
9. Ruel J, Gavaret JM, Dussault JH (1984) Abstract, 7th International Congress of Endocrinology, Quebec.
10. Savard P, Mérand Y, Bédard P, Dussault JH, Dupont A (1983) Brain Res 277: 263-268.
11. Dussault JH, Glorieux J, Letarte J, Morissette J, Guyda H (1984) Abstract, American Thyroid Association, New York.

38. Growth Hormone Disorders

Endocrinology
F. Labrie, L. Proulx, eds.

HETEROGENEITY OF GROWTH HORMONE IN THE PITUITARY GLAND

URBAN J. LEWIS
Lutcher Brown Department of Biochemistry, The Whittier Institute for Diabetes and Endocrinology, 9894 Genesee Avenue, La Jolla, CA 92037 U.S.A.

It is now clear that "growth hormone" is not a single substance. The significance of this heterogeneity is unknown but because multiple forms of the hormone have been detected in the blood, physiologic importance might be expected. We are investigating two possible roles for the various forms of growth hormone. The first is that each has a specific function and that the regulation of various activities of growth hormone is mediated through control of secretion of the individual forms. This implies that each has its own receptor or that binding of the different forms to the same receptor would initiate different secondary cellular reactions. The second possible role for the multiple forms is that growth hormone action is mediated through small peptide-segments of the various forms. Proteolytic processing of the parent prohormone would be a major site of control. Because of different conformational structures in each of the multiple forms, a variety of regions would be exposed to the immediate environment. Proteolytic attack could then produce different fragments that initiate specific cellular processes. Such a variety of forms and fragments would help explain how growth hormone can produce its numerous effects, many of which are actually opposing actions. This presentation will not dwell upon significance of the multiple forms but rather summarize what is known of their structures and point out where specific biologic importance might be indicated. Three recent reviews provide a detailed bibliography which is not possible here (1-3).

CHARACTERIZED SUBSTANCES

The 20,000 dalton variant of human growth hormone (hGH_{20K})

This form, which lacks a 15 amino acid sequence (residues 32-46), is produced by alternative mRNA processing. The deletion of this segment markedly reduces the early insulin-like effects associated with hGH. No similar variant has yet been reported for other species so a general importance for this substance is not known. The hGH_{20K} shows reduced immunoreactivity and receptor binding properties. The variant has been detected in serum, an indication that it is not only synthesized but also secreted by the pituitary gland. Alternative mRNA splicing could also produce a 20K-variant of the growth hormone that would be produced by expression of the hGH-V gene (4). This means that there are possibly two additional variants of hGH to be found in pituitary extracts.

Because hGH_{20K} has different biologic activities it can be classified as a specific hormone with distinct activities. In addition one can reason that the deletion provides a different substrate for production of a different set of fragments by proteolytic processing.

The hGH-V gene

Seeburg (4) has reported the structure of a hGH gene that, if expressed, would produce a form with 13 amino acid substitutions. The protein has yet to be identified in pituitary extracts. One of the changes in amino acid structure is the formation of a consensus sequence for glycosylation. Substitution of an asparagine for a lysine at position 140 produces an Asn-Gln-Ser sequence. This takes on added importance now that a glycosylated form of prolactin has been identified. The significance of glycosylation is not well understood. Attachment of carbohydrate has been implicated in altering proteolytic cleavage sites and in the intracellular movement and secretion of proteins. The process may well be a mechanism for modulation of hormone action. The hGH-V protein would have a significantly more alkaline isoelectric point than hGH because of a number of non-conservative substitutions. A discussion of these substitutions has been presented elsewhere (3). Receptor binding activity is only moderately affected whereas immunoreactivity was significantly decreased. The bioactivity of the hGH-V is unknown but the major structural changes suggest a hormone with properties different from hGH. These changes most certainly would alter proteolytic processing.

The disulfide dimer of hGH

The nature and significance of the large forms of growth hormone are poorly understood. Physiologic importance is suggested by alterations in their serum concentrations under varying physiologic conditions (5). The large forms are probably a mixture of dissociable aggregates of hGH_{22K} and hGH_{20K}, the interchain disulfide dimer and its aggregates and immunoreactive forms that are resistant to reducing agents. Because it is known that hGH_{20K} aggregates more readily than hGH, as is also the case for an artificially expressed sample of hGH-V, the high molecular weight material observed in serum must be examined closely for variant forms. Of the large forms, only the disulfide dimer of hGH has been isolated. It was essentially inactive in stimulating tibial cartilage of the rat but retained about 50% of the immunoreactivity of monomer hGH. A RIA value for serum hGH would not, then, give an accurate indication of bioactivity. A role for the disulfide dimer may be to provide a variation on tertiary structure for production of different cleavage products. The physiologic and structural properties of the immunologically active forms of hGH that do not dissociate in urea when reduced are unknown. It has been assumed that they are covalently linked through disulfide interchange but there is no evidence to support this.

Proteolytically cleaved forms

Several investigators have noted that limited proteolysis converts hGH almost quantitatively into a two-chain form. Location of the cleavages has been identified for some of the altered forms. Noteworthy is the fact that potentiation of growth promoting and lactogenic activities were noted for these substances. Interest in them, however, has waned because of lack of evidence that they circulate. Newer detection methods, such as the immunostaining procedure of Meuris *et al.* (6) and Sinha *et al.* (7), may revive interest in these substances if they can be demonstrated in serum.

Fragments

If the concept is correct that growth hormone serves as a prohormone for metabolically active fragments, such segments should have equal if not greater activity (on a molar basis) than growth hormone itself. Support for this view was obtained with the hGH (1-43) and hGH (32-46) peptides. The rationale for testing these peptides was that, since hGH_{20K} had diminished insulin-like activity, the deleted region might be responsible for the activity. The results (see reference 4 for bibliography of published data) indicated that the peptides were insulin potentiating, lacking any insulin-like activity. In support of this is the work by M.B. Sigel *et al.* (these laboratories, to be published) that hGH (1-43) enhances *in vitro* binding of insulin to liver membrane receptors. These results raise the question whether the insulin-like effects of growth hormone are not actually a result of potentiation of insulin activity. The literature is not consistent on this subject and Armstrong *et al.* have discussed this point (8). Although various biologic activities have been found for these peptides, they are not growth promoting. A future goal, of course, is to determine if it will be possible to administer a group of fragments of growth hormone and observe somatic growth. Another action recently reported for the hGH (32-46) peptide is that it stimulates insulin and glucagon secretion in the dog (9). Since insulin is a necessary factor for growth, stimulation of its release may be an important part of growth hormone action.

The diabetogenic activity of growth hormone is incompletely understood. There are data that indicate hGH is less active in producing glucose intolerance in the dog than is a cleavage product of the hormone. The active peptide had a molecular weight near 5,000 and was active in microgram quantities as compared to the milligrams of hGH that were needed to produce a comparable intolerance. Hart *et al.* (10) have found that the most active (tibial line assay) preparation of bovine GH that they isolated had the lowest diabetogenic activity. Our opinion is that growth hormone at high enough dosages can cause glucose intolerance but that there is another pituitary substance which is considerably more active and that this peptide is a fragment of growth hormone.

UNCHARACTERIZED FORMS

We have observed two more alkaline forms of hGH in pituitary extracts (2) but because of the shortage of human pituitary glands additional studies have not been possible.

Hart et al. (10) have reported a comparison of various biological activities of several preparations of the hormone that they isolated. The conclusion was that bovine GH as usually prepared is a mixture of different forms with varying immunological and biological properties.

Our laboratory has confirmed the work of Ellis et al. (11) which describes a biologically active (tibial line assay) immunologically unreactive form of bovine GH in the pituitary gland. The substance is not detected by radioimmunoassays for IGF-I or the fibroblast growth factor.

REFERENCES

1. Lewis UJ, Singh RNP, Sigel MB, Frigeri LG, Sinha YN, VanderLaan WP (1984) In: Saxena BB, Catt KJ, Bernbaumer L, Martini L (eds) Hormone Receptors in Growth and Reproduction. Raven Press, New York, pp 37-53
2. Lewis UJ (1984) Ann Rev Physiol 46:33-42
3. Lewis UJ, Frigeri, LG, Sigel MB, Tutwiler GF, VanderLaan WP (1984) In: Raiti S (ed) Human Growth Hormone. Plenum Press, New York, in press
4. Seeburg PH (1982) DNA 1:239-249
5. Sinha YN (1980) Endocrinology 107:1959-1069
6. Meuris S, Svoboda M, Vilamala M, Christophe J, Robyn C (1983) FEBS Letters 154:111-115
7. Sinha YN, Gilligan TA, Lee DW (1984) J Clin Endocrinol Metab 58:752-754
8. Armstrong J McD, Bornstein J, Bromley JO, MaCaulay SL, Ng FM (1983) Acta Endocrinol 102:492-498
9. Stevenson RW, Stebbing N, Rudman CG, Williams PE, Cherrington AD (1984) Program, 44th Annual Meeting of the American Diabetes Association, Abstract 572, p 149A
10. Hart JC, Blake LA, Chadwick ME, Payne GA, Simmonds AD (1984) Biochem J 218:573-581
11. Ellis S, Vodian MA, Grindeland RE (1978) Rec Prog Hormone Res 34:213-234

Endocrinology
F. Labrie, L. Proulx, eds.

HETEROGENEITY OF HUMAN GROWTH HORMONE IN THE CIRCULATION

GERHARD BAUMANN

Center for Endocrinology, Metabolism and Nutrition, Department of Medicine, Northwestern University Medical School, Chicago, Illinois 60611, USA.

Knowledge of the precise chemical nature of growth hormone (GH) in blood is of considerable biological importance because of the largely unexplained discrepancy between GH-like bioactivity in plasma and GH concentration as measured by radioimmunoassay. The bioactivity in plasma has been reported to exceed immunoassayable GH by as much as 50-200 (1). Since this cannot be attributed to somatomedins alone (1), the possibility of highly bioactive and/or poorly immunoreactive forms of GH as part of the overall growth-promoting activity of plasma must be considered.

Size heterogeneity

In the early 1970s, it was shown that fractionation of plasma on Sephadex yields two to four (usually three) immunoreactive hGH species with molecular weights of about 20,000, 45,000 and greater than 60,000 (2-4). Since no information existed about the structure of these size isomers, they were descriptively named "little", "big" and "big-big" hGH. Since hGH has a molecular weight of approximately 22,000, it appeared likely that the main species in plasma (little hGH) corresponded to that hormone. However, the relationship of the larger molecular weight species to hGH was not immediately clear - they could represent hGH precursors (prohormones), hGH aggregates, binding of hGH to plasma proteins, or material unrelated to hGH interfering in the radioimmunoassay. It was then shown that big hGH could be partially converted to little hGH by treatment with dissociating agents, such as urea (5). This finding indicated that "urea-labile" big hGH was probably an hGH dimer.

Recently, Stolar and coworkers examined the molecular nature of the big hGH forms in plasma in greater detail by high resolution techniques (6). Big-big, big and little hGH were extracted from gel-filtered plasma fractions by immunoaffinity chromatography in sufficient quantities to permit extensive characterization by polyacrylamide gel electrophoresis and isoelectric focusing. The previous interpretation of the nature of little and big hGH was essentially confirmed: these species represent monomeric and dimeric hGH. In addition, big-big hGH was recognized as a heterogeneous mixture of hGH oligomers (tri-, tetra- and pentamers). Approximately 70% of all these oligomers was readily dissociable to hGH monomers. The rest could be converted to monomers by sulfhydryl reduction, indicating that these "non-dissociable" or "urea-stable" big forms were oligomers linked by intermolecular disulfide bridges. In addition, the study by Stolar et al. revealed that each molecular size species was composed of several structurally diverse monomeric hGH forms (see below).

Studies directed at answering the question whether hGH could bind to plasma proteins indicated for the most part such was not the case (2,4). Some investigators, however, reported that radioiodinated hGH, when added to plasma, was partially converted to higher molecular weight material (7). It is presently not clear whether this is a property unique to radioiodinated hGH.

There is to date no conclusive evidence pointing toward an hGH precursor molecule as the basis for large molecular weight immunoreactive material in blood. Examination of pituitary extracts and pituitary culture media has failed to reveal a pro-hGH (8,9). Moreover, the nucleotide sequences of the hGH gene and its mRNA do not predict the existence of such a prohormone (10).

Charge heterogeneity

Charge isomerism of hGH was first recognized in pituitary extracts by Chrambach and associates (11) and Lewis and coworkers (12). Interest in the charge isomers of hGH was stimulated by the finding that certain acidic hGH forms had up to 8-fold enhanced bioactivity (11-13). These acidic forms represented hGH cleaved in the large disulfide loop to form two-chain polypeptides (11,12). On the basis of this cleavage, it was hypothesized that hGH may have to be proteolytically processed to express its full bioactivity (14). However, it has been difficult to demonstrate that proteolytic cleavage *in vivo* leads to these activated hGH forms either in the pituitary (9), or in the circulation (15), or in peripheral tissues (16). Continued studies of the heterogeneity of hGH in the pituitary have led to the identification of a number of monomeric forms, such as the 22,000 dalton single-chain form (22K), the 20,000 dalton variant (20K), 3 proteolytically cleaved 2-chain forms, an N^{α}-acetylated form, two deamidated forms, as well as other, less well-characterized forms (see 8 for review). Until recently, it was not possible to determine which of these forms reached the circulation.

Studies aimed at directly examining the question regarding the type(s) of circulating hGH relied at first on attempts to generate specific radioimmunoassays for individual hGH forms. However, it was found that crossreactivity among antibodies (including monoclonal antibodies) was too great to achieve this goal (17). Therefore, hGH was extracted from plasma by immunoaffinity chromatography and analyzed by physicochemical techniques which were capable of distinguishing between the various monomeric hGH isomers. These experiments revealed that at least three monomeric hGH forms were present in plasma shortly after a secretory stimulus [e.g., L-dopa (17)]. The predominant form was 22K which accounted for about 85% of the total hGH. The second most prevalent form was 20K (10% of total). In addition, about 5% of the total immunoreactive hGH could be attributed to one or more unidentified acidic forms. Based on the electrophoretic behavior of known pituitary forms, the acidic material could represent deamidated hGH, acetylated hGH or one of the cleaved hGH forms.

These same molecular forms were found as the monomeric building blocks for big and big-big (i.e. oligomeric) plasma hGH (6). Thus, each oligomeric species contains 22K, 20K and acidic hGH. The dimeric fraction is particularly enriched in 20K (6).

The chemical nature of hGH circulating under basal conditions, i.e. during periods of low or absent pituitary secretion, was also analyzed using the same technology. It should be emphasized that such basal conditions prevail during most of the time. Basal plasma "hGH" was found to consist of a highly variable mixture of the 3 hGH forms described above and what appear to be several immunoreactive hGH fragments (18). A fragment with a molecular weight of 16,000 was a prominent component (18). An important unanswered question is whether hGH fragments contribute to the growth-promoting bioactivity in plasma.

Type of secretory stimulus and circulating hGH forms

The possibility must be considered that the pituitary can selectively or preferentially release certain hGH forms in response to various stimuli. A number of stimuli, both physiologic and pharmacologic, have been examined in this regard. Thus far, there is little evidence for selectivity of stimuli as in all cases the distribution of hGH forms in the circulation was similar (17,19,20). Examination of the distribution of hGH forms in urine - which presumably reflects integrated plasma hGH - provides further evidence for the relative constancy of the composition of plasma hGH (21).

Physiological significance of hGH heterogeneity

It is presently not clear what the biological role of the various forms of hGH is. As assessed by radioreceptor assay, monomeric 22K and some of its cleaved congeners have the most intrinsic potency (22,23). However, this may not be the only parameter important for overall bioactivity. This is exemplified by 20K which shows full growth-promoting activity in vivo despite its poor interaction with GH receptors (24), or by the cleaved forms which show enhanced bioactivity (11-13) despite normal receptor binding (23). Some of these seeming discrepancies are probably explained by differences in metabolic clearance and hence persistence of action in vivo (25). Another exciting but presently speculative possibility centers on the generation *in vivo* of different fragments depending on the parent hormone. Some of these fragments may also be responsible for part of the excess bioactivity observed in plasma. Further dissection of the GH-like activity in the circulation will hopefully yield new insights into the bioactivity/immunoreactivity paradox.

ACKNOWLEDGMENTS

The present work was supported by grants no. AM-27047, AM-01769, MRP-1-P50-HD-10021, RR-05370, and RR-48 from the National Institutes of Health.

REFERENCES

1. Ellis S, Vodian MA, Grindeland RE (1978) Recent Progr Horm Res 34:213.
2. Goodman AD, Tanenbaum R, Rabinowitz D (1972) J Clin Endocrinol Metab 35:868.
3. Gorden P, Hendricks C, Roth J (1973) J Clin Endocrinol Metab 36:178.
4. Yalow RS (1974) Recent Progr Horm Res 30:597.
5. Wright DR, Goodman AD, Trimble KD (1974) J Clin Invest 54:1064.
6. Stolar MW, Amburn K, Baumann G (1984) J Clin Endocrinol Metab 59:In press.
7. Beitins IZ, Rattazzi MC, MacGillivray MH (1977) Endocrinology 101:350.
8. Lewis UJ, Singh RNP, Tutweiler GF, Sigel MB, VanderLaan EF, VanderLaan WP (1980) Recent Progr Horm Res 36:477.
9. Baumann G, MacCart JG (1982) J Clin Endocrinol Metab 55:611.
10. Fiddes JC, Seeburg PH, DeNoto FM, Hallewell RA, Baxter JD, Goodman H (1979) Proc Natl Acad Sci USA 76:4294.
11. Chrambach A, Yadley RA, Ben-David M, Rodbard D (1973) Endocrinology 93:848, 866.
12. Singh RNP, Seavey BI, Rice VP, Lindsey TT, Lewis UJ (1974) Endocrinology 94:883.
13. Baumann G, Nissley SP (1979) J Clin Endocrinol Metab 48:246.
14. Lewis UJ, Pence SJ, Singh RNP, VanderLaan WP (1975) Biochem Biophys Res Commun 67:617.
15. Baumann G (1976) J Clin Endocrinol Metab 43:222.
16. Baumann G, Hodgen G (1976) J Clin Endocrinol Metab 43:1009.
17. Baumann G, MacCart JG, Amburn K (1983) J Clin Endocrinol Metab 56:946.
18. Baumann G, Stolar MW, Amburn K (1983) Progr 65th Meet Endocr Soc, Abstract No. 198.
19. Stolar MW, Baumann G, Vance ML, Thorner MO (1984) J Clin Endocrinol Metab 59:In press.
20. Stolar MW, Baumann G (1984) Program 7th Intl Congr Endocrinol, In press.
21. Baumann G, Abramson EC (1983) J Clin Endocrinol Metab 56:305.
22. Gorden P, Lesniak MA, Hendricks CM, Roth J (1973) Science 182:829.
23. Baumann G, Skyler JS, Chrambach A (1975) Program 57th Meet Endocr Soc, Abstract No. 122.
24. Sigel MB, Thorpe NA, Kobrin MS, Lewis UJ, VanderLaan WP (1981) Endocrinology 108:1600.
25. Baumann G (1979) J Clin Endocrinol Metab 49:495.

Endocrinology
F. Labrie, L. Proulx, eds.

DISORDERS OF GROWTH HORMONE NEUROSECRETORY FUNCTION

BARRY B. BERCU, M.D.

All Children's Hospital, University of South Florida College of Medicine,
St. Petersburg, FL 33701

Normal growth requires the interplay of numerous biochemical events including appropriate growth hormone (GH) secretion. The regulation of pituitary GH secretion is complex involving multiple hypothalamic substances including GH releasing factor, GH inhibiting factor (somatostatin) and neurotransmitters. This system is further complicated by interactions with neurotransmitters at higher brain centers through specific neural pathways (1,2). Although the system is incompletely understood, it is possible to speculate that disruptions at any level would result in decreased GH secretion and ultimately poor linear growth velocity (GV) and short stature.

Insight into the possibility of a neuroendocrine disorder causing short stature, which we now call GH-neurosecretory dysfunction (GH-ND) (3), comes from several previous studies. First are the observations of abnormalities in GH secretion in response to a pharmacologic stimulus in patients who were irradiated for brain tumors (4) and acute lymphocytic leukemia (ALL)(5). Second was the inability of several investigators to consistently identify a bioinactive GH molecule or a defect in GH receptors in groups of children who were short and not GH deficient but who reponded to exogenous hGH (6-11). The secretion of a biologically inactive molecule can probably explain the defect in only some of these patients. Thirdly, our understanding was further aided by the opportunity to study the monkey model juxtaposed to clinical studies.

Our earlier studies included the use of insulin hypoglycemia to examine GH secretion in three groups of patients: children with ALL who received previously 2400 rads dose to the central nervous system (CNS), ALL children who did not receive prophylactic cranial radiation, and patients with Ewing's sarcoma who received 2000 rads to the CNS (12,13). The results are summarized as follows: ALL, radiation plus chemotherapy (n=18), ALL with chemotherapy only (n=5), Ewing's sarcoma, radiation plus chemotherapy (n=17); peak GH after insulin was 8.6±1.9 (mean±SE), 46.2±8.6 and 30.1±5.7 ng/ml, respectively. A blunted GH response (< 7 ng/ml) correlated highly (7/8) with patients with evidence for leukoencephalopathy. These results suggested a dose response sensitivity of the CNS to cranial radiation.

Subsequently, a controlled prospective investigation involving only radiation therapy, excluding chemotherapy, in the nonhuman primate was done.

Two groups of monkeys were studied - a CNS radiation dose of 2400 or 4000 rads given in fractions. Assessment of GH secretion after provocative testing included sequential administration of arginine, insulin and L-dopa at 0, 10, 30 and 50 weeks (14). There was consistent blunting of GH secretion after insulin but not after L-dopa or arginine. However, when the dose of insulin was doubled to 0.2 U/kg, this abnormality reversed, suggesting an abnormality in the neurosecretory control of GH. To examine endogenous physiologic GH secretion, we performed a 24 h study with blood sampling every 20 min. The 24 h GH secretory patterns were distinctly different from controls in terms of reduced number and amplitude of GH pulses as well as decreased total GH output. Using provocative tests (arginine, L-dopa, insulin at 0.2 U/kg), these irradiated monkeys could not be differentiated from controls.

Endogenous pulsatile GH secretion in patients with ALL who received 2400 rads was then examined. All quantitative parameters describing pulsatile secretion were markedly reduced, including total GH output as expressed by area under the curve (43 vs 368 units, ALL vs control). Not all individuals were very short but as a group they were significantly short when compared with their parental heights (15). This could explain the lack of catchup growth seen in these leukemic children in remission and off chemotherapy.

We speculated that disturbances in the neurosecretion in GH could result in a treatable cause for short stature not defined by the usual definitions of GH deficiency. To determine the GH secretory patterns, three groups were studied: GH deficiency, short children later defined as GH-ND and control children. GH-ND was defined as follows: height $<$ first percentile, GV $\leqslant$ 4 cm/yr or less, bone age $\geqslant$ 2 yr behind chronological age, normal findings from provocative GH testing (peak $\geqslant$ 10 ng/ml), low somatomedin-C level and abnormal 24 h secretory patterns (3). The results are summarized in the Table below:

GH SECRETORY DYNAMICS IN CHILDREN WITH GH DEFICIENCY, GH-ND AND CONTROL

Pt. Group	Peak GH after stim. tests (ng/ml)	Mean 24h GH curve (ng/ml)	GH area under curve (units)	Mean peak GH pulse amplitude (ng/ml)	#GH Pulses	Highest nocturnal pulse (ng/ml)
GH def.(n=16)	5.2 ± 0.7^{a}	1.6 ± 0.2^{a}	26 ± 6^{a}	5.4 ± 1.2^{a}	1.9 ± 0.5^{a}	9.0 ± 2.2^{a}
GH-ND(n=7)	20.6 ± 2.7^{d}	2.1 ± 0.3^{b}	42 ± 5^{b}	9.3 ± 1.2^{bc}	3.9 ± 0.6^{ce}	16.4 ± 2.0^{bd}
Control(n=22)	19.7 ± 3.7	5.5 ± 0.5	127 ± 14	17.0 ± 1.4	6.4 ± 0.3	33.4 ± 3.8

[a]GH-deficient vs control group, $P < 0.001$, [b]GH-ND vs control group, $P < 0.001$, [c]GH-ND vs GH deficient group, $p < 0.05$, [d]GH-ND vs GH deficient group, $p < 0.01$, [e]GH-ND vs control group, $p < 0.01$

In all categories quantitatively describing pulsatile GH secretion, there was a significant difference between GH deficient and GH-ND when compared to the control group. The mean values for the GH-ND group were intermediate between the GH deficient and control children. GH-ND children tended to preserve their nocturnal GH pulses although the amplitudes may be diminished. After exogenous hGH (mean dose, 0.07 U/kg), the GH-ND children more than doubled their linear GV as did GH-deficient children. One patient with GH-ND has been taken off exogenous hGH treatment and GV decelerated significantly.

These studies demonstrated that GH secretion did not increase during normal pubertal development (16), an observation now duplicated in monkeys (17). Not all peaks occurred during the first episode of Stage III and IV sleep; the maximum generally occurred at that time but it could have even occurred during the daytime. Even in classical GH deficiency as defined by blunted GH provocative testing there may be nocturnal GH peaks $\geqslant$ 10 ng/ml and even as high as 30 ng/ml (Fig.) (3,16).

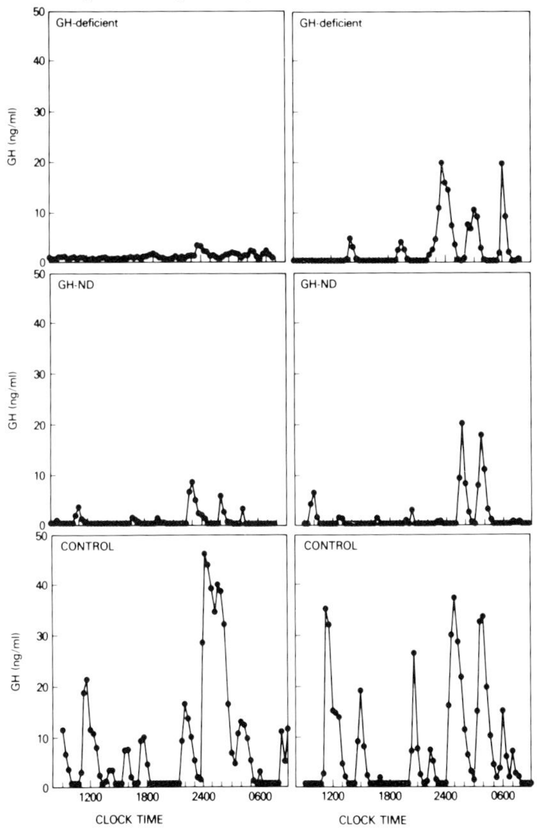

Fig. Representative 24 h GH secretory patterns in GH-deficient, GH-ND, and control children. All the patients are prepubertal except control in right lower panel (Tanner stage IV). (Ref. 3). JAMA 251:2223, 1984 (Copyright 1984, AMA)

The neuroregulation of GH secretion involves multiple neurohormones and neurotransmitters (adrenergic, dopaminergic, cholinergic, serotonergic, peptidergic). Disrupting any point in this axis could result in a decreased GH output. This is supported by the recent report of increased linear GV after dopamine agonists in children with classical GH deficiency (19). The etiologic lists showing causes for classical GH deficiency are lengthly and it is likely that there will be significant overlap with GH-ND. Permanent disruptions in neuroregulation of GH secretion could occur due to genetic influences, prenatal drug and environmental exposure. The developing CNS during perinatal life could still be vulnerable to hypoxia and birth trauma. Later in childhood, an example of an insult could be cranial irradiation. In the case of prenatal and perinatal insults, the biological expression of decreased GV and short stature may not be expressed until years later. There may also be an influence of total GH output on ultimate statural growth as suggested by increased GH secretion in tall girls (18). This could be superimposed on other genetic factors because at the other end of the scale we have demonstrated normal GH output in children who were short.

Conceptually, it is possible to conceive of overlapping circles of GH-ND, GH deficiency and normal children. The number of patients with GH-ND could exceed those with classical GH deficiency by several-fold. Further investigation is necessary to dissect the multiple etiologies of GH-ND and to better identify the spectrum of GH secretory abnormalities from absolute deficiency to a partial deficiency which must be separated from the continuum leading into normal.

REFERENCES

1. Martin JB (1978) Med Clin North Am 162:327
2. Root AW, Diamond F (1982) In: Kelley VC (ed) Practice of Pediatrics. Harper and Row, New York, pp 1-181
3. Spiliotis B, August G, Hung W, Sonis W, Mendelson W, Bercu BB (1984) JAMA 251:2223
4. Shalet SM, Beardwell CG, Morris-Jones PH, Pearson D (1976) Arch Dis Child 51:489
5. Richards GE, Wara WM, Grumbach MM, Kaplan SL, Sheline GE, Conte FA (1976) J Pediatr 89:553
6. Grunt JA, Enriquez AR (1972) Pediatr Res 6:664
7. Kowarski AA, Schneider J, Ben-Galim E, Weldon VV, Daughaday, WH (1978) J Clin Endocrinol Metab 47:461
8. Rudman D, Kutner MH, Goldsmith MA, Kenny J, Jennings H, Bain, RP (1980) J Clin Endocrinol Metab 51:1378
9. Lanes R, Plotnick LP, Spencer ME, Daughaday WH, Kowarski, AA (1980) J Clin Endocrinol Metab 50:485
10. Hayek A, Peake GT (1981) J Pediatr 99:868
11. Frazer TE, Gavin JR, Daughaday WH, Hillman RE, Weldon VV (1982) J Pediatr 101:12
12. Oliff A, Bode U, Bercu BB, DiChiro G, Graves V, Poplack DG (1979) Medical and Pediatric Oncology 7:141
13. Bode U, Oliff A, Bercu BB, DiChiro G, Glaubiger D, Poplack D. (1980) Am J Ped Hemat-Onc 2:21
14. Chrousos GP, Poplack D, Brown T, O'Neill D, Schwade JG, Bercu BB (1982) J Clin Endocrinol Metab 43:1135
15. Blatt J, Bercu BB, Gillin JC, Mendelson WB, Poplack D (1984) J Pediatr 104:182
16. Spiliotis BE, August G, Hung W, Bercu BB (1984) Ped Res 18:177A
17. Spiliotis BE, Root AW, Bercu BB (1984) 7th International Congress of Endocrinology, Quebec, Canada (Abstract)
18. Albertsson-Wikland K, Isaksson O, Rosberg S, Westphal O (1983) Acta Endocrinologica 103(suppl 256):72 (Abstract)
19. Huseman CA, Hassing JM (1984) J Clin Endocr Metab 58:419

Endocrinology
F. Labrie, L. Proulx, eds.

DISORDERS OF GROWTH HORMONE AND IGF SECRETION

THOMAS J. MERIMEE, M.D.

Professor of Medicine; Department of Medicine; Division of Endocrinology and Metabolism; University of Florida; Box J-226, JHMHC; Gainesville, FL 32610

INTRODUCTION

There are two growth factors in man highly dependent upon pituitary growth hormone (GH): Insulin-like growth factor I (IGF I) which is identical to somatomedin C, and IGF II, which does not correspond to any designated somatomedin (1,2). Both insulin-like growth factors are homologous to proinsulin, but differ from proinsulin in that they are noncovalently bound to one or more proteins of serum. The latter proteins probably restrict the action of IGF by altering its permeability through capillaries and by inhibiting subsequent access of IGF to membrane receptors (3).

There are specific receptors for both IGF I and IGF II, but tissues differ in the relative number of each; the stage of tissue maturity also varies the ratio of IGF I to IGF II receptors. IGF II receptors, for example, appear to predominate in tissues early in gestation, but IGF I receptors do so later in gestation and in the newborn and adult (4). (IGF II thus may be more important to growth and development in the fetus than in the adult.)

Defects in the action, circulation, and secretion of growth factors could occur at multiple sites, but for practical purposes can be considered either secondary to alterations in the secretion of pituitary GH or direct alterations in secretion of IGF.

I. ALTERATIONS OF IGF IN MAN (SECONDARY)

Changes in the serum concentration of IGF I and IGF II may be normal fluctuations or pathological changes due to deficient or excessive GH secretion.

IGF I concentrations in serum of less than 100 ng/ml (by immunoassay) probably occur in less than 1% of normal adults, but such values are quite common in children. 25-35% of children between the ages of 1 year and 6 years have IGF I values in this lower range, and up to 15% of older prepubital children have such values (5,6). Serum concentrations of IGF I increase during puberty and can simulate those seen in acromegaly (5,6).

Multiple metabolic states probably effect acutely both IGF I and IGF II and these conditions must be considered in determining whether a given value of IGF is abnormal. Fasting, for example, lowers IGF I and IGF II concentrations in serum to those commonly seen in hypopituitarism.

Abnormal secretion of GH (deficiency or excess) results in altered serum concentrations of IGF. In GH deficiency, GH receptor deficiency (Laron dwarfism) and panhypopituitarism serum concentrations of IGF I and IGF II are significantly depressed. In cases of excessive secretion of GH (acromegaly or gigantism) serum concentration of IGF I increases whereas IGF II remains in a normal range (5). There, thus, seems to be a difference in the dose response relationships of IGF I and IGF II to growth hormone (3).

II. PRIMARY DEFECTS OF IGF IN MAN

It appears that deficiency of IGF I can occur without a primary defect of GH secretion. It was initially thought that pygmy subjects from Africa had short stature as a result of insensitivity to IGF I or Somatomedin C. This assumption was based on the observation that although pygmy subjects had normal GH secretory responses to several stimuli, they resemble GH deficient patients in exhibiting insulinopenia after glucose ingestion and prolonged hypoglycemia after administration of insulin. Such abnormalities are common in the GH-deficient state. Somatomedin measured by bioassay was normal in pygmies. Furthermore GH treatment did not change, in this group, insulin secretion, nitrogen retention or calcium and phosphate balance.

The development of specific assays for IGF I and IGF II resolved the problem posed by these findings. Whereas IGF I levels in pygmies are low and in a hypopituitary range, IGF II levels in serum are normal. The IGF levels in pygmies are in contrast to subjects with an isolated deficiency of GH or ineffective GH receptors (Laron Dwarfs)-both of the latter groups have significantly depressed levels of both IGF I and IGF II in serum (7,8).

Figure one illustrates the effect of GH treatment on serum concentrations of IGF I and IGF II in pygmies and in subjects with GH deficiency. The ineffectiveness of GH in increasing IGF I to normal or above normal levels in pygmies, despite adequate dietary preparation is consistent with an isolated defect in secretion of IGF I.

Sporadic cases with an apparent deficiency of IGF I (two well documented) are reported also in Caucasian subjects (8). Table one summarizes the major GH and IGF data in groups thus far considered with growth retardation or dwarfism.

III. HYPOGLYCEMIA IN NONISLET CELL TUMORS: IGF

The syndrome of hypoglycemia with large nonislet cell tumors is well recognized. Megyesi using a radioreceptor assay reported that some patients with this syndrome had elevated serum concentrations of an insulin-like growth factor

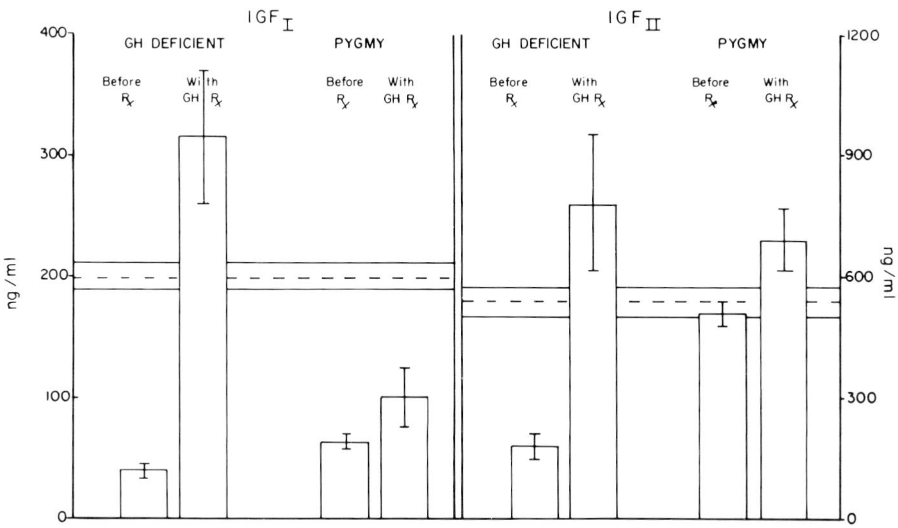

The effect of GH treatment (5 mg bid for 5 days) on IGF I and IGF II concentrations in serum. Note total absence of IGF I response to GH in the pygmy.

(9). Gordon et al reported also that 19 of 52 patients with hypoglycemia associated with an extrapancreatic tumor had elevated levels of IGF like material in plasma (10). The absence or presence of IGF tended to be consistent for a given tumor type. Two types of tumors were of special note: hemangiopericytomas were characterized by high values for IGF-like material in 6 of 7 tumors; all patients with lymphomas and hypoglycemia had normal levels of IGF. Although Daughaday has reported similar findings, there was not total agreement on samples assayed by both groups (11).

Zapf and Froesch reassayed 22 serums samples from patients with tumor-associated hypoglycemia using the radioreceptor assay first introduced by Megyesi plus the specific immunoassays for IGF I and II. They could not demonstrate increased serum levels of IGF. By immunoassay, IGF I and II tended to be decreased (12). In view of these discrepancies, the role of IGF in explaining tumor hypoglycemia remains unclear. Many investigators, however, would agree on the following:

(1) Only a minority of large tumors producing hypoglycemia have a detectable alteration of IGF (37% or 19 of 52 in series by Gordan).

(2) In the cases where IGF II is increased by receptor assay, its values may be low by immunoassay. This is compatible with production of an altered IGF II like substance (by immunoassay) that retains potency on the IGF II receptor.

TABLE 1

Summary of GH and IGF Data in Major Types of Endocrine Dwarfism

	GH	IGF I	IGF II	After GH IGF I	After GH IGF II	Metabolic Changes with GH Rx
GH-deficient subjects	absent	low	low	↑2-7 times	↑2-6 times	Yes
Laron Dwarf (absent or Defective GH receptors)	high	low	low	remains low	remains low	No
Pygmy (Hereditary)	normal	low	normal	remains low	↑15-20%	No
Pygmy Trait (Sporadic)	normal	low	normal	remains low	↑15-20%	No

BIBLIOGRAPHY

1. Rinderknecht, E., Humbel, R.E. 1978 The amino acid sequence of human insulin-like growth factor I and its structural homology with proinsulin. J. Biol. Chem. 253:2769.
2. Rinderknecht, E., Humbel, R.E. 1978. Primary structure of human insulin-like growth factor I. FEBS letters. 89:283.
3. Daughaday, W.H., Mariz, I.K., Blethen, S.L. 1980 Inhibition of access of bound somatomedin to membrane receptor and immunobinding of somatomedin in native and ethanol extracted serum. J. Clin. Endo. & Metab. 51:781.
4. Gavin, J.R., Trinedi, B., Mills, B. 1983 IGF II receptor characteristics in cultured muscle cells. Endocrine Soc. Program No. 179:395 (abs).
5. Zapf, J., Walter, H., Froesch, E.R. 1981 Radioimmunological determination of insulin-like growth factors I and II in normal subjects and in patients with growth disorders and extrapancreatic tumor hypoglycemia. J. Clin. Invest. 68:1321.
6. Luna, A., Wilson, D., Wibbelsman, C.J. Brown, R.C., Nagashima, J., Hintz, R., and Rosenfeld, R.G. 1983 Somatomedins in adolescence. J. Clin. Endo. & Metab. 57:268.
7. Merimee, T.J., Zapf, J., Froesch, E.R. 1981 Dwarfism in the pygmy: An isolated deficiency of IGF I. N. Engl. J. Med. 305:965.
8. Op Cite 1982 Insulin-like growth factors (IGFs) in pygmies and subjects with the pygmy trait: Characterization of the metabolic actions of IGF I and IGF II in man. J. Clin. Endo. & Metab. 55:1081.
9. Megyesi, K., Kahn, C.R., Roth, J., Gorden, P. 1974 Hypoglycemia in association with extrapancreatic tumors: Demonstration of elevated plasma. NSILA's by a new radioreceptor assay. J. Clin. Endocrinol. & Metab. 38:1974.
10. Gorden, P., Hendricks, C., Kahn, C.R., Megyesi, K., and Roth, J. 1981 Hypoglycemia associated with nonislet cell tumor and insulin-like growth factors. J. Clin. Endocrinol. & Metab. 1452.

11. Daughaday, W.H., Trivedi, B., and Kapidia, M. 1981 Measurement of insulin-like growth factor II by a specific radioreceptor assay in serum of normal individuals and patients with tumor-associated hypoglycemia. J. Clin. Endocrinol & Metab. 53:289.

12. Froesch, E.R., Zapf, J., and Widmer, V. 1982 Hypoglycemia associated with nonislet cell tumor and insulin-like growth factors. NEJM. (Letter) :1178.

39. Gastrointestinal Hormones

© 1984 Elsevier Science Publishers B.V.
Endocrinology
F. Labrie, L. Proulx, eds.

NEWER PEPTIDES OF THE GASTROINTESTINAL TRACT

JC BROWN, CHS McINTOSH, SC OTTE, RA PEDERSON, AMJ BUCHAN, S VINCENT

Departments of Physiology and Psychiatry, University of British Columbia, Vancouver, British Columbia, Canada V6T 1W5

INTRODUCTION

Isolation of peptides from the gastrointestinal tract presents unique problems, not the least of which is their sparcity in the source material. They either belong to the diffuse endocrine system being produced by cells of the gastrointestinal mucosa, which are relatively few in number or are present in fibres of the nervous system within the walls of the tract. Despite this problem Prof. V. Mutt of the Karolinska Institute has developed appropriate large scale extraction techniques. Almost all of the significant advances in gastrointestinal endocrinology can be attributed either directly or indirectly to the availability of this starting material. The eventual yield of an active substance after having been subjected to the necessary multiple fractionation procedures is minute. Three methods used in this laboratory, for the isolation of peptides from the Karolinska Institute starting material will be presented.

CLASSICAL PHYSIOLOGICAL APPROACH

The techniques employed in the isolation and characterization of peptides have undergone dramatic improvement since the discovery of secretin (1). The classical approach involved several well defined steps. These included, the recognition of a physiological event which in the case of secretin was stimulation of pancreatic secretion by HCl in the duodenum, exclusion of the involvement of reflexes involving the nervous system and the use of the well defined physiological phenomenon as a bioassay to monitor purification of the postulated chemical mediator. Appropriate tissue from which to isolate the postulated hormone was selected following physiological studies involving initiation of the response. This type of approach resulted in the isolation of six peptides from the mucosa of the gastrointestinal tract, secretin (1) gastrin (2), cholecystokinin-pancreozymin (CCK-PZN)(3), motilin (4), gastric inhibitory polypeptide (GIP)(5) and VIP (6).

The importance of extensive biological testing and development of a specific assay to be used to monitor purification of the peptide cannot be over-emphasized. There are two examples in the literature of peptides isolated using a bioassay for a specific biological activity which were each eventually shown to possess two distinctly different biological activities. Preparations of the hormone CCK were shown to possess pancreozymin activity and finally a single peptide with both physiological activities was isolated and characterized (7). The possible existence of other biologically active peptides in CCK-PZ containing preparations was indicated when it was recognized that purer preparations of CCK-PZ were less potent inhibitors of gastric acid secretion when comparable responses were obtained from the gall bladder (8). It was concluded that in the purification of CCK, an inhibitor of gastric acid secretion was removed. This hypothesis was pursued; a peptide with gastric inhibitory activity was isolated and the amino acid sequence reported (9,10). Rabinovitch and Dupre (11) had made similar observations on insulin release with CCK-PZ preparations. It was later shown that GIP could reproduce the insulin release response in man which had been demonstrated for CCK-PZ preparations (12). Glucose-dependent insulinotropic polypeptide was suggested as a second interpretation of the acronym GIP (13).

BIOCHEMICAL APPROACH

High performance liquid chromatography (HPLC) has become an important technique in the isolation of peptides. It now finds use in the final purification stages of many hormones and in establishing criteria of purity. When "purest" preparations of GIP were subjected to HPLC a constant minor component was observed (13). Sequence analysis of this minor component suggested that it was identical in structure to residues 3-42 of the major component (10). Side fractions obtained during the purification of GIP which by bioassay had been shown to contain CCK-like activity have been further purified on HPLC. The retention time of one of these peptides was shown to be different from CCK_8 CCK_{33} or CCK_{39}. It was therefore purified to an apparently homogeneous state on HPLC. Amino acid analyses have revealed the following composition: ASX(4), THR(1), SER(4), GLX(5), PRO(2-3), GLY(3), ALA(4), VAL(2), MET(1-2), ILE(2), LEU(4), TYR(2), PHE(1), HIS(1), LYS(4), ARG(3), TRP(?). The peptide referred to as peptide 'C' also produced powerful contractions of guinea pig ileal strips. Bioassay of HPLC fractions from the purification of peptide 'C' using the guinea pig ileum demonstrated that there were several active fractions in this preparation. Isolation problems have been significantly reduced and many peptides can be easily isolated from gastrointestinal tissue. The major problem remaining is that of determining the biological activity, if any. Partial sequence analysis can give rapid clues as to the significance of the peptide e.g. is it a degradation product of a non-biologically active protein or enzyme?

In the purification of peptide 'C' a major homogeneous fraction was obtained. Amino acid analysis showed that it was dissimilar to any of the known gastrointestinal peptides. A reasonable degree of testing revealed no biological activity. Analysis revealed that the N-terminus was blocked. Tryptic peptides were prepared and purified on HPLC. Sequence analysis of 2 of the tryptic peptides performed by Dr. J. Schilling, California Biotechnology Inc., Palo Alto revealed almost complete homology with the amino acid sequence of bovine heart cytochrome oxidase subunit VI. The peptide isolated from pig gastrointestinal mucosa was a fragment of this enzyme, and therefore highly unlikely to have a gastrointestinal regulatory function. The fact that g.i. peptides have been shown to occur as structurally related families of peptides may also offer clues as to possible functional roles for peptides which have been isolated without having a known activity.

IMMUNOLOGICAL APPROACH

GIP has been shown to be heterogeneous in tissues and plasma, using antisera raised in rabbits and guinea pigs. Little is known of the nature of these other forms. The ability to generate monoclonal antibodies, select from fusion products antibodies with high avidity, high affinity and region specificity has resulted in the development of immunoaffinity chromatography techniques, which have been applied to the isolation of immunoreactive forms (IR) of the hormone GIP. Three IR-forms have been obtained from an acetic acid extract of intestinal tissue using a monoclonal antibody to GIP, bound to sepharose CL-4B. The peptides were purified using HPLC. The amino acid composition of one of these has been shown to be: ASX(8), THR(3-4), SER(6), GLX(9), PRO(4), GLY(8), ALA(7), VAL(5), MET(2), ILE(2), LEU(6), TYR(1), PHE(2), HIS(2), LYS(6), ARG(3), TRP(+).

It is not possible to infer, from the preliminary data available, which if any of the peptides is a pro-form of GIP. The composition of the peptide reported here does not contain the amino acid composition of $GIP_{(1-42)}$. In particular the tyrosine and isoleucine content are too low. However within the sequence of this peptide it is expected that similarities with $GIP_{(1-42)}$ will be found, corresponding to the antigenic site.

CONCLUSION

Rapid advances in technology have resulted in identification and isolation of many new peptides from the gastrointestinal tract. Many of these have been isolated using HPLC and immunoaffinity purification, and have as yet no biological activity ascribed to them. Sequence analysis will provide clues to the investigator as to a possible physiological role for the peptide by comparison with sequences in known families of peptides. In addition sequence comparison will allow identification of non-biologically active peptides which may be degradation fragments of larger structural proteins.

Exquisitely specific monoclonal antibodies selected for high affinity and high avidity offer a powerful tool in peptide isolation. The rapid purification from fairly crude material of PRO-forms of hormones, "family" members with reasonable amino acid sequence homology and more exciting perhaps, the opportunity to obtain the human counterpart, become possible.

ACKNOWLEDGEMENTS

Supported by the Medical Research Council of Canada, the British Columbia Health Care Research Foundation, the Vancouver Foundation and the B.C. Division of the Canadian Diabetes Foundation. The invaluable support of Prov. V. Mutt of the Biochemistry Department II, Karolinska Institute, Stockholm, Sweden is gratefully acknowledged.

REFERENCES

1. Mutt V, Jorpes JE, Magnussoy S (1970) Eur J Biochem 15:513
2. Gregory RA, Tracy HJ (1964) Gut 5: 103
3. Mutt V, Jorpes JE (1968) Europ J Biochem 6: 156
4. Brown JC, Mutt V, Dryburgh JR (1971) Canad J Physiol Pharmacol (1971) 49:399
5. Brown JC, Pederson RA, Jorpes E, Mutt V (1969) Can J Physiol Pharmacol 47: 113
6. Said SI, Mutt V (1970) Science 169: 1217
7. Jorpes E, Mutt V, Toczko (1964) Acta Chem Scand 18: 2408
8. Brown JC, Pederson RA (1970) Scand J Gastroenterol 5: 537
9. Brown JC, Dryburgh JR (1971) Can J Biochem 49: 867
10. Jornvall H, Carlquist M, Kwauk S, Otte SC, McIntosh CHS, Brown JC, Mutt V (1981) FEBS Letters 123: 205
11. Rabinovitch A, Dupre J (1972) Clin Res 20: 945
12. Dupre J, Ross SA, Watson D, Brown JC (1973) J Clin Endocrinol Metab 37:826
13. Brown JC, Dahl M, Kwauk S, McIntosh CHS, Mueller M, Otte SC, Pederson RA (1981) In: Bloom SR, Polak JM (eds) Gut Hormones. Churchill Livingstone Edinburgh, pp 248-255

Endocrinology
F. Labrie, L. Proulx, eds.

REGULATION OF SECRETION OF GASTROINTESTINAL HORMONES

YUTAKA SEINO AND SHIGEO NISHI

Second Division, Department of Medicine, Kyoto University Faculty of Medicine, Shogoin Kawahara-cho, Sakyo-ku, Kyoto (Japan)

INTRODUCTION

Gastrointestinal (GI) hormone secretion is considered to be regulated by various factors such as nutrients, hormonal secretagogues, and neural activity. However, the details of the regulation of GI hormone secretion remain to be clarified. We have measured the effects of intraluminal, humoral, and vagal nerve factors on GI hormone secretion in man, dogs, and rats.

NUTRIENT REGULATION

Fasting state

In the interdigestive state, some peptides, e.g., pancreatic polypeptide (PP), motilin, and gastrin were found to be fluctuating intermittently in man and dogs. Plasma motilin increased in accordance with the cyclical interdigestive contractions of the GI tract in man (1) and dogs (2).

Intraluminal administration

In man, meal ingestion produced an abrupt rise in plasma gastrin, PP, gastric inhibitory polypeptide (GIP), and somatostatin, but suppressed motilin release. Oral glucose loading increased the release of plasma GIP, plasma PP significantly, and plasma gastrin slightly; whereas glucose ingestion suppressed plasma motilin levels. Meat-extract ingestion enhanced plasma PP, gastrin, and GIP secretion, but suppressed plasma motilin release. In dogs, intraduodenal glucose loading also increased plasma GIP and PP secretion, but suppressed plasma motilin levels. Following intraduodenal fat administration, plasma GIP and PP rose abruptly, but plasma motilin increased only 60 min after the fat loading. It has been reported that intraluminal nutrients such as glucose, protein, and fat stimulate fundic and pancreatic somatostatin release (3).

Intravenous administration

In man and dogs, intravenous glucose loading inhibited plasma PP and motilin release. Intravenous administration of amino acid stimulated plasma gastrin and PP secretion, but suppressed plasma motilin release. Following fat loading, the plasma PP level was reduced and plasma motilin tended to increase, but it was not statistically significant. No significant change in the plasma GIP secretion was observed after the administration of any nutrient. Using isolated rat pancreas perfusion we found that glucose and amino acid stimulate pancreatic but not gastric somatostatin secretion. According to Wasada et al. (4), fat infusion caused a significant rise in both pancreatic and gastric somatostatin secretion in dogs.

HORMONAL (GI PEPTIDES) REGULATION

The effects of various GI peptides on gastrin and gastric somatostatin release from the isolated perfused rat stomach were studied. As previously reported (3), after isolation of the stomach of fasted male Wistar rats weighing approximately 300g, and preperfusion with 4.6% dextran KRB buffer containing 5.5mM glucose, each peptide was infused into the gastric artery at a constant rate. Glucagon, secretin, and vasoactive intestinal polypeptide (VIP) evoked dose-dependent increases of somatostatin with a simultaneous dose-related decrease of gastrin release. As shown in Fig. 1, both gastrin releasing peptide (GRP) and bombesin

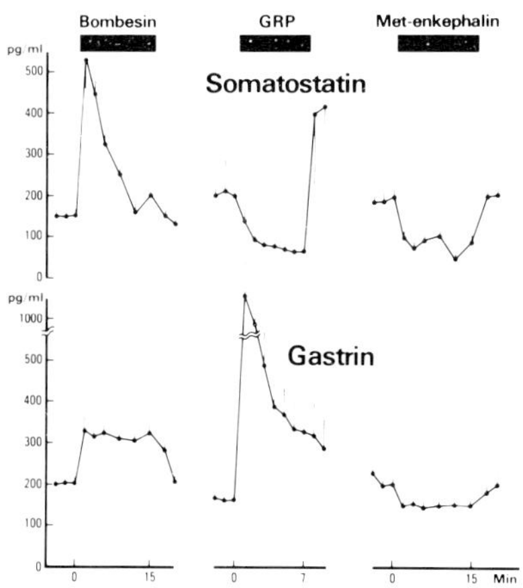

Fig. 1. Effect of bombesin, GRP, and met-enkephalin (10^{-7}M) on somatostatin and gastrin release from isolated perfused rat stomach.

stimulated gastrin secretion. However, GRP suppressed somatostatin secretion while bombesin caused a significant increase in somatostatin release. Methionine-enkephalin decreased both gastrin and somatostatin secretion.

NEURAL REGULATION

In order to elucidate the role of the vagus nerve in the regulation of gastric hormone secretion while excluding indirect effects via alterations of the circulatory or metabolic states, we have established a new *in vitro* isolated perfused rat stomach method which leaves the vagus nerves attached. Electrical stimulation of the distal end of the subdiaphragmatic vagal trunks was performed by square wave impulses (10Hz, 1ms duration, 10V). Using this procedure, the direct effect of electrical vagal stimulation on gastrin, GRP, and gastric somatostatin

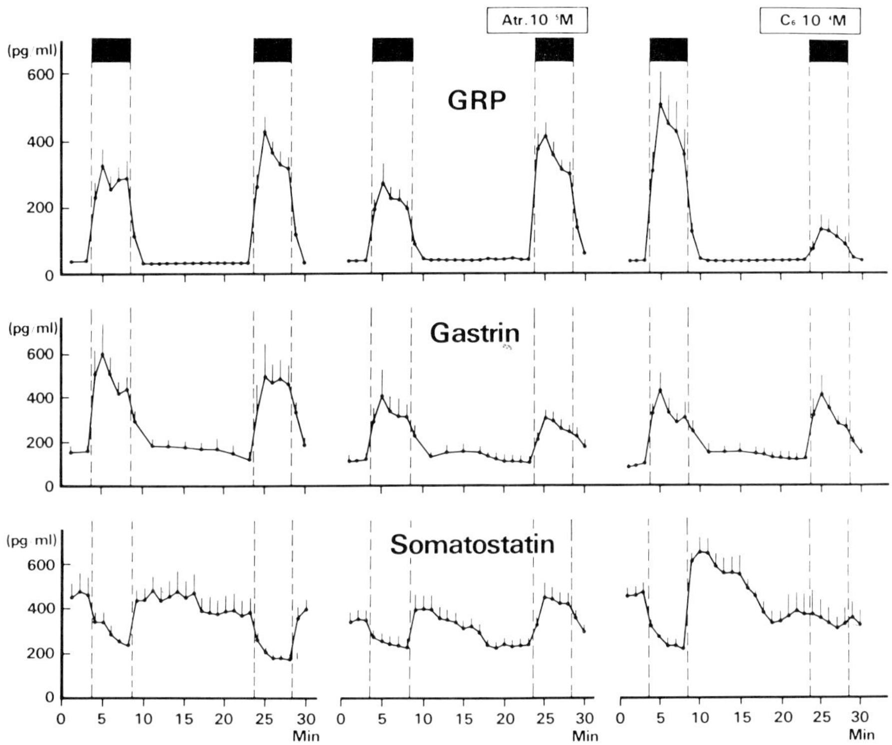

Fig. 2. Effect of the electrical vagal nerve stimulation (10Hz, 1ms, 10V) with or without atropine, with or without hexamethonium (C_6) on GRP, gastrin, and somatostatin release from isolated perfused rat stomach. Means ± S.E. are shown.

was studied. As shown in Fig. 2, vagal stimulation produced a significant rise in both GRP and gastrin, but decreased somatostatin in the perfusate. Atropine sulfate (10^{-5}M), a muscarinic blocker, augmented GRP release and reversed the decrease in somatostatin to a significant increase above basal level in response to vagal stimulation. However, the gastrin response to vagal stimulation was not affected by atropine. Hexamethonium bromide (10^{-4}M), a ganglionic blocker, suppressed both GRP and gastrin responses and completely blocked changes in somatostatin secretion induced by vagal stimulation. The infusion of naloxone (10^{-6}M), opiate-receptor antagonist, significantly reduced the basal somatostatin secretion, regardless of the presence of atropine or hexamethonium, but it did not affect either the basal GRP or gastrin secretion. The GRP, gastrin, and somatostatin responses to vagal stimulation was not changed by naloxone. In the presence of atropine, the secretion of these hormones induced by vagal stimulation was not affected significantly with naloxone infusion. On the other hand, when hexamethonium was infused, naloxone significantly reduced the GRP and gastrin responses to vagal stimulation, but did not affect the somatostatin release, which was blocked by hexamethonium.

DISCUSSION

The secretion of most of the GI hormones is regulated by nutritional stimuli coming through both intraluminal and intravenous routes. These GI peptides in turn influence the secretion of other peptides. The GIP secretion, however, is not influenced by nutrients or GI hormones, except somatostatin, via the intravenous route. Since peptides known to inhibit gastric acid secretion, such as secretin, glucagon, and VIP, cause parallel stimulation of somatostatin and inhibition of gastrin, the suppression of gastric acid by these hormones may be mediated by gastric somatostatin, probably in the local area of the antrum. Although GRP is considered to be mammalian bombesin, a discrepant result relating to gastric somatostatin secretion was observed. Recent study has shown the existence of GRP only in neurons of the mammalian stomach (6). Our findings suggest that intramural GRP neurons might play an important role in the regulation of gastrin as well as gastric somatostatin secretion, and that gastric somatostatin may be controlled not only by a cholinergic inhibitory neuron but also by a non-cholinergic, e.g., peptidergic, stimulatory neuron, both of which are under the control of preganglionic vagal fibers via nicotinic receptors. Furthermore, it is possible also that an enkephalinergic neuron may act on gastric somatostatin as a tonic stimulation, and that gastrin and GRP may, at least in part, be mediated by an enkephalinergic neuron through a hexamethonium-resistant pathway. In addition, we suggest different mechanisms of action for endogenous opiates and exogenous enkephalin, since both enkephalin and naloxone administration inhibit gastric somatostatin secretion. In conclusion, there seem to be many factors organized in a complex system which regulates the secretion of GI hormones.

REFERENCES

1. Imura H, Seino Y, Mori K, Itoh Z, Yanaihara N (1980) Endocrinol Jpn 27 (Suppl.):151-155
2. Itoh Z, Takeuchi S, Aizawa I, Mori K, Taminato T, Seino Y, Imura H, Yanaihara N (1978) Digest Dis Sci 23:929-935
3. Schusdziarra V, Unger RH (1981) In: Bloom SR, Polak JM (eds) Gut Hormones. Churchill Livingstone, Edinburg, pp 366-370
4. Wasada T, Howard B, Dobbs RE, Unger RH (1980) J Clin Invest 511-516
5. Chiba T, Seino Y, Goto Y, Kadowaki S, Taminato T, Abe H, Kato Y, Matsukura S, Nozawa M, Imura H (1978) Biochem Biophys Res Commun 82:731-737
6. Iwanaga T (1983) Biomedical Res 4:93-104

Endocrinology
F. Labrie, L. Proulx, eds.

RECEPTORS FOR SECRETIN, HELODERMIN, VIP (VASOACTIVE INTESTINAL PEPTIDE), PHI, AND GRF (GROWTH HORMONE RELEASING FACTOR) IN THE RAT PANCREAS

JEAN CHRISTOPHE, MAGALI WAELBROECK, JEAN-PAUL DEHAYE, JACQUES WINAND AND PATRICK ROBBERECHT
Department of Biochemistry, Medical School, Université Libre de Bruxelles, Boulevard of Waterloo 115, B-1000 Brussels (Belgium)

PRESENCE OF MORE THAN ONE CLASS OF RECEPTORS FOR SECRETIN AND VIP IN THE RAT PANCREAS

In dispersed rat pancreatic acini, secretin, VIP, and the parent peptides PHI and helodermin dose-dependently increase cyclic AMP to comparable high values in the presence of 0.5 mM IBMX (1-3, and see below). Besides, secretin is a secretagogue almost as efficacious as cholecystokinin (CCK-8) or carbamylcholine whereas VIP, PHI and helodermin provoke only a weak amylase release. Peptides of the secretin family are likely, therefore, to increase secretion via cyclic AMP but a fraction only of cyclic AMP pools may be concerned with the secretory process. In other terms, the efficacy of a given peptide in stimulus-secretion coupling might depend more on the type of ligand-receptor interaction involved than on the total amount of cyclic AMP produced. The functional receptors for this family of peptides, coupled to the adenylate cyclase system, are, indeed, heterogeneous. This heterogeneity will be illustrated by recent data from our laboratory on membranes and intact acini.

EXPERIMENTAL PROCEDURES

We use four methods to test the ability of secretin, VIP, and related peptides to interact with rat pancreatic receptors and the accompanying adenylate cyclase system (1-3):

1) The capacity of a peptide agonist to stimulate adenylate cyclase activity in pancreatic membranes, after receptor occupancy, is evaluated by: a) its intrinsic activity (= efficacy as related to a reference peptide), and b) the accompanying potency (Kact = EC_{50} = concentration required for half-maximal enzyme activation). When the peptide under consideration is a partial agonist with low intrinsic activity, this Kact value comes close to the affinity constant K_D ($S_{0.5}$) i.e the peptide concentration required to produce half-maximal inhibition of radioligand binding (see below) : the Kact value then reflects receptor occupancy (4).

2) The capacity of certain peptide antagonists to inhibit adenylate cyclase activation in pancreatic membranes allows to discriminate secretin-preferring and VIP- preferring receptors. For instance, the C-terminal secretin fragments

secretin-(4-27) and secretin-(7-27) hinder selectively the stimulatory effects exerted by secretin on adenylate cyclase. These inhibitory effects are exerted on both high- and low-affinity secretin receptors interacting with adenylate cyclase.

3) The intrinsic activity and Kact value of peptide agonists increasing cyclic AMP and stimulating amylase secretion is evaluated in dispersed rat pancreatic acini.

4) The app K_D ($S_{0.5}$) for peptides competing, at steady state, with ^{125}I-VIP and ^{125}I-helodermin for binding to pancreatic membranes or to intact acini. The two radioligands used are specific for, respectively, VIP-preferring and secretin-preferring receptors in the rat pancreas (see below).

IMPORTANCE OF DISULFIDE BONDS IN SECRETIN AND VIP RECEPTORS IN RAT PANCREATIC MEMBRANES

We documented previously the coexistence of high- and low-affinity secretin receptors and of low-affinity VIP receptors in rat pancreatic plasma membranes purified in the presence of 2-mercaptoethanol (1). We observed recently that an added class of receptors, with high-affinity for VIP, disappears during the preparation of these membranes (5). VIP and secretin receptors show, indeed, distinct susceptibilities towards 2-mercaptoethanol. High affinity VIP receptors are altered during pancreas homogeneization, at 5° C, in the presence of 5 mM 2-mercaptoethanol. By contrast, secretin responses are only altered by a harsher treatment e.g. when membranes, prepared in the absence of reducing agent, are exposed for 10 min at 25°C to dithiothreitol (DTT), a potent disulfide bond reagent. The importance of S-S bonds in secretin as well as in VIP responses is reflected by the fact that the same treatment with DTT does not alter the adenylate cyclase response to the hormone cholecystokinin (CCK-8) or to Gpp(NH)p and NaF (two agents acting on the guanine nucleotide regulatory site Ns). It can be inferred that the decreased responses to VIP and secretin correspond to alterations in their specific receptors. This is evident for VIP receptors tested with ^{125}I-VIP, after a preincubation with DTT : at low concentrations (1 - 2 mM) DTT reduces the number of VIP receptors; it also reduces the affinity of the remaining VIP receptors when tested at higher concentration.

SECRETIN-PREFERRING RECEPTORS

Structural requirements for secretin recognition (1)

Asp^3 is an important determinant as the neutralization of its negative charge (with Asn^3) or a simple chain elongation (to Glu^3) markedly reduces the biological activity of secretin. Increasing the hydrophobicity in position 4 by replacing Gly^4 with Ala^4 or D-Ala^4 also reduces the peptide potency. Finally, secretin-(2-27) and secretin-(3-27) exhibit very low (but still significant) potency with Kact 1000-fold and 3000-fold higher, respectively, than that of secretin (unpublished data). As stated above secretin-(4-27) is totally ineffective.

Helodermin, a peptide ligand specific for secretin-preferring receptors in rat pancreatic plasma membranes

Like secretin and VIP, helodermin, a newly isolated peptide (6) from the venom of Gila monster (Heloderma suspectum) is capable to stimulate cyclic AMP accumulation in rat pancreatic acini. Helodermin also stimulates adenylate cyclase activity in rat pancreatic membranes. These effects appear to be mediated through secretin-preferring receptors, being inhibited by secretin-(7-27), an antagonist specific for secretin receptors.

VIP-PREFERRING RECEPTORS

Importance of His^1 in VIP for VIP receptor recognition and adenylate cyclase activation.

The intrinsic activity and Kact of four VIP analogues, modified in the 1 position, both decrease in the following order (7) : VIP > ($Ac-His^1$)VIP > ($3-Me-His^1$)VIP = (Phe^1)VIP > ($D-His^1$)VIP. The position and integrity of the imidazole ring is, thus, important considering the weak efficacy and potency of the ($D-His^1$)VIP isomer, of the VIP analogue methylated on the 3-N position of the imidazole ring, and of the VIP analogue where His^1 is replaced by another aromatic group (phenylalanine). The free α-NH_2 group is also involved in adenylate cyclase activation as indicated by the low efficacy and potency of ($Ac-His^1$)VIP.

GRF can occupy VIP receptors in rat pancreatic plasma membranes. Discovery of a VIP antagonist : ($N-Ac-Tyr^1$, $D-Phe^2$)-GRF(1-29)-NH_2.

GRF exhibits considerable sequence homology with VIP, secretin, PHI, and helodermin. We compared recently (8) the stimulation of adenylate cyclase by VIP, GRF and 14 GRF(1-29)-NH_2 analogues (substituted in position 1 to 7) to the capacity of these peptides to inhibit ^{125}I-VIP binding in the same preparations of rat pancreatic plasma membranes (8). GRF(1-29)-NH_2 itself is a partial agonist as compared to VIP and secretin, with relatively low intrinsic activity on adenylate cyclase. This stimulatory effect could be due to the occupancy of either GRF- preferring receptors, secretin-preferring receptors or VIP-preferring receptors. Our data favor the third hypothesis as : 1) ($N-Ac-Tyr^1$, $D-Phe^2$)-GRF(1-29)-NH_2 inhibits both VIP- and GRF- stimulated adenylate cyclase with the same Ki (1 μM) while being unable to interfere with secretin stimulation, and 2) GRF analogues inhibit ^{125}I-VIP binding at concentrations similar to those activating adenylate cyclase.

The seven first amino acids of the N-terminal part of GRF contribute variously to the stimulation of adenylate cyclase stimulation that follows VIP receptor occupancy. An aromatic group in position 1 but not the phenolic function of Tyr^1 contribute to the activation process as Phe can replace Tyr^1. By contrast, a free α-NH_2 group (see all N-Ac-Tyr^1 derivatives) and the L-conformation of position 1 (see the effect of D-Tyr^1 replacing L-Tyr^1) are important for optimal intrinsic activity. The replacement of Ala^2 by D-Ala^2, in the native molecule as well as in the N-acetylated Tyr^1 derivative, increases the intrinsic activity. Other substitutions of Ala^2 in (N-Ac-Tyr^1)-GRF(1-29)-NH_2 by a bulkier amino acid may lead to a derivative having low (with D-Arg^2) or no intrinsic activity : (N-Ac-Tyr^1, D-Phe^2)GRF is, indeed, an interesting VIP antagonist (see above). The position of Asp^3 is also critical : (D-Asp^3)-GRF(1-29)-NH_2 presents only 22 % of the intrinsic activity of GRF. Replacement of Ala^4 by its D-isomer decreases the intrinsic activity, whereas its substitution by more hydrophobic phenylalanine increases the biological activity. Changes of Phe^6 for D-Phe^6 or pCl-Phe^6, and of Thr^7 for D-Thr^7 in the native peptide, and substitution of Phe^6 by Trp^6 in the N-Ac-Tyr^1 derivative give analogues with reduced intrinsic activity and affinity. These biological results fit adequately with Chou-Fasman structural predictions suggesting that, in the native peptide, there is no preferred conformation for residues 1 to 3 while residues 4 to 6 allow a beta sheet leading to a reverse turn between residues 6 and 10 (D.H. Coy, personnal communication).

N.B. : We tested (9), of course , the effects of the same 14 GRF analogues on adenylate cyclase activity in rat anterior pituitary homogenates. (N-Ac-Tyr^1)-GRF(1-29)-NH_2 is, this time, as potent and efficacious as the original peptide. The identity of the amino acid in position 2, in this N-acetylated derivative, is determining for enzyme activation : D-Phe^2 and D-Trp^2 derivatives act as partial agonist and the (N-Ac-Tyr^1, D-Arg^2) analogue is an efficient competitive antagonist of GRF(1-29)-NH_2. Using this antagonist, it is possible to demonstrate that, at variance with the situation prevailing in rat pancreatic membranes (8), GRF receptors and VIP receptors represent distinct entities in membranes from rat anterior pituitary, and may derive from different cell types.

SECRETIN-PREFERRING AND VIP-PREFERRING RECEPTORS IN INTACT RAT PANCREATIC ACINI. STIMULUS-SECRETION COUPLING.

Based on radioligand binding and stimulus-secretion coupling, it appears that dispersed rat pancreatic acini possess - like pancreatic membranes - functionally distinct classes of secretin-preferring and VIP-preferring receptors with each class being able to interact with secretin, VIP, PHI, and helodermin. These observations (J.P. Dehaye et al., in preparation) partially confirm those of Bissonnette et al. (10) and complete our data on pancreatic membranes (see above) :

a) Concerning secretin-preferring receptors, correlations between ^{125}I-helodermin binding, cyclic AMP levels (in the presence of IBMX), and amylase release are compatible with the existence of two subtypes. The occupancy of high affinity secretin receptors (K_D 20 nM) leads to a 3-fold increase in cyclic AMP (Kact at 8 nM) and to a 2-fold stimulation of amylase release (Kact at 4 nM). Low affinity secretin receptors, when occupied (K_D 0.3 μM) are responsible for further cyclic AMP elevation (Kact at 0.1 μM) and for most of the amylase released (a 4-fold increase over basal, Kact = 0.18 μM). Both high- and low affinity secretin preferring receptors bind ^{125}I-helodermin, have intermediate affinity for helodermin and VIP, and low affinity for PHI, secretin-(2-27), and secretin-(3-27).

(N.B. : an additional third subtype of receptors with very high affinity for secretin (Kact at 0.3 nN) induces, when occupied, a low (2-fold) elevation in cyclic AMP that is not accompanied by a secretory response. This accessory class may relate to the minority of centro-acinar cells present in acini and is not detected by ^{125}I-helodermin under our binding conditions.

b) Concerning VIP-preferring receptors, dose-response curves for ^{125}I-VIP binding inhibition and increased cyclic AMP levels are consistent with the presence of two classes of functional receptors for VIP (with K_D of 6 nM and 90 nM) whose occupancy produces, respectively, a doubling (Kact 3 nM) and a trebling (Kact 56 nM) in cyclic AMP levels. Both classes of VIP-preferring receptors show intermediate affinity for PHI, and low affinity for helodermin and secretin. A comparison with secretory curves suggests that only high-affinity VIP preferring receptors (Kact at 1 nM) are involved in modest amylase release (+ 30 %) while low affinity VIP preferring receptors remain functionally inefficient, based on this criterion. The high affinity VIP receptors are probably responsible for the synergistic action of VIP and cholecystokinin (CCK-8 : a secretatogue that increases Ca^{2+} movements) : when VIP is used simultaneously with CCK-8, the resulting amylase hypersecretion is greater than that obtained with one secretagogue only.

c) It appears that the concentrations of secretin and VIP required for half-maximal inhibition of, respectively, ^{125}I-helodermin and ^{125}I-VIP binding are 2-4 fold higher than those producing half-maximal increase in cyclic AMP levels and amylase release, suggesting spareness between receptor occupancy and changes in cyclic AMP and secretion.

TO CONCLUDE :

The functional heterogeneity of secretin and VIP receptors has been evaluated in plasma membranes and intact acini from the rat pancreas. Disulfide bonds play an important role in the functional integrity of VIP and secretin receptors. GRF binds specifically to VIP receptors in pancreatic membranes and (N-Ac-Tyr^1, D-Arg^2)GRF(1-29)-NH_2 acts as a competitive antagonist of VIP. Secretin-(4-27) and secretin-(7-27), 2 competitive secretin antagonists, are useful in discriminating secretin preferring and VIP preferring receptors. Helodermin, a peptide isolated from the venom of the lizard Gila monster, interacts specifically with secretin receptors. In dispersed acini, VIP preferring and secretin preferring receptors can be classified into subtypes when comparing dose-response curves for inhibiting radioligand binding and the concomitant increases in cyclic AMP levels and amylase secretion.

ACKNOWLEDGEMENTS:

This work was supported by a "Concerted Action" from the Ministère de la Politique Scientifique (Belgium), Grant 3.4504.81 from the Fonds de la Recherche Scientifique Médicale (Belgium) and Grant 5 ROI-AM 17010-7 from the National Institutes of Health (U.S.A.). We thank Dr. D.H. Coy (Tulane School of Medicine, New Orleans) for the generous gift of GRF and GRF analogs.

REFERENCES

1. Robberecht P, Waelbroeck M, Noyer M, Chatelain P, De Neef P, König W, Christophe J (1982) Digestion 23 : 201-210
2. Christophe J, Robberecht P (1982) In : Said SI (ed) Vasoactive Intestinal Peptide. Raven Press, New York, pp 235-252
3. Robberecht P, Chatelain P, Waelbroeck M, Christophe J (1982) In : Said SI (ed) Vasoactive Intestinal Peptide. Raven Press, New York, pp 323-332
4. Macfarlane DE (1982) Mol Pharmacol 22 : 580-588.
5. Robberecht P, Waelbroeck M, Camus JC, De Neef P, Christophe J (1984) Biochim Biophys Acta (in press).
6. Robberecht P, Waelbroeck M, Dehaye JP, Winand J, Vandermeers A, Vandermeers-Piret MC, Christophe J (1984) FEBS Lett 166: 277-282.
7. Robberecht P, Waelbroeck M, Camus JC, De Neef P, Coy D, Christophe J (1984) PEPTIDES (in press).
8. Waelbroeck M, Robberecht P, Coy DH, Camus JC, De Neef P, Christophe J (1984) Endocrinology (submitted).
9. Robberecht P, Coy DH, Waelbroeck M, De Neef P, Camus JC, Christophe J (1984) Endocrinology (submitted).
10. Bissonnette BM, Adachi H, Collen MJ, Jensen RT, Gardner JD (1982) Gastroenterology 82 : 1017.

Endocrinology
F. Labrie, L. Proulx, eds.

RELATIONSHIP BETWEEN GASTROINTESTINAL PEPTIDE PHYSIOLOGY AND CLINICAL SYNDROMES

ARTHUR SHULKES
Department of Surgery, University of Melbourne, Austin Hospital, Melbourne, Victoria, Australia 3084

The most common gastrointestinal problems are motility disorders (e.g. constipation, irritable bowel syndrome), secretory disorders (e.g. diarrhoea), peptic ulcer disease and so called psychosomatic problems. Gut hormones have potent effects on gastrointestinal secretion, motility and are probably neurotransmitters (1), but despite much research their clinical relevance remains debatable. The reasons for this current status and the prospects for the future are outlined below.

Research on gut peptides has passed through the classical secretory physiological era of Bayliss and Starling and the chemical era exemplified by Mutt and Gregory; currently we are in what Rehfeld has called the immunological era and are at the beginning of the genetic era (2). However, we still await the new era of physiology to assess the significance in health and disease of these peptides in profusion. The term 'gut hormones' is a double misnomer. The substances are not confined to the gut and not all are hormones. The term regulatory peptides has been coined because of their ubiquitous distribution and their presence in nerves and endocrine cells (3). However, the question remains what do they regulate and are there disturbances in the regulatory peptide systems which have clinical significance.

1. DISTRIBUTION

The peptides are present in nerves and endocrine cells and it is becoming increasingly apparent that "all peptides can be made everywhere" (4). Regulation of a body process can be mediated by interrelationships between several of these peptides acting as hormones and with the cholinergic, adrenergic and peptidergic nervous systems. A defect in one system can usually be compensated by another system. The first requirement in understanding the changes that occur in disease states is to determine how the peptide systems are organized and how they function physiologically.

The methods used include tissue extraction and chromatography followed by radioimmunoassay. This allows determination of abnormal levels or forms of a peptide. For instance, in patients with peptic ulcer is there a deficiency of gastric somatostatin or are the molecular forms of antral gastrin different?. The answer is no to both (5). Immunohistochemistry allows the distribution, cell type and projection of specific peptide-containing nerves to be determined.

There is a highly ordered arrangement unique to each peptide (6). A clinical example is Hirschsprung's Disease where the non-propulsive constricted segment contains less VIP and fewer VIP nerves (7). Other approaches include electron immunohistochemistry and this enables the specific granule containing the peptide to be identified (8). A new technique of hybridization histochemistry will enable the sites and rates of synthesis to be determined and thus to distinguish between disturbed synthesis and disturbed release and whether a particular cell is making the product (9).

2. MECHANISM OF ACTION

Many of the gut peptides do not act as endocrine hormones, but probably act locally either as paracrine or neurocrine agents. The co-existence in nerve terminals of gut peptides and classical transmitters is another possible control system and emphasizes the overlap of the endocrine system with the nervous system. The technique of interstitial fluid dialysis has been developed to measure paracrine and neurocrine secretions (10). Measurement of circulating levels is therefore physiologically meaningful in only a few instances and can be further compromised by the well known heterogeneity of gut peptides.

3. HETEROGENEITY: CLINICAL IMPLICATIONS

There are two major implications. Firstly, the form may not be detected by the assay. For instance, gel chromatography of plasma from a patient with peptic ulcer because of a gastrin producing tumour showed that no gastrin-17 (G-17) was present but only larger forms such as G-34 which is also biologically active. If the plasma was assayed using an antiserum which measured only G-17 the patient would have been misdiagnosed (Shulkes, Fletcher, Bladin & Hardy, unpublished observation). These G-17 specific assays are being used and Rehfeld has reported a similar case (11).

The second situation is where the form measured is not biologically active. We reported a patient with a neurotensin secreting tumour, but no biological effect could be ascribed to the 20-fold elevation in circulating NT (12). A partial explanation resides in the nature of the stored and secreted forms. High pressure liquid chromatography revealed that only N terminal (inactive) fragments were present in the tumour and plasma indicating abnormal biosynthesis and processing (12).

4. CLINICAL DISORDERS

These can be divided into primary where altered peptide secretion is the cause of the disease and secondary where altered peptide secretion is the result of the disease. Peptide secreting tumours are the only established example of primary excess peptide secretion being associated with a clinical syndrome. These include gastrinomas (peptic ulcer), VIPomas (secretory diarrhoea), somatostatinoma (diabetes, cholelithiasis), insulinoma (hypoglycaemia) and glucagonoma (dermatitis necroticans). No clinical symptoms have been established for several of the peptide products such as neurotensin and pancreatic polypeptide from pancreatic tumours and bombesin from tumours of the lung. New families of peptides are being detected by both chemical and recombinant DNA techniques. The PP/NPY/PYY and the VIP/PHI/PHM families are two examples which have immediate clinical significance. NPY normally found in adrenergic nerve fibres is elevated in the tumour and circulation of patients with phaeochromocytomas and may be of value in diagnosing these tumours (13). PHM is synthesized on the same gene as VIP and has similar stimulatory effects on intestinal secretion (14). The possibility emerges that in patients with secretory diarrhoea and normal VIP levels that PHM is the responsible agent. We cannot answer whether there is a primary role for gut peptides in duodenal ulcer disease. The potential is there: through gastrin hypersecretion, decreased secretion of acid inhibitory peptides, defective neutralization, and reduced mucosal integrity. Duodenal ulcer is a heterogenous disease and with our current state of knowledge and methodologies, it is not possible to prove or exclude the participation of gut peptides except for the uncommon gastrinoma (Zollinger-Ellison syndrome).

Many abnormalities of gut peptide secretion may be secondary to a gastrointestinal abnormality (e.g. coeliac disease, dumping). However, examination of the post prandial gut peptide profile can give information on the anatomical region of the disease and on the dynamic condition of the gut (5).

Other diseases are characterised by disturbances of the peptidergic nervous system such as Hirschsprung's or Chagas' disease (7). Whether other less gross propulsive disorders are a consequence of failure of peptidergic innervation remains to be determined. The involvement of regulatory peptides in brain diseases such as Alzheimer's Disease and schizophrenia or in obesity are other possibilities (15).

5. THERAPEUTIC USE

Several therapeutic uses of gut peptides have been proposed including somatostatin for controlling gastrointestinal haemorrhage or for suppressing the secretions of endocrine tumours (5); VIP to produce bronchodilation in asthmatics (16) or as a local vasodilator in patients suffering from penile erectile dysfunction (17).

6. PROSPECTS FOR THE FUTURE

The outstanding problem is to determine the role of the paracrine secretions. The "new" physiology technique of interstitial fluid dialysis should be of great value for measuring the secretion of locally acting substances. To determine where the peptides are being made, hybridization histochemistry and other tools of the genetic era should assist. Progress in the future will depend on development of agents which can selectively inhibit a peptide or alter its secretion or metabolism. Several such agents are now available allowing individual peptide function to be assessed and therapeutic intervention to be contemplated.

REFERENCES

1. Gregory RA (1982) Br Med Bull 38:219-220.
2. Rehfeld JF (1981) In: Bloom SR, Polak JM (eds) Gut Hormones. Churchill Livingstone, Edinburgh, pp 10-16.
3. Grossman MI (1981) In: Bloom SR, Polak JM (eds) Gut Hormones. Churchill Livingstone, Edinburgh, pp 17-22.
4. Niall HD (1982) Ann Rev Physiol 44:615-624.
5. Creutzfeldt W (1982) Scand J Gastroenterol 17 (Suppl 77):7-20.
6. Furness JB, Costa M (1982) Handb Exp Pharmacol 59:383-460.
7. Bishop AE, Polak JM, Bloom SR (1981) In: Bloom SR, Polak JM (eds) Gut Hormones. Churchill Livingstone, Edinburgh, pp 569-575.
8. Polak JM, Bloom SR (1982) Br Med Bull 38:303-307.
9. Hudson P, Penschow J, Shine J, Ryan G, Niall H, Coghlan J (1981) Endocrinology 108:353-356.
10. Bunnet NW, Walsh JH, Debas HT, Kauffman GL, Golanska EM (1983) Gastroenterology 85:1391-1398.
11. Rehfeld JF, Andersen BN, Petersen B (1983) Scand J Gastroenterol 18 (Suppl 82):19-24.
12. Shulkes A, Boden R, Cook I, Gallagher N, Furness JB (1984) J Clin Endocrinol Metab 58:41-48.
13. Adrian TE, Allen JM, Terenghi G, Bacarese-Hamilton AJ, Brown MJ, Polak JM, Bloom SR (1983) Lancet II:540-542.
14. Bloom SR, Christofides ND, Delamarter J, Buell G, Kawashima E, Polak JM (1983) Lancet II:1163-1165.
15. Edwardson JA, McDermott JR (1982) Br Med Bull 38:259-264.
16. Morice A, Unwin RJ, Sever PS (1983) Lancet II:1225-1227.
17. Ottesen B, Wagner G, Virag R, Fahrenkrug J (1984) Br Med J 288:9-11.

40. Comparative Aspects of Seasonality in Reproduction

Endocrinology
F. Labrie, L. Proulx, eds.

SEASONAL CHANGES OF GONADOTROPIC AND GONADAL FUNCTIONS IN THE FEMALE JAPANESE MONKEY

MASUMI NOZAKI AND KIYOSHI OSHIMA
Primate Research Institute, Kyoto University, Inuyama, Aichi 484 (Japan)

INTRODUCTION

Among macaques the Japanese monkey exhibits definite annual birth seasons, with breeding being precisely concentrated in a few months. In fact, conceptions in this monkey are restricted to the fall and winter months not only in the natural habitats (1) but also in controlled laboratory environments (2). Little is known, however, on the hormonal mechanisms underlying this seasonal breeding: seasonal changes of plasma levels of LH (3) and sex steroid hormones (4) in this animal have fragmentarily been reported, but information on the hormonal dynamics during the transition between the breeding and non-breeding seasons is almost completely lacking.

The present study was designed to examine seasonal changes of menstrual cycles and of basal serum LH, estrogen and progesterone levels with special reference to the transition periods.

MATERIALS AND METHODS

Ten female Japanese monkey (*Macaca fuscata fuscata*) with normal reproductive histories were used in this study. Six monkeys were individually housed in a controlled laboratory environment throughout the year. Another four monkeys were housed individually in the outdoor cages. Daily vaginal bleeding data and blood samples were collected for at least one year. Bioactive LH in serum was measured by means of radioreceptor assay (5), and LH value was expressed in terms of NIAMDD LER 907. Sex steroid hormones were measured using radioimmunoassay.

RESULTS

Three typical examples were shown in Figures 1 to 3.

Transition into the breeding season: Significant rise of the basal levels of serum LH from undetectable level initially occurred when approaching into the breeding season in late summer or fall (Figs. 1-3), which was one to two months prior to the first ovulation in the breeding season. Throughout this period, serum levels of estrogen and progesterone were low (Figs. 1-3).

Breeding season: The onset of breeding season was indicated by the rise of serum estrogen coinciding with preovulatory surge of LH, followed by progesterone elevations and menstrual bleeding (Figs. 1-2). Throughout the breeding season, fall through winter, the menstrual cycles was regularized at about one month intervals (Figs. 1-2). In this period, preovulatory surge of LH was observed 16 to 18 days prior to the onset of subsequent menstrual bleeding (Figs. 1-2). Estrogen rises in late follicular phases followed by progesterone elevations in luteal phases were also observed (Figs. 1-2).

Transition into the non-breeding season: During spring through early summer the incidence of menstrual cycles varied in individuals: some showed apparently regular cycles (Fig. 3), and another irregular. Accordingly, in most cases it was hard to tell by the incidence of vaginal bleeding when the complete cessation of the breed-

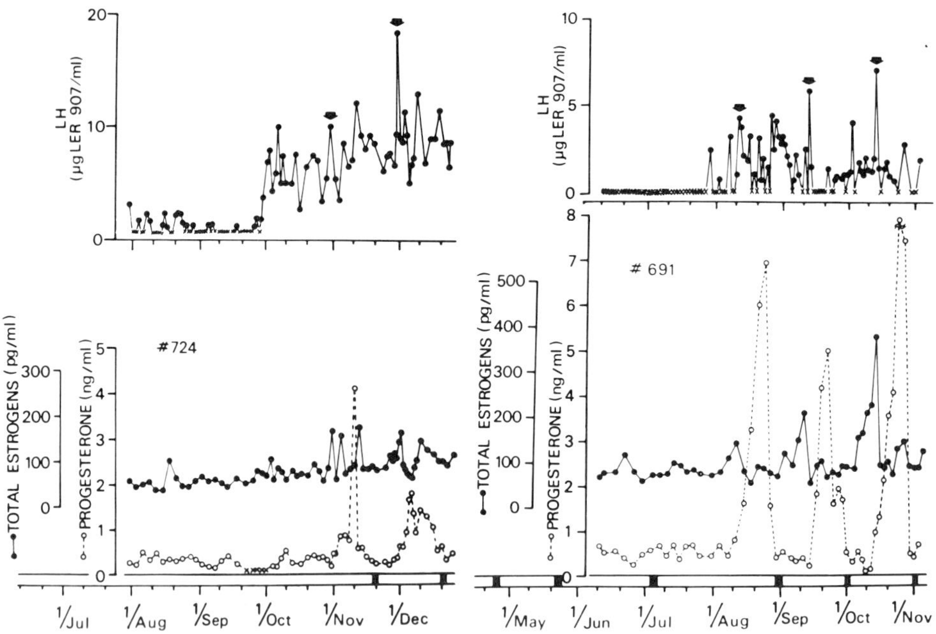

Fig. 1. (left) Serum LH, estrogen and progesterone levels and menstrual cycles in Monkey No. 724, which was housed in an outdoor cage. Black horizontal bars reflect the day of menses, and arrows in uppermost figure indicate the day of presumed ovulation. x, undetectable level of concentration.

Fig. 2. (right) Monkey No. 691, which was housed in an indoor cage. For legend, see Fig. 1.

ing season occurred. However, vaginal bleeding of outdoor groups tended to cease completely in late spring followed by continuation of no bleeding throughout the transition into the breeding season. On the other hand, in indoor groups irregular vaginal bleeding was generally observed throughout this period. In any cases, time span of serum LH, estrogen and progesterone differed greatly from those in breeding season. The most characteristic hormonal fluctuations occurred in early spring, just after the cessation of the breeding season: serum LH levels decreased to undetectable level for about 40 days (Fig. 3), and after mid-spring, subsequently serum LH levels increased and fluctuated in the range between the lowest level of the basal range in breeding season and undetectable level (Fig. 3). Throughout this period including early spring through early summer, regardless of regularity of menstrual cycles serum progesterone levels maintained in the basal range (Fig. 3), whereas serum estrogen levels were relatively high and fluctuated in the range between more than 300 pg/ml and 100 pg/ml (Fig. 3).

Non-breeding season: During mid-summer, the incidence of vaginal bleeding tended to cease in most animals and serum levels of estrogen and progesterone maintained in the basal ranges (Figs. 1-3).

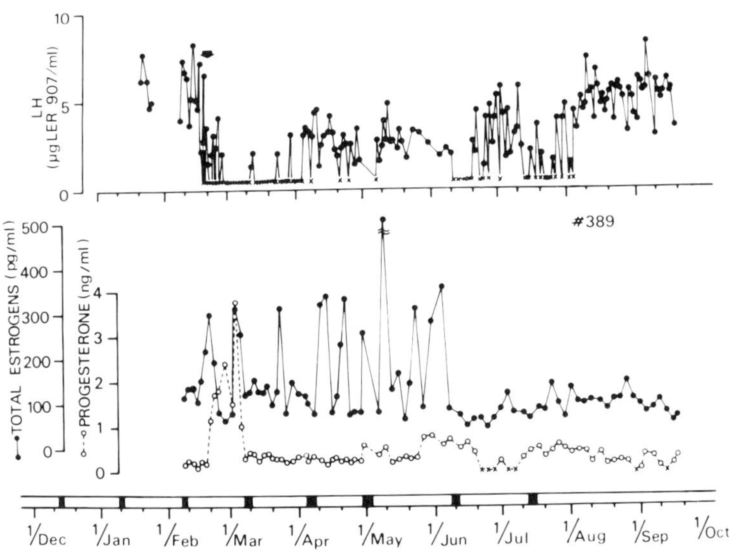

Fig. 3. Monkey No. 389, which was housed in an indoor cage. For legend, see Fig. 1.

However, in majority serum LH levels decreased to undetectable level for about one month (Figs. 1-3).

DISCUSSION

The present study has described clearly different neuroendocrine-ovarian relationships associated with the seasonal reproductive variation in female Japanese monkeys. During breeding season, the animals exhibit the cyclic endocrine patterns characteristic of ovulatory cycles. On the other hand, throughout the non-breeding season, anovulatory cycles persisted, which was characterized by low unvaring levels of serum progesterone.

During transition into the breeding season, serum LH levels began to increase one to two months before the first ovulation, as never been described in rhesus monkey (6), whereas serum LH levels completely dropped during the transition into the non-breeding season. Our data, thus describe the marked changes in serum LH levels always precede the initiation and cessation of the breeding season. This finding suggest the seasonal breeding in the Japanese monkeys is mediated througn the alternations in gonadotropin secretion.

After the cessation of breeding season, serum estrogen levels fluctuated in a wide range for about three months. Coinciding with this period, several anovulatory cycles occurred successively. These fluctuated profiles of estrogen during the transition may partly suggest development of some ovarian follicles after the cessation of breeding season, which never ovulated due to the lack of preovulatory surge of LH. Possibly positive feedback action of estrogen to brain-pituitary axis may be blocked during non-breeding season, as well as increased sensitivity of brain-pituitary axis to negative feedback action of estrogen.

REFERENCES

1. Kawai M, Azuma S, Yoshiba K (1967) Primates 8:35-74.
2. Nomura T, Ohsawa N (1976) In: Antikatzides Th, Erichsen S, Spiegel A (eds) The Laboratory Animal in the Study of Reproduction. Gustav Fisher Verlag, Stuttgart and New York, pp. 1-16.
3. Hayashi M, Oshima K, Yamaji T, Shimamoto K (1975) In: Kondo S, Kawai M, Ehara A (eds) Contemporary Primatology. Karger, Basel, pp. 152-157.
4. Aso T, Tominaga T, Oshima K, Matsubayashi K (1977) Endocrinology 100:745-750.
5. Nozaki M, Oshima K (1983) Jap J Med Sci Biol 36:237-244.
6. Walker ML, Wilson MK, Gordon TP (1984) Endocrinology 114:1074-1081.

Endocrinology
F. Labrie, L. Proulx, eds.

SEASONAL REPRODUCTION IN MARSUPIALS

M.B. RENFREE AND R.V. SHORT
Departments of Anatomy and Physiology, Monash University, Clayton, Victoria, 3168, Australia

Most marsupials are seasonal breeders, and their reproductive cycles are timed so that the young finally vacate the pouch at the most favourable time of the year. Photoperiod appears to be the primary cue in the regulation of this seasonal reproduction, but experiments designed to verify this have only been carried out in three species, the dasyurid *Sminthopsis crassicaudata* , the didelphid *Didelphis virginiana,* and the macropodid, *Macropus eugenii* (1). However, detailed investigations of the endocrine control mechanisms have only been carried out in the tammar wallaby, *M. eugenii* , a species now mainly restricted to offshore islands in the south and west of Australia.

In the tammar, births occur in the majority of females about one month after the summer solstice, with pouch emergence approximately 9 months later in late spring - early summer (1, 2). Females come into oestrus, are mated, and conceive within 24 hours of giving birth, so that they are normally pregnant for 364 days of the year. The new conceptus grows to a blastocyst of about 100 cells before entering a state of arrested development, or diapause, which lasts for 11 months. This is brought about initially by the sucking activity of the newborn pouch young, which inhibits luteal development, progesterone secretion, and hence endometrial activity and blastocyst growth (3). Removal of the pouch young before the winter solstice allows luteal reactivation and a resumption of embryonic development. This period is therefore referred to as lactational quiescence (2). However, if the pouch young is removed after the winter solstice, neither the corpus luteum nor the embryo reactivates until the summer solstice; this period is known as seasonal quiescence (Fig. 1). Follicular growth is suppressed during lactational and seasonal quiescence by the secretions of the dormant corpus luteum, since if it is removed, the animal will return to oestrus and ovulate. Thus the wallaby does not exhibit lactational or seasonal anoestrus like other marsupial and eutherian mammals, but rather lactational and seasonal luteal quiescence. The male wallaby is fertile at all times of the year, although the presence of oestrous females may stimulate testosterone secretion and hence prostatic development during the mating season (4).

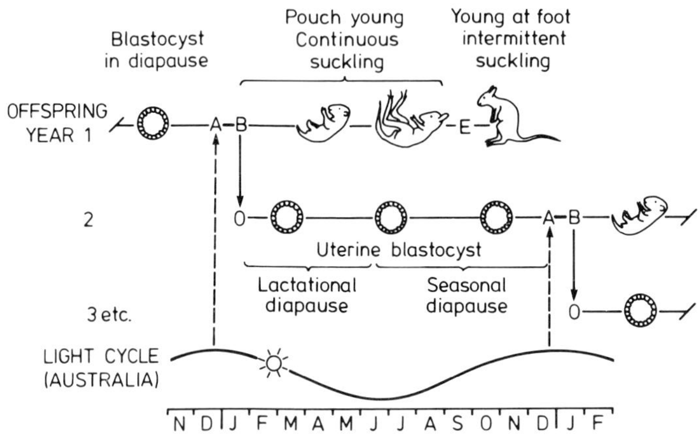

Fig. 1. The annual breeding cycle of the tammar wallaby, M. eugenii. Redrawn from (5).

During lactational quiescence, the corpus luteum is inhibited by prolactin (6); the luteal cells contain specific prolactin receptors (7), and luteal reactivation and a resumption of embryonic development occurs in response to bromocriptine treatment (8), or hypophysectomy (9), and can be prevented in hypophysectomised animals by the administration of prolactin (6). During seasonal quiescence, when the blood prolactin levels are highest (10), bromocriptine treatment will no longer cause luteal reactivation after the vernal equinox (8), although hypophysectomy is still effective (9), suggesting that photoperiod has some other as yet unexplained inhibitory effect.

Studies with animals exposed to artificial photoperiods have shown that a decrease in day length can bring about births 31-33 days later (11, 12, 13). The pineal gland appears to play a key role in mediating the effects of photoperiod on reproduction. Melatonin levels in plasma are elevated during the hours of darkness (Fig. 2), and there is a suggestion that there is a seasonal variation in the peak values (5). Denervation of the pineal by bilateral superior cervical ganglionectomy abolishes the nocturnal rise in melatonin, and allows animals to give birth during seasonal quiescence 27-28 days after removal of the pouch young (5).

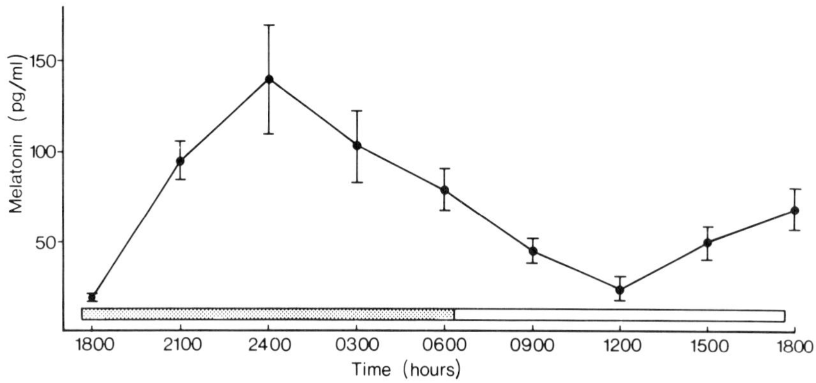

Fig. 2. Plasma melatonin concentration in intact female tammar wallabies in Perth, Western Australia, bled on August 26th, 1980. Each point represents the mean (± SEM) for 6 different animals. Shaded bar shows the duration of darkness on that date. Melatonin was measured by a specific radioimmunoassay (5).

We have further evidence that melatonin is indeed the pineal hormone that mediates the effects of photoperiod on reproduction. Tammars were given subcutaneous implants of melatonin which maintained physiological nocturnal concentrations of the hormone in plasma during the daytime (14). When non-lactating animals were implanted during seasonal quiescence, there was an almost immediate resumption of luteal activity and embryonic development, resulting in out-of-season births 25-29 days later, but when animals were implanted during lactational quiescence, there was no effect. The melatonin implants failed to depress the prolactin levels, supporting the suggestion that a fall in prolactin is not an essential requirement for the termination of seasonal quiescence (12).

It is clear from our investigations that melatonin removal by superior cervical ganglionectomy, or administration by implant, can block the animal's perception of changing photoperiod and hence eliminate seasonal quiescence. Neither of these procedures influences the duration of lactational quiescence, emphasising the basic difference in the underlying endocrine control mechanisms of lactational versus seasonal quiescence. Pituitary prolactin secretion appears to be the luteal inhibitor during lactation, but the nature of the inhibition during seasonal quiescence remains a mystery.

REFERENCES

1. Tyndale-Biscoe CH (1980) In: Cumming IA, Funder JW, Mendelsoln FAO (eds) Endocrinology 1980. Australian Academy Science, Canberra, Australia, pp 277-282
2. Tyndale-Biscoe CH, Hearn, JP, Renfree, MB (1974) J.Endocr. 63: 589-614.
3. Renfree MB (1981) Nature, Lond. 293: 100-101.
4. Catling PL, Sutherland RL (1980) J.Endocr. 86: 25-33.
5. Renfree MB, Lincoln DW, Almeida OFX, Short RV (1981) Nature 293: 138-139.
6. Tyndale-Biscoe CH, Hawkins J (1977) In: Calaby JH, Tyndale-Biscoe CH (eds) Reproduction and Evolution. Australian Academy Science, Canberra, Australia, pp 245-252.
7. Stewart F, Tyndale-Biscoe CH (1982) J.Endocr. 92: 63-72.
8. Tyndale-Biscoe CH, Hinds LA (1984) Gen.Comp.Endocr. 53: 58-68.
9. Hearn JP (1974) J.Reprod.Fert. 39: 235-241.
10. Hinds LA, Tyndale-Biscoe CH (1982) Biol.Reprod. 26: 391-398.
11. Sadlier RMFS, Tyndale-Biscoe CH (1977) Biol.Reprod. 16: 605-608.
12. Hinds LA, den Ottolander RC (1983) J.Reprod.Fert. 69: 631-639.
13. Hearn JP (1972) Aust.Mammalogy 1: 40-42.
14. Short RV, Brown AA, Mori Y, Renfree MB Unpublished observations.

Endocrinology
F. Labrie, L. Proulx, eds.

THE SEASONAL REPRODUCTIVE CYCLE OF THE RAINBOW TROUT

JOHN P. SUMPTER
Department of Applied Biology, Brunel University, Uxbridge, Middlesex, UB8 3PH, United Kingdom

INTRODUCTION

Rainbow trout are indigenous only to the Pacific coastal areas of North America, but have been introduced widely in the last hundred years, and self-sustained populations now exist in all continents except Antartica. Its present range extents from within the Arctic circle (66.6^{O}N) e.g. Alaska, Norway, down over the equator e.g. Kenya, to 55°S e.g. Argentina. The species lends itself well to domestication, which, together with the facts that it is a very popular sport fish and good eating, have led to it becoming an important farmed fish in places such as North America, Western Europe, and Japan. Selection has produced a large number of different strains, each of which breeds for a short period (on average six weeks) at a particular time each year. The range of spawning seasons extends over a nine month period, from August until April. Some strains appear unusual in that they have two distinct spawning periods each year; these will not be considered further.

THE REPRODUCTIVE CYCLE OF THE FEMALE

Differentiation of primordial germ cells into oogonia occurs at about 3 months of age. Soon afterwards the oogonia proliferate by mitosis, and some are then transformed into primary oocytes, a process that occurs throughout reproductive life. Development is then arrested at the early perinucleolus stage, by which time the oocytes have already increased in volume many thousand-fold. Rainbow trout produce a single batch of eggs each year, but spawn several times during their life. In their group synchronous ovaries at least two distinct populations of oocytes can be recognized at one time, one of primary oocytes and the other of synchronously developing secondary oocytes.

Females spawn for the first time in either their second or third year; those spawning in their second year tend to be the larger fish. In fish spawning for the first time as three-year olds, oocytes enter the secondary growth phase about I8 months prior to spawning. This phase consists of three distinct processes, namely (I) endogenous vitellogenesis, characterized by the appearance of yolk vesicles, which at one stage largely fill the cytoplasm; (2) uptake of lipid, forming oil droplets; and (3) exogenous vitellogenesis, involving the sequestration of hepatically-derived vitellogenin from the blood and its processing into the major yolk proteins lipovitellin and phosvitin, and possibly other minor components also. This latter process is responsible for further pronounced growth of oocytes, which attain a diameter of 5mm and volume approximately 250 x 10^6-fold greater than oogonia. These three processes constituting the secondary growth phase do not occur sequentially, but overlap, with endogenous vitellogenesis predominating initially and exogenous vitellogenesis finally. At the end of this phase the ovaries constitute 20% of the weight of the fish. Oocyte maturation follows, during which the germinal vesicle migrates to the periphery at the animal pole, the nuclear membrane disintegrates (often called germinal vesicle breakdown), and meiosis resumes. Ovulation of the mature eggs into the body cavity follows rapidly.

Very pronounced hormonal cycles are associated with the annual growth of the ovaries. Nothing is known about any possible changes in output of gonadotrophin - releasing factor from the hypothalamus that may accompany sexual maturation. The pituitary gland content of gonadotrophin increases steadily as maturation proceeds. Because it is not yet clear whether one, or more, gonadotrophins with distinct biological roles are present in trout (or any fish), the specificities of the existing gonadotrophin radioimmunoassays are unknown, leading to difficulties in interpretation of data obtained by their use, especially when blood gonadotrophin levels are being determined. The only statement that can be made with confidence is that the blood gonadotrophin level shows a peak around the time of ovulation. The situation regarding steroid hormones is clearer. During each reproductive cycle there are marked, regular changes in the levels of oestradiol-17β, oestrone and testosterone, peak concentrations being about 60, 30, and 300ng/ml, respectively; these very high concentrations are probably a consequence of the large ovaries. Levels of the two oestrogens rise concomitantly as the ovaries grow, to peak 2 months prior to ovulation. The testosterone level peaks later, a week before ovulation. Other steroids, such as glucuronides, are also present in appreciable amounts, their levels undergoing cyclical changes in association with ovarian development in much the same manner as the unconjugated steroids. Only the thecal layer can synthesize testosterone, which is then transported to the granulosa layer, where it is converted into oestradiol-17β. Both cell types require stimulation by gonadotrophin in order to produce their respective steroids. Although one function of these steroids, that of oestradiol (and possibly oestrone) in stimulating synthesis and secretion of vitellogenin by the liver, is well established, little else is known about their roles.

Exogenous vitellogenesis provides the majority of the mass of the eggs, and hence large quantities (upto hundreds of grams) of vitellogenin must be produced. Pituitary hormones, especially gonadotrophin, are thought to control this uptake, but details are unclear presently. The very low (ngs/ml) blood level in small

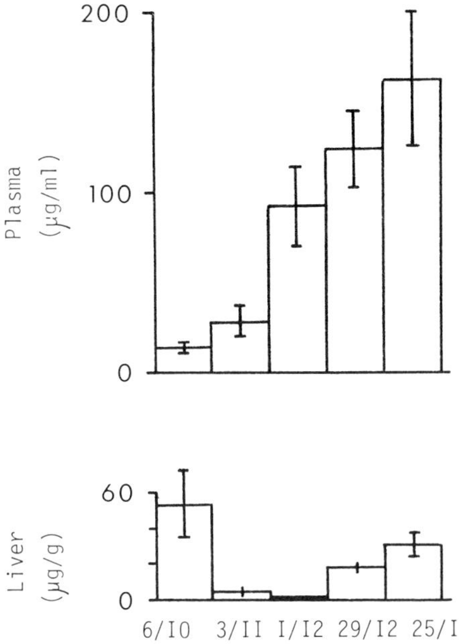

Fig. I. Vitellogenin levels in the plasma and liver of female rainbow trout when they are between I6 months (6/I0) and one year (25/I) prior to first spawning. Mean ± SEM; n = I0.

immature females rises approximately a million-fold, to tens of mgs/ml during the most intense period of exogenous vitellogenesis, when it is the major blood protein. This very marked increase is initiated considerably more than a year before first spawning (Fig. I), demonstrating that the endocrine changes underpinning the first reproductive cycle take more than a year to be completed.

Representatives of one other group of steroids, the progesterones, are found for a short time only at one specific stage of the reproductive cycle. As ovulation approaches first oestrogen, then testosterone, levels decline, to be replaced temporarily by I7α-hyroxyprogesterone and especially I7α-hydroxy-20β-dihydroprogesterone (I7α,20β-P). Within 4 days, beginning a week before ovulation, the level of I7α,20β-P rises from undetectable to 400ng/ml, and then declines after ovulation nearly as rapidly. This steroid is considered to be involved in oocyte maturation and/or ovulation.

THE REPRODUCTIVE CYCLE OF THE MALE

Males mature earlier than females, in either their first or second year. They can undergo regular annual reproductive cycles, but when mature are more susceptible to disease than females, so often die earlier. Spermatogenesis consists of a regular succession of stages which occur each year. The germ cells proliferate within cysts formed by the Sertoli cells. Primary spermatogonia are present throughout the year. Secondary spermatogonia proliferate from these stem cells by mitotic division, starting about nine months prior to the beginning of the period when milt can be stripped. The secondary spermatogonia transform into primary spermatocytes, which undergo meiosis to produce secondary spermatocytes. These in turn transform into spermatids, which undergo spermiogenesis into spermatozoa, when the cysts rupture, releasing them into the tubule lumens. At spawning the testes hydrate and the sperms are ejected into the sperm duct, a process called spermiation. Typically milt can be stripped from an individual strain of rainbow trout over a period of about 4 months. Spermatogenesis is accompanied by pronounced growth of the testes, which when fully developed comprise about I2% of body weight.

Pronounced hormone cycles accompany the annual testicular changes. Both pituitary and plasma gonadotrophin levels rise during sexual maturation, the plasma level peaking during spermiation; again, however, the technical and practical difficulties associated presently with the assay of gonadotrophin make interpretation of the data difficult. With the exception of stimulating steroidogenesis, the precise role of gonadotrophin in testicular development is unclear. The two major androgens in the blood of males are testosterone and II-ketotestosterone. The levels of both rise steadily as the testes grow, to reach peak values between I00 and I50ng/ml before the time when most milt can be stripped. The testosterone cycle may precede the II-ketotestosterone cycle by a month. Relatively little is known about the roles of these androgens. II-ketotestosterone appears to be involved in controlling development of secondary sexual characteristics, although these are not markedly developed in rainbow trout compared to other salmonid fishes. The function of testosterone in males is unknown; any hypothesis must take into account the fact that it is also a major steroid in the blood of females. It seems likely that these androgens regulate spermatogenesis in some manner, but substantiating data are lacking. Other androgens, such as IIβ-hydroxytestosterone, and a variety of glucuronides, are also present, their levels cycling annually in close synchrony with the quantitatively more important androgens. Some reports suggest that low levels of oestradiol are present in plasma of males. However, I have found either very low or undetectable levels of vitellogenin in plasma from males (ngs/ml), with no correlation between the stage of sexual maturation and the vitellogenin concentration. Because vitellogenin synthesis in trout is exquisitely sensitive to oestrogen, this would imply that oestradiol was not present in significant amounts in these males.

Low levels of I7α,20β-P (in comparison to those observed in females) are found in males. Again there is an annual cycle, with the highest levels being associated with the period when milt can be stripped. It is possible that this steroid affects the ionic composition of seminal plasma.

© 1984 Elsevier Science Publishers B.V.
Endocrinology
F. Labrie, L. Proulx, eds.

SEASONALITY OF REPRODUCTION IN A MOLLUSC: THE CENTRAL ROLE OF A NEUROENDOCRINE SYSTEM IN THE REPRODUCTION STRATEGY OF THE SNAIL *LYMNAEA STAGNALIS*

J. JOOSSE

Department of Biology, Vrije Universiteit, P.O. Box 7161, 1007 MC Amsterdam, (The Netherlands)

Among the invertebrates knowledge of the effects of seasonal factors on reproductive activity is most detailed in insects and molluscs. Like in all animals integration of information about environmental factors occurs in the central nervous system and is transmitted to (neuro-)endocrine centres involved in control of reproductive activity. The neuroendocrine centres of some snails have great advantages for experimental studies: neurones have giant size, are located peripherally under the transparant perineurium and can be identified individually. In this paper attention is focussed on the reproductive strategy of the freshwater snail *Lymnaea stagnalis*.

The natural habitat of *L. stagnalis* is in freshwater lakes and ditches. In natural conditions the snails hatch from July to September. When the shell height is about 20 mm the snails start egg laying, and in early autumn egg laying stops. Oogenesis continues at a low rate. In contrast, spermatogenesis is blocked at the meiotic stage at temperatures below 8 °C. Therefore, from November until the end of March no sperm is produced[1,2]. In June egg laying is resumed[3]. The snails die at an age of 12-14 months.

In the hermaphrodite gonad oocytes and sperm mature simultaneously, but in separate compartments of each acinus. At ovulation, oocytes (up to 200) are transported to the carrefour region of the spermoviduct where fertilization takes place. In the female duct each egg cell is packaged into an egg and these are fused to an egg mass. This whole procedure takes ca 2 h at 20 °C including fixation of the egg mass to a substrate[4]. - The snails copulate during the egg-laying season. Often a copulation is immediately followed by a reverse copulation. The greater part of sperm is digested in the bursa copulatrix. Transfer of sperm accelerates the onset of egg laying in juvenile snails[5], but decreases egg laying frequency in adult animals (Van Duivenboden, unpubl. res.).

ENDOCRINE CONTROL OF FEMALE REPRODUCTIVE ACTIVITY

Two hormones are known to be directly involved in control of female reproductive activity (see ref. 6 and 7). The endocrine Dorsal Bodies (DB) attached to the cerebral ganglia (Fig. 1) produce the Dorsal Body Hormone (DBH). This hormone stimulates vitellogenesis, and the cellular differentiation, growth and synthetic activity of the female accessory sex organs. The neuroendocrine Caudo-Dorsal Cells

(CDC) are located in the cerebral ganglia in two groups adjacent to the intercerebral commissure, which is the release site of their hormone (CDCH). This hormone induces ovulation, egg and egg mass formation and egg laying behaviour.

SEASONAL FACTORS

Based on laboratory experiments and field observations the following environmental factors appear to affect egg laying.

Temperature. Below about 12 °C egg laying does not occur in snails kept at a 12/12 LD cycle. At higher temperatures the rate of egg laying increases, with a maximum at about 22 °C.

Food availability. Starvation causes a stop of egg laying in 12/12 LD animals within 2-6 days. A considerable decrease in synthetic activity of the albumen gland, indicating a lowered DBH level, occurs within 24 h[8]. However, the reactivity to CDCH is maintained for several weeks, but absence of spontaneous egg laying means that there is a low CDC activity[9].

Photoperiod. A 16/8 LD photoperiod accelerates female sexual maturation and strongly stimulates egg laying. LD snails are more sensitive to injected CDCH and have a shorter refractory period. Together with the higher rate of egg production these differences indicate an increased release of DBH in 16/8 LD snails[4]. In studies on the interaction of the photoperiodic effects, low temperature and starvation, it appeared that LD snails maintained at 8 °C or starved during 3 weeks continued to produce egg masses, which became progressively smaller in size. Apparently, in LD snails the adverse conditions lead to a lower release of DBH, while the CDC retain their excitability. At 8/16 or 12/12 LD photoperiods both DB and CDC are inactivated. In terms of reproductive strategy this means that the snails have a dual strategy: during the reproductive season (16/8 LD photoperiod) adverse conditions lead to inactivation of the energy consuming synthetic activities in the reproductive system, which is important for survival of the individual snail, whereas the available ripe oocytes and egg mass material are released, which favours survival of the species. In this strategy the CDC system has a central role[11].

Field observations have shown that spontaneous egg laying occurs exclusively during the 16/8 LD photoperiod and at water temperatures above 12 °C in summer. During the egg laying season the snails showed nearly a 100% egg-laying response to injected CDCH (Fig. 2). During about 2 months before and after this season reactivity to CDCH started to increase and decrease, respectively. In late autumn, winter and early spring field specimens are unable to react to injected CDCH. Most probably CDCH reactivity is induced by DBH. There is evidence that it is the quantity of assimilated food that triggers the onset of the egg-laying season. Its termination very likely is determined by a synergistic action of environmental factors[3].

MICROHABITAT SELECTION FOR EGG MASS DEPOSITION

The habitat of *L. stagnalis* is highly heterogeneous. The superficial water layers are supersaturated with O_2 when the sun shines on floating plants. At the bottom there is anoxia. Temperature shows a steep gradient in the day time during the reproductive season. Egg masses are deposited nearly exclusively on solid substrates (plant leaves) in regions where maximum temperature and oxygen levels occur. For selection of this microhabitat the CDC system again plays a crucial role. In the laboratory a change from dirty to clean water of snails kept at 20 °C and 16/8 LD conditions induces CDC activity within 5-10 min and egg mass deposition after 2 h in over 90% of the snails[12]. The role of a number of component factors of this highly effective water-change stimulus has been studied[12]. Elevated O_2-content of the water, a clean jar and clean water all have a positive effect on egg laying. Clean water is the most effective factor. High O_2-content is slightly less effective, but in dirty water a sudden elevation of O_2-content still induces oviposition in about 80% of the snails. Obviously the CDC system responds to a number of environmental factors. These factors are equal to those ensuring a successful embryonic development in the egg mass.

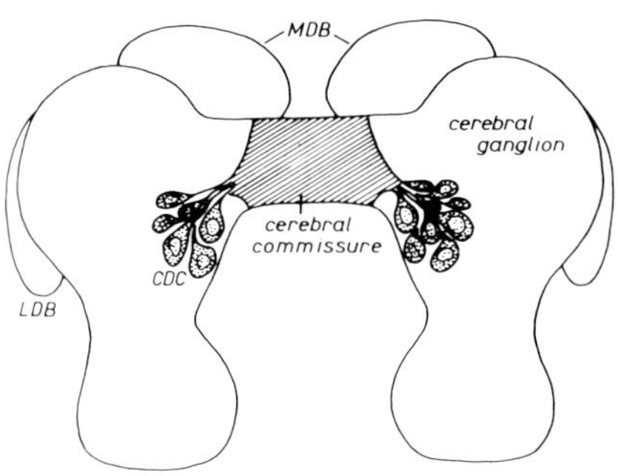

Fig. 1. Cross section through the cerebral ganglia with the position of the Medio- and Latero-Dorsal Bodies (MDB) and the Caudo-Dorsal Cells (CDC).

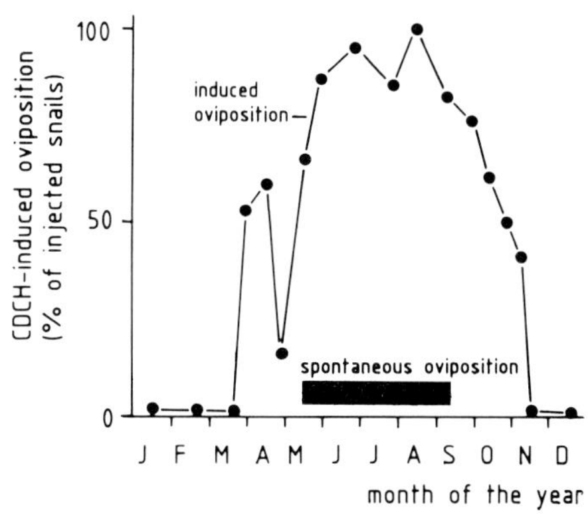

Fig. 2. Annual cycle of spontaneous and CDCH-induced oviposition (see ref. 3).

EGG LAYING BEHAVIOUR

An important question is how the snail is prevented from leaving the favourable microhabitat after its selection during the 2-3 h period of egg mass formation. The egg-laying behaviour presents the solution for this problem. CDC activity means that all cells start to fire synchronously (discharge) for ca 50 min[13]. CDCH is released and reaches a peak concentration in the blood after 1 h. Almost simultaneous with the start of the discharge, locomotion of the snail stops[14]. After about 25 min the snail starts turning around and cleans the substrate with eating movements during about 95 min and this is followed by oviposition. The resting phase keeps the animal at the selected place during preparation of the egg mass and the cleaning movements ensure a good fixation of the egg mass to the substrate.

CDCH has been characterised as a large basic peptide with a MW 4800 and a p_I of ca 9.3[15]. However, together with this peptide at least 3 other peptides are released[16]. Most probably these co-peptides modulate motor-neurons in the central nervous system involved in egg-laying behaviour.

REFERENCES

1. Joosse J (1964) Arch Néerl Zool 15:1-103
2. Joosse J, Veld CJ (1972) Gen Comp Endocrinol 18:599-600
3. Dogterom GE, Thijssen R, Van Loenhout H (1984) Gen Comp Endocrinol (in press)
4. Dogterom GE, Bohlken S, Joosse J (1983) Gen Comp Endocrinol 49:255-260
5. Van Duivenboden YA (1983) Int J Invert Reprod 6:249-257
6. Joosse J, Geraerts WPM (1983) In: Wilbur KM, Saleuddin ASM (eds) The Mollusca Vol 4(1) Physiology. Academic Press, New York, pp 317-406
7. Geraerts WPM, Joosse J (1984) In: Wilbur KM (ed) The Mollusca Vol 7 Reproduction. Academic Press, New York, pp 141-207
8. Van Elk R, Joosse J (1981) Comp Biochem Physiol 70B:45-52
9. Dogterom GE et al. (1984) Gen Comp Endocrinol (in press)
10. Bohlken S, Joosse J (1982) Int J Invert Reprod 4:213-222
11. Joosse J (1984) In: Photoperiodic regulation of insect and molluscan hormones. CIBA Symp 104. Pitman, London, pp 204-220
12. Ter Maat A, Lodder JC, Wilbrink M (1983) Int J Invert Reprod 6:239-247
13. Roubos EW (1984) Int Rev Cytol 89:295-346
14. Goldschmeding JT, Wilbrink M, Ter Maat A (1983) In: Lever J, Boer HH (eds) Molluscan Neuro-endocrinology. North-Holland Publ Co, Amsterdam, pp 251-256
15. Geraerts WPM et al. (1983) Gen Comp Endocrinol 51:471-476
16. Geraerts WPM, Tensen CP, Hogenes ThM (1983) Neurosc Letters 41:151-155

41. Regulation of Ovarian Function

© 1984 Elsevier Science Publishers B.V.
Endocrinology
F. Labrie, L. Proulx, eds.

THE ENDOCRINE CONTROL OF LACTATIONAL INFERTILITY IN WOMEN

ALAN S. McNEILLY
MRC Reproductive Biology Unit, Centre for Reproductive Biology,
37 Chalmers Street, Edinburgh EH3 9EW Scotland

INTRODUCTION

While epidemiological studies clearly show that breast feeding is associated with a delay in the resumption of normal ovarian activity and fertility post partum, this period shows considerable within individual and between population variation. Because of this and the occurrence of pregnancies during the period of lactational amenorrhoea, breast feeding has gained an unfair reputation as an unreliable period of infertility. In order to optimize the opportunity of using the natural contraceptive effects of breast feeding it is necessary to first understand the physiological and endocrinological changes during lactational amenorrhoea and during the period when ovarian activity and ovulatory cycles resume. Relatively few studies have been directed towards answering these questions and many have been cross sectional in design. While these studies have provided some insight into the overall changes in gonadotrophin, ovarian steroids and prolactin, it is not possible from such studies to understand the sequence of events which leads to the termination of the period of lactational infertility and the resumption of ovulatory cycles which have the potential to carry a pregnancy if conception occurred. Recently we have undertaken a series of longitudinal studies in breast feeding women in whom the changes in gonadotrophins, urinary steroids, prolactin and suckling activity have been recorded in detail.

ENDOCRINE CHANGES IN LACTATIONAL AMENORRHOEA.

In non-breast feeding women plasma levels of both LH and FSH recover from the suppressive effects of pregnancy by 30 days postpartum (1) and ovulatory cycles resume within 42 to 84 days postpartum. The majority of first cycles have inadequate corpus luteum function (2,3) associated with a reduced preovulatory surge of LH (3). Normal ovulatory cycles occur between 70 and 120 days postpartum.

In contrast breast feeding results in a significant suppression of follicular development assessed both by urinary excretion and plasma levels of both oestrogens and pregnanediol/progesterone (3) and by ovarian ultrasound (4) the duration of which is dependent on the strength of the suckling stimulus (5). While plasma levels of FSH return to normal within 30 days postpartum, LH levels remain at the lower limit of normal throughout the period of ovarian inactivity (6). Pulsatile secretion of LH is suppressed over 70% of the time but pulsatile secretion equivalent to that seen in the follicular phase of the menstrual cycle is observed in the remaining 30% (7) This is associated with an increase in oestrogen secretion suggesting the initiation of follicle development although oestrogens remain below the levels seen from day 10 onwards in the normal menstrual cycle. Suckling causes significant increases in prolactin during this period with significantly more prolactin release in the afternoon than morning (8). While suckling is maintained above 5 feeds and a total of 65 min (10 min/ feed) per day, follicle development is not sustained even though pulsatile LH secretion may occur (9). Breast feeding women are more sensitive to the negative feedback effects of oestrogen (10) and the amplitude of LH pulses are inappropriately low considering the low levels of endogenous oestrogen suggesting reduced hypothalamic capacity to release GnRH. Thus suckling appears to suppress the ability of the hypothalamus to sustain pulsatile secretion of GnRH and thus LH such that, when follicle development occurs in response to limited pulsatile LH secretion, the small increase in oestrogen is sufficient to switch off further GnRH secretion with resultant cessation of follicle growth.

RESUMPTION OF SUSTAINED FOLLICLE GROWTH AND OVULATION

At some stage during lactational amenorrhoea follicle growth occurs and is sustained. This is associated with a decline in the suckling stimulus with concomittent decline in prolactin (11). However, no specific changes in FSH or pulsatile secretion of LH appear to occur (7). If suckling declines rapidly then ovulation resumes although the frequency of ovulation preceeding first menstruation in breast feeding mothers varies considerably in different populations, probably depending on the different suckling patterns of these populations (12).

Even though ovulation does resume, the majority (70%) of menstrual cycles have inadequate corpus luteum (CL) function (2). The continuation of suckling and the associated marginal hyperprolactinaemia appears to prolong the occurrence of inadequate CL. Plasma FSH levels are within normal menstrual cycle range. However, basal plasma levels of LH appear to be marginally lower than normal although pulse frequency is within normal limits (6,7). Corpus luteum function improves with successive menstrual cycles as suckling declines until normal luteal function occurs. This improvement in luteal function is associated with an increase in the amount of LH released over the preovulatory and immediately postovulatory phase (13). In contrast there is little significant change in preovulatory oestrogen output suggesting normal follicular development.

The number of cycles with inadequate CL function is greater if suckling, in particular night time feeds are maintained (2,12). Since the preovulatory surge of LH in the majority of women is initiated at night (14) it is possible that the alteration in hypothalamic activity induced by night time suckling may directly affect the generation of the normal preovulatory LH surge to reduce the amount of LH released over this period. The changes within the hypothalamus remain unknown.

CONCLUSIONS

It appears that absence of a normal pulsatile pattern of LH secretion is responsible for the failure of follicle development in lactational amenorrhoea. The infrequent occurrence (30% of time) of pulsatile LH secretion initiates follicular oestrogen secretion which appears to switch off further LH release and follicular development ceases.

When suckling declines, LH secretion, if initiated, can now be sustained and follicular growth equivalent to normal menstrual cycles resumes. However, the majority of ovulations (70%) result in inadequate corpus luteum function, in particular if suckling is maintained. This inadequate CL function is related to reduced preovulatory/postovulatory release of LH but no apparent deficiency in FSH. Whether prolactin *per se* is involved in the reduced LH secretion or in affecting ovarian activity directly remains unclear (15,16).

ACKNOWLEDGEMENTS

These results summarize studies carried out with my colleagues Professor Peter Howie and Drs. Anna Glasier and Mary Houston.

REFERENCES

1. Howie PW, McNeilly AS, Houston MJ, Cook A, Boyle H (1982) Clin Endocr 17: 323-332.
2. McNeilly AS, Howie PW, Houston MJ, Cook A, Boyle H (1982) Clin Endocr 17: 609-616.
3. Poindexter AN, Ritter MB, Besch PK (1983) Fertil Steril 39: 494-498.
4. Glasier A, McNeilly AS, Baird DT (1984) Clin Endocr In press.

5. Howie PW, McNeilly AS, Houston MJ, Cook A, Boyle H (1982) Clin Endocr 17: 315-322

6. Glasier A, McNeilly AS, Howie PW (1983) Clin Endocr 19: 493-502

7. Glasier A, McNeilly AS, Howie PW (1984) Clin Endocr

8. Glasier A, McNeilly AS, Howie PW (1984) Clin Endocr In Press.

9. McNeilly, AS, Glasier AF, Howie PW, Houston MJ, Cook A, Boyle H (1983) Clin Endocr 19: 167-174.

10. Baird DT, McNeilly AS, Sawers RS, Sharpe RM (1979) J Clin Endocr Metab 49: 500-506

11. Howie PW, McNeilly AS, Houston MH, Cook A, Boyle H (1981) Br Med J 283: 757-759.

12. Howie PW, McNeilly AS (1982) J Reprod Fert 65: 545-557.

13. Glasier AF (1983) M D Thesis, University of Bristol.

14. Djahanbakhch O, McNeilly AS, Warner PM, Swanston IA, Baird DT (1984) Clin Endocr 20: 463-472.

15. McNeilly AS, Glasier A, Jonassen J, Howie PW (1982) J Reprod Fert 65: 559-569.

16. McNeilly AS (1984) In: Muller EE, MacLeod RM (eds) Neuroendocrine Perspectives volume 3. Elsevier Science Publishers, Amsterdam, pp. 279-316.

Endocrinology
F. Labrie, L. Proulx, eds.

GRANULOSA CELL-THECA CELL INTERACTIONS DURING FOLLICULAR DEVELOPMENT

J.H. DORRINGTON, H. McKERACHER, G. GARZO AND M.K. SKINNER
Banting and Best Department of Medical Research,
University of Toronto, Ontario, Canada, M5G 1L6

INTRODUCTION

In the structuring of a tissue, cells communicate to promote morphogenesis and cytodifferentiation. Cell-cell interaction can occur in a number of different ways; 1) through gap junctions formed between adjacent cells, 2) the production of cell adhesion molecules (CAM), 3) the formation of extracellular matrix (ECM) components or 4) by the secretion and transport of specific factors to neighboring cells (Fig.1). The type of cell-cell interaction which can occur in the formation of a functional unit is exemplified by the influence of mesenchymal cells on epithelial morphogenesis and differentiation (eg. uterus, prostate, mammary gland) (1).

We propose that the preovulatory follicle completes its development program as a result of similar interactions between thecal cells of mesenchymal origin and granulosa cells of epithelial origin. Since thecal cells and granulosa cells are not directly in contact they are unable to communicate through gap junctions and cell adhesion molecules. We have pursued the concept, therefore, that secreted factors such as steroids, peptides, proteins and components of extracellular matrix may be the essential local modulators of follicular development. This hypothesis is supported by the established role of androgens produced by the thecal cells in augmenting FSH-induced aromatase and cholesterol side-chain cleavage activities (2,3).

The role of proteins in local regulation was suggested by the production of an angiogenic factor by rat follicles (4) and its presence in human follicular fluid (5). Furthermore, thecal cells produced a component which promoted the proliferation of 3T3 and granulosa cells (6). DiZerega _et al_. found a protein in the venous drainage of the preovulatory ovary and in human follicular fluid which suppressed the follicular response to gonadotrophins and proposed that this inhibitory factor may be involved in atresia (7,8). In this paper we provide evidence that fibronectin is secreted by unstimulated immature granulosa cells and propose that this component of ECM may play a role in cell-cell communication and follicular development.

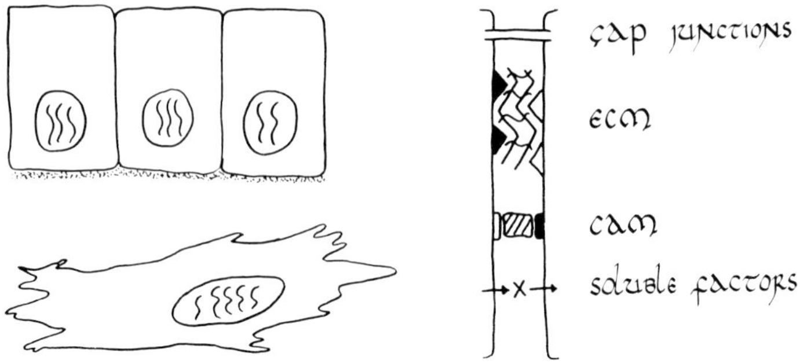

Fig.1: Mechanisms by which cells can communicate

RESULTS AND DISCUSSION

Our studies on rat granulosa cells suggest that "insulin-like" factors may be involved in modifying FSH-dependent cellular differentiation. FSH-stimulates aromatase activity, assessed by the release of tritiated water from $[1\beta\text{-}^{3}H]$testosterone, in granulosa cells isolated from DES-treated 25 day rats (9, Fig.2). Insulin, when added to a suboptimal concentration of FSH, produced a synergistic effect.

The concentration of insulin required was higher than that found in plasma, suggesting that if these effects are important physiologically then "insulin-like" factors may be produced locally within the follicle. This idea was further supported by the finding that conditioned medium obtained from cultures of rat thecal cells augmented FSH-induced aromatase activity. Thecal cell conditioned medium at a concentration of 10% produced a maximum augmentation which was comparable to that produced by insulin.

Another approach used to identify intraovarian factors was to examine, by electrophoresis, the $[^{35}S]$methionine radiolabelled proteins secreted by rat granulosa cells. A protein of molecular mass 220,000 daltons increased in intensity only in control cultures and became the major secreted protein after 72h, comprising 20% of the total radiolabelled proteins (10). This protein was identified as fibronectin by immunoprecipitation and measured by an ELISA assay. The

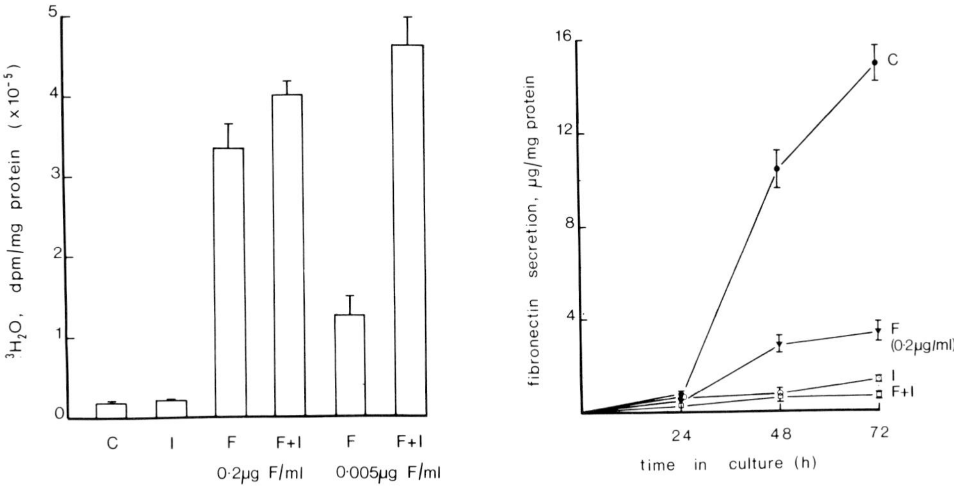

Fig. 2. Effects of NIH-FSH- 15 (F) and 5 ug insulin/ml (I) on A. aromatase activity and B. cumulative fibronectin secretion. After 48h in culture aromatase activity was assessed by incubating cells for 1h with 0.2uCi [1β-^{3}H]testosterone (0.25uM) and measuring the amount of ^3H_2O released. Each value is a mean ± SE(n=3).

hormonal regulation of fibronectin secretion was investigated using the ELISA assay. As shown in fig.3, granulosa cells from 25 day old DES-treated rats cultured under control conditions secreted low levels of fibronectin during the first 24h of culture after which there was a rapid increase in secretion until 72h. In contrast, both FSH and insulin independently suppressed the increase in fibronectin secretion found in control cultures. Testosterone and estrogen alone did not influence fibronectin secretion and did not modulate the actions of FSH and insulin.

Fibronectin is a component of ECM and plays an important role in cell adhesion, migration and cell shape. These functions are due to its ability to bind to collagen, heparin and the cell surface (11). Fibronectin can also influence normal cytodifferentiation as illustrated by its inhibitory effect on myoblast fusion and glycosaminoglycan synthesis by chondrocytes (11). In addition, fibronectin can regulate adipocyte differentiation by inhibiting normal gene expression of lipogenic proteins (12). During the early stages of follicular development fibronectin may be important for the formation of the correct granulosa cell-theca cell structural arrangement and also influence the cytodifferentiation of either cell type. The inverse relationship between fibronectin secretion and the induction of those granulosa cell functions essential for the development of the preovulatory follicle (eg. aromatase activity) indicates that fibronectin may provide a useful marker for the stage of cytodifferentiation and follicular maturation.

In summary, thecal cells and granulosa cells communicate by the production of steroids and proteins in order to promote the development of the preovulatory follicle and establish an environment in which the oocyte can develop normally.

ACKNOWLEDGEMENTS

This study was supported by a grant from the Medical Research Council of Canada.

REFERENCES

1. Cunha GR, Chung LWK, Shannon JM, Taguchi O, Fujii H. (1983) Recent Prog Horm Res 39:559-598.
2. Hillier SG, De Zwart FA (1981) Endocrinology 109:1303-1305
3. Dorrington JH, McKeracher HL, Chan AK, Gore-Langton RE (1983) J. Steroid Biochem 19: 17-32
4. Koos RD, LeMarie WJ (1983) In: Greenwald GS, Terranova PF (eds) Factors Regulating Ovarian Function. Raven Press, New York, pp 191 - 195.
5. Frederick JL, Shimanuki T, diZerega GS (1984) Science 224:389-390
6. Makris A, Klagsbrun MA, Yasumizu T, Ryan KJ (1983) Biol Reprod 29: 1135-1141
7. diZerega GS, Goebelsmann U, Nakamura RM (1982) J Clin Endocrinol Metab 54: 1091-1096
8. diZerega GS, Marrs RP, Roche PC,Campeau JD, Kling OR (1983) J Clin Endocrinol Metab 56: 35-41
9. Gore-Langton RE, Dorrington JH (1981) Mol Cell Endocrinol 22: 135-151
10. Skinner MK, Dorrington JH (1984) Endocrinology in press
11. Hynes RO (1981) In: Hay ED (ed) Cell Biology of Extracellular Matrix. Plenum Press, New York pp 295-334.
12. Spiegelman BM, Ginty CA (1983) Cell. 35: 657-666

Endocrinology
F. Labrie, L. Proulx, eds.

THE INTERACTION OF GONADOTROPHIN AND STEROIDS IN THE CONTROL OF OVARIAN CELL ACTIVITY

ABRAHAM NIMROD* AND MALENIA PEARLSMAN
Dept. of Hormone Research, The Weizmann Institute of Science, Rehovot, Israel

INTRODUCTION

The development and activity of ovarian cells is continuously modulated by the pituitary polypeptide hormones. Other hormones may also be involved in ovarian cell activation and act synergistically with the gonadotrophins. In fact, androgens have been shown to synergize with FSH in the stimulation of progestin production by cultured granulosa cells (GC) from preantral follicles (1-3). Unlike the gonadotrophins, the effect of the steroidal androgens on steroidogenesis is not mediated by cAMP, but is exerted at a step distal to the cyclic nucleotide (4). We have shown that androgen action results in increased cellular uptake of cholesterol and the activity of the mitochondrial side-chain cleavage enzyme (5). Since steroid hormones are believed to act through binding to the nucleus and modulation of gene expression, it is likely that the effect of androgen on cholesterol metabolism involves *de novo* synthesis of specific proteins.

In the present study, the involvement of protein synthesis in the FSH-androgen synergism was investigated using protein synthesis inhibitors, and an attempt was made to identify specific androgen-induced proteins using two-dimensional polyacrylamide gel electrophoresis.

MATERIALS AND METHODS

GC from hypophysectomized DES-treated immature rats were cultured as described before (5). Progesterone accumulation in the culture media was determined by radioimmunoassay of its major metabolite 20α-dihydroprogesterone (1).

Experiments using inhibitors of protein synthesis

GC were cultured for a total of 51 h, with FSH (0.5 μg/ml) included throughout the entire period. Te (0.5 μg/ml) was added 20 h after the start of the culture (zero-time) and removed 4 h later by extensive washing and a short incubation in fresh medium. Protein inhibitors (puromycin 80 μg/ml; cycloheximide 5 μg/ml or cordycepin 15 μg/ml) were added (i) before and during Te addition (-1 h to 4 h), (ii) after Te addition (4 h to 7 h) or (iii) both during and after Te (-1 h to 7 h). The inhibitors were removed by extensive washing and the GC were cultured for additional 24 h or 27 h. Progestin accumulation was then measured in the culture medium.

Present address: Biotechnology (General) Israel, Ltd.; Kiryat Weizmann, Rehovot 76362, Israel

Protein labelling by ^{35}S-methionine

Control and hormone-treated GC monolayers were first washed and incubated in Earle's solution (EBSS) for 30 min in order to deplete endogenous methionine, then challenged for 40 min with fresh EBSS containing ^{35}S-methionine. Lysates of these monolayers were taken for counting and 2-dimensional gel electrophoresis as described by O'Farrel (6).

RESULTS AND DISCUSSION

Effect of protein synthesis inhibitors

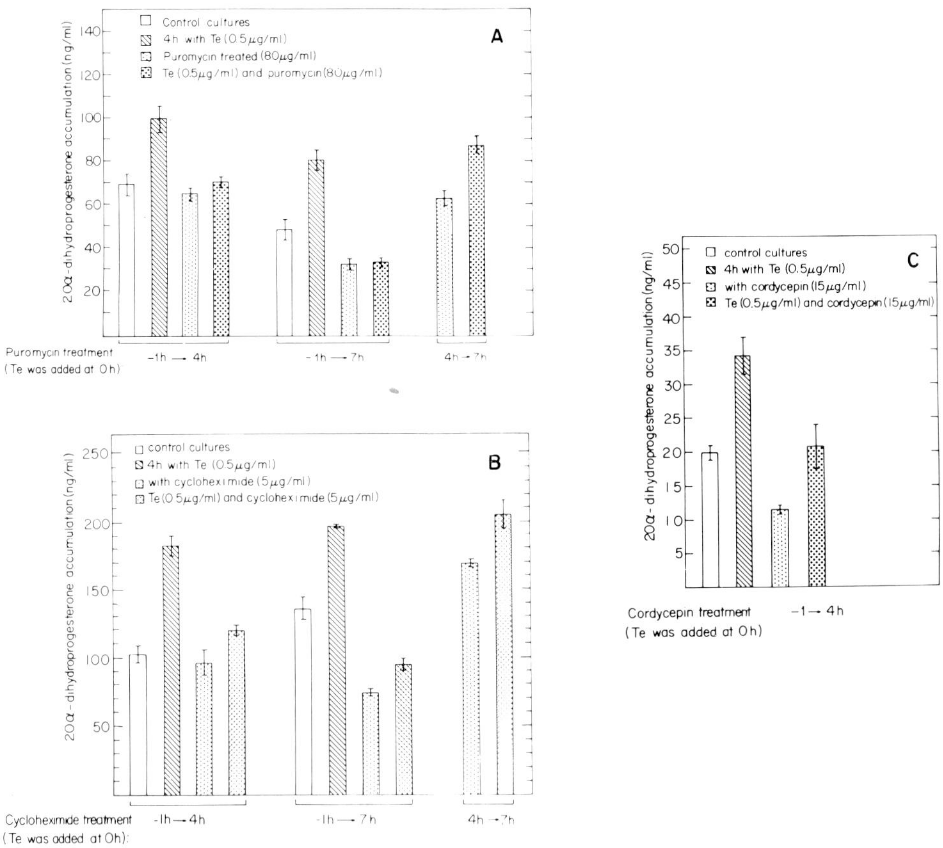

Fig. 1. Effect of protein synthesis inhibitors on the stimulation of progestin production by androgen in cultured GC. A - cycloheximide (5 µg/ml); B - puromycin (80 µg/ml); C - cordycepin (15 µg/ml). The bars and vertical bracket represent the mean ± SEM (n + 5) of progestin accumulation during 24 h or 27 h of culture with FSH after removal of Te and the inhibitors. For details see Materials and Methods.

Puromycin: At a concentration that is known to inhibit protein synthesis (80 μg/ml; ref 7), puromycin completely abolished the Te effect if added during the challenge with the steroid (-1 h to 4 h; Fig. 1A). Addition of the inhibitor after removal of the hormone (4 h to 7 h) did not affect the extent of steroidogenesis. Addition of puromycin throughout the challenge period and 3 h post-challenge (-1 h to 7 h) had reduced the steroidogenic activity of both the control and Te groups, indicating some toxic effect caused by the extended exposure to this metabolic inhibitor.

Cycloheximide: Using the same experimental regimen, cycloheximide (5 μg/ml) has also abolished the Te effect when added during Te challenge (-1 h to 4 h; Fig. 1B). Addition of the inhibitor for 3 h after Te did not abolish the androgen effect.

Cordycepin: This drug is known to inhibit the processing and synthesis of mRNA. GC exposed to 15 ug/ml cordycepin appeared unaffected morphologically. Progestin synthesis, however, was reduced by 50% in both the control and Te groups after exposure to this low concentration of the inhibitor, thus indicating some residual toxicity (Fig. 1C). Despite the reduction in steroidogenesis, the androgen effect was not abolished, thus suggesting that mRNA synthesis at that time was not crucial to the androgen effect.

Actinomycin D: This inhibitor could not be used, since at a concentration that is optimal for RNA synthesis inhibition (8 μg/ml), actinomycin D was toxic to the GC.

Collectively, the results using the metabolite inhibitors indicate that the Te effect involves de-novo protein synthesis very shortly after binding to the receptor and its activation. However, once this protein signal is transmitted, there is no further need for specific protein synthesis and the effect on steroidogenesis is subsequently expressed. Alternatively, it may be that the effect of protein synthesis inhibition on androgen action is due to interference with steroid receptor dynamics.

De-novo synthesis of proteins

^{35}S-methionine incorporation: GC were exposed to FSH, Te or both for 24 h, or cultured with FSH for 20 h and then challenged for 4 h with Te. FSH-treated cells have incorporated 50% more ^{35}S-methionine than control or Te-treated cells. However, no Te effect on total incorporation was found either after a 24 h- or 4 h-exposure (data not shown).

Electrophoretic analysis of de-novo synthesized proteins: Lysates of GC after labelling with ^{35}S-methionine were subjected to 2-D gel electrophoresis. The autoradiograms revealed no new proteins specifically induced by Te in GC exposed for 24 h to Te only (Fig. 2C), or in GC exposed to FSH and to Te for 4 h or 24 h (Fig. 2D,E). FSH caused some enhancement of 3 proteins of approximate M.W. of 80,000 dalton (a, b, c; Fig. 4B,D,E).

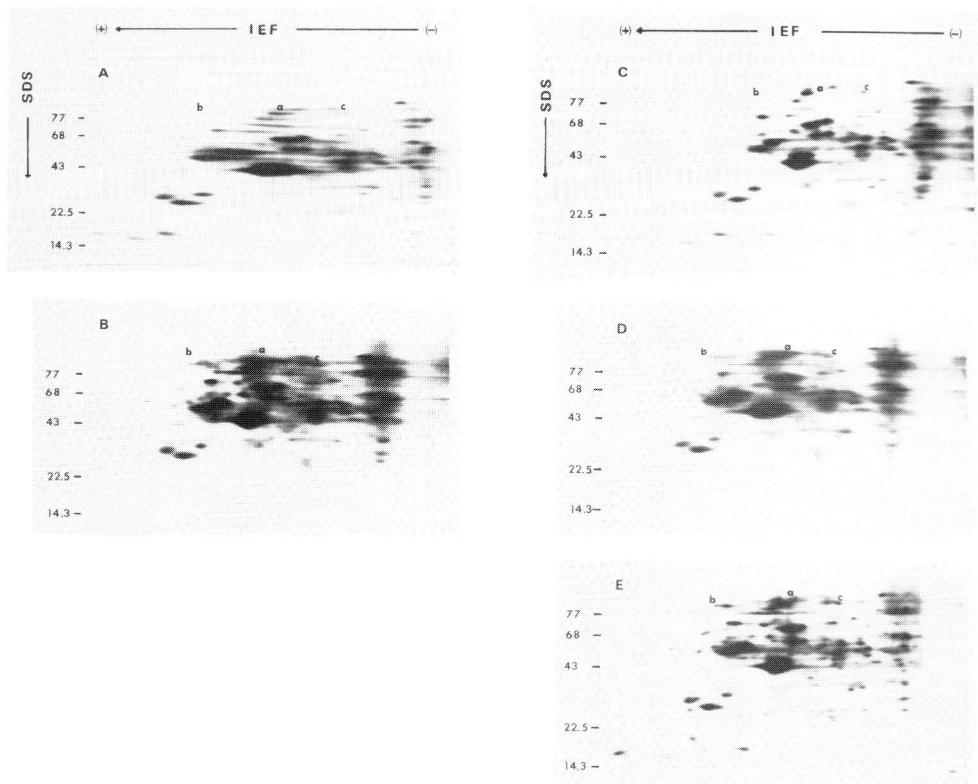

Fig. 2. Two-dimensional electrophoretograms of lyzates of GC monolayers labelled for 40 min with ^{35}S-methionine, after culture: A – for 24 h without hormones; B – for 24 h with FSH only; C – for 24 h with Te only; D – for 20 h with FSH only, then 4 h with FSH + Te; and E – for 24 h with FSH + Te.

In conclusion, no involvement of a specific androgen-induced protein was revealed. It should be emphasized that in the present experiments, protein labelling was done either immediately after a 4 h-Te challenge or after a long (24 h) exposure to the androgen. More detailed time study may be needed in order to demonstrate the specific site of androgen action in this system. The interaction of FSH (or cAMP) with the androgen may well occur before protein synthesis, i.e. at translation or at the genomic level, somehow increasing the ability of the synthetic apparatus to respond to cAMP. Alternatively, the amount of the specific androgen-induced protein may have been below detection.

REFERENCES

1. Nimrod A, Lindner HR (1976) Mol Cell Endocr 5:315-320

2. Armstrong DT, Dorrington JH (1976) Endocrinology 99:1411-1414

3. Lucky AW, Schreiber JR, Hillier SG, Schulman JD, Ross GT (1977) Endocrinology 100:128-133

4. Nimrod A (1977) Mol Cell Endocr 8:201-211

5. Nimrod A (1981) Mol Cell Endocr 21:51-62

6. O'Farrel PH (1975) J Biol Chem 250:4007-4021

7. Tsafriri A, Lieberman ME, Barnea A, Bauminger S, Lindner HR (1973) Endocrinology 93:1378-1385

© 1984 Elsevier Science Publishers B.V.
Endocrinology
F. Labrie, L. Proulx, eds.

LUTEAL PHASE DEFECTS

ANDREA R. GENAZZANI, GERARDO D'AMBROGIO, FABIO FACCHINETTI, GIORGIO ALESSANDRINI FELICE PETRAGLIA and ANNIBALE VOLPE

Department of Obstetrics and Gynecology, University of Modena, Via del Pozzo 71, 41000 - MODENA - Italy

The luteal phase of the ovarian cycle in primates is characterized by the rapid increase of Progesterone (P) plasma levels which reach a plateau around the fourth day after ovulation. This phenomenon is due to the important proliferation of granulosa cells, leading to the corpus luteum formation and is related to the positive effects of the luteinizing hormone (LH) on their mitotic index.

Large amounts of Estradiol (E_2) are also synthesized by the corpus luteum and their plasma levels pattern parallels that of Progesterone. Both of these steroids operate in negative feed-back control at the hypothalamic and pituitary levels lowering LH and follicle stimulating hormone (FSH) plasma levels. In absence of conception, the luteal phase is about 14 days long and luteolysis is the determining factor which induces gonadal steroids withdrawal. The development of corpus luteum depends on follicular maturation and its impairment affects luteal function.

The luteal phase defects represent about 3.5 % of causes of female infertility (1). Under such definition multiple clinical pathologies are comprised, all characterized by a defect in the P production by granulosa cells. On the basis of circulating P levels there have been described:

1) The Aluteal Phase is characterized by low estradiol levels in follicular phase suggestive for failure of follicular maturation, unable to induce adequate mid-cycle gonadotropin (Gn) rise and as consequence the formation of the corpus luteum.
2) The Inadequate Luteal Phase (ILP), with P plasma levels not reaching values higher than 4-5 ng/ml (2); it is caused by a lower steroidogenetic activity of corpus luteum.
3) The Short Luteal Phase (SLP), with a prompt and adequate (8-10 ng/ml) rise of plasma P levels, rapidly declining after few days (3); it is caused by precocius activation of luteolytic processes. In this case lenght of luteal phase is less than 10 days.

In the pathogenesis of luteal phase defects three main mechanisms can be taken into consideration: central, peripheral and local factors. Central factors include:

a) reduced FSH secretion in the early stage of follicle recruitment and during dominance development;
b) premature activation of a mid-cycle LH/FSH secretion in presence of either a not completely developed pre-ovulatory follicle or several follicles which differently contribute to peripheral E_2 pool;
c) increased baseline LH values leading to the polycystic ovarian disease with associated excess of intraovarian androgens;
d) hyperprolactinemia or pharmacological hypoprolactinemia due to the decreased Gn pulsatility and to the lack of prolactin (Prl) as a specific trophic factor for luteal cells, respectively.

Peripheral factors include the changes of distribution volume, transport or clearance of steroids (for example obesity, liver, thyroid and kidney disease) and all those conditions where excessive amounts of sex steroids from adrenal origin interfere with the hypothalamus-pituitary-ovarian axis.

Besides the so-called hydiopatic or genetic alterations, mainly evoked to explain aluteal cycle , local factors include those situations characterized by increased prostaglandin concentrations in peritoneal fluid (endometriosis) which are known to cause the luteinized unruptured follicle syndrome . It is therefore clear that the variable symptomatology of luteal phase defects is a function of the type of impairment. However, the more common findings are the menstrual cycle disorders, i.e. oligomenorrhea or polimenorrhea associated with dismenorrhea and modest hirsutism, acne, seborrea, etc... Due to the low circulating P levels, the E_2 overstimulation drives to the frequent occurrence of uterine fibroids and benign breast disease and when present for a long time represents a risk factor for the development of hormone dependent tumors (endometrial carcinoma). Lastly, the role of luteal phase defects appears to be more evident in the pathogenesis of the premenstrual syndrome.

The premenstrual syndrome represents one of the more common clinical findings in patients affected by luteal phase defect. It is characterized by psychological (dizzyness, depression, irritability) and somatic (weight-gain, edema, abdominal pain, headache) symptoms, mastodinia being most common. This multiple and variable symptomatology occurrs in the second half of the menstrual cycle disappearing with the occurrence of menstrual bleeding. It has been suggested that the imbalance of circulating E/P ratio is typical in patients affected by premenstrual syndrome; it could induce the complex behavioural and endocrine disorders through an impairment of opioid peptides activity in the central nervous system (CNS). The endogenous opioid peptides and the opiate receptors are widely distributed in the CNS and play important role in modulating several physiological functions (pain perception, mood, thermoregulation, regulation of anterior and posterior pituitary secretions, feeding behaviour,etc...)(4). The concentration and activity of central opioids vary in function of the circulating steroid levels as sustained by their changes during menstrual cycle (5,6), puberal development (7,8) and after gonadectomy (9, 10).

The evaluation of rise in LH plasma levels after the administration of naloxone , an opiate antagonist drug is a reliable tool to evaluate the activity of opioid receptors in CNS in human. Central opioids exert in fact a tonic inhibitory control on LH secretion.

Evaluating the LH plasma levels after naloxone administration (4 mg iv.) in the mid-luteal (10/6 days before menstrual bleeding) and late-luteal (3/1 days) phase of patients affected by luteal phase defects and premenstrual syndrome, we observed that going toward the critical period the naloxone fails to induce a significant rise of plasma LH levels, thus suggesting that the patients with premenstrual syndrome, in concomitance with their symptoms show a defective function of the central opioid tonus. The LH responsivity in these patients correlated to the P/E_2 ratio, which may be the determining factor leading to the impairment of central opioid tonus.

TREATMENT

Epimestrol (Stimovul[R], Organon, NL) is a weak estrogen molecule, which appears to increase the synthesis and storage of pituitary gonadotrophes acting on hypothalamic LH-RH and improving the positive feed-back on mid-cycle LH surge(11). The Epimestrol seem to act enhancing the maturational processes of granulosa cells and so increasing the circulating pool of E_2. For this reason the treatment with Epimestrol is performed for 10 days during the follicular phase of the cycle also in patients affected by luteal phase defects. In patients with inadequate and short luteal phase Epimestrol treatment was efficacious in restoring an adequate luteal function in the 75 % and 95 % of the cases, respectively(12). The doses used vary between 10 and 20 mg/day in function of the LH/FSH, E_2 and P plasma levels in the pretreatment cycle(13). Also the lenght of the treatment is prolonged over 10 days in the oligomenorrhoic papatients. The treatment must be performed untill an adequate luteal phase is restored; usually at least 2-3 months are necessary to obtain a stable adequate luteal function (Fig.1).

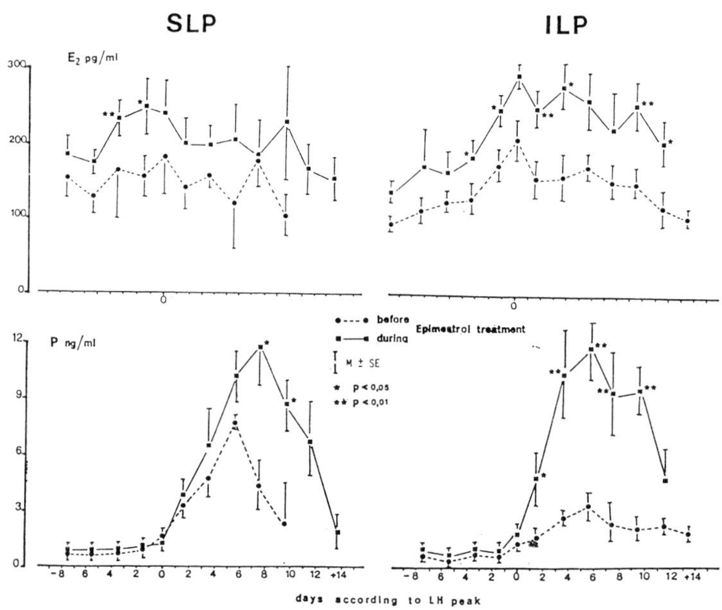

FIG.1.

Estradiol (upper part) and Progesterone (lower part) plasma levels in patients with short luteal phase (SLP) or inadequate luteal phase (ILP) before and during Epimestrol treatment.

Another kind of treatment which is more indicated in patients affected by luteal phase defects and hyperprolactinemia, is with Dopamine (DA) acting drugs. Until now Bromocriptine (Parlodel[R], Sandoz, SW) a DA agonist acting directly on postsynaptic receptors, has been usefully utilized in patients affected by luteal phase defects related to PCO, characterized by high prolactin and LH plasma levels (14). The side effects of bromocriptine and the excessively blunted PrL under treatment stimulate our group to use another DA agonist, Nomifensine (Psicronizer R, Hoechst, FRG), which acts indirectly, increasing the endogenous DA diposable at median eminence level. Such mechanism of action lead to consider the drug as less active than bromocriptine on DA receptors and unable in lowering prolactin levels in patients bearing a prolactinoma, but it is active in patients with moderate idiopathic hyperprolactinemia (15,16). A chronic treatment with Nomifensine (100-300 mg/day for 3-6 months) in patients affected by ILP or SLP with circulating prolactin levels ranging from 20 to 45 ng/ml was associated to a reduction of baseline Prl levels with, as consequence, an improved follicular maturation characterized by significantly higher E_2 mid-cycle peak plasma levels, followed by an adequate luteal phase; with this treatment a pregnancy in an hyper-PrL amenorrhoic steril patients was already reported (17).

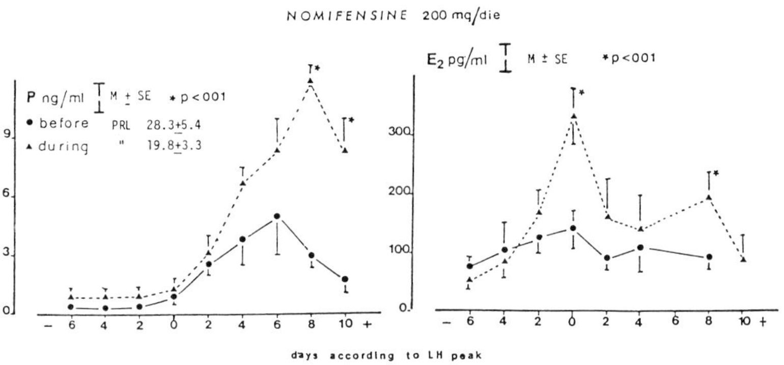

FIG.2.

Progesterone and Estradiol plasma levels in patients with inadequate luteal phase and moderate hyperprolactinemia before (solid line) and during (dotted line) chronic Nomifensine administration.

REFERENCES

1. Jones GS (1976) Fertil and Steril 21:1
2. Sherman B, Korenman S (1974) J Clin Endocrinol Metab 39:145
3. Strott C, Cargille C, Ross G, Lipsett M (1970) J Clin Endocr 30:246
4. O'Donohue TL, Dorsa DM (1982) Peptides 3: 353
5. Barden N,Mèrand Y,Rouleau D, Garon M Dupont A (1981) Brain Res 204: 441
6. Quidgley ME, Yen SSC (1980) J. Clin Endocrinol Metab 51: 179
7. Lee S,Panerai AE, Bellabarba D, Friesen HS (1980) Endocrinology 107: 245
8. Genazzani AR, Facchinetti F, Pintor C, Puggioni R,Parrini D, Petraglia F, Bagnoli F, Corda R (1983) J Clin Endocrinol Metab 57: 56

9. Genazzani AR, Facchinetti F, Ricci-Danero MG, Parrini D, Petraglia F, La Rosa R, D'Antona N (1981) J Endocrinol Invest 4: 375
10. Petraglia F, Locatelli V, Penalva A, Cocchi D, Genazzani AR, Muller EE (1984) J Endocrinol 101: 33
11. Genazzani AR, FAcchinetti F, De Leo V, Picciolini E, Franchi F, Parrini D, Kikovic PM (1978) Fertil and Steril 30: 654
12. Genazzani AR, D'Ambrogio G, Massafra C, Kikovic PM (1981) In:" Endocrinological cancer, ovarian function and disease "pp. 257-262 Excerpta Medica Amsterdam.
13. Genazzani AR, Massafra C, D'Ambrogio G, Kikovic PM (1983)In:"The Ovary" pp. 345-374, G.B. Serra (Ed), Raven Press, New York
14. Falaschi P, Rocco A, Sciarra F, Toscano V, Frajese G (1979)In:"Research on Steroids"pp.241,Klopper A, Lerner L ,Van Der Molen HJ,Sciarra F (Eds), Academic Press. London.
15. Muller EE, Genazzani AR, Murru S (1878) J. Clin Endocrinol Metab 47:1352
16. Genazzani AR, De Leo V, Murru S, Cocchi D, Camanni F, Muller EE (1982) J Clin Endocrinol Metab 54: 429
17. Genazzani AR, De Leo V, Camanni F, Muller EE (1982) J Endocrinol Invest 5:129

ACKNOWLEDGEMENTS

This study has been supported by CNR "Group of Endocrinology".

42. GRF and Regulation of GH Secretion

Endocrinology
F. Labrie, L. Proulx, eds.

GROWTH HORMONE-RELEASING FACTOR. AN UPDATE

ROGER GUILLEMIN, NICHOLAS LING, FREDERICK ESCH, PETER BOHLEN, PAUL BRAZEAU, WILLIAM WEHRENBERG, ANDREW BAIRD, BERTRAND BLOCH, CHRISTIANE MOUGIN AND FUSUN ZEYTIN

Laboratories for Neuroendocrinology, The Salk Institute for Biological Studies, 10010 North Torrey Pines Road, La Jolla, California 92037

Growth hormone-releasing factor (GRF) was originally characterized as a 44 amino acid (aa) residue, COOH-terminal amidated polypeptide that was isolated along with several biologically active fragments (37 aa, 40 aa) from an islet cell tumor of the pancreas in an acromegalic patient with no pituitary adenoma (Guillemin et al, 1982). The 40 aa fragment was also isolated and characterized in another tumor recognized in similar circumstances (Esch et al, 1982; Rivier et al, 1982). We have now characterized hypothalamic GRF from several species (human, porcine, bovine, ovine and caprine). The respective references are Ling et al, 1984; Bohlen et al, 1983, Esch et al, 1983 and manuscript in preparation for the structures of ovine and caprine GRF. Figure 1 shows the primary structures of all these GRFs of hypothalamic origin. They are all 44 amino acid, COOH-terminal amidated peptides. The primary structure of human hypothalamic GRF was shown to be identical to that of the 44 aa material originally isolated from the pancreatic tumor. Extracts of human hypothalamic tissues (stalk-median eminence fragments) collected at autopsies also showed a second peak of immunoreactive GRF in the HPLC effluent that had the elution characteristics of hpGRF-40, and the corresponding amino acid composition. In the several batches of human hypothalamic tissues processed, the amounts of hGRF-44 and hGRF-40 isolated varied, depending on whether or not the tissues had been treated with acetone (see Ling et al, 1984 for amounts). In all other studies using freshly collected hypothalamic tissues from farm animals a single form of immunoreactive GRF was isolated and characterized as the 44 aa form described in Fig. 1. Thus both forms hGRF-40 and hGRF-37 are likely degradation products as seen in the pancreatic tumor tissues originally processed or in the human hypothalamic autopsy materials. Thus, of all hypothalamic GRFs characterized so far, only rat hypothalamic GRF (see Spiess et al, 1983) is different, since it is reported to contain only 43 amino acids and to be in a free acid form (see also Fig. 1). Also, rat GRF is structurally rather different from the other GRF-peptides (see Fig. 1). It is thus possible that rodents may have a gene structure coding for GRF quite different from that of the higher mammals studied so far.

PRIMARY STRUCTURES OF HYPOTHALAMIC GRF FROM SEVERAL SPECIES

	Sequence (positions 5, 10, 15, 20, 25, 30, 35, 40)	
h GRF	YADAIFTNSYRKVLGQLSARKLLQDIMSRQQGESNQERGARARL	-NH2
p GRF	YADAIFTNSYRKVLGQLSARKLLQDIMSRQQGERNQEQGARVRL	-NH2
c, b GRF	YADAIFTNSYRKVLGQLSARKLLQDIMNRQQGERNQEQGAKVRL	-NH2
o GRF	YADAIFTNSYRKILGQLSARKLLQDIMNRQQGERNQEQGAKVRL	-NH2
r GRF	HADAIFTSSYRRILGQLYARKLLHEIMNRQQGERNQEQRSRFN	-OH

Figure 1: Amino acid sequences of mammalian hypothalamic GRFs. The letters h,p,c,b,o and r designate the human, porcine, caprine, bovine, ovine and rat species respectively.

While the various forms of GRF peptides when tested for potency (specific activity) *in vitro* always show GRF-44-NH_2 to be more potent than all other forms, it is true that when tested *in vivo* (in the rat) hGRF-40 and hGRF-44-NH_2 are statistically equipotent (see Wehrenberg and Ling, 1983). We have no explanation at the moment for the discrepancy of the potencies when tested by the two different methods.

We have also isolated, in the original tumor from which we obtained GRF, peptides corresponding to the fragments of pre-proGRF as postulated from the cDNA nucleotide sequence (Gubler et al, 1983). RIAs against such fragments show them also to be found in the hypothalamus. The C-terminal peptide of the sequence deduced for pre-proGRF has been characterized as having a pyrrolidone-carboxylic acid (pyroglutamic acid) N-terminal as well as an amidated C-terminal (Baird et al, 1984, abstract to this meeting and manuscript in preparation). Such structural characteristics are usually associated with mature forms of biologically active peptides. At the moment, no biological activity has been found for this peptide.

GRF appears to stimulate GH release by activating exocytosis of GH granules through a phosphorylation mechanism mediated by a granular receptor coupled with a cAMP-dependent protein kinase (Lewin et al, 1983). GRF does not affect the release of newly synthesized GH (<3 hrs after labelling) but only stimulates secretion of "old" GH (>12 hrs after labelling). Somatostatin, as well as somatomedin-C (IGF-1), are non-competitive antagonists of GRF on the release of GH. GRF stimulates the transcription of the GH gene 1.8- to 3.6-fold in rat pituitary cells in vitro. GRF also regulates pituitary GH transcription in vivo. There are 1.8- and 2.5-fold increases in GH gene transcription at 10 and 20 min respectively, following the injection of GRF into anesthetized rats (Barinaga et al, 1983). We have not observed any evidence of an effect of GRF on pituitary hormones other than GH, in vitro or in vivo. Continuous administration of GRF (24 hrs) in rats with an implanted cannula leads to decreasing responses to GRF in terms of GH release that can be correlated with massive depletion of pituitary GH content (Wehrenberg et al, 1984). Immunocytochemistry with several GRF antisera shows that most GRF neurons are located in the arcuate nucleus of the infundibulum, with only scattered GRF neurons in the n. ventromedialis (Bloch et al, 1983). The ontogeny of the GRF neurons in human fetuses does not correlate with previously published variations of fetal plasma GH throughout normal pregnancy. Clinical studies with synthetic GRF are proceeding in multiple clinical centers; they all show the high intrinsic activity of GRF in human subjects.

ACKNOWLEDGEMENTS

Research in our laboratories supported by NIH (HD-09690 and AM-18811) and the Robert J. Kleberg Jr. and Helen C. Kleberg Foundation.

REFERENCES

Baird A, Böhlen P, Esch F and Ling N (1984) 7th International Congress of Endocrinology, July 1-7, 1984 Quebec City, Canada (abstract).

Barinaga M, Yamonoto G, Rivier C, Vale W, Evans R and Rosenfeld MG (1983) Nature 306:84-85

Bloch B, Brazeau P, Ling N, Böhlen P, Esch F, Wehrenberg WB, Benoit R, Bloom F and Guillemin R (1983) Nature 301:607-608.

Böhlen P, Esch F, Brazeau P, Ling N and Guillemin R (1983) Biochem Biophys Res Commun 116:726-734.

Esch FS, Bohlen P, Ling NC, Brazeau PE, Wehrenberg WB, Thorner MO, Cronin MJ and Guillemin R (1982) Biochem Biophys Res Commun 109:152-158.

Esch F, Böhlen P, Ling N, Brazeau P and Guillemin R (1983) Biochem Biophys Res Commun 117:772-779.

Guillemin R, Brazeau P, Bohlen P, Esch F, Ling N and Wehrenberg WB (1982) Science 218:585-587.

Gubler, U, Monahan JJ, Lomedico PP, Bhatt RS, Collier KJ, Hoffman BJ, Böhlen P, Esch F, Ling N, Zeytin F, Brazeau P, Poonian MS and Gage LP (1983) Proc Natl Acad Sci USA 80:4311-43

Lewin, MJM, Reyl-Desmars F and Ling N (1983) Proc Natl Acad Sci USA 80:6538-6541.

Ling N, Esch F, Böhlen P, Brazeau P, Wehrenberg WB and Guillemin R (1984) Proc Natl Acad Sci USA (in press).

Rivier J, Spiess J, Thorner MO and Vale W (1982) Nature 300:276-278.

Spiess J, Rivier J and Vale W (1983) Nature 303:532-

Wehrenberg WB and Ling N (1983) Biochem Biophys Res Commun 115:525-530.

Wehrenberg WB, Brazeau P, Ling N, Textor G and Guillemin R (1984) Endocrinology 114:1613-1616.

Endocrinology
F. Labrie, L. Proulx, eds.

DISTRIBUTION AND RELEASE OF GRF

AKIRA ARIMURA, ISTVAN MERCHENTHALER, MICHAEL D. CULLER AND KATSUHIKO IWASAKI
Laboratories for Molecular Neuroendocrinology and Diabetes, Tulane University Hebert Research Center, Belle Chasse, LA 70037; Departments of Medicine and Anatomy, Tulane Medical Center, School of Medicine, New Orleans, LA 70112, USA

INTRODUCTION

The recent isolation and characterization of growth hormone releasing factor (GRF)[1,2] has prompted studies to determine the mechanisms regulating growth hormone(GH) secretion. It is generally accepted that GH secretion is under dual inhibitory and stimulatory control by the respective hypothalamic factors, somatostatin (SRIF) and GRF. The central distribution of SRIF has been extensively studied by RIA and by immunocytochemistry (ICC). As demonstrated for other hypothalamic hypophysiotropic hormones, the median eminence contains the highest concentration of SRIF, with the densely packed neurofibers abutting the primary capillaries of the hypophysial portal system. The release of SRIF into the hypophysial portal vessels appears to be under the control of neurotransmitters, such as dopamine.[3] SRIF positive cell bodies and fibers, however, are not confined to the hypothalamus but are also present in extrahypothalamic regions, including the cortex, suggesting that SRIF is not only a hypophysiotropic hormone but may also function as a neurotransmitter. This dual role has also been suggested for other hypothalamic peptides, such as LHRH, TRH and CRF, however, it is unknown whether GRF might also function as a neurotransmitter. Our studies addressed this question by examining the distribution of GRF in the rat brain by ICC. In addition, to examine the possibility that GRF may function as a neurotransmitter, we studied the effect of $hptGRF_{44}$ on SRIF release from cultured rat hypothalamic cells. Furthermore, we examined the *in vivo* GRF releasing activity of the classical neurotransmitters in urethane-anesthetized rats in which endogenous SRIF was nullified by passive immunization with SRIF antiserum.

IMMUNOCYTOCHEMICAL LOCALIZATION OF GRF

Colchicine (200-250 ug) was injected into the lateral ventricle of adult male rats under Nembutal anesthesia. Forty-eight hours later, the rats were sacrificed and the distribution of GRF-immunoreactive structures in the hypothalamus studied using PAP ICC on vibrotome sections as described.[4] Primary antiserum (R565) was generated in the rabbit against synthetic rat GRF_{43} (gift from Dr. J. Rivier) conjugated to bovine serum albumin (BSA) by glutaraldehyde. The antiserum was treated with 2 M NaI, to remove any endogenous ligand bound to the high affinity antibodies. The primary antiserum was used at a 5000X dilution with a 48 hr reaction time at 4°C.

The densest accumulation of GRF-immunopositive processes and termini was observed in the external layer of the median eminence (ME). The distribution of GRF in the ME was similar to that of SRIF and CRF. GRF-immunopositive termini occupied the central region of the ME with the densest accumulation immediately medial to the nerve containing termini. Relatively dense accumulation of GRF fibers was also observed in the dorsomedial nucleus (DMN). GRF perikarya were observed in the following regions of the colchicine treated rats: 1) arcuate nucleus; 2) perifornical regions of the hypothalamus (mostly ventral or ventromedial to the fornix); 3) scattered cell bodies in the lateral basal hypothalamus, the paraventricular and DMN. These findings are in agreement with earlier findings using antiserum to $hptGRF_{40}$[5]. No immunoreactive perikarya were observed in intact rats. The distribution of GRF perikarya in the CNS seems to be confined to the hypothalamus with only a slight difference between species. In the human, the monkey and the cat, the majority of immunoreactive cell bodies are located in the arcuate nucleus with only scattered cells found in the perifornical region.

The specificity of staining was substantiated by the finding that all staining with antiserum R565 was completely abolished by preincubation with synthetic rat GRF_{43}. Absorption with $hptGRF_{28-40}$ also abolished the staining, however, preincubation with $hptGRF_{1-29}$, $hptGRF_{1-7}$, $hptGRF_{1-7}NH_2$ or $hptGRF_{1-15}NH_2$ did not affect the staining. Thus, the antiserum R565 may recognize the C-terminal region of the GRF molecule. Other peptides tested for crossreaction were GIP, VIP, secretin, and PHI-27, none of which affected the staining, suggesting that the staining was specific for rat GRF.

The perifornical, lateral basal hypothalamic area and the arcuate nucleus project GRF fibers toward the medial basal hypothalamus. GRF staining in the median eminence was almost completely abolished in rats treated with monosodium glutamate. Staining of GRF cell bodies in the arcuate nucleus was also abolished, however, GRF cells in the perifornical and lateral basal hypothalamus were unaffected. The GRF fibers in DMN also remained unchanged. These findings suggest that GRF may function as a neurotransmitter in addition to its role as a hypophysiotropic hormone.

STIMULATION OF SRIF RELEASE FROM CULTURED RAT HYPOTHALAMIC CELLS

Pregnant CD strain rats were laparotomized on day 18 of pregnancy and the fetal rats removed under sterile conditions. The fetal hypothalami were dissected, and placed in room temperature, Ca^{++}- and Mg^{++}-free phosphate buffer. Thirty hypothalami were pooled and dispersed with 0.1% collagenase-type II in PBS. After washing, the dispersed cells were diluted with culture medium so that 4 ml, added to each culture dish, contained 1 x 10^6 cells. The cultures were maintained at 37°C under an atmosphere of 95% air; 5% CO_2. After 12 days, the cells were washed and equilibrated in Krebs Ringer bicarbonate buffer containing 0.5 mg/ml bacitracin, 0.1 mM ascorbic acid, 0.25% BSA and 0.2% glucose (KRBG). The cells were incubated in KRBG for 1 hr and for another hour in KRBG alone or KRBG containing test substances. The media from each group was collected, pooled, acidified by HCl (pH 4), and placed on a Sep-Pak C18 cartridge. The Sep-Pak was washed with 10 mM HCl and eluted with 2 ml 75% CH_3CN/10 mM HCl. The eluate was concentrated by vacuum evaporation, 50 ul 5% BSA was added, the pH adjusted to 7, and the final volume adjusted to 1.0 ml. SRIF content of the concentrate was determined by RIA.

The basal release of SRIF was 14.6±0.88 pg/dish/hr. SRIF release following addition of 0.1 mM, 1 mM and 10 mM $hptGRF_{44}$ and 10 mM ovine CRF were 15.4±4.82, 23.3±5.99, 24.6±3.95 and 18.1±4.32 pg/dish/hr, respectively. When expressed in terms of % ratio of GRF released during the second incubation period over the first incubation period, the results were 124±2.5, 139±9.7, 164±28.7, and 211± 44.3%, respectively, and the control value was 91±11.3%. Analysis of variance indicated that there was a dose-related increase in SRIF release induced by $hptGRF_{44}$. 10 nM ovine CRF also stimulated significant SRIF release.

In another experiment, using rat hypothalamic fragments *in vitro*, SRIF release was also stimulated by $hptGRF_{44}$ in a dose-related manner. 10 nM TRH and 10 nM ovine CRF also stimulated SRIF release, but the same dose of LHRH and VIP was ineffective. In Ca^{++}-free media, the basal release of SRIF from the hypothalamic fragments was considerably reduced and the ability of 10 nM $hptGRF_{44}$ to induce SRIF release was abolished suggesting that SRIF release by $hptGRF_{44}$ is Ca dependent. The results of these *in vitro* studies in addition to the ICC data support the possibility that GRF may act as a peptidergic neurotransmitter in addition to a hypophysiotropic hormone.

RELEASE OF GRF IN RATS

Adult male CD strain rats (225-300g) were anesthetized with urethane (1.5 g/kg, i.p.), and injected iv with 0.5 ml sheep anti-SRIF serum, S-773. Two hrs later, when GH levels had stabilized from the release caused by endogenous SRIF nullification, the first blood sample was collected from the jugular vein through a previously implanted cannula. The animal was placed in a Krieg's stereotaxic instrument and either 2 ul vehicle (0.9% saline/0.01% ascorbic acid) alone or 2 ul vehicle containing 10 nmole of either epinephrine, norepinephrine, dopamine, serotonin or acetylcholine was injected into the lateral ventricle. Blood samples were collected 5, 20, 35, and 50 min after the injection, and the serum GH content determined by RIA using the kit supplied from NIDDK.

Serum GH levels initially decreased after intraventricular injection of vehicle but remained relatively constant after the second blood sample (5 min postinjection). Epinephrine significantly increased GH levels 5 and 20 min postinjection and norepinephrine significantly elevated GH 5 min after injection by preventing the initial decline in GH observed with vehicle alone. Other substances tested had no effect. These findings suggest that epinephrine and, to a lesser extent, norepinephrine stimulated the release of GRF, since any possible alteration of SRIF release by these substances was nullified by pretreatment with the SRIF antiserum. Intraventricular injection of the $alpha_1$ adrenergic agonist, phenylephrine (200 nmole), suppressed GH levels, but none of the $alpha_2$ agonists, UK14,304 (75 nmole), clonidine (10 nmole), or oxymetazoline (10 nmole) or the beta agonist isoproterenol (10 nmole) altered GH levels. From these findings it is difficult to implicate a specific monoaminergic receptor in the release of GRF at the present time. The failure of clonidine, a widely used centrally acting, predominently $alpha_2$ adrenergic stimulant, to provoke GH release in our preparation is quite intriguing, since intraventricular injection of clonidine stimulates GH release in urethane-anesthetized rats which have not been treated with SRIF antiserum.[6] It is possible that this alpha agonist stimulates GH release by suppressing the release of endogenous SRIF.

SUMMARY

The present studies show that GRF neurons are confined to the hypothalamus, and that GRF may function as a neurotransmitter as well as a hypophysiotropic hormone. In addition to the results obtained using ICC localization, this concept is further supported by the finding that $hptGRF_{44}$ stimulates the release of SRIF from rat hypothalamic fragments and cultured cells. The release of GRF seems to be enhanced by epinephrine, and to a lesser extent, by norepinephrine, but which specific monoaminergic receptor is involved in GRF release will require further studies.

REFERENCES

1. Guillemin R, Brazeau P, Bohen P, Esch F, Ling N, Wehrenberg WB (1982) Science 218:585-587
2. Rivier J, Spiess J, Thorner M, Vale W (1982) Nature 300:376-378
3. Chihara K, Arimura A, Schally AV (1979) Endocrinology 104:1656-1662.
4. Merchenthaler I, Thomas CR, Arimura A (1984) Peptides, in press
5. Merchenthaler I, Vigh S, Schally AV, Petruse P (1984) Endocrinology 114:1084-1085
6. Ruch W, Jaton AL, Bucher B, Marback P, Doepfner W (1976) Experientia 32/4:529-531

© 1984 Elsevier Science Publishers B.V.
Endocrinology
F. Labrie, L. Proulx, eds.

CLINICAL STUDIES WITH GROWTH HORMONE RELEASING FACTOR

MICHAEL O. THORNER, WILLIAM S. EVANS, MARY LEE VANCE, JOÃO L. C. BORGES, ROBERT M. BLIZZARD, ALAN D. ROGOL, JULIA K. RESCHKE, LAWRENCE A. FROHMAN, CHERYLE B. WEBB, RICHARD L. FURLANETTO, JEAN RIVIER, AND WYLIE VALE
University of Virginia Medical Center, Charlottesville, VA 22908; University of Cincinnati Medical Center, Cincinnati, OH 45267; Children's Hospital of Philadelphia, Philadelphia, PA 19104; and Salk Institute, San Diego, CA 92138

Human pancreatic GH-releasing factor (1-40)-OH (hpGRF-40) and hpGRF(1-44)-NH_2 are probably identical with the human hypothalamic growth hormone releasing hormone(s)(GHRH). We have used synthetic hpGRF-40 for our clinical studies.

STUDIES IN NORMAL SUBJECTS

In men hpGRF-40 (1 ug/kg iv bolus) stimulates GH release within 5 min but does not elevate serum prolactin, TSH, LH, or ACTH (measured indirectly through plasma cortisol), or blood glucose or plasma levels of eight enteropancreatic hormones (1). When graded doses of hpGRF-40 (0.1-10 ug/kg) were given iv no differences were noted in the maximum levels of GH achieved. However, variability in response among individual subjects was noted. Doses of 3.3 and 10 ug/kg hpGRF-40 elicited a prolonged and biphasic pattern of GH release (2).

A dose of 3.3 ug/kg of hpGRF-40 given iv was used to study GH release in normal women at different phases of the menstrual cycle. The results were similar to those in normal men and no differences in the GH responsivity were found during the different phases.

INTRAVENOUS INFUSIONS OF hpGRF-40

hpGRF-40 was infused in normal young men by giving incremental doses of hpGRF-40 for 90 min increasing from 1 to 3.3 to 10 to 33 ng/kg/min (3). In addition we have performed studies using 6 h infusions of 1, 3.3, and 10 ng/kg/min and more recently we have completed a study of 24 h infusions of 2 ng/kg/min hpGRF-40 in 6 young men. Together these studies indicate: (1) the great variability in GH response between and within subjects; (2) that GH secretion occurs in a pulsatile fashion even during continuous infusion; and (3) that approximately 10% of stored pituitary GH is released with the infusions that we have used. The 24 h studies indicate that during GRF infusions GH is secreted in bursts at similar times as during a control study. The majority of the GH is secreted during the night. In a patient with a GRF secreting metastatic carcinoid tumor with levels of GRF of approximately 15 ng/ml, GH was secreted in an intermittent pulsatile fashion over a 24 h period.

PHARMACOKINETICS OF hpGRF-40

We have studied the pharmacokinetics of hpGRF-40 using a radioimmunoassay for hpGRF-40 following extraction from plasma (4). In normals, the metabolic clearance rate (MCR) and plasma disappearance rate ($T_{1/2}$) of hpGRF-40 were measured following single iv injections of 1, 3.3, and 10 ug/kg hpGRF-40. Plasma GRF levels were measured during the subsequent 180 minutes and biexponential curve analyses were performed. Increasing doses of constant infusions of hpGRF-40, 1, 3.3, 10, and 33 ng/kg/min were administered and the MCR calculated from the measurement of steady state plasma IR-GRF levels at each infusion rate. The post-infusion disappearance rate was determined by linear regression analysis of plasma IR-GRF levels during the 120 min period after cessation of the infusion.

The calculated MCR during the single injection study was 194 $\pm$ 17.5 ($L/m^2/d$) and was not significantly different from the calculated value during the constant infusion study (202 $\pm$ 16). The disappearance rate during the single injection study was divided into two linear phases: an initial equilibration phase (7.6 $\pm$ 1.2 min) and an elimination phase (51.8 $\pm$ 5.4 min). The latter was similar to the linear disappearance rate observed (41.3 $\pm$ 3.0 min) after the constant infusion. The chromatographic and biologic characteristics of plasma IR-GRF, 30 min after injection, were similar to those of synthetic hpGRF-40.

ROUTES OF ADMINISTRATION

For therapy it is likely that GRF will require administration several times each day. We undertook a preliminary investigation on the effects of intranasal and subcutaneous (sc) hpGRF-40. hpGRF-40 administered sc is less potent in stimulating GH secretion than when administered by iv route. The minimum dose to produce significant stimulation of GH secretion is 10 ug/kg sc which is 100 times the dose required by the iv route. By the intranasal route doses of 30 and 100 ug/kg stimulated GH secretion. When levels of GRF are measured in the plasma a similar hierarchy is observed. Following 10 ug/kg administered iv, sc and intranasally the levels of GRF achieved are, respectively, 66.6 $\pm$ 17.6; 1.11 $\pm$ 0.39; and 0.16 $\pm$ 0.02 ng/ml. Similarly peak levels are observed at 5 min after the iv route, 60 min after sc, and 15 min after intranasal administration.

STUDIES IN GH DEFICIENT SUBJECTS

In our initial studies hpGRF-40 (10 ug/kg iv) was administered intravenously to 12 adult patients who had presented in childhood with GH deficiency (5). In 4 the GH levels rose in response to the GRF, while serum somatomedin C concentrations increased 24 h after the single dose of hpGRF-40 in 8 of the 10 in whom it had been measured.

We have since studied 6 adult subjects who presented in childhood with idiopathic GH deficiency by challenging them with 10 ug/kg hpGRF-40 iv bolus prior to and following 5 d of treatment with 0.33 ug/kg hpGRF-40 administered iv every 3 h (6). In response to the initial 10 ug/kg challenge GH levels rose in 3 of 6. Within 12 h after initiation of intermittent iv administration of hpGRF-40 (mean ± SEM) somatomedin C levels had risen by 0.1 ± 0.05 u/ml and at the end of the 5 d period they increased from 0.24 ± 0.07 to 0.78 ± 0.32 u/ml. In response to the second challenge GH levels rose in 3 of the 4 subjects who initially failed to respond or had a minimal response (< 1 ng/ml) and increased in one of two subjects who had responded to the first dose.

Forty children with short stature were evaluated for GH reserve following pharmacological tests and after a single iv injection of hpGRF-40 (3.3 ug/kg). The children were grouped into isolated GH deficiency (IGHD), organic hypopitutarism (OH), intra-uterine growth retardation (IUGR), and constitutional delay of growth (CD) categories. In IGHD and OH patients GH concentrations did not increase to more than 7 ng/ml following pharmacologic stimulation. However, the mean (± SE) responses to hpGRF-40 were 3.4 ± 1.1 ng/ml and 8.2 ± 2.4 ng/ml in OH and IGHD categories, respectively. All chidren with IUGR and CD groups responded briskly to hpGRF-40 although there was wide variation of maximum GH levels (5-25 ng/ml).

These data indicate that hpGRF-40 can be employed to evaluate GH reserve in short children and may be useful in the diagnosis of hypothalamic pituitary disorders. The ultimate test of the utility of hpGRF-40 in children with GH deficiency or short stature is the therapeutic response (growth) when compared to the presently available natural or synthetic GH preparations. We have recently treated two children with GH deficiency with hpGRF-40 administered with a peristaltic pump (Pulsamat, Ferring Inc.) sc every 3 h. These children initially received 1 ug/kg hpGRF-40 every 3 h sc over 5 d. On a constant diet they demonstrated a reduction in nitrogen excretion and an increase in calcium excretion. Both have now completed 6 mo of therapy with hpGRF-40 (3 ug/kg every 3 h SC). In both there has been an acceleration in linear growth; one has increased from an average of 4.6 c/yr to 7.1 cm/yr and the other from 2.1 cm/yr to 14.1 cm/yr.

ACROMEGALY

Plasma IR-GRF was measured in 177 samples from unselected acromegalic patients. Not a single new patient with elevated GRF levels was found. In contrast the 3 patients with ectopic tumors secreting GRF had GRF levels in the peripheral blood in the ng/ml range in contrast to less than 100 pg/ml levels in normal subjects and other acromegalic patients. Thus, a peripheral GRF level may help to distinguish those patients with acromegaly due to ectopic GRF secretion from patients with primary pituitary tumors.

CONCLUSIONS

We believe that hpGRF has the biological effects of GHRH. It may have clinical potential in treating short stature due to GH deficiency. Analogues of GRF which are able to block the GRF receptor may prove to have a role in the treatment of diabetes and acromegaly. The future applicability of GRF in medicine and agriculture probably depends on the development of highly active smaller molecular analogues.

ACKNOWLEDGEMENTS

We thank Mrs. Donna Harris for preparing the manuscript and the Pituitary Hormone Distribution Program of NIADDK for RIA reagents. These studies were supported in part by US PHS grants: GCRC RR-847; HD13197 and AM32632 (M.O.T.); CIA 1-K03-HD-00439 (W.S.E.); 1R23-HD-17120 (M.L.V.); AM30667 and GCRC RR-0068 (L.A.F.); AM26741, AM209117, AA-03504, and HD13527 (J.R. and W.V.). We thank Dr. D. Linkie of Ferring Inc. for providing us with the Pulsamat pumps for GRF therapy.

REFERENCES

1. Thorner MO, Rivier J, Spiess J, Borges JLC, Vance ML, Bloom SR, Rogol AD, Cronin MJ, Kaiser DL, Evans WS, Webster JD, MacLeod RM, Vale W (1983) Lancet 1:24-28.

2. Vance ML, Borges JLC, Kaiser DL, Evans WS, Furlanetto R, Thominet JL, Frohman LA, Rogol AD, MacLeod RM, Bloom S, Ribier J, Vale W, Thorner MO (1984) J Clin Endocrinol Metab 58:838-844.

3. Webb CB, Vance ML, Thorner MO, Perisutti G, Thominet J, Rivier J, Vale W, Frohman LA J Clin Invest (in press).

4. Frohman LA, Thominet JL, Webb CB, Vance ML, Uderman H, Rivier J, Vale W, Thorner MO (1984) J Clin Invest 73:1304-1311.

5. Borges JLC, Blizzard RM, Gelato MC, Furlanetto R, Rogol AD, Evans WS, Vance ML, Kaiser DL, MacLeod RM, Merriam GR, Loriaux DL, Spiess J, Rivier J, Vale W, Thorner MO (1984) Lancet 2:119-123.

6. Borges JLC, Blizzard RM, Evans WS, Furlanetto R, Rogol AD, Kaiser DL, Rivier J. Vale W, Thorner MO (1984) J Clin Endocrinol Metab 59:1-6.

Endocrinology
F. Labrie, L. Proulx, eds.

SOMATOSTATIN: MECHANISMS OF RELEASE

JOSEPH B. MARTIN, WILLIAM J. MILLARD, GEORGES MCCORMICK, NORMAN KASTING AND JUNICHI FUKATA

Neuroendocrine Laboratory, Department of Neurology, Massachusetts General Hospital, Boston, MA 02114

Somatostatin was discovered and named on the basis of its effcts on inhibition of growth hormone (GH) secretion. With the discovery of growth hormone releasing factor (GRF), new questions are raised concerning the physiologic role of somatostatin in GH control. Is it important in establishing baseline levels of secretion? Does it modify secretion under physiologic conditions? How does it interact with GRF to determine pulsatile GH secretion?

This review considers several aspects of these questions which have been addressed by a variety of *in vivo* and *in vitro* experimental approaches.

I. Effects of Active and Passive Immunization on Binding of Endogenous Somatostatin

It is well known that hypothalamic lesions that destroy the somatostatin tuberinfundibular system lead to a depletion of median eminence somatostatin and to increased basal levels of GH (1). Passive immunization with highly specific polyclonal antibodies to somatostatin elicit acute GH secretion in the rat (2,3) and reverse the characteristic inhibition of GH release caused by stress and by starvation (4,5). Recent studies have extended these observations. In male rats, passive immunization elicits an increase in average basal levels of GH (Table 1); similar results occur in female rats. In both sexes average levels were determined over 4.5-6 hours after intravenous administration of 1 ml of anti-somatostatin sheep serum. Controls received normal sheep serum. Recent studies have implicated a relatively minor role for somatostatin in the regulation of GH secretion during prenatal and early postnatal development (6,7). However, the reduction in GH secretion observed in old (18-20 month) rats may be mediated in part by an elevation in endogenous somatostatin release (8). We have recently examined the effects of antisomatostatin serum in male rats given monosodium glutamate (MSG). The administration of MSG to neonatal rats results in selective destruction of arcuate neurons known to be the principle site of GRF. Rats so treated show growth retardation and markedly diminished pulsatile GH secretion (9). Furthermore, Bloch et al (10) have demonstrated using immunofluorescence techniques a severe loss of GRF in the arcuate nucleus and median eminence. Baseline levels of GH remain low after MSG treatment; administration of antiserum causes a two fold rise in average levels of GH secretion, due primarily to elevation in basal levels (Table 1). Since hypothalamic somatostatin levels are unchanged in MSG-treated rats and basal levels are elevated after anti-somatostatin serum it is likely that the peristently low levels found are due to endogenous tonic suppression of GH secretion caused by somatostatin.

In active immunization studies in the baboon, the induction of circulating antibodies to somatostatin results in elevation of basal levels of GH and in alterations in the pattern of pulsatile secretion (11).

We have also examined another model of GH secretion in an attempt to determine the roles of GRF and somatostatin in GH regulation. In these studies we have exploited the findings that blockade of alpha-adrenergic mechanisms result in suppression of GH pulsatile secretion. Administration of diethyldithiocarbamate (DDC) at a dose of 400 mg/kg completely abolishes pulsatile GH secretion. Effects are partial at lower doses. Baseline levels remain low and such animals are relatively refractory to exogeneous administration of rGRF (12). However, if DDC administration is combined with anti-somatostatin serum, there is a significant elevation of GH basal values (without pulsatile secretion) and doses of rGRF one-thousand fold less are now effective in eliciting GH secretion.

Taken as a whole, these studies permit the following conclusions:

1) Somatostatin contributes to the low levels of GH between pulses of secretion.

2) Somatostatin secretion may determine the phasic timing of episodes of GH secretion.
3) Tonic secretion of somatostatin may determine sensitivity of the pituitary to endogenous or exogeneous GRF.

II. In Vitro Studies of Hypothalamic Somatostatin from Hypothalamic Fragments or Cultures.

Reichlin has recently reviewed the extensive studies carried out to determine the factors that affect somatostatin secretion (13). From these experiments one can conclude the following:

1) GH and somatomedin C stimulate somatostatin release from hypothalamic fragments (14-16).
2) Dopamine stimulates somatostatin release (17-19).
3) Norepinephrine has variable effects on somatostatin release (17,20,21).
4) Glucagon and neurotensin stimulate somatostatin release (17,22,23).
5) Vasoactive intestinal polypeptide inhibits somatostatin release (24,25).
6) Gamma-aminobutyric acid inhibits somatostatin release (26).

III. Studies of Somatostatin Levels in Pituitary Portal Blood

The measurement of somatostatin levels in pituitary portal blood is difficult and requires anesthesia and extensive surgical manipulations. As a result it is difficult to derive physiological interpretations from such experiments. Nevertheless, such an approach provides an opportunity to measure directly the changes in somatostatin in pituitary portal blood. These studies have shown that:

1) GH stimulates somatostatin secretion (27).
2) Dopamine and norepinephrine stimulate somatostatin release (28).
3) Glucagon, neurotensin and bombesin stimulate somatostatin release (29,30).

4) Substance P and opioid peptides have no effect on somatostatin release (30).

5) Acetylcholine stimulates somatostatin release (31).

IV. Studies of Somatostatin Release into the Median Eminence using Push-Pull Cannulation Techniques.

We (32) have used push-pull perfusion to study the release of somatostatin into the median eminence of unanesthetized rats. These techniques are difficult, but have the advantage, with careful attention to experimental protocols that are non-stressful, of permitting simultaneous measurement of peripheral GH levels as an index of pituitary GH secretion. It is possible to obtain physiologic patterns of episodic GH secretion into blood while sampling continuously the concentration of somatostatin present in extracellular fluid in the median eminence.

In control rats, plasma GH levels showed a normal ultradian rhythm and relatively stable levels of immunoreactive somatostatin (IRS) (around 30 pg/15 min) appeared in the perfusate during the six hour perfusion. Intracerebroventricular administration of hGH (40 ug), neurotensin (2 ug), glucagon (25 ug) or intravenous injection of oxymetazoline (50 ug/kg bw), an alpha-adrenergic agonist, or endotoxin (150 ug/kg bw) suppressed subsequent GH surges. In these rats, however, IRS levels in the median eminence perfusate failed to change significantly compared to control rats.

In conclusion these studies suggest that:

1) GH pulses can be suppressed by several factors, including endotoxin, hGH, glucagon and neurotensin without detectable increases in median eminence somatostatin secretion.
2) GH pulses are determined primarily by GRF secretion.
3) Somatostatin may act to cause tonic suppression of GH secretion and thus to set the level of effectiveness and responsiveness to GRF.

It is evident that somatostatin has an important function in the physiologic control of GH secretion. What needs to be determined is whether this effect is primarily one of steady-state suppression, which acts to determine the effectiveness of GRF stimulation or whether it acts in a dynamic fashion to contribute to GH pulsatile release. Further studies will be required to clarify these questions.

Acknowledgements

Supported by USPHS grants AM26252 and HD17364.

ELEVATION OF PLASMA GH LEVELS FOLLOWING PASSIVE IMMUNIZATION OF RATS WITH ANTISOMATOSTATIN SERUM

Group	Normal Sheep Serum	Anti-Somatostatin Serum
Normal males	77.2 ± 10.8 (6)	122.4 ± 21.4 (6)
Normal females	42.8 ± 6.3 (6)	117.8 ± 11.5 (6)
MSG-treated males	34.9 ± 7.7 (5)	69.6 ± 14.5 (5)

Mean levels were determined for 4.5-6 hours following the iv administration of 1 ml of either normal sheep serum or anti-somatostatin serum. Numbers in parenthesis indicate group size. Mean ± SEM.

REFERENCES

1. V. Critchlow, R.W. Rice, K. Abe and W. Vale, Endocrinology 103:817, 1978.

2. A. Arimura, W. Smith, and A.V. Schally, Endocrinology 98:540, 1976.

3. L. Ferland, F. Labrie, M. Jobin, A. Arimura, and A. Schally, Biochem. Biophys. Res. Commun. 68:149, 1976.

4. L.C. Terry, J.O. Willoughby, P. Brazeau, J.B. Martin, and Y.C. Patel, Science 192:565, 1976.

5. G. Tannenbaum, J. Epelbaum, E. Colle, P. Brazeau, and J. Martin, Endocrinology 102:1909, 1978.

6. C. Oliver, P. Giraud, J.C. Lissitzky, J. Cote, F. Boudouresque, P. Gillioz and B. Conte-Devolx, Endocrinology 110:1018, 1982.

7. O. Khorram, L.R. DePalatis and S.M. McCann, Endocrinology 113:720, 1983.

8. W.E. Sonntag, L.J. Forman, N. Miki, R.W. Steger, T. Ramos, A. Arimura and J. Meites, Neuroendocrinology 33:73, 1981.

9. W.J. Millard, J.B. Martin, Jr., J. Audet, S.M. Sagar and J.B. Martin, Endocrinology 110:540, 1982.

10. R. Bloch, N. Ling, R. Benoit, W.B. Wehrenberg and R. Guillemin, Nature 307:272, 1984.

11. R.A. Steiner, J.K. Stewart, J. Barber, D. Koerker, C.J. Goodner, A. Brown, P. Illner and C.C. Gale, Endocrinology 102:1587, 1978.

12. W.J. Millard, G.F. McCormick, T.M. Badger, C.Y. Bowers, and J.B. Martin, 7th International Congress of Endocrinology, Quebec City, 1984 (Abstr).

13. S. Reichlin, In Brain Peptides, edited by D. Krieger, M. Brownstein and J.B. Martin. Plenum Press, New York, 1983 pp. 771-752.

14. B.L. Pimstone, M. Sheppard, B. Shapiro, S. Kronheim, A. Hudson, S. Hendricks, and K. Waligora. Fed. Proc. 38:2330, 1979.

15. M. Berelowitz, S.L. Firestone, and L.A. Frohman, Endocrinology 109:714, 1981.

16. M. Berelowitz, M. Szabo, L.A. Frohman, S.L. Firestone, L. Chu, and R.L. Hintz, Science 212:1279, 1981.

17. K. Maeda and L.A. Frohman, Endocrinology 106:1837, 1980.

18. S.R. Ojeda, A. Negro-Vilar, A. Arimura, and S.M. McCann, Neuroendocrinology 31:7, 1980.

19. M. Berelowitz, K. Maeda, S. Harris and L.A. Frohman, Endocrinology 107, 24, 1980.

20. A. Negro-Vilar, S. Ojeda, A. Arimura and S. McCann, Life Sci. 23:1493, 1978.

21. L.C. Terry, O.P. Rorstad, and J.B. Martin, Endocrinology 107:794, 1980.

22. A. Shimatsu, Y. Kata, N. Matsushita, H. Katakami, and N. Yanaihara, Program of the 63rd Annual Meeting of the Endocrine Society, 1981, Abstr. 198.

23. M.C. Sheppard, S. Kronheim, B.L. Pimstone, J. Neurochem. 32:647, 1979.

24. J. Epelbaum, S.V. Drouva, L. Tapia-Arancibia, E. Laplante, and C. Kordon, Ann. Endocrinol. 41:478, 1978.

25. A. Shimatsu, Y. Kato, N. Matsushita, H. Katakami, and N. Yanaihara, Program of the 63rd Annual Meeting of the Endocrine Society, 1981, Abstr. 198.

26. R. Gamse, D. Vaccaro, G. Gamse, M. DuPage, T.O. Fox and S. Leeman, Proc. Natl. Acad. Sci. USA 77:5552, 1980.

27. K. Chihara, N. Minamitani, H. Kaji, A. Arimura, and T. Fujita, Endocrinology 109:2278, 1981.

28. K. Chihara, A. Arimura, and A.V. Schally, Endocrinology 104:1656, 1979.

29. H. Abe, Y. Kato, T. Chiba, T. Taminato and T. Fujita, Life Sci. 23:1647, 1978.

30. H. Abe, K. Chihara, T. Chiba, S. Matsukura and T. Fujita, Endocrinology 108:1939, 1981.

31. K. Chihara, A. Arimura, and A.V. Schally, Endocrinology 104:1656, 1979.

32. N. Kasting, J.B. Martin, and M.A. Arnold. Endocrinology 109:1739, 1981.

43. Receptor Diseases

Endocrinology
F. Labrie, L. Proulx, eds.

RECEPTOR DEFECTS IN SYNDROMES OF EXTREME INSULIN RESISTANCE

SIMEON I. TAYLOR, PHILLIP GORDEN, AND JESSE ROTH
Diabetes Branch, NIADDK, National Institutes of Health, Building 10, Room 8N-250, Bethesda, Maryland 20205 (U.S.A.)

The insulin receptor, located on the surface of the target cell, has two important functions: to bind insulin and to couple insulin binding to insulin action. Defects in either of these receptor functions may give rise to insulin resistance. While defects in receptor function may contribute importantly to the pathogenesis of many disease states, this has been demonstrated most clearly in the syndromes of extreme insulin resistance associated with acanthosis nigricans.

Several different types of molecular defects in receptor function have been identified in patients with these clinical syndromes:

1. QUANTITATIVE DEFECTS IN THE INSULIN RECEPTOR

a. Accelerated receptor degradation. Certain patients, most of whom exhibit other evidence of autoimmune disease, may develop autoantibodies directed against the insulin receptor (1,2). In both *in vivo* and *in vitro* experiments, the earliest effect of the anti-receptor antibodies is to mimic insulin action (3,4). However, with prolonged exposure of the tissue to relatively high concentrations of anti-receptor antibodies, the tissues become resistant to insulin (4,5). Recently, we have shown that the autoantibodies markedly accelerate the degradation of insulin receptors (Fig. 1). The resultant decrease in the number of insulin receptors at the cell surface may be an important mechanism by which the anti-receptor antibodies desensitize the target cell to the effects of insulin (6).

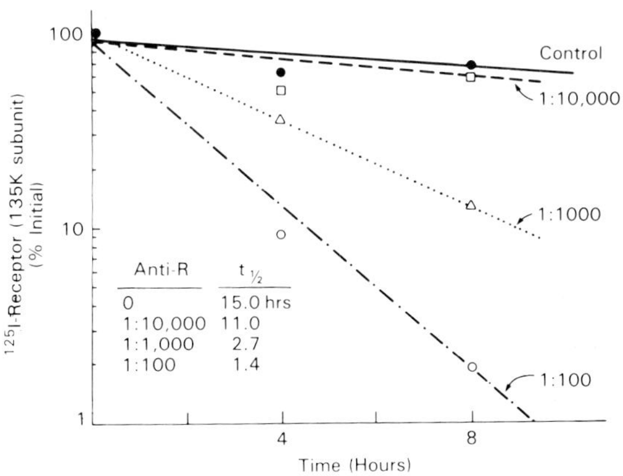

Fig. 1. Anti-receptor antibody accelerates the degradation of insulin receptors in cultured IM-9 lymphocytes. Insulin receptors on the surface of IM-9 cells were labelled with ^{125}I. Cells were incubated at 37° in the presence or absence of varying dilutions of anti-receptor antiserum B-10 (1:100, 1:1000, or 1:10,000). These data are reprinted from reference 6.

b. <u>Impaired receptor biosynthesis</u>. In certain patients with genetic forms of extreme insulin resistance, the insulin resistance results from a decrease in the number of insulin receptors at the cell surface (Fig. 2)(1,7-9). Using cultured lymphocyte cell lines derived from these patients, we have studied the biosynthesis of the receptor precursor (M_r=190 kDa) by pulse-labelling with [2-^{3}H]mannose. The processing of the precursor to the mature receptor subunits (M_r= 135 and 95 kDa) was followed during a subsequent chase period (10,11). Interestingly, these studies suggested the existence of at least two different biochemical defects in receptor biosynthesis among our patients with extreme insulin resistance. In two patients, there appeared to be a block in receptor biosynthesis at a step prior to the synthesis of the 190 kDa receptor precursor. In a third patient, the biochemical defect appeared to result in biosynthesis of an abnormal form of the receptor precursor with M_r= 148 kDa.

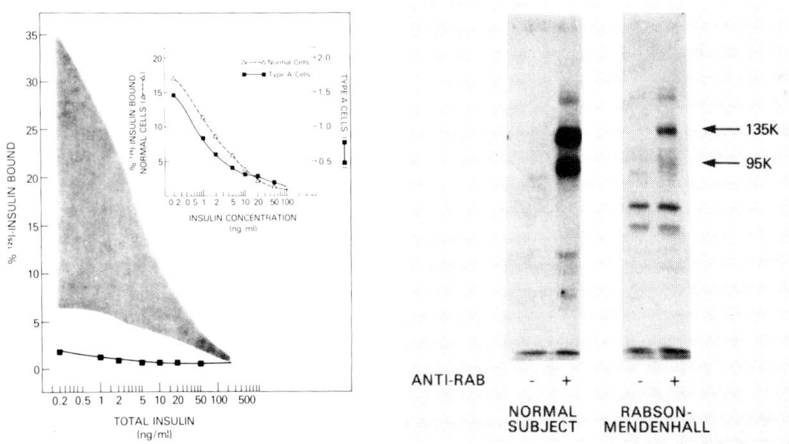

Fig. 2. Decreased number of insulin receptors on the surface of cultured lymphocytes from patients with extreme insulin resistance. In the left panel, ^{125}I-insulin binding to cultured cells is plotted as a function of the concentration of insulin (8). The shaded area represents the range of binding observed in cells from normal subjects. The inset demonstrates that there is a similar shape for the binding-competition curves obtained with cells from a normal subject and patient A-1 (a patient with Type A extreme insulin resistance). The right panel is an autoradiograph of an SDS-polyacrylamide gel of immunoprecipitates of ^{125}I-labelled insulin receptors from cultured lymphocytes of a normal subject and a patient (RM-1) with the Rabson-Mendenhall syndrome (9). In comparison to the normal subject, the cells from RM-1 have a greater than 95% reduction in the quantity of the major insulin receptor subunits (apparent molecular weight, 135 K and 95 K daltons).

2. QUALITATIVE DEFECTS IN THE INSULIN RECEPTOR.

a. Abnormal binding affinity. We have studied a patient with leprechaunism whose receptors bind insulin more tightly than do normal insulin receptors. Moreover, the receptor's ability to bind insulin has markedly reduced sensitivity to alterations in pH and temperature (Fig. 3) as well as defects in cooperative interactions among insulin binding sites (12-14). These abnormalities in insulin binding to the receptor provided the basis for assays to detect the defect in the insulin receptor. Nevertheless, because the patient's receptor actually binds an abnormally large amount of insulin under conditions of physiological temperature and pH, it seems likely that insulin resistance results from a failure to couple insulin binding to insulin action.

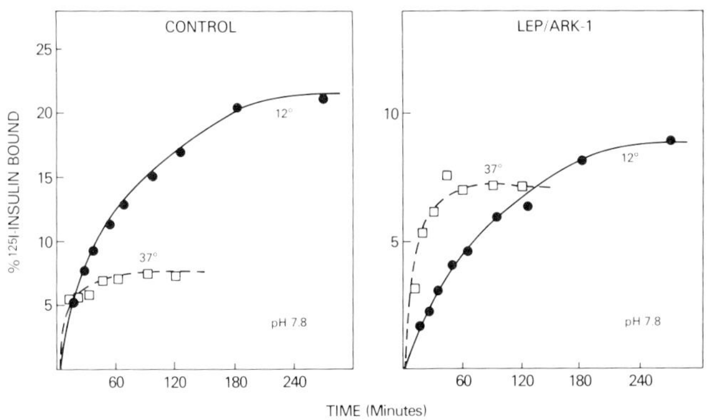

Fig. 3 Temperature insensitivity of insulin binding to receptors of a patient with leprechaunism. The time course of specific binding of ^{125}I-insulin was studied in cells from a normal subject and leprechaun/Ark-1. Whereas increasing the temperature from 12° to 37° caused a 70% decrease in steady-state insulin binding to normal insulin receptors, increasing the temperature had relatively little effect upon insulin binding to the insulin receptors of leprechaun/Ark-1. Data redrawn from reference 12.

b. Defective receptor phosphorylation. Recent studies have demonstrated that the 95 kDa subunit of the insulin receptor possesses a tyrosine-specific protein kinase activity (15). The receptor-associated protein kinase activity is stimulated by insulin and is capable of phosphorylating both the receptor itself as well as several exogenous substrates. It has been proposed that the receptor's insulin-stimulated protein kinase activity may play a key role in coupling insulin binding to insulin action although this remains controversial (16-19). Using cultured lymphocytes derived from multiple patients with extreme insulin resistance, we have not succeeded in identifying any patients with selective defects in receptor phosphorylation (20). However, two laboratories using solubilized insulin receptors from either fresh circulating monocytes (21) or erythrocytes (22) have reported insulin resistant patients whose receptors appear to have a selective defect in protein kinase activity. In addition, we have studied the effects of four anti-receptor antibodies upon the receptor-associated protein kinase activity. All of these anti-receptor antibodies were derived from patients with extreme insulin resistance and all of the antibodies had insulinomimetic effects in a bioassay using isolated rat adipocytes. Nevertheless, two antibodies stimulated and two antibodies inhibited the receptor-associated protein kinase activity (16).

REFERENCES

1. Kahn CR. Flier SJ, Bar RS, Archer JA, Gorden P, Martin MM, Roth J (1976) N Engl J Med 294:739-745
2. Taylor SI, Grunberger G, Marcus-Samuels B, Underhill LH, Dons RF, Ryan J, Roddam RF, Rupe CE, Gorden P (1982) N Engl J Med 307:1422-1426
3. Kahn CR, Baird KL, Flier JS, Jarrett DB (1977) J Clin Invest 60:1094-1106
4. Dons RF, Havlik R, Taylor SI, Baird KL, Chernick SS, Gorden P (1983) J Clin Invest 72:1072-1080
5. Karlsson FA, Van Obberghen E, Grunfeld C, Kahn CR (1979) Proc Natl Acad Sci USA 76-809-813
6. Taylor SI, Marcus-Samuels B (1984) J Clin Endocrinol Metab 58:182-186
7. Bar RS Muggeo M, Kahn CR, Gorden P, Roth J (1980) Diabetologia 18:209-216
8. Taylor SI, Samuels B, Roth J, Kasuga M, Hedo JA, Gorden P, Brasel DE, Pokora T (1982) J Clin Endocrinol Metab 54:919-930
9. Taylor SI, Underhill LH, Hedo JA, Roth J, Serrano Rios M, Blizzard RM (1983) J Clin Endocrinol Metab 56:856-861
10. Hedo JA, Kahn CR, Hayashi M, Yamada KM, Kasuga M (1983) J Biol Chem 258:10020-10026
11. Hedo JA, Taylor SI (1984) Clin Res 32:560A (abstract)
12. Taylor SI, Roth J, Blizzard RM, Elders MJ (1981) Proc Natl Acad Sci USA 78:7157-7161
13. Taylor SI, Hedo JA, Underhill LH, Kasuga M, Elders MJ, Roth J (1982) J Clin Endocrinol Metab 55:1108-1113
14. Taylor SI, Leventhal S (1983) J Clin Invest 71:1676-1685
15. Kasuga M, Karlsson FA, Kahn CR (1982) Science 215:185-187
16. Zick Y, Rees-Jones RW, Taylor SI, Gorden P, Roth J (1984) J Biol Chem 259:4896-4401
17. Simpson IA, Hedo JA (1984) Science 223:1301-2304
18. Shia MA, Rubin JB, Pilch PF (1983) J Biol Chem 258:14450-14455
19. Roth RA, Mesirow ML, Cassell DJ (1983) J Biol Chem (1983) 258:14456-14460
20. Whittaker J, Taylor SI (1983) Diabetes 32 (suppl 1): 57A (abs. #225)
21. Grunberger G, Zick Y, Gorden P (1984) Science 223:932-934
22. Grigorescu F, Flier JS, Kahn CR (1984) Clin Res 32:519A (abstract)

Endocrinology
F. Labrie, L. Proulx, eds.

THE SYNDROMES OF ANDROGEN RESISTANCE

JAMES E. GRIFFIN, MARK LESHIN, WILLIAM J. KOVACS, AND JEAN D. WILSON

Department of Internal Medicine, The University of Texas Health Science Center at Dallas, 5323 Harry Hines Boulevard, Dallas, TX 75235 (USA)

INTRODUCTION

The fundamental mechanism of sexual differentiation was elucidated by Alfred Jost who established that the castrated mammalian embryo develops as a female (1). According to the Jost formulation, chromosomal sex directs the development of either ovaries or testes. If testes develop, their hormonal secretions elicit the development of the male phenotype. If an ovary develops or if no gonad is present anatomical development is female.

Two secretions of the fetal testis are involved in male development - mullerian inhibiting substance and androgen. Mullerian inhibiting substance is a peptide hormone that acts ipsilaterally to prevent development of the fallopian tube and uterus (2). Testosterone is the principal fetal as well as the postnatal androgen in the male (3). The onset of testosterone formation by the fetal testes commences shortly after the onset of differentiation of the spermatogenic tubules and concomitant with the histological differentiation of the Leydig cells. Testosterone acts within the testis to promote maturation of the spermatogonia and is secreted into the fetal circulation where it induces development of the male phenotype.

ROLE OF TESTOSTERONE AND DIHYDROTESTOSTERONE

Dihydrotestosterone and testosterone bind to the same intracellular androgen receptor protein, but dihydrotestosterone binds with greater affinity and is more effective at promoting transformation to the DNA-binding state (4). Separate roles for testosterone in mediating virilization of the wolffian ducts and its 5α-reduced derivative dihydrotestosterone in mediating development of the external genitalia of the male were recognized on the basis of studies in animal and human embryos in which it was shown that 5α-reductase is maximal in the anlage of the prostate and external genitalia prior to virilization, whereas dihydrotestosterone formation is virtually undetectable in wolffian ducts until after virilization is advanced.

This deduction was substantiated by studies of patients with a rare disorder originally termed pseudovaginal perineoscrotal hypospadias (3). Affected 46,XY males have an external female phenotype, absence of the prostate, bilateral testes, and normally virilized wolffian structures (epididymis, vas deferens, seminal vesicle) that terminate in the vagina. At puberty the external genitalia virilize partially, axillary and pubic hair develop, and testosterone production increases to the male range. Direct evidence of a defect in 5α-reductase in this disorder, now termed 5α-reductase deficiency, was reported in 1974 in families from Dallas (5) and the Dominican Republic (6). Elevated ratios of plasma testosterone to dihydrotestosterone following administration of human chorionic gonadotropin are present prior to puberty, and normal plasma testosterone and low plasma dihydrotestosterone levels are present in adults. Elevated ratios of urinary 5β-reduced to 5α-reduced steroids, decreased *in vivo* conversion of testosterone to dihydrotestosterone, diminished 5α-reductase in tissue biopsy specimens, and deficient or abnormal 5α-reductase in fibroblasts cultured from genital skin are consistent features (3). Plasma luteinizing hormone is usually elevated but is lower than in castrated men or subjects with disorders of the androgen receptor. In some patients, virilization at puberty is accompanied by a change in gender role from female to male (7). However, other subjects who were raised as females, castrated and given subsequent estrogen replacement therapy have made successful adjustments as women. The cause of the apparent reversal in gender role is not known.

Deficiency of 5α-reductase is due to the homozygous state of an autosomal recessive gene that is manifest only in males. Homozygous 46,XX women and heterozygous 46,XY men are normal (8). The mutation has been described in a variety of ethnic groups. Consanguinity has been documented in a third, and a third are from areas with known high coefficients of inbreeding.

The molecular features of the mutation have been studied in our laboratory in cells cultured from 25 subjects from 18 families (3). In the original families 5α-reductase was deficient and has been similarly defective in 12 additional families. In 4 familes 5α-reductase was present but was qualitatively abnormal as manifested by defective binding of the enzyme to the hormone and/or the cofactor NADPH. This heterogeneity is similar to that for other inherited genetic abnormalities.

The reason that the external genitalia virilize more at puberty than during embryogenesis may be due to the presence of higher levels of plasma testosterone at puberty or to the formation of some dihydrotestosterone as a result of the residual 5α-reductase demonstrable in all patients. Price et al administered pharmacological amounts of androgen to four men with 5α-reductase deficiency and observed that virilization occurred when plasma dihydrotestosterone rose into the normal male range (9). This study favors the interpretation that the late virilization is mediated by the residual 5α-reductase present.

ROLE OF THE ANDROGEN RECEPTOR

Disorders of the androgen receptor in 46,XY individuals cause a spectrum of phenotypes that range from women with complete and incomplete testicular feminization to men with partial virilization (Reifenstein syndrome) to otherwise normal men with failure of spermatogenesis (infertile men). The endocrine pathology is similar in these disorders. Resistance to the feedback regulation of LH production by androgen commonly results in elevated plasma LH, and this in turn causes enhanced secretion of both testosterone and estradiol by the testes (3).

Keenan et al documented that the dihydrotestosterone receptor is present in fibroblasts cultured from normal genital skin (foreskin, scrotum, labia majora) and that fibroblasts grown from some women with complete testicular feminization showed no detectable receptor (10), a finding that has been confirmed (11) and that explains the profound androgen resistance in this disorder. Whether deficient binding is due to absence of the receptor or a mutant protein that cannot bind the ligand is not known. Other patients with androgen resistance have partial defects in the amount of receptor, and still others have qualitative abnormalities in the protein as evidenced by thermolability, failure of stabilization by sodium molybdate, and failure to undergo transformation to the DNA-binding state (4, 12, 13).

The androgen receptor in fibroblasts from 71 families with phenotypic and endocrine characteristics of androgen resistance have been characterized in our laboratory (3). In 14 of 24 families with complete testicular feminization binding was virtually undetectable. In 9 families with complete testicular feminization the receptor was qualitatively abnormal. In 15 families with incomplete testicular feminization binding was absent in 3, qualitatively abnormal in 6, and decreased in amount in 2. One qualitative mutation of the receptor in two 46,XY cousins with a female phenotype was of particular interest; their androgen receptor bound androgen normally but could not be transformed to the DNA-binding state because the receptor-hormone complex was unstable (4). The androgen receptor was found to be qualitatively abnormal in 12 Reifenstein families and 6 infertile men and diminshed in amount in 5 Reifenstein families and 4 unrelated infertile men. Thus, many different mutations impair the function of the receptor protein and cause a spectrum of phenotypic effects.

A category of androgen resistance that does not appear to involve either the 5α-reductase or the androgen receptor was identified by Amrhein et al in three 46,XY members of one family with the phenotype of testicular feminization, normal 5α-reductase, normal amounts of androgen receptor and normal nuclear localization of dihydrotestosterone (14). Subsequent subjects with receptor positive androgen resistance have been described with less complete impairment of androgen action (3). In 10 of 71 families studied in our laboratory (5 with testicular feminization, 4 with the Reifenstein phenotype, and one infertile male) no abnormality of the androgen receptor was demonstrable, despite endocrine evidence of profound androgen resistance. The site of the abnormality in these patients is unclear. Qualitative defects of the receptor may be too subtle to be detected by current methods, or the defect may be at some step in androgen action distal to the receptor.

CONCLUSION

Hereditary defects that impede androgen action cause resistance to the hormone during embryogenesis and in later life. In males such defects produce a variable phenotype ranging from infertile men to ambiguous genitalia to phenotypic women. The disorders can be classified into 5α-reductase deficiency, disorders of the androgen receptor, and receptor positive resistance. Analysis of the molecular basis of these defects has provided insight into normal as well as abnormal sexual development.

REFERENCES

1. Jost A (1972) Johns Hopkins Med J 130:38
2. Donahoe PK, Ito Y, Price JM, Herndon WH III (1977) Biol Reprod 16:238
3. Wilson JD, Griffin JE, Leshin M, MacDonald PC (1983) In: Stanbury JB, Wyngaarden JB, Fredricksen DS, Goldstein JE, Brown MS (eds) The Metabolic Basis of Inherited Disease. McGraw-Hill, New York, pp 1001-1026
4. Kovacs WJ, Griffin JE, Weaver DD, Carlson BR, Wilson JD (1984) J Clin Invest 73:1095
5. Walsh PC, Madden JD, Harrod MJ, Goldstein JL, MacDonald PC, Wilson JD (1974) N Engl J Med 291:944
6. Imperato-McGinley J, Guerrero L, Gautier T, Peterson RE (1974) Science 186:1213
7. Imperato-McGinley J, Peterson RE, Gautier T, Sturla E (1979) N Engl J Med 300:1233
8. Peterson RE, Imperato-McGinley J, Gautier T, Sturla E (1977) Am J Med 62:170
9. Price P, Wass JAH, Griffin JE, Leshin M, Wilson JD, Savage MO, Large DM, Bu'Lock DE, Anderson DC, Besser GM (in press) J Clin Invest
10. Keenan BS, Meyer WJ III, Hadjian AJ, Jones HW, Migeon CJ (1974) J Clin Endocrinol Metab 38:1143
11. Griffin JE, Punyashthiti K, Wilson JD (1976) J Clin Invest 57:1342
12. Griffin JE (1979) J Clin Invest 64:1624
13. Griffin JE, Durrant JL (1982) J Clin Endocrinol Metab 55:465
14. Amrhein JA, Meyer WJ III, Jones HW Jr, Migeon CJ (1976) Proc Natl Acad Sci USA 73:891

Endocrinology
F. Labrie, L. Proulx, eds.

GLUCOCORTICOID INSENSITIVITY IN MAN AND NONHUMAN PRIMATES

GEORGE P. CHROUSOS, MASAKO TOMITA, DAVID D. BRANDON, D. LYNN LORIAUX AND MORTIMER B. LIPSETT

Developmental Endocrinology Branch, National Institute of Child Health and Human Development, National Institutes of Health, Bethesda, MD 20205, USA

INTRODUCTION

Glucocorticoid insensitivity refers to the condition in which target tissues show decreased responsiveness to glucocorticoids (end-organ resistance). Since cortisol is essential for life in primates, complete glucocorticoid insensitivity would be incompatible with survival. Partial insensitivity, on the other hand, could be compensated for by elevation of circulating cortisol, a result of decreased negative feedback of glucocorticoids upon pituitary ACTH secretion. Insensitivity to glucocorticoids has been identified in man and nonhuman primates recently (1-3). In this bricf manuscript we will review the syndrome of cortisol insensitivity in man and nonhuman primates.

PRIMARY CORTISOL INSENSITIVITY IN MAN

Clinical Presentation (1,2)

The syndrome of primary cortisol insensitivity in man is a familial condition characterized by absence of signs and symptoms of Cushing's syndrome, elevated total and free plasma corticol concentrations, high urinary free cortisol excretion, high plasma ACTH and in a severly affected case (propositus) also by hypertension and hypokalemic alkalosis. The latter is due to high plasma concen-concentrations of deoxycorticosterone and corticosterone. In patients with this condition, dexamethasone, at the usual doses, fails to suppress the activity of the pituitary-adrenal axis. High dose dexamethasone therapy (3mg/d), however, corrected in our patient the hypertension and hypokalemic alkalosis, without causing signs of glucocorticoid excess.

HLA typing and biochemical testing of our extended kinship showed no association between the transmission of the condition and the HLA, suggesting that the gene responsible for the abnormality is not associated with the HLA locus.

Glucocorticoid Receptor Studies

The glucocorticoid receptor (GR) in various tissues from the severely affected patient has a low affinity for glucocorticoids (1). The hormone-receptor complex is unstable, with excess loss of specific bound ligand during thermal activation but without excess generation of meroreceptor. The molecular weight of the GR, determined by SDS-PAGE is similar to that of normal controls (~ 92,000) and the activation pattern *per se*, examined *in vitro* by heating cytosol and performing phosphocellulose chromatography, appears normal. The amount of hormone-receptor complexes bound to nuclei, however, is mildly decreased and the proportion of activated receptor in intact cells reduced. Transformation of this patient's B-lymphocytes with the Epstein-Barr (EB)-virus leads to GR induction that is much less than that observed with cells obtained from normal controls (4).

It is interesting that although the affinity defect is consistently present in the severely affected propositus of this family, two mildly affected asymptomatic members appear to have GR affinity for dexamethasone in the low normal range. (We should note that small decreases in affinity might not be detected in our assay). The GR of these patients, however, like that of the propositus, also differs from normal in the presence of increased instability of the hormone-receptor complex during thermal activation, and by a decreased induction of GR by EB-virus transformation. Thus, the GR in patients with glucocorticoid resistance is abnormal and this may lead to the glucocorticoid hyporesponsiveness.

If we assume that the asymptomatic subjects represent the heterozygote state, then the clinical picture and the receptor findings can be explained by either the presence of receptor subunits or by an abnormality in putative cytosolic factors that may normally modify the cascade of events during glucocorticoid action. Such factors have been described in the guinea pig (inhibitors) (5) or in certain mouse strains resistant to induction of cleft-palate by glucocorticoids administered to the mother during pregnancy (6). Mixing of cytosol from patients with cytosol from controls has not demonstrated the presence of excess inhibitory factors or deficiency of positive modifiers in our patients.

GLUCOCORTICOID INSENSITITY OF NEW WORLD PRIMATES

Generalized Steroid Insensitivity

New World primates also have glucocorticoid insensitivity. They have markedly elevated plasma cortisol--both total and free concentrations--increased urinary free cortisol excretion, marked increases in plasma ACTH and β-endorphin and resistance of their hypothalamic-pituitary adrenal axis to dexamethasone (3,7). Despite their high plasma cortisol levels, there is no hypertension or sodium retention and, in fact, their plasma aldosterone concentrations are increased. The kidney aldosterone receptor in these animals crossreacts poorly with cortisol, explaining the absence of sodium retention (7).

In contrast to the patients with cortisol insensitivity, in whom the defect appears isolated to the glucocorticoid axis, the New World primates also have elevated plasma concentrations of progesterone, estrogen, androgen, aldosterone, and vitamin D, without any associated symptoms (7-11). This suggests that these species have generalized, compensated steroid hormone resistance, and that their mutation(s) concern(s) some factor(s) involved in more than one steroid hormone-receptor systems.

It is of interest that the cortisol-binding globulin in the New World primates has a decreased affinity for cortisol, in addition to being present in lower concentrations (12). This finding, and the poor affinity of kidney aldosterone receptor for cortisol are probable examples of adaptive evolution in response to the mutation(s) affecting the GR.

Glucocorticoid Receptor Studies

Similarly to the patients, the GR of these primates has a decreased affinity for glucocorticoids (3), the hormone-receptor complex is "thermolabile", and the receptor fails to be induced by EB-virus transformation. The molecular weight of the GR is also indistinguishable from that of the normal human. In addition, the thermal activation pattern of the receptor, examined after either *in vivo* (intact cell) or *in vitro* (cytosol) elevations of temperature, is similar to that of controls, as assessed by either phosphocellulose or DNA cellulose binding.

New World monkeys, in addition to the glucocorticoid receptor and mineralocorticoid receptor changes, have changes of other steroid receptors such as those of progesterone (8) and estrogen (9) and possibly of androgen and vitamin D. However, the examination of these systems is either still limited to cytosolic receptors, or preliminary and further studies are warranted.

Currently, no physiological or biochemical links associate phylogenetically the alterations of the the glucocorticoid-mineralocorticoid, sex steroid, and vitamin D receptor systems. Such parallel alterations could reflect some fundamental change in the chromatin proteins or DNA sequences, putatively involved in steroidal regulation of gene transcription and common (nonclass-specific) to the different steroid hormones.

REFERENCES

1. Chrousos GP, Vingerhoeds A, Brandon D, Eil C, Pugeat M, DeVroede M, Loriaux DL, Lipsett MB (1982) J Clin Invest 69:1261-1269

2. Chrousos GP, Vingerhoeds ACM, Loriaux DL, Lipsett MB (1983) J Clin Endocrinol Metab 56:1243-1245

3. Chrousos GP, Renquist D, Brandon D, Eil C, Cutler GB, Vigersky R, Loriaux DL, Lipsett MB (1982) Proc Natl Acad Sci USA 79:2036-2040

4. Tomita M, Chrousos GP, Brandon D, Ben-Or S, Foster C, DeVougn L, Taylor S, Loriaux DL, Lipsett MB (1984) Horm Metab Res (in press).

5. Kraft N, Hodgson AJ, Funder JW (1979) Endocrinology 104:344-349

6. Katsumata M, Baker MK, Goldman AS (1981) Biochem Biophys Acta 676:245-256

7. Chrousos GP, Renquist D, Brandon D, Tomita M, Loriaux DL, Lipsett MB, (1984) Endocrinology (in press).

8. Chrousos GP, Renquist D, Brandon D, Barnard D, Fowler D, Loriaux DL, Lipsett MB (1982) J Clin Endocr Metab 55:364-368

9. Chrousos GP, Brandon D, Renquist DM, Tomita M, Johnson E, Loriaux DL, Lipsett MB (1984) J Clin Endocrinol Metab 55:364-368

10. Pugeat M, Rocle B, Chrousos PG, Dunn JF, Lipsett MB, Nisula BC (1984) J Steroid Biochem 20:473-478

11. Shinki T, Shiina Y, Takahashi S, Tanioka Y, Koizumi H, Suda T (1983) Biochem Biophys Res Commun 114:452-456

12. Pugeat M, Chrousos GP, Loriaux DL, Brandon DD, Nisula B, Lipsett MB (1984) Endocrinology (in press).

© 1984 Elsevier Science Publishers B.V.
Endocrinology
F. Labrie, L. Proulx, eds.

GONADOTROPIN RECEPTORS ALTERATIONS IN DISEASE STATES: ANTIRECEPTOR ANTIBODIES IN THE GONADOTROPIN RESISTANT OVARY SYNDROME

EDUARDO H. CHARREAU

Instituto de Biología y Medicina Experimental. Obligado 2490, 1428 Buenos Aires, Argentina and School of Science Buenos Aires University, Argentina.

INTRODUCTION

The failure of end organs to respond properly to stimulation by a homologous hormone may be due to defects in receptor function or in catalytic mechanisms subsequent to the receptor.

Although a considerable amount of data on the physiology of the gonadotropin receptors has been accumulated, this knowledge has not yet been extensively apply to human diseases. This most likely due to the fact that while it has been possible to investigate some hormone receptors in peripheral blood components the investigation of gonadotropin receptors requires the use of ovarian and testicular biopsies. In this sense the relatively low binding capacity of the human gonads would require a large amount of tissue to perform the determination reliable.

However, as summarized by Davis et al. (1), there are a number of situations described in laboratory animals which allow us to interpret a variety of clinical situations in which gonadotropin receptors may be involved.

In the human, Rajaniemi et al. (2)have determined the number and characteristics of LH receptors in samples from cystic follicles obtained from wedge resections performed in patients with polycystic ovarian disease. In these patients the receptor level was only 50% of that found in the preovulatory follicles of the early follicular phase. Their results suggest, that the first step in the mechanism of LH action on the developing follicles, the binding of this hormone to the membrane receptor does not bassically deviate from normal in polycystic ovarian disease. However when compared with normally developing follicles, the number of receptors is decreased. These results are compatible with the suggestion that the derangement of follicular development and function in this disease is due to tonic excessive LH stimulation of the follicles too early in development leading to a decreased number of receptor for LH.

Is is clear that hormonal action can be modified by alterations in either receptor number or affinity, and that a variety of factors may regulate the hormone-receptor interaction.

In this sense, hormone resistance can arise from a variety of causes in which the development of antibodies to hormone receptors is included.

A search for antibodies to LH receptor in sera of 14 patients with premature ovarian failure carried out by Austin and associates (3) was unsuccessful. Similar results were observed by Tang and Faiman (4) in samples of women who had a previous diagnosis of premature ovarian failure. However serum from one of their patients, the only one who had associated autoimmune diseases (concomitant rheumatoid arthritis, Hashimoto's thyroiditis and vitiligo), resulted individually in the greatest inhibition of FSH receptor binding. This finding points toward the possible presence of an antireceptor antibody in this patient's serum.

A functional LH agonist and LH receptor antagonist has been reported in a preliminary communication by Caldwell et al. (5) in serum from one patient with premature ovarian failure.

Furthermore in a recent careful investigation Dias et al. (6) have reported FSH receptor antibodies in serum of a male patient with primary gonadal failure, polyostic fibrous dysplasia and IgM monoclonal gammopathy.

In this presentation I wish to review our studies (7-9) on the search for circulating factors against FSH receptors in patients with the "gonadotropin resistant ovary syndrome". This syndrome was first delineated as a distinct clinical entity by Jones and de Moraes-Reuhsen in 1969, in a study of three patients with primary amenorrhea (10). Since then, a number of additional patients with the same or similar disorder have been reported. This syndrome is extremely rare and the physiopathlogy is largely unknown.

The main clinical features are amenorrhea and infertility, gonadotropins are in the menopausal range where estrogens are low or low normal. The most striking feature of this syndrome is the developmental arrest of the ovarian follicles at the stage of primordial follicles despite the presence of high endogenous levels of gonadotropin or the administration of large amounts of exogenous gonadotropins.

Thus, the disorder could result either from an abnormal FSH molecule or from some factor that blocks the action of FSH.

There are no data available in regard to the concentration or the characteristics of FSH and LH receptors in these patients.

RESULTS AND DISCUSSION

The characterization of a circulating inhibitor of FSH receptor binding was carried out in four patients with hypergonadotropic amenorrhea and myasthenia gravis which fulfill the criteria of the resistant ovary syndrome.

Sera from twenty other patients with hypergonadotropic amenorrhea, including patients with lymphocytic thyroiditis and systemic lupus erythematosus as well as patients with myasthenia gravis and normal menses failed to show inhibitory activity on FSH binding.

The presence of biological inactive gonadotropins which would be determined by the radioimmunoassays used and which would inhibit the action of these tropins including the exogenous administrated, by blocking the common receptor sites was excluded, because we found a good correspondence between the bioassay and radioimmunoassays of gonadotropins in these patients. Similar results were described by Jones and de Moraes-Reuhsen (10), Koninckx and Brosens (11) and Starup and Pedersen (12).

One might think of several different inhibitors decreasing or preventing the effect of gonadotropins.

An obvious idea was the presence of gonadotropin antibodies. In the patients with the resistant ovary syndrome here presented, antibodies against FSH and LH were investigated with negative results by studying the binding activity of the sera for the iodinated gonadotropins.

We are therefore left with a third possibility, absence or non responsiveness of the target cells. For this reason immunoglobulins were precipitated from all sera studied using ammonium sulphate or 0-5% sodium sulphate saturation and tested for their inhibitory activity on FSH binding.

Immature rat testis seminiferous tubules membranes or detergent solubilized calf testis membranes were used as a source of FSH receptor for binding studies with ^{125}I-hFSH.

Significant inhibition of binding was only apparent in patients Z, V, N, and R (Percentage FSH specific binding: control: 98.3 $\pm$ 3 (SD); Z: 30.2 $\pm$ 4.1, V: 52.2 $\pm$ 2.1, N: 36.3 $\pm$ 1.2, R: 42.3 $\pm$ 4.5, P: 97.3 $\pm$ 7.2, G: 83.1 $\pm$ 2.5.

Patient P had myasthenia gravis but normal menses while patient G had hyper-gonadotropin amenorrhea without myasthenia gravis (representative example of fifteen sera tested).

When immunoglobulins from Z, V, N, and R sera were adsorbed on immature testicular tubule membranes, FSH inhibitory activity clearly diminished, however the exposure of these immunoglobulin fractions to interstitial tissue or prostatic tissue, cause no change in FSH binding inhibitory activity, suggesting a tissue specificity for the interaction of this component.

In addition, absorption of patients IgG fractions on membrane preparations from the electric organs of Torpedo did not modify the FSH binding inhibitory activity although it was accompanied by restauration of the ^{125}I- Bungarotoxin binding.

Furthermore, the circulating inhibitor present in Z, V, N, and R sera appeared to be an immunoglobulin by multiple criteria. DEAE cellulose chromatography of the sulphate precipitates showed two peaks. The firs peak was characterized as IgG by immunoglobulin antibodies and presented inhibitory activity of FSH binding in the radioreceptor assay.

The IgG fraction isolated from DEAE cellulose columns were submitted to an additional purification procedure by selective binding to protein A-Sepharose. While no inhibitory activity could be detected in supernatants (unbound proteins) a 34% inhibition was observed with proteins eluted from protein A. Two additional experiments confirmed the immunoglublin nature of the circulating inhibitor. Sucrose gradient centrifugation of the inhibitor, partially purified by DEAE cellulose chromatography showed a unique peak in which the FSH binding inhibitor could be demonstrated. This peak behaves as a 7S protein, running in a same gradient as the human gamma globulin marker.

When IgG fractions were submitted to specific immunoprecipitation with anti-human IgG, FSH binding inhibitory activity clearly diminished and no changes were observed in the behavior of the control IgG fraction after this treatment. In addition activity is retained in the $F(ab')_2$ fraction of pepsin digested IgG.

Reichert et al. (13) have demonstrated the presence of a low molecular weight binding inhibitor in normal serum. The binding inhibitor we are dealing with, appears to be essentially different, it behaves as an immunoglobulin and appears to be specifically associated with the presence of the gonadotropin resistant ovary syndrome. The four patients with FSH binding inhibitory activity also had *myasthenia gravis*, a known autoimmune disease. This alteration in the immune system with high levels of circulating immunoglobulins could be responsible for a "non specific" inhibition of FSH binding to its receptor. However, the absence of inhibition with the same amount of immunoglobulins from normal or serum fractions from patient with *myasthenia gravis* and normal menses or serum fractions from patients with other immunological diseases, made this an unlikely possibility.

Results of double reciprocal plot analysis obtained with different levels of immunoglobulins on the binding of ^{125}I-hFSH to membrane receptors, supported the view that they are tightly bound to the receptor itself or to a receptors related membrane domain with an apparent Ki of $2.94 \times 10^{12} M^{-1}$ a thousand times higher than the affinity constant for FSH receptor binding interaction. The plasma level of this antibody was estimated as 10^{-10}M.

The "irreversible" nature of this inhibitory effect could also explain why the ovarian resistance could not be overcame by high FSH circulating levels *in vivo*. Further evidences of the biological implication of the serum inhibitor was given by the *in vitro* alteration in the production of the seminiferous tubules androgen binding protein secretion and cAMP production when this tissue is incubated in the presence of IgG fraction from patients with the resistant ovary syndrome (9).

An intrinsic failure in target cell machinery or a receptor "down regulattion" phenomenon on the ovary due to the high circulating FSH levels can not be ruled out, nevertheless the presence of circulating antibodies to FSH receptors can explain the gonadotropin resistance in these patients.

An unsettled question is the range of different immune mechanisms that may operate in patients with autoimmune diseases. Although the FSH receptor is probably the target of the autoimmune process in the resistant ovary syndrome, it is likely that the specific immune mechanisms used, differ in individual cases.

The specific question of whether the circulating antibodies are instrumental in causing the receptor defect or merely represent a secondary response to receptor damage cause by some other agent, is of great importance in understanding the pathogenesis of this disease.

Antireceptor antibodies have been implicated in the pathogenesis of several diseases, such as Grave's disease, myasthenia gravis, insulin resistant with acanthosis nigricans, allergic rhinitis and asthma. The gonadotropin resistant ovary syndrome could be a new entity responding to a similar mechanism.

However, as mentioned by Dias et al. (6) the concomitant observation of primary gonadal failure and the presence of putative antibodies to FSH receptors are not sufficient to conclude a causal relationship.

ACKNOWLEDGMENTS

I gratefully acknowledge the collaboration of Drs. V.A. Chiauzzi, S.B. Cigorraga, M.E. Escobar and M.A. Rivarola, Mrs. A.R. de la Cámara and D.B. Destéfano.

REFERENCES

1. Davis TF, Dufau ML, Catt KJ (1978) Clinics in Obstetrics and Gynecology 5: 329-362.
2. Rajaniemi HJ, Ronnberg L, Kauppila A, Ylostalo P, Vihko R (1980) J Clin Endocrinol Metab 51: 1054-1057.
3. Austin GE, Coulam CB, Ryan RJ (1979) Mayo Clin Proc 54: 394-400
4. Tang VW, Faiman C (1983) Am J Obstet Gynecol 146: 816-821
5. Caldwell BV, Luborsky-Moore JL, Kase N, Behrman HR (1978) Abstracts of the Sixtieth Annual Meeting of the Endocrine Society, Miami p 199.
6. Dias JA, Gates SA, Reichert LE (1983) Fertility and Sterility 38: 330-338
7. Charreau EH, Cigorraga SB, Chiauzzi VA, Escobar ME, Rivarola MA (1980) In: Tozzini RI, Reeves G, Pineda RL (eds) Endocrine Physiopathology of the Ovary. Elsevier, North-Holland Biomedical Press, pp 191-205
8. Charreau EH, Chiauzzi VA, Cigorraga SB, Escobar ME, Rivarola ME (1982) In: Muldoon TG, Mahesh VB, Perez Ballester B (eds). Recent Advances in Fertility Research, Part A: Developments in Reproductive Endocrinology. Alan R. Liss, New York, pp 111-121

9. Chiauzzi VA, Cigorraga SB, Escobar ME, Rivarola MA, Charreau EH (1982) J Clin Endocrinol Metab 54: 1221-1228

10. Jones GS, de Moraes-Reuhsen M (1969) Ann J Obst and Gynec 104: 597-600.

11. Koninckx R, Brosens IA (1977) Fertility and Sterility 28: 926-931

12. Starup J, Pedersen H (1978) Acta Endocrinologica 89: 744-752

13. Reichert LE, Sanzo MA, Darga NS (1979) J Clin Endocrinol Metab 49: 866-872

44. Therapeutic Problems

Endocrinology
F. Labrie, L. Proulx, eds.

SILENT THYROIDITIS

THOMAS F. NIKOLAI, M.D.

Section of Endocrinology, Marshfield Clinic, 1000 N. Oak Ave., Marshfield, Wisconsin 54449 United States and the Marshfield Medical Foundation

In the past decade a new form of lymphocytic thyroiditis called silent thyroiditis has been described. It has also been called by other terms such as thyrotoxicosis with painless thyroiditis; silent, painless, atypical, or occult subacute thyroiditis; postpartum thyroiditis; hyperthyroiditis; lymphocytic thyroiditis with spontaneously resolving hyperthryoidism; and transient hyperthyroidism with lymphocytic thyroiditis. Although originally described as a silent or painless form of subacute granulomatous thyroiditis, more recently it has been shown to be a form of lymphocytic thyroiditis by multiple investigators. The cardinal features of this disease include a transient hyperthyroidism, elevated levels of serum T4 and T3, a suppressed radioactive iodine uptake, and lymphocytic thyroiditis on biopsy. This disease is usually first recognized by finding a suppressed radioactive iodine uptake in the patient who is thought to have hyperthyroidism of Graves' disease. Multiple episodes may occur in the same individual. About 10% of affected patients are found to have the disease in the immediate postpartum period, hence the term postpartum thyroiditis. Whether silent thyroiditis and postpartum thyroiditis are the same disease is not definitely established. However, they have the same clinical course and the pathology of the thyroid is the same in both.

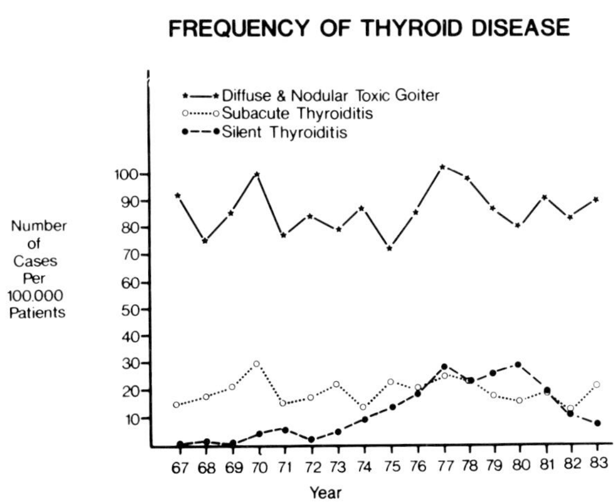

Fig. 1. Frequency of different forms of hyperthyroidism, 1967-1983.

The incidence of silent thyroiditis is unknown. A gradual increase in the observed frequency of silent thyroiditis from 1969 through 1980 compared to other causes of hyperthyroidism and subacute thyroiditis has occurred in central Wisconsin of the United States (Fig. 1). Silent thyroiditis has only been reported in the United States, Canada, Japan, and Sweden. Most of the cases reported in Canada and the United States come from around the Great Lakes area. Postpartum thyroiditis has been shown to have an incidence of 5-12% in three surveys reported in Japanese, American, and Swedish women. The male-to-female ratio of reported cases of silent thyroiditis is 1.5-2:1, somewhat lower than for most thyroid diseases. Cases have been found in all decades of life but most often occur in the middle ages.

Initial reports described silent thyroiditis as a silent or painless form of subacute granulomatous thyroiditis. This has since been disproved by multiple reports showing only lymphocytic thyroiditis by percutaneous core needle biopsy or fine needle biopsy of the thyroid. In addition, viral antibody titers which are often positive during the course of subacute thyroiditis are negative in silent thyroiditis.

Fifty percent of patients with a history of silent thyroiditis followed up one to ten years later have shown a persistence of or the development of antithyroid antibodies, thyroid enlargement, and/or permanent hypothyroidism. This rarely occurs in subacute thyroiditis. These findings suggest that silent thyroiditis is an early manifestation of chronic lymphocytic or Hashimoto's thyroiditis.

Thyroid histology in silent thyroiditis is quite variable ranging from focal lymphocytic infiltration and follicle disruption to extensive lymphocytic

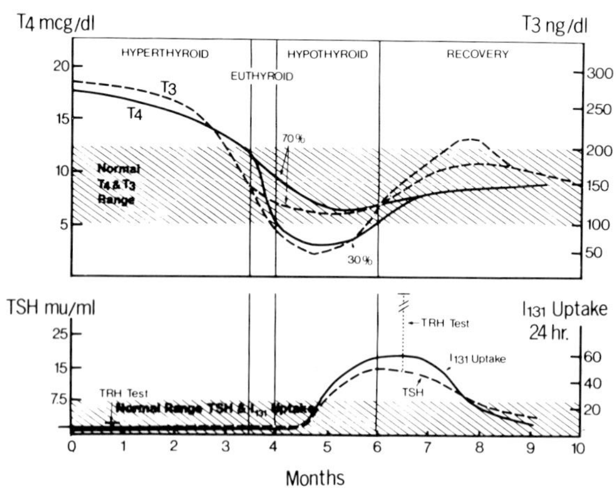

Fig. 2. Schematic representation of the course of silent thyroiditis.

infiltration, follicle disruption and collapse, and fibrosis. The finding of severe fibrosis, lymphoid follicles, and Askanazy cells characteristic of Hashimoto's thyroiditis are infrequently found or absent. However, our pathologists could not distinguish the histopathologic changes of silent thyroiditis from Hashimoto's thyroiditis when specimens from the two diseases were mixed.

The clinical course of silent thyroiditis is quite variable. About 10% of the patients are asymptomatic and are found by routine thyroid testing. The hyperthyroidism is usually of a mild-to-moderate degree although 20-30% of affected individuals have more severe hyperthyroidism causing moderate-to-severe disability. The signs and symptoms are those of classic hyperthyroidism but atrial fibrillation, angina pectoris, diffuse myalgias, muscle weakness, hypokalemia, periodic paralysis, and postpartum depression have been reported. The classic features of Graves' disease such as pretibial myxedema, exophthalmos, and acropachy do not occur. The majority of patients have enlarged thyroid glands up to two or three times normal size. The enlargement is usually symmetrical. The thyroid tissue is substantially firmer than normal. Silent thyroiditis has also been found in nodular thyroids and in single nodules and ectopic thyroid tissue. Thyroid pain and tenderness are infrequent and quite mild. The hypothyroidism that occurs in a recovery phase in about 30% of patients is usually transient. In postpartum thyroiditis only a hypothyroid phase may occur.

Thyroid function tests reflect the clinical course of the disease as outlined in Fig. 2. During the transient hyperthyroid phase the serum T4 and T3 are elevated and the radioactive iodine uptake, TSH, and TRH stimulation tests are suppressed. In the hypothyroid phase the serum T4 and T3 are decreased. The TSH, radioactive iodine uptake, and TRH stimulation tests gradually become normal during the latter part of the hypothyroid phase and may even become elevated reflecting recovery of the thyroid gland. Anti-microsomal and anti-thyroglobulin antibody levels are positive in 60% and 25% respectively of affected patients during the hyperthyroid phase. Those with higher thyroid antibodies appear to have a more severe disease and are more likely to have a hypothyroid phase. The sedimentation rate is elevated in only 50% of the patients, not above 50 mm./hour. This is another distinguishing feature from subacute thyroiditis as almost all patients with subacute thyroiditis with hyperthyroidism have sedimentation rates above 50 mm./hour.

The diagnostic features of silent thyroiditis are listed in Table I. They include clinical thyrotoxicosis with elevated serum T4 and T3 levels, a suppressed radioactive iodine uptake (below 3%), a non-tender thyroid (enlarged in only 50%), a negative history for intake of iodine-containing material or thyroid hormone, and lymphocytic thyroiditis on thyroid biopsy. The ratio of

TABLE I

DIAGNOSTIC FEATURES OF SILENT THYROIDITIS
1) Clinical hyperthyroidism
2) Non-tender thyroid gland
3) Elevated serum T4 and T3
4) Suppressed radioactive iodine uptake
5) Lymphocytic thyroiditis by biopsy
6) Negative history for iodine and thyroid hormone intake

TABLE II

CLASSIFICATION OF THYROTOXICOSIS ACCORDING TO RADIOACTIVE IODINE UPTAKE
Depressed Radioactive Iodine Uptake
1) Silent thyroiditis
2) Subacute granulomatous thyroiditis
3) Thyrotoxicosis due to excessive thyroid hormone intake
-- iatrogenic
-- factitious
4) Graves' disease with high iodine intake
5) Iodide-induced hyperthyroidism (jodbasedow's disease)
6) Metastatic follicular or papillary follicular carcinoma of the thyroid
7) Struma ovarii
Elevated Radioactive Iodine Uptake
1) Diffuse toxic goiter (Graves' disease)
2) Toxic multinodular goiter (Plummer's disease)
3) Toxic uninodular goiter (toxic adenoma)
4) Hashitoxicosis
5) Excessive TSH production
-- TSH-producing pituitary adenoma
-- metastatic trophoblastic tumor
-- TRH excess syndrome
-- selective pituitary resistance to thyroid hormone

serum T3 (ng./dl.) over serum T4 (mcg./dl.) has been used as an index for separating thyrotoxicosis of thyroiditis from that due to overproduction of thyroid hormone as in diffuse or multinodular toxic goiter. A ratio above 20 is frequently present when overproduction of thyroid hormone occurs because of excessive production of T3. However, this ratio is not sensitive enough to be used clinically.

As silent thyroiditis and Graves' hyperthyroidism often cannot be separated unless the radioactive iodine uptake is done, a new classification for thyrotoxicosis (Table II) has been developed which separates thyrotoxicosis due to low or suppressed radioactive iodine uptake from thyrotoxicosis due to elevated or normal radioactive iodine uptake.

Types of hyperthyroidism with low radioactive iodine uptake that are difficult to differentiate from silent thyroiditis are Graves' hyperthyroidism with acute iodide ingestion and iodine-induced thyrotoxicosis (Jodbasedow's disease). A history of excessive iodine intake and the finding of urinary excretion of inorganic iodide greater than 1000-1500 mcg./24 hours, or a serum inorganic iodide level of greater than 1.5 mcg./dl. are helpful in making this differentiation. Observation for one or two months probably is the best method of making the differentiation between these diseases. Factitious hyperthyroidism is very difficult to distinguish from silent thyroiditis. The combination of a high index of suspicion, a non-palpable thyroid gland, and the response of the thyroid to exogenous TSH stimulation will help here.

Unless silent thyroiditis is recognized, inappropriate treatment such as that for Graves' hyperthyroidism may result. Once recognized, therapy should be individualized. In those patients with mild hyperthyroidism, observation or treatment with mild sedatives, tranquilizers, or beta-blocking agents are sufficient. Corticosteroid therapy has been shown to dramatically shorten the course of hyperthyroidism to 7-10 days. Thiourea therapy is not effective in the hyperthyroid phase.

About 10-15% of patients have recurring episodes of transient hyperthyroidism with up to five and six episodes seen in a few patients. Radioactive iodine (I-131) ablation of the thyroid and thyroidectomy can be used in those who continue to have recurrences. As 50% of the patients have been shown to develop goiters and/or hypothyroidism on long-term follow up, patients who have had an episode of silent thyroiditis should have thyroid evaluation at 1-2 year intervals.

REFERENCES

1. Nikolai TF, Brosseau J, Kettrick MA et al (1980) Arch Intern Med 140:478
2. Nikolai TF, Coombs GJ, McKenzie AK (1981) Arch Intern Med 141:1455
3. Woolf PD (1980) Endocr Rev 1:411
4. Amino N, Mori H, Iwatani Y et al (1982) N Engl J Med 306:849
5. Nikolai TF, Coombs GJ, McKenzie AK, Beltaos E (1982) Arch Intern Med 142:2281

© 1984 Elsevier Science Publishers B.V.
Endocrinology
F. Labrie, L. Proulx, eds.

THYROID HORMONE RESISTANCE

BRUCE D. WEINTRAUB, MARGARIDA MENEZES-FERREIRA, PATRICIA PETRICK, CHARLES EIL, and PAOLO BECK-PECCOZ
NIADDK, National Institutes of Health, Bethesda, Maryland, USA

Thyroid hormone resistance refers to a heterogeneous group of sporadic or familial syndromes in which patients demonstrate variable degrees of refractoriness to the action of endogenous or exogenous thyroid hormones. Refetoff et al. (1,2) initially reported a family in which 3 of 6 children demonstrated deaf-mutism, delayed bone maturation and stippled epiphyses, goiter, elevated total and free serum T_4 and T_3, and elevated ^{131}I uptake. Despite elevated thyroid hormone levels, these patients displayed no clinical features of hyperthyroidism and also failed to respond to large exogenous doses of T_4 or T_3. These patients also demonstrated pituitary resistance to thyroid hormone, with inappopriately normal or elevated TSH in the face of elevated serum free T_4 and T_3. Since this initial description a number of other cases of generalized resistance to the action of thyroid hormone have been reported (3-5). Most of the cases have been familial but sporadic cases have also been described. In the familial cases both autosomal recessive and autosomal dominant patterns of inheritance have been suggested, with variable expression of the disease in affected members of the same family (3-5).

It was subsequently recognized that certain patients appeared to have selective pituitary resistance to the action of thyroid hormone. Gershengorn and Weintraub (6) initially described a patient with elevated free T_4 and T_3 and inappropriately elevated TSH in the basal state and a marked TSH response to TRH. However, unlike patients with generalized resistance to thyroid hormone, this patient displayed clear clinical and biochemical features of peripheral hyperthyroidism. Moreover exogenous T_3 caused only a partial suppression of TSH and increased peripheral hyperthyroidism. Many additional sporadic cases of selective pituitary resistance have been reported (5), as well as one familial description of six affected females in three generations (7). In addition a single case of selective peripheral but not pituitary resistance to the action of thyroid hormone was recently reported by Kaplan et al. (8).

These syndromes of thyroid hormone resistance are believed to result from one or more cellular defects in the action, transport or metabolism of T_4 and/or T_3. However, despite a number of studies the molecular basis of these disorders has not yet been elucidated. In particular, studies of equilibrium T_3 binding to its nuclear receptor have been highly variable with minimal or no differences in patients compared to controls. We have recently observed that fibroblasts from patients with generalized resistance display kinetic abnormalities in $[^{125}I]T_3$ nuclear uptake, and that such a method may be more powerful than equilibrium analysis for establishing the diagnosis in cultured cells (10). Such abnormalities have not elucidated the primary cellular defect, and could result from either abnormalities intrinsic to the T_3 nuclear receptor, as suggested by certain investigators (11), or from abnormalities of thyroid hormone transport, as suggested by others (12). Finally, it must be stressed that thyroid hormone resistance may emerge as a heterogeneous disease with different primary mechanisms in different cases or families.

Patients with generalized or selective pituitary resistance must be distinguished from those with TSH-secreting pituitary tumors, who also display inappropriately measurable or elevated serum levels of TSH in the face of increased total and free serum thyroid hormone, a syndrome we have termed "inappropriate secretion of TSH" (5-6). Other conditions may be confused with inappropriate secretion of TSH, as listed in Table I. Although none show all features of the syndrome, certain laboratory tests (indicated in parentheses) may be similar.

TABLE I

CONDITIONS CONFUSED WITH INAPPROPRIATE SECRETION OF TSH

1. Methodologic Interference
    A. Serum anti-rabbit IgG or anti-bovine TSH antibodies (TSH)
    B. Serum anti-iodothyronine antibodies (TT_4, TT_3, FT_4, FT_3)
2. Increase in Normal Serum Iodothyronine Binding Proteins (TT_4, TT_3)
3. Abnormal Serum T_4 Binding Proteins (TT_4, FT_4)
4. Treated Hypothyroid Patients Prior to Equilibrium (TT_4, TT_3, FT_4, FT_3, TSH)
5. Neonatal Period (TT_4, FT_4, TSH)
6. Inhibition of Peripheral T_4 to T_3 Conversion (TT_4, FT_4, TSH).

Once the above conditions are excluded, the distinction between neoplastic and nonneoplastic conditions causing inappropriate secretion of TSH is determined by a constellation of clinical, biochemical and radiological criteria as indicated in Table II. The most useful discriminator between neoplastic and nonneoplastic TSH production is measurement of the serum free alpha subunit (5).

TABLE II

CLINICAL AND LABORATORY FEATURES OF PATIENTS WITH INAPPROPRIATE SECRETION OF TSH

Parameter	Pituitary Adenoma	Thyroid Hormone Resistance	
		Isolated Pituitary	Generalized
Occurrence	sporadic	sporadic > familial	familial > sporadic
Metabolic status	hyperthyroid	hyperthyroid	hypo - or euthyroid

Goiter	present	present	present
Thyroid hormones	increased	increased	increased
TSH, basal	increased	increased	increased
TSH response to TRH	minimal increase	marked increase	marked increase
Alpha subunit	increased	normal	normal
Pituitary mass	usually present	normal	normal
TSH suppression by:			
thyroid hormones	minimal or none	yes	yes
dopamine agonists	minimal or none	yes	yes
glucocorticoids	yes	yes	yes

The optimal therapy for patients with inappropriate secretion of TSH rests on accurate diagnosis. Because the occurrence of this syndrome is uncommon there has been limited experience in the treatment of both neoplastic and nonneoplastic diseases. Moreover the reports are primarily anecdotal in nature, and there have been no controlled trials of different therapeutic approaches. A variety of therapeutic modalities have been employed as shown in Table III (our preferences are underlined).

TABLE III
THERAPEUTIC MODALITIES FOR PATIENTS WITH INAPPROPRIATE SECRETION OF TSH

Treatment	Pituitary Adenoma	Thyroid Hormone Resistance	
		Isolated Pituitary	Generalized
Surgical	<u>Transsphenoidal microsurgery</u>	Thyroidectomy	Not indicated
	Transfrontal craniotomy		
Irradiation	Conventional supervoltage	^{131}I	Not indicated
	Proton beam and Heavy Particle		
Pharmacologic	Dopamine agonists	<u>Dopamine agonists</u>	<u>T_4 or T_3</u>
	Corticosteroids	T_3	
	Somatostatin	Somatostatin	
	Thyroid hormone analogs	<u>Thyroid hormone analogs</u>	
	Beta-adrenergic blockers	Beta-adrenergic blockers	
	Antithyroid drugs	Antithyroid drugs	

Patients with TSH-secreting pituitary tumors should be treated with transsphenoidal surgery when possible, and a selective adenomectomy is most desirable. Patients with selective pituitary resistance are best treated with agents that selectively suppress TSH. Dopamine agonists such as bromocriptine and pergolide generally suppress TSH to some extent, but restoration of euthyroidism has been more difficult to achieve. A promising new approach is the use of thyroid hormone analogs that demonstrate selective pituitary action *in vivo*. Recently Beck-Peccoz et al. (13) reported successful treatment of a patient resistant to bromocriptine with 3,5,3' triiodothyroacetic acid (TRIAC), which caused TSH suppression and restoration of euthyroidism. Patients with the unusual familial type of selective pituitary resistance have responded to small doses of exogenous T_3 with restoration of euthyroidism (7). However, we have not observed such a response in the more common sporadic cases. Although some patients with generalized resistance may be well compensated and not require exogenous thyroid hormone, we believe that most cases should be treated. This is particularly important in children who may require further elevations in serum thyroid hormone to assure normal intellectual and physical development. Certain patients show enhanced cardiac response compared to other tissues, and these can be treated with a combination of thyroid hormone and beta-adrenergic blockers.

With the greater availability of sensitive and specific TSH radioimmunoassays, increasing numbers of these patients are being recognized. The question of routine measurement of serum TSH in patients with hyperthyroidism associated with diffuse goiter, elevated ^{131}I uptake, and no features of Graves' Disease, is beyond the scope of this discussion and relates to complicated issues of cost-effectiveness. Nonetheless, all endocrinologists should be familiar with these syndromes, since recognition of affected patients is important clinically and will certainly provide basic insights into the action of thyroid hormone.

REFERENCES

1. Refetoff S, Dewind LT, DeGroot LJ (1967) J Clin Endocrinol Metab 27:279
2. Refetoff S, DeGroot LJ, Bernard B, Dewind LT (1972) Metabolism 21:723
3. Refetoff S, (1982) Am J Physiol 243:E88
4. Lamberg B-A, Liewendahl K (1980) Ann Clin Res 12:243
5. Weintraub BD, Gershengorn MC, Kourides IA, Fein H (1981) Ann Int Med 95:339
6. Gershengorn MC, Weintraub BD (1975) J Clin Invest 56:633
7. Rosler A, Litvin Y, Hage C, Gross J, Cerasi E (1982) J Clin Endocrinol Metab 54:76
8. Kaplan MM, Swartz SL, Larsen PR (1981 Am J Med 70:1115
9. Eil C, Fein HG, Smith TJ, Furlanetto RW, Bourgeois M, Stelling MW, Weintraub BD (1982) J Clin Endocrinol Metab 55:502
10. Menezes-Ferreira MM, Eil C, Wortsman J, Weintraub BD (1983) Endocrinol 113 (suppl): T_7 (Abstract)
11. Bernal J, Refetoff S, DeGroot LJ (1978) J Clin Endocrinol Metab 47:1266
12. Wortsman J, Premachandra BN, Williams K, Burman KD, Hay IA, Davis PJ (1983) Ann Int Med 98:904
13. Beck-Peccoz P, Piscitelli G, Cattaneo MG, Faglia G (1983) J Endocrinol Invest 6:217

Endocrinology
F. Labrie, L. Proulx, eds.

THERAPEUTIC DECISION-MAKING IN ASYMPTOMATIC HYPERCALCEMIA AND PRIMARY HYPERPARATHYROIDISM

H. HEATH III
Endocrine Research Unit, Mayo Clinic, Mayo Foundation, and Mayo Medical School, Rochester, Minnesota, 55905, (USA)

BACKGROUND

The real dilemma in primary hyperparathyroidism (1°HPT) today is not how to diagnose it or how to treat it, but whether to detect and treat it at all. The wide use of automated chemical analyzers has transformed 1°HPT from a rare disease severely affecting the bones, kidneys, and other organs, to a common one [25 cases per 100,000 population annually in Western countries (1)] that is often asymptomatic. Most cases are now found by "screening" of serum calcium, and half or more are asymptomatic or have no unequivocal complications.

The diagnosis of 1°HPT is no longer a difficult exercise with proper use of history, physical examination, and readily-available laboratory tests, including selective use of parathyroid hormone assays (2). I have detailed elsewhere an approach to diagnosis (1). In about half of diagnosed cases, the decision to treat is easy, because of disease severity, symptoms, or complications. Physician anxiety seems highest in the "asymptomatic" remainder. A distinction must be maintained between asymptomatic persons who have no detectable adverse effects of the disease, and those who are asymptomatic yet have medically detectable complications of the disease (1). Since severe urolithiasis, renal failure, and hyperparathyroid bone disease are now uncommon (3), attention has turned recently to other possible adverse effects of 1°HPT, such as osteopenia, arterial hypertension, and psychological problems.

THE SKELETON IN PRIMARY HYPERPARATHYROIDISM

Dauphiné, et al. (4) found the prevalence of vertebral crush fracture to be several-fold increased in hyperparathyroid patients. The basis for this may be abnormal bone loss. Several groups have found significantly decreased bone density or mass in 1°HPT (5-11). Sites manifesting osteopenia included the hands, forearm, lumbar spine, proximal femurs, calcanei, and total body. Techniques included neutron activation (5), radiography (6), single photon absorptiometry (7-11), dual photon absorptiometry (10), and computed tomography (11). The cause of bone loss in primary hyperparathyroidism is probably parathyroid hormone excess [possibly compounded by failure to raise plasma levels of calcitonin (12)] that stimulates osteoclastic bone resorption.

While it is almost inarguable that 1°HPT causes bone loss, several urgent questions remain. Is the loss sufficient to cause clinical osteoporosis and fractures? Dauphiné, et al. (4) suggest that it does, but confirmatory evidence from prospective studies is needed. Can osteopenia be prevented medically? Estrogen therapy (13,14) might be of value in selected cases, but the long-term effects on bone are unknown. Does osteopenia remit when 1°HPT is cured? One doubts it, and suggests that prevention may be more feasible than reversal. Postmenopausal women are most likely to acquire 1°HPT, and most likely to develop osteoporosis. For this reason, the risk of osteopenia deserves serious consideration in decision-making about treatment of "mild" 1°HPT.

HYPERTENSION IN HYPERPARATHYROIDISM

Older studies suggesting that arterial hypertension was common in 1°HPT were suspect because so many of the patients had renal failure. However, it is now clear that raised blood pressure is strongly associated with this disease. Our epidemiogic study found a relative risk of about 2.0 for hypertension in a population-based group of hyperparathyroid subjects (15). Christensson, et al. (16) showed significantly higher blood pressure in 68 persons found by ambulatory health screening to be hyperparathyroid than in age- and sex-matched controls. Nainby-Luxmore, et al. (17) reported a similar case-comparison study, and found 1°HPT to be associated with a shift of blood pressure upward by about 15/20 mm Hg. Studies of pathogenesis have been inconclusive. It is also unclear whether treatment of 1°HPT ameliorates the hypertension; available evidence is discouraging.

PSYCHOLOGIC AND OTHER SYMPTOMS

Various reports suggest improved mental and physical well-being in elderly patients with 1°HPT after surgical cure (e.g., 20,21). My colleagues and I can recite similar antecdotes, but hard evidence is unavailable to support these concepts. For the present, I am convinced from clinical experience that even "mild" 1°HPT can cause a variety of puzzling symptoms that remit upon cure of the disease. Sometimes an operation provides the only answer.

SUMMARY

1°HPT often presents with clear indications for treatment (urolithiasis, etc.). In the remainder of cases, more subtle adverse effects are still possible. Clearly, "asymptomatic" disease can be nonetheless harmful. The major candidate adverse effects are osteopenia, hypertension, and various psychologic and somatic complaints. Whether these are benefited by treatment of 1°HPT is unproved, but intuitively, one thinks they should be. We are left with a cost-benefit equation containing an excess of undefinable variables.

Treat, or follow (20,21)? One can lay down no laws, but I believe that well-documented 1°HPT generally deserves surgical treatment. In the meantime, research is needed to more clearly define the long-term risks of the disease and allow us to better figure the cost-benefit equation in a given case.

REFERENCES

1. Heath H III, Purnell DC (1982) In: Heath DA, Marx SJ (eds) Butterworth's International Medical Reviews, Clinical Endocrinology. 2. Calcium Disorders. pp 189-216

2. Heath H III (1984) ENDO, Am Assoc Clin Chem 2:1-10

3. Scholz DA, Purnell DC (1981) Mayo Clin Proc 56:473-478

4. Dauphiné RT, Riggs BL, Scholz DA (1975) Ann Intern Med 83:365-367

5. Cohn SH, Roginsky MS, Aloia JF, Ellis KJ, Shukla KK (1973) J Clin Endocrinol Metab 36:750-755

6. Genant HK, Heck LL, Lanzl LH, Rossmann K, Vander Horst J, Paloyan E (1973) Radiology 109:513-524

7. Dalen N, Hjern B (1974) Acta Endocrinologica 75:297-304

8. Pak CYC, Stewart A, Kaplan R, Bone H, Notz C, Browne R (1975) Lancet 2:7-8

9. Tougaard L, Hau C, Rodbro P, Ditzel J (1977) Acta Endocrinologica 84:314-319

10. Seeman E, Wahner HW, Offord KP, Kumar, R, Johnson WJ, Riggs, BL (1982) J Clin Invest 69:1302-1309

11. Pozzi-Mucelli RS, Kanter AS, Genant HK, Cann CE, Ettinger B, Kolb FD (1983) J Comput Assist Tomogr 7:555

12. Lambert PW, Heath H III, Sizemore GW (1979) J Clin Invest 63:602-608

13. Gallagher JC, Nordin BEC (1972) Lancet 1:503-507

14. Marcus R, Madvig P, Crim M, Pont A, Kosek J (1984) Ann Int Med 100:633-640

15. Heath H, Hodgson SF, Kennedy MA (1980) N Engl J Med 302:189-193

16. Christensson T, Hellstrom K, Wengle B (1977) Eur J Clin Invest 7:109-113

17. Nainby-Luxmoore JC, Langford HG, Nelson NC, Watson RL, Barnes TY (1982) J Clin Endocrinol Metab 55:303-306

18. Alveryd A, Bostrom H, Wengle B, Wester PO (1976) Acta Chir Scand 142:491-494

19. Peskin GW, Greenburg AG, Salk RP (1978) Am J Surg 136:45-48

20. Hodgson SF, Heath H III (1981) Mayo Clin Proc 56:521-522

21. Van't Hoff W, Ballardie FW, Bicknell EJ (1983) Br Med J 287:1605-1608

© 1984 Elsevier Science Publishers B.V.
Endocrinology
F. Labrie, L. Proulx, eds.

ANTIANDROGEN TREATMENT OF ACNE

FRIEDMUND NEUMANN, SEMIRAMIS AYDINLIK, AND URSULA LACHNIT-FIXSON
Research Laboratories of Schering AG Berlin (West) and Bergkamen, Federal Republic of Germany

Sebaceous gland function and sebocyte proliferation is androgen-dependent, as has been shown in numerous studies using different models. All the important enzymes of androgen biosynthesis have been demonstrated in the skin. For example, the skin and its appendages are able to synthesize active androgens from biologically inactive or less active precursor molecules. Studies using the Costovertebral gland of hamsters have revealed specific dihydrotestosterone binding receptors in the cytosol as well as in the nuclear fraction. It is also known that increased sebaceous gland function is the most important factor in the etiology of acne.

Excessive keratinization of the infrainfundibulum - a process which is also androgen-dependent to a certain degree - followed by comedo formation and bacterial infection are secondary events.

There is a relationship between the sebum secretion rate and the severity of acne.

Basing on this knowledge, it was natural to use antiandrogens for the treatment of this disease. The antiandrogen which has been developed and which is available in Europe and several other countries for the treatment of androgen-induced or mediated disorders of the skin such as acne, seborrhoea, hirsutism, and androgenetic alopecia is cyproterone acetate.

Cyproterone acetate (CPA) is a steroid hormone having 3 main properties: It is antiandrogenic, it is a quite potent progestogen and it inhibits gonadotropin secretion. CPA is not androgenic at any dose and is not estrogenic. It does, however, have some glucocorticoid-like effects in rodents (but not in women) when given in high doses. As regards the molecular mechanism of action, CPA competes with androgens (dihydrotestosterone) for cytosol receptor sites and inhibits the translocation of the androgen receptor complex into the nucleas.

Principally, this antiandrogen affects all androgen-dependent organs and functions.

For the disease under discussion (acne), the effect on sebaceous gland function is most important.

The inhibitory effect of CPA on sebaceous glands has been demonstrated in several models using species such as mice, rats, hamsters and gerbils and, of course, also in men and women. Figure 1 gives only one example. It is interesting that the main metabolite, 15-OH-CPA, is even more active than the parent compound.

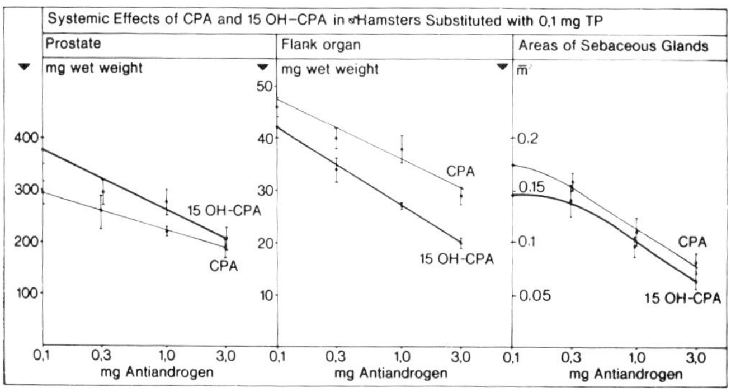

Fig.1. Effect of three weeks' systemic administration of cyproterone acetate (CPA) and its main metabolite, 15-hydroxyprogesterone acetate (15-OH-CPA), on the weight of the prostata and flank organ and on the size of the sebaceous gland areas in the ear of castrated male hamsters under replacement with 0.1 mg/day/animal s.c. testosterone propionate.

For the use of CPA in the treatment of acne (and other androgen-mediated disorders of the skin), the activity pattern of this anti-androgen is of paramount importance. Because CPA is a potent antiandrogen and a potent progestogen as well, it was possible to develop a preparation comparable to an oral contraceptive, but with a therapeutic effect. This preparation (Diane^{R}) contains 2 mg CPA and 50 µg ethinylestradiol.

The following tables (1 and 2) show the results of a multicentric phase III study with a total of 12,228 treatment cycles. No pregnancy occurred during the period of treatment. The cycle control (bleeding abnormalities) is excellent (Table 1), the therapeutic effect is convincing (Table 2), even in patients with severe acne of several years' standing who had not responded to other therapeutic regimens (antibiotics, benzoyl peroxyde, glucocorticoids).

TABLE I

INTERMENSTRUAL BLEEDINGS UNDER TREATMENT WITH DIANE[R] IN 1.354 WOMEN

Event	No. of treated cycles*	(%)
No intermenstrual bleeding	11.350	(92.8)
Breakthrough bleeding	243	(2.0)
Spotting	543	(4.4)
Spotting and breakthrough bleeding	92	(0.8)
Total	12.228	(100)

*No. tabl. omitted

TABLE II

THERAPEUTIC EFFECTIVENESS OF DIANE[R]

Disease	Localization	% Healing/ Improvement
Moderate acne	Face	93
	Décolleté	94
	Back	95
Moderate seborrhoea	Oily skin	92
	Oily scalp	91
	Dandruff	86
Moderate hirsutism	Face	70
	Bust	50
	Abdomen	50
	Legs	55

This preparation is well tolerated and has a beneficial effect on the lipoprotein pattern (increase of HDL). The side effects are (with one exception) qualitatively and quantitatively comparable with the side effects of other oral contraceptives.

Table 3 shows the time needed for the excepted effects of Diane[R] treatment to appear.

TABLE III

TIME TABLE FOR EXPECTED EFFECTS OF DIANE^R TREATMENT

Seborrhoea	Pronounced improvement after 2-3 cycles, normalization after the 4th cycle
Pronounced acne vulgaris	Improvement after 3-4 cycles
Alopecia androgenetica	Improvement only after 9 cycles at the earliest
Facial hirsutism	Reduction after 6-10 cycles
Hirsutism (non-facial)	Marked improvement generally only after the additional administration of cyproterone acetate (Androcur^R)

Since recently, we have preliminary clinical data from a multicentral double blind study with a preparation containing a lower estrogen dose. This preparation contains 2 mg cyproterone acetate and only 35 µg ethinylestradiol.

As regards the therapeutic effectiveness and cycle control, there are no significant differences between Diane® and this preparation. However, the early manifestation of therapeutic effectiveness was more pronounced with the reduced version.

Also, under estrogen reduced preparation estrogen dependent complaints were less common than with Diane®.

CONCLUSIONS

Diane^R is a potent hormonal preparation for acne therapy which is widely used in Europe and other countries. Some side effects are less frequent with the new preparation containing only 35 µg ethinylestradiol in combination with 2 mg CPA.

REFERENCES

1. Hammerstein J, Lachnit-Fixson U., Neumann F, Plewig G (eds) (1980). Androgenization in women. Acne, seborrhoea, androgenetic alopecia and hirsutism. Lectures and discussion of a symposium, Berlin, 23th-24th February, 1979. Excerpta Medica, Amsterdam
2. Molinatti GM, Martini L, James VHT (eds) (1983). Androgenization in women. Raven Press, New York
3. Volkaer R, Fanta D (eds) (1981). Combined antiandrogen-estrogen therapy in dermatology. Proc. of the Diane symposium, Brussels, 11th September, 1980. Excerpta Medica, Amsterdam

45. Neurohypophysial Peptides

Endocrinology
F. Labrie, L. Proulx, eds.

THE MOLECULAR BASIS OF NEUROHYPOPHYSEAL HORMONE EXPRESSION

DIETMAR RICHTER, HARTWIG SCHMALE, RICHARD IVELL & MONIKA REHBEIN

Institut fur Physiologische Chemie, Abteilung Zellbiochemie, Universitat Hamburg, 2000 Hamburg 20, Martinistr. 52, FRG.

INTRODUCTION

The biosynthesis of the related neurohypophyseal hormones vasopressin and oxytocin has been traced from the level of the genome in the magnocellular neurones of the hypothalamus through to release of the physiological peptides by neurosecretory nerve endings in the posterior pituitary. Although a number of details remain to be clarified, the biosynthetic pathway for both hormones is now defined and involves the prior synthesis of composite precursors. In addition to vasopressin and oxytocin, each precursor also includes a neurophysin polypeptide which is thought to play a carrier or protective role in helping the hormones to reach intact their site of release in the posterior pituitary. The vasopressin, but not the oxytocin precursor contains additionally a glycoprotein moiety at its C-terminus.

THE VASOPRESSIN AND OXYTOCIN GENES AND THEIR DERIVED HORMONE PRECURSORS

Isolation and sequencing of DNA complementary to the specific mRNAs encoding oxytocin and vasopressin (1,2), provided the key with which it was possible to identify and characterize the genes for the two hormones (3-5). DNA hybridization analysis indicates that each gene appears to exist in only a single copy. The two genes are clearly homologous both in sequence and in organization, confirming their derivation from a common ancestral gene, probably early in vertebrate evolution. Each comprises three exons separated by intervening sequences (Fig.1), each exon encoding one of the principal functional units of the hormone precursor.

The first exon encodes the hormone, either vasopressin or oxytocin, preceded by a signal peptide which directs the whole precursor into the endoplasmic reticulum and the secretory pathway. It also encodes the first few variable amino acids of the neurophysin molecule associated with the hormone during neurosecretion. The 5' untranslated region of the genes, which precedes the protein-coding region is completely non-homologous between the two genes; since this region is thought to be important for the regulation of transcription it would emphasize the independent regulatory control of the vasopressin and oxytocin genes.

The second exon encodes the central 67 amino acids of the neurophysin polypeptides. The DNA for this highly conserved

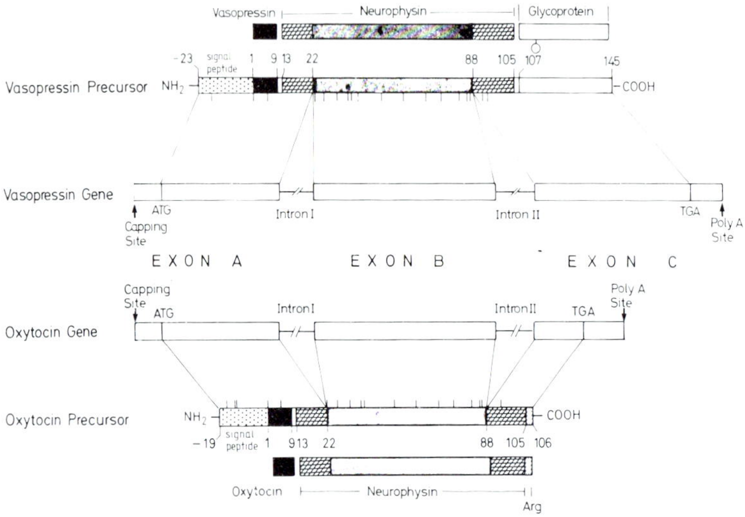

Fig. 1. Comparison of the vasopressin and oxytocin genes from the rat and their protein products.

sequence is so closely homologous between the oxytocin and vasopressin genes that a "gene conversion" must be invoked as explanation. Although still poorly understood, gene conversion appears to act via mutual recombination or correction between closely related gene sequences on the same or different chromosomes, so as to ensure conservation of an important DNA sequence (6). This observation tends to strengthen the argument that the neurophysins may well have an additional function besides their role as carrier proteins.

The third exon in both genes begins by encoding the variable C-terminus of the neurophysins, but whereas in the oxytocin gene this is followed by a stop codon to denote the end of the precursor, the vasopressin gene encodes an additional polypeptide moiety of 39 amino acids which is glycosylated and whose function is not yet known. Interestingly, the oxytocin gene predicts an extra basic amino acid residue following immediately after the known neurophysin sequence. This basic amino acid corresponds precisely with the cleavage signal separating the neurophysin and glycoprotein in the vasopressin precursor. Could it be that the ancestral oxytocin gene also possessed the C-terminal glycoprotein, but that following gene duplication the DNA sequence encoding the glycoprotein DNA was discarded leaving the terminal basic amino acid in this precursor as a rudiment of the ancestral cleavage signal?

With DNA probes specific for either hormone precursor in hand, it is now possible to study their regulation. So far our data show that in rats put under osmotic stress the level of mRNA encoding the vasopressin precursor is differently affected depending on the hypothalamic region studied. The mRNA levels increased 5-fold and 2-fold over the control animals in the supraoptic and paraventricular nuclei, respectively whereas no stimulation was observed in the suprachiasmatic nuclei (J.P. Burbach, M.J. De Hoop, E.R. De Kloet, H. Schmale and D. Richter, submitted). It is not yet clear whether the osmotic stress directly acts on the expression of the vasopressin gene or whether the different levels of mRNA are due to different RNA degrading activities. It would be extremely interesting to find other physiological parameters which may affect specifically the vasopressin mRNA level in the suprachiasmatic nuclei whose neurons project to other brain areas.

POST-TRANSLATIONAL PROCESSING OF THE COMPOSITE PRECURSORS

The genes predict that oxytocin and vasopressin are synthesized as parts of longer composite precursor polypeptides, so-called polyproteins. The structure of these polyproteins has been independently elucidated by in vitro translation of hypothalamic mRNA (7) as well as by in vivo pulse chase experiments (8). Processing of the polyproteins involves firstly removal of the N-terminal signal sequence accompanying transit of the nascent precursor into the endoplasmic reticulum. Subsequently, in the Golgi and in the neurosecretory granules, the hormones are cleaved from their neurophysins and the C-terminal glycopeptide of the vasopressin precursor is set free. Precisely where and in what order these events occur is still not clear; results of translating hypothalamic mRNA in frog oocytes suggest that different sets of enzymes are involved, one recognizing pairs of basic amino acids and subsequently the glycine residue involved in C-terminal hormone amidation, the other recognizing particular single basic amino acids such as that between neurophysin and glycoprotein (7).

THE GENETIC BASIS OF HEREDITARY DIABETES INSIPIDUS IN BRATTLEBORO RATS

The Brattleboro rat has autosomically inherited diabetes insipidus attributable to a deficiency in the hormone vasopressin. Not only does this strain lack vasopressin but the corresponding neurophysin and the glycoprotein are also absent (9,10).

To analyze this defect the vasopressin gene was isolated from Brattleboro genomic DNA and the sequence determined (11). Comparison with the vasopressin gene from normal rats indicated that the genes were identical except for a single nucleotide deletion in the second exon (Fig. 2).

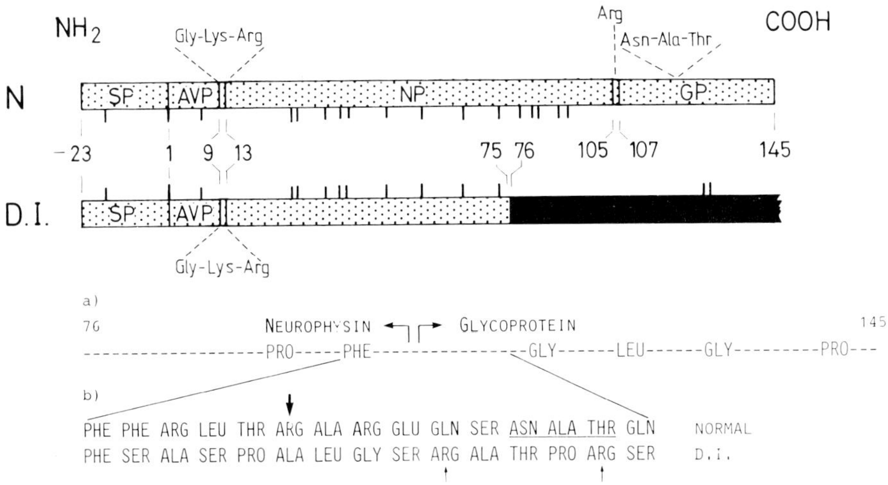

Fig. 2. Vasopressin precursor structures deduced from the gene sequences of normal and diabetes insipidus (Brattleboro) rat. For details see ref. 11.

This base deletion has as consequence:

(i) that all the protein-coding DNA in the 3′ direction of the point mutation is frame-shifted by one base, predicting therefore a precursor with a C-terminus completely different from that in normal rats (Fig. 2);

(ii) that, although the mutant mRNA is correctly transcribed and spliced, it has no stop codon: polysomes once formed, probably remain jammed on the mRNA, with the result that protein synthesis of this altered precursor could be inhibited;

(iii) although the vasopressin nonapeptide is correctly encoded, the C-terminal part of the neurophysin carrier is not, and hence subsequent processing and packaging of the hormone is also likely to be influenced.

Thus, although vasopressin mRNA is produced in Brattleboro hypothalami, it appears neither in vitro nor in vivo to yield a detectable translation product.

EXPRESSION OF THE OXYTOCIN AND VASOPRESSIN GENES IN PERIPHERAL TISSUES

The synthesis of both vasopressin and oxytocin has recently been shown to occur also in cells other than the hypothalamic

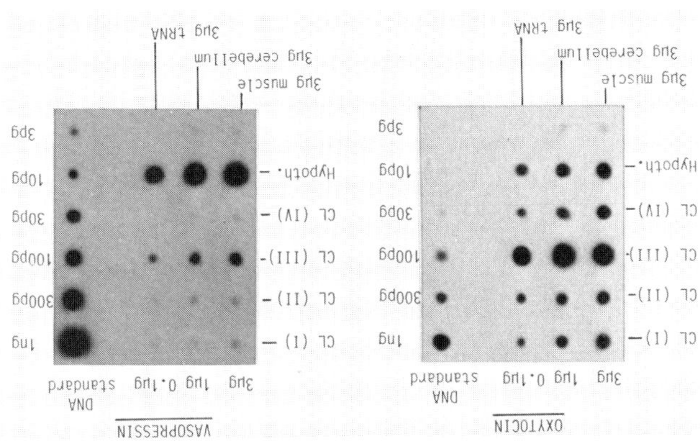

Fig. 3. Dot blot analysis of bovine mRNA from hypothalamus and various corpora lutea. Left: hybridized with the 3' oxytocin-specific probe; right: hybridized with the 3' vasopressin-specific probe (4).

magnocellular neurones. Production of the two hormones has been documented in lung carcinomas (12) and in the ovarian corpus luteum (13). In the latter tissue we have been able to show that the oxytocin gene is very highly expressed depending upon the phase of the luteal cycle, producing in the cow up to 250 times more oxytocin mRNA per organ than a single hypothalamus (ref 14; Fig. 3).

The different size of this mRNA - compared to that from hypothalamus - which can be attributed to a reduced poly(A) tail, indicates a tissue-specific regulation of oxytocin gene expression at the post-transcriptional level. In contrast, the vasopressin gene is expressed some three orders of magnitude less efficiently in this tissue. A detailed investigation of this system should lead to a greater understanding of the regulatory control of oxytocin gene expression.

Acknowledgement

We thank H. Christiansen and B. Pohl for excellent technical assistance and the Deutsche Forschungsgemeinschaft for financial support.

REFERENCES

1. Land H, Schutz G, Schmale H, Richter D (1982) Nature 295: 299-303
2. Land H, Grez M, Ruppert S, Schmale H, Rehbein M, Richter D, Schutz G (1983) Nature 302:342-344
3. Schmale H, Heinsohn S, Richter D (1983) EMBO J. 2:763-767
4. Ivell R, Richter D (1984) Proc.Natl.Acad.Sci. 81:2006-2010
5. Ruppert S, Scherer G, Schutz G (1984) Nature 308:554-557
6. Baltimore D (1981) Cell 24:592-594
7. Richter D (1983) In: Moldave K, Cohen W (eds) Progress in Nucleic Acid Research and Molecular Biology. Academic Press, New York pp 248-266
8. Russell JT, Brownstein MJ, Gainer H (1981) Neuropeptides 2: 59-66
9. Sokol HW, Valtin H (eds) (1982) The Brattleboro Rat. Ann. N.Y.Acad.Sci. 394:1-828
10. Watson SJ, Seidah N, Chretien M (1982) Science 217:853-855
11. Schmale H, Richter, D (1984) Nature 308:705-709
12. Yamaji T, Ishibashi M, Yamada N, Kondo Y (1983) Endocrinol.Japon. 30:451-461
13. Wathes DC, Swann RW, Birkett SD, Porter DG, Pickering BT (1983) Endocrinology 113:693-698
14. Ivell R, Richter D, manuscript submitted.

Endocrinology
F. Labrie, L. Proulx, eds.

ORGANIZATION OF THE PARAVENTRICULAR NUCLEUS

M.KAWATA AND Y.SANO

Department of Anatomy, Kyoto Prefectural University of Medicine, Kawaramachi-Hirokoji, Kamikyo-ku, Kyoto 602 (Japan)

INTRODUCTION

The hypothalamic paraventricular nucleus (PVN) in mammals, like the supraoptic nucleus (SON), has long been recognized as major sources of oxytocin and vasopressin which are released from the capillaries of the posterior lobe of the pituitary. Recent immunohistochemical studies have revealed that some neurons in the PVN produce releasing or release-inhibiting hormones which regulate the secretion of the anterior pituitary hormones. Moreover, the neurons in the PVN are now known to send their axons to the various regions of the central nervous system including the brainstem and spinal cord, particularly associated with the autonomic function. Thus, the PVN has been implicated in the regulation of autonomic as well as neuroendocrine system (1-3). These discoveries necessitate an investigation of the principal cellular organization of the PVN (4,5).

We here focused on the intrinsic organization of this integrative nucleus, with particular emphasis on the cytoarchitecture, peptide localization, projection sites, aminergic input, glial cell distribution and vascularity within the PVN.

MATERILAS AND METHODS

Eighty rats (Wistar, Long-Evans) of both sexes including six male Brattleboro rats, fifteen cats(*Felis catus*), ten dogs (*Canis familiaris*), and eight monkeys (*Macaca fuscata*) of both sexes were used in this study.

Each of the histological and immunohistochemical procedures employed in this study has been described in detail (6-9), therefore will be outlined here briefly.

Several types of rapid Golgi and Golgi-Kopsch impregnations were carried out. The morphology and localization of neurons containing peptides, such as oxytocin, vasopressin, neurophysin I, neurophysin II, ovine and rat corticotropin-releasing factor (CRF), somatostatin, cholecystokinin and Met-enkephalin were examined with the modified peroxidase-antiperoxidase method.

Aminergic input to the PVN was analyzed by means of the fluorescence histochemistry modified by glyoxylic acid method and the immunohistochemistry in conjunction with dopamine-β-hydroxylase (DBH) and serotonin antisera. Horseradish peroxidase and diamidino-phenylindole (DAPI) were injected into the posterior pituitary or several levels of the spinal cord in order to trace the intra- and extrahypothalamic projection from the PVN. Vascularity and the distribution of the glial cells were investigated by perfusing India ink through the left cardiac ventricle and by applying the immunohistochemistry with the antiserum to S-100 protein, respectively.

Results

The PVN was divided into two major populations of neurons: the more lateral magnocellular neurons and the more medial parvocellular ones. It was found by the Golgi analysis that magnocellular neurons project their dendrites medially and axons laterally, whereas parvocellular neurons send their dendrites and axons vertically in each opposite direction. Immunohistochemical studies clarified that the preferential distribution of oxytocin- and vasopressin-containing neurons are recognized: oxytocinergic neurons are located ventromedially and vasopressinergic neurons are distributed dorsolaterally in the rat, while quite the reverse was found in the cat, dog, and monkey. Cell bodies of somatostatin, CRF, cholecystokinin, and Met-enkephalin neurons were located in the caudal periventricular, rostral periventricular, dorsolateral and posterolateral portions of the PVN, respectively. A large number of DBH-positive nerve fibers was mainly observed in the dorsolateral portion of the PVN, which correspond to the area where vasopressinergic neurons predominate. A relatively small number of serotonergic nerve fibers was distributed in the parvocellular medial portion in contrast to the sparse occurrence in the magnocellular lateral portion. Interestingly, DBH-positive nerve fibers in the Brattleboro rat were increased in number and the topographic arrangements observed in the control was minimal, while serotonergic nerve fibers were not recognized at all in the magnocellular lateral portion.

With the use of the retrograde tracer method, it was found that the neurons projecting to the posterior lobe show a different population and localization of the neurons projecting to the

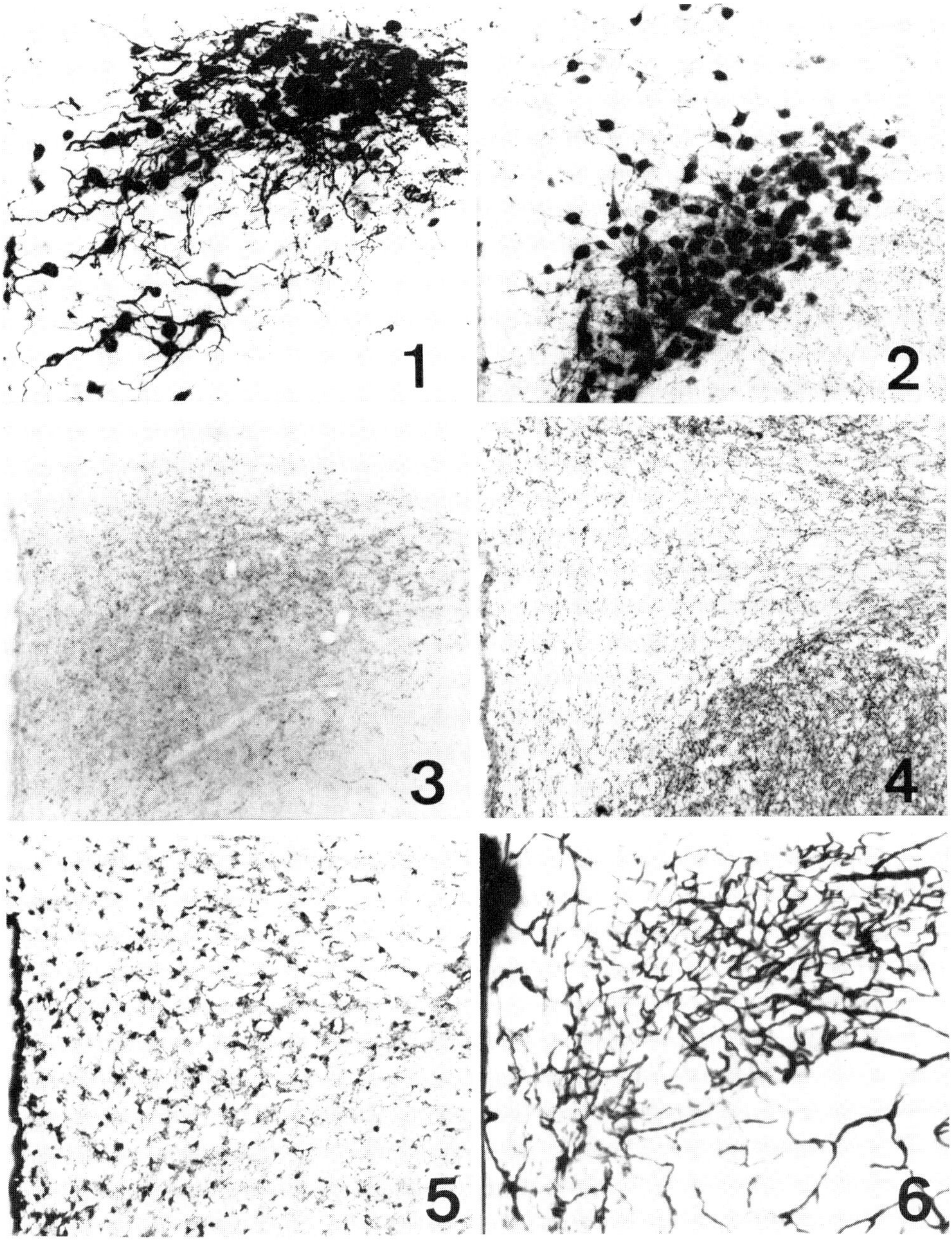

Fig.1-6. Paraventricular nucleus of the rat hypothalamus. Stained with (1) anti-vasopressin, (2) anti-oxytocin, (3) anti-DBH, (4) anti-serotonin, (5) anti-S 100 protein, (6) India ink.

extrahypothalamic areas, such as dorsal medulla and spinal cord: the former was localized in the rostro-central part and the latter was in the caudal part of the PVN. S-100 protein-containing glial cells were sparsely distributed in the magnocellular portion. However, a large number of these cells was observed in the parvecellular portion. The PVN was extremely vascularized and a high density of capillaries occurred only in the magnocellular portion.

ACKNOWLEDGEMENTS

We would like to thank Dr.Y.Ibata, Department of Anatomy, Kyoto Prefectural University of Medicine, Drs.H.Yamashita and K.Inenaga, Department of Physiology, University of Occupational and Environmental Health, School of Medicine, and Dr.K.Hashimoto, Department of Medicine, Okayama University Medical School, for advice during this work.

REFERENCES

1. Swanson LW, Sawchenko PE (1980) Neuroendocrinology 31:410-417
2. Swanson LW, Sawchenko PE (1983) Ann Rev Neurosci 6:269-324
3. Sawchenko PE, Swanson LW (1982) J Comp Neurol 205:260-272
4. Armstrong WE, Warach S, Hatton GI, McNeill TH (1980) Neuroscience 5:1931-1958
5. Van den Pol AN (1982) J Comp Neurol 206:317-345
6. Kawata M, Sano Y (1982) Anat Embryol 165:151-167
7. Kawata M, Hashimoto K, Takahara J, Sano Y (1982) Cell Tissue Res 230:239-246
8. Kawata M (1983) In: Sano Y, Ibata Y, Zimmerman EA (eds) Structure and Function of Peptidergic and Aminergic Neurons. JSSP-VNU, Tokyo-Utrecht, pp33-53
9. Yamashita H, Inenaga K, Kawata M, Sano Y (1983) Neurosci Lett 37:87-92

Endocrinology
F. Labrie, L. Proulx, eds.

DESIGN OF MORE SPECIFIC ANTAGONISTIC ANALOGS OF THE NEUROHYPOPHYSIAL HORMONES

W. H. SAWYER and M. MANNING

Department of Pharmacology, College of Physicians and Surgeons of Columbia University, New York, NY, and Department of Biochemistry, Medical College of Ohio, Toledo, OH, (USA)

INTRODUCTION

Antagonists of the actions of neurohypophysial peptides can be valuable tools for probing the physiological functions of these hormones. They may also have therapeutic uses. Effective antagonists of the vasopressor response to arginine-vasopressin (AVP) have been widely exploited in recent years to define the contribution endogenous AVP makes to cardiovascular regulation. Antagonists of the antidiuretic and oxytocic responses to AVP and oxytocin (OT) have not yet proved as useful, partly due to their relative lack of receptor specificity. We will briefly review the history of the development of antagonists of AVP and OT and some of our recent efforts to improve the specificity of antagonists of the antidiuretic response to AVP. We will also discuss problems that arise from the probable existence of receptors for these hormones that do not fall into the known categories of their peripheral receptors.

DEVELOPMENT OF EFFECTIVE ANTAGONISTS

Vincent du Vigneaud and his group produced the first antagonistic analog of OT merely eight years after they had first established the molecular structure of OT. This was OT in which they had methylated the 2-tyrosine hydroxyl. It was a weak antagonist of the vasopressor response and a weak oxytocic agonist. Later du Vigneaud's group found that dialkyl substituents on the β-carbon of the 1-hemicystine of OT produced more effective antagonists. When we combined such dialkyl substitutions and alkylation of the 2-tyrosine in single molecules we found their effects on antagonism were additive. Among many analogs of OT and AVP combining these changes are the most potent known antagonists.

Peripheral receptors for the neurohypophysial hormones fall into at least three classes. These are the uterine-type OT receptors, the V_1-type AVP receptors on vascular smooth muscle and hepatocytes, and the antidiuretic V_2-type receptors on renal tubules (1). V_1-receptors are most susceptible to blockade by synthetic analogs and many potent and specific V_1-antagonists have been reported. Although we have made a number of effective in vivo antagonists of oxytocic responses (2,3) these remain distressingly nonspecific in that most are potent V_1-antagonists as well. Our first effective V_2-antagonists were also far from specific. The best of these, $d(CH_2)_5[Tyr(Et)^2]VAVP$, for example, was actually about four times better as a V_1-antagonist than as a V_2-antagonist (Table I).

TABLE I

INFLUENCE OF THE 2-AMINO ACID ON THE SPECIFICITY OF A SERIES OF ANTAGONISTIC AVP ANALOGS.

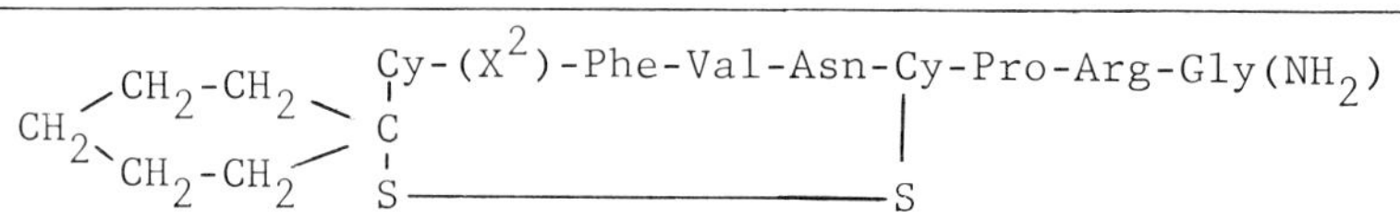

$d(CH_2)_5[X^2]VAVP$

X^2	Antagonistic potencies, ED's (nmoles/kg)* Antidiuretic	Vasopressor	Oxytocic	Potency AD/VP	Ref.
Tyr(Et)	1.9	0.49	13	0.26	11
D-Tyr(Et)	1.1	0.45	2.6	0.41	12
D-Tyr	2.2	0.29	6.9	0.13	12
D-Phe	0.67	0.58	8.9	0.87	13
D-Ile	0.70	8.2	44	12	13
D-Leu	1.2	26	61	22	13

*The ED ("effective dose") is the dose that reduces the response to 2x units of agonist to equal the response to 1x units.

IMPROVING ANTAGONISTIC SPECIFICITY

We have synthesized and characterized several hundred new AVP analogs in our efforts to improve the specificity of V_2-antagonism. This effort seems justified since specific antagonists make more incisive pharmacological probes and, if used clinically, should have fewer unwanted side-effects. If we only consider the classical peripheral V_1, V_2 and OT receptors it appears that we have been rather successful in enhancing specificity (Tables I and II).

Our definition of specificity of antagonists, however, ignores the possibility that AVP may act on other receptor types. It has recently been reported that AVP causes ACTH release and enhances ACTH release in response to CRF by acting on receptors that are clearly neither of the V_1 nor V_2 types (4,5). Receptors in the

TABLE II

INFLUENCE OF THE 4-AMINO ACID ON ANTAGONISTIC SPECIFICITY OF AN ANTIDIURETIC ANTAGONIST

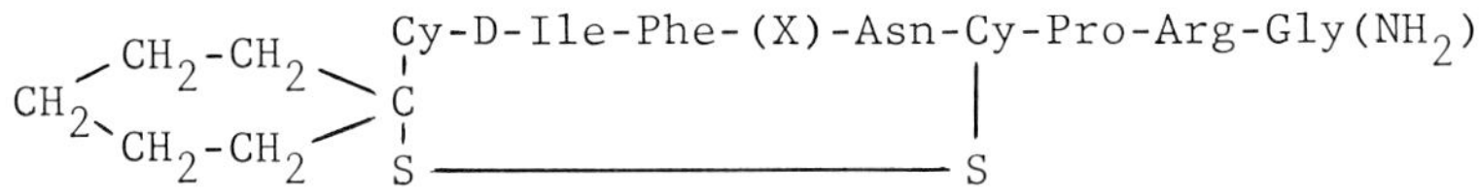

$d(CH_2)_5[D\text{-}Ile^2, X^4]AVP$

X^4	Antagonistic potencies, ED's (nMoles/kg) Antidiuretic	Vasopressor	Oxytocic	Potency AD/VP	Ref.
Val	0.70	8.2	44	12	13
Thr	0.88	11	9.5	12	14
Abu	0.41	12	19	29	14
Ile	0.67	26	9.4	39	14
Ala	1.7	66	57	39	14
(Gln, Leu, Ser, Orn, nVa, Asn, Cha, Lys, Phe				less than 12)	14

central nervous system may also be of several types. Those that mediate the effects of AVP on conditioned avoidance behavior in rats appear quite unique in that desglycinamide analogs of AVP with little or no V_1 or V_2 activity are behaviorally active (6). In fact, an AVP metabolite, pyroglutamyl-asparaginyl-cystinyl-prolyl-arginine, is many times more active than AVT itself (7). Behavioral activity of this peptide is blocked by a "specific" V_1-antagonist although the receptors involved can certainly not be considered to be of the V_1-type.

Still other types of brain receptors for AVP may exist. AVP can excite hippocampal neurons by acting on uterine-type OT receptors (8). AVP receptors mediating effects on baroreceptor sensitivity (9), antipyresis (6) and activation of adrenergic output from the nucleus tractus solitarius (10) have not been well characterized but they do appear to differ among themselves and from the brain receptors that mediate behavioral effects.

The apparent diversity of AVP receptor types, particularly in the brain, makes it important that we attempt to refine antagonistic specificity further. As these receptors become better characterized pharmacologically it may be possible to design more selective antagonists that act peripherally but have no central effects. This could be of obvious advantage if antagonists of AVP and OT are to be used clinically.

CONCLUSIONS

Although we have made progress in the design of specific antagonists of the V_1 and V_2 receptors we have yet to design truly specific OT blockers. There are probably several other types of AVP receptors that do not fall into the V_1 or V_2 classification. These should be further characterized pharmacologically and considered in further attempts to design more specific antagonists of the peripheral responses to AVP and OT.

ACKNOWLEDGEMENTS

Unpublished findings of the authors reported here were from studies supported by Research Grants from the National Institutes of Health, AM 01940 and GM 25280.

REFERENCES

1. Sawyer WH, Grzonka Z, Manning M (1981) Mol Cell Endocrin 22:117-134
2. Sawyer WH, Haldar J, Gazis D, Seto J, Bankowski K, Lowbridge J, Turan A, Manning M (1980) Endocrinology 106:81-91
3. Bankowski K, Manning M, Seto J, Haldar J, Sawyer WH (1980) Int J Peptide Protein Res 16:382-391
4. Knepel W, Homolka L, Vlaskovska M, Nutto D (1984a) Endocrinology 114:1797-1804
5. Knepel W, Homolka L, Vlaskovska M, Nutto D (1984b) Neuroendocrinology 38:344-350
6. Kovàcs GL, de Wied D (1983) Neuroendocrinology 37:258-261
7. de Wied D, Gaffori O, van Ree JM, de Jong W (1984) Nature, London 308:276-278
8. Mühlethaler M, Sawyer WH, Manning M, Dreifuss JJ (1983) Proc Natl Acad Sci (US) 80:6713-6717
9. Imai Y, Nolan PL, Johnston C (1983) Circ Res 53:140-149
10. Matsuguchi H, Sharabi FM, Gordon FJ, Johnson AK, Schmid PG (1982) Neuropharmacology 21:687-693
11. Manning M, Lammek B, Kolodziejczyk M, Seto J, Sawyer WH (1981) J Med Chem 24:701-706
12. Manning M, Olma A, Klis WA, Kolodziejczyk M, Seto J, Sawyer WH (1982a) J Med Chem 25:45-50
13. Manning M, Klis WA, Olma A, Seto J, Sawyer WH (1982b) J Med Chem 25:414-419
14. Manning M, Nawrocka E, Misicka A, Olma A, Klis WA, Seto J, Sawyer WH (1984) J Med Chem 27:423

Endocrinology
F. Labrie, L. Proulx, eds.

IS OXYTOCIN A NEUROTRANSMITTER IN THE VERTEBRATE HIPPOCAMPUS ?

M. MÜHLETHALER , M. RAGGENBASS and J.J. DREIFUSS
Department of Physiology, University Medical Center, 1211 Geneva 4, Switzerland

Vasopressin and oxytocin synthesized in neuronal cell bodies located in the hypothalamus are carried to the neurohypophysis, from which they are released into the general circulation. In addition, vasopressin- and oxytocin-like immunoreactivity is present in nerve fibers projecting to various areas within the central nervous system including the hippocampus. A calcium-dependent, depolarization-induced release of these peptides can be demonstrated from some areas of the brain where vasopressinergic and oxytocinergic axones have been shown to terminate synaptically on neuronal elements, a finding suggesting that oxytocin and vasopressin might, in addition to their well known hormonal effects, exert neurotransmitter-like actions in the brain (1).

We have shown in 1982 that both vasopressin and oxytocin increase the rate of firing neurones in hippocampal slices obtained from rats (2), a finding now confirmed by others (3). Here we briefly summarize data showing that the structure-activity relationship in the hippocampus to perfusion of medium containing neurohypophysial peptides or structural analogues has a great similarity to that of the oxytocin receptors responsible for smooth muscle contraction in the uterus, but differs markedly from that of receptors mediating vasopressin effects. In a second part, evidence is provided showing that in the hippocampus oxytocin acts directly on a class of interneurones which in turn inhibit pyramidal neurones.

Characterization of a neuronal response as being oxytocic.

Extracellular recordings were obtained from spontaneously active, single neurones located in the CA1 area of the ventral hippocampus. Oxytocin exerted a powerful excitatory effects on these cells. In Fig. 1A we computed the increase in firing rate from the resting level to the peak level reached in the presence of oxytocin. The lowest effective concentration was 10^{-9} M and stimulation was maximal at 10^{-6} M. The curve for vasopressin was found to run in parallel, but was displaced to the right by a factor of ten (4). Since this greater sensitivity to oxytocin was noticed for every cell tested, we may assume that oxytocin and vasopressin act on the same cells.

A great number of structural analogues are available which possess agonistic and/or antagonistic effects on peripheral target tissues responsive to neurohypophysial hormones. However, since no specific oxytocic antagonist is available, we compared the effect of oxytocin in the hippocampus with that of several partial or full agonists. These compound included arginine-vasopressin (IV), arginine vasotocin (III), as well as four unnatural analogues (I,V, VI,VII). The potency of each of these compounds in the hippocampus was determined by applying it at 10^{-6} M for 5 min and by counting the total number of action potentials generated in response to peptide application. To facilitate comparison, the effect of each compound was expressed relative to that of vasopressin applied at the same concentration. The results, shown in Fig. 1B, relate the potency of each compound with its endocrine activity. It is apparent that the relative potency in the hippocampus of the seven compounds correlated well with their myotonic activity on the uterus. No correlation was obtained with their antidiuretic or vasopressor activities (see ref. 4 for details).

These data suggest that an excitatory effect of oxytocin and vasopressin in the hippocampus might depend upon the presence in this area of the brain of receptors similar to the receptors for oxytocin found in the uterus.

Contrasting effects of oxytocin on pyramidal and non-pyramidal neurones.

Non-pyramidal neurones can be distinguished from pyramidal neurones according to electrophysiological criteria (5). We therefore endeavoured to assess which type of neurones might represent the initial target of oxytocin and vasopressin action in the hippocampus. Neurones that we presumed to be non-pyramidal had a mean rate of spontaneous activity of about 10-30 spikes/s and often fired in short bursts. Stimulation of the alveus did not elicit an antidromic action potential, whereas stimulation of stratum radiatum evoked a burst of orthodromic action potentials which outlasted the duration of the population spike; the first spike of this synaptically-evoked burst often occurred before the onset of the population spike. All cells so identified were excited by oxytocin.

To decide whether this excitatory effect on presumptive non-pyramidal neurones was direct or indirect, we performed a few experiments in conditions of synaptic uncoupling. Due to the increase in the concentration

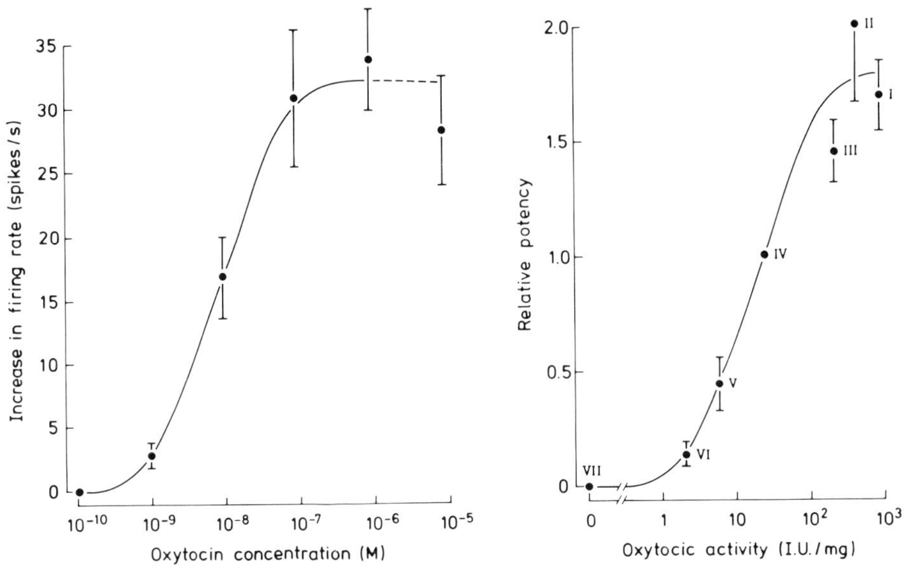

Fig. 1. Effect of oxytocin and of structural analogues on the firing of hippocampal neurones. Left : Each point shows mean increase in firing rate at the oxytocin concentration indicated. Right : Relative potency in the hippocampus of oxytocin (II) and of six structural analogues plotted on the abciss according to their oxytocin agonistic activity on uterine smooth muscle. Each point shows the mean increase in firing rate induced by the compound relative to the increase induced by arginine vasopressin (IV). Note that relative potency increases with increasing oxytocic activity (log scale).

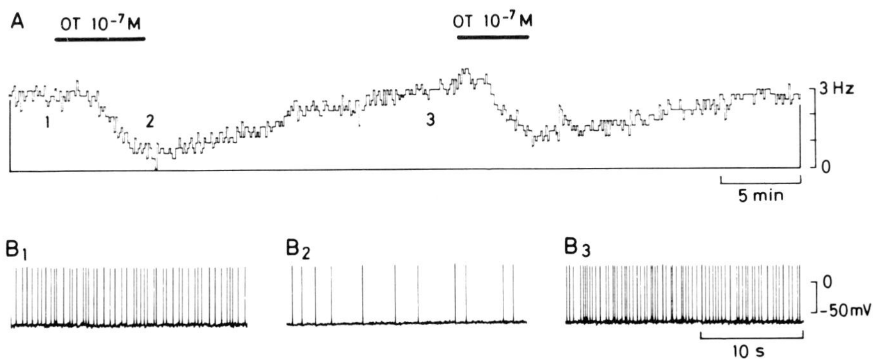

Fig. 2 Effects of oxytocin (OT) on the firing rate of a spontaneously active pyramidal neurone. A : OT added to the medium during the periods indicated by the thick horizontal lines caused a reversible decrease in firing. B : Oscilloscope tracings at the times indicated by numbers in A. Intracellular recording with potassium-acetate filled microelectrode.

of extracellular divalent cations non-pyramidal neurones tended to loose their spontaneous activity, but a majority were reactivated in response to oxytocin.

We next tested the effects of neurohypophysial peptides on pyramidal neurones recorded with intracellular microelectrodes. Oxytocin, 10^{-7} M, caused a membrane hyperpolarization which averaged 2.9 mV in half of the neurones tested; a reversible decrease in firing rate was seen in half of those that were spontaneously active; and in cells in which spontaneous inhibitory postsynaptic potentials were apparent, oxytocin produced an increase in their rate of occurrence. An example of a pyramidal neurone whose firing was slowed by oxytocin is shown in Fig. 2.

These data are best interpreted by assuming that oxytocin and vasopressin directly excite a class of inhibitory interneurones in the hippocampus, whereas the effect of these peptides on pyramidal neurones would be indirect and inhibitory. Interneurones are proportionally rare in the hippocampus, but the axon of some ot these cells has extensive local ramifications (6).

Although the density of fibres immunoreactive for neurohypophysial peptides may appear moderate, the interneurones which respond to these peptides therefore conceivably affect the activity of a great number of pyramidal neurones.

This work was supported in part by Swiss NSF grant 3.560.083.

REFERENCES

1. Buijs RM, van Heerikhuize JJ (1982) Brain research 252:71-76
2. Mühlethaler M, Dreifuss JJ, Gähwiler BH (1982) Nature 296:749-751
3. Tiberiis BE, McLennan H, Wilson N (1983) Neuropeptides 4:73-86
4. Mühlethaler M, Sawyer WH, Manning MM, Dreifuss JJ (1983) Proc. Natl. Acad. Sci. USA 80:6713-6717
5. Ashwood TJ, Lancaster B, Wheal HV (1984) Brain Research 293:279-291
6. Somogyi P, Nunzi MG, Goria A., Smith AD (1983) Brain Research 259:137-142

46. Hormones and Aging

Endocrinology
F. Labrie, L. Proulx, eds.

AGING AND ADRENAL

HIROSHI IBAYASHI and KEN-ICHI KATO
The Third Dept of Internal Medicine, Faculty of Medicine,
Kyushu University, Fukuoka 812, Japan

INTRODUCTION

In view of the hormonal regulation of homeostasis, considerable attention has been focused on the effect of aging on the adrenocortical function in man. Several studies have shown that adrenocortical function decreases with aging, and have suggested alterations in adrenocortical control mechanisms in the aged subjects.

Histologically, the human adrenal cortex is divided into three zones: an outer zona glomerulosa, a middle zona fasciculata, and an inner zona reticularis. The zona glomerulosa is the main producer of aldosterone, while the zonae fasciculata and reticularis are exclusively responsible for the production of cortisol and adrenal androgens. The zona reticularis, as the senescent zone of the cortex, was also early noted to have prominent deposition of pigmented lipids (lipofuscin). To this lipofuscin special attention has been devoted as a morphological finding of aging process.

The present studies demonstrate the age-related changes in the steroid secretory capacity of adrenal gland in the healthy human subjects, with special reference to alteration in the secretion of adrenal androgens with aging.

MATERIALS AND METHODS

Healthy males and females, aged 20-116 years, were volunteered for this study. The adrenal glands for the in vitro experiments and primary monolayer cultures were obtained at operation from patients with advanced breast cancer.

Plasma steroid hormone concentrations were measured by specific RIAs with LH-20 microcolumn chromatography. Colorimetric methods were used for measurement of malondialdehyde (MDA) formation in the human adrenal microsomes by lipid peroxidation, and for measurement of α-tocopherol content in the adrenals. The extraction and reincorporation of α-tocopherol in the microsomal particles were performed by the method of Ernster et al. NADPH-dependent lipid peroxidation was assayed by incubating microsomal fraction with ADP, $FeCl_3$ and NADHP at 25°C or 30°C, as previously reported[8]. The activities of microsomal steroid-synthesizing enzymes, 17α-hydroxylase, $C_{17,20}$lyase, 21-hydroxylase and 3β-hydroxysteroid dehydrogenase-isomerase (3β-HSD) were assayed using ^{3}H-labeled steroids as the substrates.

Statistical significance was evaluated using Student's t-test or the paired t-test.

RESULTS AND DISCUSSION

Plasma aldosterone concentrations in the males showed a significant decrease with aging. The response of plasma renin activity (PRA) after furosemide injection was definitely low in the aged men compared with that of the young controls. Abe and Omata[1] (1984) reported a age-dependent decline in plasma active renin concentration (PARC). These findings suggested that the reduced aldosterone secretion rate in the aged might be mainly due to decreased production of renin with advancing age.

While urinary 17-OHCS showed a slight decrease from 20 years of age, urinary 11-deoxy-17KS represented a marked decline in both sexes. No significant changes in plasma cortisol levels during aging were observed; however, plasma adrenal androgens, such as dehydroepiandrosterone (DHEA), DHEA sulfate and androstenedione showed a significantly age-related and linear decline from 20 years of age. The plasma levels of pregnenolone (P_5) and P_5 sulfate, which are the stem-steroids in the biosynthetic pathway of cortisol, demonstrated a definite decrease with a similar reduction in plasma concentrations of intermediate steroids, such as progesterone (P_4) and 17α-OH P_4, in the aged males[3,5] (Table 1). The plasma levels of adrenal androgens would be an usuful parameter for estimation of individual aging process.

Despite no significant differences in responses of plasma cortisol and aldosterone to ACTH stimulation between young and aged groups, the responses of plasma DHEA and DHEA sulfate demonstrated a marked decrease in the aged, although that of 17α-OHP$_4$ was significantly higher. These results suggested the decrease in the activities of the enzymes responsible for the biosynthesis of adrenal androgens, especially $C_{17,20}$lyase, in the aged adrenal glands (Fig. 1).

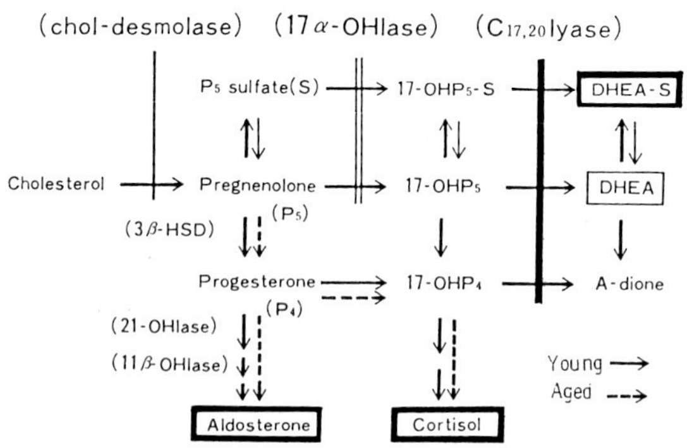

Fig. 1. Age-related changes in the biosynthesis of adrenocortical steroid hormones in humans

To elucidate the basis for the decline in secretory capacity of adrenal androgens in the aged, we investigated the alterations in the activities of steroid-synthesizing enzymes in the human adrenal microsomes following the in vitro treatments by lipid peroxidation, in connection with the prominent deposition of lipofuscin in the aged adrenocortical reticular cells. The in vitro lipid peroxdation of adrenal microsomes caused a rapid and marked decrease in the activities of microsomal $C_{17,20}$lyase and 17α-hydroxylase, although 3β-HSD activity showed no significant changes (Fig. 2).

The in vitro experiments of the extraction and reincorporation of α-tocopherol, one of potent biological antioxidants[2], showed that microsomal α-tocopherol had the protecting effect in a dose-dependent manner against the lipid peroxidation of adrenal microsomes and prevented the losses of androgen-synthesizing enzyme activities resulting from lipid peroxidation. A critical level of α-tocopherol

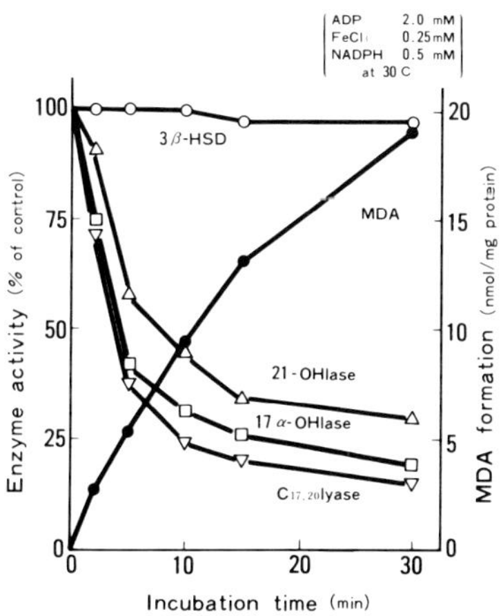

Fig. 2. Effect of lipid peroxidation on activities of microsomal steroid-synthesizing enzymes

content in microsomes to prevent the lipid peroxidation was estimated to be approximately 0.5 µg per mg of microsomal protein. Recently, Quinn and Payne[7] (1984) reported an oxygen-mediated damage of microsomal P-450 enzymes in cultured murine Leydig cells. Further investigations will be needed to clarify the mechanisms responsible for decrease in activities of 17α-hydroxylase and $C_{17,20}$lyase in the aged adrenal glands.

We found a direct effect of prolactin on adrenal androgen secretion from cultured human adrenal cells in the presence of ACTH. Plasma prolactin levels, however, were not affected with advancing age in either sex[4].

Parker and Odell[6](1984) have recently identified a new cortical androgen stimulating hormone (CASH) from the human pituitary gland which stimulates the production of adrenal androgens. Further studies of age-related changes in pituitary CASH secretion should be anticipated along these lines.

Table 1: Urinary and plasma steroid hormone levels with aging (20-116 years)

17-OHCS(mg/day)	male (n=168) female(n=165)	y=5.7-0.03x y=4.1-0.02x
11-deoxy-17KS(mg/day)	male (n=42) female(n=42)	y=5.4-0.05x(r=-0.79)** y=4.9-0.05x(r=-0.81)**
Aldosterone(ng/dl)	male (n=94)	y=12.2-0.06x(r=-0.34)**
Cortisol(μg/dl)	male (n=121) female(n=97)	y=13.6-0.04x(r=-0.22) y=10.3+0.02x(r=0.16)
Dehydroepiandrosterone (DHEA, ng/dl)	male (n=96) female(n=86)	y=353.4-3.77x(r=-0.67)** y=349.2-3.52x(r=-0.66)**
DHEA sulfate(μg/dl)	male (n=156) female(n=85)	y=195.2-1.94x(r=-0.81)** y=137.5-1.20x(r=-0.74)**
Androstenedione(ng/dl)	male (n=114) female(n=131)	y=197.4-1.40x(r=-0.59)** y=161.4-1.23x(r=-0.68)**
19-OH-androstenedione (ng/dl)	young male(n=18) aged male (n=20)	28.3±11.5(SD) 11.8±7.5(SD)**
Pregnenolone (P_5, ng/dl)	male (n=72)	y=294-2.90x(r=-0.79)**
P_5 sulfate(μg/dl)	male (n=72)	y=14.6-0.17x(r=-0.90)**
Progesterone(P_4, pg/ml)	male (n=99)	y=649.2-4.6x(r=-0.67)**
17-OH-P_4(ng/dl)	male (n=151)	y=208.7-1.3x(r=0.53)**

y: steroid hormone level x: years of age
**: statistical significance of correlation, $p<0.01$

REFERENCES

1. Abe K and K Omata (1984) Japanese J. Gerontol. 21:95-100
2. Hornsby PL and JF Crivello (1983) Mol Cell Endocrinol 30:123-147
3. Ibayashi H (1983) Japanese J Int Med 72:1125-1142
4. Ibayashi H (1983) Folia Endocrinol Japon 59:1783-1789
5. Kato K et al (1984) Japanese J. Gerontol 21:101-106
6. Parker LN et al (1983) Endocrinology 113:2092-2096
7. Quinn PG and AH Payne (1984) J Biol Chem 259:4130-4135
8. Takayanagi R et al (1980) Biochem J 192:853-860.

receptor and cytosol androgen receptor are also significantly reduced by megestrol acetate[17]. That these effects on androgen receptor are mediated by the blockade of androgen is indicated by the partial repair of this phenomenon when testosterone is administered simultaneously with megestrol. The effects of anti-androgen administration on decreasing the major biochemical mediators of androgen action would be expected to result in a decrease in prostate growth if in fact such mediators are critical for prostate growth. In an effort to address this possibility, we studied urinary outlet obstruction in patients with BPH over a 20-week period in a double blind study using placebo or Megace® 120 mg a day[18]. We noted a significant increase in both mean and maximum urinary flow rates in the megestrol-treated compared to placebo patients[18]. These studies suggest that the biochemical effects of megestrol in blocking androgen action may be responsible for the clinically effective decrease in outlet obstruction observed with the drug.

Any putative endocrine factor in the pathogenesis of BPH must be reconciled with the fact that the ratio of stroma to epithelium is increased in BPH from 2:1, found in normal prostates, to a ratio of 5:1 in BPH[19]. A comparison of stroma and epithelium in regard to biochemical mediators of androgen and estrogen action reveals that stroma contains increased levels of 5α-reductase, nuclear DHT, nuclear estrogen and estrogen receptor. Although we have emphasized the important role of androgen in BPH and the clinical effectiveness of anti-androgens in decreasing outlet obstruction, there are no direct studies to demonstrate that increase in DHT in the prostate stimulates excessive stromal growth.

Estrogen appears to be important in the pathogenesis of BPH as indicated by the fact that:

(1) Dog BPH produced by androgen is augmented by estrogen administration[3]; estrogen increases the formation of nuclear androgen receptor.

(2) Estrogen receptors have been identified in the prostate, primarily in the stroma[9,20].

(3) Stromal nuclei have the highest concentration of estradiol in the prostate[9].

In pursuit of the relationship of estrogen to increased stromal growth seen in BPH, we have studied the effects of an anti-estrogen on stromal growth, measuring _in vitro_ incorporation of ^{3}H-proline into prostate stroma obtained from patients treated for ten days with tamoxifen, 40 mg per day. These studies showed that tamoxifen, an inhibitor of estrogen receptor, significantly decreases stromal protein synthesis and decreases both nuclear androgen receptor and cytosol progesterone receptor in whole prostates of humans treated with the drug for ten days as compared to control patients.

CPK (creatine phosphokinase), an estrogen-dependent enzyme found in estrogen target tissues, was also decreased in prostate tissue following tamoxifen administration. No changes were noted following tamoxifen in whole tissue 5α-reductase, endogenous prostatic steroids, total plasma testosterone or the formation of 6α- and 17βandrostanetriols.

The perspective on prostate disease has changed within the last few years. There is a possibility that DHT is not the sole or major factor in the pathogenesis of BPH. This perspective is not only due to any potentially important recent data of Walsh concerning DHT concentrations in the prostate, but also to the fact that estrogen may have an important, if not dominant, role in the pathogenesis of BPH. The data obtained recently in our laboratory strongly support this possibility and indicate that at least growth of the stroma as well as whole tissue nuclear androgen receptor and cytosol progesterone receptor together with CPK are under estrogen control and can be significantly modulated by blocking estrogen action.

REFERENCES

1. Moore RA (1944) Surgery 16:152
2. Geller J, Albert J (1982) In: Korenman SG (ed) Endocrine Aspects of Aging. Elsevier North-Holland, New York, pp 137-161
3. DeKlerk DP, Coffey DS, Ewing LL, Mc Dermott IR, Reiner WG, Robinson CH, Scott WW, Strandberg JD, Talalay P, Walsh PC, Wheaton LG, Zirkin BR (1979) J Clin Invest 164:842-849
4. Siiteri PK, Wilson JD (1970) J Clin Invest 549:1737-1745
6. Bruchovsky N, Callaway T, Lieskovsky G, Rennie PS (1980) In: Wittliff JL, Dapunt O (eds.) Steroid Receptors and Hormone Dependent Neoplasia. Masson, New York pp 121-131
7. Hammond GL (1978) J Endocrinol 78:7-19
8. Walsh PC, Hutchins GM, Ewing LL (1983) J Clin Invest 72:1772-1777
9. Krieg M, Bartsch W, Thomsen M, Voigt K-D (1983) J Steroid Biochem 19:155-161.
10. Krieg M, Bartsch W, Janssen W, Voigt KD (1979) J Steroid Biochem 2:615-624
11. Morfin RF, DiStefano S, Bercovici JP, Flock HH (1978) J Steroid Biochem 9:245-252
12. Bruchovsky N, Lesser B (1976) In: Singhal RL, Thomas JA (eds.) Cellular Mechanisms Modulating Gonadal Hormone Action. Advances in Sex Hormone Research. University Park Press, Baltimore, pp 1-55
13. Issacs et al: Changes in the metab of DHT in human BPH (1983) J Clin Endocrinol Metab 56:139-146
14. Barrack E, Bujnovsky P, Walsh P (1983) Cancer Res 43:1107-1116
15. Robel - (unpublished data)
16. Geller J, Albert J, Geller S, Loza D, Cantor T, Yen S (1976) J Clin Endocrinol Metab 43:1000-1008
17. Geller J, Albert J and Geller S (1982) The Prostate 3:11-15
18. Geller J, Nelson CG, Albert J, Pratt C (1979) 14:467-474
19. Bartsch G, Doxenbichler G and Rohr HP (1983) J Ster Biochem 19:147-154
20. Ekman P, Barrack ER, Greene GL, Jensen EV, Walsh PC (1983) J Clin Endocrinol & Metab 57:166-176

Endocrinology
F. Labrie, L. Proulx, eds.

ANDROGENS, SEXUALITY AND THE AGEING MALE

JOHN BANCROFT

MRC Reproductive Biology Unit, Centre for Reproductive Biology, 37 Chalmers Street, Edinburgh EH3 9EW, Scotland, G.B.

There is general agreement that male sexuality declines with age. The most striking change is in frequency of coital activity with the partner (1). It is now well recognised that ageing has effects on erectile function *per se*, and erectile problems increase sharply in the later years (2). Other aspects of male sexuality, in particular sexual interest and nocturnal erections may decline less sharply (3).

A decline in testicular hormones with advancing age has been widely reported. Most early studies were consistent in reporting a decline in total and free testosterone in the plasma from the sixth decade onwards, typically associated with an increase in SHBG and to a lesser extent in oestrogen (4,5). Considerable individual variation in the degree of such changes has been obvious. More recent studies have concentrated on exceptionally healthy older men (6,7) and have found no ageing effect on testosterone apart from a slight increase in the amount of testosterone binding. These workers have attributed the earlier findings to the effects of ill health, alcohol, etc. and concluded that ageing *per se* does not affect testosterone production. It would be more correct to say that *age per se* is not the relevant factor, but ageing is a variable process and their subjects, because of their fitness, had presumably been little affected by it.

Evidence of levels of androgens and sexual activity in the same men has been less available. Davidson *et al*. (8) studied 220 men aged 41 to 93 and found that plasma testosterone was correlated with a number of measures of sexuality. But these correlations were small and disappeared when they controlled for age, indicating that whilst both variables were associated with age, their direct causal relationship to each other was less obvious. Tsitouras *et al*. (9) in a further sample from the Baltimore Ageing Project, divided 183 healthy men aged 60 to 79 into 3 groups according to their level of sexual activity in the previous year. They found that the most active group had significantly higher testosterone levels than the least active. Once again we cannot assume that it is a causal relationship but it does entitle us to look more closely at the role of androgens in male sexuality.

Our studies of hypogonadal men have shown that androgens are necessary for normal levels of sexual appetite and ejaculation (10,11). The relationship with sexual activity is more complex as it depends in part on the partner and

and her preparedness to initiate. The role of androgens in erectile function is also more complex. We have investigated this in two ways, measuring erections in the laboratory to erotic stimuli such as films and fantasy and measuring erections during sleep. Erectile responses to film do not appear to be androgen dependent (12,13). In our study erections in response to fantasy did appear to be androgen dependent but this was not replicated by Davidson and his colleagues (13).

Sleep erections on the other hand do appear to be androgen dependent. We assessed 4 hypogonadal men in the sleep laboratory before and after testosterone replacement and compared them with 7 eugonadal men assessed in the same way. The three parameters assessed, i.e. maximum circumference change, total duration of erection and latency to first erection all showed significant improvement in the hypogonadal men receiving testosterone undecanoate but no change in the eugonadal men receiving testosterone injections (14). This finding has also been reported by Davidson's team (13). Thus we have evidence that androgens influence sleep erections but are not necessary for erections to certain types of erotic stimuli and therefore presumably for the integrity of the erectile mechanisms _per se_. It remains a possibility that androgens are necessary for normal tactile sensitivity and this may be relevant to decline in reflexive erections with advancing age. As yet there is no evidence on this point.

The next question is how much testosterone is required to maintain male sexuality. This is of crucial importance to our older men. If there is a threshold above which further testosterone will have no behavioural effect, and if that threshold is below the "normal" range, then the large majority of older men will have more than enough testosterone for their sexual purposes. If however this threshold is less certain, varies considerably from man to man, and in many cases is well within the "normal" range, then the reduction we see in older men may be of some behavioural importance.

In a further group of 8 hypogonadal men we used a design whereby each subject either had 4 progressively rising or 4 progressively falling doses of testosterone undecanoate administered double-blind (14). We were thus able to compare behavioural measures for these 4 dose levels having controlled for order effect. We found that there was a dose response relationship in our measures of sexual interest and in the reported incidence of morning erections. There was no clear indication from this data that a plateau or theshold had been reached with the higher doses. What would therefore happen if one increased the supply of testosterone in men with initial plasma testosterone levels well within the normal range? We examined this in a further group of 20 men, 10 of whom presented with erectile problems and 10 with loss of sexual interest. They were all eugonadal and their mean ages were 45.4 yr + 44.6 yr respectively.

They all received testosterone esters by injection and placebo injections in a double-blind crossover design for 6 weeks each. From our previous results we predicted that the low interest group would show improvement with testosterone whereas the erectile impotence group would not. That was exactly what we found (15). Thus increasing circulating testosterone can affect sexual desire even in eugonadal men, but it should be emphasised that the gains in this study were relatively modest. It is worth noting at this point that Tsitouras et al.(1982) found an association between testosterone levels and sexual activity (and hence presumably sexual interest) but not between testosterone and erectile impotence reinforcing our findings that erectile function and dysfunction are independent of testosterone. This conclusion has to be qualified as erectile failure may results as a secondary psychological reaction to androgen dependent loss of sexual interest.

Thus there would seem to be a good case for a relative lack of testosterone contributing to the decline in sexual interest and sleep erections in older men, even in those whose testosterone levels remain within the normal range. We believe that further research on this issue should concentrate less on correlational studies between circulating hormones and behaviour, which assess only very crudely the relevant hormonal parameters, and more on controlled evaluation of hormone administration along the lines described above.

There are various clinical considerations required, in particular possible adverse effects of androgens on the prostate and less certainly on the cardio-vascular system. But there may be a proportion of older men who could benefit substantially from some extra testosterone and what is needed are better clinical indicators of those likely to respond.

The method of administration poses problems. Testosterone by injection is the most certain way of elevating circulating levels but this produces a massive rise for a few days after an injection and then a progressive fall to baseline levels within 7 to 14 days (16). Oral administration of testosterone undecanoate (Restandol, Organon) should theoretically be preferable but in eugonadal men we have found the absorption to be rather variable (17). We need more evidence of the pharmacodynamics of testosterone administration before we can be sure of the optimum method.

REFERENCES

1. Martin CE (1977) Sexual activity in the ageing male In: Handbook of Sexology Money J, Musaph H (eds). Elsevier/North Holland, pp 813-824

2. Kinsey AC, Pomeroy WB, Martin CE (1948) Sexual behaviour in the human male. Saunders, pp 236

3. Hegeler S, Mortensen M (1978) Sexuality and Ageing. British J Sexual Medicine 5 (32):16-19

4. Vermeulen A, Rubens R, Verdonck L (1972) Testosterone secretion and metabolism in male senescence. J Clinical Endocrinology 34:730-735

5. Stearns EL, MacDonnel JA, Kaaufman BJ, Lucman TS, Winter JS, Faiman C (1976) Declining testicular function with age. American J Medicine 57:761-766

6. Harman SM, Tsitouras PD (1980) Reproductive hormones in ageing men I Measurement of sex steroids, basal luteinizing hormone and Leydig cell response to human chorionic gonadotrophin. J Clinical Endocrinology & Metabolism 51:35-40

7. Sparrow D, Bosse R, Rowe JW (1980) The influence of age, alcohol consumption and body build on gonadal function in men. J Clinical Endocrinology & Metabolism 51:508-511

8. Davidson JM, Kwan M, Greenleaf WJ (1982) Hormonal replacement and sexuality in men. Clinics in Endocrinology & Metabolism 11 (3)599-623

9. Tsitouras PD, Martin CE, Harman SM (1982) Relationship of serum testosterone to sexual activity in healthy elderly men 37:288-293

10. Skakkebaek NE, Bancroft J, Davidson DW, Warner P (1980) Androgen replacement with testosterone undecanoate in hypogonadal men: a double-blind controlled study. Clinical Endocrinology 14:49-61

11. Davidson JM, Camargo CA, Smith ER (1979) Effects of androgens on sexual behaviour in hypogonadal men. J Clinical Endocrinology & Metabolism 48:955-958

12. Bancroft J, Wu FCW (1983) Changes in erectile responsiveness during androgen replacement therapy. Archives Sexual Behavior 12:59-66

13. Kwan M, Greenleaf WJ, Mann J, Grapo L, Davidson JM (1983) The nature of androgen action on male sexuality: a combined laboratory self-report study on hypogonadal men. J Clinical Endocrinology & Metabolism 57:557-562

14. O'Carroll R, Bancroft J (1984a) Effects of androgen replacement on sexual behaviour and nocturnal erections in hypogonadal men. Submitted for publication

15. O'Carroll R, Bancroft J (1984b) Testosterone therapy for low sexual interest and erectile dysfunction in men: a controlled study. British J Psychiatry. In press (August)

16. Sokol RZ, Palacios A, Campfield LA, Saul C, Swerdloff RS (1982) Comparison of the kinetics of injectable testosterone in eugonadal and hypogonadal men. Fertility & Sterility 37:425-430

17. Bancroft J, O'Carroll R, Davidson DW. In Preparation

Endocrinology
F. Labrie, L. Proulx, eds.

EXPERIMENTAL ASPECTS OF AGE-RELATED CHANGES IN THE ENDOCRINE SYSTEM

B.J. MERRY AND A.M. HOLEHAN
Wolfson Institute, University of Hull, Hull HU6 7RX England

With advancing maternal age in mammals there is a gradual decline in fertility and finally a cessation of reproduction, but it is possible in the female rodent to delay the onset of reproductive senescence and so provide a manipulative system for studying the endocrinology of reproductive decline. It is well established that caloric restriction in rodents extends maximum lifespan and retards growth and sexual maturity. Continuous adjustment of food intake so that the body weight is maintained at 50% that of fully-fed rats will delay puberty to later than 60 days after which greater than 70% of females exhibit normal oestrous cycles. Maximum lifespan is extended from 36 to 47 months and reproductive senescence is delayed by over one year. After 200 days oestrous cycles in fully-fed rats become irregular and increase in length, the most common abnormality being an extension of the period of cornification (persistent oestrus) with an increased frequency of recurrent pseudopregnancy occurring in the second year of life. No obvious change in the regularity of the cycles of dietary restricted rats occur until about 730 days and a gradual lengthening of the cycle is not observed. It is clear that the observations on vaginal cytology indicate a slowing down in the rate of reproductive ageing in the dietary restricted rat(1).

Rats retained on a restricted diet throughout postweaning life are fertile, bearing multiple live litters to an age far exceeding that of the fully-fed control females (Table 1). Control animals show a rapid decline in fertility from 270 days and were infertile by 500 days, while in the dietary restricted female maximum fertility was achieved about 500 days with some virgin females breeding and rearing litters as late as 900 days.

HORMONAL CHANGES

As the irregularities in oestrous cyclicity have been attributed to changes in ovarian endocrine secretion and reduced capacity of the hypothalamo-pituitary system to respond to gonadal hormone feedback, it would appear that these factors remain undisturbed in restricted rats for a longer period. This is in agreement with the hormonal profile reported for dietary restricted female rats(2), which show no significant difference in the overall pattern of oestradiol-17β across the oestrous cycle but the total amount of the hormone released is 46% that of the control animals. A comparison of hormone profiles in dietary restricted and fully-fed rats at an age when control females are showing an increase in cycle length reveal significantly higher levels of FSH associated with an early release of the preovulatory peak of LH in the restricted females. Such an alteration in the hormonal profile has, as one consequence, a reduced exposure of the follicular ovum to high levels of oestradiol-17β. Some of the alterations in hormonal levels similar to those of women during late reproductive life have been reported for the ageing rat during the oestrous cycle. Serum levels of oestradiol, oestrone and testosterone were elevated earlier in the cycle of old rather than of young rats, and in old rats with oestrous cycles prolonged to 6 days, the plasma level of oestradiol rises early in relation to the time of ovulation[3].

TABLE I

EFFECT OF DIETARY RESTRICTION ON BREEDING PERFORMANCE IN RATS

Age (days)	No. of Rats	% Pregnant	Litter Size
Control rats			
150	45	100	12.5 ± 0.4
210	20	100	8.3 ± 0.5*
270	20	75†	6.3 ± 0.5*
420	30	20†	1.0 ± 0.4*
450	28	0	---
Experimental rats			
300	60	13	6.0 ± 0.7
330	50	30†	10.0 ± 0.2
510	50	80†	5.0 ± 0.5
840-930	32	25†	4.5 ± 0.8

* Significantly different from value at 150 days, $P<0.01$ (ANOVA)
† Significant nonhomogeneity of percentages, $P<0.01$ (method of Brandt & Snedecor)

ABNORMAL DEVELOPMENT

It is well documented that the incidence of abortions, stillbirths and congenital anomalies increases as maternal age advances [4]. Although reproductive lifespan is extended by one year in dietary restricted rats a reduced incidence of congenital malformations has been recorded in offspring born to underfed females (Table 2).

A delay of ovulation in rats results in gross and chromosomal abnormalities during early developmental stages and it has been proposed that the oocyte undergoes preovulatory ageing as a result of prolonged oestrous cycles during late reproductive life[4]. Butcher and Pope[5] have investigated the effect of spontaneously delayed ovulation on subsequent developmental anomalies in one year old rats with lengthened or irregular oestrous cycles. The occurrence of developmental anomalies at all stages of gestation in aged rats was significantly greater when conception occurred during a 6-day cycle than when the cycle was 4 or 5 days in length.

TABLE 2
EFFECT OF DIETARY RESTRICTION ON BIRTH DEFECTS

Group	Total No. Pups	No. Malformed	% Malformed
Fully-fed rats	7076	71	1.01
Dietary restricted	1021	0	0.00

It is possible in young adult rats to induce an experimental delay of 48 hours in the timing of ovulation by injecting sodium pentobarbital[5]. This delay in ovulation results in follicular ageing associated with developmental defects, a decrease in the implantation and fertilisation rate linked with a three-fold increase in polyspermy. Associated with extended oestrous cycles is an early rise in the plasma levels of oestradiol-17β in relation to the timing of ovulation. Binding of the endogenous oestrogen with a specific antisera during this period of the cycle prevented the increase in developmental defects[5], but the incidence of developmental defects resulting from delayed ovulation was restored by administration of diethylstilbestrol which did not cross-react with the antisera. Therefore, a role for oestrogen in ageing oocytes within the follicles seems feasible in normally fed rats. It is proposed by Butcher and Page[4] that the early rise in oestrogen appears to have two detrimental actions. One effect is the retention of the preovulatory follicle in an environment of elevated oestrogen, a possible consequence of which is a disruption of the oocyte RNA stacking arrangement[6]. The other effect is a changed intrauterine environment which produces a decreased implantation rate.

The alteration in the hormonal profile of dietary restricted rats in comparison with fully-fed control females has, as one consequence, a reduced exposure of the follicular ovum to high levels of oestradiol-17β. In the context of the data presented by Butcher and Page[4] on the effect of oestradiol-17β on preovulatory ageing and subsequent abnormal development, the reduced incidence of birth defects observed in the offspring from dietary restricted rats can be partly explained.

HYPOTHALAMIC AGEING

It has been long established that if rats are ovariectomized at 6 months of age and then given young ovarian transplants at advanced ages (24-27 months), the young ovarian grafts stimulated a series of apparently normal oestrous cycles[7]. The prolonged absence of oestrogen apparently conserves the hypothalamic sensitivity to the steroid. In contrast, old intact rats and mice which have ceased to cycle do not respond to young ovarian grafts. Finch[8] has presented data that long-term ovariectomy retards the normal hypothalamic age changes whereas short-term exposure to high levels of oestradiol accelerates their onset. The theory has been proposed that one mechanism of reproductive ageing involves a cumulative impact of ovarian steroids on the hypothalamus and pituitary,[8]. The reduced circulating levels of oestradiol-17β observed in the dietary restricted rats would be compatible with the observations of Aschheim[7] and Finch[8] in retaining to a greater age normal oestrous cyclicity.

REFERENCES

1. Merry BJ, Holehan AM (1979) J Reprod Fert 57:253-259
2. Holehan AM (1984) The effect of ageing and dietary restriction upon reproduction in the female CFY Sprague Dawley rat. Ph.D. Thesis, University of Hull
3. Lu KH, Chang RJ, Kledzik GS (1979) Prog 61st Ann Meet Endocrine Soc Abstr No. 134:106
4. Butcher RL and Page RD (1981) In: Schwartz NB, Hunzicker-Dunn M (eds) Dynamics of Ovarian Function. Raven Press, New York, pp 253-271
5. Butcher RL, Pope RS (1979) Biol Reprod 21:491-495
6. Peluso JJ, Hutz R, England-Charlesworth C (1981) In: Schwartz NB, Hunzicker-Dunn M (eds) Dynamics of Ovarian Function. Raven Press, New York, pp 303-308
7. Aschheim P (1983) In: Meites J (ed) Neuroendocrinology of Aging. Plenum Press, New York and London, pp 73-101
8. Finch CE, Felicio LS, Flurkey DM, Gee DM, Mobbs C, Nelson JF, Osterburg HH (1980) Peptides Suppl 1, 1:163-175

47. Calcitonin and the Central Nervous System

Endocrinology
F. Labrie, L. Proulx, eds.

TISSUE SPECIFIC PATTERNS OF RNA PROCESSING REGULATION AND DEVELOPMENTAL SPECIFICITY OF NEUROENDOCRINE GENE EXPRESSION

MICHAEL G. ROSENFELD[1], SUSAN G. AMARA[1], and RONALD M. EVANS[2]

[1]Eukaryotic Regulatory Biology Program (M-013), University of California, San Diego, La Jolla, CA 92093
[2]Molecular Biology and Virology Laboratory, The Salk Institute, San Diego, CA 92138 (USA)

ABSTRACT

Alternative RNA processing events act in a tissue-specific fashion to generate two mature transcripts from a single neuroendocrine gene (calcitonin), predicting production of novel neuropeptides. A trans-acting mechanism serves to adjudicate these developmental decisions.

We have documented that the rat calcitonin gene can generate two mRNAs encoding discrete polypeptide products as a result of tissue-specific alternative RNA processing events (1-4). One of these RNAs encodes the precursor to the calcium-regulating hormone, calcitonin, and generates calcitonin and two other peptides in thyroidal C cells, the other RNA encodes the precursor of a novel neuropeptide referred to as calcitonin gene-related peptide (CGRP); two other peptides are predicted as products of CGRP mRNA expression. The two RNAs share a region of 5′ homology, predicting an N′-terminal region of 72 amino acids common to the precursors of calcitonin and CGRP. Sequence analysis of the rat calcitonin/CGRP gene confirmed that both CGRP and calcitonin mRNAs are derived from a single genomic locus; the rat calcitonin/CGRP gene contains all of the information present in the two mRNAs. The gene contains six exons; in the case of calcitonin mRNA, the first three exons are spliced to the fourth (calcitonin-coding) exon to generate the mature mRNA. In the case of CGRP mRNA, the first three exons are ligated to the fifth (CGRP-coding) and sixth (CGRP-3′-noncoding) exons to generate CGRP mRNAs; the fourth (calcitonin-coding) exon is spliced out with the two adjacent intervening sequences. The point of divergence between the two mRNAs corresponds precisely to intervening sequence/exon boundaries. Using a combinatorial analysis involving histochemical mapping using antisera against a synthetic peptide corresponding to the C′-terminal portion of CGRP, S_1 nuclease resistance assay, and sequence analysis of cDNA clones, the expression of CGRP mRNA in the brain and in other tissues (4) was established. A detailed analysis revealed a tissue-specific pattern of these alternative RNA processing events. Thus, in thyroid C cells both calcitonin and CGRP mRNAs are produced in a ratio of 95:97:1, respectively. In the brain, CGRP mRNA is at least 200-fold more prevalent than calcitonin mRNA, which, if present at all, is below levels of detection by available assays. Calcitonin and CGRP are co-produced in the identical thyroidal C cells. In medullary thyroid carcinomas, the relative concentration of CGRP mRNA:calcitonin mRNAs varies widely (from <2% to >90% CGRP mRNA).

Distribution of CGRP in the central nervous system and somatic tissues

CGRP is distributed in a unique pattern, distinct from all known peptides. In the central nervous system CGRP is present in fibers and neurones believed to subserve motor, sensory and integrative functions. Thus, CGRP is present in a subset of the small cells of the trigeminal ganglion (approx. 5%) and in the spinal sensory ganglia (30-50%); these cells are believed to relay pain and temperature information. In the spinal ganglia, CGRP neurones are the predominant small cell type; substance P-containing neurones are, for example, a subset of CGRP neurones. CGRP is also distributed in almost every portion of the pathways mediating the sensory and motor aspects of ingestive behavior; for example, CGRP is present in a subset taste buds and in the motor nucleus innervating muscles which function in deglutition (4). CGRP has been identified at the neuromuscular junction of the striated muscle of the upper esophagus, as well as skeletal muscle; this is the initial peptide identified at neuromuscular junctions in mammalian species (Polak et al., unpublished observations). CGRP is present in a subset of cells of one of the two motor nuclei of the vagus nerve (n. ambiguus). Finally, CGRP is widely distributed in non-sensory nerve fibers surrounding both arteries and veins throughout most tissue.

CGRP is also present in the endocrine system, being present in thyroid C cells, bronchiolar cells, in a subset of adrenal chromaffin cells, and is the peptide in the baskets of neural fibers which surround the pancreatic islets. Thus, CGRP is one of the most widely distributed of known peptides. Based upon its anatomic distribution and upon initial physiological studies using chemically-synthesized peptide, CGRP is suggested to exert regulatory effects on nociception, ingestive behavior, and cardiovascular homeostasis (4,5); exerts unique effects on blood pressure and catechloamine release, inhibits basal and stimulated gastric acid release; it is tempting to speculate that CGRP also exerts a role in mineral metabolism.

A second gene encodes a CGRP-related protein

A second rat gene, related to the CGRP gene, has been identified and characterized in the rat. This gene is expressed in rat, generating two mRNAs which apparently share 5′ sequence homology, but diverge in the 3′ portion of their coding domains. The sequence of one cDNA predicts a precursor peptide which will generate give peptide products by proteolytic processing events. Two of the N′ terminal predicted peptide products are homologous to the 'common region' shared by calcitonin and CGRP precursor peptides. The third N′ terminal peptide is unique to this mRNA. The fourth predicted peptide product differs by a single amino acid from CGRP primary structure. The CGRP-related mRNA is expressed in the brain, while the alternative RNA product is expressed in the thyroid gland. Therefore, similar RNA processing events seem to operate in expression of the CGRP-related gene, and a series of novel peptides are the apparent result.

Similar RNA processing events operate in expression of the human calcitonin/CGRP gene

We have isolated and sequenced the cDNA clones from human CGRP and calcitonin mRNAs, and the human calcitonin/CGRP gene. Based upon sequence analysis of these clones we have established that the human calcitonin/CGRP gene can also generate two discrete mRNAs encoding the precursors to calcitonin and CGRP peptides (6). Based upon alternative RNA processing events, documenting the operation of this type of post-transcriptional regulation in the human neuroendocrine system. The structure of the human CGRP precursor peptide predicts the excision of a 37 amino acid peptide differing in 4 amino acids from the primary sequence of rat CGRP. Both RNA and peptide products of the human calcitonin/CGRP gene are expressed in the human pituitary gland, consistent with the possible regulated expression of these peptides in many species (6).

Analysis of the human CGRP mRNA reveals sufficient homologies with salmon calcitonin to suggest that calcitonin and CGRP exons are derived from a common primordial gene, and that the calcitonin/CGRP gene arose either by duplication and sequence divergence of the calcitonin (CGRP) exon itself, or via gene duplication and rearrangement events, whereby the CGRP-coding regions of one gene became fused into the coding region of the calcitonin gene. The intriguing consequence of these evolutionary events was the generation of a gene with the structural and/or sequence information conferring a tissue-specific pattern of RNA processing regulation, implying that there is a biological advantage to production of CGRP, rather than calcitonin, in specific tissues. The common evolutionary origin of calcitonin and CGRP exons also raise the possibility that, in human, salmon calcitonin might represent a ligand for CGRP receptors. Thus, some of the reported effects of salmon calcitonin on ingestive behavior and analgesia (7-10) might, in part, reflect actions at CGRP receptors. It will be important to determine whether human calcitonin mimics all of the effects of salmon calcitonin in humans.

Mechanism of alternative RNA processing events

The calcitonin/CGRP gene is an example of a complex transcription unit. We have documented that this gene utilizes a single transcriptional initiation site (CAP site); but that the calcitonin and CGRP mRNAs utilize distinct poly(A) sites at the end of the fourth and sixth exons, respectively. Thus, the alternative pattern of exons at the 3′ ends of the two mRNAs is associated with differential usage of at least two alternative poly(A) sites (11). These observations indicate that regulated poly(A) site selection associated with alternative RNA splicing reactions is a physiologically significant developmental mechanism for determining neuropeptide expression and is likely to be important in establishing the phenotype of specific groups of neurons. The mechanisms involved appear to operate in expression of animal cell DNA viruses (12) and in the case of many eukaryotic genes. Thus far, the structural basis for the poly(A) site selection events is unknown. Thus, the canonical calcitonin sequence preceding the poly(A) endonucleolytic site is AAUAAA and AUUAAA in the case of calcitonin and CGRP mRNAs, respectively; however, it is unlikely that this sequence difference alone accounts for the observed alternative RNA processing events. We have established that transcription proceeds across the entire gene irrespective of which mRNA is produced. Thus, it is the differental endonucleolytic cleavage, as opposed to transcriptional termination events, which dictate the observed patterns of RNA processing. Selection of the endonucleolytic site could reflect the action of either a positive or negative factor; evidence for the existence of cell-specific, trans-active factor(s) which adjudicate the poly(A) site selection in expression of the calcitonin/CGRP gene has been provided by studies of the expression of the gene transfected into the heterologous cell types. Characterization of the trans-acting factor(s) which dictates poly(A) selection, and determining whether it recognizes structural elements on nascent RNA transcripts or genomic DNA, will permit assessment of the potential significance of modulation of poly(A) site utilization as a general mechanism for regulating productive processing of neuroendocrine and

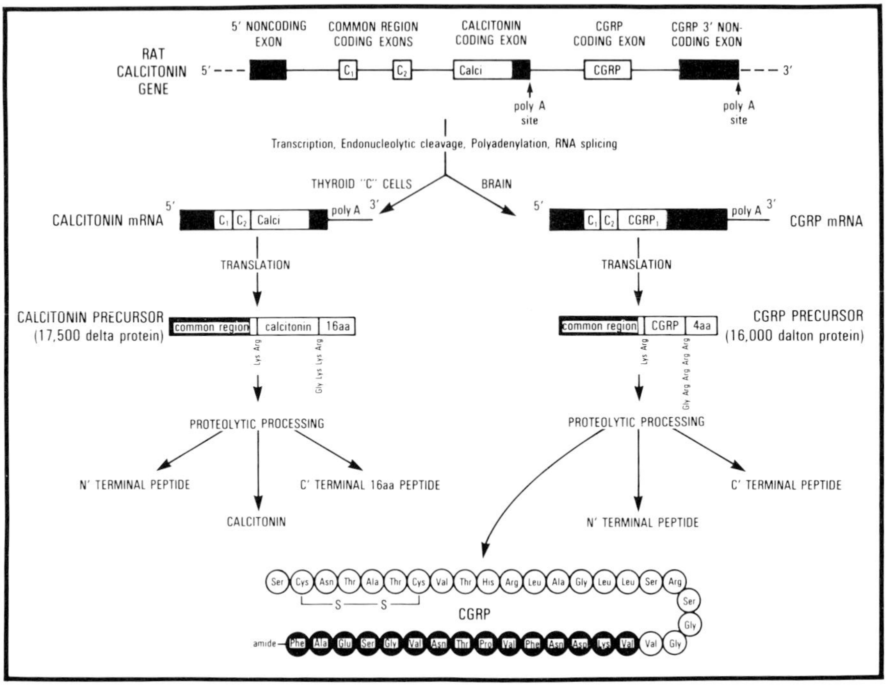

brain transcription units.

REFERENCES

1. Rosenfeld MG, Amara SG, Roos BA, Evans RM (1981) Nature 291:63-65

2. Rosenfeld MG, Lin CR, Amara SG, Stolarsky LS, Ong ES, Evans RM (1982) Proc Natl Acad Sci USA 79:1717-1721

3. Amara SG, Jonas V, Rosenfeld MG, Ong ES, Evans RM (1982) Nature 298:240-244

4. Rosenfeld MG, Mermod J-J, Amara SG, Swanson LW, Sawchenko PE, Rivier J, Vale WW, Evans RM (1983) Nature 304:129-135

5. Fisher LA, Kikkawa DO, Rivier JE, Amara SG, Evans RM, Rosenfeld MG, Vale WW, Brown MR (1983) Nature 305:534-536

6. Jonas V, Lin CR, Kawashima E, Semon D, Swanson LW, Mermod J-J, Evans RM, Rosenfeld MG (1984) 'Alternative RNA processing events generate calcitonin and CGRP mRNAs in the human pituitary', manuscript submitted

7. Braga P, Terri S, Santagostino A, Olgiatio VR, Pecile A (1978) Life Sciences 22:971-979

8. Yamamoto M, Tachukawa W, Maeno H (1980) Neuropharmacology 20:83-86

9. Twery MJ, Obie JF, Cooper CW (1982) Peptides 3:749-752

10. Freed WJ, Perlow MJ, Wyatt RS (1979) Science 206:850-853

11. Amara SG, Evans RM, Rosenfeld MG (1984) 'Alternative poly(A) site selection as a molecular mechanism for tissue-specific expression of neuroendocrine genes', manuscript submitted.

12. Ziff EB (1980) Nature 287:491-499.

© 1984 Elsevier Science Publishers B.V.
Endocrinology
F. Labrie, L. Proulx, eds.

THE CALCITONIN GENE PEPTIDE FAMILY AND THE CENTRAL NERVOUS SYSTEM

IAIN MACINTYRE

Endocrine Unit, Royal Postgraduate Medical School, Ducane Road, London, UK.

The work I shall discuss represents a collaboration by my own team at the Royal Postgraduate Medical School with Howard Morris' team at Imperial College, Emson and colleagues at the MRC Neurochemical Pharmacology Unit, Cambridge, Fink of the MRC Brain Metabolism Unit, Edinburgh and Azria of the Pharmaceutical Research and Development Group of Sandoz Ltd., Basle.

INTRODUCTION

The prediction of a new peptide in the rat (rCGRP) rested on nucleotide sequence data; its actual existence was suggested by immunofluorescent localisation[1,2]. However, these latter techniques are inconclusive and leave the question of the existence of CGRP in man completely undecided. Rosenfeld and colleagues also concluded that CGRP is absent from rat thyroid[2] where calcitonin is expressed, while the latter peptide was not found in the CNS where CGRP was abundant. These differences were thought to arise from differential tissue-specific processing of the transcript from the rat calcitonin gene. We have recently reported the first isolation and characterisation of human CGRP[3]. Here we describe the distribution of the peptide in man and rat and outline preliminary pharmacological studies of both peptides. The results differ in several important respects from those reported for the predicted rat peptide.

THE ISOLATION OF HUMAN CGRP

The primary structure of hCGRP was determined unequivocally by a novel mass spectrometric approach, fast atom bombardment (FBA) mapping[4,5] after isolation from human medullary thyroid carcinoma[3]. There are four differences from the sequence predicted for the rat peptide. In addition the C-terminal amide and the amino terminal 2-7 disulphide bridge were conclusively established. The latter two features were only surmised in the predicted structure of the rat peptide. This work proved the existence of hCGRP and was, in fact, the first isolation of CGRP from any species. The structural differences meant charge changes in important areas of the molecule and suggested the possibility of differences in the pharmacological properties of hCGRP from the rat peptide. Detailed studies show that these predicted differences exist.

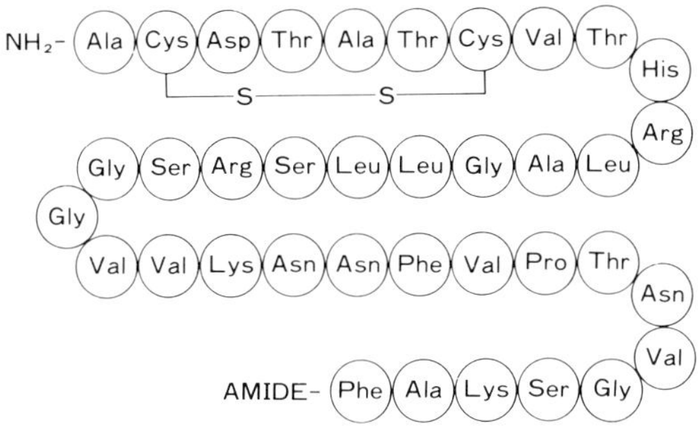

Fig.1 Sequence of human CGRP

DISTRIBUTION OF CGRP

Fig. 2a & 2b shows the wide distribution of rCGRP (Wimalawansa, Emson & Girgis, unpublished); the peptide is abundant in rat thyroid in contra-distinction to earlier reports[2]. The high concentration in the posterior horn of the spinal cord is established conclusively. The main findings also hold true for man (Fig.3) (Girgis, Yates & Fink, unpublished). These results were largely based on a novel amplified enzyme-linked immunoassay system (Self & Johannsson, unpublished) with a sensitivity of 1pg hCGRP per tube after overnight incubation. Presumably hCGRP is also the product of the calcitonin gene as shown by the human gene sequence (Lipps and colleagues, personal communication). Antibody-based localisation studies are in progress and fully confirm these findings (Emson, unpublished results).

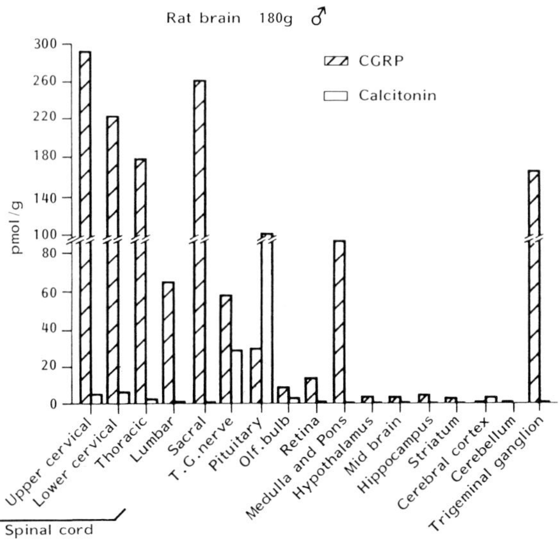

Fig.2a Tissue distribution of CT and CGRP in rat brain.

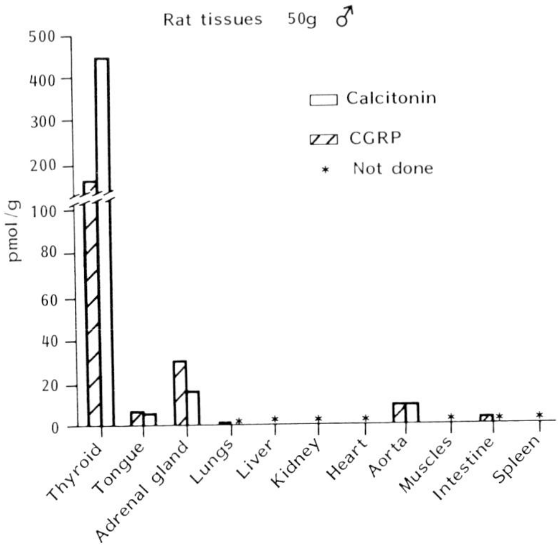

Fig.2b Tissue distribution of CT and CGRP in the rat

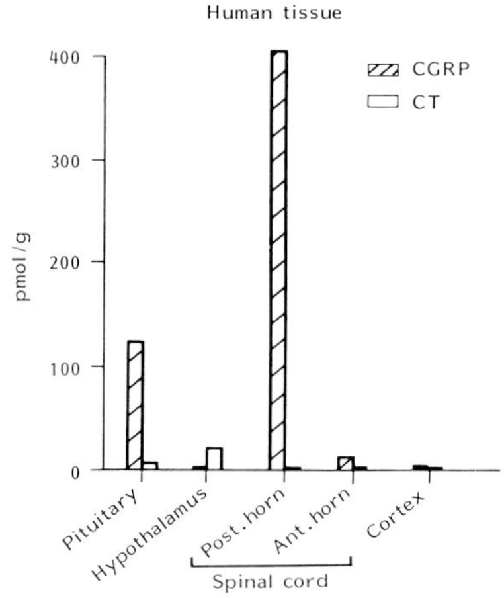

Fig.3. CT and CGRP in human nervous tissue

PHARMACOLOGY

hCGRP has potent effects on the isolated rat auricle (Fig.4) and guinea pig ileum (Tippins, Morris, Panico, Etienne, Bevis, Girgis, MacIntyre, Azria & Attinger, in press). We have also recently found that the peptide has powerful plasma calcium modulating effects in rat (Fig.5), rabbit (Fig.6) and chick preparations . It is impossible to exclude a physiological effect of hCGRP on plasma calcium regulation.

Further since hCGRP circulates in medullary carcinoma of the thyroid[3] it is possible that it circulates in lower concentrations in health. However, it remains to be determined whether CGRP has a true hormonal function in man in addition to a CNS neuromodulator or neurotransmitter role. Nevertheless, the multiple biological effects of hCGRP in test systems suggest physiological counterparts in the CNS, CVS and GI systems and perhaps even in the regulation of plasma calcium. It is too early to speculate on a possible role in disease but the elevated plasma levels in medullary carcinoma raise the possibility of involvement of the peptide in some of the symptoms of that condition.

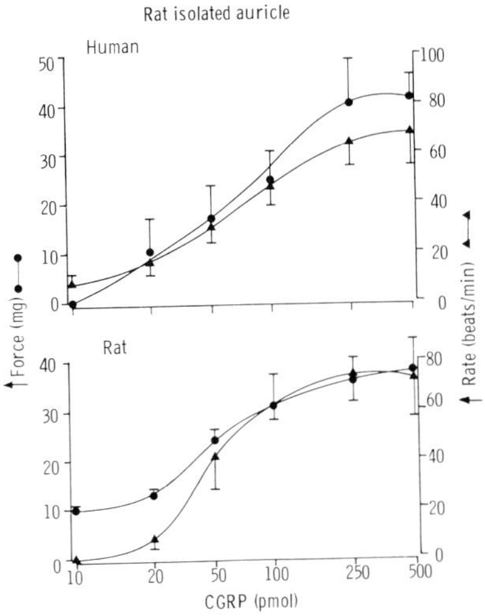

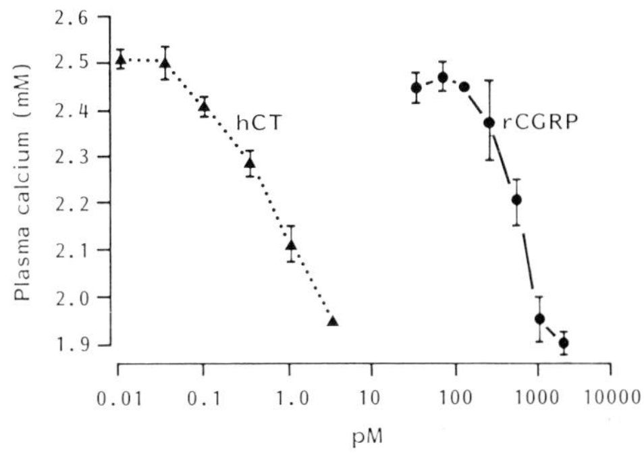

Fig.4 Dose-response curves of rat and human CGRP on rat isolated auricle

Fig.5 Dose-response curves of CGRP and hCT on plasma

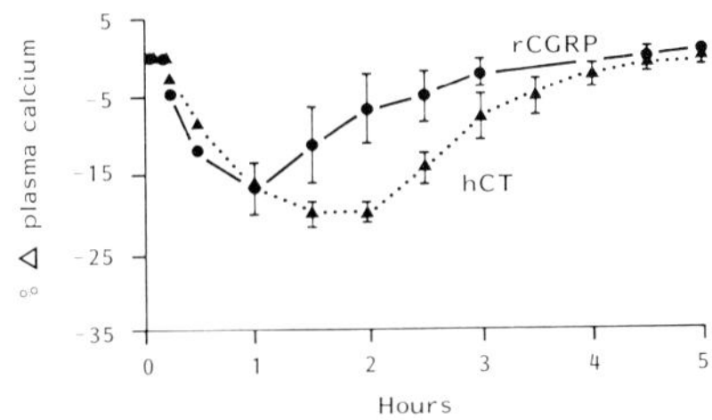

Fig.6. Time course of the effect of rCGRP (5ug/kg) and hCT (5ug/kg) on plasma calcium in the rabbit.

REFERENCES

1. Amara SG, Jonas V, Rosenfeld MG, Ong ES & Evans RM (1982) Nature 298: 240-244.
2. Rosenfeld MG, Mermod J-J, Amara SG, Swanson LW, Sawchenko PE, Rivier J, Vale WW & Evans RM (1983) Nature 304:129-135.
3. Morris HR, Panico M, Etienne T, Tippins J, Girgis SI & MacIntyre I (1984) Nature 308:746-748.
4. Morris HR, Panico M, Karplus A, Lloyd PE & Riniker B (1982) Nature 304:643-645.
5. Morris HR, Panico M & Taylor GW (1983) Biochem biophys Res Commun 117:299-305.

© 1984 Elsevier Science Publishers B.V.
Endocrinology
F. Labrie, L. Proulx, eds.

CALCITONIN BINDING SITES IN THE BRAIN

MASAO KOIDA AND HIROMICHI NAKAMUTA

Department of Pharmacology, Faculty of Pharmaceutical Sciences, Setsunan University, Nagaotoge-cho 45-1, Hirakata 573-01, Japan

RONALD C. ORLOWSKI AND GLENN L. STAHL

Armour Pharmaceutical Co., Kankakee, Ill. 60901, USA

Salmon calcitonin (sCT) by intracerebroventricular injection induces a variety of behavioral effects in mammals; analgesia (1), anorexia (2,3), decreased gastric acid secretion (4), tail-whipping (5), etc. It is also known that the sCT-specific binding sites occurring in mammalian brains exhibit the properties expected of the "physiological" or "pharmacological" receptor (6-10). On the basis of the available evidence, it seems that the binding sites have some of the qualities of a receptor.

IN VITRO BINDING STUDIES

^{125}I-sCT binds to the membrane fraction of the rat brain in ways that are saturable, CT-specific, pH- and temperature-dependent, and of low reversibility. The affinity decreases in the order sCT (IC_{50}: 1~nM) > (Asu^{1,7})eel CT > porcine CT (pCT), sCT(11-32) > sCT(22-32) > human CT (hCT) > sCT(1-11) = 0. The order of the CTs is the same as that of the hypocalcemic activity assayed in rats. Scatchard analysis locates the sites of the lowest K and the highest B_{max} in the hypothalamus. The midbrain or brainstem follows within these parameters. In the subcellular fractions, the density decreased in the order of $P_3 > P_2 > P_1$, and among the subfractions P_2 was the highest in the synaptosomal fraction. The in vitro autoradiographic studies (11,12) appear to provide more detailed mapping of the sites among the brain regions. Most of the anterior hypothalamic nuclei exhibit the high grain density which may mediate the anorectic effect. A series of other spots also heavily labeled such as brainstem, nucleus tractus spinalis nervi trigemini, some laminae of the spinal cord, etc., may be related to the antinociceptive action of sCT.

From a photoreactive derivative (13) of ^{125}I-sCT, the radioactivity is transferred by UV light to some macromolecules of the hypothalamus, including some material corresponding to BSA in size. Labeling of this material was depressed by sCT(11-32) to a large extent. Since no in vivo activity has been detected with this fragment (refer to Table 1), it is considered that only a small population of the binding sites would function as the receptor through which sCT induces anorexia.

IN VIVO BINDING STUDIES (5)

After intracerebroventricular injection into rats, most of the anorectic dose of ^{125}I-iodo-sCT gradually enters the systemic circulation to cause a long-lasting hypocalcemia. It was also found that the peptide can survive in the brain for a long time as reflected by a long duration of anorexia. Three hours after injection, about 1% of the radioactive dose was retained by the hypothalamus, more than one half of which was recovered as iodo-sCT by HPLC.

IN VITRO EFFECTS

sCT (1 μM) inhibits the activity of adenylate cyclase in brain slices or in brain homogenate (8), while the Ca-uptake by hypothalamic slices in inhibited by a much lower concentration (10 nM) of sCT (3,14). The latter effect appears to be specific to sCT and also to the brain region (14).

IN VIVO EFFECTS

Spontaneous intake of food and water in rats is suppressed in parallel fashion by central injection of sCT in a dose dependent manner. The peptide specificity of the effect and some of the dose-effect relationships are summarized in Table 1. Food intake is also inhibited by subcotaneous injection of sCT (15,16), though water intake remains unaffected. When a daily dose of 1.6 nmol/kg is repeated, a strong tolerance to this effect develops and within 3 days rats can acquire complete tolerance to the subsequent dose. Even after that, however, the animals will be able to respond normally to the first central challenge of sCT (62 pmol/rat). This suggests that the site of action leading to anorexia would differ depending on the route of administration.

The suppressive effect of sCT on gastric acid secretion (4), intestinal motility (17) or stress-induced feeding (3) may be a better measure of the CNS actions of the CTs, since these effects have been reported to be detectable with a dose less than one hundredth of the effective anorectic dose of sCT in Table 1, but the struc-

ture-activity relationship remains to be established.
In contrast, antinociception would be a different type of measure. In sofar as tested by the method of Randall & Selitto (18), no antinociception has been detected in rats on complete anorexia by sCT (19). On the other hand, pCT even in a low dose (20 pmol/ rat) was able to develop a distinct antinociception.

TABLE 1

THE ANORECTIC ACTIVITY OF CTs AND sCT FRAGMENTS IN RATS

Treatment[a)]	Dose (pmol/rat)	n	Food intake (g) for 3 hr	6 hr	24 hr	Water intake (g/24 hr)
saline		6		7.2	20	31
sCT	1.9	6		7.2	20	35
	6.2	7		4.0	15	27
	19	6		0.3**	7.3**	17**
	62	12		0**	0.8**	2.9**
[Asu^{1,7}]eel CT	1.9	7		4.7	19	36
	6.2	6		1.5**	13	22
	19	7		0.2**	6.4**	12**
	62	10		0.1**	1.3**	6.3**
saline		11	2.1	7.2	20	30
sCT(1-11)	1240	12	3.2	7.0	17	25
sCT(11-32)	3720	9	3.7	8.3	19	32
sCT	19	5	0**	0.2**	7.4**	18**
sCT plus sCT(11-32)	19 1240	7	0.2**	0.9**	8.6**	16**
pCT	3720	11	0.6*	5.8	17	25
hCT	3720	7	1.4	5.0	23	34
sCT	62	12		0**	0.8**	2.9**
Iodo-sCT	62	6		0**	0.8**	5.1**
Photoreactive sCT	62	9			4.6**	

a) injected intracerebroventricularly.
* and ** indicate significant inhibition as compared with the saline-treated control ($P < 0.05$ and $P < 0.01$, respectively)

CONCLUSION

It is concluded that some CTs given centrally interact with the receptors in the anterior hypothalamic nuclei, possibly affecting the Ca-flux, which then leads to inhibition of feeding behavior.

ACKNOWLEDGEMENTS

Research was supported in part by Grant in Aid for Scienctic Research to M. K. (No. 557514 and No. 58570931) from the Ministry of Education, Science and Culture, Japan.

REFERENCES

1. Pecile A, Ferri S, Braga PC, Olgiati VR (1975) Experientia 31:332-333
2. Freed WJ, Perlow MJ, Wyatt RJ (1979) Science 206:850-852
3. Levine AS, Morley JE (1981) Brain Res 222:187-191
4. Morley JE, Levine AS, Silvis SE (1981) Science 214:671-673
5. Morimoto T, Okamoto M, Koida M, Nakamuta H, Stahl GL, Orlowski RC (1984) unpublished.
6. Koida M, Nakamuta H, Furukawa S, Orlowski RC (1980) Japan J Pharmacol 30:575-577
7. Nakamuta H, Furukawa S, Koida M (1981) Japan J Pharmacol 31: 53-60
8. Rizzo AJ, Goltzman D (1981) Endocrinol 108:1672-1677
9. Fischer JA, Sagar SM, Martin JB (1981) Life Sci 29:663-671
10. Fischer JA, Tobler PH, Kaufmann M, Born W, Henke H, Cooper PE (1981) Proc Natl Acad Sci USA 78:7801-7805
11. Olgiati VR, Guidobono F, Netti C, Pecile A (1983) Brain Res 265:209-215
12. Henke H, Tobler PH, Fischer JA (1983) Brain Res 272:373-377
13. Moseley JM, Findley DM, Martin TJ, Gorman JJ (1982) J Biol Chem 257:5846-5851
14. Koida M, Yamamoto Y, Nakamuta H, Matsuo J, Okamoto M, Morimoto T, Seyler JK, Orlowski RC (1982) Japan J Pharmacol 32:981-986
15. Perlow MJ, Freed WJ, Carman JS, Wyatt RJ (1979) Pharmacol Biochem Behav 12:609-612
16. Twery MJ, Obie JF, Cooper CW (1982) Peptides 3:749-755
17. Bueno L, Fioramonti J, Ferre JP (1983) Peptides 4:63-66
18. Randall LO, Selitto JJ (1957) Arch int Pharmacodyn Ther 3: 409-419
19. Morimoto T, Okamoto M, Koida M, Nakamuta H, Orlowski RC (1984) unpublished.

© 1984 Elsevier Science Publishers B.V.
Endocrinology
F. Labrie, L. Proulx, eds.

CALCITONIN: A CANDIDATE FOR A NEUROMODULATOR OF PAIN INHIBITING SYSTEMS

ANTONIO PECILE, FRANCESCA GUIDOBONO, VALERIA SIBILIA, CARMELA NETTI
Dept. of Pharmacology, Chemotherapy and Medical Toxicology, University of Milan, 32 Via Vanvitelli, 20129 Milan, Italy

The presence of immunoreactive-calcitonin (CT) (1, 2) and of specific binding sites (2, 3) in various areas of the brain indicate that CT may be a neuromodulator in the CNS. Among the various physiological functions of the peptide in nervous tissue, the most striking is its inhibition of pain perception in both animals (4) and humans (5). The antinociceptive activity of CT is opioid-independent since a) it is naloxone insensitive, b) CT given with morphine has analgesic activity which is the sum of the actions of both drugs, c) repeated injections of CT do not decrease the pain threshold in the rabbit (6), and d) long-term treatment in rats also still evokes pronounced analgesia (Fig. 1) without development of tolerance. Thus CT may well be considered to be, like other neuropeptides (i.e. neurotensin and caerulein), a candidate of endogenous non-opiate peptidergic system, for which the mechanism of pain control is still poorly understood. Since there is strong evidence that there are inhibitory serotonergic (5HT) and nor-adrenergic (NE) pathways that control nociceptive input (7), we examined the possible inter-relationship between CT and those biogenic amines known to be involved in pain modulatory systems. We used either CNS chemical lesions or pharmacological manipulation to characterize the neural mechanisms that underly pain inhibition by CT.

Role of biogenic amines in CT analgesia

The possible involvement of the 5HT system on salmon CT (sCT) analgesia was investigated by lowering central 5HT with drugs, such as the selective neurotoxin 5,6 dihidroxytryptamine (5,6DHT) or p-clorophenylalanine (pCPA) or the receptor blocker metergoline. The destruction of 5HT neurons did not affect the antinociceptive effects of sCT nor did pretreatment with metergoline or with the inhibitor of 5HT biosynthesis, pCPA.On the basis of the above, we decided to study the role of the catecholaminergic (CA) system in the antinociceptive activity of sCT. Treatment with 6hydroxydopamine (6OHDA) which selectively destroys CA-containing neurons strongly decreased sCT analgesia, as did treatment with α and β blockers or with propranolol alone, whereas phentolamine alone had no effect (8). Since the effect of propranolol was significant but transient (30 min.), we examined the possibility that only one type of β adrenoreceptors might be involved. For this purpose we studied the effects of a selective β_1 blocker atenolol, which was able to lower significantly for up to 60 min the effects of CT on pain threshold (Fig. 2), suggesting that the CA system, through β_1 receptors, is important in the antinociceptive activity of CT.

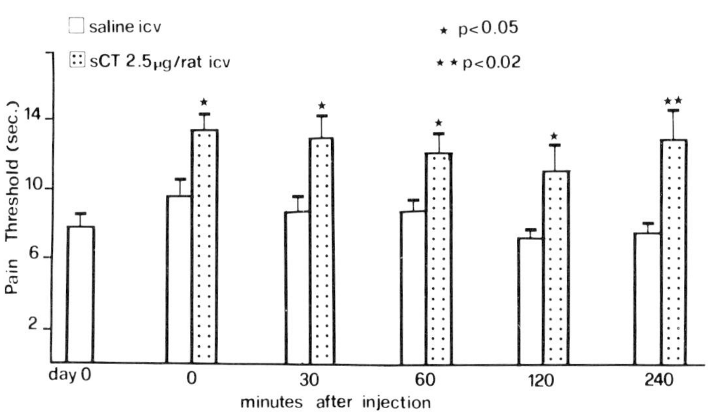

Fig. 1. Hot-plate latencies (mean ± SE) after chronic treatment with sCT injected intracerebroventricularly (icv) for 14 days (250 ng/rat/day). The plate was set at 53°C, licking of the hind paw was taken as end point; a 20 sec cut-off time was used. Day 0 baseline latency was measured before the start of the experiment. The analgesic response was evaluated at different times after the administration of sCT, 2.5 μg/icv/rat.

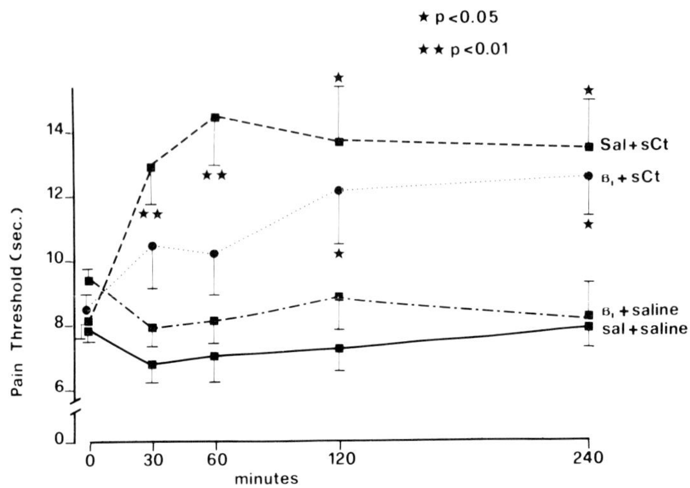

Fig. 2. Analgesic effects of sCT (2.5 μg/icv/rat) after pretreatment with a β_1 blocker, atenolol (5 μg/icv/rat, 15' before sCT). Hot plate latencies are means ± SE.

These findings are consistent with our previous evidence (6) that non-opiate mechanisms are involved in pain inhibition by sCT, since long-term treatment did not produce dependence or tolerance. Furthermore the results obtained with monoamine neurotoxins and with drugs that lower the tone of 5HT or CA systems indicate participation of NE but not of the 5HT system in the antinociceptive effects of the peptide.

Since only β blockers significantly inhibited the sCT-induced analgesia, the β receptors may have a predominant role in pain modulation by sCT. It is well recognized that activation of the NE system may modulate pain transmission (9) and could be involved in opioid analgesia and in non-opioid-induced analgesias of acute stress and classical conditioning procedures. It is proposed that sCT antinociception might act by modulating the CA neural pathway, either by direct spinal action or by activating the descending bulbospinal CA system. To know at which of these levels it acts, we are evaluating the effects of electrolytic lesions, starting with these in the ventromedial PAG. Preliminary results have shown that the antinociceptive activity of sCT is still demonstrable in lesioned rats. Further neuroanatomical studies are in progress. The analgesic effect of CT might be of physiological relevance. Recently it has been reported that the rat CT gene encodes also for a novel peptide (CGRP) (10) which is formed in relatively greater amounts in the central and peripheral nervous system and is endowed, like CT, with antinociceptive activity when centrally administered (11). The distribution for binding sites for CGRP and CT differs in some regions of rat brain (JA Fischer, personal communication) but both bind in considerable amounts in the mesencephalon and the spinal cord, areas involved in pain processing mechanisms. Thus calcitonins and CT related peptides may be a "family" of neuropeptides partecipating as neuromodulators in the multiple systems of perception control.

ACKNOWLEDGEMENTS

This work was supported by CNR grant CT82 and by "Gruppo Italiano per lo studio della calcitonina".

REFERENCES

1. Pavlinac DM, Lenhard LW, Parthermore JG, Deftos LJ (1980) J Clin Endocrinol Metab 50:717
2. Fischer JA, Tobler PH, Kaufmann M, Born W, Henke H, Cooper PE, Sagar SM, Martin JB (1981) Proc Natl Acad Sci USA 78:7801
3. Olgiati VR, Guidobono F, Netti C, Pecile A (1983) Brain Res 265:209
4. Pecile A, Ferri S, Braga PC, Olgiati VR (1975) Experientia 31:332
5. Fraioli F, Fabbri A, Gnessi L, Moretti C, Santoro C, Felici M (1982) European J Pharmacol 78: 381
6. Braga PC, Ferri S, Santagostino A, Olgiati VR, Pecile A (1978) Life Sci 22:971
7. Basbaum AI, Fields HL (1984) Ann Rev Neurosci 7: 309
8. Pecile A, Guidobono F, Sibilia V, Netti C (1984) In: Cohn D, Fujita T, Potts jr J, Talmage R (eds) Endocrine Control of Bone and Calcium Metabolism. Elsevier Science Publishers BV, Amsterdam, vol 8A, pp 176-179
9. Reddy SV, Yaksh TL (1980) Brain Res 189: 582
10. Rosenfeld MG, Mermod JJ, Amara SG, Swanson LW, Sawchenko PE, Rivier J, Vale WW, Evans RM (1983) Nature (London) 304: 129
11. Bates RFL, Buckley GA, Mc Ardle CA (1984) Br J Pharmacol 82:295P

48. Corticotropin-Releasing Factor and Regulation of ACTH Secretion

Endocrinology
F. Labrie, L. Proulx, eds.

DISTRIBUTION OF CORTICOTROPIN RELEASING FACTOR (CRF) IN THE CENTRAL NERVOUS SYSTEM

SANDOR VIGH, ISTVAN MERCHENTHALER, PETER PETRUSZ, ANDREW V. SCHALLY, BELA FLERKO

Department of Anatomy, University Medical School, Pecs, Hungary (S.V.,I.M.,B.F.); the Endocrine and Polypeptide Laboratories, Veterans Administration Medical Center, and Department of Medicine, Tulane University, School of Medicine, New Orleans, La. 70146, USA (A.V.S.) and Department of Anatomy, University of North Carolina, Chapel Hill, N.C. 27514, USA (P.P.)

INTRODUCTION

The chemical characterization and synthesis of a 41-amino-acid ovine hypothalamic peptide with high intrinsic ACTH releasing activity have recently been reported (14). The biological potencies of synthetic ovine CRF have been tested by various laboratories *in vivo* (11,13,14) and *in vitro* (11,13,16). This peptide meets many of the physiological criteria to characterize it as a natural CRF. Synthetic CRF causes a dose-related release of ACTH and β-endorphin *in vivo* and *in vitro* (13,14), does not increase plasma corticosterone levels in hypophysectomized rat, demonstrating that it does not stimulate the adrenal gland directly (13). Furthermore, administration of rabbit anti-CRF serum reduces plasma ACTH levels in adrenalectomized rats and intact stressed animal (10).

The availability of synthetic ovine CRF has allowed the generation of antibodies for CRF radioimmunoassay (RIA) and immunocytochemistry (ICC) (15). Distributional maps of the CRF containing neurons and pathways in the rat brain had been provided by Olschowka et al. (9), Swanson et al. (12) and Merchenthaler (3). The quantitative distribution of CRF in hypothalamic and extrahypothalamic areas has also been studied by RIA (1). In addition, it has been shown that intracerebroventricular administration of CRF elicits specific autonomic and behavioral responses (3). All these results suggest that CRF, like other neuropeptides, may function not only as a hypophysiotropic hormone controlling ACTH release, but also as a neuromodulator mediating several neuroendocrine and autonomic functions. The present study describes and summarizes the ICC localization of CRF-immunoreactive structures throughout the central nervous system of the rat.

MATERIAL AND METHODS

Adult male rats (Sprague Dawley), colchicine treated animals of the same strain, long term adrenalectomized or hypophysectomized rats and rats with various stereotaxic knife cuts were used. The details of the experimental conditions, the unlabeled peroxidase immunocytochemical method and the recently developed silver intensification technique employed were described elsewhere (2,4-8). The primary antiserum to ovine CRF (SV-22) was raised in rabbit and characterized by agar gel diffusion, RIA and ICC (7,15). Briefly, the characteristics of the antibodies obtained in immunodiffusion, the distinct immunocytochemical localization, the results of the RIA cross-reactivity tests, the absorption and the dual staining tests, and the presence of CRF immunoreactivity in Brattleboro rats indicate that our antisera detected CRF-like immunoreactivity distinct from TRH, LH-RH, somatostatin-14, somatostatin-28, Lys-vasopressin (LVP), Arg-vasopressin (AVP), rat neurophysin II, substance P, vasoactive intestinal peptide (VIP), cholecystokinin (CCK) and all the pituitary hormones.

RESULTS AND DISCUSSION

The absorption of the antiserum with synthetic CRF prevented all immunostaining; however, absorption with all the peptides mentioned above had no effect on the intensity and the distribution of the staining. Immunoreactive CRF was present in perikarya, neuronal processes and terminals in all major subdivisions of the rat central nervous system. The results of these studies are schematically represented in Fig. 1.

Telencephalon

The neocortex contained mostly bipolar, vertically oriented cell bodies. Although there were CRF-immunopositive perikarya in all parts of the neocortex, these cell bodies were much more frequent in the prefrontal, insular and cingular areas.

Scattered CRF-positive cells were found in the olfactory bulb, the anterior olfactory nucleus, the accessory olfactory bulb and in small numbers among the granular cells of the main olfactory bulb.

In the hippocampus, CRF-immunopositive cells were seen in the indusium griseum, the CA_3 and CA_1 fields of Ammon's horn, the fasciola cinerea, the septal half of the dental gyrus and the subiculum.

Many CRF-stained cells were found in the central nucleus of the amygdala. In the septal region, most CRF-containing cell bodies were seen in the bed nucleus of the stria terminalis, both in its dorsal and ventral parts. Numerous CRF cells were present in all of the above mentioned areas. Scattered fibers were

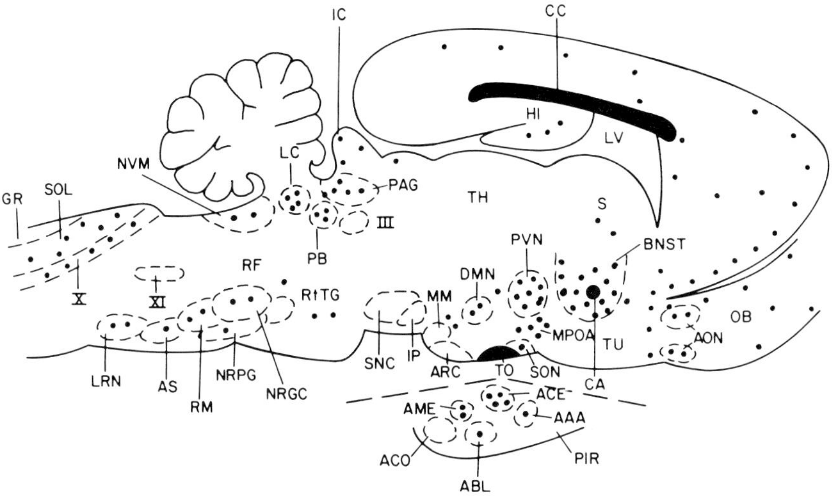

Fig. 1. Schematic drawing summarizing the distribution of CRF-immunopositive perikarya (solid circles) in a parasagittal segment of the brain as seen in colchicine-treated rats. Abbreviations: AAA: anterior amygdaloid area, ABL: basolateral amygdaloid nucleus, ACE: central amygdaloid nucleus, ACO: anterior cortical nucleus, AME: medial amygdaloid nucleus, AON: anterior olfactory nucleus, ARC: arcuate nucleus, BNST: bed nucleus of the stria terminalis, CC: corpus callosum, DMN: dorsomedial nucleus, GR: nucleus gracilis, HI: hippocampus, IC: inferior colliculus, IP: interpeduncular nucleus, LC: locus ceruleus, LRN: lateral reticular nucleus, LV: lateral ventricle, MM: medial mammillary nucleus, MPOA: medial preoptic area, NRGC: nucleus reticularis gigantocellularis, NRPG: nucleus reticularis paragigantocellularis, NVM: nucleus vestibularis medialis, OB: olfactory bulb, PAG: periaqueductal gray, PB: parabrachial nucleus, PIR: piriform cortex, PVN: paraventricular nucleus, RF: reticular formation, RM: raphe magnus, RtTG: reticulotegmental nucleus of the pons, SCN: substantia nigra, SOL: solitary tract, SON: supraoptic nucleus, TH: thalamus, TO: tractus opticus, TU: tuberculum olfactorium.

observed in the stria terminalis, the ventral amygdalofugal pathway, the caudat putamen and the globus pallidus.

Diencephalon

The great majority of the CRF-immunoreactive perikarya were localized in the parvocellular part of the PVH, although scattered cell bodies within this nucleus were observed among the magnocellular perikarya as well (Fig. 2). The CRF-positive fibers originating from the PVH form a medial, an intermediate, and a lateral fiber pathway. The lateral and intermediate CRF tracts leave the dorsolateral part of the PVH and course laterally and medially to the fornix, then run ventrally toward the optic tract (Fig. 3). Just dorsal to the optic tract they turn in caudal direction and run parallel with and very close to the basal surface of the hypothalamus; individual fibers then turn medially to terminate in the external layer of the median eminence (ME) (Fig. 4). Only a few fibers originate from the medial-ventral part of the PVH (medial pathway). These fibers run in ventral direction along the walls of the 3rd ventricle and terminate in the ME. Both hypophysectomy and particularly adrenalectomy resulted in a dramatic increase in immunostaining of the paraventriculo-infundibular (PV-IN) CRF system (Fig. 3 and 5). In colchicine treated animals outside of the PVH, numerous CRF-immunopositive perikarya were found in the medial preoptic and periventricular preoptic nuclei. Scattered perikarya were seen in the anterior, basolateral and posterior hypothalamus, the dorsomedial, the supraoptic, dorsal periventricular and premammillary nuclei. ICC observations in rats with various knife cuts provided evidence that some of the CRF-containing cell bodies in the above mentioned areas had afferent connections to the ME.

The origin and course of CRF immunoreactive fibers terminating in the ME are summarized schematically in Fig. 6. In addition, scattered fibers with CRF immunoreactivity were present throughout the hypothalamus and in the midline nuclei of the posterior thalamus, including the nucleus reuniens, the rhomboid nucleus, the paratenial and the paraventricular nucleus.

Mesencephalon

CRF-containing perikarya were seen in the periaqueductal gray, predominantly in its ventral portion, in the dorsal nucleus of the raphe and the dorsal parts of the central tegmental area, throughout its rostrocaudal extent. Scattered CRF-positive cells were found in the superior and inferior colliculi. CRF fibers were coursing dorsally-dorsomedially from the level of the supramammillary nuclei to the periaqueductal gray of the mesencephalon.

Metencephalon

The largest group of CRF-immunopositive perikarya in the metencephalon was located in the locus ceruleus, the dorsal and ventral parabrachial nuclei.

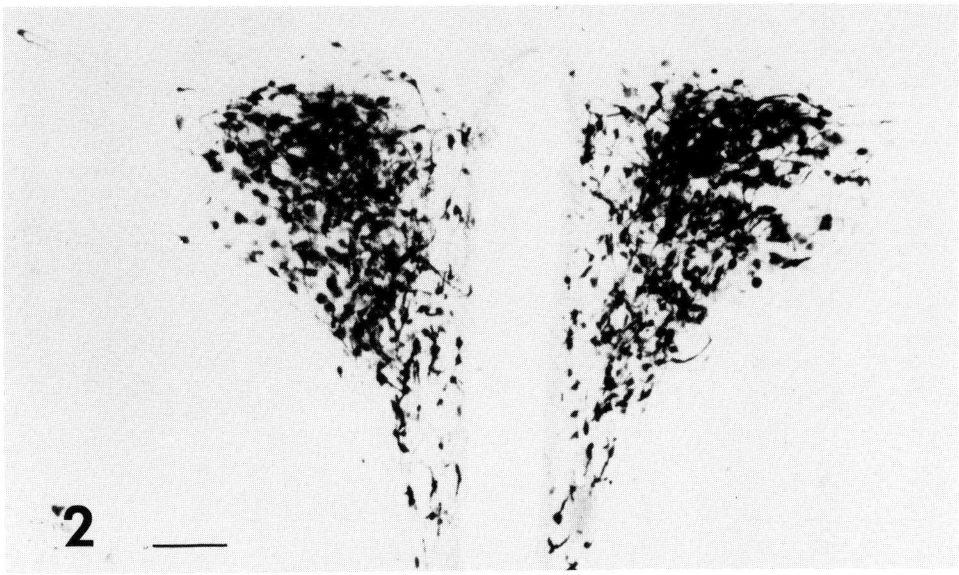

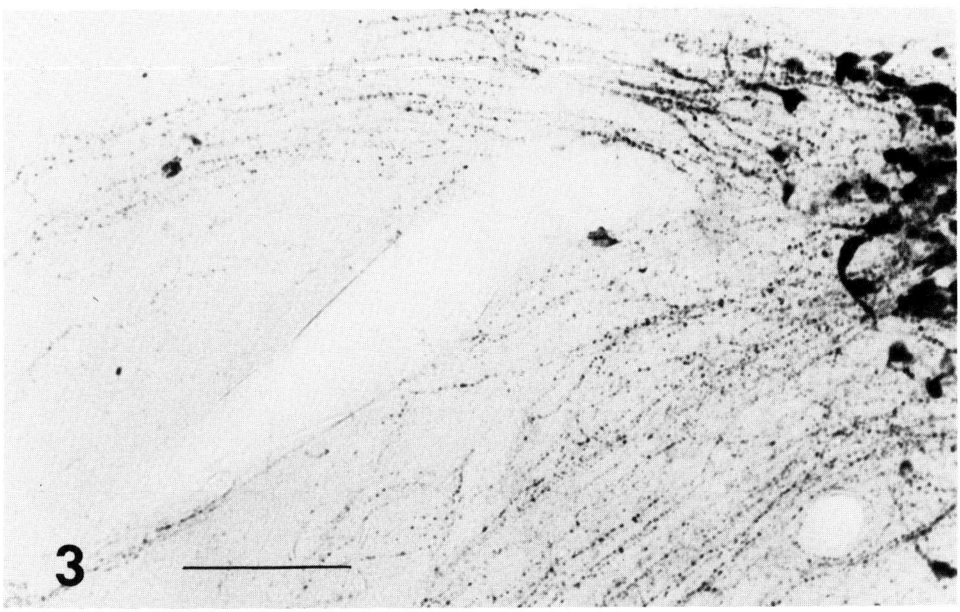

Fig. 2. CRF immunopositive cell bodies in the PVN of a colchicine treated rat. Silver-gold intensified section. Fig. 3. The central part of the paraventriculoinfundibular CRF system. Perikarya in the PVN send their processes in either ventral (cannot be seen) or lateral direction, forming a curved fan of fibers. Long term adrenalectomized rat, silver-gold intensification. Bar represents 100μ.

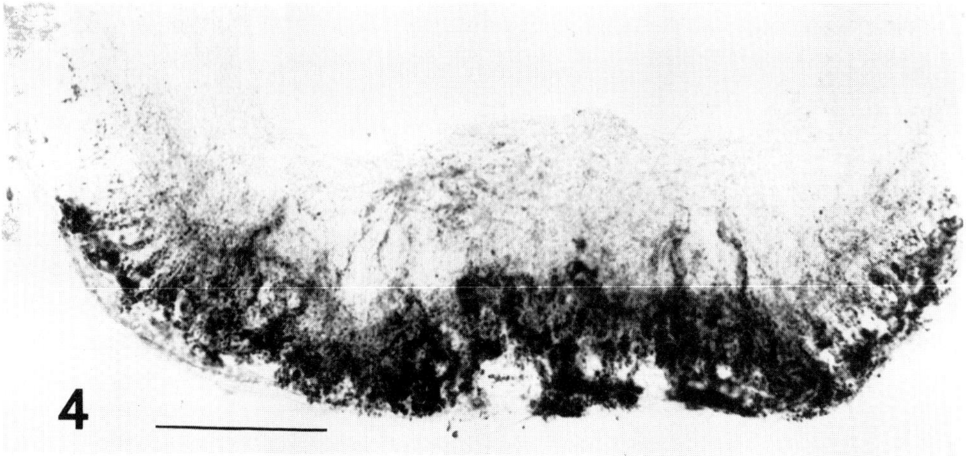

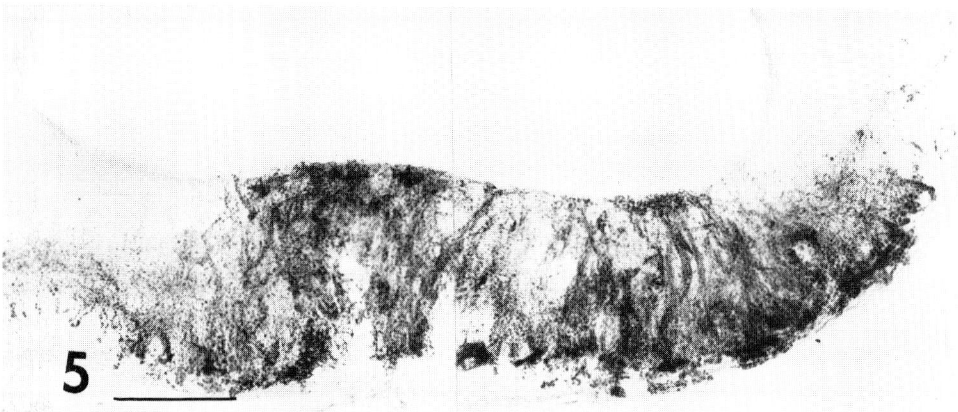

Fig. 4. Distribution of CRF immunoreactivity in the anterior region of the ME of a control rat. The majority of the fibers and terminals are seen in the external zone. Fig. 5. Distribution of CRF immunoreactivity in the anterior region of the ME of a long-term adrenalectomized rat. Increased immunostaining can be seen in both zones of the ME. Bar represents 100 μ.

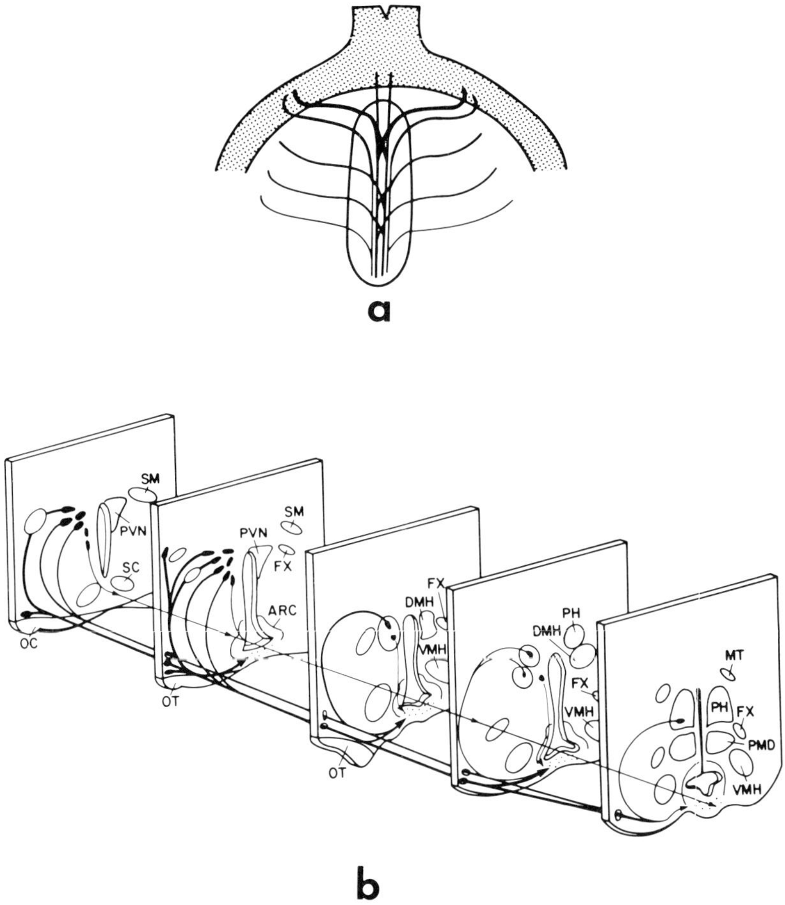

Fig. 6. (a) Schematic illustration of CRF afferents as they approach the ME at the base of the hypothalamus. The ME is represented by the oval area in the middle. CRF-containing fibers approach the ME from anterior and antero-lateral directions. The majority reach the ME through the lateral-basal retrochiasmatic area (thick lines), but scattered fibers can be seen as far caudally as the level of the pituitary stalk. The ipsilateral fibers form terminals in the entire length of the ME. Many of them cross the midline and give terminals on the contralateral side in regions close to the midline. (b) Schematic illustration of the major sources and pathways of CRF fibers terminating in the ME. CRF afferents from the PVN form a fan of fibers consisting of a medial, a more diffuse intermediate, and a lateral tract. Axons arising from the DMN and the periventricular hypothalamic nuclei join the curved fan of fibers formed by the paraventriculo-infundibular CRF system. Lines of different thickness reflect the differences in the relative number of fibers within the tracts. ARC: arcuate nucleus; DMH: dorsomedial nucleus; FX: fornix; MT: mamillothalamic tract; OC: optic chiasm; OT: optic tract; PMD: dorsal premammillary nucleus; PH: periventricular nucleus; PVN: paraventricular nucleus; SC: suprachiasmatic nucleus; SM: stria medullaris; VMH: ventromedial nucleus.

CRF-positive cell bodies, in small number, were also found in the medial vestibular nucleus, in a region lateral to the superior olivary complex, the paragigantocellular reticular nucleus, the inferior central nucleus of the raphe and the laterodorsal tegmental nucleus. Fibers with CRF-immunoreactivity were seen in all of these regions. A dens plexus of the CRF-fibers was found lateral to the locus ceruleus, in the mesencephalic nucleus of the trigeminal nerve, and in the dorsal and ventral parabrachial nuclei.

In the cerebellum, CRF-immunopositive fibers were observed in the molecular layer of the cortex, apparently in close association with the dentritic tree of the Purkinje cells.

Myelencephalon

The majority of the CRF-immunopositive cells and fibers were seen in the nucleus of the solitary tract and the dorsal vagal complex. CRF-positive fibers were traced from the pontine reticular formation to the medullary reticular formation.

Spinal cord

In control rats no CRF-containing cell bodies were found. Following local colchicine treatment or long-term hypophysectomy, CRF-positive cell bodies were detected in laminae V-VII and X at thoracic and lumbal levels, as well as in the intermediolateral column (Fig. 7). Labeled fibers were seen in the regions mentioned above, and in the dorsal part of the lateral funiculus close to the spinothalamic tract.

The distribution of CRF-like immunoreactivity in the brain and spinal cord as indicated by Swanson et al. (12) anatomically and probably also functionally can be divided into three major parts: 1. the hypothalamo-infundibular system which projects to the ME. The main function of this system is the regulation of ACTH and β-endorphin release from the pituitary gland; 2. the existence of CRF immunoreactive cell bodies and fibers in the extrahypothalamic areas of the subcortical brain regions and in the spinal cord suggests a role for CRF as a neuronal modulator or neurotransmitter; 3. cerebral cortex, mainly those parts belong to the limbic system.

It seems likely that CRF, like other neuropeptides, has several functions, only one of which is the release of ACTH and β-endorphin from the pituitary. The characteristic distribution of CRF in close association with a large number of autonomic centers suggests that CRF is an important regulatory peptide, mediating several stress responses. The presence of CRF in the central visceral nuclei of the cranial nerves and its association with the sympathetic intermediolateral column provides additional evidence for its involvement in the

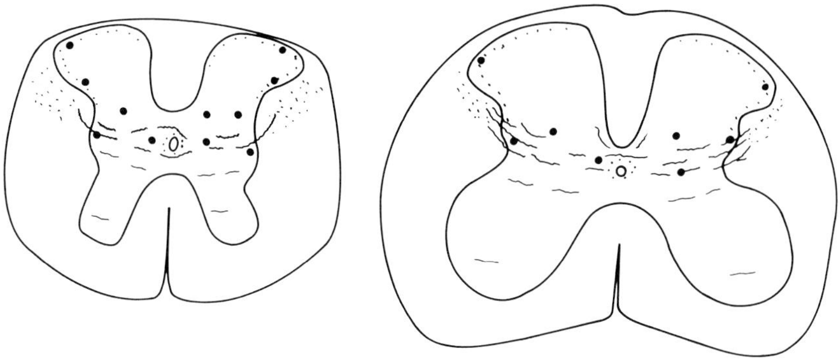

Fig. 7. Schematic drawing summarizing the distribution of CRF-immunoreactive cell bodies and fibers in low thoracic (left) and lumbal (right) levels in the spinal cord of hypophysectomized rats.

regulation of autonomic functions. Its presence in the marginal zone of dorsal horn, in lamina X of the spinal cord, in the sensory nuclei of most of the cranial nerves and in the midline of the thalamus suggests a role in the processing of nociceptive afferents in these regions, CRF can modify noxious stimuli prior to activation of the ascending pathways.

REFERENCES

1. Fischman AJ, Moldow RL (1982) Peptides 3:149
2. Liposits I, Lengvari S, Vigh S, Schally AV, Flerko B (1983) Peptides 4:941
3. Merchenthaler I (1984) Peptides 5:53
4. Merchenthaler I, Gorcs T, Petrusz P (1982) J Histochem Cytochem 30:607
5. Merchenthaler I, Hynes MA, Vigh S, Schally AV, Petrusz P (1983) Brain Res 275:373
6. Merchenthaler I, Hynes MA, Vigh S, Schally AV, Petrusz P (1984) Neuroendocrinology in press
7. Merchenthaler I, Vigh S, Petrusz P, Schally AV (1982) Am J Anat 165:385
8. Merchenthaler I, Vigh S, Petrusz P, Schally AV (1983) Regul Pept 5:295
9. Olschowka JA, O'Donohue L, Mueller GP, Jacobowitz DM (1982) Neuroendocrinology 35:305
10. Rivier C, Brownstein M, Spiess J, Rivier J, Vale W (1982) Endocrinology 110:272
11. Sueiras-Diaz J, Coy DH, Vigh S, Redding TW, Huang WY, Torres-Aleman I, Schally AV (1982) Life Sci 31:429
12. Swanson LW, Sawchenko PE, Rivier J, Vale W (1983) Neuroendocrinology 36:165
13. Turkelson CM, Arimura A, Culler MD, Fishback JB, Groot K, Kanda M, Luciano M, Thomas CR, Chang D, Chang JK, Simizu M (1982) Peptides 2:425
14. Vale W, Spiess J, Rivier C, Rivier J (1981) Science 213:1394
15. Vigh S, Merchenthaler I, Torres-Aleman I, Sueiras-Diaz J, Coy DH, Carter WH, Petrusz P, Schally AV (1982) Life Sci 31:2441
16. Vigh S, Schally AV (1984) Peptides 5:241

Endocrinology
F. Labrie, L. Proulx, eds.

VASOPRESSIN AND THE 41-AMINO ACID CORTICOTROPIN RELEASING FACTOR INVOLVEMENT IN THE CONTROL OF CORTICOTROPIN SECRETION

GLENDA GILLIES, ELIZABETH LINTON AND PHILIP LOWRY
Protein Hormone Unit, St Bartholomew's Hospital, West Smithfield, London EC1A 7BE (UK)

INTRODUCTION

The rôle of vasopressin (VP) in the control of adrenocorticotropin (ACTH) secretion has been debated for 30 years. Gel filtration of hypothalamic extracts from normal[1] and Brattleboro[2] rats, coupled with the isolated rat anterior pituitary cell column bioassay have led to the conclusion that CRF is not a single, simple peptide, but consists of VP and at least 2 other factors, which synergise with each other for full biological activity[1]. The results from many laboratories now suggest that the recently characterised 41-amino acid CRF (CRF-41)[3] plays a significant rôle in the physiological control of ACTH release at the level of the corticotrope, along with VP.

METHODOLOGY AND RESULTS

Chromatography

With the development of an ovine CRF (oCRF-41) radioimmunoassay (RIA)[4], one of the bioactive CRF's found after gel filtration chromatography (BioGel P2 and Sephadex G-50) of rat hypothalamic extracts was found to be related to this peptide. This peak synergised with the other ACTH-releasing peaks, including the VP peak. Trypsinization experiments provided evidence that the CRF peak eluting at the void volume was a precursor for a smaller molecular weight CRF, and another CRF was identified which eluted near oxytocin in both chromatographic systems[5].

In vitro experiments

Ovine CRF-41, although a more potent releaser of ACTH than VP in our bioassay, was found not to be as active as a rat stalk-median eminence extract (rSME). A combination of synthetic oCRF-41 and VP however resulted in a log dose-response curve parallel to that for rSME[6]. It has been reported that the rat 41-amino acid CRF (rCRF-41) has similar hypophysiotropic potencies to that of oCRF pituitary monolayer cultures[7], but in the isolated cell column bioassay rCRF-41 was more active than oCRF-41.

In vitro immunoneutralization of the CRF-41 and VP components of ACTH-releasing activity in rSME showed that bioactivity was reduced to 50% and 40% respectively. When both antisera were combined 20% of bioactivity remained[8]. This is further evidence of synergism between these 2 peptides.

In vivo experiments

From in vivo experiments Yates et al[9] deduced that VP interacted with the hypothalamo-pituitary-adrenal axis by direct action on the anterior pituitary, by stimulating CRF release from the hypothalamus and by potentiating the action of CRF at the level of the anterior pituitary. It has now been shown that exogenous synthetic CRF-41 and VP synergise in their ACTH-releasing effect in humans[10]. Results from experiments with VP antagonists have been equivocal[11,12] and this may be due to the fact that the anterior pituitary receptor mediating the action of vasopressin on ACTH release seems to be of neither the classical V_1 (pressor) nor V_2 (antidiurectic) type[13]. As selective blockers for these receptors are not yet available, we elected to use VP antibodies to study the peptide's involvement in ACTH release in vivo.

In collaboration with Dr F Tilder's group at Amsterdam's Free University, rats were pre-treated with the immunoglobulin (IgG) fractions from antisera to oCRF-41, VP and to a combination of both. We observed a reduction of the plasma ACTH response to 28%, 53% and 16% respectively 5 minutes after formalin stress and to 13%, 37% and 12% respectively 5 minutes after restraint stress[14]. The antibody pre-treatment did not attenuate the stress-induced rise in plasma prolactin in the same animals, demonstrating that both VP and an oCRF-41-like peptide play a physiological rôle in the control of the ACTH but not prolactin response during stress.

Released CRF

Hypothalami from female Wistar rats were cut into $1mm^3$, mixed with pre-swollen BioGel P2, packed into a plastic column and perfused at the rate of 0.17 ml/min[15]. Ten minute fractions were collected and assessed immediately for bioactivity and VP and CRF-41 immunoactivity in basal and 56 $mMK^{\pm}$ stimulated fractions. The release of VP immunoactivity paralleled that of CRF bioactivity, but CRF-41 immunoactivity was below the detection limit of RIA. However, the involvement of both VP and CRF-41 in the bioactivity was indicated by immunoneutralization of released CRF with CRF-41 and VP antisera alone and in combination. Comparison of the VP content versus CRF bioactivity for a hypothalamic extract, released CRF and synthetic VP is given in Table I and suggests that a significant difference in composition and/or lability of factors exists between released and extracted CRF.

SUMMARY

Considerable evidence now suggests that both the 41-amino acid hypothalamic CRF and VP are physiological CRF's which interact and synergise with each other, and possibly also with other hypothalamic factors, to control the release of ACTH from the pituitary. The relative rôles which these peptides play in a variety of circumstances remains to be established.

Investigation on the nature of released ACTH-releasing activity in vitro has employed 56 mMK+ stimulation of hypothalamic pieces and suggests that a significant difference in composition may exist between released and extracted activity. This non-specific depolarising stimulus would release all components with ACTH-releasing activity, which may not reflect the ratio in which they are released physiologically. More information on the relative rôles of CRF-41 and VP may be gained using specific stimuli (neuro-transmitters, steroids, drugs) for CRF release on superfused hypothalamic pieces and cultured neurons, along with the development of a more sensitive CRF-41 immunoassay.

TABLE I

COMPARISON OF EXTRACTED AND RELEASED CORTICOTROPIN RELEASING ACTIVITY WITH ARGININE VASOPRESSIN (AVP) CONTENT.

	AVP content pg/ml	ACTH released in bioassay (ng)	Inter-assay coefficient of variation (bioassay) n = 6
0.25 SME/ml	250-300	1.4-2.2	20.8%
Synthetic AVP	1000	0.5-1.3	37%
Released CRF diluted 1:5	35	1.165	-

ACKNOWLEDGEMENTS

This work was supported by the British Medical Research Council and the Joint Research Board of St Bartholomew's Hospital, London.

REFERENCES

1 Gillies G E, Lowry P J (1979) Nature 276: 463-465

2 Gillies G E, Lowry P J (1980) J Endocrinol 84: 65-70

3 Vale W, Spiess J, Rivier C, Rivier J (1981) Science 213: 1394-1397

4 Linton E A, Lowry P J (1982) Neuropeptides 3: 45-52

5 Gillies G E, Puri A, Linton E A, Lowry P J (1984) Neuroendocrinol 38: 17-24

6 Gillies G E, Linton E A, Lowry P J (1982) Nature 299: 355-357

7 Rivier J, Spiess J, Vale W (1983) PNAS 80: 4851-4855

8 Linton E A, Gillies G E, Lowry P J (1983) Endocrinol 113: 1878-1883

9 Yates F E, Russell S M, Dallman M F, Hedge G A, McCann S M (1971)

Endocrinology 88: 3-15

10 Liu J H, Muse K, Contreras P, Gibbs D, Vale W, Rivier J, Yen S S C (1983) J Clin Endocrinol Metab 57: 1087-1089

11 Mormède P (1983) Nature 305: 345-346

12 Rivier C, Vale W (1983) Nature 305: 325-328

13 Baertschi A J, Gähwiler B, Antoni F A, Holmes M C, Makare G B (1984) Nature 308: 85-86

14 Linton E A, Berkenbosch F, Hodgkinson S C, Tilders F J H, Vermes I, Lowry P J (1984) submitted for publication

15 Gillies G E, Puri A, Hodgkinson S C, Lowry P J (1984) J Endocrinol in press

Endocrinology
F. Labrie, L. Proulx, eds.

EFFECT OF CORTICOTROPIN-RELEASING FACTOR (CRF) ON SOME ENDOCRINE FUNCTIONS

CATHERINE RIVIER AND WYLIE VALE

Peptide Biology Laboratory, The Salk Institute, 10010 North Torrey Pines Road, La Jolla, California 92037

Corticotropin-releasing factor (CRF) was initially purified and isolated on the basis of its ability to stimulate the secretion of ACTH and -endorphin by the pituitary (1-3). The physiologic role played by endogenous CRF in regulating ACTH release has been supported by experiments showing that administration of anti-CRF serum or CRF antagonists would lower resting plasma levels of ACTH in adrenalectomized rats, and inhibit the stress-induced rise of ACTH secretion in intact animals (4-6).

The effect of CRF on ACTH release can be observed following various routes of administration (7). In addition to ACTH and -endorphin (3), the intravenous (iv) injection of CRF stimulates the secretion of adrenal corticosteroids and progesterone, but does not significantly modify plasma levels of LH or PRL in acute experiments (Fig. 1). This is in contrast to results obtained after intracerebroventricular (icv) administration of CRF, which markedly inhibits the secretion of LH and GH (8, 9).

Since the continuous exposure to stimuli often results in desensitization to the trophic signal (10), we have studied the effect of injection of CRF in a repeated or continuous manner. Intact rats which received two injections of 0.15 or 0.75 nmol CRF showed a blunting of the ACTH response when CRF was again injected 0.5-6 h later (11). This blunting also occurred in adrenalectomized animals, suggesting that this partial desensitization was not solely due to corticosteroid feedback. Further support for this hypothesis came from results such as those illustrated in Fig. 2, in which 1.5 nmol CRF was injected intermittently (iv every two hours) to intact male rats. Following an initial blunting of the ACTH response similar to the one observed in twice-injected rats (11), pituitary responsiveness was at least partially maintained for 24 hours despite the continuous presence of elevated plasma corticosterone levels. The maintenance of pituitary responsiveness with episodic exposure to CRF, as opposed to the desensitization observed with continuous exposure to the peptide, is reminiscent of results obtained with another releasing factor, GnRH (13, 14). These results indicate that though continuous exposure to CRF is accompanied by a certain degree of desensitization, it still results in plasma ACTH and corticosteroid levels which are significantly elevated over baseline.

Administration of CRF by Alzet minipumps, which delivered 0.75 nmol CRF/hr for 7 or 14 days, resulted in elevated plasma levels of ACTH and corticosterone throughout the period of exposure to the releasing factor (12). Apart from

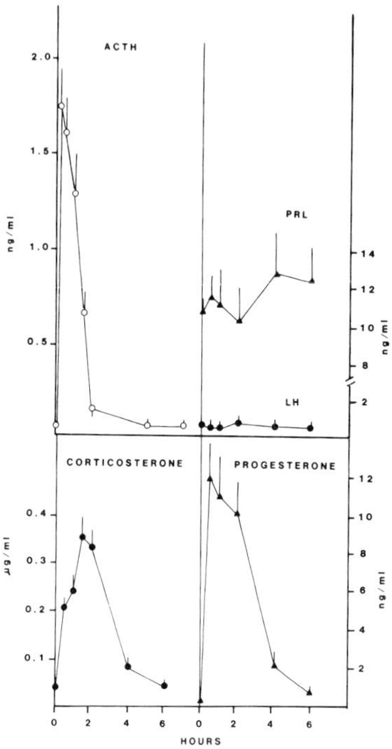

Fig. 1. Effect of the iv injection of 0.3 nmol oCRF to freely moving male rats. Plasma ACTH levels were measured 5 min, and plasma PRL, LH, corticosterone and progesterone 10 min, after administration of the peptide. Each point represents the mean ± SEM of 5 animals.

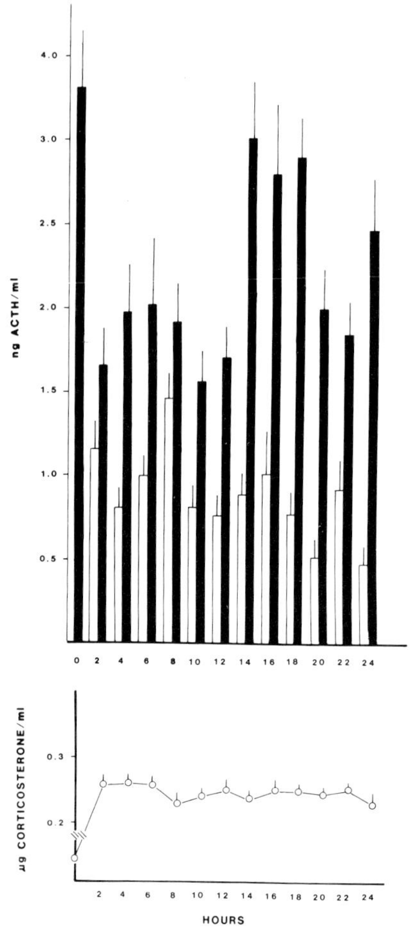

Fig. 2. Effect of the repeated (every 2 hrs) iv injection of 1.5 nmol oCRF to freely moving male rats. Open bars represent levels before each injectionµ closed bars represent levels 5 min after each injection. Each bar represents the mean ± SEM of 5 rats.

ACTH and corticosterone, the long-term infusion of CRF also modified the release of testosterone, LH and PRL (12). Since the CRF-induced lowering of plasma testosterone levels was not observed in adrenalectomized animals, we considered the possibility that adrenal steroids might affect the pituitary's responsiveness to GnRH. As illustrated in Fig. 3, both dexamethasone and progesterone can diminish this GnRH-induced release of LH. This suggests that stimulation of the adrenal corticosteroid production by ACTH during prolonged infusion of CRF may interfere with the normal function of the pituitary-gonadal axis through changes in the ability of the gonadotrophs to respond to GnRH.

These results indicate that the acute and chronic administration of CRF is

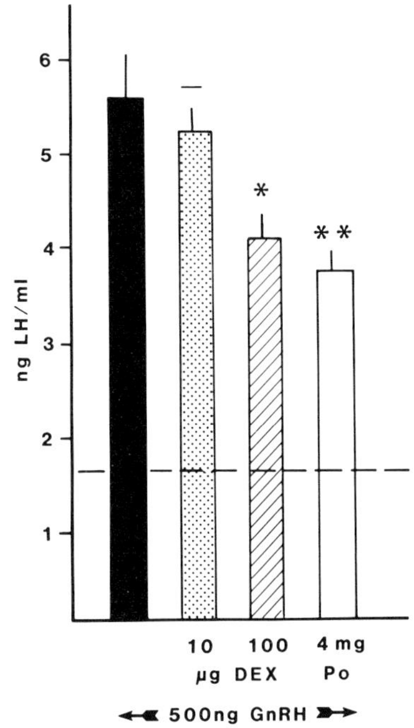

Fig. 3 Effect if dexamethasone (DEX) and progesterone (Po) on GnRH-induced secretion in freely moving male rats. The steroids were injected ip 4 hrs before the peptide. Blood samples were obtained 10 min after administration of GnRH. Each point represents the mean ± SEM of 5 animals: --, control levels; -, p>0.05 *, p<0.05; **, p<0.01.

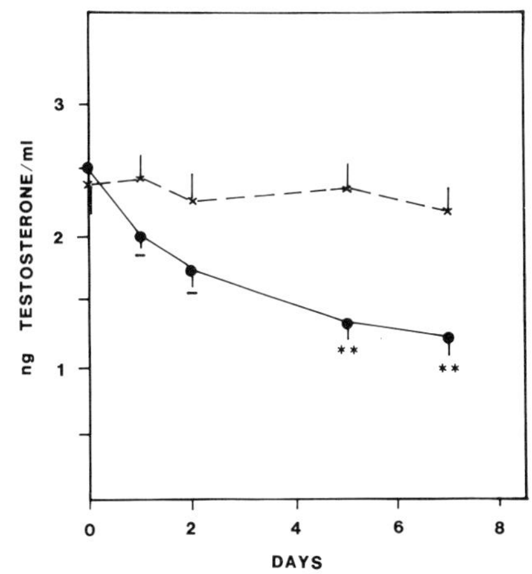

Fig. 4 Effect of infusion of 0.75 nmol oCRF/hr on testosterone secretion by adult male rats. Blood samp- obtained by decapitation. Each point represents the mean ± SEM of 5 animals: --, control rats; ___, CRF-treated rats; -, p >0.05; ** p<0.01.

accompanied by profound alterations in the release of a number of hormones. The persistently high levels of circulating ACTH and corticosterone measured during the long-term administration of CRF suggests that in the presence of elevated levels of CRF, a new set point for ACTH and corticosterone secretion is reached. It is possible that certain states of adrenal-hyper-responsiveness, such as Cushing's disease and alcoholic pseudo-Cushing's, might be associated at some stage with higher output of CRF. Additionally, the ability of CRF to inhibit some reproductive parameters in long-term experiments may be linked to the recognized deleterious effects of stress on fertility.

ACKNOWLEDGEMENTS

Research supported by NIH grants AM-26741 and HD-13527; the Rockefeller Foundation; and the March of Dimes-Birth Defects Foundation. This research was conducted in part by the Clayton Foundation for Research - California Division. CR and WV are Clayton Foundation Investigators. The authors thank Susan Logan and Gloria Swart for manuscript preparation.

REFERENCES

1. Vale W, Spiess J, Rivier C, Rivier J (1981). Science 213:1394-1397
2. Spiess J, Rivier J, Rivier C, Vale, W (1981) Proc Natl Acad Sci USA 78:6517-6521
3. Rivier C, Brownstein M, Spiess J, Rivier J, Vale W (1982) Endocrinology 110:272-278
4. Rivier C, Rivier J, Vale W (1982) Science 218:377-379
5. Rivier C, Vale W (1983) Nature 305:325-327
6. Rivier J, Rivier C, Vale W (1984) Science 224:889-891
7. Rivier C, Vale W (1984) Fed Proc, Proc Kroc Foundation Conference on CRF, Santa Barbara, CA, February 20-24
8. Rivier C, Vale W (1984) Endocrinology 114:914-919
9. Rivier C, Vale W (1984) Endocrinology (in press)
10. Catt K T, Dufau M L (1977) Ann Rev Physiol 39:529
11. Rivier C, Vale W (1983) Endocrinology 113:1422-1426
12. Rivier C, Vale W (1984) J Clinical Investigation in press
13. Belchetz P E, Plant T M, Nakai Y, Keogh G T, Knobil E (1978) Science 202:631-633
14. Smith M A, Vale W W (1981) Endocrinology 108:752-759

Endocrinology
F. Labrie, L. Proulx, eds.

CLINICAL STUDIES WITH OVINE CORTICOTROPIN-RELEASING HORMONE

DAVID N. ORTH, C. ROWAN DeBOLD, G. STEPHEN DeCHERNEY, RICHARD V. JACKSON, WILLIAM R. SHELDON, Jr., WENDELL E. NICHOLSON, DONALD P. ISLAND, A. NANCYE ALEXANDER, HOWARD UDERMAN, WILLIAM S. EVANS and MICHAEL O. THORNER

Departments of Medicine, Vanderbilt University Medical Center, Nashville, Tennessee 37232 and University of Virginia Medical Center, Charlottesville, Virginia 22908, U.S.A.

INTRODUCTION

Ovine corticotropin-releasing hormone (oCRH) was isolated from hypothalamic extracts and subsequently synthesized (1). It stimulates release of immunoreactive corticotropin (IR-ACTH) and β-endorphin (IR-βEND) from animal pituitaries in vitro and in vivo (1-3). Our studies were designed to elucidate the physiology and pharmacokinetics of oCRH in man.

MATERIALS AND METHODS

Subjects

Normal volunteers who had previously given their informed consent were studied. Their medical histories were unremarkable, and their physical examinations, serum chemistries, blood cell counts, urinalyses and EKGs were normal.

Study Protocol

Synthetic oCRH, generously provided by Drs. Jean Rivier and Wylie Vale, was administered in late afternoon. Subjects fasted after a light lunch and remained supine or semirecumbant during the study. Intravenous lines were established in both forearms. Saline was infused at the rate required to replace blood volume. Blood was obtained at -15, 0, 2, 5, 10, 15, 30, 60, 90 and 120 min and at hourly intervals thereafter. oCRH was injected iv in the opposite forearm. Pulse and blood pressure were monitored frequently during the study. The dose-response studies were double-blinded; others were single-blinded.

Radioimmunoassays

IR-ACTH was measured in unextracted EDTA-plasma, using antiserum IgG-ACTH-1 (IgG Corporation, Nashville, TN) (4), as was IR-cortisol (Micromedic Systems, Horsham, PA). Other IR-proopiomelanocortin peptides were measured by published assays (5), and IR-oCRH was measured (6) using antiserum IgG-oCRH-1 (IgG Corp.).

Statistical Analysis

Results were compared using analysis of variance and Duncan's multiple range test (7).

RESULTS AND COMMENTS

Dose-Response of Plasma IR-ACTH and IR-Cortisol

Doses of oCRH from 0.001 to 30 μg/kg body wt were administered as an iv bolus or, for the highest dose, a 20-sec infusion. The threshold dose appeared to be 0.01-0.03 μg/kg, the half-maximal dose 0.3-1 μg/kg, and the maximally-stimulating dose 3-10 μg/kg (8). Although higher IR-ACTH responses were observed after 30 μg/kg oCRH, many of these subjects appeared to be stressed. However, plasma levels of the other stress-related hormones, IR-GH and -PRL, did not rise, nor did those of IR-FSH, -LH, or -TSH, even after the highest oCRH dose. Plasma IR-ACTH rose within 2 min of oCRH injection and reached a peak after 10-15 min. Plasma IR-cortisol rose after 10 min or more and reached a peak at 30 min. Increasing the oCRH dose increased both the magnitude and duration of the response (8).

Side Effects

Facial flushing, tachycardia, and hypotension of increasing frequency, severity, and duration were observed after oCRH doses of 3 μg/kg or more (8). Shortness of breath, unassociated with wheezing, ischemic EKG changes or later increase in serum creatine phosphokinase, also occurred frequently. We have given more than 300 doses of oCRH to more than 100 individuals with no serious consequences.

Other Proopiomelanocortin Peptides

The plasma level of IR-lipotropins (IR-LPHs), which reflects both βLPH and γLPH, and of IR-βEND, which reflects both βLPH and βEND, rose and fell concomitantly with those of IR-ACTH (9). At no time after oCRH injection was there a significant difference between the molar concentrations of any of these peptides in circulating plasma.

Duration of Response

The response to oCRH was biphasic and prolonged: IR-ACTH reached a peak at 15 min, fell until 90 min, and rose to a second peak at 2-3 h (10). IR-cortisol levels reflected levels of IR-ACTH, but no second peak was seen after the highest oCRH dose, presumably due to maximally-stimulating levels of ACTH in plasma for 6 h after oCRH injection. Plasma IR-ACTH and cortisol were elevated 8 and 10 h, respectively, after the 30 μg/kg dose (10).

Pharmacokinetics of oCRH

The prolonged effect of oCRH is due to its long half-life in circulating plasma. IR-oCRH displayed similar pharmacokinetics over the full range of effective doses administered (6). It had a triexponential disappearance curve, with an initial distribution $t_{1/2}$ of 6.1 ± 0.5 (mean ± SEM) min and subsequent metabolic $t_{1/2}$s of 55 ± 3.8 and 198 ± 54 min. The initial volume of distribution was 6.2 ± 0.6 l, about 1.9 times the estimated plasma volume, and the metabolic clearance rate was 2.4 ± 0.2 ml/min·kg (146 ± 12 l/m^2·day). After 2, 30 and 90 min, the apparent molecular size and bioactivity of plasma IR-oCRH were identical to those of the injected peptide, indicating that oCRH survives intact in blood for a long time (6).

Effect on Circadian Rhythm

After oCRH doses of 3 and 30 μg/kg given in late afternoon, the next morning's normal circadian rise in plasma IR-ACTH and IR-cortisol was progressively diminished (10). This was due to the prolonged hypercortisolemia stimulated by oCRH, since Addisonian patients (11) or normal subjects whose cortisol secretion was acutely blocked with metyrapone (unpublished observations) had a normal rise in plasma IR-ACTH the morning after oCRH administration. Their plasma IR-ACTH responses were also far greater, indicating that cortisol secreted as the early result of oCRH administration inhibits further ACTH release in response to oCRH still circulating in blood.

Effect of Sex and Hour of Administration

Responses of men and women were not significantly different. The IR-ACTH rise was identical whatever time of day oCRH was given, but the IR-cortisol increment was greater in the evening, when basal plasma IR-cortisol was lower (unpublished observations).

Interaction with Vasopressin

The increment in plasma IR-ACTH after oCRH 1 µg/kg iv or synthetic arginine vasopressin (AVP) 10 pressor units im, which represent similar molar doses, was identical, but the effect of oCRH lasted longer and the total amount of ACTH released was greater (12). AVP caused a 2.6-fold potentiation of the plasma IR-ACTH response to oCRH when given 15 min earlier, and a 4-fold potentiation when given simultaneously. The latter response was still of somewhat lesser magnitude and of considerably briefer duration than the response to hypoglycemic stress (12). oCRH 1 or 10 µg/kg given at the time of threshold hypoglycemia (40 mg/dl) did not cause a greater plasma IR-ACTH response, suggesting that the response to hypoglycemic stress is maximal and probably involves prolonged exposure to relatively high concentrations of CRF, AVP and, possibly, other ACTH secretagogues.

Responses of Patients with Cushing's and Nelson's Syndromes

The response to oCRH of patients with untreated pituitary ACTH-dependent Cushing's disease is highly variable (13,14), but is markedly reduced or absent after successful transsphenoidal microadenomectomy (14). Thus, the microadenomas appear to be responsive to oCRH, raising the possibility that endogenous CRH may be involved in the etiology of some cases of Cushing's disease. Patients with Cushing's syndrome due to adrenal tumor do not respond. However, the highly variable response of Cushing's disease patients and the fact that some patients with ectopic ACTH syndrome respond to oCRH (15) suggest that oCRH may not provide a very useful differential diagnostic test in Cushing's syndrome (16). The magnitude of the response in patients with untreated Cushing's disease does not appear to correlate with the duration or severity of the disease or with basal plasma cortisol levels. Responses to oCRH return to normal over many months after successful microadenomectomy. Most patients with Nelson's syndrome respond to oCRH and, although the actual increment in plasma IR-ACTH is great, the percent rise is normal (13).

Combined Anterior Pituitary (CAP) Function Test

The combination of oCRH 1 µg/kg, hpGRH(1-40) 1 µg/kg, GnRH 100 µg and TRH 200 µg, given as successive 20-sec iv infusions to normal subjects, resulted in the same increments in plasma IR-ACTH, -cortisol, -GH, -FSH, -LH, -TSH and -PRL as when the factors were given individually (17). The increases of IR-GH and -PRL were greater and that of IR-LH was smaller in these women in the early follicular phase of the menstrual cycle than in the men. Hormone levels were at or near their peaks by 60 min. The CAP function test has been useful in assessing pituitary hormone status in the first 8 patients studied (18) and provides a short, safe, and practical test of combined anterior pituitary function.

SUMMARY

Synthetic oCRH, administered in an appropriate dose, alone or in combination with hpGRH(1-40), GnRH and TRH, is a safe and useful investigative and diagnostic agent in man.

ACKNOWLEDGMENTS

We thank Drs. Jean Rivier and Wylie Vale, Peptide Biology Laboratory, Salk Institute, La Jolla, CA, for the synthetic oCRH and IgG Corporation, Nashville, TN, for IgG-ACTH-1 and IgG-oCRH-1 antisera. These studies were supported in part by NIH grants 1-R01-AM33334, 5-R01-AM26741, 5-M01-RR00095, 1-F32-CA06939 (CRDeB) and 1-F32-AM06758 (GSDeC), 5-T32-AM07061 (WRS), and by an Australian NHMRC Fellowship (RVJ).

REFERENCES

1. Vale W, Spiess J, Rivier C, Rivier J (1981) Science 213: 1394-1397
2. Rivier C, Brownstein M, Spiess J, Rivier J, Vale W (1982) Endocrinology 11: 272-278
3. Vale W, Rivier C, Brown MR, Spiess J, Koob G, Swanson L, Bilezikjian L, Bloom F, Rivier J (1983) Recent Prog Horm Res 39: 245-270
4. Nicholson WE, Davis DR, Sherrell BJ, Orth DN (1984) Clin Chem 30: 259-265
5. Wilson MG, Nicholson WE, Holscher MA, Sherrell BJ, Mount CD, Orth DN (1982) Endocrinology 110: 941-954
6. Nicholson WE, DeCherney GS, Jackson RV, DeBold CR, Uderman H, Alexander RN, Rivier J, Vale W, Orth DN (1983) J Clin Endocrinol Metab 57: 192-196
7. Steel RGD, Torrie JH (1960) Principles and Procedures of Statistics. McGraw-Hill, New York, pp 99-131
8. Orth DN, Jackson RV, DeCherney GS, DeBold CR, Alexander AN, Island DP, Rivier J, Rivier C, Spiess J, Vale W (1983) J Clin Invest 71: 587-595
9. Jackson RV, DeCherney GS, DeBold CR, Sheldon WR, Alexander AN, Rivier J, Vale W, Orth DN (1984) J Clin Endocrinol Metab 58: 740-743
10. DeBold CR, DeCherney GS, Jackson RV, Sheldon WR, Alexander AN, Island DP, Rivier J, Vale W, Orth DN (1983) J Clin Endocrinol Metab 57: 294-298
11. DeBold CR, Jackson RV, Sheldon WR, Island DP, Orth DN (1983) Endocrinology 112 (Suppl): 264 (Abstract)
12. DeBold CR, Sheldon WR, DeCherney GS, Jackson RV, Alexander AN, Vale W, Rivier J, Orth DN (1984) J Clin Invest 73: 533-538
13. Orth D, DeCherney G, DeBold C, Sheldon W, Jackson R, Atkinson A, Hadden D, Kennedy L, Chretien M, Gilbert F, Krieger D, Roman S, Rothman G, Cook D (1984) Program 7th International Congress of Endocrinology (Abstract)
14. Orth DN, DeBold CR, DeCherney GS, Jackson RV, Alexander AN, Rivier J, Rivier C, Spiess J, Vale W (1982) J Clin Endocrinol Metab 55: 1017-1019
15. Lytras N, Grossman A, Perry L, Tomlin S, Wass JAH, Coy DH, Schally AV, Rees LH, Besser GM (1984) Clin Endocrinol (Oxf) 20: 71-84
16. Orth DN (1984) N Engl J Med 310: 649-651
17. Sheldon WR, DeBold CR, DeCherney GS, Island DP, Thorner MO, Evans WS, Orth DN (1984) Clin Res 32: 273A (Abstract)
18. DeBold CR, Sheldon WR Jr, DeCherney GS, Island DP, Thorner MO, Evans WS, Orth DN (1984) Program 7th International Congress of Endocrinology (Abstract)

49. The Astwood Symposium on Thyroid Hormone Action

Endocrinology
F. Labrie, L. Proulx, eds.

TRANSPORT AND MOLECULAR ACTION OF TRIIODOTHYRONINE (T_3) AT THE NUCLEAR LEVEL

J.H. OPPENHEIMER, D.B. JUMP, C.N. MARIASH, H.L. SCHWARTZ, S. SEELIG and H.C. TOWLE
Departments of Medicine, Pediatrics, and Biochemistry, University of Minnesota, Minneapolis, MN 55455 U.S.A.

Most of the currently recognized actions of thyroid hormone can be explained as a consequence of the interaction of the principal thyroid hormone triiodothyronine (T_3) with a specific intranuclear receptor [1]. In the following review we shall consider studies from our laboratories dealing with some of the cellular events preceding and following the occupation of the nuclear receptors.

PRE-RECEPTOR TRANSPORT

We shall first discuss the transport of thyroid hormone to the nuclear site of initiation. Recent evidence from one of our laboratories (JHO) has indicated that the two-way exchange of T_3 both between plasma and cells and between nucleus and cytosol involves the operation of stereospecific transport systems or channels [2]. These conclusions are based on experiments in which we have used as the biochemical probes the two enantiomers of T_3, the naturally occurring levo (L) and its synthetic mirror image, the dextro (D) form. Although D-T_3 is bound to specific nuclear receptors almost as tightly as L-T_3, D-T_3 exhibits only one sixth of the biological activity of L-T_3. The discrepancy between thyromimetic action and nuclear binding was shown to be due to the fact that **in vivo** the nucleus accumulated L-T_3 much more readily than D-T_3 [3]. This was postulated to be due to the operation of a transport system [2].

In order to characterize the energetics of the transport systems we have estimated the concentration of free hormone in plasma and cytosol and in the nuclei of liver, kidney, heart, and brain. Our general approach in estimating the free hormone concentration was as follows. Measurements of plasma free T_3 were performed by standard equilibrium dialysis. Similarly, we determined the concentration of free T_3 in cytosol from the product of total cytosolic T_3 measured by direct radioimmunoassay and the dialysis fraction ascertained by equilibrium dialysis. For estimating the free nuclear T_3 we applied the Law of Mass Action which assumes that hormone in the nucleus is in reversible equilibrium with T_3 in the free form. Since the ratio bound to free receptors is known from published **in vivo** studies in rats [5,6] and since the association constant of the nuclear receptors can be determined, the free nuclear T_3 concentration can be calculated.

Our calculations are summarized in Table 1 and are expressed in terms of free T_3 ratios (cytosolic/plasma and nuclear/cytosolic) both for L- and D-T_3. It is apparent that the higher the ratio the higher the energy requirement. Our results lead to two major conclusions: 1. The cytosolic/plasma free T_3 ratio and stereospecificity varies from tissue to tissue; 2. The nuclear/cytoplasmic free T_3 ratio appears to be substantially greater for L than for D in every tissue. Moreover, the identification of gradients of free T_3 from cytosol to the nucleus raises the distinct possibility that the transport of other hormones and metabolites from cytosol to nucleus may also be mediated by stereospecific energy requiring systems.

TABLE I

FREE T_3 CYTOSOLIC/PLASMA AND FREE T_3 NUCLEAR/CYTOSOLIC RATIOS

Tissue	Free T_3 Cytosolic/Plasma ratios		Free T_3 Nuclear/Cytosolic ratios	
	L	D	L	D
Liver	2.8	21.6	58.2	3.70
Kidney	1.17	63.3	55.9	1.54
Heart	1.49	2.07	80.6	24.9
Brain	0.9	0.32	251.0	108.6

POST-RECEPTOR EVENTS

We should now like to turn to the events which follow the nuclear occupation of the receptor. At present, the best method for assessing the consequence of receptor occupation by T_3 is the measurement of the activity or concentration of specific mRNA sequences regulated by T_3. Previous studies in our laboratory clearly have shown that approximately 8% of the high abundancy mRNA's in liver cells are influenced by thyroid hormone [7]. This conclusion is based on an analysis of individual translational products of poly(A+)-containing RNA's derived from livers of animals subjected to various thyroid hormone manipulations. Of the 231 identifiable translational products, some 19 changed, 11 increasing with thyroid hormone and 8 diminishing, and one exhibiting a biphasic alteration. We have also been able to successfully document the unique patterns of mRNA activity spectra which occur in response to other hormones and stimuli [8-10]. Quantitation has been made possible by the use of computerized videodensitometry [11]. These studies allowed us to draw the following conclusions in regard to thyroid hormone action: 1. Approximately 40% of the high abundancy mRNA sequences which respond in the liver to T_3 are mediated by T_3 as a result of an antecedent stimulation of pituitary growth hormone [8]; 2. There is a striking similarity in the mRNA activity patterns produced by a high carbohydrate, fat-free diet and the hyperthyroid state [8,10]; similarly there is a strong relationship in the directional shifts induced by hypothyroidism and starvation [9]. The effect of carbohydrate are largely exerted directly at the hepatocellular levels since they can be reproduced by the addition of glucose and T_3 to the medium of cultured hepatocyte [12].

Of special interest was the mRNA coding for "spot 14", a protein with molecular weight 17,000 and pI 4.9 ($mRNA_{S14}$). By translational assay this mRNA responded rapidly after the administration of T_3 and increased to levels approximately 20-fold above baseline hypothyroid levels within 4 hours [13]. Carbohydrate administration augmented [8] and starvation reduced [9] the translational activity of this mRNA. Efforts in one of our laboratories (HCT) resulted in the preparation of a library of cDNA's in plasma PBR 322 to hepatic mRNA sequences stimulated by T_3 and carbohydrate administration [14]. One of the transformed colonies contained a cDNA to $mRNA_{S14}$. The response of $mRNA_{S14}$ as determined by hybridization (dot-blot) analysis was correlated highly with the results of translational analysis [15]. Increased activity of $mRNA_{S14}$ thus was due to increased mass rather than to enhanced translational activity. Serial measurements indicated that $mRNA_{S14}$ rose after only 20 minutes following T_3 administration. In addition, $mRNA_{S14}$ showed marked circadian variation which, in more recent studies by Kinlaw et al have been shown to persist even in the face of full occupation of nuclear receptors. In our original survey, the highest levels of $mRNA_{S14}$ were identified in liver with substantially lower concentrations in heart, brain, spleen and testes [15]. More recent studies by Jump et al, however, have shown levels of $mRNA_{S14}$ in fat which equal or exceed those in liver. High levels of $mRNA_{S14}$ have also been identified in lactating mammary gland. The finding of $mRNA_{S14}$ in three lipogenic tissues and the response of this sequence both to carbohydrate and to T_3 is compatible with the concept that this mRNA codes for a protein involved in fatty acid synthesis, metabolism or storage.

In separate studies in one of our laboratories (HCT) the gene for spot 14 was shown to consist of two exons and one intervening sequence [16]. Two mRNA's differing by 170 bases at the 3' end are transcribed from the gene. Their nucleotide sequence has been identified. The translated portion of the protein has been identified exclusively with the first exon and a TATA box variant located some 27 base pairs upstream from the 5' initiating site. Comparison of the nucleotide and predicted amino acid sequence with those products registered in computer banks revealed surprisingly little homology. Further analysis of the 5,000 base precursor HnRNA indicated a response to T_3 administration within 10 minutes after T_3 clearly preceding a rise in mature $mRNA_{S14}$ [16].

In other studies, induction of $mRNA_{S14}$ was demonstrated in cultured isolated hepatocyte [17]. The decrease in the level of stimulated $mRNA_{S14}$ levels following the complete cessation of uridine incorporation by actinomycin was not influenced by T_3. These studies as well as the temporal analysis of accumulation of $mRNA_{S14}$ in the intact animal strongly suggest that T_3 increases the level of $mRNA_{S14}$ by augmenting its synthesis. Whether increased synthesis results from stabilization of the precursor HnRNA or reflects augmented rates of transcription remains to be determined. Regardless of this, the rapidity of response of $mRNA_{S14}$ makes it probable that T_3 exerts its effect directly at the S14 gene level without the necessity of the generation of an antecendent regulatory protein by T_3.

REFERENCES

1. Oppenheimer JH (1979) Science 203:971-979.
2. Oppenheimer JH, Schwartz HL (1983) Program of the Endocrine Society 65th Annual Meeting, Abstract 484, p 201.
3. Schwartz HL, Trence D, Oppenheimer JH, Jiang NS, Jump DB (1983) Endocrinology 113:1236-1242.
4. Oppenheimer JH, Squef R, Surks MI, Hauer H (1963) Proc Soc Exp Biol & Med 113:837-840.
5. Oppenheimer JH, Schwartz HL, Surks MI (1974) Endocrinology 95:897-903.
6. Crantz FR, Silva JE, Larsen PR (1982) Endocrinology 110:367-375.
7. Seelig SA, Liaw C, Towle HC, Oppenheimer JH (1981) Proc Nat Acad Sci 78:4733-4737.
8. Liaw C, Seelig S, Mariash CN, Oppenheimer JH, Towle HC (1983) Biochemistry 22:213-221.
9. Carr FE, Seelig S, Mariash CN, Schwartz HL, Oppenheimer JH (1983) J Clin Invest 72:154-163.
10. Carr FE, Bingham B, Oppenheimer JH, Kistner C, Mariash CN (1984) Proc Nat Acad Sci 81:974-978.
11. Mariash CN, Seelig SA, Oppenheimer JH (1982) Analytical Biochemistry 121:388-394.
12. Topliss DJ, Mariash CN, Seelig S, Carr FE, Oppenheimer JH (1983) Endocrinology 112:1868-1870.
13. Seelig SA, Jump DB, Towle HC, Liaw C, Mariash CN, Schwartz HL, Oppenheimer JH (1982) Endocrinology 110:671-673.
14. Narayan P, Liaw CW, Towle HC (1984) Proc Nat Acad Sci (in press).
15. Jump DB, Narayan P, Towle H, Oppenheimer JH (1984) J Biol Chem 259:2789-2797.
16. Liaw CW, Towle HC (1984) J Biol Chem (in press).
17. Mariash CN, Jump DB, Oppenheimer JH (1984) Clinical Research 32:486A.

Endocrinology
F. Labrie, L. Proulx, eds.

INFLUENCE OF THYROID HORMONE ON MESSENGER RNA LEVELS IN THE RAT HEART

W.H. DILLMANN
Department of Medicine, University of California, San Diego, California (U.S.A.)

The heart is a major target organ for thyroid hormone action and thyroid hormone induced changes in cardiac protein formation have been described (1). In spite of the important role which changes in mRNA level play in mediating alterations in protein formation influences of thyroid hormones on cardiac mRNA levels have been only incompletely characterized. We have therefore investigated the influence which changes in thyroid hormone status exert on specific mRNAs in the rat heart. Thyroid hormones induced changes in the level of the mRNAs coding for the two isoforms of myosin heavy chain (MHC), that is MHC-alpha and MHC-beta, are of particular interest to us and will be described first.

It has been documented that rat ventricular myosin contains three myosin isoforms, myosin V_1, V_2 and V_3. Myosin V_1 contains two MHC-alpha, MHC-V_2 contains one MHC-alpha and one MHC-beta and MHC-V_3 contains two MHC-beta. In the normal rat heart MV_1 predominates, whereas in hypothyroid hearts MV_3 predominates. Myosin heavy chains have a molecular weight of 200,000 and represent the most abundant polypeptide in that molecular weight area in the rat heart. We quantitated the levels of MHC-alpha and MHC-beta in the heart of normal and hypothyroid rats, using _in vitro_ translation of RNA isolated from the heart of normal, hypothyroid and T_3-injected hypothyroid rats. In more recent studies a specific cDNA probe corresponding to MHC-alpha mRNA was used for a more precise quantitation of the levels of this mRNA after T_3 administration to hypothyroid animals. In addition we quantitated thyroid hormone-induced changes in other mRNA species which are of unknown coding capacity using _in vitro_ translational, separation of the $[^{35}S]$-labeled translational products and subsequent quantitation by digital matrix photometry.

The techniques used for these studies have been described previously in detail (2,3). A brief outline of the methodological approach will be provided. To quantitate the translational activity of MHC mRNA in the heart of normal and hypothyroid rats we proceeded in the following way. RNA was prepared from fresh hearts of normal, hypothyroid and T_3-injected hypothyroid rats. The unfractionated RNA was translated in a modified rabbit reticulocyte lysate system in the presence of $[^{35}S]$-methionine. $[^{35}S]$-Methionine incorporated into MHC was quantitated by separating the MHC from other translational products on 10% polyacrylamide SDS gels. Proteins were visualized by staining and the MHC band was cut from the gel and thoroughly destained. Translational aliquots containing the same amount $[^{35}S]$-MHC was then used for peptide mapping. Peptide mapping of MHC was performed according to the procedure of Cleveland (4). Myosin heavy chain cut from the first gel was placed in the well of a second polyacrylamide gel and then incubated with staphylococcus aureus V8 protease or chymotrypsin. Myosin heavy chain was digested during the electrophoretic run. After electrophoresis the generated peptides were identified by fluorography.

Comparison of the peptide map of MHC synthesized in vitro from RNA obtained from hypothyroid, euthyroid or T_3-treated hypothyroid animals showed that peptide maps from normal and hypothyroid animals differ from each other in several unique peptide fragments which were present only in the in vitro formed MHCs from normal or hypothyroid animals (2). The MHC peptide maps of T_3-injected hypothyroid animals were identical to those found in normal rats. These studies therefore indicate that changes in myosin isoenzyme predominance are accompanied by corresponding changes in the predominance of MHC-alpha and MHC-beta mRNA. In the hypothyroid rat ventricle MHC-beta mRNA predominates, whereas in the normal rat ventricle MHC-alpha is the predominant mRNA.

To quantitate with a more precise method the mass of MHC mRNA itself we used the following approach. cDNA was synthesized from normal rat heart RNA by conventional methods and inserted into the Pst side of PBR322. The rat cDNA library was screened by hybridization with drosophila MHC DNA (gift of Dr. Roizeck) and two colonies containing MHC sequences were selected. One colony containing a 1000 nucleotide insert was selected as a probe to quantitate MHC mRNA. The MHC insert was labeled at one end by filling the 3' recessed strand in the presence of 4 [^{32}P] dNTPs and the labeled cDNA was used to hybridize to RNA. Hypothyroid rats received a single injection of 200 ug T_3/100 g body weight and cardiac RNA was prepared 0, 1, 2, 5 and 12 hours later. Total RNA from each group was hybridized to [^{32}P] cDNA digested with S_1 nuclease and the digested products were separated by electrophoresis under denaturing conditions. Hybridization of RNA from hypothyroid rats generated one band (MHC-beta RNA) which was smaller than the band observed in normal animals (MHC-alpha RNA). At 1 and 2 h. after T_3, only MHC-beta RNA was observed, while MHC-alpha RNA was significantly induced by 5 h. and MHC-beta RNA significantly reduced by 5 h. MHC-alpha RNA became the major mRNA by 12 h. after T_3.

Direct determination of the level of isozymic MHC mRNAs with a specific cDNA probe shows therefore a rapid T_3 response (5 h.). This is surprising in view of the long half-life (5,4 days) of MHC polypeptide and the duration of myosin isoenzyme turnover. The time response of the two isozymic MHC RNAs after T_3 administration appears reciprocal indicating that the expression of the two MHC genes may be coordinately regulated by T_3.

To determine the influence of T_3 on cardiac mRNAs other than MHC, RNA was translated in vitro [^{35}S]-methionine labeled proteins were separated by two-dimensional gel electrophoresis using isoelectric focusing in the first dimension and SDS slab gel electrophoresis in the second dimension and quantitated by digital matrix photometry. The following results were obtained. A total of 421 translational products were identified by fluorography and changes in the predominance of 12 of these were influenced by thyroid status of the animals. Predominance of 8 species was increased in euthyroid animals, whereas 4 translational products were increased in hypothyroid animals. The majority of the thyroid hormone related alterations occurred in spot pairs of similar molecular weight, but slightly different isoelectric points. In contrast, the relative predominance of mRNAs coding for the major contractile proteins, like light chain 1, light chain 2, tropomyosin, actin and MHC was not altered by the thyroid status of the animals. The relative levels of these abundant mRNA species remained unaltered in spite of thyroid hormone related increases in total RNA levels. In order to determine the time course with which the T_3 induced changes occur, hypothyroid rats were injected with .2 mg T_3/100 g BW, then cardiac RNA was prepared 1, 2, 3, 5, 12 and 24 hours after T_3 injection. RNA was quantitated by _in vitro_ translation and digital matrix photometry as described above. Quantitation of specific translational products indicated that 1 h. after T_3 injection the mRNAs coding for mRNAs represented by spot 71, 72 (Mr 81,000, pI 5.54, 5.50) were already significantly increased. These mRNA species are not detectable in the hypothyroid rat heart. A marked decrease in the predominance of spot 247 is detected 12 h. after T_3 administration. The predominance of spot 247 is increased in hypothyroid rat hearts. 24 Hours after T_3 administration the decrease in spot 247 predominance persisted and the predominance of spot 253 became markedly decreased. The time response of mRNA levels varies therefore for specific mRNAs and two of these mRNAs which are properly represented isozymic forms show a very rapid 1 h. response after T_3 administration.

In the hypothyroid and the diabetic heart a decrease in glucose consumption occurs, in addition thyroid hormone levels are decreased in diabetic animals and insulin levels are lowered in hypothyroid rats. We wanted to determine if diabetes and hypothyroidism can exert similar influences on specific cardiac mRNA species. RNA was isolated from the heart of normal, hypothyroid and diabetic hearts and quantitated by _in vitro_ translation by the methods outlined above. Out of the 12 mRNA directed products which were altered in hypothyroid rats, two were exclusively influenced by thyroid hormone lack, the other mRNA showed similar changes in hypothyroid and diabetic hearts. Of the 13 mRNAs which change in diabetic hearts, two were exclusively altered by insulin lack. Thyroid hormone influence and insulin-induced changes in the level of specific mRNAs show therefore a large overlap in the rat heart. Only 2 out of 12 mRNAs respond exclusively to hypothyroidism and 2 out of 13 mRNAs show diabetes specific changes. Because of the exclusive thyroid hormone responsiveness of 2 mRNAs hypothyroid induced changes are most likely not the result of decreased insulin levels of hypothyroid rats.

Recent investigations by us and others have shown that myosin isoenzyme distribution and the thyroid hormone responsiveness of Ca++-activated myosin ATPase is different in the ventricle and in the atrium of the rat heart. We therefore determined if differences in the thyroid hormone responsiveness of specific mRNAs occur in these two parts of the rat heart. RNA was quantitated as described above and we found in confirmation of our previous studies that 12 specific mRNAs were modulated by the thyroid status in the rat ventricle. Of the 8 mRNAs preferentially increased in the normal ventricle only 4 were similarly affected in the normal atrium. However, 4 new mRNA species which were not affected by thyroid hormone in the ventricle were significnatly more predominant when atrial tissue was obtained from normal animals. Similarly of the 4 mRNA species preferentially decreased in the normal ventricle, only 2 were affected in the atrium and 2 new mRNAs were significantly decreased in normal atrium which were not affected in normal ventricles. It appears therefore that the response of specific mRNAs to thyroid hormone is different for atrial and ventricular tissue.

SUMMARY

Our results indicate that the *in vivo* effects of thyroid hormone on cardiac mRNA levels are very complex. In addition to a general increase in total RNA and mRNA levels increases or attenuations in the predominance of a small number of specific mRNAs are observed when euthyroid and hypothyroid animals are compared. Two of the specific mRNAs (spot 71, 72) show a very rapid 1 h. response after thyroid hormone administration. Furthermore, these studies indicate that the thyroid hormone responsiveness of specific parameters is highly tissue specific and is even different for two distinct parts of the same organ like the atrium and the cardiac ventricle. In addition these studies clearly show that myosin heavy chain, which is a major contractile protein in the heart, is thyroid hormone responsive. The two isoforms of myosin heavy chain, MHC-alpha and MHC-beta seem to be altered in a reciprocal fashion by the thyroid status.

REFERENCES

1. Carter WJ, Van der Weijden BWS, Faas FH (1980) Metabolism 29:910
2. Dillmann WH, Barrieux A, Reese GS (1984) J. Biol. Chem. 259:2035
3. Dillmann WH, Barrieux W, Neeley WE and Contreras P (1983) J. Biol. Chem. 258:7738
4. Cleveland DW, Fischer SG, Kirschner MW and Laemmli UK (1977) J. Biol. Chem. 252:1102

© 1984 Elsevier Science Publishers B.V.
Endocrinology
F. Labrie, L. Proulx, eds.

ONTOGENESIS OF THYROID HORMONE RECEPTOR

J. BERNAL, A. PEREZ-CASTILLO, T. PANS & F. PEKONEN

Depto Endocrinologia Experimental, Inst. de Investigaciones Biomedicas, C.S.I.C., Facultad de Medicina, U.A.M., 28034 Madrid, Spain, and Minerva Foundation, 00101 Helsinki, Finland

INTRODUCTION

The importance of thyroid hormones in the regulation of developmental processes is well recognized. Little is known, however, on the specific events triggered by thyroid hormones and the timing of action during maturation. For instance, it is not clear to what extent thyroid hormones influence prenatal human brain development. Among the possible approaches to this question is the study of the ontogenesis of thyroid hormone nuclear receptor, which might give clues on the development of sensitivity of a particular tissue during maturation. This paper is a brief account of the work done up to the present on the ontogenesis of thyroid hormone receptor in the laboratory rat and in man.

ONTOGENESIS OF THYROID HORMONE RECEPTOR IN RAT TISSUES

DeGroot et al (1) and Coulombe et al (2) have shown that the concentration of receptor in rat liver is low in the newborn rat and increases progressively, reaching maximum levels at 30-50 days of age. At this time, receptor levels were 2-4 times higher than at birth. An increase of T3 receptor from birth to adulthood has also been shown for the rat pituitary (3). Other organs show a different pattern: in rat cerebrum and lung receptor concentrations were higher 2 days after birth than in adult animals (4,5,6). Our data agree with these. We have studied the ontogenesis of receptor in rat liver, lung,and heart from the 16th day of fetal life to the 30th day of postnatal life. The brain, in addition, was studied from day 14 of gestation. T3 binding was also studied in nuclear extracts from whole fetuses at days 12 and 13. No receptor was detected at day 12, and minimal amounts were present in whole fetuses at day 13. The receptor was clearly detected in 14-days old brains (70 fmol/mg DNA) and increased to day 16 (200 fmol/mg DNA), remaining at this level until birth. There was a further increase (2-3 times) after birth, with a peak at day 6. The lung showed a similar pattern. In contrast, in liver and heart the receptor increased linearly with time from low levels at day 16 (fetal) to about 10 times at day 30 (postnatal).

ONTOGENESIS OF THYROID HORMONE RECEPTOR IN THE HUMAN FETUS

Little data is available in human fetal tissues. T3 receptor has been demonstrated in the lung at 12-19 weeks of gestation (7). We have recently examined the nuclear T3 receptor in tissues of aborted fetuses from the 10th to the 18th week of gestational age (8). In preliminary experiments, a nuclear binding protein with the specificity of the T3 receptor was detected in nuclear extracts from a 16 week-old fetal brain. The receptor was present in low concentrations in the 10 week-old fetal brain, increasing through the 16-18 weeks (fig 1). Shown in the same figure is the change in total DNA per brain during the same period. Total DNA increased, indicating rapid cell proliferation. This period of brain development corresponds to the critical one of neuroblast multiplication (9).

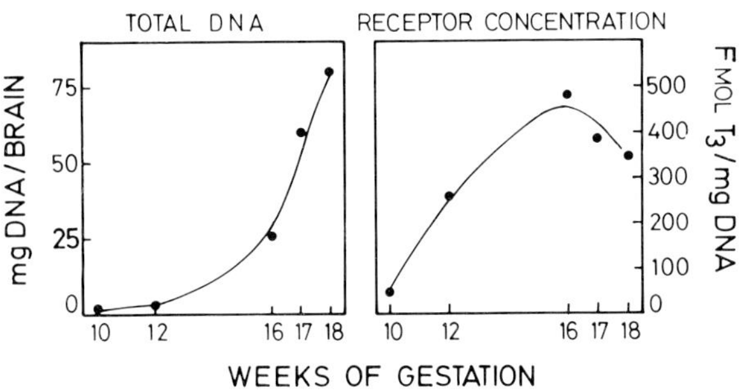

Fig 1. Total DNA and T3 receptor concentration in fetal human brain at different gestational ages. From (8).

The receptor was also present in other fetal organs at 16 and 18 weeks of gestation. This is shown in fig 2 for brain, liver, heart and lung. A comparison of receptor levels in human fetal tissues with adult rat organs leads to the suggestion that there are changes of receptor concentration during development, with increments in concentration in the liver and heart, and decrements in the lung, as also occurs in the rat.

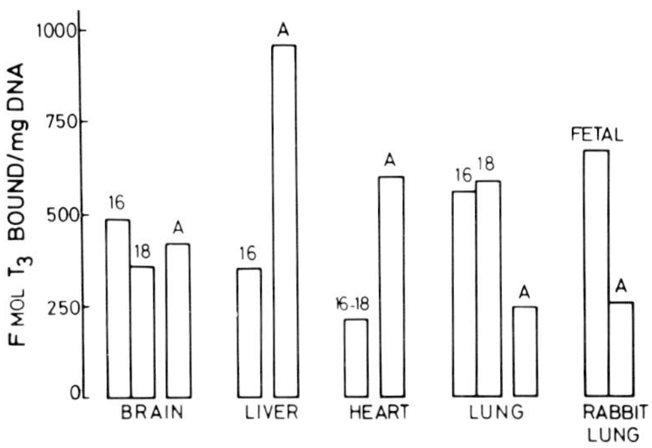

Fig 2. T3 receptor concentrations in human fetal tissues at 16 and 18 weeks of gestational age. Data are from (8). A: receptor levels in adult rat organs (10).Data for the rabbit lung are from reference 11.

THYROID HORMONES IN FETAL TISSUES

The presence of receptor does not, by itself, ensures that fetal tissues are thyroid hormone dependent. Taking into account the low levels of T3 present in the fetal circulation, it would be expected that tissue T3 concentrations and receptor occupancy might be very low. In rat tissues receptor occupancy has been shown to increase during the neonatal period (1). Results of T4 and T3 determinations in fetal human tissue extracts are shown in fig 3. T4 was present in all tissues examined. T3, however, was only present in the brain, in other tissues being below the limit of detection. These results suggest that T3, in fetal brain, arises mainly, if not exclusively, from local 5' deiodination of T4. It is likely that receptor occupancy in fetal tissues is dependent on a differential pattern of maturation of 5' deiodinases. In this way, the receptor might be operative in some tissues (brain) whereas in others its appearance during fetal life might have the significance of an anticipatory mechanism.

In conclusion, receptor development in the laboratory rat and in man follows a definite pattern according to the tissues. In some, such as lung, receptor concentrations are high during the fetal periods and decrease later. In others, such as liver and heart, the receptor increases with further development. It is likely that receptor occupancy at early stages of development depends on the previous development of tissue deiodinases (12).

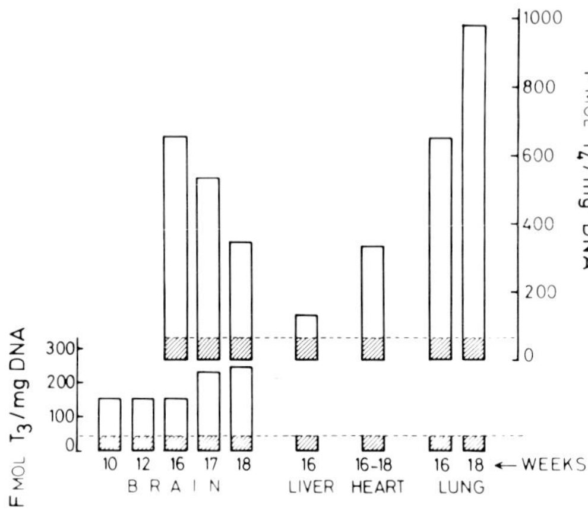

Fig 3. T4 and T3 concentrations in human fetal tissues. From (8).

REFERENCES

1. DeGroot LJ, Robertson M, Rue PA (1977) Endocrinology 100:1511
2. Coulombe P, Ruel J, Dussault JH (1979) Endocrinology 105:952
3. Coulombe P, Ruel J, Faure R, Dussault JH (1983) Am J Physiol 245:E81
4. Schwartz HL, Oppenheimer JH (1978) Endocrinology 103:943
5. Valcana T, Timiras PS (1978) Mol Cell Endocrinol 11:31
6. Ruel J, Coulombe P, Dussault JH (1982) Pediatr Res 16:238
7. Gonzales LW, Ballard PL (1981) J Clin Endocrinol Metab 53:21
8. Bernal J, Pekonen F (1984) Endocrinology 114:677
9. Dobbing J, Sands J (1970) Nature 226:639
10. Oppenheimer JH, Schwartz HL, Surks MI (1974) Endocrinology 95:897
11. Lindenberg JA, Brehier A, Ballard PL (1978) Endocrinology 103: 1725
12. Kaplan MM, Yaskoski KA (1981) J Clin Invest 67:1208

© 1984 Elsevier Science Publishers B.V.
Endocrinology
F. Labrie, L. Proulx, eds.

POST-RECEPTOR MECHANISMS IN THYROID HORMONE ACTION

LESLIE J. DEGROOT, FRED TOFFEL, ANDRZEJ KUBICA, AND JULIUS BRTKO

Thyroid Study Unit, Department of Medicine, The University of Chicago, 5841 South Maryland Ave., Chicago, IL 60637 (USA)

Thyroid hormone action may occur through a single mechanism, but it now seems likely that there are multiple pathways of expression of hormone action. Current interest centers on hormonal action through receptors present in the cell nucleus, but compelling evidence suggests there are actions mediated directly at the cell membrane (1) and probably directly in the mitochondria (2). Assuming that the nuclear receptors are involved in a major portion of thyroid hormone action, it may also be questioned whether there is a hierarchical response flowing from one primary action, from which all other actions ultimately follow, or multiple discrete and separate actions of hormone. Most efforts to analyze hormone action have been predicated on the basis of primacy of action of hormone at one particular site, although in fact nothing guarantees that this is the correct approach.

Given the concept of essential unity of action and primacy of one response, and speaking of nuclear receptors only, what mechanisms may be postulated through which thyroid hormone might work after it binds to the receptor? Several can be readily cataloged; others, perhaps more important, may well be present. For example:

A. Thyroid hormone could cause transfer of receptor from one compartment such as cytosol, to another such as the nucleus, and thereby initiate function of a receptor whose intrinsic action may only take place when present in the new compartment.

B. Hormone could cause transfer of receptor from one physical state to another, for example, from the free state to being bound to a macromolecule such as chromatin, by changing the affinity of binding of receptor to chromatin.

C. Thyroid hormone might define a binding specificity such that receptor could bind nonspecifically to any site on chromatin in the absence of hormone, but in its presence would bind only to specific sites on the gene.

D. Hormone might cause dissociation of an inhibitor of receptor function, in analogy to the action of cyclic-AMP on kinases.

E. Hormone might cause an allosteric activation of an (unknown) enzymatic function of the receptor.

F. Hormone might alter the function of the receptor as an acceptor for phosphorylation, or ADP ribosylation, or some other post-transcriptional modification of the protein, thus allowing a negative or positive activating effect.

G. Analogous to the allosteric activating effect, hormone might make the receptor active in initiating transcription on a promoter site, whereas unoccupied receptor might be inactive.
Unfortunately, thinking of these possible routes of action does not get us much closer to knowledge of the actual response.

If one presumes that the central action is through some effect on chromatin and its constituent genes and regulatory proteins, one might propose a sequence of actions such as the following: "Zero order", indicating a direct effect on the physical structure of a gene; First order, indicating a derivative of the zero order response, such as increased function of polymerase; Second order response, which might represent increased transcriptional products; Third order, which might represent increased products of translational activities; and Fourth order, which might represent the increased metabolic responses caused by new protein synthesis. Such a sequential examination makes sense if one believes that the hormone acts through a single focus which is of primary importance and has primacy in response. In reviewing post-receptor mechanisms, it is perhaps useful to review the observations on such responses, starting in the reverse order, looking at generalized metabolic responses and working closer to the presumed central primary site of action, although certainly any such classification of responses cannot but be a bit artificial.

Fourth order responses are herein meant to be the gross metabolic responses seen in the whole animal or in tissues or organs affected by thyroid hormone and include heightened oxygen metabolism, growth, anabolism, and under the effects of extreme hormone levels, catabolism. These will not be examined in more detail, since such responses have been well documented now for more than half a century.

Third order responses, meaning alterations in enzyme and protein products of translational activity, have also been clearly documented as mechanisms in the sequence of response to thyroid hormone action over the past 3-5 decades. Perhaps hundreds of enzyme responses have been cataloged (3,4). Both secretory and non-secretory, and doubtless structural, proteins undergo increased (or decreased) synthesis. Recent studies have emphasized increased formation of membrane sodium-potassium ATPase (5), rat liver phosphoenol pyruvate carboxykinase (6), and glucokinase, and much attention has centered on the production of pituitary growth hormone (7), and malic enzyme (8), and alpha-glycerophosphate dehydrogenase (9) in liver. Cardiac myosin isozyme distribution is altered so that low activity myosin ATPase is observed in hypothyroid animals and highly active myosin ATPase predominates in T_3 treated animals (10). Increased enzyme function, presumably representing increased amount of enzyme, is seen in several of these systems within 3-4 hours after animals receive the hormone, and presumably represents the T_3-induced response of both increased transcriptional and translational activity, since agents like alpha-amanitin and cycloheximide prevent these responses. Nikodem et al. amplified these results by using 2-D electrophoresis of liver proteins and showed that, within 24 hours after T_3 administration, approximately 67 of 500 identifiable liver protein subunits had increased concentration in response to T_3 administration (11).

Alterations also occur in nuclear protein content. Bernal showed that thyroidectomized animals had an increased amount of a particular nuclear globulin and that T_3-treated animals contained a nuclear protein not present in hypothyroid animals (12, 13). Both changes were reversed by the addition or subtraction of thyroid hormone.

The activity of cytosolic, and nuclear protein kinases is altered within a few hours after administration of thyroid hormone, and changing patterns of cytosolic protein phosphorylation are evident (14) (Fig. 1). Cytosolic protein kinase activity active with protamine as substrate gradually decreased over a period of 24-48 hours after T_3 administration. Protein kinase active with casein as substrate gradually increased over this period (15), and it is this enzyme which mediates most of the T_3 induced protein phosphorylations (16). Stimulation of both phosphorylation and dephosphorylation of specific proteins is evident within 5-12 hours after T_3 administration (14). Phosphorylation of pyruvate kinase and acetyl Co-A carboxykinase is increased by the action of thyroid hormone. Since the increased kinase activity observed 5-12 hours after T_3 administration is inhibited by either alpha-amanitin or cycloheximide, these changes appeared to be due to prior transcriptional activity. Nevertheless, it is of importance that thyroid hormone alters the phosphorylation pattern of numerous specific rat liver proteins, probably through the action of casein kinase. This may be a major route through which hormone exerts its "third order" actions, in addition to direct effects on new protein synthesis.

Preceding the production of new proteins must be the production of new mRNA's, and this "second order" action of thyroid hormone has been clearly demonstrated. New mRNA synthesis is evident in liver within 3-8 hours after administration of thyroid hormone (17) (Fig. 2). Increments in specific mRNA's, including those for growth hormone (18), $\alpha_{2\mu}$-globulin (19), albumin (20), and malic enzyme (21), have also been documented. Increased pituitary growth hormone mRNA is evident within 1-1/2-3 hours after administration of T_3 to hypothyroid animals (18). Most recently, evidence has been presented for an increase in the mRNA for an unidentified liver protein occurring within 10 minutes of T_3 administration to an hypothyroid rat (22). This dramatically early accumulation of new mRNA is reported to be inhibited by cycloheximide, which might suggest that it is dependent upon prior protein synthesis, but more likely indicates that its

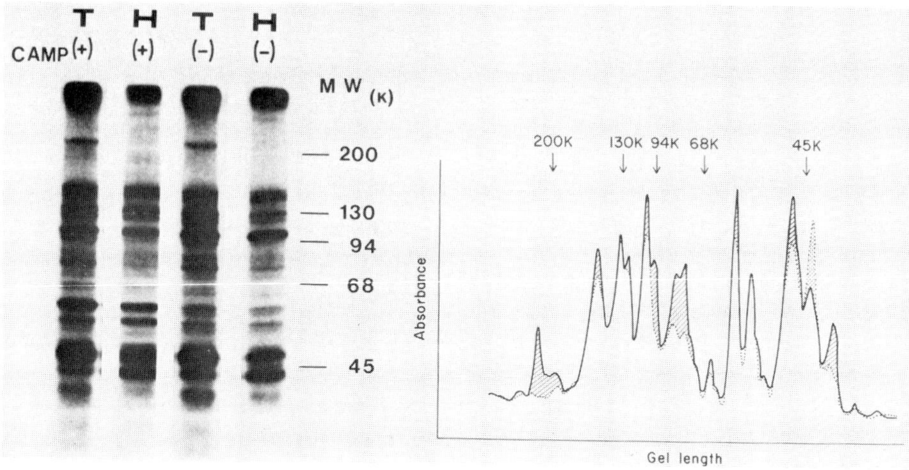

Fig. 1. Left, Autoradiogram of ^{32}P-labeled phosphoproteins separated by SDS-PAGE. Cytosols obtained from Tx rats given 20 µg T3/100 g BW. Day for 3 days (T) or vehicle (H) were incubated with [γ-^{32}P] ATP in the absence (—) or presence (+) of 1 µM cAMP. After incubation at 30 C for 2 min, SDS-stop solution was added. The mixture was boiled for 5 min, and the aliquots containing 105 µg protein were subjected to SDS-PAGE (see Materials and Methods for details). The dried gel was exposed to Kodak X-Omat R film for 3 days at -80 C with an intensifier screen. Right, Densitogram of the autoradiogram. The optical density of the developed X-ray film was scanned with a Zeineh soft laser scanning densitometer. (———) = the pattern of phosphoproteins of T3-treated sample (T); (. . . . .) = H sample. The scanned samples were cytosols incubated with [γ-^{32}P] ATP in the presence of 1 µM cAMP. [hatched box] = increase caused by T3 treatment; [dotted box] = decrease caused by T3 treatment. The markers with numbers indicate the mobilities of standard molecular weight markers.

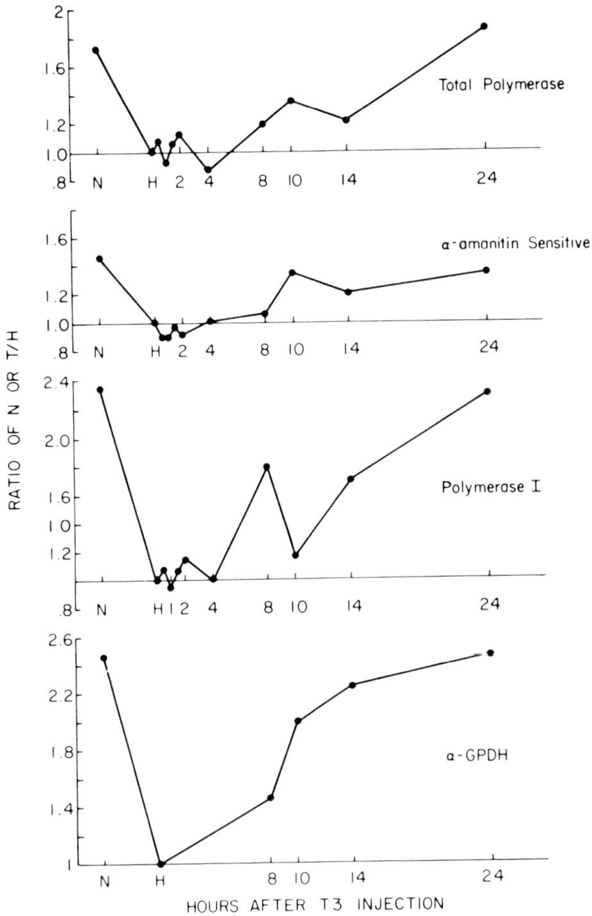

Fig. 2. Stimulation of generalized mRNA synthesis by triiodothyronine. Normal (N), hypothyroid (T), and T3-injected (T) rats were studied. The T3-treated groups are indicated on the ordinate by the hours after T3 injection. Total nuclear polymerase, α-amanitin-sensitive polymerase II producing mRNA, polymerase I-producing ribosomal RNA, and mitochondrial α-glycerophosphate dehydrogenase levels were measured. There is clear stimulation of polymerase function and increased activity of mitochondrial enzyme at 8-10 hours after administration of T3 to these animals. Polymerase I and II levels are both increased.

production is dependent on some rapidly turning over protein(s). While it is inferred that an increase in mRNA can be equated with increased transcription, effects of T_3 on mRNA turnover or stability, which might secondarily increase the steady state level of mRNA, have only been fully excluded in the studies by Samuels and co-workers ( ) on the GH_3 cell line.

Increased quantities of mRNA implies increased transcription, and this "first order" event has been clearly documented. Some reports suggest that liver polymerase and brain polymerase may be increased in activity within 1-1/2 hours after administration of T_3 to hypothyroid animals (23, 24). While this remains uncertain, increased liver nuclear polymerase activity, using either endogenous or exogenous template, clearly occurs within 3-8 hours after administration of thyroid hormone (25). An even earlier response of some polymerase functions must occur, because of the above mentioned evidence for the production of new mRNA's of unknown type within 10 minutes and of growth hormone mRNA within 1-1/2 hours of T_3 administration. Possibly there is an early stimulation of a polymerase for a few proteins, including polymerase subunits, leading to a later increase in total polymerase enzyme activity. Rat liver DNA template availability to E. Coli polymerase in vitro is not increased within the first few hours after T_3 administration, but is increased in normal animals as compared to hypothyroid animals (25). Thus, probably transcription of specific genes is increased early and DNA template availability is more globally enhanced at a later date.

In addition to actions on polymerase and mRNA production, thyroid hormone has several other effects on nuclear proteins in the early interval after its administration to an hypothyroid animal. Nuclear protein kinase activity with casein and with protamine substrates is increased within 1.5 hours (15) (Fig. 3). It is not known whether this response is inhibited by cycloheximide. T_3 administration to hypothyroid animals is reported to induce, within 30 minutes, increased phosphorylation of NHP when the nuclei are subsequently incubated with ATP in vitro (26). While we have been unable to confirm this observation, Nikodem et al. have found increased phosphorylation of certain classes of nuclear proteins (27), and we have found increased in vivo phosphorylation of liver nuclear protein within 3-5 hours of administration of T_3 (28).

Recently we have studied in vitro phosphorylation of a fraction of acid soluble nuclear proteins 1.5 hours after in vivo T_3 administration. We find that phosphorylation of chromatin protein, which is solubilized by brief micrococcal nuclease digestion, and recovered by acid and salt extraction, is enhanced. This fraction contains histones, HMG proteins, and other unidentified species. The response is not inhibited by prior cycloheximide administration. We have not yet identified a specific target phosphoprotein whose phosphorylation is specifically enhanced, but this class of proteins is believed to be associated with

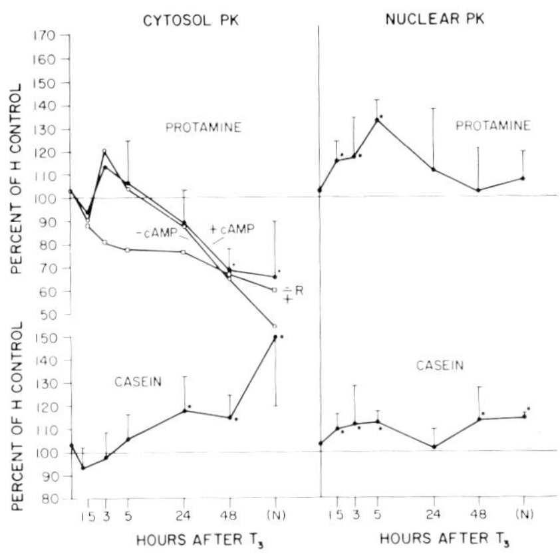

Fig. 3. Protein kinase activity prepared from cytosol (Panels A and B) or from nuclei (Panels C and D) are displayed with values for T3 treated animals and normal animals in relationship to the coincidentally assayed hypothyroid animals, taken as 100%. The percent of control activity is displayed on the ordinate. On the abscissa the numbers indicate hours after injection of T3 to hypothyroid animals, and N indicates the activity in normal animals. Assays were conducted with protamine substrate (Panels A and C) or casein substrate (Panels B and D). In Panel A, activity is shown for assays with or without cAMP present. Also shown in Panel A is the activity ratio of samples assayed with and without cAMP for each time point after T3 treatment and in normal animals.

actively transcribed genes and could include proteins involved in regulation of transcription (29).

These data suggest of course that T_3 could have a "zero order" effect on a protein kinase, separate from other putative direct actions via control of transcription. We have also found that T_3 administration inhibits nuclear ADP ribosylation activity within 30 minutes, again via a cycloheximide-insensitive reaction (30). Jackowski and Kun have already reported that T_3 administration over four days causes decreased ribosylation of cardiocyte NHP, and suggest that this mechanism may increase the availability of promoter sites for initiation of transcription (31).

It has been reported that thyroid hormone causes specific phosphorylation of histone fraction F1 (32), and increased DNAse digestibility of chromatin has been reported in response to thyroid hormone, both after in vivo administration (33) and after addition of hormone to liver nuclei in vitro (34). Whether all of these phenomena, including phosphorylation and ADP-ribosylation, and chromatin structural alterations, are related to alterations in template availability or polymerase function is uncertain. Polymerase subunits are known to be substrates for kinases (35), and phosphorylation of polymerase has been reported to increase its activity (36). Phosphorylation of nuclear proteins may alter the ability of the polymerase to read genes by altering nucleosomal structure, or may alter the tightness with which proteins cover regions of genes to be translated, or have one of many other theoretical actions. These responses could be "zero order" in the classification scheme noted above, and subsequent effects on polymerase could be "first order".

"Zero order" direct effects of thyroid hormone receptor on the promoter or enhancer region for a gene are attracting speculative interest, but few facts are available. It is suggested in the progesterone receptor system, that receptor binds to a specific (presumed) promoter site about 300 base pairs upstream from the TATA box and site of initiation of transcription for the ovalbumin gene (37). Glucocorticoid receptor has been shown to bind to specific sites on DNA 200-300 bp above the cap site, and to act as an enhancer in the human metallothionecin (38) and mouse mammary tumor virus systems (39). In these systems there is the interesting observation that the binding to the promoter is apparently specific, but the effect can be on any following gene. While it is logical to assume that other small molecules such as Vitamin D and thyroid hormone may follow a similar pathway of action, no evidence for a direct effect of occupied T_3 receptor on gene function has so far been adduced.

Current data suggests thus that nuclear actions of thyroid hormone, ignoring for purposes of this discussion the action on the cell membrane and mitochondria, may be at the transcriptional level, but could involve both direct effects on polymerase function, and possibly independent actions via alterations in chromatin structure, protein phosphorylation, and ribosylation or other reactions. Current data also suggests that altered transcription will involve not one but many genes, and that both positive and negative regulation will occur (40). It also seems plausible that thyroid hormone will not activate a unique set of genes, but will, rather, cause some change in many normally expressed genes, and will probably interact with other stimuli including nutritional (41) and hormonal factors. It is usual in the scientifically unenlightened state for the assembled facts to suggest several coincident independent events in any particular system under study. Often deeper insight provides a cohesive, unitary explanation. Possibly the continued analysis of thyroid hormone action will follow this path.

ACKNOWLEDGMENTS

Supported by United States Public Health Service Grants AM13377 and AM27384

REFERENCES

1. Segal J, Schwartz H, Gordon A (1977) Endocrinology 101:143
2. Sterling K, Milch PO, Brenner MA, Lazarus HI (1977) Science 79:966
3. DeGroot LJ, Larsen PR, Refetoff S, Stanbury JB (eds) The Thyroid and Its Diseases. Fifth edition. John Wiley & Sons, New York (1984) 907 pages.
4. Sestoft L (1980) Clin Endocrinol 13:489
5. Lo C-S, Edelman IS (1976) J Biol Chem 251:7834-7840
6. Muller MJ, Thomsen A, Sibrowski W, Seitz HJ (1982) Endocrinology 111:1469-1475
7. Seo H, Vassart G, Brocas H, Refetoff S (1977) Proc Natl Acad Sci USA 74: 2054-2058
8. Mariash CN, Oppenheimer JH (1983) Endocrinology 112:80
9. Oppenheimer JH, Coulombe P, Schwartz HL, Gutfeld NW (1978) J Clin Invest 987-997
10. Dillmann WH, Berry S, Alexander NM (1983) Endocrinology 112:2081-2087
11. Nikodem VM, Trus BL, Rall JE (1981) Proc Natl Acad Sci USA 78:4411-4415
12. Bernal J, Coleoni AH, DeGroot LJ (1978) Endocrinology 102:452-459
13. Rodriguez-Pena A, Bernal J (1982) Acta Endocrinol 99:567-572
14. Nakamura H, DeGroot LJ (1983) Endocrinology 112:670-680
15. DeGroot LJ, Rue PA, Nakamura H (1984) J Endocrinol Invest (in press)
16. Nakamura H, Rue PA, DeGroot LJ (1983) Endocrinology 112:1427-1433
17. DeGroot LJ, Rue PA, Robertson M, Bernal J, Scherberg N (1977) Endocrinology 101:1690-1700
18. Seo H, Brocas H, Vassart G, Refetoff S (1978) Endocrinology 103:1506-1509
19. Kurtz DT, Sippel AE, Feigelson P (1976) Biochemistry 15:1031-1036
20.
21.

22. Seelig S, Jump DB, Towle HC, Liaw C, Mariash CN, Schwartz HL, Oppenheimer JR (1982) Endocrinology 110:671-673

23. Jothy S, Bilodeau J-L, Champsaur H, Simpkins H (1975) Biochem J 150: 133-135

24. Berti LN, Sato C, Gomez CJ, Krawiec L (1981) Horm Metab Res 13:691-695

25. DeGroot LJ, Rue PA (1980) Endocrinology 107:1989-1997

26. Taningher M, Molinari MP, Cesarone CF (1977) Endocrinology 101:1221-1227

27. Nikodem VM, Huang DR, Trus BL, Rall JE (1983) Horm Metab Res 15:550-554

28. Coleoni AH, DeGroot LJ (1980) Endocrinology 106:1103-1107

29. Toffel F, DeGroot LJ (1984) Abstract submitted to the 60th Annual Meeting of the American Thyroid Association, New York, NY, September, 1984

30. Kubica AK, DeGroot LJ (1983) Abstract presented at the XIII Annual Meeting of the European Thyroid Association, Madrid, Spain, July, 1983

31. Jackowski G, Kun E (1983) J Biol Chem 258:12587-12593

32. Zoncheddu A, Viarengo A (1974) Separatum Experientia 30:737

33. Nikodem VM, Rall JE (1982) Biochem Biophys Res Commun 106:1148-1154

34. Re RN, LaBiche RA, Bryan SE (1983) Biochem Biophys Res Commun 110:61-68

35. Hirsch J, Martelo OJ (1976) J Biol Chem 251:5408-5413

36. Kranias EG, Schweppe JS, Jungmann RA (1977) J Biol Chem 252:6750-6758

37. Lai EC, Riser ME, O'Malley BW (1983) J Biol Chem 258:12693-12701

38. Karin M, Haslinger A, Holtgreve H, Richards RI, Krauter P, Westphal HM, Beato M (1984) Nature 1:913

39. Govindan MV, Spiess E, Majors J (1982) Proc Natl Acad Sci USA 79:5157-5161

40. Seelig S, Liaw C, Towle HC, Oppenheimer JH (1981) Proc Natl Acad Sci USA 78: 4733-4737

41. Martial JA, Seeburg PH, Guenzi D, Goodman HM, Baxter JD (1977) Proc Natl Acad Sci USA 74:4293-4295

50. Neuropeptides and Amines: Functional Interactions

© 1984 Elsevier Science Publishers B.V.
Endocrinology
F. Labrie, L. Proulx, eds.

ENKEPHALINS IN THE ADRENAL MEDULLA: REGULATION OF SYNTHESIS AND PROCESSING BY CATECHOLAMINES AND cAMP IN BOVINE CHROMAFFIN CELLS IN PRIMARY CULTURE AND BY THE SPLANCHNIC INNERVATION IN THE ADRENAL OF THE RAT

CHRISTOPHER D. UNSWORTH, *STEVEN P. WILSON and O. HUMBERTO VIVEROS

Department of Medicinal Biochemistry, The Wellcome Research Laboratories, Research Triangle Park, NC 27709 and *Department of Pharmacology, Duke University Medical Center, Durham, NC 27710 (U.S.A.)

INTRODUCTION

Adrenal medulla chromaffin cells contain large amounts of opioid peptides[1,2,3,4] (OP) derived from proenkephalin A[5] that are costored and cosecreted with catecholamines (CA) from chromaffin vesicles (for review, see reference 6). Chromaffin cell OP depleted via reflex neurogenic stimulation in guinea pigs[7] or by nicotine in bovine adrenomedullary cells[8] and in human pheochromocytes in cultures[9] return to normal or above-normal levels within a few days. These findings are apparently in contradiction with reports that have shown increases in adrenomedullary OP in the rat after splanchnic denervation[1,5,10], suggesting that in this species the splanchnic innervation represses rather than stimulates the synthesis of OP. Reserpine treatment *in vivo*[7] and a variety of CA depleting drugs in cultured chromaffin cells[9,11,12] reduce CA content, but increase OP levels, apparently by increased *de novo* synthesis and processing of enkephalin precursors[12,13]. These results led to the suggestion that an intracellular catecholamine pool may contribute to the regulation of OP biosynthesis and processing in chromaffin cells. Activation of adrenomedullary nicotinic receptors is followed by a rise in cAMP *in vivo*[14] and in cultured cells[15], suggesting that OP content may be, at least in part, regulated through cyclic nucleotides. The present studies were undertaken to elucidate the role of cAMP, CA and splanchnic innervation in the regulation and processing of adrenomedullary OP.

CYCLIC AMP AND OPIOID PEPTIDES OF BOVINE CHROMAFFIN CELLS IN CULTURE

The effect of cAMP analogs and compounds that elevate endogenous levels of cAMP was studied in primary cultures of bovine adrenal medulla cells maintained in a chemically defined medium[16]. Native opioid peptide activity (NOP), comprised mainly of met- and leu-enkephalin, was determined in acetic acid extracts of the cultures by an opiate radioreceptor assay[11]. Total opioid peptide activity (TOP) was measured in the extracts after sequential digestion with trypsin and carboxypetidase B[3,8]. Cryptic opioid peptides (COP, extended enkephalin containing peptides inactive in the receptor assay) were estimated as the difference between TOP and NOP. Addition of 8Br cAMP or Forskolin (that markedly enhances chromaffin cell cAMP levels, Abou-Donia, Zimmerman and Viveros; unpublished) increased both NOP and COP in similar proportion (Table I). Inhibitors of cyclic nucleotide phosphodiesterase and addition of dibutyryl-cAMP had similar effects on NOP and COP[12]. These actions can be totally dissociated from changes in protein and CA content suggesting they are not simply a reflection of an increase in total protein synthesis or secondary to CA depletion. The proportional and simultaneous increase in NOP and COP suggest that cyclic nucleotides induce a concomitant activation of *de novo* synthesis of proenkephalin and of processing. The increase in *de novo* synthesis is further supported by the recent finding that cAMP addition to chromaffin cell cultures increases the levels of proenkephalin mRNA[17].

TABLE I

EFFECT OF DIFFERENT TREATMENTS ON CHROMAFFIN CELL NATIVE OPIOID PEPTIDE, CRYPTIC OPIOID PEPTIDE AND CATECHOLAMINE CONTENT

Addition to Medium	NOP	COP	NE	E	DA
	--pmol/5x10^5 cells--		--------nmol/5x10^5 cells---------		
	Experiment 1				
None	18.8 ± 0.5	48.2 ± 1.2	8.9 ± 0.2	27.5 ± 0.3	0.45 ± 0.02
8-Bromo-cAMP, 0.5 mM	22.8 ± 0.7[a]	62.4 ± 3.5[a]	6.3 ± 0.3[b]	19.4 ± 0.4[b]	1.36 ± 0.20[a]
Forskolin, 10 μM	23.4 ± 0.1[b]	62.8 ± 1.8[b]	6.8 ± 0.2[b]	12.9 ± 0.2[b]	1.55 ± 0.04[b]
Tetrabenazine, 100 μM	36.9 ± 0.5[b]	49.4 ± 2.6	0.5 ± 0.04[b]	2.5 ± 0.2[b]	<0.03
	Experiment 2				
None	20.7 ± 0.6	31.9 ± 1.3	12.8 ± 0.2	19.6 ± 0.1	0.35 ± 0.01
α-Methyltyrosine, 1 mM	29.8 ± 0.4[b]	36.7 ± 2.3	8.7 ± 0.2[b]	15.8 ± 0.3[b]	0.03 ± 0.003[b]
	Experiment 3				
None	24.2 ± 2.5	60 ± 5	14.7 ± 0.1	12.2 ± 0.2	1.90 ± 0.04
Brocresine, 150 μM	51.9 ± 0.9[b]	55 ± 8	9.2 ± 0.2[b]	8.7 ± 0.3[a]	n.d.

NE, norepinephrine; E, epinephrine; DA, dopamine; NOP, native opioid peptides; COP, cryptic opioid peptides; n.d., not detectable.
Chromaffin cell cultures were maintained in the absence or the presence of the indicated drugs for 3 days. Data are expressed as means ± S.E.M.; a, $p < 0.01$ compared to no additions; b, $p < 0.001$ compared to no additions.

CATECHOLAMINES AND OPIOID PEPTIDES OF CULTURED CHROMAFFIN CELLS

Depletion of endogenous CA by tetrabenazine (a blocker of vesicular uptake of CA), α-methyl-p-tyrosine (an inhibitor of tyrosine hydroxylase) and brocresine (an inhibitor of DOPA-decarboxylase) produced increases in NOP levels with no change in COP (Table I) even when assayed repeatedly between 4 hr and 3 days after drug addition[12]. The effects of these agents on increasing NOP and decreasing CA is dose- and time-dependent and the increases in OP levels induced by different concentrations of tetrabenazine were approximately proportional to the CA depletion. Tetrabenazine treatment induced exponential losses of each CA in the cells with approximate half-times of 2.5, 17 and 20 hr for dopamine, norepinephrine and epinephrine, respectively. Norepinephrine and epinephrine in the culture medium were elevated 40- and 20-fold, respectively, over those of untreated cultures 24 hr after tetrabenazine. Single or repetitive additions of norepinephrine and epinephrine, to give concentrations similar to those achieved in the medium of tetrabenazine-treated cells (15 μM and 7.5 μM, respectively) failed to modify chromaffin cell OP levels 3 days later. The increase in cell OP levels induced by reserpine was not blocked by phentolamine (1 μM), propranolol (10 μM), or haloperidol (10-100 μM). These results suggest that extracellular CA and cell-surface CA receptors do not mediate the effects of tetrabenazine or reserpine on chromaffin cell OP levels. The effect of CA depleting agents does not seem to be mediated by changes in chromaffin cell cAMP levels since these were never found to change after tetrabenazine (Abou-Donia, Zimmerman and Viveros, unpublished). A further difference between the cAMP-dependent and -independent effects on chromaffin cell OP is that CA-depleting agents never increase COP, suggesting that the primary effect is an increase in processing that is matched by an increase in precursor synthesis. That the effects of CA depletion on increased OP involves *de novo* synthesis is also suggested by an increased rate of incorporation of radiolabeled amino acids into enkephalins[13] and by the blockade of the increase of OP stores following reserpine by inhibitors of mRNA translation and ribosomal protein synthesis[7,11].

ROLE OF NEUROGENIC STIMULATION AND SPLANCHNIC INNERVATION ON RAT ADRENAL MEDULLA OPIOID PEPTIDES

Reflex neurogenic stimulation of the adrenal medulla was obtained by maintaining rats in hypoglycemic shock for 3 hr through insulin administration (Fig. 1). Similar to previous findings in the guinea pig[7], 3 hr of neurogenic stimulation produced a marked depletion of NOP, presumably due to exocytotic cosecretion since CA were also markedly decreased. The initial decrease in NOP is followed by a rapid increase attaining control levels 48 hr later and further increasing to 2.5-fold control levels the third day of after insulin. COP also increased above control levels preceding the rise in NOP.

The effect of two different surgical procedures to decentralize the rat adrenal is presented in Fig. 2. To obtain complete adrenal decentralization the left celiac and superior mesenteric ganglia were surgically removed. CA and OP fell immediately on both the innervated and denervated glands. The pattern of OP and CA changes in the left denervated gland resembled those produced by the short stress of insulin hypoglycemia. The changes observed in the right innervated gland are suggestive of a maintained compensatory increase in splanchnic nerve discharge in response to surgical stress and the extensive vascular and visceral sympathetic denervation. When left adrenal denervation was obtained by just sectioning the left major splanchnic nerve below the diaphragm (a relatively minor surgical procedure) there was a very small decrease in left or right adrenomedullary levels of CA or OP and at no time was there an increase in NOP or COP in the denervated gland (Fig. 2). These results suggest that the apparent increase in OP as a consequence of adrenal

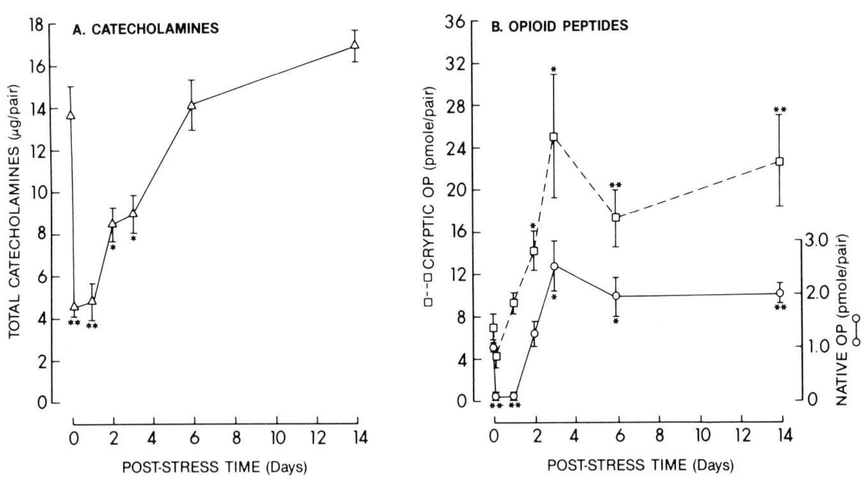

Fig. 1. Effect of maintained splanchnic nerve stimulation on catecholamines and opioid peptides of the rat adrenal medulla. Reflex splanchnic stimulation was induced by insulin hypoglycemia for 3 hr. Hypoglycemia was terminated by administration of a 40% sucrose solution by stomach tube and access to food. Adrenal medullas were carefully dissected from cortices under a stereoscopic microscope in the cold before homogenization in 0.5 M acetic acid. Data are means ± S.E.M.; t-test comparisons against no insulin treatment (0 time): *p <0.02, **p <0.005.

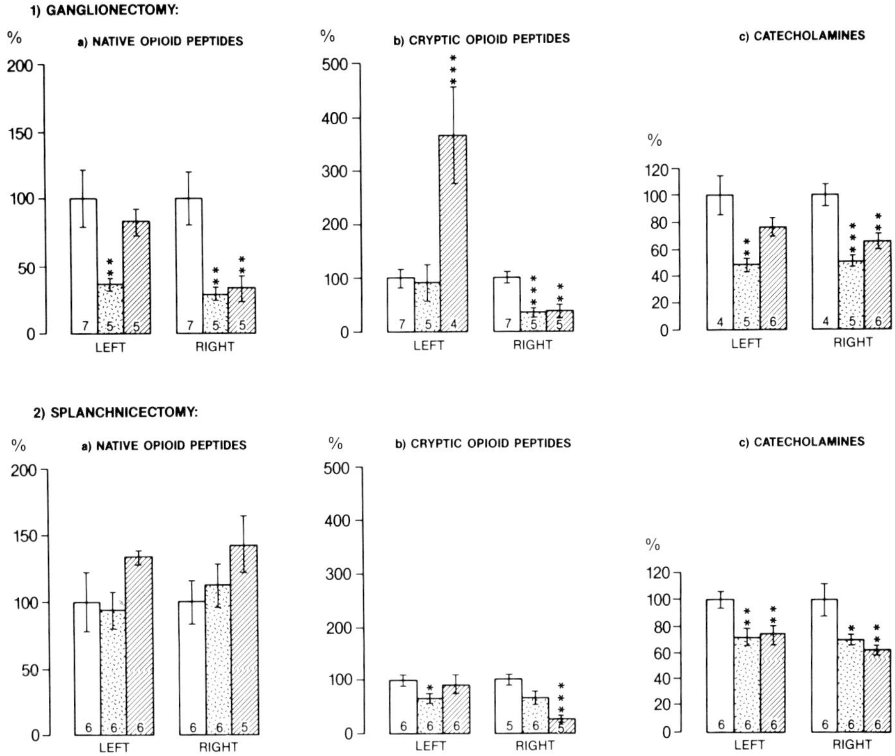

Fig. 2. Effects of two types of adrenal denervation on rat adrenomedullary catecholamines and opioid peptides. Left adrenal glands were denervated by removal of the left celiac and superior mesenteric ganglion or by sectioning the left splanchnic nerve between diaphragm and celiac ganglion. Medullas were dissected from cortices before homogenization and assay. Clear bars: unoperated controls; stippled bars: 24 hr post-surgery; cross-hatched bars: 48 hr post-surgery. Data are means ± S.E.M.; t-test comparison against corresponding unoperated controls: *$p < 0.05$, **$p < 0.02$, ***$p < 0.005$.

denervation reflects the differential response of the innervated and denervated glands to different intensities and length of neural stimulation rather than the splanchnic innervation exerting a tonic inhibitory influence on the expression of OP in the rat adrenal medulla.

In conclusion, OP synthesis and processing in adrenomedullary chromaffin cells in culture can be modified by a number of factors including cAMP-dependent and -independent mechanisms. Since neurogenic stimulation produces both a decrease in adrenomedullary CA levels (due to secretion) and a nicotinic receptor mediated activation of adenylcyclase the same mechanisms shown to affect OP synthesis and processing in culture may regulate these processes *in vivo*.

REFERENCES

1. Schultzberg M, Lundberg JM, Hokfelt T, Terenius L, Brandt J, Elde RP, Goldstein M (1978) Neuroscience 3:1169-1186
2. Viveros OH, Diliberto EJ Jr, Hazum E, Chang K-J (1979) Mol Pharmacol 16:1101-1108
3. Lewis RV, Stern AS, Rossier J, Stein S, Udenfriend S (1979) Biochem Biophys Res Commun 89:822-829
4. Yang H-YT, Digiulio AM, Fratta W, Hong JS, Majane EA, Costa E (1980) Neuropharmacology 19:209-215
5. Udenfriend S, Kilpatrick DL (1983) Arch Biochem Biophys 221:309-323
6. Viveros OH, Diliberto EJ Jr, Daniels AJ (1983) Federation Proc 42:2923-2928
7. Viveros OH, Diliberto EJ Jr, Hazum E, Chang K-J (1980) In: Costa E, Trabucchi M (eds) Adv Biochem Psychopharmacol Vol 22, Neural Peptides and Neuronal Communication. Raven Press, New York, pp 191-204
8. Wilson SP, Chang K-J, Viveros OH (1982) J Neurosci 2:1150-1156
9. Wilson SP, Chang K-J, Viveros OH (1981) Peptides 2 (Suppl 1):83-88
10. LaGamma EF, Adler JE, Black IB (1983) Soc Neurosci Abstr 9:306
11. Wilson SP, Abou-Donia MM, Chang K-J, Viveros OH (1981) Neuroscience 6:71-79
12. Wilson SP, Unsworth CD, Viveros OH (1984) J Neurosci (in press)
13. Wilson SP, Chang K-J, Viveros OH (1980) Proc Natl Acad Sci USA 77:4364-4368
14. Guidotti A, Costa E (1974) J Pharmacol Exp Ther 189:665-675
15. Schneider AS, Cline HT, Lemaire S (1979) Life Sci 24:1389-1394
16. Wilson SP, Viveros OH (1981) Exp Cell Res 133:159-169
17. Schwartz JP, Quach TT, Panula P, Costa E (1983) Soc Neurosci Abstr 9:745

Endocrinology
F. Labrie, L. Proulx, eds.

EFFECTS OF VASOACTIVE INTESTINAL POLYPEPTIDE (VIP) ON N1E-115 NEUROBLASTOMA CELLS

BRITTA HEDLUND
Department of Biochemistry, Arrhenius Laboratory, University of Stockholm, S-106 91 Stockholm, Sweden

SUMMARY

Responses of N1E-115 neuroblastoma cells to vasoactive intestinal polypeptide (VIP were studied. Application of VIP produced an approx. 10 mV tetrodotoxin resistant depolarization lasting 10-25 seconds. VIP did also stimulate cyclic AMP synthesis with 20 nm VIP giving maximal response. It is suggested that N1E-115 neuroblastoma cells which posses VIP receptors and muscarinic acetylcholine receptors may be a useful system to study VIP-receptors and VIP-receptor mediated responses and VIP-ACh interactions.

INTRODUCTION

The 28 amino acid residues long peptide; vasoactive intestinal polypeptide (VIP) originally isolated from porcine small intestine (1), is widely distributed both in the central and peripheral nervous system (2-5). It is a potent secretagogue and its effects on enzyme secretion in the pancreas and potentiating effects on salivary secretion are well studied (6-10). In the central nervous system VIP is an important neuropeptide with actions in the hypothalamus (11-13).

Among the cell reponses mediated by VIP are excitation of for example cortical, hippocampal and spinal neurons (3, 14, 15), and stimulation of adenylate cyclase (AC) (16, 17). The VIP mediated depolarizations have in most cases been tetrodotoxin (TTX) resistant, indicating that the responses does not involve sodium (14, 15, 18). The effects of VIP on different secretory responses have been suggested to be mediated via increased cAMP levels, which would promote an increase in the intracellular concentration of calcium, the primary mediator of secretory responses (6, 10). This effect has, in similarity to a variety of other tissues (19), been suggested to be regulated by guanine nucleotide binding proteins (20).

Neuroblastoma cells have been shown to possess a variety of neurotransmittor receptors (21, 22), and they have been used as a model system to study different phenomena, such as short- and long-term desensitization of muscarinic receptors (23, 24). High levels of VIP have also been found in clonal neuroblastoma and astrocytoma cell lines (25). For example, in N1E-115 neuroblastoma cells approx. 0.6 ng VIP/10^6 cells was found (25), and there has also been a report of VIP stimulated cAMP synthesis in neuroblastoma x glioma cells (26). The aim of this study was to determine whether N1E-115 neuroblastoma cells responded to VIP, and whether VIP stimulated cAMP synthesis could be observed. The results indicated that the cells respond to VIP and that they can provide a useful system to study VIP-receptors and VIP-mediated cell responses and interactions of e.g. muscarinic and VIP receptors.

METHODS

N1E-115 neuroblastoma cells, passage 13-16, a gift from Prof. Xandra O. Breakefield, Yale University, were used in these experiments. They were grown in a humidified atmosphere at 37°C in Dulbecco's Modified Eagle Medium (DMEM) supplemented with 5% fetal calf serum (FCS). Eight to nine days before an experiment the cells were subcultivated onto petridishes, using DMEM supplemented with 2% FCS. The medium was changed the day before an experiment.

Electrophysiological recordings, using 80-120 Mohm electrodes filled with 4 M KAc, were carried out using a conventional electrophysiological setup, described in detail elsewhere (27, 28). The petridish was placed on the stage of an inverted Olympus microscope, and the culture medium replaced with Hepes-buffered DMEM. All recordings were carried out at room temperature (22-25°C). An observed resting membrane potential of at least -30 mV was accepted as a good penetration. VIP was applied via pressure ejection applying a pressure of 20 kPa. The pipette contained 10 μM VIP dissolved in Hepes-buffered DMEM. All other agents were applied directly to the bath in a total volume of 100 μl.

VIP stimulated AC was studied using a Krebs-Ringer's buffer containing 137 mM NaCl, 2.7 mM KCl, 1.8 mM $CaCl_2$, 1 mM $MgCl_2$, 2 g/l glucose, 10 mM teophyllin, 1000 U/ml bacitracin, pH = 7.4. After 10 minutes preincubation with buffer at 37°C, the cells were incubated with VIP and/or GTP for indicated time periods at 37°C. After this the buffer was removed and 1 ml 0.4 M perchloric acid (PCA) added. The cells were then pelleted and saved for later protein determination and the PCA in the supernatant removed via addition of 100 μl 10 M KOH. The pH of the supernatant was adjusted to 6-8 via addition of glacial acetic acid, and the amount of cAMP determined using a kit from the Radiochemical Centre, Amersham, UK.

RESULTS AND DISCUSSION

Neuroblastoma cells respond to application of VIP with a depolarizing response accompanied with an approx. 20% decrease in membrane resistance (Figure 1). Of 20 cells tested 15 responded to VIP. The mean resting membrane potential of the cells recorded from was -45 ± 7 mV (mean ± SD) (n = 20), and the observed response had an amplitude of 12 ± 3 mV (n = 15) and a length of 16 ± 6 sec (n = 15). The response had the characteristics of a slow postsynaptic potential, which has been suggested for peptides (29). Using the data described in (30) the concentration of VIP at the cell surface was estimated to approx. 1 nM, which is a concentration within the range where VIP is assumed to be physiologically active (9). Picomolar to nanomolar concentrations of VIP have also in other systems been shown to produce a response (31).

Attempts were also made to determine a reversal potential for the response. Cells were held at different membrane potentials and the response to VIP recorded. In four cells studied, the cells could be depolarized to + 40 mV without changing the polarity of the response (Data not shown). The response was TTX resistant and was completely blocked by addition of $CoCl_2$ in the five cells tested (Figure 1), indicating that in all of these cells, the inward current is mainly carried by calcium. Slow excitatory postsynaptic potentials accompanied by a decrease in membrane resistance have also been suggested to be mediated via an increase in membrane calcium and/or sodium conductance (29). It may be that there, in some cells, is a component of sodium conductance in the VIP

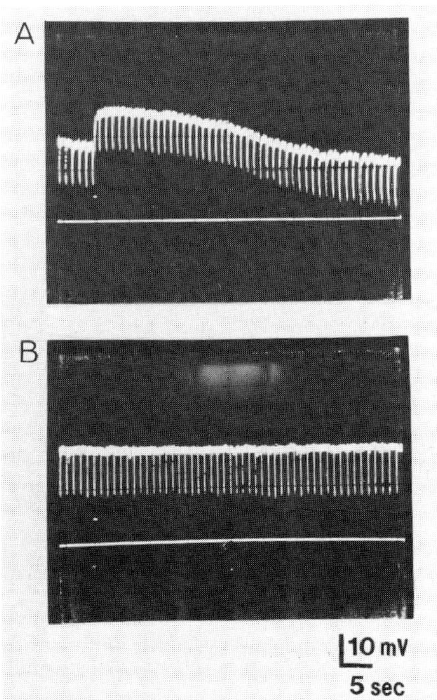

Fig. 1. Responses of one representative N1E-115 neuroblastoma cell to A) a 200 msec pressure pulse VIP. B) a 200 msec pressure pulse VIP in the presence of $CoCl_2$ (10 mM).

response. This is however a matter for further investigations, as well as in detail characterize VIP receptor stimulated ion conductances and determine eventual cross reactivity with other peptides.

As can be observed in Figure 2, VIP did also stimulate cAMP synthesis, with a maximum after two minutes. Maximal effect was obtained using approximately 20 nM VIP (Figure 2). The stimulatory effect of VIP was prolonged in the presence of GTP (0.1 mM) (Data not shown). These data are in accordance with the multitude of studies showing the presence of VIP-stimulated adenylate cyclase (AC) in a variety of tissues (16, 17, 20).

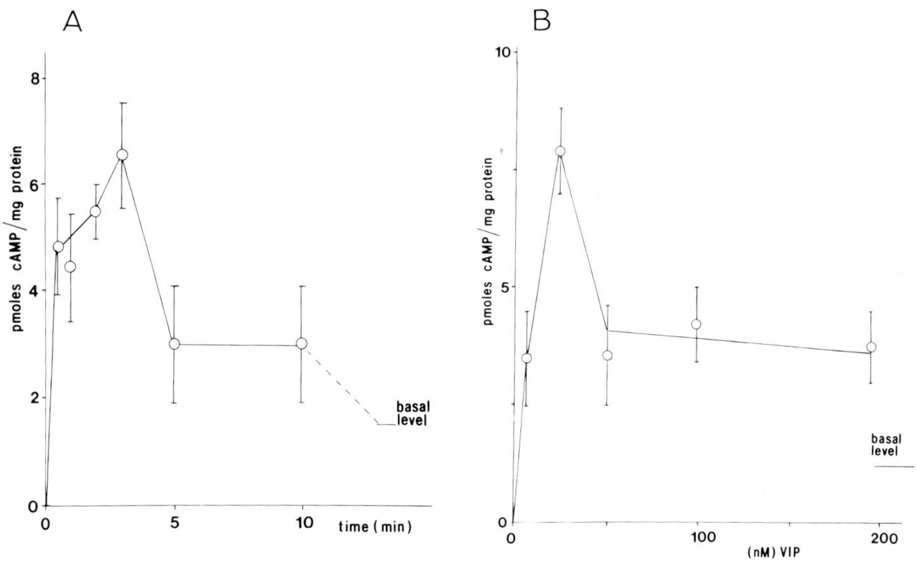

Fig. 2. VIP stimulated cAMP synthesis in N1E-115 neuroblastoma cells.
A) Cells were incubated with VIP (20 nM) for different time periods.
B) Cells were incubated for 2 minutes with different concentrations of VIP.

There are no reports that VIP will activate a membrane conductance and cAMP synthesis in the same cell. Where effect on the cAMP levels have been observed, no effects on the membrane potential could be detected (6). Increased intracellular concentrations of calcium have been suggested to inhibit AC activity (6), and if the VIP receptor had the ability both to activate AC and to activate a calcium conductance, the latter effect would prevent the first from beeing observed (6). Potent secretagogues of enzyme secretion, such as hormone of the pancreozymin family, do however cause marked membrane potential changes together with an increased AC activity (6). These data indicate that VIP can activate either a membrane calcium conductance or AC or both. It remains to be tested what effects an increased intracellular calcium concentration will have on the AC activity in this system. The effects on the membrane conductance lasted however approx. 20 seconds, whereas increased cAMP levels were observed after time periods of minutes. One possible explanation is therefore that the membrane conductance change proceeds the activation of AC, and that both can be observed in the same cell, but at different times.

VIP has also been found to interact with other neurotransmittors, such as interactions with acetylcholine in the submandibular salivary gland (32, 33) and with noradrenaline in the cerebral cortex (34). Interactions between muscarinic receptors and VIP-receptors on activation of AC, and regulatory effects of GTP have been observed in GH_3 pituitary cells (13). It has also been reported that similar interactions between acetylcholine and other hormonal substances may take placce in neuroblastoma cells, and that these can be specifically desensitized (35). The VIP response in neuroblastoma cells is atropine resistant, but som preliminary data indicate that interactions betwen muscarinic receptors and VIP-receptors take place. N1E-115 neuroblastoma cells may therefore provide a useful, well controlled system to study VIP-receptors, VIP-receptor mediated reactions and possible interactions with other neurotransmittor receptors.

ACKNOWLEDGEMENTS

Part of this work was carried out at the University of Stockholm, part of it at Yale University. The study was supported by grants to Dr. Tamas Bartfai, University of Stockholm, from the Swedish Medical Research Council and by a grant (MS-07609) from the NINCDS to Prof. Gordon M. Shepherd, Yale University. I am most grateful to Prof. Xandra O. Breakefield, Yale University, for the gift of N1E-115 neuroblastoma cells, for providing tissue culture facilities and for valuable discussions. VIP was a gift from Prof. Viktor Mutt, Karolinska Institutet, Stockholm.

REFERENCES

1. Said, SI and Mutt, V (1970) Polypeptide with broad biological activity: Isolation from small intestine. Science 169:1217-1218.

2. Fuxe, K, Hökfelt, T, Said, SI and Mutt, V (1977) Vasoactive intestinal polypeptide and the nervous system: immunohistochemical evidence for localization in central and peripheral neurons, particularly intracortical neurons of the cerebral cortex. Neuronsci Lett 5:241-246.

3. Phillis, JW, Kirkpatrick, JR and Said, SI (1979) Vasoactive intestinal polypeptide excitation of central neurons. Can J Physiol Pharmacol 56:337-340.

4. Kelly, JS (1980) Electrophysiology of peptides in the central nervous system. Br Med Bull 38:283-290.

5. North, RA and Egan, TM (19829 Electrophysiology of peptides in the peripheral nervous system. Br Med Bull 38:291-296.

6. Schulz, I and Stolze, HH (1980) The exocrine pancreas: The role of secretagogues, cyclic nucleotides, and calcium in enzyme secretion. Ann Rev Physiol 42:127-156.

7. Pearson, GT, Singh, J, Daoud, MS, Davison, JS and Petersen, OH (1981) Control of pancreatic cyclic nucleotide levels and amylase secretion by noncholinergic, nonadrenergic nerves. J Biol Chem. 256:11025-11031.

8. Petersen, OH (1982) Mechanisms of action of hormonal and neuronal peptides on exocrine gland cells. Br Med Bull 38:297-302.

9. Lundberg, JM (1981) Evidence for coexistence of vasoactive intestinal polypeptide (VIP) and acetylcholine in neurons of cat exocrine glands. Acta Physiol Scand, suppl 496.

10. Putney, JW (1979) Stimulus-permeability coupling: Role of calcium in the receptor regulation of membrane permeability. Pharmacol Rev 30:209-245.

11. Emson, PC, Fahrenkrug, J, Schaffalitzky de Muckadell, OB, Jessell, TM and Iversen, LL (1978) Vasoactive intestinal polypeptide (VIP): vesicular localization and potassium evoked release from rat hypothalamus. Brain Res 143:174-178.

12. Kerwin, RW, Pay, S, Bhoola, KD and Pycock, CJ (1980) Vasoactive intestinal polypeptide (VIP)-sensitive adenylatee cyclase in rat brain: regional distribution and localization on hypothalamic neurons. J Pharmacol Exp Ther 32:561-566.

13. Onali, P, Carola, E, Olianas, MC, Schwartz, JP and Costa, E (1983) In GH_3 pituitary cells, acetylcholine and vasoactive intestinal peptide antagonistically modulate adenylate cyclase, cyclic AMP content, and prolactin secretion. Mol Pharmacol 24:189-194.

14. Dodd, J, Kelly, JS and Said, SI (1979) Excitation of CA1 neurons of the rat hippcampus by the octacosapeptide, vasoactive intestinal polypeptide (VIP). Br J Pharmacol 66:125P.

15. Phillis, JW and Kirkpatrick, JR (1979) Actions of various gastrointestinal peptides on the isolated amphibian spinal cord. Can J Physiol Pharmacol 57:887-899.

16. Amiranoff, B and Rosselin, G (1982) VIP receptors and control of cyclic AMP production in Advances in Peptide Hormone Research Series, Ed SI Said, Raven Press, New York, pp 307-320.

17. Deschodt-Lanckman, M, Robberecht, P and Cristophe, J (1977) Characterization of VIP-sensitive adenylate cyclase in guinea pig brain. FEBS Lett 87:76-80.

18. Phillis, JW (1982) Neuronal excitation by vasoactive intestinal polypeptide in Advances in Peptide Hormone Research Series, Ed SI Said, Raven Press, New York, pp 299-305.

19. Rodbell, M (1980) The role of hormone receptors in GTP-regulatory proteins in membrane transduction. Nature 284:17-22.

20. Amiranoff, B, Laburthe, M and Rosselin, G (1980) Potentiation by guanine nucleotides of the VIP-induced adenylate cyclase stimulation in intestinal epithelial cell membranes. Life Sci 26:1905-1911.

21. Matsuzawa, H and Nirenberg, M (1975) Receptor mediated shifts in cGMP and cAMP levels in neuroblastoma cells. Proc Natl Acad Sci 72:3472-3476.

22. Bartfai, T, Breakefield, XO and Greengard, P (1978) Regulation of synthesis of guanosine 3':5'-cyclic monophosphate in neuroblastoma cells. Biochem J 176:119-127.

23. Shifrin, GS and Klein, WL (1980) Regulation of muscarinic acetylcholine receptor concentration in cloned neuroblastoma cells. J Neurochem 34:993-999.

24. Siman, RG and Klein, WL (1979) Cholinergic activity regulates muscarinic receptors in central nervous system cultures. Proc Natl Acad Sci 76:4141-4145.

25. Said, SI and Rosenberg, RN (1976) Vasoactive intestinal polypeptide: Abundant immunoreactivity in neural cell lines and normal nervous tissue. Science 192:907-909.

26. Propst, P, Moroder, L, Wünsch, E and Hamprecht, B (1979) The influence of secretin, glucagon and other peptides, of amino acids, prostaglandin endoperoxide analogues and diazpam on the level of cAMP in neuroblastoma x glioma hybrid cells. J Neurochem 32:1495-1500.

27. Masukawa, LM, Hedlund, B and Shepherd, GM (1984) Electrophysiological properties of identified cells in the in vitro olfactory epithelium of the Tiger salamander. J Neurosci, submitted for publication.

28. Hedlund, B (1984) Effects of atropine treatment on the responsiveness of N1E-115 neuroblastoma cells to applied acetylcholine. J Neurosci, submitted for publication.

29. Hartzell, HC (1981) Mechanisms of slow postsynaptic potentials. Nature 291, 539-544.

30. Smith, TG and Cunningham, MF (1983) Pressure ejection system for quantitative focal application of neuroactive substances from micropipettes. Med & Biol Eng & Comput 21:138-144.

31. Williams, JT and North, RA (1979) Vasoactive intestinal polypeptide excites neurones of the myenteric plexus. Brain Res 175:174-177.

32. Hedlund, B, Abens, J and Bartfai, T (1983) Chronic atropine treatment induced supersensitivity of VIP receptors and muscarinic receptors in the rat salivary gland. Science 220:519-521.

33. Lundberg, JM, Hedlund, B and Bartfai, T (1982) Vasoactive intestinal polypeptide enhances muscarinic ligand binding in cat submandibular gland. Nature 295:147-149.

34. Magistrelli, PJ, Schorderet, M (1984) VIP and noradrenaline act synergistically to increase cyclic AMP in cerebral cortex. Nature 308:280-282.

35. Green, DA and Clark, RB (1982) Specific muscarinic cholinergic desensitization in the neuroblastoma-glioma hybrid NG108-15. J Neurochem 39:1125-1131.

© 1984 Elsevier Science Publishers B.V.
Endocrinology
F. Labrie, L. Proulx, eds.

PEPTIDE AND AMINE INTERACTIONS IN CENTRAL NERVOUS SYSTEM AND PITUITARY FUNCTIONS: FUNCTIONAL AND CLINICAL ASPECTS

William H. ROSTENE and Guillaume CHARPENTIER
INSERM U.55, Hôpital Saint-Antoine, 184, rue du Faubourg Saint-Antoine, 75012 Paris, and Service de Médecine Interne, Endocrinologie-Diabétologie, Hôpital de Corbeil, 91100 Corbeil (France)

INTRODUCTION

In spite of extensive research, current notions about peptide-amine interactions remain far from satisfactory and many discrepancies are due to the complex neural circuits which control physiological responses, to the various ways in which a peptide exhibits its effects on aminergic transmission, and finally to the importance of the endocrine environment of the target cell.

We will try to illustrate in an original and refreshing way, by means of one particular neuropeptide, the Vasoactive Intestinal Peptide (VIP), how a peptide can influence the activity of aminergic systems (serotoninergic (5-HT), cholinergic and dopaminergic (DA)) in central nervous system (CNS) and anterior pituitary functions.

VIP-AMINE INTERACTIONS IN THE CNS

Interactions at the presynaptic level

One possibility for a neurotransmitter/modulatory role of VIP is that the peptide may regulate aminergic neurotransmission at the presynaptic level. A recently unexpected effect of VIP is the effect of the peptide on specific enzymatic activities which lead to the synthesis of important neurotransmitter substances. VIP stimulates the activity of serotonin-N-acetyltransferase, a rate-limiting enzyme in the synthesis of melatonin in rat pineal glands *in vitro*, independently of noradrenergic neurotransmission (1) but dependent on the dark-light cycle (2). An interesting observation is that the pineal gland is innervated by the superior cervical ganglion in which VIP stimulates the activity of tyrosine hydroxylase, enzyme involved in the synthesis of catecholamines (3). The fact that VIP regulates the activity of the pineal gland is of particular importance, since melatonin has been reported to influence brain 5-HT levels (4) and to be involved in the control of pituitary functions (5).

We recently observed that *in vitro* addition of VIP to brain homogenates increases the activity of cholineacetyltransferase (CAT), the enzyme involved in the synthesis of acetylcholine (6). The CAT activity is enhanced in the anterior hypothalamus and in the hippocampus. Increased activity occurs rapidly

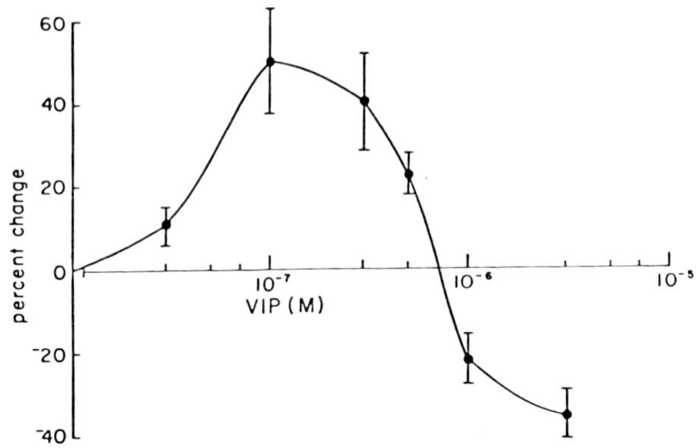

Figure 1: Dose-dependent effect of VIP on CAT activity in the rat hippocampus. Results are expressed as percentage of change versus control and represent the mean ± SEM of 4 individual values for each VIP concentrations. From (6).

after VIP addition and shows a biphasic effect with increasing concentrations of VIP with a maximum at 10^{-7}M (Fig.1). Kinetic analysis indicates that the increased activity of CAT by VIP is due to an enhanced affinity of the enzyme for one of the substrates choline, but not acetyl CoA (6). Therefore VIP-cholinergic interaction can be demonstrated in the brain, but in contrast to the periphery (7), at a presynaptic level.

A peptide may also affect aminergic neurotransmission through an effect on release. Many examples of such effect are available in the CNS. In the case of VIP, it was recently shown that the peptide stimulates *in vitro* the release of newly synthetized ^{3}H-5-HT from male rat suprachiasmatic nuclei (SCN) (8).

Interactions at the postsynaptic level

A peptide may also exert its neurotransmitter/modulatory role at the postsynaptic level in regulating transmitter receptor sensitivity. By means of isolated membrane preparations (9) and/or *in vitro* binding of ^{3}H-5-HT on brain slices coupled with visualization by quantitative autoradiography (10), we recently showed that VIP alters the binding of ^{3}H-5-HT to 5-HT_1 receptors in the hypothalamic SCN and in the dorsal hippocampus and possibly nowhere else in the brain of normal male rats.

VIP is able to decrease the number of 5-HT_1 binding sites in the SCN as determined by densitometric measurements following *in vitro* incubation of 10^{-7}M VIP in the presence of increasing concentrations of ^{3}H-5-HT (Fig.2). This obser-

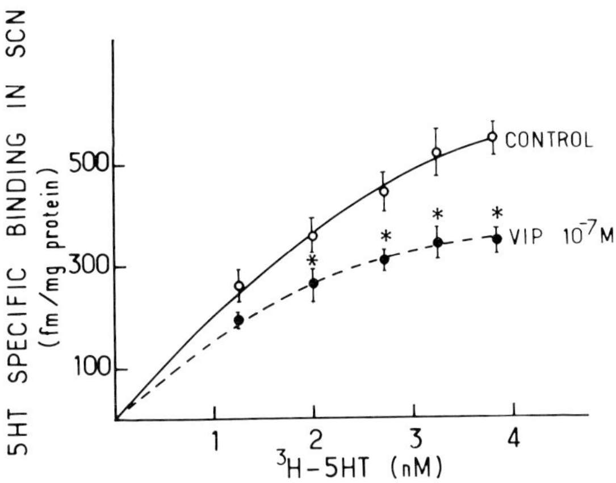

Figure 2: Effect of VIP (10^{-7}M) on specific binding of ^{3}H-5-HT in the rat suprachiasmatic nucleus (SCN). Increasing concentrations of ^{3}H-5-HT were incubated with or without VIP. Specific binding was determined as the difference between total and non-specific (in the presence of 1 μM unlabeled 5-HT) binding obtained by direct densities measurements on autoradiograms. Each point is the mean ± SEM of 6 determinations. * $p<0.01$ vs respective control point. From (13).

vation may serve as neurobiological support for the possible involvement of VIP and 5-HT in the regulation of many rhythms including circadian patterns of pituitary hormones (11). In contrast to the SCN, the effect of *in vitro* VIP incubation is to specifically increase the number of 5-HT_1 binding sites in a dose-dependent manner in a discrete region of the dorsal hippocampus, the dorsal subiculum, a structure known to be the major site through which the hippocampal neural activity influences the rest of the brain (10).

Since the hippocampus is the target brain structure for adrenal steroids (12), we investigated the possibility that such steroids may regulate neurotransmitter receptor sensitivity and thus influence the responsiveness of hippocampal neurons to intrinsic and afferent innervation. Bilateral adrenalectomy (ADX) for 6 days counteracts the stimulatory effect of VIP on 5-HT_1 binding sites in the dorsal subiculum and this effect is restored in ADX rats bearing a corticosterone implant (13, Fig.3). The modulatory permissive role of adrenal steroids in VIP activity in the hippocampus may have various aspects, since ADX can either mask the increase of 5-HT_1 binding sites induced by VIP such as in the dorsal subiculum, or unmask an effect which is not observed in normal animals such as in various hippocampal subfields (13).

A schematic representation of the possible interactions of VIP with aminergic systems such as 5-HT at both pre- and postsynaptic levels is

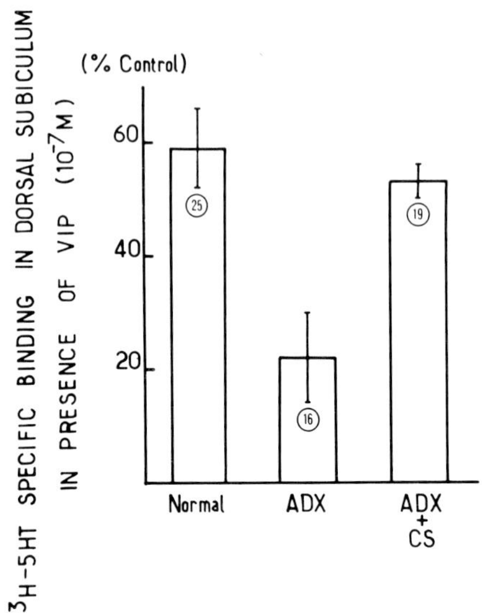

Figure 3: Effect of adrenalectomy (ADX) and corticosterone (CS) restoration on VIP (10^{-7}M) effect on 5-HT_1 binding sites in the dorsal subiculum of the rat hippocampal formation. Number of determinations in parenthesis. Redrawn from (13).

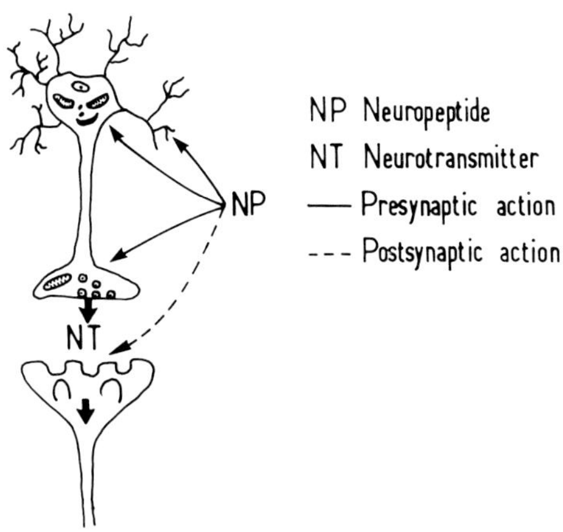

Figure 4: Schematic representation of possible interactions between a neuropeptide (NP) and a "classical" neurotransmitter (NT) at both pre- and postsynaptic levels.

illustrated on Fig.4.

VIP-AMINE INTERACTION IN THE ANTERIOR PITUITARY

There is now a general consensus on the fact that VIP is able to stimulate prolactin (PRL) release by a direct action on the pituitary gland (11). In vitro data were corroborated by in vivo experiments in rats and humans of both sexes, suggesting that VIP acts as a specific PRL-releasing factor.

Since the release of PRL by the anterior pituitary is under the controi of various brain substances mainly DA (14), VIP-DA interactions in vitro and in vivo were tested in rats and humans showing that DA counteracts VIP-stimulation of PRL release, an effect which probably takes place on the coupling of VIP receptors with adenylate cyclase activity (see review 11). In vivo stimulation of PRL release by VIP in normal subjects is much higher for the same dose of VIP than in prolactinomas, which suggests a relative impairment of the VIP response in prolactinomas (15, 16). An interesting observation is that the stimulatory effect of VIP is restored when patients are treated with DA in order to lower PRL secretion (17). In the same experiments, in five microadenomas "non-responder" in vivo to VIP, the peptide is only able to stimulate adenylate cyclase activity if the levels of the enzyme are previously decreased by DA (Fig.5). This kind of approach may tell us whether VIP can be used as a marker

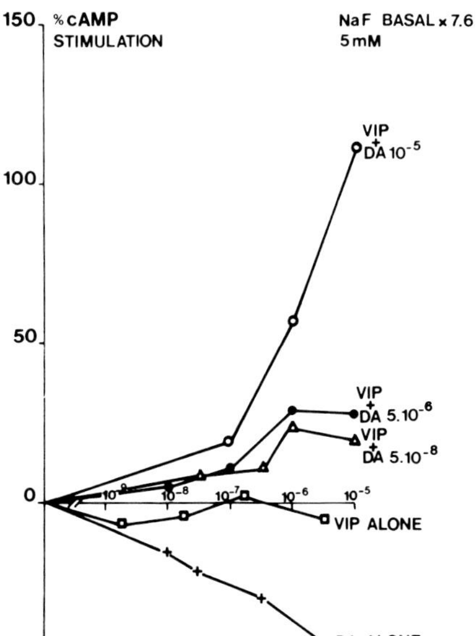

Figure 5: In vitro adenylate cyclase activity in a human PRL-secreting adenoma ("non-responder" to VIP in vivo) by DA and VIP. Results are expressed as percentage of cyclic AMP produced per min in response to increasing concentrations of DA or VIP.

to confirm a diagnostic of prolactinoma.

In conclusion, modulatory peptides can thus exhibit both in animals and humans under various endocrine conditions multiple effect on aminergic transmission which result in refined physiological responses.

ACKNOWLEDGEMENTS

We are indebted to Mrs D. LHENRY for her skillful secretarial assistance, and D. HUI BON HOA for her technical help.

REFERENCES

1. Kaneko T, Cheng PY, Oka H, Oda T, Yanaihara N, Yanaihara C (1980) Biomed Res 1: 84-87
2. Yuwiler A (1983) Science 220: 1082-1083
3. Ip NY, Ho CK, Zigmond RE (1982) Proc Natl Acad Sci USA 79: 7566-7569
4. Anton-Tay F, Chou L, Anton S, Wurtman RJ (1968) Science 162:277-278
5. Moszkowska A, Scemama A, Lombard MN, Hery M (1973) J Neural Transm 34:11-22
6. Luine VN, Rostène WH, Rhodes J, Mc Ewen BS (1984) J Neurochem 42:1131-1134
7. Lundberg JM, Hedlund B, Bartfai T (1982) Nature 295:147-149
8. Hery M, Faudon M, Hery F (1984) Peptides, in press
9. Rostène WH, Fischette CT, Mc Ewen BS (1984) J Neurosci 3: 2414-2419
10. Rostène WH, Fischette CT, Rainbow TC, Mc Ewen BS (1983) Neurosci Lett 37: 143-148
11. Rostène WH (1984) Progress in Neurobiology, in press
12. Mc Ewen BS (1982) In: Ganten D, Pfaff DW (eds) Current Topics in Neuro-endocrinology, Springer Verlag, Berlin, pp. 1-22
13. Rostène WH, Fischette CT, Dussaillant M, Mc Ewen BS (1984) Neuroendocrinology, in press
14. Rostène WH (1982) In: Tixier-Vidal A, Richard P (eds) Regulations Cellulaires Multihormonales en Neuroendocrinologie, vol. 110, INSERM, Paris pp. 173-188
15. Kato Y, Shimatsu A, Matsushita N, Ohta H, Imura H (1984) Peptides, in press
16. Charpentier G, Bercovici JP, Jednak P, Talbot JN, Mutt V, Rosselin G (1982) Biomédecine 36:106-107
17. Tater D, Charpentier G, Besson G, Rosselin G, Bercovici JP (1983) CR Acad Sci Paris 297:331-334

51. Electrophysiological Aspects of Hormone Secretion

Endocrinology
F. Labrie, L. Proulx, eds.

CHARACTERIZATION OF NORADRENERGIC AFFERENTS TO HYPOTHALAMIC MAGNOCELLULAR NEURONS

L.P. RENAUD, T.A. DAY, J.C.R. RANDLE, C.W. BOURQUE AND A.V. FERGUSON
Neurosciences Unit, Montreal General Hospital Research Institute and McGill University, 1650 Cedar Avenue, Montreal, Quebec, Canada H3G 1A4

INTRODUCTION

The hypothalamic supraoptic (SON) and paraventricular (PVN) nuclei contain both vasopressin (VP) and oxytocin (OXY) secreting magnocellular neurons (1). The SON and PVN also receive a dense catecholaminergic innervation (2,3). Recent anatomical studies indicate that the origin of these fibers to the SON is almost exclusively from noradrenaline containing neurons in the A1 cell group of the ventrolateral medulla while the PVN receives fibers from noradrenaline cells located in the A1, A2 and A6 catecholamine cell groups (4). The role of noradrenergic afferents in regulating the release of VP and OXY in the neurohypophysis is controversial, with both facilitatory and inhibitory actions proposed. To clarify the functional nature of these endogenous noradrenergic pathways and the actions of exogenously applied noradrenaline on neurosecretory neurons, we have conducted both in-vivo and in-vitro experiments. The results of these investigations support the notion of a central facilitatory action on VP release for noradrenergic afferents mediated through an α-adrenergic mechanism.

METHODS

In-vivo experiments

Extracellular recordings were obtained from SON and PVN neurosecretory neurons in pentobarbital anesthetized male Sprague-Dawley rats. A transpharyngeal approach to the brain permitted insertion of monopolar stimulating electrodes into the A1 and A2 regions to activate these afferent pathways and placement of a bipolar electrode in the posterior pituitary to identify neurosecretory cells by antidromic activation. Putative VP-secreting cells were differentiated from OXY-secreting neurons by their phasic activity and/or response to baroreceptor activation achieved through a rise in blood pressure following intravenously administered metaraminol (5). Spike train analyses were performed with a PDP 11/34 computer. All stimulation and recording sites were verified in 50 m histological sections processed for catecholamine histofluorescence (6) and then Nissl stained.

For neuropharmacological studies, noradrenaline, its agonists and antagonists were pressure applied from solutions contained in triple barrelled micropipettes rigidly attached to the side of the recording electrode.

In-vitro experiments

Recordings were obtained from SON neurons in perfused hypothalamic explants (7). Noradrenaline and adrenergic agonists were applied either by pressure from an adjacent pipette or into the perfusion media; antagonists were administered by addition to the perfusion media. Extracellullar recordings examined changes in firing frequency during drug applications; intracellular recordings also assessed membrane potential and resistance changes. Cells marked by intracellular Lucifer-yellow injections confirmed recordings from SON neurons.

RESULTS

In-vivo recordings

SON neurons: In 18 experiments data obtained from ipsilateral SON neurosecretory cells revealed that electrical stimulation within 200-300 microns of the center of the A1 cell group consistently enhanced the activity of putative VP-secreting cells (Table 1). In marked contrast was the absent or inhibitory response noted among putative OXY-secreting neurons. In 5 animals pretreated with 6-hydroxydopamine injected into the area above the SON in sufficient quantities (6.8 μg base in 0.25 μl saline) to deplete catecholamine histofluorescence, comparatively few VP-secreting cells responded.

TABLE 1: Effects of electrical stimulation of A1 on the excitability of SON neurons in (a) untreated animals and (b) those subjected to 6-OHDA treatment.

	No. of cells	Response to A1 stimulation: Excited	Inhibited	No Effect
(a) Untreated (n=18)				
Putative VP-cells	28	100%	0	0
Putative OXY-cells	23	0	9%	91%
(b) 6-OHDA treatment (n=5)				
Putative VP-cells	10	10%	0	90%
Putative OXY-cells	10	0	0	100%

PVN neurons: In a separate series of experiments, PVN neurosecretory neurons were examined for responses to electrical stimulation in A1 and A2 regions. Data indicated a pattern of response to A1 stimulation analogous with that recorded in SON (Table 2).

TABLE 2: Effect of A1 region stimulation on the excitability of PVN neurosecretory cells.

	No. of cells	Response to A1 stimulation: Excited	Inhibited	No effect
(a) Untreated (n=13)				
Putative VP-cells	18	78%	0	22%
Putative OXY-cells	15	13%	13%	73%
Unclassified	33	48%	0	52%
(b) 6-OHDA treated (n=8)				
Putative VP-cells	14	0	0	100%
Putative OXY-cells	27	0	0	100%
Unclassified	24	0	0	100%

In contrast to the specificity of the A1 input to VP-secreting cells, stimulation in A2 was noted to enhance the excitability of both VP and OXY-secreting neurons in PVN (Table 3).

TABLE 3: Effect of A2 region stimulation on excitability of PVN neurosecretory cells.

	No. of cells	Response to A2 stimulation: Excited	Inhibition	No effect
(a) Untreated (n-13)				
Putative VP-cells	10	60%	0	40%
Putative OXY-cells	20	70%	10%	20%
Unclassified	22	45%	5%	50%
(b) 6-OHDA treated (n=5)				
Putative VP-cells	9	11%	0	89%
Putative OXY-cells	10	0	0	100%
Unclassified	13	8%	0	92%

Neuropharmacology: In the SON, pressure application of noradrenaline revealed the presence of a concentration dependent change in the excitability of neurosecretory cells (Table 4) such that predominantly excitatory responses were observed with lower concentrations, while cells were more likely to show a depression of activity at higher concentrations.

TABLE 4: Response of SON neurosecretory cells to pressure application of noradrenaline in different concentrations.

Concentration of noradrenaline solution	No. of cells	Response		
		Excited	Inhibited	No Effect
50-100 μM	16	62.5%	27.5%	0
150-500 μM	52	65.4%	17.3%	17.3%
1-100 mM	8	12.5%	25.0%	62.5%

Moreover, the application of the α-1 adrenergic antagonist prazosin reversibly diminished or blocked noradrenaline induced excitations while noradrenaline induced depressions were reduced or blocked by application of the β-adrenergic antagonists timolol and propranolol.

In-vitro

Extracellular recordings from 141 SON cells revealed an increase in the excitability of 85% of cells following the application of noradrenaline and the α-adrenergic agonist methoxamine; effective concentrations ranged between 10-200 μM. These excitations were effectively blocked by prazosin in concentrations as low as 12 nM. During intracellular recordings, noradrenaline induced membrane depolarizations were accompanied by increased firing, but little or no consistent change in membrane resistance was observed.

COMMENTS

These data reveal that (a) electrical activation of two endogenous noradrenergic pathways arising in A1 and A2 enhances the firing of putative VP-secreting cells, (b) that a similar enhancement in the activity of neurosecretory cells can be achieved with the exogenous application of noradrenaline in low concentration and (c) that these excitatory effects are mediated through an α-adrenergic mechanism. These observations support earlier proposals that suggest a facilitatory role for noradrenaline on the release of VP. The observed depressant actions of exogenously applied noradrenaline at higher concentrations are in agreement with previous data (8) that indicate this pattern of response to be mediated through β-adrenergic receptors.

ACKNOWLEDGEMENTS

We are grateful to the Canadian MRC, FRSQ and Quebec Heart Association for their financial support, and to Gwen Peard for typing the manuscript.

REFERENCES

1. Vandesande F, Dierickx K (1975) Cell Tiss Res 164:153-162
2. Fuxe K (1965) Acta Physiol Scand 64: Suppl 247:37-85
3. Ungerstedt U (1971) Acta Physiol Scand 367:1-48
4. Sawchenko PE, Swanson LW (1982) Brain Res Rev 4:275-325
5. Harris MC (1979) J Endocr 82:115-125
6. Furness JB, Heath JW, Costa M (1978) Histochemistry 57:285-295
7. Bourque CW, Renaud LP (1983) J Neurosci Meth 7:203-214
8. Barker JL, Crayton JW, Nicoll RA (1971) J Physiol 218:19-32

© 1984 Elsevier Science Publishers B.V.
Endocrinology
F. Labrie, L. Proulx, eds.

PATTERNS OF ELECTRICAL ACTIVITY AND HORMONE RELEASE FROM NEUROSECRETORY CELLS

G. LENG and R.J. BICKNELL
A.F.R.C. Institute of Animal Physiology, Babraham, Cambridge CB2 4AT (U.K.)

In the lactating rat, during suckling, oxytocin is released as a discrete bolus at intervals of 5-10 min to cause each reflex milk-ejection. In the dehydrated rat, after water deprivation or saline drinking, vasopressin is released at a sustained high level for prolonged antidiuresis. Thus the functional requirements for secretion of these two hormones differ in respect of the temporal characteristics of release required. Recent research has shown that the electrical activity of oxytocin and vasopressin neurones, which is the primary determinant of hormone release, is ideally matched to these demands: when oxytocin is released during milk-ejection, and when vasopressin is released during dehydration, the necessary hormone release is achieved with a highly efficient patterning of electrical impulses.

VASOPRESSIN RELEASE

It has been known for many years that rat vasopressin neurones in the magnocellular neurosecretory nuclei discharge "phasically" when activated by dehydration (1). A typical vasopressin neurone will discharge action potentials in bursts of 20-40 s duration at 6-15 spikes/s, separated by silent periods of similar duration. In 1979 Dutton and Dyball (2) demonstrated that this phasic patterning led to enhanced vasopressin secretion: they showed that release from the isolated rat neurohypophysis *in vitro*, evoked by electrical stimulation, was greater when the stimuli were presented in a phasic pattern. Two processes appear to strongly influence the amount of hormone released by each action potential: these processes are "facilitation" and "fatigue".

Facilitation

Dutton and Dyball (2) originally proposed that clustering of action potentials in bursts during phasic firing enhanced vasopressin release via facilitation of calcium entry into the secretory terminal, and subsequent experiments have partially supported this hypothesis. Most recently, Shaw et al (3) demonstrated that the amount of vasopressin release per stimulus pulse evoked by bursts of pulses presented at a fixed frequency of 10Hz increases with burst length for bursts of up to 20 s. However, facilitation does not fully account for the enhanced efficiency of phasic patterning: we noted that phasic patterns of discharge from vasopressin neurones did not contain a marked preponderance of short inter-spike intervals when compared with the non-phasic discharge patterns of other hypothalamic neurones, yet confirmed the superior efficiency of phasic discharge (4).

Fatigue

From subsequent studies of the temporal profile of vasopressin release in an *in vitro* perifusion system during sustained electrical stimulation we demonstrated the existence of a reversible "fatigue" of stimulus-secretion coupling. During 20 min of 13Hz electrical stimulation of isolated rat neurohypophyses vasopressin was not released at a steady rate, but following an initial peak the release rate declined dramatically. Analysis of this data suggested that about 50% of the vasopressin released by 20 min of stimulation was released within the first 2 min. This fatigue proved to be reversible: a repeat stimulation after a 20 min recovery period without stimulation would produce a second, high but transient peak of release (5).

In fact, the time course of the fatigue is considerably more rapid than that which could be inferred from the earlier study. In recent experiments (Fig.1) single rat neurohypophyses were stimulated at 13Hz for 18, 36, 54 and 72 s, separated by 24 min periods without stimulation: the order of presentation of stimuli was varied between experiments according to a latin square, and the total vasopressin and oxytocin released by each period of stimulation was measured by RIA (see ref.6 for full details). From these data we calculated the amounts of the two hormones released in each successive 18 s of a 72 s burst, and found that for vasopressin but not for oxytocin, the efficiency of hormone release declines rapidly even between 18 and 36 s from the start of a burst. Furthermore, recovery from fatigue could be achieved with as little as 30 s of silence.

OXYTOCIN RELEASE

The oxytocin neurones in the magnocellular neurosecretory nuclei, when activated by suckling, discharge in synchrony prior to each milk ejection in a brief high frequency burst (2-4 s at 40-80 Hz). This pattern - the "reflex milk-ejection burst" - is optimally effective both in terms of the effiency of release from the neurohypophysis and subsequently in its effect upon the mammary glands.

About 0.5 - 1 mU (1-2 pmol) oxytocin is released into the circulation by each milk-ejection burst. The response of the rat mammary gland to oxytocin is non-linear and this amount of oxytocin produces a response that is close to the top of the steep portion of the dose response curve. For effective contraction of mammary epithelium, it is important that the oxytocin arrives as a bolus: 1 mU of oxytocin injected over 30 s, for instance, produces a negligible change in intramammary pressure. Thus the pattern in which oxytocin is released from the neurohypophysis during reflex milk-ejection is matched to the requirements of

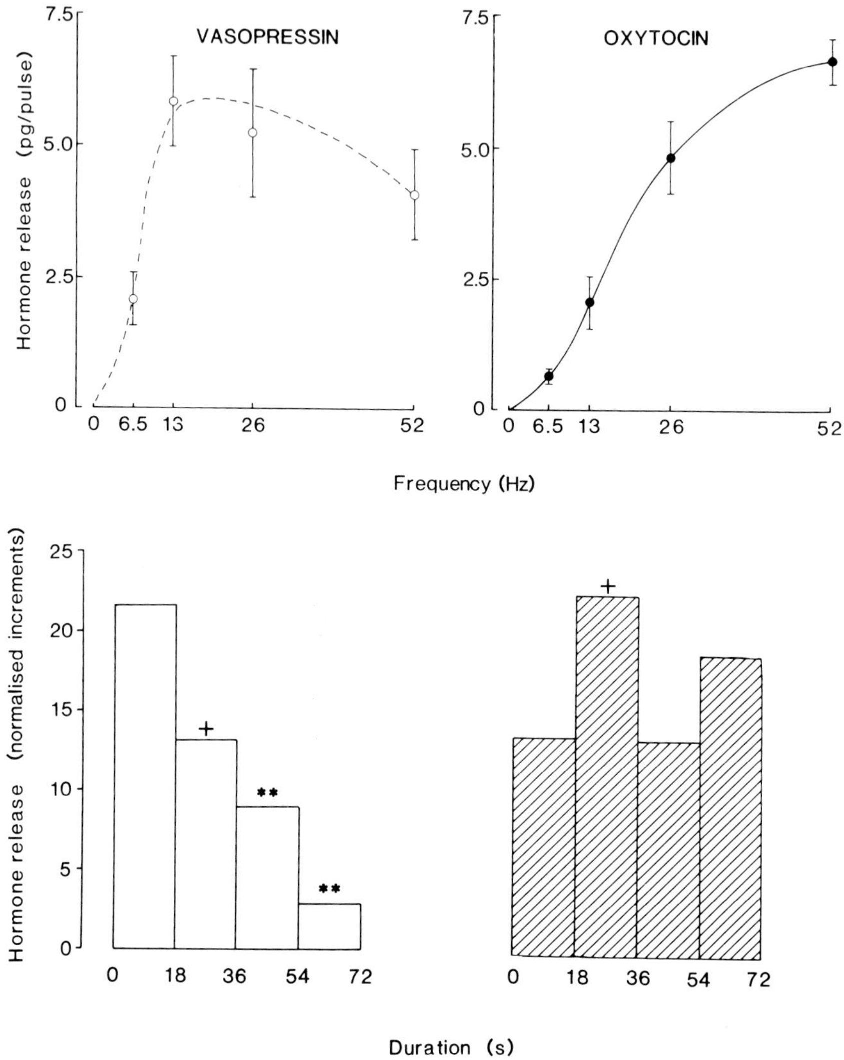

Fig. 1. Vasopressin (left) and oxytocin (right) released from isolated rat neurohypophyses _in vitro_, measured by RIA.

Top: Glands were stimulated with 156 pulses presented at 52 Hz, 26 Hz, 13 Hz and 6.5 Hz. Data are means $\pm$ S.E.M. of 4 experiments.

Bottom: Glands were stimulated for 18, 36, 54 and 72 s at 13 Hz. The histograms show the calculated release in each 18 s of a 72 s period of stimulation. The data (from 14 experiments, see ref. 6) are normalised to compensate for variation in the amounts of hormone released in each experiment.

Significantly different from release in 0-18 s, + p 0.1; ** p 0.01

the mammary gland. As with vasopressin, it also appears that oxytocin release evoked by reflex milk-ejection bursts of stimuli is at optimal efficiency.

To demonstrate this, we again looked at hormone release from the isolated rat neurohypophysis, and compared the effectiveness of a 3 s train of stimuli at 52 Hz with a 6 s train at 26 Hz, a 12 s train at 13 Hz and a 24 s train at 6.5 Hz: both oxytocin and vasopressin were measured by RIA. As before, the order of presentation of the stimulations was varied according to a latin square. For oxytocin, 3 s at 52 Hz produced a dramatically greater release than the lower frequencies of stimulation, whereas in agreement with Dutton and Dyball (2), 13 Hz was the most effective frequency for releasing vasopressin (Fig.1). If we compare the hormone release per pulse at 13 Hz with that at 52 Hz, oxytocin release is about 3 times greater at the higher frequency whereas vasopressin release is abot 50% less.

CONCLUSIONS

The electrical discharge patterns displayed by oxytocin and vasopressin neurones during physiological activation of hormone secretion are optimally efficient for release of the respective hormones. We remain a long way from understanding why particular patterns of stimulation are more effective than others for releasing hormone from the neurohypophysis - the more so because of the different behaviour of the oxytocin and vasopressin nerve terminals. These differences are not reflected in any ultrastructural or biochemical correlates that have as yet been documented. We have speculated that fatigue of vasopressin release during continued electrical stimulation is the result of inactivation of calcium entry into the terminals possibly as a direct result of raised intracellular calcium (7). According to this hypothesis calcium flux across the membrane rather than intracellular calcium would be the ultimate stimulus for secretion. This hypothesis remains to be tested.

REFERENCES

1. Wakerley JB, Poulain DA, Brown D (1974) Brain Res 148:425-440
2. Dutton A, Dyball REJ (1979) J Physiol 290:433-440
3. Shaw F, Bicknell RJ, Dyball REJ (1984) Neuroendocrinology, in press
4. Bicknell RJ, Leng G (1981) Neuroendocrinology 33:295-299
5. Ingram CD, Bicknell RJ, Brown D, Leng G (1982) Neuroendocrinology 35:424-428
6. Bicknell RJ, Brown D, Chapman C, Hancock PD, Leng G (1984) J Physiol 348:601-613
7. Nordmann JJ (1983) Progr Brain Res 60:281-304

© 1984 Elsevier Science Publishers B.V.
Endocrinology
F. Labrie, L. Proulx, eds.

CENTRAL ELECTROPHYSIOLOGIC CORRELATES OF PULSATILE LUTEINIZING HORMONE SECRETION

R.C. Wilson*, J.S. Kesner, J.M. Kaufman, T. Uemura, T. Akema and E. Knobil

Departments of Neurobiology and Anatomy* and Physiology and Cell Biology
University of Texas Medical School at Houston, P.O. Box 20708, Houston, Texas
U.S.A. 77225

INTRODUCTION

In the rhesus monkey, as in other mammals, luteinizing hormone (LH) is secreted from the pituitary gland in discrete pulses as a consequence of the periodic secretion of hypothalamic luteinizing hormone releasing hormone (LHRH) into the pituitary portal circulation (2,3,4). Pulsatile LHRH release is governed, in turn, by a neuronal "pulse generator" resident in the arcuate region of the medial basal hypothalamus (MBH) (6,7).

As an initial step toward the identification and study of the hypothalamic LHRH pulse generator, we have attempted to record spontaneous changes in hypothalamic electrical activity coincident with the initiation of LH pulses. Because LHRH release in quantities sufficient to elicit an LH pulse undoubtedly requires the synchronous discharge of multiple neurosecretory neurons, we have employed multiple unit recording techniques to facilitate the detection of changes in neuronal firing. Our preliminary attempts to monitor the activity of the LHRH pulse generator using single electrodes acutely placed into the MBH of ovariectomized rhesus monkeys occasionally yielded evidence of striking increases in multiple unit activity (MUA) synchronous with LH pulses in the peripheral circulation (5). As described in the present report, our subsequent studies, using multiple chronically implanted electrodes, have confirmed our original observations and have permitted the characterization of this phenomenon. A definitive account of these studies has been published elsewhere (9).

METHODS

Twenty-one adult female rhesus monkeys, fitted with indwelling cardiac catheters, were used. The animals were ovariectomized to increase the amplitude of LH pulses in the peripheral circulation. To maximize the probability of establishing and maintaining contact with hypothalamic areas exhibiting pulse generator activity, each animal was chronically implanted with bilateral electrode arrays consisting of nine 50µm nichrome wires. These were placed stereotaxically in the region of the arcuate nucleus of the MBH. MUA recordings were obtained in animals anesthetized by a continuous infusion of thiopental and in awake monkeys restrained in primate chairs.

Details of the construction of electrodes and of the implantation and recording procedures have been provided elsewhere (9).

RESULTS

In 16 of the 21 animals studied, characteristic increases in MUA associated with the initiation of LH pulses in the plasma were recorded. Ninety-seven such episodes were analyzed in 16 anesthetized monkeys and 233 in 5 awake animals. Typically, in awake animals restrained in primate chairs, these periodic MUA increases or volleys took the form of square waves with an initial "overshoot" on the ascending limb. This overshoot ranged in magnitude from 50-500% of baseline and declined precipitously within 1-2 min to enter a plateau phase of still marked increased activity lasting 5-15 min. Variations of this pattern were occasionally observed including the absence of a plateau phase with the initial overshoot returning directly to baseline and the appearance of additional spikes of activity during the plateau phase, most typically just prior to its termination. The onset of circhoral MUA volleys was invariably followed, within 2-5 min, by a rise in plasma LH concentration. Barbiturate anesthesia decreased the frequency of the MUA volleys to one every 2-3 h and prolonged the duration of the plateau phase to approximately 30 min.

In individual animals these characteristic MUA patterns were obtained from 1 to 9 of the 18 electrodes in the bilateral array and were reproduced in as many as 29 recording sessions over a period of 11 months, the longest interval studied to date. Comparable patterns of neuronal activity were not observed independently of synchronous LH pulses.

DISCUSSION

From the foregoing observations, we conclude that the dramatic increase in neural traffic associated with the initiation of each LH pulse reflects the activation of a hypothalamic pulse generator which controls LHRH secretion. The morphologic identity of the pulse generator remains to be determined. Clusters of LHRH - containing neurons are one possible source of this electrophysiologic activity and, in the rhesus monkey, are found scattered throughout the MBH (8). Although pulse generator activity must culminate in LHRH release, it is quite possible that the pacemaker function may originate in, and be recorded from, other MBH neuronal systems which then impinge on LHRH cells. Participation of an adrenergic component in the operation of the pulse generator, for example, is suggested by the inhibition of pulsatile LH release following pharmacologic blockade of α-adrenergic receptors (1).

Regardless of the source of the GnRH pulse generator activity observed in the present study, direct electrophysiologic access to the central component of the hypothalamo - hypophyseal - ovarian system opens new avenues for the study of the neural control of reproductive processes such as the advent of puberty, the normal menstrual cycle and a variety of physiological and pathological amenorrheic states. Ultimately, the processes underlying the synchronization of the neurosecretory elements of the pulse generator and the mechanisms which account for the timing of its rhythmic activation and deactivation must be characterized before the neuroendocrine control system which governs reproduction in the higher primates is finally understood.

REFERENCES

1. Bhattacharya, A.N.; Dierschke, D.J.; Yamaji, T.; Knobil, E.: The pharmacologic blockade of the circhoral mode of LH secretion in the ovariectomized rhesus monkey. Endocrinology 90:778-786 (1972).

2. Carmel, P.W.; Araki, S.; Ferin, M.: Pituitary stalk portal blood collection in rhesus monkeys: evidence for pulsatile release of gonadotropin releasing hormone (GnRH). Endocrinology 99:243-248 (1976).

3. Clarke, I.J.; Cummins, J.T.: The temporal relationship between gonadotropin releasing hormone (GnRH) and luteinizing hormone (LH) secretion in ovariectomized ewes. Endocrinology 111:1737-1739 (1982).

4. Dierschke, D.J.; Bhattacharya, A.N.; Atkinson, L.E.; Knobil, E.: Circhoral oscillations of plasma LH levels in the ovariectomized rhesus monkey. Endocrinology 87:850-853 (1970).

5. Knobil, E.: Patterns of hypophysiotropic signals and gonadotropin secretion in the rhesus monkey. Biol. Reprod. 24:44-49 (1981).

6. Krey, L.C.; Butler, W.R.; Knobil, E.: Surgical disconnection of the medial basal hypothalamus and pituitary function in the rhesus monkey. I. Gonadotropin secretion. Endocrinology 96:1073-1087 (1975).

7. Plant, T.M.; Krey, L.C.; Moossy, J.; McCormack, J.T.; Hess, D.L.; Knobil, E.: The arcuate nucleus and the control of gonadotropin and prolactin secretion in the female rhesus monkey (*Macaca mulatta*). Endocrinology 102:52-62 (1978).

8. Silverman, A.J.; Antunes, J.L.; Abrams, G.M.; Nilaver, G.; Thau, R.; Robinson, J.A.; Ferin, M.; Krey, L.C.: The luteinizing hormone-releasing hormone pathways in rhesus (*Macaca mulatta*) and pigtailed (*Macaca nemestrina*) monkeys: new observations on thick unembedded sections. Journal Comp. Neurol. 211:309-317 (1982).

9. Wilson, R.C.; Kesner, J.S.; Kaufman, J.M.; Uemura, T.; Akema, T.; Knobil, E.: Central electrophysiologic correlates of pulsatile luteinizing hormone secretion in the rhesus monkey. Neuroendocrinology 39:in press.

Endocrinology
F. Labrie, L. Proulx, eds.

INTRACELLULAR RECORDINGS FROM NORMAL PITUITARY CELLS: REGULATION OF ELECTRICAL EVENTS LEADING TO HORMONE RELEASE BY HYPOPHYSIOTROPHIC PEPTIDES

W.T. MASON, C.D. INGRAM, R.J. BICKNELL AND D.W. WARING
A.F.R.C. Institute of Animal Physiology, Babraham, Cambridge CB2 4AT, U.K.

INTRODUCTION

Our studies are directed towards isolation of specific populations of normal pituitary cells and investigation of the relationship between their secretory and electrical properties using intracellular and patch clamp recordings of single ion channels. This report considers some of our findings with normal gonadotrophs, somatotrophs and lactotrophs, and discusses the possibility that hormone secretion by these pituitary cell types may not be dependent on action potentials *per se*, but rather occurs due to conductance fluctuations of membrane ion channels induced by hypothalamic releasing hormones.

MATERIALS AND METHODS

Preparation of cell cultures

Gonadotrophs were obtained by trypsin dispersion of ovine adenohypophyseal pars tuberalis, where they are the sole hormone-containing type (1,2). Somatotrophs and lactotrophs were prepared by collagenase dispersion of bovine pars distalis, and isolation on Percoll density gradients. Of the various fractions obtained, a dense (60% Percoll) fraction was highly enriched for somatotrophs and a lighter fraction (50/60% interface) contained mainly lactotrophs. Levels of purification were assessed by immunocytochemistry for growth hormone and prolactin and by radioimmunoassay of the fractions for pituitary hormones.

Electrophysiology

Intracellular recordings were made at 35-37° C using pipettes filled with either 4M KAcetate/0.1 M KCl, or 150 mM KCl. Both produced electrodes of 80-150 MΩ. Cells were continuously perifused with recording medium containing (mM) 125 NaCl, 15 $NaHCO_3$, 5 KCl, 1.3 $MgCl_2$, 5 $CaCl_2$, 5 glucose and 5 HEPES, pH 7.4 equilibrated with 5% CO_2/95% O_2. Noise analysis was performed on a PDP 11/23 computer. Data were filtered at 200 Hz and digitized at 500 Hz. Power spectra were constructed using a fast Fourier transform algorithm from blocks of 4096 points of data averaged over 10 to 50 blocks.

Single channel recordings were made at room temperature (18-23° C) using previously described techniques (3) which employed 7-20 MΩ electrodes filled with recording medium. These studies were performed in a static bath and peptides were added as a bolus to give the desired final concentration.

RESULTS

Gonadotrophs

Ovine gonadotrophs studied with intracellular recording had a resting potential (V_m) of -74.5 ± 3.2 mV (mean±s.e.m., n=56). Upon injection of depolarizing current, 95% of these cells generated a Ca^{2+}-dependent spike of about 30 mV. Under conditions in which they released luteinizing hormone (LH), both basal and gonadotrophin releasing hormone (GnRH)-induced (50-200 nM), we never observed spontaneous spike discharge in over 100 gonadotrophs examined. However, GnRH added in this concentration range did induce large increases in the extent of membrane voltage fluctuations (Figure 1A).

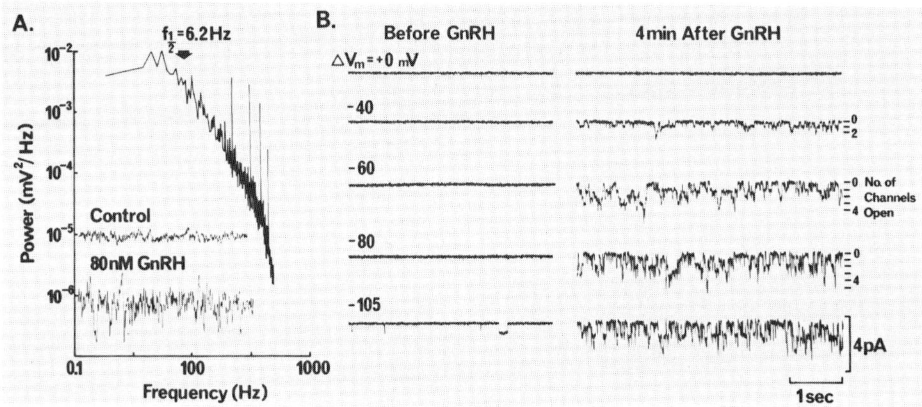

Fig. 1. (A) Power spectra of intracellularly-recorded GnRH-induced voltage noise, yielding $f_{\frac{1}{2}}$ of 6.2 Hz, or a mean event lifetime of 26 ms. (B) Patch clamp recordings of a gonadotroph, with the patch voltage clamped to the indicated levels. Note that in the presence of GnRH, hyperpolarization of the patch leads to an increased probability of channel opening.

The variance ratio associated with GnRH-induced voltage fluctuations compared to that measured prior to GnRH exposure was 3.1 ± 0.5 ($p<0.01$, n=26). Segments of voltage noise were also used to evaluate difference power spectra (GnRH minus control). These revealed a half power frequency ($f_{\frac{1}{2}}$) of 5.6 ± 0.5 Hz, or an event duration for GnRH-induced fluctuations of about 30 msec. GnRH-induced noise increase was abolished by Ca^{2+} channel blockers including Mn^{2+}, Co^{2+} and nifedipine. Injection of Lucifer Yellow CH followed by immunocytochemistry for LH confirmed the identity of recorded cells as gonadotrophs.

These results indicate that GnRH acts to open Ca^{2+} dependent ion channels which are manifest as discrete conductance fluctuations leading to increased voltage noise. This suggests that ovine gonadotrophs may release LH in response to GnRH in a fashion independent of action potentials.

Single channel analysis of GnRH action has revealed that GnRH acts to increase the opening of an inward current channel with a unit conductance of 5-7 pS. This channel is mediated not by direct GnRH-channel interaction, but rather via a secondary internal messenger system. GnRH in the patch pipette did not affect channel activity, whereas GnRH applied to the bath caused multiple channel openings (Figure 1B). This channel is not a 'pure' Ca^{2+} channel, but rather a non-selective cation channel with Ca^{2+} estimated to carry approximately 60% of total current under recording conditions.

Somatotrophs

Bovine somatotrophs had a V_m in the range of -60 to -80 mV, and, like gonadotrophs, they responded with only a single spike to current injection. When human pancreatic growth hormone releasing factor (GRF 1-44) was applied to somatotrophs at 20-100 nM, the variance of voltage noise increased by a factor of 2.3 ± 0.8 ($p < 0.01$, n=6). This noise increase arose from slow, depolarizing fluctations in potential which were Ca^{2+} dependent and blocked by Co^{2+} (4 mM). Power spectra were fit by a single Lorentzian with a half-power frequency of 4.2 Hz, indicating a mean conductance duration of around 40ms.

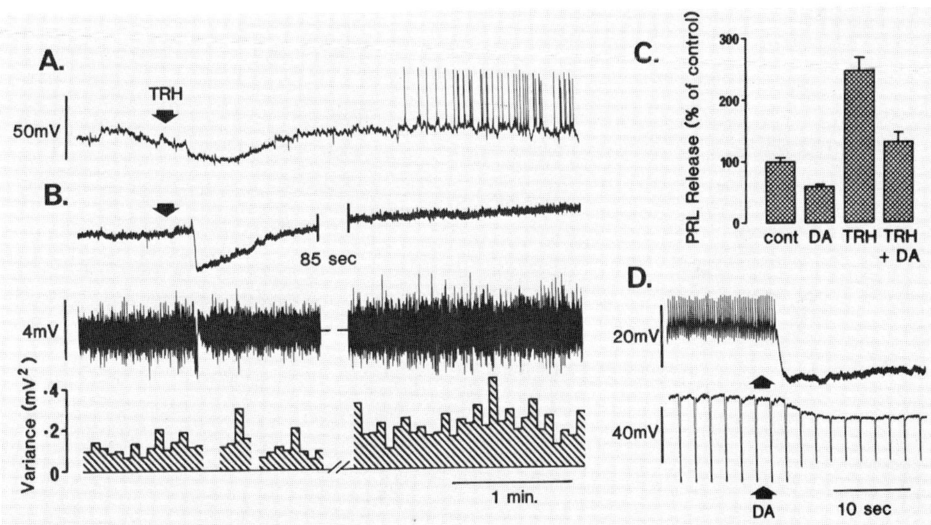

Fig. 2. Record of V_m from a putative lactotroph. TRH induces a transient hyperpolarization followed by depolarization and spiking activity. (B) Upper trace shows d.c. intracellular record of biphasic V_m response to TRH, and lower traces are high gain a.c. coupled record of V_m noise increase caused by TRH and computed variance of these data. Mean of noise variance (control) was 0.248 mV^2 and that of the TRH-induced noise was 0.448 mV^2. (C) Effect of 10 uM DA and 1 uM TRH on prolactin release from cell cultures under recording conditions. (D) Inhibition of spontaneous action potentials by application of DA. Record below shows conductance decrease during DA application and spike abolition, measured with constant current pulses.

Lactotrophs

Bovine lactotrophs had a V_m similar to gonadotrophs and somatotrophs, but their electrical properties were notably different. Lactotrophs also generated voltage fluctuations in response to thyrotrophin releasing hormone (TRH) (Figure 2B), some of which led to spikes. The differences included: (1) Repetitive action potentials in response to current injection, (2) 50% of the cells generated spikes both spontaneously and in response to TRH. This response was preceded by a biphasic change in V_m (Figure 2A), (3) dopamine (DA) was a potent inhibitor of spiking activity, inducing a hyperpolarization and conductance increase (Figure 2D). TRH-induced noise increases and spiking were also accompanied by release of prolactin, and hormone release was inhibited by DA (Figure 2D).

DISCUSSION

Our results with normal pituitary cells suggest that action potentials may not necessarily be a prerequisite for stimulation of hormone release by hypophysiotrophic hormones. Rather, they suggest that releasing hormones act to open ion channels which are permeable to Ca^{2+}, and that this Ca^{2+} entry may be sufficient to activate hormone release. Data from gonadotrophs suggest these channels are not regulated via direct hormone-channel interaction.

Lactotrophs generate action potentials in response to TRH, but they also exhibit large numbers of potential fluctuations, indicative of increased ion channel activity. These small potential fluctuations appear responsible for spike initiation.

In conclusion, the common mechanism which underlies the action of hypothalamic releasing hormones on anterior pituitary cells we have examined is their ability to induce the opening of Ca^{2+} permeable ion channels which is reflected in increased membrane voltage fluctuations and single channel activity. In lactotrophs, these may lead to spiking activity, although what proportion of Ca^{2+} entry required for hormone release flows as a result of spikes as compared to the opening of ion channels without spiking remains a topic for further research.

Acknowledgments. This work was generously supported by grants from the Nuffield Foundation (UK), Burroughs Wellcome Foundation (USA) and by a grant from the Meat and Livestock Commission to C.D. Ingram. We have pleasure in acknowledging the help of Dr. T.D. Lamb in noise analysis procedures.

REFERENCES

1. Gross DS, Turgeon JL and Waring DW (1984) Endocrinology 114:2084-2091.
2. Mason WT, Waring DW (1984) J. Physiol. 350:73P.
3. Hamill OP, Marty A, Neher E, Sakmann B, Sigworth FJ (1981) Pflugers Arch. 391:85-100.

MEET-THE-PROFESSOR

© 1984 Elsevier Science Publishers B.V.
Endocrinology
F. Labrie, L. Proulx, eds.

INFERTILITY IN THE FEMALE

B. LUNENFELD, D. VARDIMON, B. GOLDSTEIN

World Health Organization Collaborating Center for Research on Fertility Promoting Agents, Institute of Endocrinology, Chaim Sheba Medical Center, Tel-Hashomer 52621 (Israel) and University of Bar-Ilan, Department of Life Sciences, Ramat-Gan (Israel)

INTRODUCTION

Infertility should be viewed as a description or symptom rather than a diagnosis. It describes a class of symptoms characterized by a couple's inability to achieve parenthood. Primary or secondary infertility may vary in its expression- - affecting the male, female or both partners: its cause may be uni or multifactorial and its etiology may be due to genetic, hormonal, iatrogenic or developmental factors; may be of psychosomatic origin or due to sequella of post inflammatory, infectious or viral disease.

In recent years a variety of causative mechanisms have been more clearly defined and may be important in prevention and therapy. Infertility is thus most usefully regarded as a synonym of decreased ability or inability of procreation and is not the title of a single disease entity. The extent of childless marriage, whether voluntary or involuntary, varies considerably both from society and over periods of time. The magnitude and geographic distribution of infertility remains largely unknown. Analysis of existing data, based on indirect indices of infertility suggests that a core level of around 5% of couples suffer from infertility, although there is some indication that this figure may be as low as 1% and as high as 40% in different communities.

A base rate or "core" of infertility represents the biological variation of human populations with respect to chromosomal, congenital and endocrinological abnormalities affecting both men and women. To these base rates must also be added the occurrence of certain acquired disorders present to a greater or lesser degree in most communities, probably related to the socioeconomic status of the geographical area and the population investigated. Such disorders would include fallopian tube occlusion, peritubal adhesions or uterine synechia following pelvic inflammatory disease, abortion or postpartum sepsis. It is, perhaps, when certain of these acquired conditions reach epidemic proportions, or when there appears to be an unusual clustering of cases among certain population groups or occupations, that infertility becomes a major health problem.

The infertile couple should be diagnosed and treated as a single unit, since each partner contributes a share to the fertility potential of the other. The decrease of the fertility potential of any one of the two partners will adversely affect the fertility of the couple. Although there are few reasons to completely halt the investigation of the status of one partner while completing that of the other, the entire workup must proceed with an eye to the findings of both.

The possibilities for classifying and treating the infertile couple are virtually unlimited; thus the striking lack of uniformity in the process by which these couples are evaluated and treated. Because of the historical variability of the infertility workup, comparison of data from different investigations and treatment schemes have seldom been appropriate, and our ability to properly assess the relative merits of each has been poor. Coordinated multicentered research using standardized procedures helps to clarify many issues, as well as to improve diagnostic precision and the results of subsequent management in terms of effectiveness, cost and risk.

HISTORY AND PHYSICAL EXAMINATION

The infertile couple should be investigated and treated as a unit. Evaluation should begin with a detailed history and a complete physical examination of both partners. On the first visit, marital and sexual history should be carefully recorded. Family history and physical examination should be oriented towards the identification of systemic diseases (tuberculosis, etc.), endocrinopathies (Cushing's syndrome, etc.), and genetic abnormalities (Turner's syndrome, etc.).

The female's physical examination should include a careful evaluation of the breast, particularly for detecting the presence of galactorrhoea, which must be differentiated from other breast secretions since it is indicative of possible breast tumors. The vaginal examination should be directed towards detecting congenital abnormalities (vaginal septum, absence of the uterus), tumor or infection. Special attention should be given to the possibility of previous pelvic inflammatory disease, or lower abdominal surgery, which may be suggestive of a possible mechanical cause for the infertility. When such evidence exists, mechanical factors must be investigated prior to treatment. Hysterosalpingography is the method of choice for determining the presence of lesions within the uterine cavity as well as tubal obstruction or other abnormalities. The detection of extrauterine, peritubal or periovarian lesions (adhesions, endometriosis, etc.), is performed by laparoscopy. However, due to the inherent deficiency of each of these methods, and since they complement each other, in many instances it will be necessary to use both.

LABORATORY INVESTIGATIONS

After the clinical evaluation described above, further evaluation of endocrine causes of infertility essentially depends upon three factors: blood prolactin, presence or absence of endogenous sex steroids and gonadotrophins. Prolactin estimations are advisable since it can disturb infertility in the female when secreted in excess. Excessive secretion of prolactin may be idiopthic; it may result from functional hypothalamic disorders or it may follow the use of different drugs including contraceptives. Prolactin producing pituitary tumors enlarging the sella turcica, or more frequently, a microadenoma, can also be the result of this disorder. Therefore, patients with elevated prolactin levels must have a thorough radiological skull examination with frontal and lateral tomograms of the sella turcica and a visual field examination to rule out a space-occupying lesion in the hypothalamic pituitary region.

In cases where thyroid-releasing hormone (TRH) is excreted in excess, as in primary hypothyroidism, prolactin will be elevated and some of the effects will be similar to those where the hypothalamic pituitary dysfunction was prolactin induced. Treatment of the underlying cause by supplementation with thyroid hormones or their analogues will, in most cases, correct the metabolic disturbance and suppress the excessive TRH and the consequent hyperprolactinemia. (Table I). Infertility due to idiopathic hyperprolactinemia and adenoma without suprasellar extension may be treated successfully with prolactin inhibitors. (Table I).

In amenorrheic women, FSH determinations should be performed. Elevated levels are indicative of gonadal failures.

Low or undetectable levels are due to hypothalamic or pituitary insufficiency. Patients pertaining to this category are amenorrheic, with little or no evidence of endogenous estrogen activity. They will not bleed following the administration of gestogen. This group can be successfully treated with gonadotropins, while some of them can also be treated by pulsatile administration of releasing hormones. (Table I).

Women who have anovulatory cycles as determined by basal body temperature but spontaneous uterine bleeding, along with amenorrheic patients with endogenous estrogen activity, who respond to the administration of gestagens by withdrawal bleeding, are classified as having hypothalamic-pituitary dysfunction. For these women, the treatment of choice is drugs which compete with estrogen receptors, such as clomiphene citrate and tamoxifen. (Table I).

In a situation where adrenal or ovarian steroids, especially androgens, are secreted in excess, interference in the complex feedback mechanism regulating the ovarian cycle may result. The severity of the cycle disturbances will be relative to the quality and amount of the steroids secreted and the responsiveness of the target cells. Patients pertaining to this etiological entity will be women with a variety of menstrual cycle disturbances and usually with some clinical signs of androgenization, virilization and a tendency toward obesity. It is essential that these cases be investigated to determine the source of androgens and the nature of the secreting tissue (autonomous source, enzyme deficiency, benign hypertrophy).

We have tried to demonstrate that infertility has manifold origins, each with its own characteristic pattern. Recognition of well defined underlying causes will permit the choice of optimal and cost effective management of the patient.

TABLE I

ETIOLOGICAL DIAGNOSIS AND SUGGESTIONS FOR TREATMENT OF CHOICE OR ALTERNATIVE TREATMENT

Etiological diagnosis	Treatment of choice	Alternative treatment
Hypothalamic or pituitary insufficiency	Menotropines (HMG) followed by HCG	Pulsatile administration of LHRH
Hypothalamic or pituitary dysfunction	Clomiphene citrate (CC) (Serophen, Clomid, Ikaclomin) Tamoxifen (Valodex)	CC + HCG CC + Estrogen HMG/HCG
Excessive secretion of prolactin	Ergoline derivatives (ED) (Bromocryptine, Lysuride, Metergoline)	ED + CC ED + HMG/HCG HMG/HCG
Primary hypothyroidism	Thyroid hormones or their analogues (TH)	TH + CC TH + HMG/HCG
Inappropriate secretion of ovarian androgens	Cyproterone acetate and estrogen for 6 months followed by CC or HMG/HCG or pure FSH	Wedge resection LH RH antagonist followed by HMG/HCG
Inappropriate secretion of adrenal androgens	Corticosteroids (COR)	COR + CC COR + HMG/HCG

ACKNOWLEDGEMENTS

This study was supported in part by the World Health Organization (WHO) special program of research, development and research training in human reproduction.

Endocrinology
F. Labrie, L. Proulx, eds.

DISORDERS OF WATER METABOLISM

ALAN G. ROBINSON
Division of Endocrinology and Metabolism, School of Medicine, University of Pittsburgh, Pittsburgh, PA 15261, USA.

Synthesis and Release

The hormones of the neurohypophysis, oxytocin and vasopressin, are synthesized in specialized magnocellular neurons which are grouped into the supraoptic nuclei and the paraventricular nuclei of the hypothalamus. The projections of the magnocellular neurons which are important for water balance are via the supraopticohypophyseal tract to the posterior pituitary. Other neurons project to the median eminence, third ventricle, spinal cord, brainstem, and forebrain. Projections to the median eminence may be involved in the release of ACTH. The function of projections elsewhere has not been elucidated, but may be involved in a variety of CNS functions. Acetylcholine is a major neurotransmitter in the release of vasopressin. Separate angiotensin II receptors have also been described. Neurotransmitters involved in release of vasopressin all have their input at the level of the hypothalamus and therefore diseases of the neurohypophysis are diseases of hypothalamic dysfunction rather than diseases localized in the sella at the level of the posterior pituitary.

It is now confirmed that vasopressin is synthesized as part of a large precursor molecule (containing vasopressin, vasopressin-neurophysin, and a glycopeptide) which is packaged into neurosecretory granules. During transport to the posterior pituitary the precursor is converted to the three products. The granules are stored in axon terminals until a stimulus is perceived at the perikaryon. As the entire contents of the granule are released by exocytosis, there is concurrent release of vasopressin, vasopressin-neurophysin, and the glycopeptide.

Physiologic Control - Osmoreceptors and Volume Receptors

The two regulatory systems which are primarily involved in the physiologic control of vasopressin are osmoreceptors and volume receptors. The osmoreceptors are exquisitely sensitive to changes in osmolality and a 1% increase in osmolality of the extracellular fluid will cause a measureable increase in vasopressin. At 280 mOsm/kg vasopressin begins to be released and increases arithmetically with further increases in osmolality. There is also an exquisite sensitivity of the kidney to respond to vasopressin with water retention. Vasopressin concentrations in plasma between 1-5 pg/ml produce urine osmolalities throughout the entire physiologic range from less than 100 mOsm/kg to a maximum urinary concentration of 1000 mOsm/kg. While levels of vasopressin may increase further, this will not be translated into increased urine osmolality because of the maximum on the ability of the kidney to concentrate urine. Thirst is similarly controlled by osmoreceptors. In humans the threshold for thirst is reported to be higher than that for vasopressin and not stimulated until plasma osmolality is as high as 295, an osmolality which should produce sufficient vasopressin to cause maximum concentration of the urine. Therefore, most humans probably drink sufficient water by habit and by social custom that the urine osmolality goes through wide swings of dilution and concentration without the person ever experienceing marked thirst.

Volume receptors are predominantly high pressure baroreceptors in the carotid sinus and aortic arch, but there may also be some input from low pressure volume receptors in the left atrium or venous system. Afferents from the volume receptors ascend through the brainstem and have an adrenergic input on the magnocellular neurons - predominantly inhibitory, i.e. decreased input results in increased release of vasopressin. Volume receptors require as much as a 10% decrease before release of vasopressin is stimulated. However, once the threshold for release of vasopressin is reached there is then an exponential increase in vasopressin with further decreases in volume. Thus, the final concentration of vasopressin achieved with marked volume receptor stimulation is much greater than the maximum obtained with osmolar stimulation.

Multiple pathophysiologic mechanisms may affect the neurohypophysis including trauma, tumors, infiltrative lesions, vascular lesions, pulmonary diseases, infectious diseases, and a variety of drugs.

<u>Hypofunction of the Posterior Pituitary</u>

Diabetes insipidus is a disease of hypofunction of the neurohypophysis. In classic diabetes insipidus lack of vasopressin produces a dilute urine, polyuria, and secondary polydipsia. Nephrogenic diabetes insipidus has similar symptomatology, but is produced by insensitivity of the kidneys to vasopressin. Primary polydipsia enters the differential diagnosis, but is produced by a primary stimulus to the thirst center, increased water intake, inhibition of secretion of vasopressin, and secondary polyuria. These three causes of polyuria are differentiated either by indirect or by direct tests.

All of the indirect tests are based upon some correlation of plasma osmolality with urine osmolality, thus using the patients own renal concentrating mechanism as an internal bioassay for vasopressin. Plasma osmolality is increased either by hypertonic NaCl or by a dehydration test. With the standard dehydration test complete hypothalamic diabetes insipidus shows little concentration of urine and responds markedly to vasopressin;

patients with partial diabetes insipidus show some concentration of their urine, and respond further to administered vasopressin; patients with nephrogenic diabetes insipidus show some concentration of their urine, but respond to pharmacologic levels of vasopressin; patients with primary polydipsia show some concentration of their urine, but do not respond to vasopressin. This differential is most often confusing in nephrogenic diabetes insipidus and partial central diabetes insipidus. Robertson found that partial diabetes insipidus and primary polydipsia may also be indistinguishable because both may have limited ability to concentrate urine due to washout of the renal medulla and both may have sufficient ability to secrete vasopressin to maximally concentrate their urine with a dehydration test. However, in children Czernichow utilized a standard 14 hour dehydration test and found no overlap between partial diabetes insipidus and primary polydipsia.

Direct tests utilize some method of increasing plasma osmolality but rely upon measured levels of vasopressin in addition to the urine parameters. Nephrogenic diabetes insipidus can always be distinguished from central diabetes insipidus because the levels of vasopressin are easily measureable and elevated. For partial diabetes insipidus and primary polydipsia the levels of vasopressin may be low in both cases and they may still be difficult to distinguish unless there is an extremely sensitive assay of vasopressin which can be referred to a carefully constructed nomogram of POsm versus vasopressin.

Special cases of diabetes insipidus which require extra care are postoperative diabetes insipidus which may evolve to a "triphasic response" of diabetes insipidus -SIADH - diabetes insipidus. This results from necrosis of a disconnected posterior pituitary. Diabetes insipidus with inadequate thirst which requires a fixed amount of fluid replacement. Absent osmoreceptor with intact volume receptor, a form of diabetes insipidus which has previously been called "essential hypernatremia".

Replacement of water is a treatment of diabetes insipidus and in sufficient amount will correct any metabolic abnormality. The most physiologic hormone replacement is DDAVP which can be given intranasally or as a subcutaneous injection. Certain pharmacologic agents enhance the effect of vasopressin. Chlorpropramide in doses of 100-500 mg/d may a useful therapy in patients with partial diabetes insipidus.

Hyperfunction of the Posterior Pituitary

Hyperfunction of the posterior pituitary is known as the syndrome of inappropriate secretion of antidiuretic hormone. Many central nervous system disorders will produce this abnormality, probably increasing release of vasopressin by decreasing the tonic inhibition which impinges upon the neurohypophysis from the medulla and brainstem. Water is retained to dilute the body electrolytes. Expansion of the extracellular fluid stimulates natriuresis. Water retention with dilution and the progressive natriuresis produce hyponatremia. Excess secretion of vasopressin may also be caused by ectopically produced vasopressin, most commonly by broncogenic carcinoma of the lung, but also pancreatic carcinoma, thymoma, hepatoma, and several other disorders. In the past the diagnosis of SIADH was based upon indirect tests and a concentrated urine which was inappropriate for the degree of hyponatremia. Measurement of vasopressin in plasma has provided a more direct diagnosis of SIADH. Robertson has reported that the patients may have either erratic secretion of vasopressin, low fixed secretion of vasopressin, or reset osmostat. Determining the type of vasopressin secretion may have therapeutic implications. A fixed baseline of vasopressin secretion may only be noted when extra fluid is taken and modest fluid restriction may suffice to treat the disorder. Reset osmostat may allow excretion of an administered water load at an abnormally low sodium. These patients are not at great danger to develop severe hyponatremia and can be treated conservatively. In patients with erratic secretion or extremely high levels of vasopressin only severe fluid restriction may suffice to normalize sodium and pharmacologic agents which inhibit the renal response to vasopressin as demeclocycline or agents which increase sodium absorption as orally administered urea may be useful.

Supported by NIH AM16166, RR00056, and NS17138 grants.

BIBLIOGRAPHY

1. Cross, B.A. and Leng, G. (1983). The Neurohypophysis: Structure, Function, and Control, Progress in Brain Research Vol. 60. Elsevier, Amsterdam.

2. Czernichow, P. and Robinson, A.G. (1984) (eds.) Diabetes Insipidus. S. Karger AG, Basel, Switzerland.

3. Czernichow, P. and Robinson, A.G. (1980) Neurohypophysis. In: Collu, R., Ducharme, J.R., Guyda, H. (eds) Comprehensive Endocrinology Series - Pediatric Endocrinology. Raven Press, NY pp 571-596.

4. Robertson, G.L. (1981) Diseases of the Posterior Pituitary. In: Felig, P., Baxter, J.D., Broadus, A.E., Frohman, L.A. (eds.) Endocrinology and Metabolism. McGraw-Hill, NY pp 251-277.

5. Robertson, G.L., Aycinena, P., and Zerbe, R.L., (1982). Neurogenic Disorders of Osmoregulation. Am. J. Med. 72:pp 339-353.

6. Robinson, A.G. and Verbalis, J.G. (1984). Clinical Disorders of the Neurohypophysis. In: Smith, C.W. (ed.) The Peptides, Chemistry and Biology of Neurohypophyseal Hormones. Academic Press, NY.

© 1984 Elsevier Science Publishers B.V.
Endocrinology
F. Labrie, L. Proulx, eds.

THE NORLANT[R] SUBDERMAL IMPLANT SYSTEM: A LONG-ACTING, LOW-DOSE, PROGESTIN-ONLY CONTRACEPTIVE METHOD FOR WOMEN

C. WAYNE BARDIN

The Population Council, Center for Biomedical Research, 1230 York Avenue, New York, New York 10021

Following the demonstration that capsules of polydimethylsiloxane could serve as a delivery system for lipophilic drugs (1,2), Segal and Croxatto suggested that steroid-filled polydimethylsiloxane capsules might serve as a long-acting, reversible method of steroid contraception (3). There followed a series of animal and clinical studies in which a variety of progestins were tested in the laboratories of the Population Council and in the clinics of the Council's International Committee for Contraception Research (ICCR) (4).

By 1975, sufficient information had accumulated to permit the ICCR to initiate a random double-blind trial to compare the three progestin-containing implants which had appeared promising in Phase 1 and Phase 2 clinical trials. In the early stages of the study, one progestin was withdrawn for toxicological reasons, and by one year polydimethylsiloxane capsules containing levonorgestrel appeared superior to the remaining candidate. From these initial studies, the Norplant[R]* Subdermal Implant System was developed. This is a long-acting, low-dose, progestin-only contraceptive method for women. Levonorgestrel is delivered at 30 µg/day from six polydimethylsiloxane capsules which are implanted beneath the skin. Once in place, effective drug levels rise within 24 hours and are maintained for over five years. The relatively constant blood levels over this extended period of time suggest that the release rate approaches zero order kinetics. The Phase 3 clinical trials conducted since 1975 with this contraceptive system indicate that its effectiveness approaches that of sterilization, but reversibility is much easier. In view of the recent approval of the Norplant[R] implant system for sale in Finland, the country of manufacture, it is pertinent to review the performance of this newest form of hormonal contraception.

CONTRACEPTIVE EFFECTIVENESS

Nine hundred ninety two women were enrolled in Phase 3 clinical trials by the Population Council. They included women enrolled in two open studies conducted

---

*Norplant[R] is the Population Council's registered trademark for contraceptive subdermal implants.

in Chile and in two multi-centered studies in 1975-76 and 1978-79 (5). By January, 1983, 129 of these individuals had completed five years use of a single set of implants, and a few individuals completed eight years. The cumulative experience at five years was 2,381 women years of use. The cumulative number of pregnancies at five years was 11. In these women, the annual gross pregnancy rate (per 100 users) ranged from 0.2 - 1.3 per 100 women years. The cumulative gross pregnancy rate at five years was only 2.7 per 100 users. In other words, the pregnancy rate for implant users after five years of use had risen to that observed for pill use for one year under optimal conditions. It is of note that four pregnancies occurred among women who have used the implant between 4.5 and 6.5 years. In this period of time, the Pearl pregnancy index was 2.0 per 100 women years as opposed to 1.3 before 5 years. The rise in the gross pregnancy rate after three years and the rise in the Pearl index between 4.5 and 6.5 years suggest there is a slight decrease in effectiveness of the implants during the latter two years. The effectiveness, however, still remains far superior to the pill and most IUDs.

MECHANISM OF ACTION

In view of the low dose of levonorgestrel delivered by the Norplant^R implants and the high contraceptive effectiveness it was of interest to determine the mechanism of action of this contraceptive system. Blood samples were obtained from women with subdermal implants two or three times per week, and serum progesterone levels were measured in order to detect cycles in which there was presumptive evidence for ovulation. Depending on the year, up to half of the cycles were judged to be "possibly ovulatory." Subsequent studies demonstrated that cervical mucus was extremely thick; post-coital tests indicated that viable spermatozoa could not penetrate this mucus. These observations suggested that the Norplant^R implants have at least two mechanisms of action: they inhibit ovulation and, in addition, have a direct action on the uterus.

Since other progestin-only methods which do not block ovulation (i.e., the progestin-only mini pill and a progesterone-containing IUD) have been associated with a high incidence of ectopic pregnancy, it was important to determine the incidence of this complication in implant users. After more than 2,500 women years of use accumulated in ICCR trials through January, 1983, only two ectopic pregnancies were observed. The ectopic pregnancy rate was, therefore, 0.8 per 1,000 women years which was less than the incidence of ectopic pregnancy among all women in the United States between the ages of 15 and 45 (6,5). This pregnancy rate was not higher than that associated with non-medicated or copper-bearing IUD use in the United States or the United Kingdom (7-9).

CONTINUATION RATES

In the cohort of women enrolled in the ICCR studies in 1978-79, almost half of the initial acceptors were still using the implants four years after they were inserted. The annual continuation rates were 81 per 100 women during each of the first two years, rising to 85 and 87 per 100 women in years three and four, respectively. The increased annual continuation rates after two years reflect the early termination of individuals because of bleeding abnormalities or the desire to have another child. The high discontinuation rates were most noticeable among women under age 25 and in those who had used implants as a birth spacing method. Even though the number of women who stopped using the method was high in these groups, they nonetheless had high continuation rates compared with women using oral contraceptives. More recent studies performed outside ICCR clinics in Egypt, Thailand, Indonesia, and Ecuador report first year continuation rates equal to or much better than those in the ICCR clinics (10-13).

MENSTRUAL PROBLEMS

Since hormone administration is continuous in this and all other forms of progestin-only contraception, women note some disruption of normal menstrual function. The major abnormality in the first year was an increase in the number of bleeding and spotting days. However, the total blood loss during the first year was not increased and blood loss in the second year and years thereafter tended to decrease. Nonetheless, a certain percentage of implant users terminate this form of contraception because of menstrual problems. Experience with the Norplant^R system, however, has demonstrated that the number of women who elect to discontinue because of menstrual abnormalities has tended to decline in each successive group that has been enrolled in an implant study. This is probably because each group has been better informed about the method and understands that irregular bleeding is to be expected in some individuals. This increased experience probably accounts for the decrease in the termination rates attributed to menstrual problems in the 1978-79 cohort when compared to the 1975-76 group (5).

It is of note that differences in rates of termination for menstrual problems were striking between the various clinics in which the studies were conducted. In Chile, the cumulative gross termination rate from menstrual irregularities was just above three per 100 users at three years in the 1978-79 cohort. At a Finnish clinic, the three year cumulative termination rate for menstrual problems was 18, while in the Dominican Republic it was 25. This observation suggests that local clinic factors operate to influence the discontinuation rate of Norplant^R implants as with other contraceptives.

OTHER MEDICAL REASONS FOR REMOVAL

After discontinuation because of menstrual problems and infection at the site of insertion were excluded, removals arising from complaints about physical and mental well being accounted for a small number of discontinuations. Pathological conditions discovered upon examination by staff which led to removals also fell into this category. By the end of the fourth year, 13 women per 100 had implants removed for these medical reasons. Rates for removal were higher in the Dominican Republic than in other countries, as was the case for discontinuation because of bleeding (5).

CLINICAL PHARMACOLOGY

Implant users were compared to IUD users with regard to lipid and lipoprotein measurements, clinical chemistries, and selected hormone assays. In the implant group, mean serum glucose was significantly elevated (84.1 ± 1.5 vs 89.1 ± 1.4) and inorganic phosphorous significantly reduced (3.4 ± 0.1 vs 3.0 ± 0.1). In both instances, all individual measurements were within the range of values observed in normal women. Testosterone and triiodothyronine levels in the implant group were lower than in IUD users, but no individual values were outside the normal range. Mean values for all other parameters were not different between the groups (6).

RETURN TO FECUNDABILITY AFTER DISCONTINUATION

In the 1978-79 cohort, 45 of the acceptors (12%) discontinued use of Norplant^R implants by January, 1983 in order to have another child. Life-table analysis of pregnancy rates after implant removal indicated that the rates were 75 and 90 per 100 women at 12 and 24 months, respectively. This one year rate was not significantly different from that after removal of IUDs (5).

CONCLUSIONS

Results summarized in this report indicate that the Norplant^R implants combine a high degree of use-effectiveness in preventing pregnancy with excellent continuation rates. No unexpected serious side effects have been observed in women who have used this method to date. As with other progestin-only methods, the active agent is administered continuously; this results in menstrual irregularities which are the major reason for discontinuation. Increased experience with the method suggests that menstrual problems are usually tolerated in view of its other desirable features. The method's great effectiveness indicates that it is ideal for women who have had all the children they desire but do not want an irreversible type of contraception. The method is also useful for women who want contraception for child spacing since the return to fertility after implant removal is similar to that after discontinuation of other non-hormonal methods.

REFERENCES

1. Folkman, J and Long, DM (1964) J Surg Res 4:139-142

2. Dziuk, PJ and Cook, B (1966) Endocrinology 78:208-211

3. Segal, SJ and Croxatto, HB (1967) In: XXIII Meeting of the American Fertility Society, Washington, D.C..

4. Segal, SJ (1983) Stud Fam Plan 14:159-163

5. Sivin, I, Diaz, S, Alvarez-Sanchez, F, and Robertson, D (1983) Stud Fam Plan 14:184-191

6. Sivin, I, Croxatto, HB, Diaz, S, Robertson, DN, and Pavey, M (1983) Contraception 27:281-288

7. Tietze, C and Lewit, S (1970) Stud Fam Plan 1:1-40

8. Sivin, I (1979) Contraception 2:151-173

9. Vessey, MP, Yeates, D, and Flavel, R (1979) Lancet 8 September:501-503

10. Shaaban, M, Salah, M, Zarzour, A, and Abdullah, A (1983) Stud Fam Plan 14:163-169

11. Satayapan, S, Kanchanasinith, K, and Varakamin, S (1983) Stud Fam Plan 14:170-176

12. Marangoni, P, Cartagena, S, Alvarado, J, Diaz, J, and Faundes, A (1983) Stud Fam Plan 14:177-180

13. Lubis, F, Prihartono, J, Agoestina, T, Affandi, B, and Sutedi, H (1983) Stud Fam Plan 14:181-184

Endocrinology
F. Labrie, L. Proulx, eds.

ANOREXIA NERVOSA: A COMPULSIVE BEHAVIOUR DISEASE

IVOR H. MILLS

Department of Medicine, University of Cambridge, Addenbrooke's Hospital, Cambridge, CB2 2QQ, England

Ancrexia nervosa is a condition which occurs mainly in young women between the ages of 15 and 25 years. It began to increase rapidly from the early 1960's when the slim image for women became fashionable. As a result of this changed image, many young women start dieting but after a week or so most of them give it up. The ones who persist are self-selected for their determination and they all have perfectionist types of personality.

Initially their dieting may be well controlled but at a certain point a sudden change occurs and they are aware that they can no longer control their dieting: "the diet took over". From this point on, their weight loss is more rapid and amenorrhoea sets in.

The factor which determines who will become anorexic and who will not becomes clear from a study of perfectionist individuals. They have high standards in what they set out to do and will not easily give up under difficult circumstances. In many ways they resemble the Pattern A (coronary prone) people. They drive themselves to try and achieve the impossible in terms of time scale, volume of work and quality of work. They respond excessively to a competitive environment and attempt to outstrip their peers. It is not surprising, therefore that 75% of them are working for important examinations when they start their crash dieting (1). The other 25% are caught up in social problems which they persist in trying to solve even though others can see that it is impossible, e.g. trying to bring divorced parents together again.

Their single-mindedness leads to their relinquishing social commitments and eventually they become unable to make normal social contacts.

The more one talks to patients with anorexia nervosa, the more one realises it is not possible to reason with them. Their ideas are fixed on dieting, losing weight, fitting smaller clothes, etc. The severe ones may be convinced that their weight is too low after a prolonged discussion but a few hours later the intense anorexic ideas will have returned. This led to the concept that anorexia nervosa is a compulsive behaviour disease.

A compulsive behaviour disease is one in which abnormal behaviour is driven by a part of the brain which is not amenable to reason. From the association with excessive mental drive to achieve almost impossible goals it seems likely that it develops when a person drives herself over the top of the Yerkes-Dodson curve relating arousal to achievement. Few people are able to drive arousal that far because fatigue supervenes to terminate the work. The perfectionist individual, however, manages to drive herself despite fatigue.

The intensity of the compulsive drive can be scored by means of the Compulsion Score developed and validated by Mills & Medlicott (2). The scores for normal controls, pure anorexics, anorexics who also binge and other compulsive behaviour individuals are shown in Table I (after Medlicott & Mills, to be published).

TABLE I

COMPULSION, ALCOHOL, AND DEPRESSION SCORES

Group	n	Compulsion Score	Alcohol Score	Depression Score
Controls	42	13.1 ± 1.1	0.7 ± 0.3	7.9 ± 0.9
Pure anorexics	34	32.1 ± 1.9**	0.6 ± 0.3	13.8 ± 0.8**
Bingeing anorexics	28	35.8 ± 1.9**	5.8 ± 1.2**	17.0 ± 0.6**
Other compulsives	28	28.0 ± 2.2**	1.6 ± 0.6	11.1 ± 1.1*

* $P < 0.01$
** $P < 0.005$

It is clear from this table that the anorexics who also binge have a tendency to be attached to drinking alcohol in excess and have just as high a compulsion score as the pure anorexics who are not attached to alcohol. Both are severely depressed although it may be masked by their high arousal: the depression may be made worse by fighting the compulsive drive.

Antidepressants are effective in treating about 50% of patients with anorexia nervosa as out-patients. About 30% require a single admission to hospital and 10% have repeated admissions: 10% leave the clinic uncured.

As inpatients re-feeding stimulates metabolism and the serum tri-iodothyronine rises progressively. In a few patients it rises into the thyrotoxic range and they are unable to put on weight even on 3500 k cal per day (3).

Investigations of the mechanisms of the compulsive drive in anorexia and other diseases led us to test a variety of substances affecting neuronal transmission in the brain. Apart from the benefit of antidepressants, we were disappointed in our search (2). We then considered that the opiate system in the brain might be responsible especially since it stimulates the hippocampus by disinhibition. We, therefore, proceeded to treat anorexic patients with continuous intravenous naloxone over long periods of time (4). The rise in weight gain on a constant diet was very striking and it disappeared promptly on stopping naloxone infusions.

The mechanism of this weight gain appears to be by inhibition of lipolysis because plasma levels of β-hydroxybutyrate and non-esterified fatty acids fell promptly when naloxone was started and rose promptly when it ceased (4).

The short term naloxone therapy does not have a great deal of effect on the compulsive drive from the brain. Longer term treatment led to a more stable state after discharge from hospital (2). Of 13 patients treated with doses between 112 mg over 5 weeks and 2.8 g over 25 weeks, 10 were almost stable or gained weight over the next six months.

The part of the brain that might be responsible for compulsive behaviour might be the hippocampus, partly because it is the region through which all new information is processed to get into the memory mechanism and partly because the hippocampus when overstimulated goes into long-term potentiation which lasts for many months (5).

The hippocampus contains enkephalinergic neurones which arise from the lateral entorhinal and perrhinal cortex. Dynorphin is released in the hippocampus and produces long-lasting excitation (6) and this could be the basis of long-term potentiation.

REFERENCES

1. Mills IH, Wilson RJ, Eden MAM, Lines JG (1973) In: Robertson RF (ed) Symposium - Anorexia Nervosa and Obesity. Royal College of Physicians of Edinburgh, Edinburgh, Pub no. 42, pp 31-43
2. Mills IH, Medlicott L (1984) In: Pirke KM, Ploog D (eds) The Psychobiology of Anorexia Nervosa. Springer-Verlag, Berlin, pp 161-171
3. Moore R, Mills IH (1979) Clin Endocrinol 10:443-449
4. Moore R, Mills IH, Forster A (1981) J Roy Soc Med 74:129-131
5. Popper KR, Eccles JC (1977) The Self and its Brain. Springer International, Berlin
6. Henriksen SJ, Chouvet G, McGinty J, Bloom FE (1982) In: Verebey K (ed) Opioids in Mental Illness. Ann NY Acad Sci 398. New York Academy of Sciences, New York, pp 207-219

Endocrinology
F. Labrie, L. Proulx, eds.

OSTEOPOROSIS

R. L. LINDSAY, M.B.Ch.B., Ph.D., M.R.C.P., Helen Hayes Hospital, West Haverstraw, New York, and Department of Medicine, Columbia Presbyterian Medical Center, New York City, New York.

Osteoporosis being increasingly recognized as a major public health problem. The real incidence of crush fractures among the aging population is not known. However, estimates of affected individuals range up to 5 million or more in the USA with a female to male ratio of 10 to 1. Currently, approximately 300,000 female neck fractures occur each year in the USA, with a 5-15% annual death rate following fracture. Presently, it has been estimated that the USA spends $4 billion caring for patients with osteoporosis.

Recent evidence from the United Kingdom[1,2] and the USA[3] suggests that the prevalence of osteoporosis is increasing, with an increasing incidence of fractures. In the USA the incidence of femoral neck fracture, for example, appears to be increasing by about 40% per decade with an increase in age independent incidence among the at-risk population from 1.8% to 2.05% from 1970 to 1980.

It has been suggested that femoral neck fracture and vertebral crush fracture may represent end points of different disease processes[4]. These fractures differ in female to male ratio (10.1 vertebral in comparison to 2:1 for femoral neck). Not all patients who have had femoral neck fracture necessarily have vertebral fractures and the loss of trabecular bone appears greater among patients presenting with vertebral fracture than among those with hip fracture[4]. More recently, we have demonstrated that such differences in trabecular bone mass may also be present among female relatives of osteoporotic patients, and can be observed in young women at the time of maximum bone mass. The differences in expression of the disease may result from differences in the pathogenesis of trabecular or cortical bone loss. Loss of trabecular bone appears to be more dependent on loss of ovarian function, while the reduction in cortical bone may be more dependent on malabsorption of calcium which occurs in both sexes with age, but obviously will be superimposed on the effects of the menopause in women.

Generally, however, in the pathogenesis of osteoporosis of aging, several risk factors, both causative and associative, can be recognized (Table 1). The disorder most commonly affects caucasian or asiatic women, generally of higher social class. A positive family history of the disorder is often obtained as well as a history of menopause (or oophorectomy) poor diet and faulty lifestyle. In the pathogenesis of osteoporosis, dietary factors of importance may include low calcium intake, excessive intake of phosphorus, protein and alcohol. Lack of exercise is probably the main lifestyle factor of causative importance. Cigarette smoking and high caffeine intake may be risk factors only by association, rather than cause and effect. Obesity appears to be protective, pobably by increasing conversion of adrenal androgens to estrogens with postmenopausal women.

Non-invasive techniques for measurement of bone mass have become increasingly available over the past 10 years, and will become more so during the next decade. However, their clinical usefulness for the individual patient as an early diagnostic measure remains to be determined. The techniques vary in site of measurement, cost and radiation dose as well as accuracy and precision. Currently, they should be used only as an adjunct to clincial judgement in the asymptomatic individual.

It has become evident that the sexual dichotomy in presentation of the disorder may result from the lower bone mass at maturity combined with an excessive loss of bone following ovarian failure, an exaggeration of the

TABLE 1
NON-INVASIVE TECHNIQUES FOR MEASUREMENT OF BONE MASS

Technique	Site	Cortical/Trabecular Ratio	Accuracy	Precision	Radiation
Radiogrammetry	Metacarpal	99:1	?	±2%	5-8 mrem
Radiodensitometry	Metacarpal	99:1	?	2-15%	5-8 mrem
Single-Photon Absorptiometry	Mid-Radius	95:5	4%	2-4%	5 mrem
	Distal Radius	75:25	5%	2-4%	5 mrem
Dual-Photon Absorptiometry	LV 2-4	40:60	5-7%	2-5%	5-15 mrem
	Femur Neck	75:25	?	?	5-15 mrem
	Total Skeleton	80:20	2-4%	2-4%	10-40 mrem
Computerized Tomography	Vertebral Body	5:95	?*	?*	200 mrem
Neutron Activation Analysis	Total Body	80:20	3-5%	2-3%	1 rem
	Trunk	30:70	±10%	5%	400 mrem

*Precision and accuracy of CT vary depending on methodology - dual energy scanning improves accuracy (by some correction for marrow fat), but precision does not appear to change. Radiation dosage doubles, however.

individual loss of bone mass with age. Among oophorectomized or postmenopausal woman the rate of bone loss depends on sex hormone status[5] and several studies have now shown that bone loss may be prevented by therapy with estrogens[6,7,8] or certain progestogens[9]. Since the postmenopausal phase of acceleration of bone loss last only 3-8 years, the earlier therapy is begun, the greater the benefits achieved, although some small reversal of bone loss can be achieved if therapy is begun with the first 3-4 years after menopause[6]. One prospective study and several retrospective studies have shown that sex steroids prevent fracture.

The mode of action of these sex hormones in prevention of bone loss remains to be elucidated. The currently most acceptable hypothesis suggests that estrogens function by manipulation of the triad of hormones normally associated with the control of calcium homeostasis (Figure 1). However, a direct non-genome dependent action of estrogen on bone cannot be ruled out. In addition to the prevosion of estrogen therapy to those women particulary at risk for the disorder, advice should include increased calcium intake (to 1.5-2g/day if no contra-indication) and exercise (gravity resistive exercise such as walking, running or competitive sports for the younger individual).

Figure 1: The Calcitonin Hypothesis of Estrogen Action

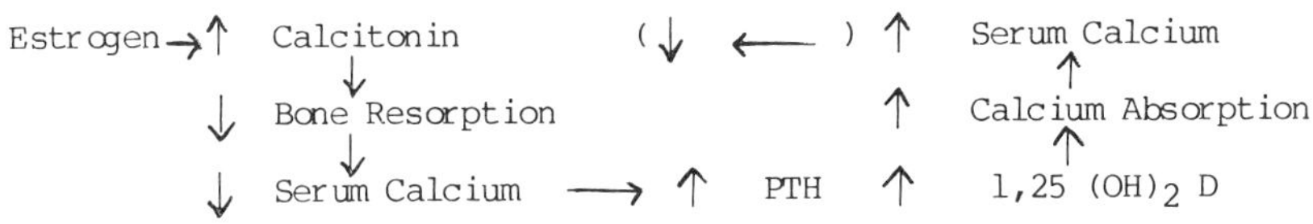

After fracture therapy becomes more difficult, and no good studies currently are available to guide the clinician, prevention of further bone loss in this group of patients is not necessarily synonymous with fracture prevention, and it must be realized that fracture frequency will decline with the passage of time, even in the absence of a successful therapuetic regimen. Standard techniques of treatment usually rely on a polypharmaceutical approach with combinations of calcium estrogen fluoride, vitamin D and other agents. No good data about the effectiveness of any of these approaches are available. However, currently we adopt the simplest approach using calcium (total intake 2g/day) estrogen and exercise (if possible). The utilization of other agents is still under clinical study. It is possible that therapy should be tailored to the metabolic status of the skeleton, with the use of agents to stimulate bone increases if there is histological evidence of low remodeling rate and depression of bone turnover being reserved only for those 10-20% of patients with a high remodeling rate.

Newer approaches to therapy depend on the manipulation of the bone remodeling cycle to obtain a larger number of synchronous cycles in which the activity of osteoclasts can be reduced, on the assumption that osteoblasts, replacing the suppressed osteoclast population, will lay down more new bone than has been resorbed, with a resultant positive bone balance.

REFERENCES

1. Fenton-Lewis A, Brit Med J 283 1217-1220.

2. Wallace WA, Lancet 1983; 1413-1414.

3. Lindsay R, Dempster DW, Clemens TL, International Symposium on Osteoporosis, Copenhangen 1984 (In press).

4. Riggs BL, Wahner HW, Dunn WL et. al., J Clin Invest 67; 328-335.

5. Lindsay R, Gutts JRT, Hart DM, Clinical Endocrinology 6 87-93; 1977.

6. Lindsay R, Hart DM, Aitken JM, et. al., Lancet: 1038-1041; 1976.

7. Hassman A, Gallagher JC, Simpson M, et al., Brit Med J 2, 789; 1977.

8. Recker R, Seville PD, Heaney RP, Ann Intern Med 87, 649-655; 1977.

9. Lindsay R, Hart DM, Purdie D, et. al., Cli Sci Mol Med 54;193-195.

10. Frost H, Clin Orthop 143, 227-244.

Endocrinology
F. Labrie, L. Proulx, eds.

ENDOCRINE HYPERTENSION: FOCUS ON MINERALOCORTICOID EXCESSES

EDWARD G. BIGLIERI

Clinical Study Center, San Francisco General Hospital Medical Center, San Francisco, CA 94110

INTRODUCTION

Excessive production of known and unknown hormones from the adrenal gland is the usual cause of primary endocrine hypertension. The steroids of the adrenal cortex are the proximate cause of elevated blood pressure in diverse types of adrenal disorders.

The principal group of hormones producing elevated blood pressure are the mineralocorticoid hormones (MCH) of the zona glomerulosa (ZG) and zona fasciculata (ZF). Aldosterone, the most potent MCH, is produced in the ZG. In excess, it produces the syndrome of primary aldosteronism, the index type of MCH hypertension. Hypernatremia, hypokalemia, and the suppression of the renin system are the hallmarks of an MCH effect.

I. ZONA GLOMERULOSA MCH EXCESS

a) Primary aldosteronism

Primary aldosteronism is caused by a unilateral aldosterone producing adrenocortical adenoma (APA). In addition to the electrolyte disturbances mentioned before, aldosterone production is increased but cortisol levels are normal. The overnight recumbent plasma aldosterone concentration is elevated (>20 ng/dl) and decreases or fails to increase in response to the upright posture in 95% of the 65 patients studied in our center. Precursor steroids in the aldosterone pathway in the ZG are frequently elevated. The elevated plasma 18-hydroxycorticosterone (18-OHB) levels in patients with APA show virtually no overlap with the 0800h levels in hyperaldosteronism due to idiopathic hyperaldosteronism (IHA, hyperplasia). Values greater than 65 ng/dl are seen in all 30 proven cases of APA, and less than 65 in 15 patients with IHA. High salt intakes, administration of DOC acetate, or fludrocortisone, saline infusions (2 liters over 2 hrs) suppress urinary and plasma aldosterone levels to <6 μg/24h or, 4 ng/dl only in essential hypertension but not in primary aldosteronism. In addition, a single oral dose (25 mg) of a converting enzyme inhibitor (captopril) does not distinguish APA from IHA. An additional unique characteristic of patients with APA is the observation that prolonged spironolactone (SPL) treatment does not increase but often decreases aldosterone production by tumors even though renin and plasma potassium levels rise. Increases occur in IHA.

Patients with adenoma, rarely respond to the above test maneuvers. However, because of rare exceptions all patients with primary aldosteronism should have computed tomography. Computed tomography localizes the unilateral adenoma in 80% of cases with chemical findings of APA. If biochemical and hormonal levels and radiologic techniques fail to localize an adenoma bilateral adrenal vein catherization must be performed.

This approach has identified a new subset of primary aldosteronism due to primary hyperplasia. The biochemical and hormonal characteristics are similar to APA and not IHA. Computed tomography does not identify an adenoma and adrenal vein sampling does not lateralize aldosterone production. Reduction of adrenal tissue (subtotal or unilateral adrenalectomy) has produced sustained cures. PAH is usually bilateral, rarely unilateral.

Hyperaldosteronism with hyperplasia

IHA forms the bulk of this group with growing hormonal evidence that the drive is extra-adrenal. Possible pituitary peptides may stimulate the ZF to produce aldosterone, but whether these peptides are hypertensinogenic is not known. Total or subtotal adrenalectomy, while correcting the hyperaldosteronism, does not cure the hypertension. The strong clinical similarities between IHA and essential hypertension suggest that IHA may be part of the essential hypertensive spectrum.

Glucocorticoid remediable hyperaldosteronism is a familial disorder that clearly links the pituitary to an adrenal aberration. Glucocorticoid treatment (1-2 mg dexamethasone/day) corrects the clinical, biochemical, and hormonal abnormalities. Although ACTH levels are normal, its suppression improves and administration of supraphysiologic amounts aggravate the manifestations of this disorder.

ZONA FASCICULATA MCH EXCESS (Table 1)

The ZF is the site of cortisol production. When in great excess, cortisol also has major MCH activity. The 17-deoxypathway in the ZF, also under ACTH control, produces deoxycorticosterone (DOC), 18-hydroxyDOC (18-OHDOC), and corticosterone (B), the MCHs of the ZF. However, aldosterone and 18-OHB levels are normal. These steroid patterns are also seen after 3 days of superphysiologic doses of ACTH. The inhibition of aldosterone by ACTH is in part due to renin suppression; decrease in MCH receptors, and intra-adrenal inhibition of ZG synthesis after 3 days of continuous superphysiologic doses of ACTH.

Congenital Adrenal Hyperplasia (CAH)

The 11β-hydroxylase deficiency (11β-OHD) and 17α-hydroxylase deficiency (17α-OHD) are the two forms of CAH with hypertension. 11β-OHD in the ZF affects the transformation of 11-deoxycortisol to cortisol, and DOC to 18-OHDOC and B. The steroids proximal to the defect, DOC and 11-deoxycortisol, increase. DOC produces the MCH effects of this disorder. The elevated ACTH levels increase androgen production so that hirsutism and virilization occur.

The 17α-OHD also presents with MCH hypertension but a defect in 17-hydroxylation blocks androgen and estrogen formation in both the adrenal and ovary. Thus, these patients present with hypogonadism, primary amenorrhea, and eunicoid habitus. The inability to make cortisol, increases ACTH secretion and stimulation of the MCH pathway of the ZF - DOC, B, 18-OHDOC (and only in this instance 18-OHB). These steroids produce mineralocorticoid hypertension, suppress renin, and the ZG production of aldosterone. ACTH suppression with glucocorticoid therapy corrects the hypertension and MCH excess in these two forms of CAH.

Primary cortisol resistance

This disorder has only recently been recognized. Glucocorticoid receptors are defective and their affinity for cortisol reduced. High levels of cortisol and ACTH occur. The steroid pattern produced is similar to those observed in patients with 17α-OHD. The MCH pathway in the ZF is stimulated to produce excess DOC and B. Renin levels are reduced with subsequent low normal aldosterone production. Very high doses of dexamethasone are required to ineffectively suppress ACTH so that SPL and other anti-hypertensive agents are required for control.

Ectopic ACTH Syndrome and Cushing's Disease

The ectopic ACTH syndrome is associated with hypertension, hypokalemia, and normal aldosterone production. The intense stimulation of the ZF results not only in cortisol excess but in excesses of the MCH pathway - DOC, 18-OHDOC, and B. Less pronounced elevations are seen in Cushing's disease. The normal levels of aldosterone and 18-OHB could be a consequence of intra-adrenal inhibition and 11- and 18-hydroxylation by cortisol.

III. OTHER MINERALOCORTICOID HORMONES

The 11β-hydroxysteroid reductase deficiency implies the inability to convert 11-hydroxy steroids to 11-keto steroids - a defect in metabolism. This defect identifies a group of hypertensive children who first presented with MCH hypertension. Other steroids were normal. ACTH administration aggrevated, but salt restriction and SPL reduced the hypertension. Glucocorticoid treatment has questionable results on both the hypertension and steroid secretion. The search for a causative MCH for this defect has been unsuccessful. Yet, the evidence is strong for a MCH responsive to ACTH, and linked with sodium. The only marker available is the inability to convert tetrahydrocortisol to tetrahydrocortisone. The link between this diagnostic defect and the mechanism for the hypertension is unknown.

TABLE 1

	CORTISOL μg/dl	DOC ng/dl	18-OHDOC ng/dl	B ng/dl	ALDOSTERONE ng/dl	18-OHB μg/dl
ZONA GLOMERULOSA MCH EXCESS						
APA (n=15)	11.7±1.0	19.3±3.6	8.8±1.6	365± 57	52.5± 9.9	137.4±22.2
IHA (n=10)	10.2±	7.9±1.3	3.8±0.6	160± 28	16.4± 1.5	28.4± 4.1
PAH (n=4)	12.5±3.0	18.8±2.5	7.2±3.3	400±132	33.7± 3.2	64.4±15.6
APA-Ca (n=3)	12.0±1.0	46.5±2.1	---	216±60	105.2±56.0	---
ZONA FASCICULATA MCH						
ACTH AND CORTISOL EXCESS						
CUSHING´S DISEASE (n=4)	27.1± 1.2	17.9±3.1	8.3±2.5	490±70	8.0±1.5	20.8±7.4
ECTOPIC ACTH (n=3)	70.0±20.8	80.9±35.0	14.8±2.8	1570±500	4.7±1.0	14.3±6.6
3rd DAY ACTH	49.6±12.6	477.3±44.2	79.8±14.0	2960±510	12.0±1.7	37.7±5.5
CORTISOL RESISTANCE (n=1)	(27.4)	(53.8)		(2870)	(2.0)	
ACTH WITHOUT CORTISOL EXCESS						
CAH (11β-OHD) (n=7)	3.1±0.6	417±33.6	1.0±0.1	70±20	2.1±0.6	5.0±1.8
CAH (17α-OHD) (n=4)	N.D.	243.8±35.9	192.0±38.1	11300±2800	4.0±0.8	255.8±90.4
NORMAL RANGE	10.6±1.4	7.8± 0.6	5.6±0.8	238±31	8.5±1.2	19.5±3.3

CAH = congenital adrenal hyperplasia; 11β-OHD = 11β-hydroxylase deficiency; 17α-OHD = 17α-hydroxylase deficiency; ( ) single value from literature; PAH = primary adrenal hyperplasia; APA-Ca = APA carcinoma; ND = not detected

REFERENCES

1. Biglieri EG, Baxter JD (1981) In: Felig P, Baxter JD, Broadus AE, Frohman LA (eds). The endocrinology of hypertension. McGraw-Hill, New York, pp 551-598.

2. Biglieri EG, Kater CE (1982) In: Genest J, Kuchell O, Hamet P, Cantin M (eds). Hypertension: Physiopathology and Treatment. McGraw-Hill Co., New York, pp 939-947.

3. Bravo EL, Tarazi RC, Dustan HP, Fouad FM, Textor SC, Gifford RW, Vidt DG (1983) Changing clinical spectrum of aldosteronism. Am J Med 74:641-651.

Endocrinology
F. Labrie, L. Proulx, eds.

EUTHYROID HYPERTHYROXINEMIA

J.R. STOCKIGT
Ewen Downie Metabolic Unit, Alfred Hospital, Melbourne, Australia 3181

The term euthyroid hyperthyroxinemia (1) is used when total and/or free T_4 are increased in the absence of hyperthyroidism (Table I). The T_4 excess may be transient or persistent, associated with low, normal or high levels of triiodothyronine. Apart from alterations in the concentration of thyroxine binding globulin (TBG), increased T_4 binding to albumin, prealbumin or autoantibodies can cause hyperthyroxinemia. These abnormalities can cause assay artifacts that lead to spurious results with some T_4 assays. Binding may be altered by a change in protein concentration (i.e. capacity), as occurs with TBG, or the affinity between protein and ligand may be abnormal, as is now recognized for albumin and prealbumin.

THYROXINE BINDING GLOBULIN EXCESS causing hyperthyroxinemia is routinely detected by many simple techniques, but the T_3RU may not normalize extreme variations in T_4 if calculated as resin/total counts. The modified calculation of resin/serum counts gives a larger correction factor at extremes of TBG (2,3) and should now be adopted. Detailed reviews of TBG-related binding variations can be found elsewhere (4,5).

FAMILIAL DYSALBUMINEMIC HYPERTHYROXINEMIA (FDH) is an important cause of persistent T_4 excess with normal serum T_3 in non-goitrous, clinically-euthyroid subjects. Total T_4 is about double mean normal (6-9). T_4 and T_3 as well as TSH, are responsive to stimulation and suppression (8). Early accounts failed to identify the abnormality because concentrations of TBG, prealbumin and albumin were normal. About 25-50% of albumin molecules have an abnormal binding site with T_4 affinity 20-50 times higher than normal (10,11). Recent studies (12) suggest an excess of a normal minor albumin component with high T_4 affinity. The T_3RU is normal-high because affinity for T_3 is not

TABLE 1

EUTHYROID HYPERTHYROXINEMIA

1. Binding Abnormalities
   *Excess TBG
   Dysalbuminemia (FDH)
   Prealbumin-Associated (PAH)
   *Autoantibody-Associated
2. *Hormone-Resistance Syndromes
3. Drug-Related Effects
   Amiodarone
   Contrast Agents
   Propranolol
   Amphetamine
4. Ingestion of Thyroxine
5. Acute Psychiatric Illness
6. Hyperemesis Gravidarum
7. Unknown Cause

* T_3 usually increased also

increased and binding is inhibited by barbitone. Free T4 by equilibrium dialysis and free and total T3 are normal. The "unbound analog" free T4 methods give hyperthyroid values because the analogs bind to FDH albumin (13,14). The abnormality of FDH becomes more obvious at artificially-high hormone concentrations (Fig 1), making the "T4-loaded uptake test" specific for FDH (15).

In PREALBUMIN-ASSOCIATED HYPERTHYROXINEMIA (PAH), T4 excess of 150-180 nM is associated with normal levels of T3. Electrophoretic and immunoprecipitation studies show increased T4 binding to prealbumin (16,17), but prealbumin is only mildly elevated (350-500 mg/l c.f. normal 200-400 mg/l), suggesting abnormally high affinity for T4 (17). The structural basis for the difference is so far unknown. A distinction between PAH and FDH can be based on differences in binding capacity (18), because FDH albumin has a T4 capacity of about 200 μM, while prealbumin capacity is about 3 μM. With T4 in 50-fold excess of normal, both FDH and PAH show lower than normal free counts. At 1000-fold excess T4, prealbumin sites are filled, making PAH indistinguishable from normal, while excess binding persists in FDH (Fig 1).

AUTOANTIBODY-ASSOCIATED HYPERTHYROXINEMIA Autoantibodies that bind T4, T3 or rT3 occur most often with autoimmune thyroid disease. High T_4 may result from an assay artifact, but may also reflect an increase in response to abnormal binding (19). Assays after alcohol extraction give the true circulating level, but may over-estimate the available hormone because the in vivo effect of abnormal binding is ignored. A free T_4 measurement should compensate for this abnormality, but analog tracer methods can give spuriously-high values in the presence of autoantibodies (20).

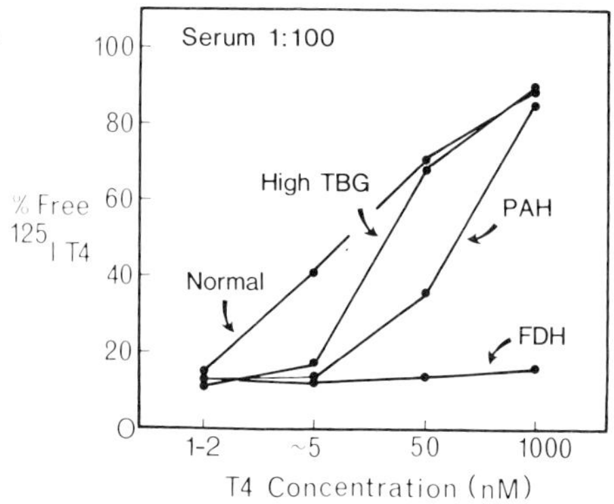

Fig. 1. Effect of T_4 loading on dextran-charcoal uptake of ^{125}I T_4 in normal, TBG excess, PAH and FDH sera. Serum diluted 1:100 in phosphate buffer, 0.04M pH 7.4, giving an endogenous T_4 concentration of 1-2 nM. Mean of >4 subjects at each point.

HORMONE RESISTANCE SYNDROMES are associated with excess T_3 and T_4, both total and free (21-23). In generalised resistance, T_3 and T_4 excess is associated with goiter, inviting a misdiagnosis of hyperthyroidism (21). Free T_4, irrespective of method, will reinforce this impression. Selective pituitary resistance usually presents as hyperthyroidism, with excess of both T_3 and T_4, with intact TSH response to TRH (22,23). A defect in the intra-pituitary deiodination of $T_4 \cdot T_3$ has been postulated, and exogenous T_3 (23) has been advocated as treatment. Because pre-emptive plasma binding simulates resistance, binding abnormalities must be excluded before hormone resistance can be proven.

DRUG-RELATED HYPERTHYROXINEMIA can occur with amiodarone, after exposure to oral cholecystographic contrast agents, with beta blockers such as propranolol (24), or with amphetamines (25). Amiodarone and the oral cholecystographic contrast agents are competitive substrates for outer ring deiodinase and T4 excess may occur from diminished clearance (26), as well as increased production resulting from iodine loading. The response differs from typical Jod-Basedow as T3 generally remains normal, because of impaired T4-T3 conversion (27). However, true hyperthyroidism, with marked excess of both T4 and T3, is reported (28,29). It is not known why T3 excess occurs, but those with thyroid autonomy in iodine-deficient areas appear to be especially at risk (29).

INGESTION OF T4. During oral L-thyroxine replacement, many euthyroid patients have elevated levels of T4 with normal T3 (30). It has been suggested that deiodination of ingested T4 shows autoregulatory variation (31), but the mechanism is not yet established. The time between dose and sampling is usually disregarded when assessing T4, but maximum levels 2-4 h after ingestion of 100-300 μg may be 20-50% higher than the steady state levels (32).

Reports of TRANSIENT HYPERTHYROXINEMIA IN ACUTE PSYCHIATRIC ILLNESS indicate that initial samples may often show T4 excess (33). Acute stress-induced release of T4, not attributable to TSH, occurs in experimental animals and is blockable by alpha adrenergic antagonists (34). Possible acute hormone release, either from the thyroid or from the liver (35), deserves further study.

HYPEREMESIS GRAVIDARUM was associated with temporary T4 excess in most of 33 pregnancies so affected (36), a change not due to increased binding. Excess T3 was found in less than half, but the TSH response to TRH was often diminished.

PERSISTENT HYPERTHYROXINEMIA WITHOUT DEFINABLE CAUSE occurs in some euthyroid individuals or kindreds (37-39) with T4 in the range 150-250 nM, associated with high free T4 in some cases. Defective peripheral T4-T3 deiodination, perhaps due to diminished cell entry, has been suggested (39), but others have been unable to confirm this finding (40).

No single test proves the diagnosis of hyperthyroidism; e.g. high T4 and T3, both total and free, occur with goiter in thyroid hormone resistance. If resistance is generalised, euthyroidism is the rule; if selective pituitary resistance is present, hyperthyroidism occurs. With our present knowledge, the distinction is clinical! While high T_4 levels should not alone be taken as evidence of hyperthyroidism, T_3 may decrease transiently in hyperthyroid patients during severe illness, so that true hyperthyroidism can be temporarily associated with isolated T_4 excess (41). As suggested by Borst et al (1), such dilemmas are often best resolved by passage of time.

REFERENCES

1. Borst GC et al. Ann Intern Med 1983;98:366-378.
2. Schussler GC et al. New Engl J Med 1978;299:510-515.
3. Felicetta JV et al. Metabolism 1979;28:756-761.
4. Refetoff S et al. J Clin Invest 1972;51:848-867.
5. Robbins J et al. Rec Prog Hormone Res 1978;34:477-519.
6. Hennemann G et al. Lancet 1979;1:639-642.
7. Lee WNP et al. J Clin Endocrinol Metab 1979;49:292-299.
8. Stockigt JR et al. J Clin Endocrinol Metab 1981;53:353-354.
9. Lalloz MRA et al. Clin Endocrinol 1983;18:11-24.
10. Docter R et al. Clin Endocrinol (Oxf) 1981;15:363-371.
11. Barlow JW et al. J Clin Endocrinol Metab 1982;55:244-250.
12. Docter R. Lancet 1984;1:50.
13. Stockigt JR et al. Clin Endocrinol (Oxf) 1981;15:313-318.
14. Rajatanavin R et al. Ann Intern Med 1982;97:865-867.
15. White EL et al. Thyroid Research VIII. Aust Acad Sci 1980:513-516.
16. Moses AC et al. New Engl J Med 1982;306:966-969.
17. Lalloz MRA et al. Clin Endocrinol (Oxf):in press.
18. Stockigt JR et al. New Engl J Med 1982;307:824.
19. Beckett GJ et al. Clin Endocrinol (Oxf) 1983;19:295-303.
20. Beck-Peccoz P et al. J Clin Endocrinol Metab 1984;58:736-739.
21. Bantle JP et al. Arch Intern Med 1982;142:1867-1871.
22. Weintraub BD et al. Ann Intern Med 1981;95:339-351.
23. Rosler A et al. J Clin Endocrinol Metab 1982;54:76-82.
24. Cooper DS et al. Am J Med 1982;73:867-871.
25 Morley JE et al. Ann Intern Med 1980;93:707-709.
26. Lambert MJ et al. J Clin Endocrinol Metab 1982;55:1058-1065.
27. Sogol PB et al. Endocrinology 1983;113:1464-1469.
28. Leger AF et al. J Nucl Med 1983;24:582-585.
29. Martino E et al. Ann Intern Med;in press.
30. Salmon D et al. Arch Intern Med 1982;142:571-573.
31. Lum SMC et al. J Clin Invest 1984;73:570-575.
32. Symons RG et al. Clin Endocrinol 1983;19:539-546.
33. Spratt DI et al. Am J Med 1982;73:41-48.
34. Langer P et al. Acta Endocrinologica 1983;104:443-449.
35. Cavalieri RR et al. J Clin Invest 1966;45:939-949.
36. Bouillon R et al. Am J Obstet Gynecol 1982;143:922-926.
37. Maxon HR et al. Acta Endocrinologica 1982;100:224-230.
38. Jansen M et al. Lancet 1982;2:849-851.
39. Wortsman J et al. Ann Intern Med 1983;98:904-909.
40. Hennemann G. Personal communication.
41. Engler D et al. J Clin Endocrinol Metab 1978;46:77-82.

Endocrinology
F. Labrie, L. Proulx, eds.

PRIMARY BREAST CANCER PROGNOSTIC FACTORS

WILLIAM L. McGUIRE AND GARY M. CLARK

Department of Medicine/Oncology, University of Texas Health Science Center at San Antonio, 7703 Floyd Curl Drive, San Antonio, Texas 78284

INTRODUCTION

Estrogen receptor (ER) has been well documented as an important predictor of long disease-free intervals and survival for patients with primary breast cancer (4). In advanced breast cancer it has been hypothesized that the presence of progesterone receptor (PgR) might be a more sensitive marker for predicting response to endocrine therapy (1,5). We have recently found that PgR was more important than ER in predicting disease-free survival for a group of patients with Stage II breast disease that was treated according to a randomized protocol.

This report examines the generality of that result by extending our analysis to include patients from other institutions. The additional patients were not treated according to a rigid clinical protocol, but rather received treatments in much the same way as the majority of breast cancer patients in a community practice. Of interest was whether the relationship between steroid receptors and disease-free survival that we have previously reported would hold with this new group of patients with different demographic and treatment profiles. The relationships between steroid receptor levels and both disease-free and overall survival were examined in detail.

MATERIALS AND METHODS

The patients on the randomized adjuvant therapy protocol have been described in previous publications (2,3). These patients were randomized to receive one of three treatment modalities: 1) cytoxan, methotrexate, 5-fluorouracil (CMF); 2) CMF plus tamoxifen (CMFT); 3) CMFT plus bacillus Calmette-Guerrin vaccination. Patients who were not enrolled on a clinical trial were treated on an individual basis including: 1) neither chemotherapy nor endocrine therapy; 2) chemotherapy alone; 3) endocrine therapy alone; 4) combined chemotherapy and endocrine therapy. All patients had a radical or modified radical mastectomy with the biopsy specimen from the primary tumor sent to San Antonio for ER and PgR assays.

RESULTS AND DISCUSSION

A total of 619 patients were included in these analyses, 189 treated according to a clinical protocol and 430 treated on an individual basis. The patients on the randomized study tended to have smaller tumors and were more likely to be ER+ and PgR+ than patients not on study. There were no significant differences in the distribution of age, menopausal status, or the number of positive nodes.

We examined several subsets of the potential prognostic factors using Cox's multiple regression technique. This procedure can incorporate several prognostic factors simultaneously. If a particular variable is deemed statistically significant, the implication is that if all other factors in the model are held constant, then a change in the value of the variable in question will significantly affect the survival.

For disease-free survival, only four prognostic factors were significant when analyzed simultaneously: the number of positive nodes, PgR, ER, and the size of the primary tumor. For overall survival, the significant prognostic factors were: the number of positive nodes, ER, PgR, chemotherapy. Patients who had ER- and PgR- tumors with more than 3 positive nodes comprised a particularly poor prognostic group. It was of interest that once other variables were taken into account, participation in the randomized trial was not a significant factor. Table I presents the p-values for the prognostic factors in these models as well as p-values for the variables not in the model.

The number of positive nodes was the single most important factor in each of these models. Both steroid receptors were also significant factors in each model. PgR was slightly more important than ER for predicting disease-free survival, but ER was more important than PgR for predicting overall survival. Patients who received chemotherapy tended to have longer survival, but this variable did not help to predict time of recurrence.

TABLE I
MULTIVARIATE SURVIVAL ANALYSES

Disease-Free Survival		Overall Survival	
Factors in the Model	P-Value	Factors in the Model	P-Value
Positive Nodes	< .0001	Positive Nodes	< .0001
PgR Status	.008	ER Status	.0003
ER Status	.014	PgR Status	.002
Size of Primary Tumor	.022	Chemotherapy	.004
Factors not in the Model		Factors not in the Model	
Endocrine Therapy	.14	Endocrine Therapy	.08
Chemotherapy	.21	Size of Primary Tumor	.13
Age	.44	Age	.56
Menopausal Status	.98	Menopausal Status	.68

We have recently found that PgR was more important than ER in predicting disease-free survival. But these conclusions were based on results from a controlled clinical trial. It was of interest to know whether patients who were treated according to a strict protocol in a clinical trial might constitute a prognostically different population than patients who received individualized therapies. Patients on the clinical trial tended to have smaller primary tumors, were more likely to be ER+ and PgR+, and all received chemotherapy. When the potential prognostic factors were examined one at a time, participation in a clinical trial was nearly a significant predictor of overall survival ($p = .09$). However, when examined from a multivariate point of view, there was no significant difference in survival or disease-free survival between patients who were on study and those who were not.

PgR status enhanced the predictive power of ER for both survival and time to recurrence. This underscores the importance of our previous suggestion that PgR be routinely measured and incorporated into future adjuvant therapy trials.

ACKNOWLEDGMENT

This work was supported in part by NIH Grant CA 30195.

REFERENCES

1. Horwitz KB, McGuire WL, Pearson OH, Segaloff A (1975) Predicting response to endocrine therapy in human breast cancer: a hypothesis. Science 29:726-727
2. Hubay CA, Pearson OH, Marshall JS, Rhodes RS, Debanne SM, Mansour EG, Hermann RE, Jones JC, Flynn WJ, Eckert C, McGuire WL (1980) Antiestrogen, cytotoxic chemotherapy and Bacillus Calmette-Guerrin vaccination in stage II breast cancer: a preliminary report. Surgery 87:494-501
3. Hubay CA, Pearson OH, Marshall JS, Stellato TA, Rhodes RS, Debanne SM, Rosenblatt J, Mansour EG, Hermann RE, Jones JC, Flynn WJ, Eckert C, McGuire WL (1981) Adjuvant therapy of stage II breast cancer: 48 month follow-up of a prospective randomized clinical trial. Breast Cancer Res Treat 1:72-82.
4. Knight WA, Livingston RB, Gregory EJ, McGuire W L (1977) Estrogen receptor as an independent prognostic factor for early recurrence in breast cancer. Cancer Res 37:4669-4673
5. McGuire WL (1978) Hormone receptors: their role in predicting prognosis and response to endocrine therapy. Semin Oncol 5:428-433.

© 1984 Elsevier Science Publishers B.V.
Endocrinology
F. Labrie, L. Proulx, eds.

CLINICAL USE OF LHRH AGONISTS

WILLIAM F. CROWLEY, JR., M.D.

Reproductive Endocrine Unit, Massachusetts General Hospital, Boston, MA 02114

INTRODUCTION

Two experimental observations may illustrate the diverse clinical applications of LHRH and its analogues. In the now classic studies of Knobil, arcuate nucleus-lesioned and pre-pubertal (1,2) Rhesus monkeys (both LHRH deficient) were replaced with exogenous LHRH. Continuous administration of LHRH was unable to restore physiologic levels of gonadotropin secretion. Episodic delivery of LHRH at a frequency designed to mimic the endogenous gonadotropin pulsations restoring appropriate gonadotropin secretion to these animals. Moreover, increasing the duration of exposure to LHRH resulted in decreasing levels of gonadotropin secretion (3) and fit the general criteria of desensitization of pituitary gonadotropin secretion.

A second experimental observation was made in LHRH deficient adult males with hypogonadotropic hypogonadism employing a long-acting LHRH analogue, D-Trp6-Pro9-Net-LHRH (LHRHa) (4). Alternate day administration was capable of producing a stable gonadotropin elevation for 8 hours, whereas daily administration of the same dose blocked pituitary responsiveness to LHRHa administration. It became clear that intermittent stimulation by LHRH was absolutely essential for consistent secretion whereas continuous receptor occupancy by either LHRH or its long-acting analogues produced an effective and selective blockade of gonadotropin secretion.

Not only is it evident that intermittency of hypothalamic stimulation is required for physiologic functioning of the gonadotroph, it also appears that such pulsatility is most likely achieved by intermittent administration of natural sequence LHRH since the rapid metabolism of this peptide is an essential component of the neuroendocrine control of reproduction. Continuous receptor occupancy can be achieved by either a pure LHRH antagonist or by the paradoxical effect of long acting LHRH agonists. The hypothalamic-pituitary-gonadal axis can be represented by the analogy of a computer. The hardware of this system (hypothalamic neurons, the gonadotrophs, and the gonads) will not function if the "software" component, i.e. the hypothalmic secretory program of LHRH is not functioning properly. Physiologic secretion of gonadotropins and fertility are critically dependent upon a precise program of episodic hypothalamic secretion.

With these observations, two broad categories of application of LHRH and its analogues readily emerge. The first of these clinical uses are in the "fertility program" of the reproductive system. The second broad category of clinical applications is the antifertility effects, which can be evoked by administration of LHRH agonists or antagonists.

PRO-FERTILITY APPLICATIONS OF LHRH

Using portable infusion pumps which can be programed to any desired frequency of intermittent stimulation (Ferring), "hypothalamic replacement therapy" is administered in both men and women with LHRH deficiency (5,6). The selection of the frequency of LHRH administration is based upon physiologic data. The dosage of LHRH has been adjusted by determining the amplitude of pituitary gonadotropin pulsations as well as the degree of gonadal responsiveness.

In men with idiopathic hypogonadotropic hypogonadism (IHH), physiology of LHRH in the human male and hypothalamic replacement therapy were investigated (6). Each of these males was carefully selected for study after having failed to undergo puberty by age 18 and demonstrated a serum testosterone in the prepubertal range. Each subject had no evidence of other neuroendocrine or pituitary disease by insulin tolerance and TRF testing as well as a normal CT scan of the hypothalamic-pituitary area. A gonad capable of responding was documented by both hCG stimulation and testicular biopsy prior to therapy. These patients were treated with natural sequence LHRH at a 2-hour frequency. This was based on previous studies of adult males (7). The dose of LHRH was empirically adjusted utilizing the serum testosterone level and spanned a range of 25 to 300 ng/ke.

The clinical results of this replacement therapy were quite striking as all of the signs and symptoms of puberty were encountered. A uniform response of increased libido, potency, erections, and the appearance of an ejaculate was noted in all subjects. Tripling of testicular size occurred by the 3-6 month period and appearance of mature sperm in the ejaculate was noted in two-thirds of the patients. The gonadotropin dynamics previously reported in these subjects (6) are interesting; it appears that supraphysiologic gonadotropin levles are required to initiate gonadal steroidogenesis in these men with essentially prepubertal gonads prior to LHRH treatment. Moreover, these patients are capable of impregnating their wives and achieving a total normal fertility with this treatment (6).

Deficiencies of endogenous LHRH secretion in females manifest themselves as two basic clinical diagnoses. Amenorrhea has a predominantly "hypothalamic" etiology. The common hypothalamic defect in this heterogeneous group is one of faulty endogenous LHRH secretion. Chronic anovulation, another manifestation of endogenous LHRH deficiency represents 10-15% of infertile women. Both of these diagnoses might prove amenable to replacement therapy with exogenous LHRH. The use of clomiphene citrate, an anti-estrogen capable of stimulating endogenous LHRH secretion is associated with an increased frequency of multiple gestation and mild ovarian hyperstimulation (8). Human gonadotropin injections (Pergonal) often result in multiple gestations as well as the ovarian hyperstimulation syndrome, and necessitates extensive monitoring by ultrasound and estrogen levels (9). In attempting to understand the pathophysiology of the disorder in hypothalamic amenorrhea and anovulatory infertility and its difference from normal, we have performed detailed studies of ovulatory women in the menstrual cycle in which frequent gonadotropin samples were obtained over the course of a 24-hour period, to define more precisely the aberrancies of hypothalamic LHRH secretion seen in amenorrheic and anovulatory women. We have determined that the vast majority of patients with hypothalamic amenorrhea have either disorders of the frequency and/or amplitude of LHRH-induced gonadotropin pulsations. These patients represent the female counterpart of hypogonadotropic males and as such should prove equally amenable to treatment with pulsatile LHRH. The precise dosage, frequency, and route of LHRH administration is considerably more complicated in the female than in the male. These factors have made the task of inducing ovulation in females with pulsatile LHRH considerably more complex than inducing puberty in males. In our own experience, intravenous LHRH administration is more effective than the subcutaneous route in these women. A dosage of LHRH of 1-5 ug intravenously or 5-10 ug subcutaneously represents the most "physiologic" replacement dosages. In the first published case of an LHRH deficient female (Kallmann's syndrome), LHRH replacement was capable of simulating all of the events of a normal menstrual cycle ( ). It is clear from studies in LHRH deficient patients with an intact pituitary and ovaries that the entire process of folliculogenesis, ovulation, and formation and demise of the corpus luteum can besustained with a fixed input of exogenously administered LHRH. In 15 patients with a variety of hypothalamic disorders varying from congenital LHRH deficiency to hypothalamic amenorrhea, our experience indicates that pulsatile LHRH administration represents a generally successful form of therapy which may well complement or replace treatment with gonadotropins.

Anti-Fertility Effects of GnRH Analogues

Utilizing LHRH agonists to block the LHRH receptor on the pituitary membrane, it has been possible to effect a selective chemical castration therapy in a wide variety of circumstances. The first two indications were the use of LHRH agonists to inhibit ovulation as a new method of contraception (10) and its use in precocious puberty (11). By means of single daily injections of an LHRH analogue, D-=Trp6-Pro-Net-LHRH, we have demonstrated dramatic clinical responses of children with centrally mediated precocious puberty. In 52 such patients treated to date, there has been a uniform suppression of endogenous gonadotropin pulsations. A suppression of gonadal steroidogenesis to pre-pubertal levels has been observed accompanied by dramatic clinical responses including uniform cessation of menses, a striking arrest or regression of breast growth in females, and a decrease to 50% of pretherapy levels of the testicular volume in the males. It is clearly possible to the pituitary-gonadal axix over extended time periods by using daily LHRHa administration. All of the patients withdrawn from LHRHa therapy following 2 months, 10 months and 3 years of continuous LHRHa administration have demonstrated a prompt return of reinitiation of the pubertal process (12). More recently we have investigated the impact of this selective removal of gonadarche from the pubertal process upon both growth and adrenal maturation since this therapeutic probe now permits us to pursue such a novel line of investigation. Similar approaches and successes have also been reported with LHRHa induced suppression of the pituitary in endometriosis (13); polycystic ovarian disease (14); metastatic prostate (15) and breast cancer (16); and uterine fibroids (17).

Thus, it appears that LHRH and its analogues represent a major therapeutic advance in reproductive medicine with an impact upon Pediatrics, Urology, Medical Oncology and Gynecology.

REFERENCES

1. Belchetz PE, Plant TM, Nakai Y, Keogh EJ and Knobil E. Hypophyseal response to continuous and intermittent delivery of hypothalamic gonadotropin-releasing hormone. Science 202: 631-33,1978.

2. Wildt L, Marshall G and Knobil E. Experimental induction of puberty in the infantile rhesus monkey. Science 207:1371-1375, 1980.

3. Knobil E. Neuroendocrine control of the menstrual cycle. Rec. Prog. Hormone Res. 36:53-88, 1980.

4. Crowley WF, Vale WW, Rivier J and McArthur JW. LHRH in hypogonadotropic hypogonadism. In: LHRH Peptides as Female and Male Contraceptives, PAFRF Series on Fertility Regulation, GI Zatuchni, JD Shelton and JJ Schiarra (eds), Harper & Row, Philadelphia, 1981, pages 321-333.

5. Crowley WR, Beitins IZ, Vale W, Kliman B, Rivier J, Rivier C, and McArthur JW. The biologic activity of a potent analogue of gonadotropin-releasing hormone in normal and hypogonadotropic men. N.Eng. J. Med. 302:1052-1057, 1980.

6. Hoffman AR and Vrowley WF. Induction of Puberty in men by long-term pulsatile administration of low-dose gonadotropin-releasing hormone. N. Eng. J. Med. 307:1237-41, 1982.

7. Santen RJ, Leonard JM, Sherins RJ, Gandy HM and Paulsen CA. Short and long term effects of clomiphene citrate on the pituitary-testicular axis. J. Clin. Endocr. Metab. 33:970-9, 1971.

8. Greenblatt RB, Roy S, Mahesh, VB, Barfield WE and Jungok EC. Induction of ovulation. Am. J. Obstet. Gynecol. 84:900-912, 1962.

9. Brown JB, Evans JH, Adey FD, Taft HP and Townsend L. Factors involved in the induction of fertile ovulation with human gonadotropins. J. Obstet. Gynecol. Brit. Comm. 76:289-306, 1969.

10. Bergquist C, Nillius SJ and Wide L. Inhibition of ovulation in women by intranasal treatment with a luteinizing hormone-releasing hormone agonist. Contraception 19:497-506, 1979.

11. Crowley WF, Comite F and Cutler G. Therapeutic use of pituitary desensitization with a long-acting LHRH agonist: A potential new treatment for idiopathic precocious puberty. J. Clin. Endocr. Metab. 52:370-372, 1981.

12. Mansfield MJ, Loughlin JS, Crawford JD, Bode HH, Beardsworth DE, Rivier J, Vale W, Kushner DC and Crowley WF. Treatment of central precocious puberty with a long-acting analogue of luteinizing hormone releasing hormone: Effects upon somatic growth and skeletal maturation in an eighteen month trial. N. Eng. J. Med. 309:1286-93, 1983.

13. Meldrum DR, Chang RJ, Lu J, Vale W, Rivier J, Judd HL. "Medical oophorectomy" using a long-acting GnRH agonist-- A possible new approach to the treatment of endometriosis. J. Clin. Endocr. Metab. 54:1081-1083, 1982.

14. Chang RJ, Laufer LR, Meldrum DR, Defazio J, Lu JK, Vale WW, Rivier JE and Judd HL. Steroid secretion in polycystic ovarian disease after ovarian suppression by a long-acting gonadotropin releasing hormone agonist. J. Clin. Endocr. Metab. 56:897-903, 1983.

15. Borgmann V, Hardt W, Schmidt-Gollwitzer M, Adenauer H, Nagel R. Sustained suppression of testosterone production by the luteinizing hormone-releasing hormone agonist buserelin in patients with advanced prostate carcinoma. A new therapeutic approach? Lancet 1:1097-1099, 1982.

16. Klijn JGM and deJong FH. Treatment with LHRH analogue (buserelin) in pre-menopausal patients with metastatic breast cancer. Lancet 1:1213-1216, 1982.

17. Filicori M, Hall DA, Loughlin JS, Rivier J, Vale W and Crowley WF. A conservative approach to the management of uterine leiomyoma: Pituitary desensitization by a luteinizint hormone releasing hormone analogue. Am. J. Obstet. Gynecol. 147:726-727, 1983.

Endocrinology
F. Labrie, L. Proulx, eds.

INTENSIVE TREATMENT OF INSULIN-DEPENDENT DIABETES: HOW AND WHY

WILLIAM V. TAMBORLANE and STEPHANIE A. AMIEL

Departments of Pediatrics, Internal Medicine and the Clinical Research Centers, Yale University School of Medicine, New Haven, CT.

It has long been recognized that normal or near-normal glucose control is rarely observed in Type 1 diabetic patients with conventional once or twice daily insulin injections, adjusted according to urine and occasional blood glucose determinations. Indeed, the inaccuracy of urine glucose measurements to reflect glycemic excursions made the pursuit of stringent therapeutic goals potentially dangerous. However, recent advances in self-blood glucose monitoring and insulin delivery have made it feasible to achieve and maintain striking improvements in glucose regulation for prolonged periods of time.

PHYSIOLOGIC INSULIN DELIVERY SYSTEMS

In non-diabetics insulin release can be roughly divided into two major components: basal secretion between meals and during the night and augmented secretion with each meal. Basal secretion is important in restraining hepatic glucose production in the fasting state and may also play an important role in priming the liver for prandial bursts of insulin secretion. In addition, basal insulin requirements appear to fluctuate during the night, reaching a nadir at 3:00 a.m. and increasing between 4:00 and 8:00 a.m. Augmented secretion is needed for the disposal of ingested carbohydrate by the liver as well as insulin-sensitive peripheral tissues.

It is often difficult to maintain adequate basal insulin levels with a single daily dose of intermediate-acting insulin. Underinsulinization in the basal state results in hepatic over production of glucose through the night and fasting hyperglycemia. Deficient basal insulin replacement also leads to marked post prandial hyperglycemia, since endogenous glucose production is not suppressed by feeding. While a second injection before supper can overcome some of these difficulties, problems with nocturnal hypoglycemia may then be exaggerated. With a presupper dose of intermediate-acting insulin, peak plasma insulin levels may be observed between 2:00 and 4:00 a.m., the time of lowest insulin requirements. Furthermore, until recently few patients received rapid-acting insulin when they most needed it - with each meal.

Intensive treatment strategies employ insulin delivery systems designed to mimic more clearly normal insulin secretory patterns than is possible with conventional treatment regimens. In a multiple daily injection (MDI) program, long-acting insulin (ultralente) is usually given either in single or divided doses to stimulate basal insulin secretion and rapid-acting insulin is given prior to each meal. Finer tuning can be accomplished with continuous subcutaneous insulin infusion (CSII) systems. With CSII, rapid-acting (regular) insulin alone is administered by a small, battery powered infusion pump. The most recent devices can be programmed to deliver basal replacement at a single or variable (depending on time of day) infusion rate. Additional insulin is administered via the pump as a bolus infusion over a few minutes at each meal time.

Both MDI and CSII require frequent patient self-monitoring of blood glucose levels for careful adjustment of basal and premeal insulin doses. The finger is pricked with a spring-operated lancet device and a drop of blood is placed on a glucose oxidase-impregnated reagent strip. The strip is read using either a color chart or a reflectance meter. The meter method frees the patient from direct responsibility for interpretation of results and may be slightly more accurate. The chart method is often more convenient.

EFFECTS OF INTENSIVE TREATMENT OF TYPE I DIABETES

CSII and MDI have proven to be effective means to achieve marked reductions in blood glucose for prolonged periods (1-3). Lowering blood glucose levels with intensive treatment has been associated with correction of a variety of metabolic abnormalities which characterize poorly controlled diabetes and which may play an important role in the development of diabetic complications (Table 1). In addition, intensive treatment has been shown to increase nerve conduction velocity (4) and reduce vitreous fluorescein leakage (5), microalbaminuria (6) and capillary basement membrane thickness (7), abnormalities which may represent preclinical manifestations of microangiopathy and neuropathy. Improved metabolic control in adolescent diabetics is often accompanied by a sharp acceleration of growth velocity (8). Patients have also reported a number of subjective benefits from having more control of their diabetes. They frequently report a general sense of increased well-being, decreased depression, increased control over life events and a better attitude concerning their disease.

On the other hand, intensive insulin treatment is not without risks. The major risk of MDI and CSII is hypoglycemia. The major safeguard against this problem is frequent blood glucose monitoring. One of the objectives of self-monitoring is to detect asymptomatic hypoglycemia so that insulin doses can be adjusted before a serious hypoglycemic episode occurs. Occasional nocturnal sampling (3:00 a.m.) may be required.

TABLE I

EFFECTS OF INTENSIVE TREATMENT OF TYPE I DIABETES

Metabolic

1. Reduces:
   - Total cholesterol and triglycerides
   - LDL cholesterol
   - Ketones and FFA
   - Fasting and post prandial branched chain amino acids
   - Urinary calcium and phosphate excretion . Glucagon, epinephrine and growth hormone
2. Increases:
   - HDL cholesterol
   - IGF-I
   - Insulin sensitivity

Functional

1. Reduces:
   - Vitreous flurescein leakage
   - Microalbuminuria
2. Increases nerve conduction velocity

Anatomic:

1. Reduces muscle capillary basement membrane width
2. Increases growth velocity (adolescents)

MICROANGROPATHY

It had been hoped that long-term utilization of MDI and CSII would permit resolution of the question of the role of hyperglycemia in the pathogenesis of the vascular complications of diabetes. Unfortunately, this issue remains unresolved. Two small, short-term clinical trials have failed to demonstrate a beneficial effect of CSII on established retinopathy. In the Kroc (9) and Steno (10) Studies, Type 1 diabetic patients with non-proliferative (background) retinopathy were randomly assigned to CSII or unchanged conventional treatment. CSII-treated patients achieved and maintained significantly lower blood glucose and glycosylated hemoglobin levels. Despite improved diabetic control for 8-12 months, CSII did not slow the progression of established retinopathy. Indeed, the frequency of deterioration tended to be greatest in the CSII treatment group in both studies.

In both the Kroc and Steno Studies, the new lesions which accounted for the progression of retinopathy consisted mostly of soft exudates. Soft exudates are thought to represent microinfarcts of the nerve fiber layer. It is concievable that the metabolic improvement induced by CSII reduces retinal perfusion causing infarction of previously compromised areas. The loss of localized areas of the retina may simply be the price paid for preservation of normal retinal tissue. It should also be kept in mind that the long-term outcome may be quite different. A preliminary 2-year follow-up report by the Steno Group suggests that CSII treatment may lead to improvement in retinopathy after a more prolonged period of observation (11). Furthermore, it remains to be established whether intensive treatment regimens might prevent the development of retinopathy (or nephropathy), if initiated early in the course of the disease. The Diabetes Control and Complications Trial (DCCT) sponsored by the National Institutes of Health has been undertaken to answer these critically important questions.

ACKNOWLEDGEMENT

We are indebted to Sonja Kornienko for her expert assistance in the preparation of the manuscript.

REFERENCES

1. Tamborlane WV, Sherwin RS, Genel M, Felig P (1980) Am J Med 68:190
2. Champion MC, Shephard GAA, Rodger NW, Dupre J (1980) Diabetes 29:206
3. Peterson CM, Jones R, Dupuis A, Levine B, Bernstein R, O'Shea M (1979) Diabetes Care 2:329
4. Pietri A, Ehle AL, Raskin P (1980) Diabetes 29:668
5. White NH, Waltman SR, Krupin T, Santiago J (1982) Diabetes 31:80
6. Viberti GC, Pickup JC, Jarrett RJ, Keen H (1979) N Engl J Med 300:638
7. Raskin P, Pietri AO, Unger R, Shannon WA (1983) N Engl J Med 309:1546
8. Rudolf MCJ, Sherwin RS, Markowitz R, Bates SE, Genel M, Hochstadt J, Tamborlane WV (1982) J Pediatr 101:333
9. Kroc Collaborative Study Group (1983) Diabetes 32 (suppl 1): 37
10. Lauritzen T, Steno Study Group (1983) Lancet 1:200
11. Lauritzen T, The Steno Study Group (1983) Lancet 1:1445

© 1984 Elsevier Science Publishers B.V.
Endocrinology
F. Labrie, L. Proulx, eds.

CLINICAL AND THERAPEUTIC ASPECTS OF HYPERPROLACTINAEMIA

MICHAEL BESSER
Department of Endocrinology, St. Bartholomew's Hospital, London, EC1A 7BE, UK.

In the 15 years since the establishment of prolactin as a distinct human pituitary hormone, hyperprolactinaemia has become widely recognised as a frequent cause of reproductive dysfunction in women and rather less commonly of impotence in men. The availability of potent medical means of lowering pathologically elevated prolactin levels using the dopamine agonists related to the ergot alkaloids has not only provided an efficient, highly successful method for reversing the hypogonadism associated with hyperprolactinaemia but also has led to a medical means of shrinking many pituitary tumours.

Clinical features and causes of hyperprolactinaemia

The clinical features of the hyperprolactinaemic syndromes are now well recognised. Galactorrhoea is commonly found in only a minority of patients, be they men or women; most authors quote an incidence of about 30%. In women breast atrophy is not a feature despite the occurrence of oestrogen deficiency in some patients. In men the breast often appears normal and gynaecomastia is minimal, if present at all. Often there is a fat accumulation in the breast. The classic menstrual disorder is amenorrhoea and this is more likely to occur when a pituitary tumour is clearly demonstrable and particularly when there is an abnormality of the pituitary fossa on the plain skull film. However, even when pituitary tumours can clearly be demonstrated, oligomenorrhoea is often seen and occasionally regular menstruation with infertility due to anovulation or a deficient luteal phase. Men frequently have no features of hypogonadism on examination but simply complain of relative or absolute impotence, with lowering of libido.

The majority of patients appear to have either pituitary tumours or hypothalamic and pituitary stalk lesions. Small tumours of the hypothalamus such as gliomas and craniopharyngiomas may be clinically and radiologically indistinguishable from pituitary tumours and if the hyperprolactinaemia is treated with bromocriptine amenorrhoea and other features of hypogonadism as well as galactorrhoea may disappear and normal gonadal function ensue just as if there were a primary pituitary tumour secreting prolactin. Care must be taken to avoid diagnosing such patients as having pituitary tumours since such masses do not shrink under dopamine agonist therapy. Such cases are examples of "pseudoprolactinoma".

Prolactinomas - pituitary tumours secreting prolactin - are the most common type of pituitary adenoma; they probably constitute at least 40% of tumours previously described as "functionless". High resolution CT scanning, using iv contrast, and reformation in two planes, is usually able to identify accurately and clearly a pituitary tumour.

CLINICAL MANAGEMENT OF PROLACTINOMAS AND IDIOPATHIC HYPERPROLACTINAEMIA

While medical treatment clearly is the treatment of choice for patients in whom no pituitary lesion can be demonstrated, the so-called "idiopathic" cases, the optimal treatment of demonstrable prolactinomas remains controversial. While medical treatment is highly effective, transsphenoidal hypophysectomy has in the past been the preferred primary treatment in some centres, but surgical cure of the hyperprolactinaemia is reported in only 40 - 80% of cases and recurrence of hyperprolactinaemia is said to occur in half of these (1,2).

Medical management of small prolactinomas

Dopamine agonist therapy in patients with microadenomas (tumours smaller than 1cm in maximum diameter), small macroadenomas (lesions larger than 1cm but not producing any mass effects), and idiopathic cases, is highly successful in lowering the elevated prolactin levels and restoring gonadal function to normal both in men and in women. Most experience in the use of dopamine agonist ergot related drugs has been with bromocriptine. Return of circulating prolactin levels to the normal range occurs in over 90% of patients irrespective of the degree of elevation of prolactin before treatment.

Usually within 2 months of the return of regular menstruation, ovulation and adequacy of the luteal phase is encountered and galactorrhoea disappears. In men, potency returns to normal and if reduced, the seminal volume also is normalised. Sperm concentrations do not usually change. The dose of bromocriptine usually required lies between 5 and 10mg per day although occasionally maximum suppression of prolactin can only be achieved with doses of up to 40mg/day. This drug has been shown to directly inhibit secretion by the pituitary lactotrophs through activation of dopamine receptors on the tumour and its action is blocked by dopamine antagonists.

Medical management of patients with large prolactinomas

Recently it has become clear that not only are elevated circulating prolactin levels returned to normal by dopamine agonist therapy but in at least two thirds of patients with large tumours there is clear evidence that the tumour mass shrinks concomitantly. There is no consistent evidence that functionless pituitary tumours shrink under this treatment, whether they are associated with hyperprolactinaemia (pseudoprolactinomas) or not. Conventional doses of bromocriptine, sufficient to lower prolactin levels to normal, or equivalent doses of other dopamine agonists are all that is required. Neighbourhood compressive features resolve as the tumour shrinks, and often patients report symptomatic changes within 48 - 72 hours. Objective evidence of tumour shrinkage such as obtained from CT scanning can be seen within 10 - 14 days although improvement may not be seen for 3 or 4 weeks. If there is no clinical or radiological evidence of tumour shrinkage by 3 months we then refer the patient for surgery. Once the tumour has shrunk back into the fossa, definitive ablative therapy can be pursued. In addition to reduction of the tumour mass, in about half of the patients the accompanying hypopituitarism resolves. With macroadenomas surgery is infrequently successful in lowering prolactin to normal even transiently and in the majority of patients recurrence occurs (1,2).

RADIOTHERAPY IN CONJUNCTION WITH DOPAMINE AGONISTS

The use of bromocriptine alone only rarely results in permanent lowering of prolactin levels if treatment is stopped. Clearly there is a case for some additional treatment given in conjunction with dopamine agonist therapy to provide longterm control. Although originally introduced to prevent prolactinoma enlargement during pregnancy (3), we have now shown that modern megavoltage radiotherapy is safe and effective both in preventing tumour growth and in producing a gradual reduction of circulating prolactin levels to normal (3,4). Interim dopamine agonist therapy is used in the patients until prolactin levels return to the normal range. The ovulation rate, as indicated by circulating progesterone concentrations, is 97% and the successful conception rate 86% using this combination of radiotherapy and interim dopamine agonist therapy.

MANAGEMENT OF PATIENTS WITH PROLACTINOMAS DURING PREGNANCY

The normal pituitary gland and tumours enlarge during pregnancy. The risk of tumour enlargement in patients with microadenoma is small, probably of the order of 1%, but the incidence in patients with macroprolactinomas is considerably higher. The reported incidence varies between 10 - 25%. Careful radiotherapy prevents tumour enlargement without adversely affecting fertility. Since prolactin levels fall only slowly after such therapy, despite its protective effect on tumour growth during pregnancy, interim dopamine agonist therapy is used following the radiotherapy and on this regimen successful conception is achieved (4). Should the patient present with evidence of tumour growth in pregnancy, the clear treatment of choice is to start dopamine agonist therapy forthwith. Oestrogen-induced tumour growth is particularly susceptible to shrinkage on bromocriptine at conventional dosage. Bromocriptine is then continued throughout the pregnancy and radiotherapy is given in the puerperium.

CONCLUSIONS

In the majority of patients who have hyperprolactinaemia due to a pituitary cause, the mammotroph cells of evident tumours or in the apparently simply hyperplastic gland, retain dopamine receptors, activation of which lowers prolactin levels to normal. Bromocriptine and similar ergot related dopamine agonist drugs therefore restore prolactin levels to normal; in association with this, gonadal function returns rapidly to normal both in males and females. If bromocriptine is stopped, however, prolactin levels usually rise once more to the pretreatment levels. On dopamine agonist therapy the mass of the pituitary tumour shrinks in at least two thirds of patients, even if these tumours are massive and extend into the neighbouring structures outside the pituitary fossa. With the shrinkage of the tumour, resolution of the neighbourhood compressive syndromes is seen and in many patients the hypopituitarism resolves. The combination of modern megavoltage radiotherapy with interim dopamine agonist therapy is a highly effective way of providing immediate control of the clinical hyperprolactinaemic syndrome. The radiotherapy provides a gradual reduction in prolactin levels so that dopamine agonist therapy may eventually be stopped. Hypopituitarism is a rare association of the radiotherapy; if it does occur, except for growth hormone deficiency which is seen early but is unimportant, it is not seen until many years after the treatment and after the passage of sufficient time to allow successful completion of planned families and towards the end of the period of normal fertility. In patients without evidence of pituitary tumour or who have microadenomas, dopamine agonist therapy alone appears to be the treatment of choice.

REFERENCES

1. Randall RV, Laws ER, Abboud CF, Ebersold MJ, Kao PC, Scheithauer BW 1983 Mayo Clin Proc 58: 108-121
2. Serri O, Rasio E, Beauregard H, Hardy J, Somma M 1983 N Engl J Med 309: 280-283
3. Thorner MO, Besser GM, Jones A, Dacie J, Jones AE 1975 Brit Med J 4: 694-697
4. Grossman A, Cohen BL, Charlesworth M, Plowman PN, Rees LH, Wass JAH, Jones AE, Besser GM 1984 Brit Med J 288: 1105-1109

Endocrinology
F. Labrie, L. Proulx, eds.

HIRSUTISM
FROM PHYSIOPATHOLOGY TO A STRATEGY FOR DIAGNOSIS AND TREATMENT

F. KUTTENN, M. VINCENS, I. MOWSZOWICZ, F. WRIGHT and P. MAUVAIS-JARVIS

Hirsutism in women may be defined as excessive hair growth in anatomical sites where such growth is considered to be a secondary male characteristic. It is related to an increased activity of the androgen-dependent structure = the pilosebaceous follicle.

The skin is a target-organ for androgens since it contains specific enzyme(s) and receptor(s) for androgen action. The skin is capable of transforming testosterone (T) into DHT due to the 5α-reductase present in the microsomes (24). Human skin can also convert weak androgens : dehydroepiandrosterone and especially androstenedione (A) into T, and then DHT. DHT either binds its receptor (7,20) and the DHT-receptor complex is fixed to the chromatin to trigger specific androgen action, or DHT may be converted into 3α- and 3β-androstanediols (diols) (4,10,16,17) the end-products of the 'active' androgen metabolism. They pass into the circulation and are then excreted in the urine (18).

Hirsutism can therefore have 2 origins (i) an androgen overproduction by the ovaries or the adrenal glands, (ii) an hypersensitivity of the skin to androgens with an increased utilization of these androgens even circulating at a normal level. This is what we called 'Idiopathic Hirsutism' (IH).

The first possibility has been extensively reviewed (2,8,10). The raised metabolic clearance rate of T due to its increased metabolism into DHT and 3α-diol in extra hepatic tissues supports the second possibility (9,10,16). A low concentration of TeBG may facilitate the increased androgen metabolism. However, an intracellular mechanism has been put forth with the identification of a very high (male-type) 5α-reductase activity in skin from hirsute patients with normal plasma androgens (10). Moreover it is in this IH group without obvious sign of androgen overproduction that this activity is the highest. Whether this increased 5α-reductase activity is primary or has been induced by a temporary androgen overproduction during the fetal life or at puberty remains to be determined. In contrast to 5α-reductase, the androgen binding capacity is found similar in the skin of hirsute patients and normal men and women

(21), and without any difference in the different types of hirsutism. An increased androgen binding cannot be held responsible for skin hypersensitivity and the receptor assay is therefore of no value to evaluate hypersensitivity to androgens.

Plasma levels of T and A are good indexes of Androgen Production, whereas the Utilization of Androgens by the skin can be evaluated in two ways = directly by the *in vitro* measurement of T 5α-reductase capacity in the skin (10), or indirectly by the assay of plasma-or-urine 3α-diol glucuronide (6,26).

Several groups have proposed the assay of free T in the evaluation of hirsutism, arguing that free T is the key to androgen action. Even if physiopathologically interesting, free T shows a very wide range without noticeable correlation with either total plasma androgens or intensity of hirsutism (1,15). It cannot give any idea of the final target cell receptivity which is the ultimate and determining factor of androgen-induced hair growth (3,10,12,14,15). Lastly, free T remains of little value in orienting the etiologic diagnosis and of no help in the choice of treatment.

Even the active intracellular androgen DHT when assayed in plasma, provides little information (10,15). In fact, the active DHT, that which is produced in target cells from the 5α-reduction of T, does not enter the blood for the most part, except after being metabolized into diols (16).

DIAGNOSTIC STRATEGY

The etiologic diagnosis of hirsutism should be made through a very comprehensive clinical inquiry, all the steps of which are important. The history of the patient (menstrual cycles, family antecedents, therapy ?) and the clinical examination (degree of hyperandrogeny, enlarged ovaries) already orient the diagnosis towards an ovarian or an adrenal origin. And the most important biological investigation is the plasma T assay, which, alone, has irreplaceable diagnostic value (19).

1. If plasma T is normal, and the menstrual cycle regular and ovulatory, it is 'idiopathic hirsutism'. High 5α-reductase activity in the skin and high plasma-or-urine 3α-diol glucuronide, contrasting with normal plasma T, would confirm the diagnosis.
2. Plasma T between 0.8 and 1.2 ng/ml, with long irregular cycles, enlarged ovaries, suggests the Polycystic Ovary Syndrome (PCO). Plasma A is higher than 2.5 ng/ml. If LH is high and dramatically

responds to LHRH, it is PCO type I. LH slightly above normal with a strong response to LHRH evokes PCO type II (25). In fact, the LHRH test is certainly more interesting for the physiopathologic understanding than necessary for the diagnosis of PCO.

3. Plasma T level higher than 1.5 ng/ml first suggests the existence of an ovarian or adrenal tumor, but two other diseases may be responsible for such a high T level : the exceptional ovarian hyperthecosis, and adrenal hyperplasia due to an enzymatic defect.

Uronephrogram with tomography, ultrasonography, scanning can help the diagnosis of an adrenal tumor. But coelioscopy, or even laparotomy, are of no help at all in ovarian tumor diagnosis because tumors can be very small. Finally, ovarian and adrenal venous catheterization with selective blood sampling for steroid assays, as described by Kirshner and Jacobs (8) is generally the most successful to localize the oversecretion and the tumor.

4. Late Adrenal Hyperplasia (LAH) due to an enzymatic deficiency is a cause of delayed onset of hirsutism.

Patients with adrenal hyperplasia are generally described as having a particular morphotype: short, android, with delayed puberty and long irregular cycles. In fact, plasma T level may be high ($\geqslant$ 1.2 ng/ml) but it shows a very wide range and is sometimes normal. Cortisol may be low, but is often normal. ACTH should be high but is also often normal. Even 17 OHP, the immediate precursor up-stream the enzymatic block, is not constantly elevated (3), however its dramatic increase after ACTH stimulation provides the diagnosis (23). Thanks to this test LAH has been diagnosed in 24 patients among 400 hirsute women examined in our department over the last 5 years (13). In fact, most of these 24 patients showed only clinical characteristics of 'IH' : isolated hirsutism, regular ovulatory menstrual cycles..

For the etiologic diagnosis, two biological investigations are therefore determinant : (1) the assay of plasma T which differentiates between overproduction of androgens or skin hypersensitivity to androgens, (2) the ACTH test, the only means to detect with certainty an adrenal enzymatic block.

TREATMENT

Because hirsutism results from either an androgen overproduction or from hypersensitivity of the skin to androgens, its treatment must therefore suppress the pathological processes involved in order to be effective. Androgen overproduction, if any, must be suppressed by surgery of ovarian or adrenal tumors, substitutive cortisol therapy in the case of adrenal hyperplasia due to an enzymatic defect, or inhibition of ovarian gonadotropin stimulation in the case of polycystic ovaries of hyperthecosis. Antiandrogens must be used as much as possible. They act on the target cell and inhibit the action of remaining circulating androgens. The anti-androgens currently used are estrogens, progesterone and anti-androgenic progestogens.

Estrogens act at 3 different levels : They have a negative feed-back effect on gonadotropin secretion and thus suppress the androgen ovarian secretion. They increase the synthesis of TeBG, thus reducing the amount of free circulating testosterone. They are competitive inhibitors of DHT binding to its receptor. As a consequence and used on a long term basis, estrogens also inhibit the androgen dependent enzyme 5α-reductase. They are used in association with progestogens in estrogen-progestogen 'pills'. This treatment is effective in ovarian hirsutism. It is often disappointing in idiopathic hirsutism. Estrogen-progestogen associations also have the contra-indications of synthetic estrogens - obesity, hypertension, diabetes, hyperlipidaemia.

Progesterone is a classic antiandrogen acting as a competitive inhibitor at both levels : 5α-reductase and binding to the receptor. However, due to its extensive hepatic metabolism when administered orally, it is essentially used by percutaneous administration and is therefore mainly a complementary treatment for the minor sign of hyperandrogeny - seborrhea, acne -associated with hirsutism.

Cyporoterone acetate (CPA) is a progestin and an antigonadotropic agent which inhibits ovarian androgen secretion. It is also a peripheral antiandrogen as a competitive inhibitor of DHT binding to its receptor. Its use in hirsutism has dramatically transformed the prognosis of this disease.

Hammerstein has proposed an inversed sequential pill (CPA 100 mg/day from the 5th to the 14th day of the cycle associated with Ethinyl-estradiol (EE) 50 μg from the 5th to the 25th day). This treatment still has the contra-indications of synthetic estrogens (5). Another combination, the 'Diane' pill, associates 50 μg EE with only 2 mg CPA, which is actually too low a dosage to be efficient in terms of antiandrogenic, antigonadotropic action, as well as progestogen activity to counteract the effect of 50 μg EE.

We have proposed to administer CPA in moderate sequential doses (50 mg x 21 days per cycle) associated with percutaneous natural 17β -estradiol (E_2 perc.) (21,22). At this dose, CPA suppresses androgen ovarian secretion and peripheral effects as shown by dramatic decreases in plasma T, A, LH, E_2 and the constant absence of plasma P. CPA has a contraceptive effect due to its antigonadotropic action as well as to its luteomimetic action on cervical mucus and endometrium. E_2 perc. has no antigonadotropic effect, it just provides a physiologic estrogen input to maintain target organ eutrophy and regular bleeding without the metabolic side-effects of orally administered synthetic estrogens.

In the past 6 years, 350 hirsute patients have been treated in our department with CPA + E_2 perc. for 3-year periods. Clinical results are spectacular: seborrhea and acne decrease dramatically within one month of treatment, decrease in hirsutism appears after 3 months. By the end of 9 months of treatment, all patients declare 'being transformed'. After 20 months, they no longer have hirsutism.

The administration of cyproterone acetate in moderate sequential doses therefore provides considerable efficiency without side effects. Its association with percutaneously administered estradiol is another guarantee of metabolic safety. The rapid and dramatic improvement in hirsutism makes this therapy a first choice method in the treatment not only of hirsute women with contra-indication to synthetic estrogens but also in other cases of hirsutism.

REFERENCES

1. Andre CM, James VHT (1974) Plasma androgens in idiopathic hirsutism. Steroids 24:295
2. Bardin CW, Lipsett MB (1976) Testosterone and androstenedione blood production rates in normal women and women with idiopathic hirsutism or polycystic ovaries. J Clin Invest 46:891
3. Bouchard Ph, Kuttenn F, Mowszowicz I, Schaison G, Raux-Eurin MC, Mauvais-Jarvis P (1981) Congenital adrenal hyperplasia due to partial 21 hydroxylase deficiency. A study of five cases. Acta Endocrinol (Copenh) 96:107
4. Gomez EC, Hsia SL, Frost P (1972) Cutaneous transformation of testosterone into 5α-androstane-3β-diol. J Clin Endocrinol Metab 34:417
5. Hammerstein J, Meckies J, Leo-Rossberg I, Moltz L, Zielke F (1975) Use of cyproterone acetate (CPA) in the treatment of acne, hirsutism and virilism. J Steroid Biochem 6:827
6. Horton R, Hawks D, Lobo R (1982) 3α, 17β-androstanediol glucuronide in plasma. A marker of androgen action in idiopathic hirsutism. J Clin Invest 69:1203.

7. Keenan BS, Meyer WJ III, Hadjian AJ, Migeon CT (1975) Androgen receptor in human skin fibroblasts: characterization of a specific 17β-hydroxy-5α-androstan-3-one protein complex in cell sonicates and nuclei. Steroids 25:535

8. Kirschner MA, Jacobs JB (1971) Combined ovarian and adrenal vein catheterization to determine the site(s) of androgen overproduction in hirsute women. J Clin Endocrinol Metab 33:199

9. Kirschner MA, Bardin CW (1972) Androgen production and metabolism in normal and virilized women. Metabolism 21:667

10. Kuttenn F, Mowszowicz I, Schaison G, Mauvais-Jarvis P (1977) Androgen production and skin metabolism in hirsutism. J Endocrinol 75:83

11. Kuttenn F, Rigaud C, Wright F, Mauvais-Jarvis P (1980) Treatment of hirsutism by oral cyproterone acetate and percutaneous oestradiol. J Clin Endocrinol Metab 51:1107

12. Kuttenn F, Mowszowicz I, Mauvais-Jarvis P (1980) Androgen metabolism in human skin. In: Mauvais-Jarvis et al (eds) Percutaneous absorption of steroids. Acad. Press, New York, p 99

13. Kuttenn F, Coullin Ph, Girard F, Billaud L, Mowszowicz I, Mauvais-Jarvis P Late onset adrenal hyperplasia (LAH): Endocrinological and HLA studies in 24 families. Submitted for publication

14. Leichter SB, Jacobs LS (1976) Normal gestation and diminished androgen responsiveness in an untreated patient with 21 hydroxylase deficiency. J Clin Endocrinol Metab 42:575

15. Lobo RA, Goebbelsmann U, Horton R (1983) Evidence for the importance of peripheral tissue events in the development of hirsutism in polycystic ovary syndrome. J Clin Endocrinol Metab 57:393

16. Mahoudeau JA, Bardin CW, Lipsett MB (1971) The metabolic clearance rate and origin of plasma dihydrotestosterone in man and its conversion to the 5α-androstanediols. J Clin Invest 50:1338

17. Mauvais-Jarvis P, Bercovici JP, Crepy O, Gauthier F (1970) Studies on testosterone metabolism in subjects with testicular feminization syndrome. J Clin Invest 49:31

18. Mauvais-Jarvis P, Charransol G, Bobas-Masson F (1973) Simultaneous determination of urinary androstanediol and testosterone as an evaluation of human androgenicity. J Clin Endocrinol Metab 38:142

19. Mauvais-Jarvis P, Kuttenn F, Mowszowicz I (1981) Hirsutism. In: Monographs on Endocrinology. Springer Verlage, New York

20. Mowszowicz I, Riahi M, Wright F, Bouchard Ph, Kuttenn F, Mauvais-Jarvis P (1981) Androgen receptor in human skin cytosol. J Clin Endocrinol Metab 52:338

21. Mowszowicz I, Melanitou E, Doukani A, Wright F, Kuttenn F, Mauvais-Jarvis P (1983) Androgen binding capacity and 5α-reductase activity in pubic skin fibroblasts from hirsute patients. J Clin Endocrinol Metabol 56:1209

22. Mowszowicz I, Wright F, Vincens M, Rigaud C, Nahoul K, Mavier Ph, Guillemand S, Kuttenn F, Mauvais-Jarvis P (1984) Androgen metabolism in hirsute patients treated with cyproterone acetate. J Steroid Biochem 20:757

23. Pham-Huu-Trung MT, Gourmelen M, Girard F (1973) The simultaneous assay of cortisol and 17α-OHprogesterone in the plasma of patients with congenital adrenal hyperplasia. Acta Endocrinol (Copenh) 74:316

24. Voigt W, Fernandez EP, Hsia SL (1970) Transformation of testosterone into 17β-hydroxy-5α-androstan-3-one by microsomal preparations of human skin. J Biol Chem 245:5594

25. Rebar R, Judd HL, Yen SSC (1976) Characterization of the inappropriate gonadotrophic secretion in polycystic ovary syndrome. J Clin Invest 57:1320

26. Wright F, Mowszowicz I, Mauvais-Jarvis P (1978) Urinary 5α-androstane-3α, 17β-diol radioimmunoassay : a new clinical evaluation. J Clin Endocrinol Metab 47:850

Endocrinology
F. Labrie, L. Proulx, eds.

CLINICAL USEFULNESS OF VITAMIN D METABOLITE ASSAYS

ROGER BOUILLON

Laboratorium experimentele geneeskunde, Rega Instituut,
Minderbroedersstraat 10, B-3000 Leuven, Belgium

A normal calcium and bone metabolism requires the regular supply and an intact metabolism of vitamin D. The more detailed knowledge about the different vitamin D metabolites has already introduced their measurement in clinical medicine. The methodology for vitamin D metabolite assays became better established (1,2) and is summarized in table 1.

TABLE 1: AVAILABILITY AND CLINICAL USEFULNESS OF ASSAY METHODOLOGY FOR VITAMIN D METABOLITES

	VITAMIN D_3 OR D_2	$25\text{-}OHD_{2/3}$	$1,25\text{-}(OH)_2D$	$24,25\text{-}(OH)_2D$
SPECIFIC BIOASSAY	NO	±	YES	NO
ABSORPTIOMETRIC ASSAY AFTER HPLC	YES*	YES	NO	NO
MASS FRAGMENTOGRAPHIC ASSAY	YES	YES	YES	YES
CPB ASSAY USING DBP	(YES)	YES*	NO	YES
USING NATURAL RECEPTORS	NO	NO	YES*	-
RADIOIMMUNOASSAY	(YES)	YES	YES*	(YES)*
CLINICAL USEFULNESS	LOW	HIGH	HIGH	UNKNOWN

* PREFERRED METHOD

The concentration of *vitamin D_3* in normal serum is usually low (a few nanograms/ml) and increases only transienly after the ingestion of relatively large (pharmaceutical) amounts or after intensive UV irradiation. Due to its short serum half-life it is not a reliable estimate of steady state vitamin D nutrition and thus represents only an indicator of very recent access to vitamin D_3. Few clinical data have been accumulated with regard to its concentration in disease states but it seems unlikely to become an important clinical tool.

TABLE 2: SUMMARY OF THE SITUATIONS ASSOCIATED WITH INCREASED OR DECREASED CONCENTRATION OF VITAMIN D METABOLITES

VITAMIN D ↓

Decreased	Increased
? Vitamin D deficiency ? anefric patients	recent exposure to UV light recent oral intake of D

25-OH D ↓

Decreased	Increased
Privatational Rickets/ osteomalacia Malabsorption of short bowel S Biliary cirrhosis Anticonvulsant therapy Nephrotic syndrome RISK GROUPS: (1) infants born in winter (2) children and women of immigrants in WE (3) elderly population	Hypervitaminosis D

$1,25-(OH)_2D_3$

Decreased	Increased
substrate deficiency Privatational Rickets Intestinal Malabsorption Parenteral Nutrition Nephrotic Syndrome	*substrate excess*
enzyme deficiency *inborn*: Vit.D-dependent rickets *organic*: renal insufficiency *functional*: hypoparathyroidism pseudohypoparathyroidism tumoral osteomalacia hypomagnesemia tumoral hypercalcemia hyperthyroidism Addison's disease insulin deficiency	*enzyme excess* *functional*: hyperparathyroidism hypothyroidism glycocorticoid excess? acromegaly sarcoidosis pregnancy
DBP deficiency: fetal life nephrotic syndrome liver cirrhosis	*DBP excess*: estrogens *end organ resistance* true vitamin D resistance (II) osteopetrosis
? old age +/- osteoporosis ? rhabdomyolysis ? X-linked hypophosphatemia	? idiopathic hypercalciuria ? tumoral calcinosis

TABLE 3: USEFULNESS OF VITAMIN D ASSAY IN THE DIFFERENTIAL DIAGNOSIS OF RICKETS

	Ca	P	25-OHD	24,25-$(OH)_2D$	1,25-$(OH)_2D$	PTH
Vitamin D-deficient rickets	N-↓	↓	↓↓	↓↓	↓ N ↑	↑
Vitamin D-dependent rickets (I)	↓	↓	N	N	↓	↑
True vitamin D resistance (II)	↓	↓	N	↓-N	↑↑	↑
Calcium-deficient rickets	↓	↓	N	N	↑	↑
Phosphate-deficient rickets	N	↓↓	N	N	N (↓)	N

TABLE 4: USEFULNESS OF VITAMIN D ASSAYS IN THE DIFFERENTIAL DIAGNOSIS OF HYPERCALCEMIA

	25-OHD	1,25-$(OH)_2D$	PTH
1. Primary Hyperparathyroidism	N	↑	↑
2. Vitamin D intoxication	↑↑	N or ↓	↓
3. Pseudohyperparathyroidism (tumoral hypercalcemia)	N	(↓)	↓
GRANULOMATOUS DISEASES			
4. Sarcoidosis	N	↑	↓
5. Coccidioimycosis			
PRIMARY INVOLVEMENT OF BONE RESORPTION			
6. Bone Metastases or hematological cancers			
7. Hyperthyroidism	N	↓	↓
8. M. Addison			
9. Immobilisation + increased bone turnover			
10. Milk-alkali Syndrome	N	?	?
11. Familial hypocalciuric or benign hypercalcemia	N	N	N

Vitamin D_2 or D_3 are rapidly hydroxylated to *25-hydroxyvitamin D* (25-OHD) without much feed-back regulation and then circulates in blood with a prolonged half-life (2-3 weeks), tightly bound to the specific vitamin D-binding protein (DBP). 25-OHD, therefore, becomes the ideal parameter to evaluate the body reserve of vitamin D. Its serum concentration in a healthy population depends on many factors, but especially on exposure to UV light and to a lesser extend also on nutritional intake. Geography (lattitude), season, work (in-door versus out-door) and cultural habits, are thus of primary importance. Increased skin pigmentation also decreases the efficacy of vitamin D_3 synthesis and thus indirectly decreases the 25-OHD concentration as is evident by comparing its concentration in white and black populations of North America and in natives and immigrants in Western Europe. Abnormally high 25-$(OH)_2$D concentrations, above 100 ng/ml, are associated with vitamin D toxicity and only occur after ingestion of pharmaceutical amounts of vitamin D (Table 2).

Classical vitamin D-deficient rickets or osteomalacia are only found in patients with 25-OHD levels below 5-6 ng/ml. Since, however, such bone lesion only develop after a very prolonged period of vitamin D deficiency it should not be unexpected to find such low 25-OHD level in patients without evident bone disease. These situations can be defined as subclinical vitamin D deficiency and can be compared with a state of iron deficiency before the development of clinical anemia. A detailed list of diseases or risk situations for vitamin D deficiency is given in table 2. Adequate prevention of vitamin D deficiency in infants has been introduced long before measurements of 25-OHD could demonstrate this necessity. The major risk group for 25-OHD deficiency is now the sick or institutionalized elderly population which frequently suffer from osteopenia and bone fractures and to which this vitamin D deficiency may contribute.

The concentration of the most active form of vitamin D, *1,25-$(OH)_2$D* varies according to calcium and phosphorus intake and is feed-back regulated by a number of hormones (2). Abnormally high or low concentrations are found in many disorders (table 2), which frequently have a disturbed parathyroid hormone secretion as intermediate mechanism. The total 1,25-$(OH)_2$D concentration in serum also depend on the concentration of its transport protein which decreases during liver and kidney diseases but increases during estrogen treatment or pregnancy. The clinical usefulness of this measurement is largely found in the differential diagnosis of rickets and hypercalcemia (table 3 and 4). Whether the measurement of the other vitamin D metabolites can contribute to clinical medicine awaits further research.

1. Haddad JG (1983) In: Bikle DD (eds) Assay of calcium-regulating hormones. Springer Verlag, New York, pp 49-63

2. Bouillon R, Van Baelen H, De Moor P (1980) J Steroid Biochem 13:1029-1034

Endocrinology
F. Labrie, L. Proulx, eds.

DIAGNOSIS AND TREATMENT OF THE SOLITARY THYROID NODULE

YOSHIHIDE FUJIMOTO
Department of Endocrine Surgery, Tokyo Women's Medical College, Tokyo (Japan)

The frequency of the solitary thyroid nodule in adults has been estimated to range from 1 to 5%. The incidence of thyroid carcinoma was estimated as 3.7 cases per 100,000 individuals in the United States. Population survey on the prevalence of thyroid carcinoma carried out in a non-endemic area, Japan, over 6 years revealed a rate of as high as 1 per 1,000 individuals (1).

In the evaluation of thyroid nodules, the most common diagnostic problem concerns whether it is malignant or not. A history of exposure to external irradiation, progressive enlargement of the nodule and recent onset of horseness, all indicate increased possibility of thyroid malignancy. The careful physical examination remains a fundamental procedure. Patient's age, sex and race are also considered.

An effective employment of specific diagnostic procedures is important. In our experience over 25 years, we have developed a practical approach, in which physical examination, ultrasound scanning and roentgenography of the neck are all we need for an evaluation of a majority of nodular thyroid lesions, except for follicular carcinoma.

We have been using ultrasonography since 1961 (2). The new equipment recently developed with high quality can provide us not only with the differentiation between cystic and solid nodules, but also with fine morphological details of thyroid lesions. Ultrasonography has one more advantage: it can determine whether the actual lesion is uninodular or multinodular.

As to the roentgenographic examination, we performed a fundamental study on the evaluation of usefulness and the technical problems, using surgical specimens resected from 200 patients (100 benign and 100 malignant tumors), and using a phantom, respectively, in 1970 (3,4). We found that psammomatous calcification and some other figures of calcific deposits indicated not only the presence of thyroid cancer but also biological behavior of the malignant neoplasms. Like other diagnostic procedures, these two methods need a great deal of experience in both performing the procedure and reading of the findings obtained.

Currently a fine needle aspiration biopsy cytology (ABC) is the most high-lighted as a quickly performable, cost-effective, noninvasive method and also as a tool giving direct information on the underlying pathology. It surely is true when highly trained technicians are available for the aspiration, processing and reading of cytology. ABC is useful particularly in the diagnosis of papillary carcinoma and anaplastic carcinoma. The results in our series are shown in Figure 1.

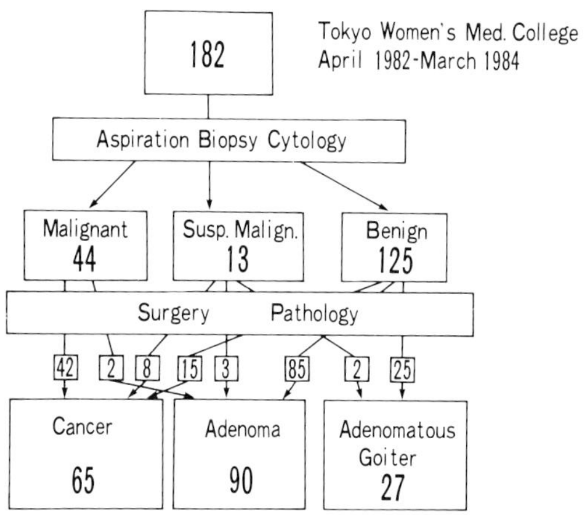

Fig. 1. Accuracy of ABC diagnosis as compared with pathological diagnosis

Thyroid scintigraphy appears to have been overutilized. I-123 or Tc-99m scan can detect a 'hot' nodule, although its frequency ranges only 2 to 5% of all solitary nodules in our country. Selection of patients for surgery, based on the finding of 'cold' nodule on Tc-99m scan and Tl-201 accumulation to the nodule, is simple, but the method is expensive and does not always correspond to the pathology of malignancy.

Diagnostic thyroid suppression therapy may be applied only for patients who have probable benign nodules.

We reviewed the results of our diagnostic ways carried out in 453 patients with nodular thyroid lesions who visited our clinic during the last two-year period. They were referred to our surgical clinic mostly by physicians, so the patients had nearly all already been selected in terms of indication for surgical treatment. The patients were classified into four groups according to clinical impression, based mostly on physical findings (Table 1). 'Malignant?' nodule means that mobility of a nodule is more or less limited and usually the nodule has an irregular surface. 'Benign?' nodule means a completely round and readily movable one. 'Adenomatous nodule?' is the one whose surface is not completely smooth or the shape is not completely round, but is readily movable.

TABLE 1

A REVIEW OF PREOPERATIVE DIAGNOSTIC PROCEDURES AND TREATMENT IN OUR SERIES OF 453 PATIENTS (2-year period)

	PHYSICAL EXAMINATION								
	BENIGN? 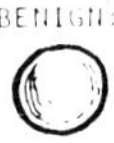		MALIGNANT? 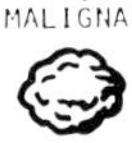		ADENOMATOUS NODULE ? 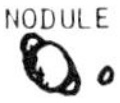		ADENOMATOUS GOITER ? 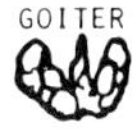		TOTAL
NO. OF PATIENTS	205		100		61		87		453
	CLINICAL AND LABORATORY EXAMINATIONS *ULTRASONOGRAPHY *SOFT TISSUE ROENTGENOGRAPHY OF THE NECK *ASPIRATION BIOPSY CYTOLOGY (SCINTICANNING WITH ^{99m}Tc, ^{201}Tl, ^{67}Ga)								
PREOPERATIVE SUSPICION	BEN.	MAL.	BEN.	MAL.	BEN.	MAL.	BEN.	MAL.	
	191	14	10	90	47	14	84	3	
CONSERVATIVE FOLLOW	48	0	6	2	20	1	72	0	149
REFUSE OF SURGICAL Rx	21	1	0	6	2	1	1	1	33
SURGERY OR OPEN BIOPSY									
ADENOMATOUS GOITER	12	0	0	4	16	2	11	1	46
CYSTIC NODULE	0	0	4	0	0	0	0	0	4
ADENOMA	105	7	0	7	7	0	0	0	126
PAPILLARY CA	0	4	0	52	1	7	0	0	64
FOLLICULAR CA	4	2	0	7	0	3	0	1	17
MEDULLARY CA	1	0	0	1	0	0	0	0	2
ANAPLASTIC CA	0	0	0	7	0	0	0	0	7
MALIG. LYMPHOMA	0	0	0	3	1	0	0	0	4
SUBACUTE THYROIDITIS	0	0	0	1	0	0	0	0	1

After the specific diagnostic procedures, the thyroid nodules were again classified as those suspected of being 'benign' and those suspected of being 'malignant'. Table 1 shows how accurate those preoperative suspicions were and how the patients were treated. As for the diagnosis, seven malignant tumours were preoperatively falsely suspected of bening nodules, and 21 benign nodules were falsely diagnosed as malignant tumors.

Preoperative diagnostic processing was reviewed in detail in each of four patient groups. Figure 2 shows the result of a group of 'benign' thyroid nodules. Those were the most representative solitary thyroid nodules and therefore the selection of a proper treatment was most important in that group. A total of 205 patients were divided by ultrasonography into 79 with cystic nodules and 126 with solid tumors. Seventy-nine patients with cystic nodules were either conservatively treated or proved to have benign nodules after surgery. One hundred and twenty-six patients with solid nodules were further examined by neck X-ray and ABC; and 14 were conservatively treated, 21 refused surgery, and 91 underwent operation (80 patients or 88% had benign and 11 patients or 12% had malignant tumours).

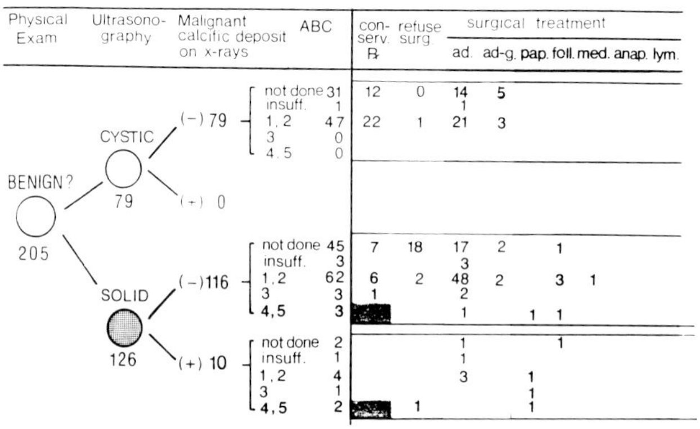

Fig. 2. Preoperative diagnostic processing in a group of suspective 'benign' nodules

The ratio of benign and malignant nodules in the patients who underwent operation is important and is shown in Figure 3. The patients were grouped by physical findings and the size of the nodules.

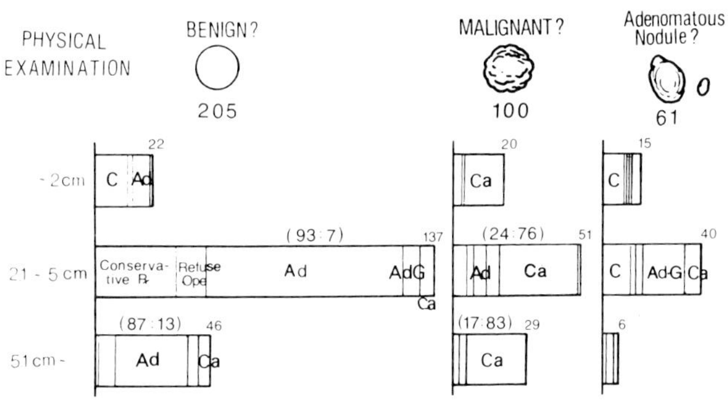

Fig. 3. Ratio of benign and malifnant nodules in the operated patients (nodules were grouped by their size)

REFERENCES

1. Maruchi N, Furihata R, Makiuchi M (1971) Population surveys on the prevalence of thyroid cancer in a non-endemic region, Nagano, Japan. Int J Cancer 7:575

2. Fujimoto Y, Oka A et al (1967) Ultrasound scanning of the thyroid gland as a new diagnostic approach. Ultrasonics 5:177

3. Fujimoto Y, Akisada M (1970) Roentgenologic-histologic patterns of calcification in thyroid nodules. Endocrinol Jpn 17:263

4. Akisada M, Fujimoto Y (1973) Soft Tissue Roentgenography in Diagnosis of Thyroid Cancer. Igaku-Shoin and Prenum Press, Tokyo, New York

Endocrinology
F. Labrie, L. Proulx, eds.

MANIFESTATIONS OF PANCREATIC ENDOCRINE TUMOURS

S.R. BLOOM and J.M. POLAK

Departments of Medicine and Histochemistry, Royal Postgraduate Medical School, Du Cane Road, London W12 0HS (United Kingdom)

Over the last few years the major advance in endocrine tumours of the pancreas has been the discovery that they produce a wide range of regulatory peptides. Output of one particular peptide usually dominates clinically to produce a particular syndrome. The reason why the pancreas should be such a rich source of endocrine tumours is still unknown. Often when a tumour producing one syndrome is resected, secondaries develop in which another cell type is dominant and the clinical picture changes. It has, therefore, been suggested that all pancreatic endocrine tumours should be referred to as islet tumours so that their multiple hormone production be more readily recognised. For clarity each individual tumour syndrome will be dealt with here as a separate entity. Since treatment of these tumours follows a similar pattern, this aspect is covered together at the end of this short update.

INSULINOMAS

Unlike the other pancreatic endocrine tumours, insulinomas are usually benign. Thus surgical resection gives rise to a life-long cure in approaching 90% of cases. Since insulin is a very potent hormone, clinical symptoms are noticed early when the tumours are still extremely small. This can give rise to great difficulty in their localisation. Since the symptoms of low sugar involve adrenergic discharge and mental changes, distinction from the common functional disorders can be very difficult. Thus the insulinoma syndrome is overdiagnosed and the most frequent clinical problem is its exclusion. The diagnosis is based on inappropriately high insulin secretion in the face of prevailing hypoglycaemia and requires a normogram to be constructed for each particular insulin radioimmunoassay. In order to achieve the necessary hypo-glycaemia and demonstrate a failure of inhibition of insulin secretion, the patient is made to undergo a prolonged fast (i.e.

48 hours) and daily exercise is continued. It is useful simultaneously to demonstrate a rise in urinary ketones to confirm fasting in those cases where hypoglycaemia does not develop. Rarely insulinomas secrete intermittently, the diagnosis is then difficult to establish and the patient has to be followed until symptoms become more severe. In the uncommon malignant insulinomas, frequent feeding and suppression of insulin release with diazoxide and a thiazide diuretic is required. The cytotoxic agent, streptozotocin, is only occasionally helpful.

GASTRINOMA

Measurement of plasma gastrin in patients with duodenal ulcer is now performed quite frequently as the radioimmunoassay is readily available. Since gastrin is often elevated, secondary to mild hypochlorhydria (this can co-exist with duodenal ulcer), the problem is to detect the relatively rare case of genuine gastrinoma. Indeed the highest measured gastrin levels (for example 100 fold elevated) are usually associated with achlorhydria. Thus if gastrin measurement is used as a screen for gastrinomas in patients with duodenal ulcer, an elevated value must be followed up by measurement of gastric acid secretion. If this is at the upper end of the normal range or elevated in the presence of high gastrin, then the presence of a gastrin-producing tumour becomes extremely likely. Controversy now exists as to how important it is to resect the tumour. The availability of the H_2 receptor blocking agents and potassium ATPase inhibitors makes it possible to completely inhibit gastric acid secretion. The only significant effect of gastrin is on the parietal cell of the stomach. Thus the main aim of surgery is to effect curative removal of the tumour. Unfortunately when patients who have had an apparently successful tumour resection are followed up, there is an ever increasing incidence of recurrence and it has been calculated that by 30 years all tumours will have recurred. Thus, unlike insulinomas, gastrinomas appear to be universally malignant. Since they are also slow-growing, the benefit of surgery, especially is difficult can sometimes be questionable.

GLUCAGONOMA

Since the recognition of the characteristic rash - necrolytic migratory erythema, associated with glucagonomas, the frequency with which they are diagnosed has greatly increased. In our experience dermatologists, even not having seen a glucagonoma previously, achieve a greater than 50% diagnostic accuracy from the skin appearance alone. Glucagon levels in the plasma are usually considerably elevated and thus a single blood sample will confirm or refute the diagnosis. Because the tumours present late they are usually easy to localise. Though permanent surgical cure is possible only in a minority of patients, debulking the tumour and reducing the plasma glucagon level gives prolonged remission of symptoms, as the tumour is usually very slow growing. The cause of the rash is uncertain but treatment with both the zinc and amino acids (high protein diet) are helpful, suggesting a possible dermal deficiency syndrome. Interestingly, these patients usually only have mild non-ketotic diabetes, though severe weight loss is an important feature in them all.

VIPoma

Pancreatic tumours associated with severe watery diarrhoea and hypokalaemia are almost always associated with elevated plasma vasoactive intestinal peptide (VIP) concentrations. Pharmacologically this peptide is a potent stimulus to small intestinal juice production, increases bile output from the liver, raises blood sugar, lowers blood pressure and causes flushing of the skin. All these features are seen in the VIPoma syndrome. If untreated the patients die of torrential diarrhoea and so the nickname 'pancreatic cholera' is sometimes used. Many cases are still missed due to lack of general awareness and nonavailability of local VIP assays. As with glucagonomas, the measurement of a single blood sample gives the diagnosis. Plasma VIP is not raised in other causes of watery diarrhoea with the exception of ganglioneuromas, one of the commonest childhood tumours, where VIP production is an important feature and explains the previously recognised high incidence of diarrhoea. If surgical resection is not possible, most of these tumours respond to streptozotocin. Tumour debulking can be helpful as some are slow-growing. Temporary remission of symptoms can be achieved with high dose steroid administration. Work with cell cultures has shown that adrenal medullary cells produce VIP in the absence of steroids and this is suppressed when they are reintroduced.

Recently a new peptide - peptide histidine isoleucine (PHI), has been isolated from the procine intestine. PHI, like VIP, will stimulate intestinal juice secretion pharmacologically. It is widely distributed in nerves throughout the body and this distribution was found to parallel VIP. Tumours producing VIP were always found to produce a PHI-like peptide and conversely all tumours producing PHI produced VIP. It was therefore not surprising when it was discovered that the messenger RNA coding for prepro VIP also coded for PHI (in man the last amino acid is methionine and the peptide has to be re-named PHM). Since PHM is co-produced with VIP, the old term VIPoma is no longer fully descriptive of the mechanism of diarrhoea in these tumours. Indeed since PHM has a longer half life in the circulation, it may sometimes be the more relevant mediator of the diarrhoea.

SOMATOSTATINOMAS

The islet of Langerhans contains B cells, A cells and also two other cell types, the D cell producing somatostatin and the PP cells producing pancreatic polypeptide (PP). Thus it is not surprising to find some tumours produce large quantities of somatostatin. In about half the cases the patients suffer from a syndrome of diabetes mellitus, gall stones and low acid output. In addition there is weight loss. Surprisingly the symptoms are often found to have existed for many years so it seems likely that these tumours are very slow growing. At presentation their bulk can be considerable, however, and they are usually very difficult to completely resect.

PPomas

If somatostatin produces relatively mild clinical symptoms, pancreatic polypeptide (PP) produces none. Indeed elevation of plasma PP is usually picked up as an incidental finding in patients suffering from excess production of one of the other pancreatic tumour hormones. PP elevation is useful as a general marker for the presence of these tumours and helps confirm the diagnosis. If PP elevation is borderline, the atropine suppression test can be helpful. Normal PP cells are considerably influenced by the background vagal tone and inhibition of this by administration of atropine greatly reduces the PP output. In contrast the output from tumour cells is not altered by the administration of atropine.

NEUROTENSINOMAS

In about 10% of VIPomas neurotensin is also found to be elevated in the plasma and extracts of tumour. Neurotensin has recently been found to increase the secretion of juice from the intestinal wall and, in large doses, encourages defaecation. It may thus be a contributory factor to the diarrhoea syndrome. Occasional tumours have been found which produce only neurotensin, however, and these patients are asymptomatic. It thus seems likely that neurotensin's effect is relatively weak or that neurotensin receptor down regulation rapidly occurs in the face of continuously elevated hormone levels.

GRFomas

Growth hormone-releasing factor (GRF) was first isolated from pancreatic tumours associated with acromegaly. Although quite frequently produced by pancreatic endocrine tumours in a small amount, it is very rarely responsible for their diagnosis by producing acromegaly. It is possible, however, that it encourages tumour growth, though the direct effects of GRF on tissues other than the pituitary are not yet established.

OTHER ENDOCRINE TUMOURS

Pancreatic endocrine tumours producing neuropeptide Y (NPY), ACTH, and calcitonin gene-related peptide (CGRP), or corticotrophin-releasing factor (CRF) occur quite rarely. Storage of 5-hydroxytryptamine (5HT) allows the histological diagnosis of a carcinoid tumour but carcinoid syndrome resulting from excess 5HT secretion is uncommon. Some gut hormones, for example, secretin, motilin or peptide tyrosine tyrosine (PYY) do not appear to be produced by pancreatic endocrine tumours.

TUMOUR LOCALISATION

Once the clinical syndrome and elevated hormone levels have been established, tumour localisation and assessment of the possibility of surgical removal is required. Non-invasive techniques such as ultrasound and computerised axial tomography allow detection of larger pancreatic tumours and significant hepatic metastases. Nuclear megnetic resonance scanning gives less good definition and is not yet useful in this context. Arteriography, particularly highly selective arteriography with background subtraction almost always allows localisation of the pancreatic primary and will detect even small hepatic secondaries. The advent of digital angiography will offer additional help. Rarely, when tumours are too small to be found by angiography, help can be obtained by measurement of hormone levels in selective venous samples. Access to the portal vein by the transhepatic route allows samples from numerous pancreatic venous tributaries and sometimes a sudden increase in hormone concentration indicates the site of the tumour. Unfortunately the procedure is risky even in the best hands and is very time-consuming. False tumour localisation may also occur due to random hormone fluctuations or aberrant venous drainage.

TREATMENT

Complete or partial surgical excision should usually be undertaken as even if malignant these tumours are slow growing and prolonged palliation can result. If this is not possible, the only useful cytotoxic agent is streptozotocin. This produces significant tumour regression in approximately 95% of VIPomas, 30% of insulinomas and a lower proportion of the remaining tumour types. Occasionally this remission is dramatic and many years of palliation result. The main toxicity of streptozotocin is renal with the production of a nephrotic syndrome-like picture. The sensitivity to the drug rises dramatically with pre-existing renal damage and the dose should be reduced more than proportionately to renal function. Marrow and liver toxicity also occur but are far less frequent. The addition of other agents such as 5-florouracil and DTIC have not been effectively tested. On their own, significant tumour regression is rare. If the main hormone production, and thus clinical symptoms, results from hepatic secondaries, these can be necrossed by hepatic artery embolisation, a procedure which can be performed under local anaesthetic and may result in useful remission of many months.

CONCLUSION

The availability of radioimmunoassays for a range of regulatory peptides has allowed the diagnosis of a number of differenttumour types and clinical syndromes. Frequently, however, the tumours are mixed. Unfortunately these tumours are sufficiently rare to have made it difficult to develop effective treatment regimes, particularly with cytotoxic agents. Recently, the development of a long-acting somatostatin analogue (SMS 201-995) has allowed useful palliation in otherwise terminal cases and may also act to stop tumour cell growth. It may be that similar natural agents, which inhibit differentiation and cell growth offer the most promising avenue for future therapy.

REFERENCES

1. Mallinson CN, Bloom SR, Warin AP, Salmon PR, Cox B (1974) A glucagonoma syndrome. Lancet II:1-4

2. Long RG, Bryant MG, Mitchell SJ, Adrian TE, Polak JM, Bloom SR (1981) Clinicopathological study of pancreatic and ganglioneuroblastoma tumours secreting vasoactive intestinal polypeptide (VIPomas) Brit Med J 282:1767-1771

3. Polak JM, Bloom SR, Adrian TE, Heights P, Bryant MG, Pearse AGE (1976) Pancreatic polypeptide in insulinomas, gastrinomas, VIP and glucagonomas. Lancet I:328-330

4. Blackburn AM, Bryant MG, Adrian TE, Bloom SR (1981) Pancreatic tumours produce neurotensin. J Clin Endocrinol Metab 52:820-822

5. Guillemin R, Brazeal P, Bohlen P, Esh F, Ling N, Wehrenberg WB (1982) Growth hormone-releasing factor from a human pancreatic tumour that caused acromegaly. Science 218:585-587

6. Wood SM, Bloom SR Pancreatic and gastrointestinal hormone-secreting tumors. In: Donal RA (ed) A Guide to Diagnosis. Dekker, New York. Chpt 32:533-551

7. Welbourn RB, Wood SM, Polak JM, Bloom SR (1981) Pancreatic endocrine tumours. In: Bloom SR, Polak JM (eds) Gut Hormones, 2nd edition. Churchill Livingstone, Edinburgh, pp 547-554

NEW TECHNICAL DEVELOPMENTS

Endocrinology
F. Labrie, L. Proulx, eds.

METHODS FOR DETECTING GENE POLYMORPHISM

GRAEME I. BELL
Chiron Corporation, 4560 Horton Street, Emeryville, CA 94608

The use of cloned DNA and oligodeoxyribonucleotide probes to isolate genes and examine allelic sequence variation has increased our understanding of the molecular basis of several heritable diseases, provided tools for prenatal diagnosis and carrier identification and, in addition, extended our knowledge of the chromosomal location and linkage of human genes (1). These studies have often exploited the nucleotide sequence differences which exist between alleles or intergenic spacer DNA. A nucleotide sequence difference is described as being polymorphic if it occurs in the population with a frequency of greater than 1%. Sequences present at less than 1% frequency are termed variants (2). As many of the basic methods (3) and strategies (1,2) used for detecting nucleotide sequence variation have been described, this report will focus on recent modifications which simplify these procedures and increase their utility.

The isolation and sequence comparison of alleles reveals all the nucleotide differences between them. Extensive sequence comparisons are often necessary to identify mutations which alter the expression of a gene or the structure of its mRNA or protein. Genes have traditionally been isolated from phage λ- or cosmid-based genomic DNA libraries by in situ hybridization with a ^{32}P-labeled probe to a gene (3). Seed (2,3) has recently described a strategy for isolating genes from λ libraries that exploits homologous recombination between phage containing the gene of interest and a miniplasmid bearing a DNA segment homologous to that gene. Phage having the integrated miniplasmid can be purifed by growth under the appropriate selective conditions. This procedure should be particularly useful when a number of alleles of a gene are being isolated. The isolated DNA can be sequenced using strategies based upon the base-specific chemical degradation procedure (5-8), or the enzymatic chain termination procedure using M13 or double-stranded DNA templates (9-13). If the gene has been sequenced previously, a series of oligodeoxyribonucleotides can be prepared and used to rapidly generate the sequence of other alleles with the chain termination technique .

Although it may often be desirable to compare the sequences of various alleles this type of analysis is not amenable to examining large numbers of individuals. The indirect analysis of gene sequences using restriction endonucleases and the blotting procedure developed by Southern (14) can be used to survey large numbers of individuals for sequence variation. However, this procedure only monitors those sequences that comprise the recognition sequence of a restriction endonuclease or regions characterized by insertions, deletions or other chromosomal rearrangements. Sequence variation is indicated by differences in the sizes of hybridizing restriction fragments, i.e. restriction fragment length polymorphism (RFLP). Since first described, a number of modifications and variations to this technique have been described. Genomic DNA, often prepared from white blood cells (15), is digested with a restriction endonuclease and the resulting DNA fragments separated by electrophoresis in a vertical or horizontal agarose slab gel. After denaturation and neutralization of the DNA in the agarose gel, it can be tranferred by diffusion (3,14) or electrophoretically (16) to a nitrocellulose filter (3), nylon membrane [Genescreen (NEN), Biodyne (Pall), Zeta Probe (Bio-Rad)] or derivatized filter paper (17). The denatured DNA can also be immobilized by drying the agarose gel (8-21) This latter procedure has been used in hybridization studies with oligodeoxyribonucleotide probes; larger probes do not diffuse as well through the dried gel.

^{32}P-labeled DNA probes can be prepared by nick-translation (3), the combined exonuclease-polymerase activities of T4 DNA polymerase (3) and by using a mixture of hexadeoxynucleotides to prime the synthesis of labeled DNA from a denatured restriction endonuclease fragment (22,23). Strand specific DNA probes can be prepared using recombinant M13 templates (24) and the hybridization primer, and stand-specific RNA probes using the *Salmonella typhimurium* bacteriophage SP6 promoter (25) [Riboprobe (Promega Biotec)].

The prehybridization and hybridization conditions described by Wahl et. al (17) are widely used. The hybridization temperature is usually 42°C but a higher temperature may be required when using GC-rich probes. Nonhybridized probe is removed by washing the filter in 0.1xSSC and 0.1% SDS for one hour at 50°C. If the background is unacceptable the filter can be washed longer in this solution at 50°C or a higher temperature as many hybrids are stable in 0.1xSSC at 65°C.

The hybridizing DNA fragments are identified by autoradiography in the presence of intensifying screens at -76°C. The length of exposure is determined by the specific activity of the probe, which is usually greater than $2x10^8$ cpm/µg. Regions of hybridization can usually be detected on an overnight exposure.

Procedures using ^{32}P-labeled oligodeoxyribonucleotide probes to identify genes which have specific mutations have recently been described (18-20). Since the probe usually hybridizes to other sequences, it is necessary to digest the DNA with a restriction endonuclease which will generate a characteristic fragment in a region with low background hybridization. Knowledge of the sequence of the normal and mutant gene is also necessary for designing the sequence of the probe.

Several developments have recently been reported which may further simplify the procedures for detecting gene polymorphism. Church and Gilbert (26) have devised a strategy for genomic sequencing based upon a combination of sequencing and blotting procedures which can be used to determine the sequence of a specific gene in the presence of the other genomic sequences. In addition, several groups (27,28) have described rapid and sensitive colorimetric methods for visualizing DNA probes hybridized to DNA or RNA immobilized on nitrocellulose. Leary et al (27) prepared biotin-labeled DNA probes by nick-translation in the presence of biotinylated analogs of TTP. After hybridization, they incubated the nitrocellulose filter with a complex of avidin and biotinylated horseradish peroxidase or alkaline phosphatase which binds to the hybridized biotin-labeled DNA. Subsequenct incubation of the filter in the presence of substrates for these enzymes results in the deposition of a colored precipitate at sites of hybridization. Renz and Kurz (28) used a similar strategy except that they crosslinked horseradish peroxidase or alkaline phosphatase to the single-stranded DNA probe and used this material as a probe. Apparently the bound protein does not affect the ability of the probe to hybridize to complementary sequences. The sensitivity of these colorimetric procedures for visualizing hybrids approaches that achieved with radioactive probes and thus could eliminate the need for radioactivity in the blotting procedure.

1. Caskey CT, White RL (eds) (1983) Recombinant DNA Aplications to Human Disease. Cold Spring Harbor Laboratory, Cold Spring Harbor
2. Cooper DN, Schmidtke J (1984) Hum Genet 66:1-16.
3. Maniatis T, Fritsch EF, Sambrook J (1982) Molecular Cloning, A Laboratory Manual. Cold Spring Harbor Laboratory, Cold Spring Harbor
4. Seed B (1983) Nucleic Acids Res 11:2427-2445
5. Maxam A, Gilbert W (1980) Methods in Enzymology 65:499-560.
6. Cooke NE, Coit D, Shine J, Baxter JD, Martial JA (1981) J Biol Chem 256: 4007-4016
7. Ruther U (1982) Nucleic Acids Res 10:5765-5772
8. Frischauf AM, Garoff H, Lehrach H (1980) Nucleic Acids Res 8:5541-5549
9. Sanger F, Coulson AR, Barrell BG, Smith AJH, Roe BA (1980) J Mol Biol 143:161-178.
10. Wallace RB, Johnson MT, Suggs SV, Dembek P, Itakura K (1981) Gene 16:21-26.
11. Hong GF (1982) Bioscience Reports 2:907-912
12. Hong GF (1982) J Mol Biol 158:539-549
13. Deininger PL (1983) Anal Biochem 135:247-263
14. Southern EM (1975) J Mol Biol 98:503-517
15. Bell GI, Karam JH, Rutter WJ (1981) Proc Natl Acad Sci USA 78:5759-5763
16. Bittner M, Kupferer P, Morris CF (1980) Anal Biochem 102:459-471
17. Wahl GM, Stern M, Stark GR (1979) Proc Natl Acad Sci USA 76:3683-3687
18. Conner BJ, Reyes AA, Morin C, Itakura K, Teplitz RL, Wallace RB (1983) Proc Natl Acad Sci USA 80:278-282
19. Kidd VJ, Wallace RB, Itakura K, Woo SLC (1983) Nature 304:230-234

20. Studencki AB, Wallace RB (1984) DNA 3:7-15
21. Purrello M, Balazs I (1983) Anal Biochem 128:393-397
22. Feinberg A, Vogelstein B (1983) Anal Biochem 132:6-13
23. Feinberg A, Vogelstein B (1984) Anal Biochem 137:266-267
24. Hu N, Messing J (1982) Gene 17:271-277
25. Little PFR (1984) Nature 309:191
26. Church GM, Gilbert W (1984) Proc Natl Acad Sci USA 81:1991-1995
27. Leary JJ, Brigati DJ, Ward DC (1983) Proc Natl Acad Sci USA 80:4045-4049
28. Renz M, Kurz C (1984) Nucleic Acids Res 12:3435-3444

© 1984 Elsevier Science Publishers B.V.
Endocrinology
F. Labrie, L. Proulx, eds.

DEVELOPMENTS IN AFFINITY CHROMATOGRAPHY OF STEROID HORMONE RECEPTORS

JAN MESTER, GERARD REDEUILH, THIERRY BUCHOU, JACK-MICHEL RENOIR,
PIERRE FORMSTECHER AND ETIENNE-EMILE BAULIEU
Lab. Hormones, Inserm U33, 78 r. du Général-Leclerc, 94270 Bicêtre, France

INTRODUCTION

Affinity resins suitable for purification of several different kinds of steroid hormone receptors have been synthesized during the last decade. This report deals with the improvements we have made in the purification of the progesterone receptor (PR) and estrogen receptor (ER). By our procedures it is possible to purify not only the "transformed" and partially proteolyzed forms, but also the large (8S), non-activated receptors. The two methodologically different principles employed are probably applicable also to other steroid hormone binding proteins.

PROGESTERONE RECEPTOR

Purification using a "classical type" affinity resin

Experimental procedures. The affinity resin (NADAc-Sepharose) was synthesized as described (1). We have used routinely five batches of the resin, with steroid residue concentrations between 0.1 and 0.3 μmol/ml wet gel.

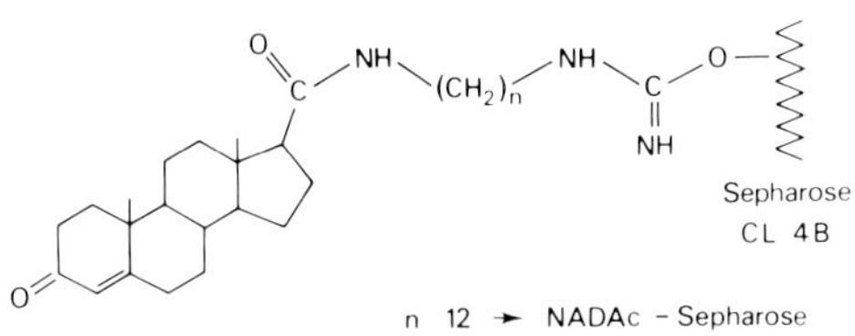

Fig.1 Affinity resin for PR purification

The cytosol fraction of the homogenate of estrogen-stimulated chick oviducts was recovered as described (1). All further operations were carried out at 4-6°C.

Charging of cytosol onto affinity gel: The resin was packed into columns of 2 cm diameter (20 to 30 ml gel/column), and the cytosol was loaded at a rate of 0.3 ml per ml gel.hour. The total volume of cytosol was 5ml/ml of gel. The concentration of PR was 3 to 4 nM in terms of progesterone binding sites.

Washing of the loaded gel is crucial for both yield and purity of the final product. We have developed procedures of maximum stringency possible without loss of or damage to the PR. These consist of a sequence of: 1. high-salt buffer (0.3M KCl), 3 gel bed volumes; 2. low-salt buffer, 10 gel bed volumes; 3. urea (2.5M for the non-activated PR, or 3M for the activated PR), 3 gel bed volumes; 4.low-salt buffer, 10 gel bed volumes. Washing is done as fast as possible. At the stages of washing with high-salt buffer and with urea, care has to be taken that the actual concentration of all components throughout the gel reaches that in the buffer. In practice, we allow one gel bed volume enter the gel before adding the rest of the solution and resuspending thoroughly with a glass rod.

Effects of the urea washing step are illustrated in the Table I and Fig.2. The improvement in purity is about 3.5-fold for 8S-PR and about 2-fold for 4S-PR, so that the specific activities obtained are about 40% of those attainable when the receptor is purified to homogeneity. (The 4S-PR are single subunits A(79K) and B (108K) (2) while the 8S-PR is a complex containing a hormone-binding subunit, A or B, and probably two non-hormone-binding subunits of M_r~90K (3). The 8S-PR is stable in the presence of ≦2.5M urea (4).)

TABLE I

PURIFICATION OF PR BY AFFINITY CHROMATOGRAPHY INCLUDING (a) OR EXCLUDING (b) THE UREA WASHING STEP

Receptor form	Purification factor		Yield (%)	
	a	b	a	b
non-activated (8S)	950 ± 260	260 ± 50	25 ± 4	33 ± 5
activated (4S)*	117 ± 16	55 ± 29	22 ± 4	25 ± 4

*) Activation by $(NH_4)_2SO_4$ precipitation; the purification factor shown does not include the approx. 10-fold purification obtained in the activation procedure.

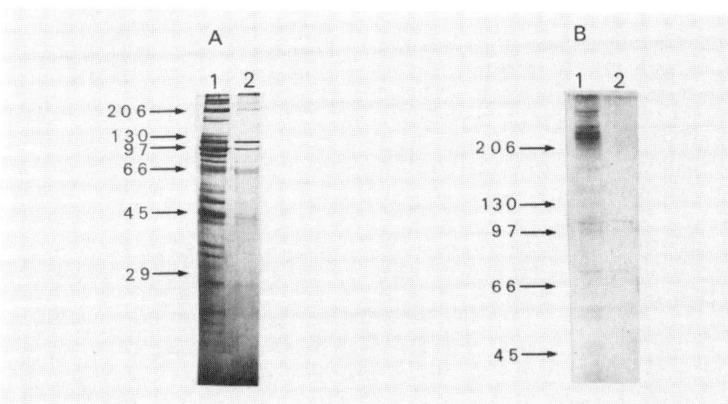

Fig.2. SDS-PAGE of the PR eluted from NADAc-Sepharose. A:8S-PR; B:4S-PR as in Table I. Urea washing step was omitted for samples shown in lanes A1 and B1, included for those in lanes A2 and B2. M_r's of marker proteins are indicated by arrows.

Elution of the PR retained specifically on NADAc-Sepharose gel is achieved by an overnight incubation with 10^{-6}M progesterone (1). The yield is usually over 70% of receptor retained on the affinity gel.

Recycling: In order to remove any remaining proteins, the gel is washed immediately after use with 6M urea (5 vol.). To remove traces of free steroid, exhaustive washing is carried out with H_2O, H_2O/CH_3OH (1/1), CH_3OH, H_2O/CH_3OH (1/1) and H_2O; the gel is stored with NaN_3 at 4°C. No loss of receptor-binding capacity has been noted after more than 50 cycles with the same batch of the resin.

ESTROGEN RECEPTOR

Use of estradiol (E_2)-biotin in purification by biotin-avidin interaction

In contrast with affinity resins, which necessitate an empirical approach, a soluble ligand allowing subsequent separation of the receptor makes it possible to work under controlled conditions since the affinity of the steroid derivative can be measured and its concentration chosen by the experimentator. Another potential advantage concerns purification of those receptors which are present in the tissue complexed with an endogenous ligand as exchange in liquid phase is easier to accomplish than "stripping" the ligand under mild conditions. E_2 linked to a soluble dextran macromolecule has been used previously in our laboratory to purify the trypsinized calf uterus ER by exploiting the difference in size between the ER-E_2-dextran and ER-E_2 complexes (5). Here we describe a series of E_2-biotin conjugates designed for ER purification by biotin-avidin interaction (Fig.3); their synthesis is reported elsewhere(6). All these compounds competed with E_2 for ER binding sites (Fig. 4a). They also bound to avidin as demonstrated by their capacity to displace the 4-hydroxyazobenzene-2'-carboxylic acid dye (7; not shown). When avidin was added to the solution containing the Va or Vb derivative (shorter spacer chains), it reduced dramatically their relative binding activity (RBA) for ER; in contrast, avidin caused only a moderate decrease of RBA of the two long-spacer-chain compounds VIa and VIb (Fig 4b). This is probably a consequence of the fact that both the E_2-binding site on ER and the biotin-binding site on avidin are buried in deep clefts, so that only when separated by a long spacer chain, both E_2 and biotin moieties can be simultaneously bound to the respective proteins.

The binding of the E_2-biotin derivatives to ER was a reversible process as demonstrated by exchange with $^3HE_2$. Two ER forms tested, the 4S (trypsinized) and 8S (molybdate-stabilized) behaved identically in binding experiments.

Binding of (biotinyl-E_2)-ER to immobilized avidin: Calf uterus cytosol was incubated to equilibrium with the compound VIb (10^{-6}M) in the presence of Na_2MoO_4 to stabilize the 8S form of ER. Unbound biotinyl-E_2 was removed by charcoal adsorption and centrifugation, and the supernatant was charged onto an avidin-Sepharose column.

Biospecific elution: The avidin-Sepharose column with retained ER-E_2-biotin complex was extensively washed with a sequence of buffers including a 2.5M urea step. Exchange with 20 μM $^3HE_2$ was then accomplished by a 30 min incubation at 37°C, and the ER content in the eluate was determined by filtration on a column of Ultrogel AcA 34 (8). Yield was about 40 to 50% of the retained ER, and the purification factor about 500 to 1500-fold, resulting in ER purity of 5 to 7% (assuming one binding site/60000 d; 9). Hydrodynamic characteristics of the purified ER were indistinguishable from those of the non-activated ER in crude calf uterus cytosol ($s_{20,w}$ =8.0; R_s=7.4 nm) Further purification of the ER eluted from avidin-Sepharose can be obtained by DEAE-Sephacel chromatography (6).

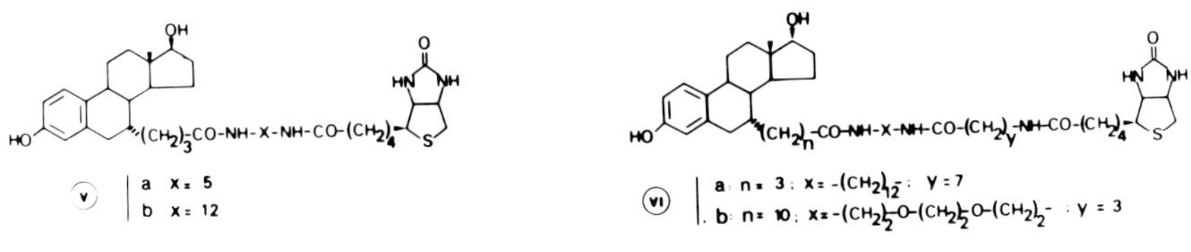

Fig. 3. Structures of the E_2-biotin conjugates.

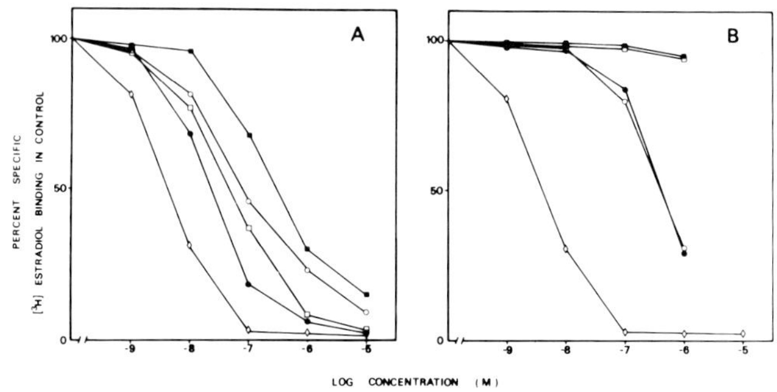

Fig.4. Competition of the compounds Va(□), Vb(■), VIa(o), VIb(•) and of E_2(◇) for $^3HE_2$ binding to ER, in the absence (A) or presence (B) of avidin (2 μM).

REFERENCES

1. Renoir JM, Yang CR, Formstecher P, Lustenberger P, Wolfson A, Redeuilh G, Mester J, Richard-Foy H, Baulieu EE (1982) Eur J Biochem 127: 71
2. Schrader WT, Birnbaumer ME, Hugues MR, Weigel NL, Grody WW, O'Malley BW (1981) Rec Progr Horm Res 37: 583
3. Renoir JM, Buchou T, Mester J, Radanyi C, Baulieu EE(1984) Biochemistry (in press)
4. Buchou T, Mester J, Renoir JM, Baulieu EE (1983) Biochem Biophys Res Commun 114: 479
5. Hubert P, Mester J, Dellacherie E, Neel J, Baulieu EE (1978) Proc Natl Acad Sci USA 75: 3143
6. Redeuilh G, manuscript in preparation
7. Green NM (1970) Methods in Enzymology 18: 418
8. Redeuilh G, Richard-Foy R, Secco C, Torelli V, Bucourt R, Baulieu EE, Richard-Foy H (1980) Eur J Biochem 106: 481
9. Katzenellenbogen JA, Carlson KE, Heiman DS, Robertson DW, Wey LL, Katzenellenbogen BS (1983) J Biol Cem 258: 3487

THE REVERSE HEMOLYTIC PLAQUE ASSAY FOR DETECTION OF HORMONE SECRETION BY INDIVIDUAL CELLS

PHILIP F. SMITH AND JIMMY D. NEILL

Department of Physiology and Biophysics, University of Alabama in Birmingham, University Station, Birmingham, AL 35294

INTRODUCTION

Functionally distinct subpopulations of pituitary (AP) cell types have been described using cell separation techniques (1,2). However, the extent and physiological significance of functional heterogeneity on a single cell level is not known. A method for detecting secretion by single cells, the reverse hemolytic plaque assay (RHPA), has been adapted in our laboratory for detection of hormone secretion by dispersed anterior pituitary cells incubated as a monolayer with ovine erythrocytes (RBCs)(3). This assay, based on complement-mediated lysis of protein A-coated RBCs in the presence of an antiserum directed against a secretory protein, results in a zone of hemolysis, a plaque, surrounding each cell which has secreted that protein. In the present study, we describe some aspects of heterogeneity among pituitary cells which have been garnered with the RHPA.

MATERIALS AND METHODS

Antisera used in the RHPA were prepared in this laboratory (oLH, rat GH and rat Prl) or received as a gift from Dr. J.L. Roberts (ACTH; Bridgette). Antiserum used for immunocytochemistry (ICC) was either a gift of the National Pituitary Agency (anti-rat LHβ) or was purchased commercially (anti-ACTH, Immunonuclear Corp., Stillwater, Minn.).

The details of the RHPA have been described previously (3). In brief, Cunningham chambers were constructed on poly-l-lysine coated microscope slides. Trypsin-dispersed pituitary cells (500,000 cells/ml) were mixed with protein-A coated oRBCs, and infused into the chambers. After cell attachment (45 min), chambers were washed before antiserum (1:40 - 1:200 dilution in DMEM-0.1% BSA) and secretagogues (where appropriate) were infused. Slides were incubated for 2 h, then washed and infused with complement (guinea pig serum) (GIBCO; 1:20 - 1:50 dilution in DMEM-BSA). After the plaques developed (30 min), slides were fixed in 1% glutaraldehyde, and the percentage of pituitary cells which formed plaques was recorded.

Plaque assays were performed in sequence for ACTH and LH secretion to detect possible dual secretion of these hormones by the same cell. The RHPA was modified (Frawley and Neill, unpublished) to permit sequential additions of RBC and antisera by attaching pituitary cells to poly-l-lysine coated slides in the absence of RBC and then incubating them for 24 h in DMEM containing 10% fetal bovine serum. Then, Cunningham chambers were constructed over the pituitary cells using gridded coverslips (4). A mixture of protein-A coated RBCs, ACTH-antiserum, guinea pig serum and CRF (10^{-7}M) was infused into the chambers. After a 2 h incubation (37°C, 5% CO_2) the chambers were flushed with DMEM-BSA and a second mixture containing LH antiserum and GnRH (10^{-7}M) was added and incubation continued for a second 2 h period. Selected grids were photographed at the end of the first sequence and again after the second. By comparing photographs of the first and second sequences the percentage of ACTH secreting cells which also secreted LH was determined.

To perform ICC on plaque-forming cells, we infused 0.2 M Na acetate/0.5 M NaCl (pH 2.5) at the end of the plaque reaction for 10 min at 4°C to elute antibodies bound to the RBC. Plaques were then fixed and processed for immunocytochemistry using the ABC method (Vector Labs) with diaminobenzidine as a substrate.

RESULTS

In the RHPA for each of the 4 hormones, presorption of antiserum with the appropriate hormone blocked plaque formation. Furthermore, in the case of GH, ACTH, and LH, the size of plaques formed was related in a dose-dependent manner to the concentration of secretagogue present. Table 1 shows the percentage of pituitary cells from proestrus rats which secreted GH, Prl, ACTH or LH as measured in the plaque assay. These proportions correspond closely with the percentage of hormone-containing cells of each type derived from ICC on aliquots of the same cells. However, in some physiological conditions, the percentage of LH-secreting cells was substantially less than the percentage of LH-containing cells (diestrus-I in the female rat or during the neonatal period in the male rat). Non-secretory pools of cells were also observed in the corticotrope and lactotrope populations under certain conditions. Another

TABLE 1

PERCENTAGE OF PITUITARY CELLS FROM PROESTRUS RATS THAT FORMED PLAQUES WHEN ASSAYED FOR SECRETION OF THE LISTED HORMONES

Hormone Secreted	Percentage (%)
Prl	55
GH (GHRH 10^{-7}M)	30
LH (GnRH 10^{-7}M)	5
ACTH (CRH 10^{-7}M)	4

striking result of these studies was the wide range of secretory responses seen in cells from a single pituitary gland. This was most evident in the gonadotrope population from proestrus rats where the range in plaque size (which is directly related to amount of hormone secreted; Smith and Neill, unpublished observation) was over 1000 fold.

Figure 1 illustrates the results from a sequential plaque assay; it demonstrates a typical grid field photographed after performing assays for LH and ACTH on the same pituitary cells. Using cells from neonatal male rats we found that only a small percentage of ACTH-secreting cells (<5%) also secreted LH.

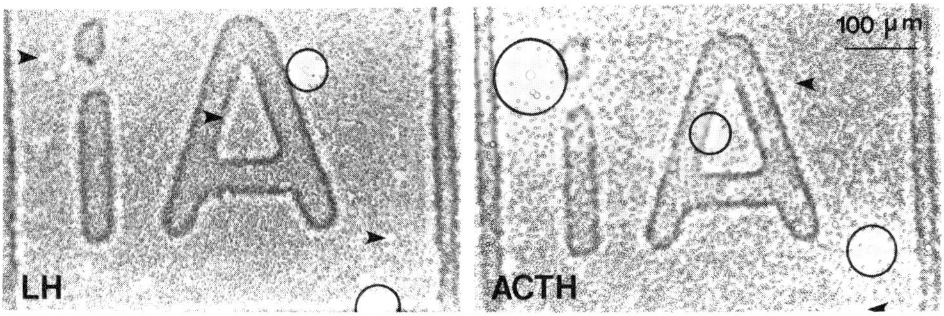

Fig. 1. Sequential plaque assay using gridded coverslip. 1st sequence - LH; 2nd sequence - ACTH. Plaques are outlined by circles. Plaque-forming cells can be seen in the center of each plaque and are indicated by arrows in the companion sequence.

PAP-ICC was performed on ACTH and LH plaques from neonatal male rats to further study the overlap in these populations. The majority of LH-secreting cells were unstained with ACTH antiserum (Fig. 2A). However, a small number of LH-secreting cells contained ACTH. Furthermore, approximately half of the LH-containing cells did not secrete LH in response to GnRH. Most ACTH-containing cells also secreted ACTH (Fig. 2B).

DISCUSSION

Using the RHPA we have been able to identify individual cells secreting Prl, GH, LH or ACTH. The percentages of pituitary cells secreting these hormones in general correspond closely with the percentages of hormone-containing cells of each type. However, under certain experimental conditions a significant proportion of cells may be unresponsive even to maximally stimulatory doses of the appropriate secretagogue. Further evidence for pituitary cell heterogeneity is seen in the range of responses among individual cells from the same pituitary.

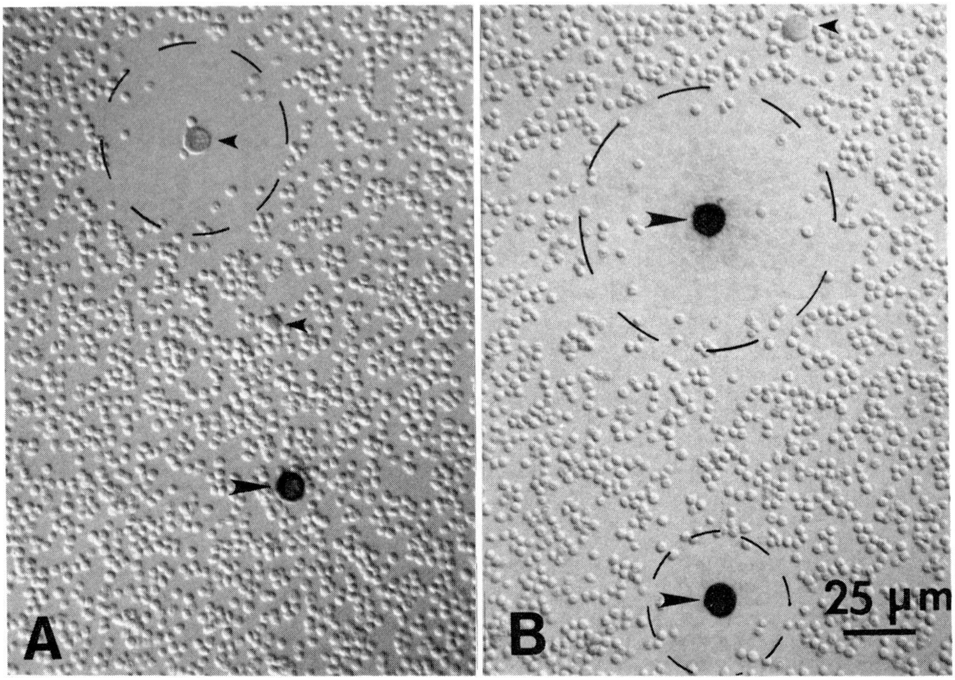

Fig. 2A&B. Combined plaque assay - ICC. Fig. 2A. Plaque assay for LH; ICC for ACTH. Fig. 2B. Plaque assay for ACTH; ICC for ACTH. Small arrows indicate unstained cells; large arrows indicate immunoreactive cells; plaques are outlined for clarity.

This may be as large as three orders of magnitude in some cell types. These findings (as well as those describing cells with multihormonal secretory capacity) demonstrate that the pituitary output of a given hormone is the result of responses by a number of functionally distinct subpopulations. The reverse hemolytic plaque assay coupled with other biochemical and morphological techniques which can be applied to individual cells will permit more detailed studies of the nature of the differences among cells.

REFERENCES

1. Denef C, Hautekeete E, Dewals R (1978) Endocrinology 103:736-747
2. Hymer WC, Page R, Kelsey RC, Augustine EC, Wilfinger W, Ciolkosz M (1980) In Jutisz M, McKerns (eds) Synthesis and Release of Adenohypophyseal Hormones. Plenum Press, New York, pp. 125-166
3. Neill JD, Frawley LS (1983) Endocrinology 112:1135-1137
4. Lin PF, Ruddle FH (1981) Exp Cell Res 134:485-488

Endocrinology
F. Labrie, L. Proulx, eds.

IN SITU cDNA:mRNA HYBRIDIZATION: A TECHNIQUE TO STUDY GENE EXPRESSION IN INDIVIDUAL CELLS

J.L. ROBERTS, J.N. WILCOX, AND C.E. GEE
Center for Reproductive Sciences and Department of Biochemistry, Columbia University, New York, New York, 10032, U.S.A.

INTRODUCTION

A major area of interest in our laboratory is the study of peptide hormone gene expression in complex tissues such as the pituitary and brain. In order to measure changes in peptide hormone mRNAs in response to different hormonal manipulations, the standard approach has been to extract total RNA from a homogenate of a tissue sample and quantitate the amount of a specific mRNA by filter or solution hybridization using the appropriate cDNA as a probe. A major drawback of this approach is that it can only assess overall tissue content of the specific mRNA. If the tissue contains a heterogenous population of cells expressing the gene of interest, each population being regulated differently, such information would not be apparent in assessing overall tissue content of a specific mRNA since the observed level of the specific mRNA would be an average of all cell types. One way around this problem is to dissect the tissue into smaller and smaller regions in which the regulation of the gene of interest is more homogeneous. This is not possible in the brain in many cases since it is by its very nature an extremely complex tissue. We have therefore been developing the technique of *in situ* cDNA:mRNA hybridization with the ultimate goal of making this technique a semi-quantitative assay for mRNA levels in individual cells.

In situ cDNA:mRNA hybridization is conceptually similar to filter and solution hybridization techniques except that the cDNA probes are allowed to hybridize to mRNAs *in situ*, within cells, on tissue sections. After hybridization the tissue sections are processed for autoradiography and cDNA:mRNA hybrids visualized by the distribution and density of silver grains over individual cells. A large number of manuscripts dealing with this general technique have appeared over the past five years (1-7). They encompass a broad range of animals, tissues and probes used but are primarly concerned with answering anatomical questions. In this presentation we would like to discuss our studies attempting to develop the *in situ* hybridization technique to study and quantitate individual cell levels of various peptide hormone messenger RNAs in the brain and pituitary.

MATERIALS AND METHODS

Male or female Sprague-Dawley rats were anesthetized with pentobarbitol, the systemic circulation rinsed with saline and perfused for 20 min with 4% paraformaldehyde in PBS. The pituitary and brain tissue were removed and immersed in sterile 15% sucrose PBS for 60 min at 4°C. The tissues were then embedded in M1 compound (Lipshaw, Detroit, Mich.) and frozen in liquid nitrogen. Ten micron sections were obtained on a cryostat and thaw mounted on gelatin coated slides. The sections were immediately refrozen and stored in slide boxes containing dessicant at -70°C for up to 4 wks prior to hybridization. Just prior to the *in situ* hybrizidation procedure the slides were removed from the freezer, immediately covered with 10ug/ml proteinase-K solution and incubated for 10 min at 30°C followed by a 10 min wash in 0.2xSSC (1xSSC: 0.15M NaCl, 0.015M Na Citrate, pH 7.0). Tissue sections were then prehybridized in the hybridization buffer (HB: 5xSSC, 1xDenhardt's, 50% formamide) without probe for 1-2 h at 30°C in airtight hybridization boxes containing filter paper saturated with 4xSSC and 50% formamide. At the end of the prehybridization step the HB was blotted off and replaced with 25ul of HB containing 1ng tritiated POMC cDNA probe (specific activity $5x10^6$ CPM/ug DNA), coversliped and incubated in the hybridization boxes at 30°C for 15-20 h. At the end of the hybridization step unhybridized probe was washed off in two 10 min washes in 2.0xSSC followed by an overnight wash in 3 liters of 0.5xSSC with gentle stirring. The sections were then dehydrated in graded alcohols containing 0.3M NH_4Ac and dried in a vaccum dessicator. For visualization of the cDNA:mRNA hybrids the slides were dipped in a 1:1 solution of NTB2 nuclear emmulsion (Kodak, Rochester, NY) and ultra-pure water, dried and allowed to expose in the dark at 4°C with dessicant for 2-4 wks. After development, the slides were counterstained with hemotoxylin and eosin to visualize the cells. Recent studies have suggested that ribonuclease remains active in paraformaldehyde fixed tissue so some changes had been made in the original protocol used by Gee and Roberts (3,4). The time in the sucrose solution was reduced to allow less time for ribonuclease to act prior to freezing of the tissue. Another modification was thawing the tissue sections directly in the proteinase-K solution instead of thawing them at 30°C followed by rehydration in graded alcohols prior to the proteinase-K step. Ribonuclease becomes active at higher temperatures in the presence of water, thus treating the sections with proteinase-K upon thawing therefore degrades ribonuclease before it becomes active. This was found to enhance the *in situ* autoradiographic signal about 10 fold.

RESULTS AND DISCUSSION

We have used the *in situ* cDNA:mRNA hybridization technique to visualize cells in the rat pituitary containing beta LH, prolactin, kallikrein and POMC mRNA. Initial studies indicated that this technique could also be used to demonstrate the presence of POMC mRNA containing cells in the periarcuate region of the rat hypothalamus co-localized with POMC peptides. However, *in situ* hybridizations in the brain yielded variable results and high backgrounds. It is important to realize that the brain is different from the pituitary and that these techniques need be optimized individually for each tissue and cDNA probe used . We have refined the *in situ* hybridization technique and now obtain strong, reproducible signals in the brain using POMC cDNA probes. We are currently surveying the anatomical distribution of cells containing POMC mRNA. Earlier work indicated that there might be a population of cells in the amygdala and cortex containing POMC mRNA of lower molecular weight than found in the pituitary and hypothalamus (8). To date we have not found any cells outside of the basal hypothalamus that contain POMC mRNA as determined by *in situ* hybridizations.

While the *in situ* technique can be very useful in answering anatomical questions its greatest value to neuroendocrinology lies in its ability to resolve mRNA:cDNA hybrids at the level of the individual cell and therefore its potential as a semiquantitative assay for mRNA levels in individual neurons of the brain. However, to use this technique quantitatively requires that the system be optimized for the greatest signal to noise ratio possible. Small probes (50-100 bases) and a mild deproteination step with either HCl or proteinase-K enhances the *in situ* autoradiographic signal. These factors are probably related to the diffusion of relatively large molecules through a complex tissue matrix in which the mRNA is located. We have observed high non-cellular backgrounds in the brain associated with highly myelinated structures like the optic tract. This has the effect of increasing general backgrounds in the brain making interpretation of silver grain deposition difficult. This problem is partly allieviated by increasing the temperature of the 0.5xSSC wash after hybridization. We have experimented with incorporating non-specific nucleic acids and proteins into prehybridization and hybridization buffers decrease backgraounds and the specific signal as well.

Assuming we have dealt with all of the problems associated with getting a good autoradiographic signal with a high signal to noise ratio using the *in situ* cDNA: mRNA hybridization technique we are faced then with the problem of what to quantitate. Counting silver grains in all hybridizing cells is only quantitating mRNA levels in the tissue not at the level of the individual cell and gives no advantage over filter hybridization procedures. Some secondary method must be employed to subdivide the population of hybridizing cells into functional subgroups. With this problem in mind we are now pursuing studies designed to make the *in situ* technique compatable with immunocytochemistry on the same tissue section. We have determined that the *in situ* technique is compatable with retrograde fluorescent tracing techniques used to map axonal projections in the brain. Fast blue injected into a POMC terminal field is taken up by axons terminating in that region and transported back to the cell body of origin in the arcuate nucleus. After sectioning and hybridization to a POMC cDNA probe, some arcuate cells can be observed to contain both the fluorescent dye and silver grains from the cDNA hybridization. Using this technique it shall be possible to begin to study regulation of a specific mRNA in subsets of cells that project to any given region of the brain.

REFERENCES

1. Brahic M and Haase AT (1978) Proc Natl Acad Sci USA 75:6125
2. Hudson P, Penschow J, Shine J, Ryan G, Niall H and Coghlan J (1981) Endocrinology 108:353
3. Gee CE and Roberts JL (1983) DNA 2:155
4. Gee CE, Chen CL, Roberts JL, Thompson R and Watson SJ (1983) Nature 306:374
5. Clissod PM, Arnstein HRV, and Chesterton CJ (1977) Cell 11:353
6. Harding JD, MacDonald RJ, Przybyla A, Chirgwin JM, Pictet, RL and Rutter WJ (1977) J Biol Chem 252:7391
7. Moen RC and Palmiter RD (1980) Dev Biol 78:450
8. Civelli O, Birnberg N and Herbert E (1982) J Biol Chem 257:6783

Endocrinology
F. Labrie, L. Proulx, eds.

MONOCLONAL ANTIBODIES AGAINST THE INSULIN RECEPTOR

RICHARD A. ROTH AND DAVID O. MORGAN
Stanford University Medical School, Stanford, CA 94305

INTRODUCTION

The development of the monoclonal technique by Köhler and Milstein (1) greatly facilitated the study of plasma membrane receptors for hormones, neurotransmitters and other ligands (2). This technique allowed the production of large quantities of homogeneous antibodies to small amounts of antigens in impure preparations. However, the production of a particular monoclonal antibody can be an arduous task. To further aid anyone undertaking such a project, we will outline some of our experiences in the production of monoclonal antibodies to the insulin receptor.

MATERIAL AND METHODS

Insulin binding assays, fusions and purification of the receptor were performed as previously described (3-5).

Immunizations

Two Balb/C mice were injected in the peritoneum with 3 μg of purified receptor emulsified in complete Freund's adjuvant at day 0, 14 and 28. Four days prior to fusion, they were injected in the peritoneum with 5 μg of purified receptor without Freund's adjuvant.

Plate binding assays

Fifty μl of affinity purified rabbit anti-mouse IgG (Cappel), 40 μg/ml in 20 mM Na-PO_4, pH 7.4, 150 mM NaCl (PBS), was added to each well of a polyvinyl chloride microtitration plate (Dynatech). After 16 hrs at 4°C, the wells were washed three times with PBS containing 1% bovine serum albumin (BSA). Fifty μl supernatant was added to the wells and after 2 hrs at 24°, the plates were washed three more times. Fifty μl of labeled receptor (10,000 cpm) was added, left 2 hrs at 24°, and the plates were washed 3 more times. The wells were then cut off and counted. Receptor was labeled by either crosslinking to ^{125}I-insulin with disuccinimidyl suberate (5) or by iodination with chloramine T.

RESULTS

Immunization strategies

As previously reported (3), mice immunized with intact IM-9 cells produced antisera which inhibited insulin binding to IM-9 cells and precipitated the insulin-receptor complex. Mice injected with purified insulin receptor produced antisera which also inhibited insulin binding and precipitated the receptor with a higher titer than those mice which were injected with intact IM-9 cells (Fig. 1). The spleen cells of these mice were therefore fused to a myeloma cell by the protocol of de St. Groth and Sheidegger (6).

Screening procedures

Prior studies have indicated that inhibition of ^{125}I-insulin binding to IM-9 cells was a sensitive method to detect antibodies to the insulin receptor (3,4). However, this assay was quite laborious and would detect only antibodies to the insulin binding site of the receptor. Therefore, another assay was sought. Antisera to the receptor and the monoclonal antibody to the insulin binding site of the receptor could be detected by their ability to bind ^{125}I-insulin-receptor complexes after precipitation with rabbit anti-mouse Ig coated *Staphylococcus aureus* (Figs. 1 and 2). This assay was still fairly cumbersome and was not that sensitive.

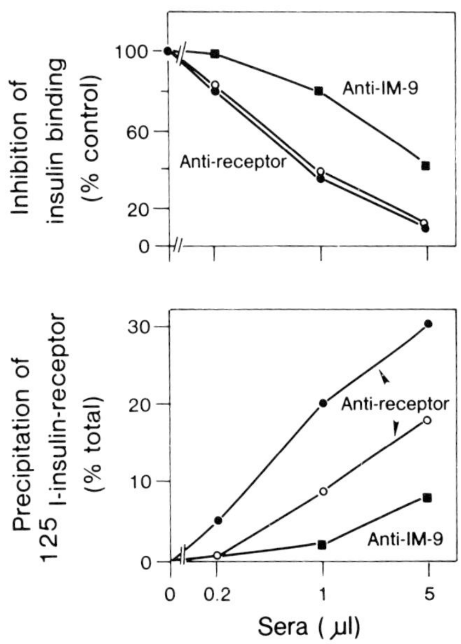

Fig. 1. Inhibition of ^{125}I-insulin binding to IM-9 cells (top) and precipitation of ^{125}I-insulin crosslinked to the receptor (bottom) by antisera of mice injected with either purified receptor (O,●) or IM-9 cells (■).

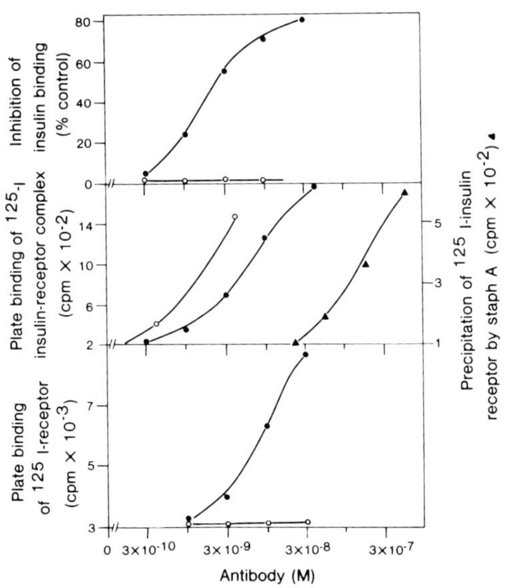

Fig. 2. Comparison of assays for monoclonal antibodies against the insulin binding site (●) and another site (O). Top panel, inhibition of insulin binding. Middle panel, precipitation of ^{125}I-insulin receptor complex by plate assay (O,●) or staph A (▲). Bottom panel, precipitation of iodinated receptor by plate assay.

Another assay for anti-receptor antibodies was, therefore, devised. This assay entailed coating microtiter wells with affinity purified anti-mouse Ig and then letting the monoclonal antibodies in the hybridoma supernatants bind this antibody. The presence of an anti-receptor antibody bound to the wells could then be detected by adding labeled receptor to the wells. The receptor could be labeled by cross-linking with ^{125}I-insulin or by iodination. This assay was much less work than the staph A precipitation assay and was more sensitive (Fig. 2).

The plate binding assay was therefore used to screen the hybridomas from the fusions. One hybridoma producing monoclonal anti-receptor antibody was detected by this technique (Fig. 2). This antibody did not inhibit insulin binding to IM-9 cells nor did it bind to the iodinated receptor (Fig. 2).

DISCUSSION

A monoclonal antibody can be an extremely useful tool for both purifying a hormone receptor and studying its function in the intact cell. Although numerous successes have been reported in the production of monoclonal antibodies to hormone receptors (2), it is still not a straightforward project to make a monoclonal antibody to a particular receptor. Before undertaking such a project, one should consider the various immunization schemes, fusion protocols and screening procedures. The choice of each of these may be crucial in determining whether a useful monoclonal anti-receptor antibody is obtained.

Our past experience has indicated that mice with the highest titer of antisera are most likely to yield a hybridoma making a particular monoclonal antibody (7). Thus, one should optimize the immunization protocol before beginning fusions. One can vary antigen dose, timing and location of injection. In addition, one should consider various strains of mice other than Balb/C (SJL, C3H) since these can, in certain cases, give better immune responses. The source of antigen is also important. A species that is less related to the mouse will be more likely to be antigenic in the mouse. However, the monoclonal antibody that is ultimately obtained may only react with receptor of the species used for immunization.

It is apparent that a considerable amount of antigen may be needed to test out the various immunization schemes. Thus, one should consider whether purified antigen is preferable over crude antigen. Although we observed a higher titer of anti-receptor antibodies with mice that were injected with purified receptor than with intact IM-9 cells, the yield of hybridomas making anti-receptor antibodies was not substantially different in the two groups of mice. Also of interest was the finding that the monoclonal antibody that was obtained from the mouse injected with purified receptor did not inhibit insulin binding. Thus, this antibody is similar to those monoclonal anti-insulin receptor antibodies isolated by Kull et al who also utilized purified receptor as immunogen (8). These antibodies are in contrast to the 3 inhibiting monoclonal antibodies identified from the fusions utilizing mice injected with intact IM-9 cells.

Finally, one must carefully consider the screening procedure to be utilized since the antibody one isolates is often best in assays that mirror the assay used to identify it (7). Thus, the screening assay should reflect the ultimate planned use of the antibody. In addition, the assay must be rapid, sensitive and unambiguous. In our early work we screened the antibodies for their ability to inhibit insulin binding. This assay is very sensitive but quite laborious and would not detect all anti-receptor antibodies. The plate binding assay described in the present paper overcomes all these shortcomings. Its usefulness is demonstrated by its ability to identify a new hybridoma producing an anti-receptor antibody. This assay could also be adapted to screening for the production of antibodies to receptors other than the insulin receptor.

ACKNOWLEDGMENTS

This work was supported by NIH Research Grant AM-26918, a NIH RCDA AM-01171 to RAR, and an Alberta Heritage Foundation Grant to DOM. The assistance of Mary Mesirow is gratefully acknowledged.

REFERENCES

1. Köhler G, Milstein C (1975) Nature 256:495-497

2. Eisenbarth GS, Jackson RA (1982) Endocrine Rev 3:26-39

3. Roth RA, Wong KY, Maddux BA, Goldfine ID (1981) Biochem Biophys Res Commun 101:979-987

4. Roth RA, Cassell DJ, Wong KY, Maddux BA, Goldfine ID (1982) Proc Natl Acad Sci USA 79:7312-7316

5. Roth RA, Mesirow ML, Cassell DJ (1983) J Biol Chem 258:14456-14460

6. Fazekas De St Groth S, Scheidegger D (1980) J Immunol Meth 35: 1-21

7. Roth RA (1984) In: DePirro R, Lauro R (eds) Handbook on Receptor Research. Field Educational Italia-Acta Medica, in press

8. Kull FC Jr, Jacobs S, Su YF, Cuatrecasas P (1982) Biochem Biophys Res Commun 106:1019-1026

Endocrinology
F. Labrie, L. Proulx, eds.

NON-ISOTOPIC IMMUNOASSAYS

W.P. COLLINS
Diagnostics Research Unit, Department of Obstetrics and Gynaecology, King's College School of Medicine, Denmark Hill, London SE5 8RX (UK)

INTRODUCTION

The application of techniques based upon the principles of immunoassay has enabled rapid advances to be made in the practice of diagnostic and therapeutic medicine. Radioimmunoassay (RIA) was the first of these methods to be developed, which measured the analyte in a simple manner, with good sensitivity, accuracy and precision. The essential components of RIA are: (i) a limited concentration of specific antibodies; (ii) a reference preparation - preferably identical with the substance to be measured; (iii) an antigen labelled with a radioactive isotope; and (iv) a method of separating the antibody-bound and free fractions. Most established laboratories have automatic scintillation counters, trained staff, and good facilities for data reduction and statistical analysis.

ASSAY DEVELOPMENT

RIA is undergoing refinement through the introduction of simpler techniques to separate the antibody-bound and free fractions, the development of non-extraction methods for haptens, and the use of monoclonal antibodies. Other developments have involved: (i) labelling an antibody instead of the antigen in a move from limited to excess reagent systems (i.e. immunoradiometric assay; IRMA), and (ii) the use of different labels to radioisotopes for both immuno and immunometric assays. The concept of two-site IRMAs (with a capture antibody on a solid-phase, and a second labelled antibody to a different epitope of the analyte) has enabled the development of more sensitive, practical methods for the measurement of protein hormones.

LIMITATIONS OF RIA AND IRMA

The increasing availability and usefulness of isotopic methods has raised several problems which include: (i) the radioactive half-life and radiolysis of the labelled reagent, which limits assay sensitivity, and; (ii) health hazards associated with the use and disposal of radioactive compounds and the solvents and photofluors necessary for liquid scintillation counting, which are incompatible with the development of tests for use nearer the patient. To date, at least 10 alternative labels to radioisotopes have been advocated (bacteria, erythrocytes, latex particles, gold sols; enzymes, substrates and cofactors; dyes, fluorescent, phosphorescent and chemiluminescent compounds).

PARTICLE IMMUNOASSAY

Red blood cells or latex particles are linked to the antigen or antibody; the separation system does not require the intervention of the assayist and the end-point may be semi-quantitative (by serial dilution of the sample) or quantitative. A threshold value is used to give positive or negative results for pregnancy tests. Semi-quantitative methods are performed in tubes with hemi-spherical bases, and the quantitative procedure in open ended, horizontal glass capillaries. In the latter system the distance between the parallel lines of precipitated labelled reagent (read through an eyepiece with a graticule) is proportional to the concentration of analyte. The tests take approx. 2 hours and have the advantages of simplicity and low cost. Alternatively latex particles are being used in the development of methods, which use nephelometry or particle size analysis to distinguish between the antibody-bound and free fraction. Gold and silver sols have also been used as labels in simple tests for the semi-quantitative or quantitative measurement of proteins and haptens.

ENZYME IMMUNOASSAY

Enzyme immunoassay (EIA) may be subdivided into separation systems (e.g. enzyme linked immunosorbent assay - ELISA) or non-separation assays (e.g. enzyme multiplied immunoassay - EMIT) for the measurement of haptens. The latter approach capitalizes on the finding that relatively small enzymes are inactivated when the labelled antigen is bound to antibody - leaving the free fraction available for measurement. The enzymes that have been used most extensively are horseradish peroxidase, alkaline phosphatase from calf intestinal mucosa, β-D-galactosidase from Escherichia coli and glucose oxidase from Aspergillus niger. A variety of end points have been used including pH change, colorimetry, fluorimetry, chemiluminometry and electrometry. The potential sensitivity of detection is good > 10^{18} moles). Recently, the production of purified enzymes by affinity chromatography, together with the use of monoclonal antibodies and solid-phase systems has enabled the development of improved methods (immunoenzymometric assays) for the measurement of protein hormones. To date, EIA has not been widely applied to the measurement of haptens for the followings reasons: (i) compared to radioisotopes the label has a large molecular weight which often interferes with the antibody binding reaction; (ii) the synthesis of labelled antigen is difficult to control and the product needs to be characterised for enzyme and antibody-binding activities; (iii) the homogeneous systems are relatively insensitive due to non-specific interference from the biological sample; and (iv) the end-point determination is more complex and time consuming than for RIA. Nevertheless, the availability of automatic equipment for taking spectrophotometric or fluorescent measurements from microtitre plates, together with the appropriate software for data reduction, makes this approach attractive for the routine analysis of a large number of samples. Dipsticks have also been produced which use an enzyme as a label for the detection of protein hormones, and an apo-enzyme for the measurement of haptens.

FLUORESCENCE AND PHOSPHORESCENCE IMMUNOASSAYS

To date, the most commonly used fluorophores have been derivatives of fluorescein, rhodamine or umbelliferone. Recently, erythrosin has been used as a label for the measurement of haptens by phosphorescence immunoassay. The most sensitive fluorescence immunoassays (FIAs) and phosphorescence immunoassays, where the antigen is labelled with a fluorophore, have been most successfully applied to the measurement of analytes that are present in amounts > 1 ng/ml of biological fluid. Attempts to increase sensitivity have involved the attachment of fluorophore to polylysine which is subsequently linked to the analyte to form a labelled antigen and by the use of immunofluorometric assay (IFMA). Recently, methods involving the use of time-resolved fluorimetry have been introduced for the measurement of protein hormones. Europium chelates covalently linked to monoclonal antibodies constitute the label and become fluorogenic when attached to an organic moiety surrounded by detergent in an aqueous solution. Assays for the measurement of TSH and hCG have good sensitivity, accuracy and precision. Limited reagent methods with a second, labelled antibody are being developed for the measurement of haptens.

CHEMILUMINESCENCE IMMUNOASSAY

Many organic compounds including cyclic hydrazides and acridinium esters are chemiluminescent upon oxidation. Bioluminescence is a special case of chemiluminescence which is found in living organisms. The reactions are catalysed by an enzyme (luciferase), which oxidises a specific substrate (luciferin). Both reactants vary with the species. Recently solid phase chemiluminescence immunoassays (CIAs) have been described for the measurement of plasma steroids, urinary steroid glucuronides, LH and human chorionic gonadotrophin (hCG). Derivatives of isoluminol have been used to form the labelled antigens, and an enhancer has been identified to improve the signal without the use of sodium hydroxide. Immunochemiluminometric assays (ICMAs) using monoclonal antibodies labelled with acridinium ester are preferred for the measurement of protein hormones. All methods have improved sensitivity, and equivalent accuracy and precision to a corresponding RIA or IRMA. In addition, CIA or ICMA has the following advantages: (i) the labelled antigens or antibodies are very stable; (ii) the health hazards and waste disposal problems of radioisotopes are eliminated; (iii) non-separation methods using chemical energy transfer or differential activation of the non-bound fraction may be developed and (iv) the cost of equipment is relatively low. The end point can be extremely rapid < 30 secs as in chemiluminescence, or continuous as in bacterial or firefly bioluminescence. Aspects of CIA or ICMA under active development are (i) the synthesis of alternative chemiluminescent labels with a higher quantum yield; (ii) the identification of enhancers and inhibitors; (iii) the development of improved chemiluminometers; (iv) the purification of reagents for bioluminescence; and (v) the production of enzyme labels.

CONCLUSIONS

It is anticipated that increases in the use of radioactivity for immunoassay will be resisted and the pressure to find alternative biochemical labels may become more intense. The current use of alternative procedures, however, is likely to be limited due to the large investment in equipment by centralised laboratories for scintillation counting and data processing. The tendency towards the use of non-invasive immunochemical tests (e.g. on saliva or early morning urine) in the ward, outpatient clinic or home should encourage the development and facilitate the acceptance of non-isotopic procedures.

REFERENCES

This article is a summary of a book on Alternative Immunoassays (Ed. W P Collins), to be published by John Wiley and Sons Ltd., Chichester, 1984.

© 1984 Elsevier Science Publishers B.V.
Endocrinology
F. Labrie, L. Proulx, eds.

POLYPEPTIDE MICROSEQUENCE ANALYSIS WITH THE COMMERCIALLY AVAILABLE GAS-PHASE SEQUENCER

FREDERICK S. ESCH
Laboratories for Neuroendocrinology, The Salk Institute, 10010 North Torrey Pines Road, La Jolla, California 92037

INTRODUCTION

Technological advances in polypeptide sequencing procedures have progressed at a remarkable rate since the spinning cup or liquid phase sequencer was introduced in 1967 (1). However, the large quantities of sample required (often > 50 nmol) and the inability to sequence short peptides (< 50 amino acids) were major limitations in the liquid phase technology until the introduction of Polybrene (2,3), a quaternary ammonium salt polymer, in 1978. Polybrene interacts with polar components of peptide chains to prevent peptide losses from the spinning cup during organic solvent extractions and thus permits the sequence analysis of small quantities (1-10 nmol) of both proteins and peptides; indeed, even short hydrophobic peptides can be sequenced to completion. Subsequent improvements in instrumental design, in the purification of reagents and solvents employed in the Edman chemistry and in the reverse-phase liquid chromotographic analysis of phenylthiohydantion (>PhNCS) amino acids led to the development of a subnanomole sequencing capability (4). Unfortunately, the extensive and sophisticated instrumental modifications required for this increased sensitivity precluded the widespread utilization of this modified sequencer. In 1981 a new type of sequanator was described (5) and subsequently made commercially available in 1982 which incorporates many of these improvements in a novel design whereby the coupling buffer and cleavage acid are employed in gaseous rather than liquid phases. This ensures that polypeptide samples are never present in liquids in which they are appreciably soluble and thus minimizes "peptide washout" during a degradation cycle.

Instrumental Design. The gas phase sequencer is marked by its simplicity of design and the miniaturization of its component parts. The elaborate spinning cup assembly of its predecessor has been replaced by a small, glass cartridge-type reaction cell (2.5 x 5 cm) manufactured to hold a glass fiber disc on which the polypeptide is degraded. Miniaturized zero dead volume, Kel-F valve blocks eliminate cross-contamination of reagents and solvents. The reservoirs and valve blocks are located to minimize the length of connecting tubing to the reaction cartridge. The automatic phenylthiohydantoin conversion accessory eliminates manual intervention in the final phase of the Edman chemistry, contributing to the overall efficiency and ease of operation of the instrument. The >PhNCS amino acids are delivered to a miniature fraction collector into tubes compatible with commercially available HPLC autosamplers so that transfer losses of the >PhNCS amino acids are never incurred. The overall miniaturization of the instrument has decreased reagent and solvent consumption to $\leq$ 10% of that used by the spinning cup technology. The levels of UV-absorbing impurities from these chemicals are likewise decreased in reverse-phase liquid chromatography (RPLC) chromatograms of >PhNCS amino acid residues from the sequencer. The attenuation of these background artifacts is of vital importance for ultrasensitive microsequence analyses and may be the most significant contribution of this new technology.

Operation of the Sequencer. The sequential degradation of polypeptides on the Applied Biosystems Inc. (Foster City, CA) Model 470A gas phase sequencer is controlled via an HP9915 microprocessor (Hewlett-Packard). The software is very "user friendly" and has recently been modified so that all drying steps are accomplished with argon rather than a vacuum system. This has eliminated the inconvenience and expense of maintaining a liquid nitrogen trap to protect a vacuum pump from the corrosive chemicals employed in the degradation. Routine maintenance is minimal and generally involves keeping reagent and solvent reservoirs filled and briefly cleaning the glass cartridge/reaction cell after each sequenator run. For optimal performance it is advisable to closely monitor reagent and solvent deliveries in each sequenator run as per the manufacturer's recommendations. Highly reproducible deliveries are vital for obtaining high repetitive yields and maximal sequence information. It is also worth noting the lot numbers of chemicals employed in each sequence analysis as such a record can be of great aid in troubleshooting poor sequencer performance.

PhNCS Amino Acid Analysis. Microsequence analysis with $\leq$ 100 pmol quantities of polypeptides demands an exquisitely resolutive, reliable, ultrasensitive methodology for the identification and quantitation of >PhNCS amino acid residues. We have employed the RPLC conditions and instrumentation suggested by Applied Biosystems Inc. and indicated in Figure 1 and have found them to be quite effective. The 30 minute gradient program adequately resolves all the >PhNCS amino acids yielding sharp peaks which permit quantitation to $\leq$ 1 pmole of each <PhNCS amino acid. The resolution of the various residues from themselves and from the UV-absorbing artifacts of the Edman degradation may be readily accomplished by methodically manipulating the initial concentration of acetonitrile present in the program, the slope of the gradient program and the pH and ionic strength of the buffer employed. The inclusion of the internal standard,

>PhNCS aminoisobutyric acid, is a helpful reference, particularly in peptide degradations where the background level of >PhNCS amino acids is low or non-existent. A light box for viewing chromatograms from successive cycles of a degradation is a highly useful method of data evaluation, particularly when the data have been obtained with a multi-pen recorder possessing a very consistent chart-drive motor.

Instrumental Performance. As of March 1984 we have structurally characterized nine growth hormone releasing peptides from seven different sources using the gas phase sequencer (Table I). Three peptides containing 44(hpGRF-44), 40(hpGRF-40) and 37(hpGRF-37) amino acids in identical sequences from their amino termini were characterized from a human pancreatic tumor (Tumor I) surgically removed from an acromegalic patient who presented no indication of pituitary abnormality (5,6). The 40 and 37 amino acid peptides are probably proteolytic degradation products of the larger, mature hpGRF-44. The subnanomole capability of the sequencer was vital in the structural characterization of hpGRF-40 obtained from yet another human pancreatic tumor (Tumor II in Table I) where only 1800 pmols of peptide were available for amino acid analysis, Edman degradation and carboxyl terminal determination (7). Recent refinements in our sequencing procedures have significantly increased our repetitive yields and have permitted the identification of the N-terminal 43 of 44 amino acids of the ovine, caprine and human hypothalamic GRFs (manuscripts in preparation) using only 500 pmols of each peptide (Table I). These improvements have permitted the complete structural characterization of each of these molecules with <800 pmols of each peptide.

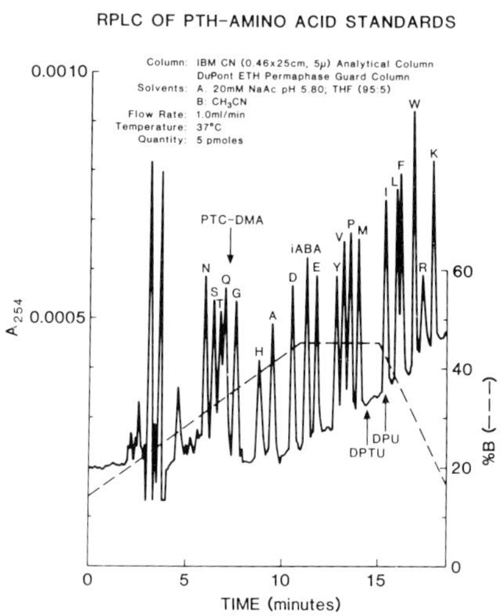

Figure 1. RPLC of 5 pmol >PhNCS amino acid standards. iABA represents the internal standard >PhNCS aminoisobutyric acid; The elution positions of typical UV-absorbing artifacts generated during a degradation are indicated in the Figure as: PTC-DMA (phenylthiocarbamyl-dimethylamine), DPTU (N, N'-diphenylthiourea) and DPU (N, N'-diphenylthiourea). Chromatography was performed at 37°C and 1.0 ml/min with an IBM CN analytical column (0.46 x 25cm, 5 μ particle size) and an Uptight precolumn filled with DuPont ETH Permaphase. Solvent A consisted of 20mM sodium acetate, pH 5.80:THF (95:5) and solvent B was acetonitrile.

Table I
GAS PHASE SEQUENCE ANALYSIS OF GROWTH HORMONE RELEASING PEPTIDES AND THEIR CYANOGEN BROMIDE DIGESTION FRAGMENTS.

Peptides	Amount Analyzed (pmols)	No. Amino Acids	No. Residues Identified	Initial Yield	Average Repetitive Yield
Intact hpGRF-44[a]	1500	44	40	37.3%	89.7%
CNBr Fragment: hpGRF-44(1-27)[a]	540	27	25	57.4%	88.9%
CNBr Fragment: hpGRF-44(28-44)[a]	490	17	17	64.3%	89.1%
Intact hpGRF-40[a]	4060	40	40	73.4%	88.7%
CNBr Fragment: hpGRF-40(1-27)[a]	1381	27	25	100.5%	88.9%
CNBr Fragment: hpGRF-40(28-40)[a]	950	13	13	44.7%	87.8%
Intact hpGRF-37[a]	2000	37	35	34.8%	87.2%
CNBr Fragment: hpGRF-37(1-27)[a]	777	27	25	83.2%	87.4%
CNBr Fragment: hpGRF-37(28-37)[a]	732	10	10	26.0%	88.3%
Intact hpGRF-40[b]	500	40	33	40.0%	91.4%
CNBr Fragment: hpGRF-40(28-40)[b]	90	13	13	27.1%	85.0%
Intact pGRF-44	2000	44	42	13.8%	91.4%
CNBr Fragment: pGRF-44(28-44)	680	13	12	17.3%	84.3%
Intact bGRF-44	1780	44	43	38.5%	91.7%
Intact oGRF-44	500	44	43	59.4%	92.3%
Intact gGRF-44	500	44	43	35.4%	92.5%
Intact hhGRF-44	500	44	43	40.0%	90.9%

[a]Tissue source: Tumor I
[b]Tissue source: Tumor II

hhGRF-44 +	hpGRF-44:	YADAIFTNSYRKVLGQLSARKLLQDIMSRQQGESNQERGARARL-NH_2
	hpGRF-40:	YADAIFTNSYRKVLGQLSARKLLQDIMSRQQGESNQERGA
	hpGRF-37:	YADAIFTNSYRKVLGQLSARKLLQDIMSRQQGESNQE
	pGRF-44:	YADAIFTNSYRKVLGQLSARKLLQDIMSRQQGERNQEQGARVRL-NH_2
bGRF-44 +	gGRF-44:	YADAIFTNSYRKVLGQLSARKLLQDIMNRQQGERNQEQGAKVRL-NH_2
	oGRF-44:	YADAIFTNSYRKILGQLSARKLLQDIMNRQQGERNQEQGAKVRL-NH_2

References

1. Edman P, Begg G (1967) Eur J Biochem 1:80-91
2. Tarr GE, Beecher JF, Bell M, McKean DJ (1978) Anal Biochem 84:622-627
3. Klapper DG, Wilde CE, Capara JD (1978) Anal Biochem 85:126-131
4. Hunkapiller MW, Hood LE (1978) Biochemistry 17:2124-2133
5. Guillemin R, Brazeau P, Böhlen P, Esch F, Ling N, Wehrenberg W (1982) Science 218:585-587
6. Esch FS, Böhlen P, Ling N, Brazeau P, Wehrenberg W, Guillemin R (1983) J Biol Chem 158:1806-1812
7. Esch FS, Böhlen P, Ling NC, Brazeau PE, Wehrenberg WB, Thorner MO, Cronin MJ, Guillemin R (1982) Biochem Biophys Res Commun 109:152-158

© 1984 Elsevier Science Publishers B.V.
Endocrinology
F. Labrie, L. Proulx, eds.

PURIFICATION OF HUMAN INSULIN RECEPTOR WITH HIGH INSULIN-BINDING AND KINASE ACTIVITIES

Y. FUJITA-YAMAGUCHI

Beckman Research Institute of the City of Hope, Duarte, CA 91010 (U.S.A.)

INTRODUCTION

For the study of a protein, whether it involves characterization of its structure and/or its biological function, one must first isolate the protein in pure form. It is easy to isolate proteins which are water-soluble and/or abundant in tissues. In contrast, it is more difficult to purify proteins which are membrane-bound and minor components in tissues, as in a case of the peptide hormone receptors.

By a combination of conventional methods, 4 to 5 purification steps are generally required to isolate a protein in pure, uncontaminated form. It is almost impossible to purify peptide hormone receptors by such conventional methods, since, being not abundant in starting materials, more and more steps are required to isolate them. Therefore, it is necessary to establish very simple, efficient purification schemes for isolation of the receptors, that is, an application of affinity chromatography which takes advantage of the binding specificity of the hormone (or monoclonal antibodies) to the receptor. The receptor can be easily separated from a greater portion of unwanted material by the use of an affinity column, hormone (or monoclonal antibody)-bound matrix.

Recently developed techniques such as microsequencing and gene engineering technologies have provided a new strategy for determination of an entire amino acid sequence of the proteins which are available in very small quantities: 1) Purify a desired protein enough to determine its partial amino acid sequence. 2) Design and synthesize DNA probes complementary to the amino acid sequence. 3) Use the DNA probe specific to the desired protein to identify cDNA encoding the protein. 4) Determine DNA sequence of the cDNA isolated, from which its primary sequence will be deduced. If we can purify enough "peptide hormone receptors" to determine their partial amino acid sequence, it would be possible to obtain its total amino acid sequence (1). Then, one could express cDNA encoding the receptor in bacteria and produce substantial amounts of the receptor, which could be a great help in understanding the mechanism of hormone-receptor interaction and following events.

In attempting to determine the primary structure of the insulin receptor, we have purified a biologically active insulin receptor (2,3). This preparation also has provided a good "in vitro" system for studying the mechanism of insulin action (4,5).

PURIFICATION OF INSULIN RECEPTOR

Since the first purification of the receptor from rat liver by Jacobs *et al.* in 1977 (6), purification of insulin receptor had been reported from different laboratories (7-9). However, their results were controversial because no one had purified insulin receptor with specific activity of 20μg of insulin bound per mg of protein, which would be expected if insulin receptor with Mr=300,000 binds one molecule of insulin. The low specific activities achieved by them could be due to contaiminants in the preparation or to inactivation of the receptor.

Among the methods originally proposed, we have realized that insulin-sepharose affinity chromatography is the most practical and efficient method to purify insulin receptor, since we take advantage of the high affinity and specificity of the receptor to insulin. This approach has been pioneered by Cuatrecasas (10) and used by his colleagues (6) and others (9) but unfortunately resulted in purifying the receptor with poor insulin binding activity. We have reevaluated the synthesis of insulin-Sepharose and elution conditions, and have developed a new elution method (pH5 with high salt) without using urea to purify insulin receptor (2).

Placental membranes (0.8-1.2g of protein) prepared from two fresh human placentae (wet weight, 800-1200g) are usually used for purification of the receptor. Insulin-binding activity is monitored throughout the purification. Table I summarized a typical receptor purification.

Insulin receptor was purified 2400-fold with a yield of 40% from human placental membranes by sequential affinity chromatography on wheat germ agglutinin-Sepharose and insulin-Sepharose. Approximately 50μg of purified receptor was obtained from 2 placentae. The receptor was eluted from insulin-Sepharose using mild conditions (50 mM acetate buffer, pH 5, containing 1M NaCl and 0.1% Triton X-100) so that it was stable and retained full insulin binding activity. Specific activity of the purified receptor determined by Scatchard analysis was 28 μg of insulin bound per mg of protein, whereas the receptor eluted by previously used conditions (pH 6.0 with 4.5 M urea) resulted in only 6 μg of insulin bound per mg of protein. This indicated that four to five-fold increases in specific activity can be obtained by using the new conditions, and that the low specific activity obtained by Jacobs *et al.* is due to inactivation of the receptor.

TABLE 1

PURIFICATION OF HUMAN INSULIN RECEPTOR FROM PLACENTAL MEMBRANES

	TOTAL PROTEIN (mg)	INSULIN BINDING ACTIVITY (Specific Activity)[a] (μg/mg)	TOTAL ACTIVITY (μg)	PURIFICATION (-fold)	YIELD (%)
Placental membranes	870[b,c]				
Triton X-100 Extract	323[b]	0.0116	3.75	1	100
WGA-Sepharose	23.1[b]	0.087	2.01	7.5	54
Insulin-Sepharose	0.052[d]	28.5	1.48	2457	40

[a] Insulin binding activity was calculated from the Scatchard plots (13) and expressed as μg of insulin bound/mg of protein.
[b] Determined by a modified Lowry's method (14).
[c] Prepared from 2 small placentae.
[d] Determined by amino acid analysis (15).

CHARACTERIZATION OF THE PURIFIED INSULIN RECEPTOR

SDS-gel electrophorsis of the purified receptor showed two major protein bands with Mr 125K (α) and 90K (β) and a minor band with Mr 50K under reducing conditions (2). All three components were immunoprecipitated by anti-insulin receptor sera (3). Peptide mapping of isolated subunits revealed that the α subunit is distinct from the β subunit and that the 50K subunit is a degradation product of the β subunit. Further analysis by two-dimentional SDS-gel electrophoresis provided conclusive evidence that a disulfide-linked complex (α_2,2β) is the basic structural unit of insulin receptor (11).

The purified receptor shows a curvilinear Scatchard plot, suggesting the presence of negative cooperativity among insulin binding sites (2). The purified receptor is capable of phosphorylating tyrosine residues in the β subunit (autophosphorylation) (3) as well as in exogeneous substrates such as histone 2B, casein, anti-pp60^{Src} antibody, and a synthetic peptide which resembles an autophosphorylation site of pp60^{Src}(12). Insulin stimulates the phosphorylation reaction by 3- to 5- fold. Kinetic analysis using the synthetic peptide reveals that insulin increases Vmax of phosphorylation reaction with little change in the Km value (12).

REFERENCE

1. Suggs SV, Wallace RB, Hirose T, Kawashima EH, Itakura K. (1981) *Proc. Natl. Acad. Sci.* USA 78: 6613-6617.

2. Fujita-Yamaguchi, Y, Choi S, Sakamoto Y, Itakura K (1983) *J. Biol. Chem.* 258: 5045-5049.

3. Kasuga M, Fujita-Yamaguchi Y, Blithe DL, Kahn CR (1983) *Proc. Natl. Acad. Sci.* USA 80: 2137-2141.

4. Tamura S, Fujita-Yamaguchi Y, Larner J (1983) *J. Biol. Chem.* 258: 14749-14752.

5. Tamura S, Brown TA, Whipple JH, Fujita-Yamaguchi Y, Dubler RE, Cheng K, Larner J (1984) *Biochem. Biophys. Res. Commun.* 119: 465-472.

6. Jacobs S, Schechter Y, Bissel K, Cuatrecasas P (1977) *Biochem. Biophys. Res. Commun.* 77: 981-988.

7. Williams PF, Turtle JR (1979) *Biochim. Biophys. Acta* 579: 367-374.

8. Harrison LC, Itin A (1980) *J. Biol. Chem.* 255: 12066-12072.

9. Siegel TW, Ganguly S, Jacobs S, Rosen OM, Rubin CS (1981) *J. Biol. Chem.* 256: 9266-9273.

10. Cuatrecasas P (1972) *Proc. Natl. Acad. Sci.* USA 69: 1277-1281.

11. Fujita-Yamaguchi Y (1984) *J. Biol. Chem.* 259: 1206-1211.

12. Kasuga M, Fujita-Yamaguchi Y, Blithe DL, White MF, Kahn CR (1983) *J. Biol. Chem* 258: 10973-10980.

13. Scatchard G (1949) *Ann. N.Y. Acad. Sci.* 51: 660-672.

14. Bensadoun A, Weinstein D (1976) *Anal. Biochem.* 70: 241-250.

15. Del Valle U, Shively JE (1979) *Anal. Biochem.* 96: 77-83.

© 1984 Elsevier Science Publishers B.V.
Endocrinology
F. Labrie, L. Proulx, eds.

ANALYSIS OF SPECIFIC mRNA's BY RNA BLOT AND DOT HYBRIDIZATION

F. CARTER BANCROFT

Molecular Biology and Virology Department, Sloan-Kettering Institute, New York, NY 10021

In recent years, there has been a great deal of interest in developing convenient and reliable methods to follow a specific messenger RNA (mRNA) in animal cells or organs during induction by hormones, differentiation, etc. Interest in this area has been stimulated by the advent of recombinant DNA technology and the consequent availability of pure probes for the RNA products of specific genes.

Of the techniques developed, the ones most widely employed involve either transfer of size-fractionated RNA molecules from a separation gel to a nitrocellulose sheet ("blotting"), or direct application of nucleic acids to such a sheet ("dotting"). These blot/dot techniques fall into two categories, representing assays of two different levels of expression of a gene. The techniques most commonly employed (RNA gel blot, and RNA and cytoplasmic dot hybridization) measure the amount of the mRNA product of the gene in cells or tissue; i.e., the _steady state_ level of the mRNA. The other type of technique (nuclear run-on transcription) measures the incorporation of radioactive precursors into an mRNA; i.e., the rate of _synthesis_ of the mRNA. The second assay is clearly preferable for direct measurements of specific gene expression. However, its technical difficulty and expense have tended to limit its use.

These two types of techniques have two features in common. Both are based on the use of specific hybridization between an mRNA sequence and its complementary DNA (cDNA) copy, to detect that mRNA in a mixture of RNA's. In addition, both are performed by immobilizing unlabeled nucleic acids on a nitrocellulose sheet, followed by exposure of the nitrocellulose under annealing conditions to a solution of ^{32}P-labeled nucleic acids. However, in a steady state assay, the sample (unlabeled mRNA) is immobilized, while in a synthesis assay the sample (labeled mRNA) is in solution. The two categories of techniques are described separately below.

Assays for the Steady State Level of an mRNA

Until fairly recently, the standard blot/dot-type assay was RNA gel blot hybridization ("Northern gels"). This involves size separation of RNA by gel electrophoresis, followed by transfer (blotting) of the RNA to an appropriate substrate to which the RNA becomes immobilized. A specific RNA band is visualized by hybridization with a labeled cDNA plasmid. The substrate originally employed was chemically modified paper (1). However, the demonstration by Thomas (2) that in high salt RNA will bind to nitrocellulose has led to widespread use of nitrocellulose sheets for immobilization of RNA samples. The techniques employed in labeling the cDNA probes by nick translation and performing RNA gel blot hybridization have been described in detail (3).

The technique described above requires gel analysis of each sample. In addition, purification of RNA from samples of cells or tissues can be a difficult and time-consuming process. For many types of endocrine regulation studies, it would be useful to employ a convenient technique for the simultaneous analysis of an mRNA in multiple samples. For example, with such a technique it would be feasible to analyze in replicate samples such parameters as the time course or dose-response curve of the effect of single or multiple hormones on the levels of one or more specific mRNA's. We therefore developed a dot technique for analyzing relative levels of a specific mRNA in unfractionated cytoplasmic preparations, termed cytoplasmic dot hybridization (4). In this technique, a detergent is employed to prepare cytoplasm from cells or tissue. Each cytoplasmic sample is denatured by heating in the presence of formaldehyde, and dotted onto a nitrocellulose sheet. A sheet containing graded dilutions of a number of samples is then hybridized to an appropriate ^{32}P-labeled cDNA plasmid. Control experiments have shown that this technique is both specific and quantitative, can be employed with either pituitary cells in culture or pituitary tissue, and is as sensitive as RNA dot hybridization (4).

As shown previously, the formaldehyde denaturation step is required for the detection of a strong signal with this technique (4). In addition, the baking step is required for retention on the nitrocellulose of the RNA in cytoplasmic samples. A "quick-blot" technique for immobilizing cytoplasmic RNA has been described recently, in which the baking step is omitted (5). However, we have been unable to detect a GH mRNA signal in GH_3 cells with this technique, probably because of loss of RNA from the nitrocellulose during either the application of samples or the washing steps (M. Johnson and C. Bancroft, unpublished observations).

An example of the use of cytoplasmic dot hybridization is shown in Fig. 1. In this experiment, the possibility of an interaction between Dexamethasone and various concentrations of insulin in regulating growth hormone mRNA in GH_3 cells was investigated. It is seen that with the cytoplasmic dot technique, relative levels of an mRNA in 24 separate cultures can be quantitated simultaneously.

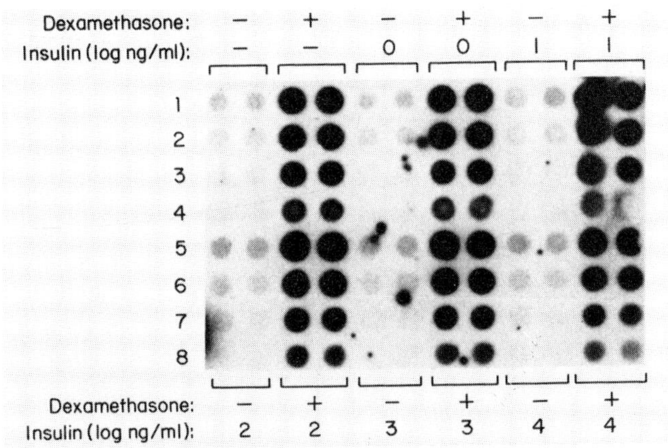

Fig. 1. Multihormonal analysis by cytoplasmic dot hybridization. Duplicate cultures of rat pituitary (GH_3) cells were incubated with the indicated concentrations of hormones, and relative growth hormone mRNA levels measured. Four two-fold serial dilutions of cytoplasm prepared from 3-5 x 10^5 cells from each culture were analyzed.

This technique has been shown to be applicable to a wide variety of eukaryotic cells and tissue. For example, it has been used to analyze alcohol dehydrogenase mRNA in fruit flies (6), vitellogenin mRNA in chick liver (7), prolactin and growth hormone mRNA in rat pituitary cells (8,9), PDGF-induced mRNA's in mouse fibroblasts (10), and oncogene-related mRNA's in human neuroblastomas (11). Interestingly, this technique has also been employed to analyze RNA viruses in plant tissues (12). In addition, the cytoplasmic dot protocol has proven useful in a number of systems for the analysis of purified RNA by RNA dot hybridization.

Dot Assay for the Synthesis of an mRNA

As noted above, in this type of assay, the unlabeled DNA probe is immobilized onto nitrocellulose, while the labeled RNA to be analyzed is in solution. By employing a sheet containing dots of various cloned DNA sequences, it is possible to monitor simultaneously the amounts of labeled RNA in the solution complementary to each of the cloned DNA probes employed. Kafatos et al (13) first used this type of assay, to analyze levels of 17 different labeled silkmoth chorion mRNA sequences. More recently, Hofer et al (14) have employed this approach to analyze transcription of a mouse globin gene. Nuclei from cells incubated with or without an inducer (DMSO) were incubated in vitro with ^{32}P-UTP to label total nuclear RNA. The RNA was then hybridized to a nitrocellulose sheet containing a series of DNA clones corresponding to various regions of the globin gene and its flanking DNA sequences. This yielded information both about the induction by DMSO of globin gene transcription, and about which portions of the gene and its downstream flanking regions are transcribed.

REFERENCES

1. Alwine JC, Kemp DJ, Stark GR (1977) Proc Natl Acad Sci 74:5350
2. Thomas, PS (1980) Proc Natl Acad Sci 77:5201
3. Maniatis T, Fritsch EF, Sambrook J (1982). Molecular Cloning: A Laboratory Manual. Cold Spring Harbor Laboratory
4. White BA, Bancroft FC (1981) J Biol Chem 257:8569
5. Bresser J, Doering J, Gillespie D (1983) DNA 2:243
6. Anderson SM, McDonald JF (1983) Proc Natl Acad Sci 80:4798
7. Burch JBE, Weintraub H (1983) Cell 33:65
8. White BA, Bancroft FC (1983) J Biol Chem 258:4618
9. Wark JD, Tashjian AH Jr (1983) J Biol Chem 258:12118
10. Cochran BH, Reffel AC, Stiles CD (1983) Cell 33:939
11. Kohl NE, Kanda N, Schreck RR, Burns G, Latt SA, Gilbert F, Alt FW (1983) Cell 35:359
12. Maule AJ, Hull R, Donson D (1983) J Virol Methods 6:215
13. Kafatos FC, Jones CW, Efstradiatis A (1979) Nucleic Acids Res 7:1541
14. Hofer E, Hofer-Warbinek, Darnell JE Jr (1982) Cell 29:887

Endocrinology
F. Labrie, L. Proulx, eds.

ISOLATION FROM PORCINE FOLLICULAR FLUID OF A PROTEIN EXHIBITING POTENT INHIBIN LIKE BIOLOGICAL ACTIVITY

J RIVIER, R McCLINTOCK, J SPIESS, J VAUGHAN, D DALTON, A CORRIGAN, R AZAD AND W VALE

The Salk Institute, Peptide Biology Laboratory, 10010 N. Torrey Pines Road, La Jolla, California 92037

INTRODUCTION

The existence of a water soluble substance of gonadal origin that can selectively suppress FSH secretion has been suspected for more than fifty years[1]. The quest to chemically characterize these molecules referred to as inhibin (IN) in the male and folliculostatin (FS) in the female has not succeeded to date[2,3]. A 31-peptide which structure was recently reported by Ramasharma, *et al.*[4] may not have the biological properties expected of IN or FS, one of several of the physiological regulators of FSH secretion[2,3].

We report here a preparative scale purification method for folliculostatin from porcine follicular fluid (pFF) using reverse phase HPLC (RP·HPLC) solely. Other reports on the partial purification of IN or FS have generally used more conventional approaches such as gel permeation and electrophoresis after ammonium sulfate fractionation by selective precipitation[2].

MATERIAL AND METHODS

Starting Material was non-charcoal treated pFF made available to us by the Contraceptive Development Branch of NICHD.

In vitro FS Assay was based upon the ability of FS to lower basal FSH secretion by cultured rat anterior pituitary cells. This assay is a long-term version of the method developed in 1972[5] and further refined[6]. Parallel dose response curves (3-5 points) gave us a relative potency versus an internal standard composed of crude pFF. Peptide concentration was determined by amino acid analysis after acid hydrolysis.

RP·HPLC were as described in reference 7-10. Exact conditions are reported in Table I. Most runs were performed at elevated temperatures (Steps 1, 2 at 50°C, Step 3 at 60°C, Steps 4 and 5 at 30°C); these temperatures could be obtained preparatively by running hot water (80°) around the metal tubing feeding the cartridge whereas analytically columns were immersed in a thermostated water bath.

RESULTS

Problems associated with the RP·HPLC of proteins has been addressed by us and others using mostly model substances commercially available. It was found that proteins generally elute within a narrow window of concentration of organic modifier suggesting that the observed separation may be in part due to the differences in the solubility of the proteins under those conditions rather than the result of their partitioning during the chromatographic process. We therefore investigated which solvent compositions gave maximal precipitation of undesired proteins while keeping FS activity in solution and used two HPLC solvents (CH_3CN and propanol) in our study. pFF was first diluted (1/1) with triethyl ammonium phosphate buffer (TEAP) which had been shown to have unusual solvating properties and could be used to adjust pHs[7]. Upon addition of either of the organic modifiers to the clear FS containing solution, massive precipitation occurred when reaching 36% to 42%. The supernatant from this precipitation step contained only one-fifth of this overall FS activity, but could be applied directly, upon dilution, onto RP·HPLC supports with little detrimental effect to the preparative HPLC cartridges[10] (Step 1, Table I) thus allowing for a concentration step (Step 2, Table I) followed by two highly resolutive semi-preparative runs and two desalting/concentration steps. All except the last two steps were run at 60°C since it resulted in better separation without loss of activity which is in agreement with the proposed mechanisms of elution (see above). We also realized that the chromatographic behavior of the mixture was sensitive to slight variations in pH as a result of ion pairing effects or of conformational changes in the proteins which both could have altered the separation. The range of pH used varied from 7.0 to 5.0 with TEAP and 2.1 with .1% TFA. In the latter case we observed two zones of activity, one of which only is reported here for it may represent the most potent of the two entities. The second zone eluted slightly later and is being further purified.

Based on gel permeation experiments and a preliminary amino acid composition we suspect this isolated FS activity to have a molecular weight (M.W.) ranging from 10,000-12,000. This proposed M.W. is clearly smaller than that proposed by others[11] and may be the result of our investigating the FS activity found in the upper phase of our first precipitation step or that the conditions used may have selectivity cleaved an active portion of the molecule from a larger precursor. We plan to investigate such hypotheses with the availability of selective antibodies which could be raised using synthetic replicate of a total or partial sequence. Interestingly, FS activity found in the ammonium sulfate supernatant of a 50% cut was found to have similar physicochemical and biological properties to those described here for the material processed after precipitation by organic solvents. The presence or absence of carbohydrate moieties in our preparation has not yet been fully investigated.

TABLE I

Purification of folliculostatin from 1450 ml of Porcine Follicular Fluid

HPLC(a) Step	Flow Rate ml/min	Solvent Composition(b) A	Solvent Composition(b) B	Load Fragments	Load Volume (ml)	Gradient	RV(c) ml	SA(d)
1	50	0.1% TEAP pH 7	80% CH_3CN 0.1% TEAP	970	3600	35-85% B in 45 min.	650-1025	0.92
2	50	0.1% TEAP pH 6.5	80% CH_3CN 0.1% TEAP	1450	1850	30-85% B in 45 min.	1000-1150	0.72
3	3	0.1% TEAP pH 5.0	60% CH_3CN 0.1% TEAP	300	90	50-80% B in 25 min.	48-55.5	138
4	2.5	0.1% TFA	60% Propanol 0.1% TFA	280	20	35-65% B in 20 min.	27.5-29.7	9640
5	0.8	0.1% TFA	60% Propanol 0.1% TFA	440	4.0	35-95% B in 45 min.	14.8-15.9	27000

(a) Silicas were from Vydac. Steps 1 and 2 used 5 x 30 cm cartridges filled with 15-20 μm C_4(10). Steps 3 and 4 used 1 x 30 cm columns filled with 5 μm C_4. Step 5 used a 0.46 x 25 cm column filled with 5 μm C_{18}.

(b) TEAP buffer was 0.1% H_3PO_4 titrated to pH with redistilled triethylamine. Except for Steps 1 and 2, the active fractions (diluted with an equal volume of H_2O) were loaded 1.5 ml at a time into a 2 ml injector loop.

(c) Retention volume (RV) of the active zone was measured in ml from the start of the gradient (not including loading volume). Fractions were stored at 3-5°C. Aliquots for assays (0.1-1% of total fraction volume, never less than 5 μl) were measured with micropipettes and plastic tips and were transferred into polypropylene tubes containing bovine serum albumin (10 μl;10 mg/ml) and dried in a Savant rotary evaporator. Losses prior to assays and inconsistent results could be minimized in this manner. In order to determine recoveries of biological activity throughout the purification scheme, a record must be kept of the original volume of follicular fluid (1 ml being defined as 1 fragment) that is applied per chromatographic run so that a specific activity can be deduced. When 300 fragments were loaded (Step 3), five identical runs were performed to process the total 1450 fragments. Manual column fractionation was based on OD patterns.

(d) Specific activity (SA) is defined as the % recovery of activity multiplied by the purification factor; the purification factor being the original protein concentration divided by the final protein concentration.

CONCLUSION

A 27,000 fold purification of FS was achieved using RP·HPLC and ca. 300μg of protein were isolated from 1450 ml of pFF. The highly purified material exhibited half maximal inhibition at 77 pg/ml in one *in vitro* assay. As we had observed with other natural products obtained in small amounts, biological potency did not remain constant with time, but seemed to reach a lower plateau within a few days. Whether this observation is the result of adsorption to container, self aggregation or chemical alteration (oxidation, partial hydrolysis, etc.) of the active moiety, may have to await the availability of a synthetic replicate.

The high potency, dose response parallelism with, and similar V_{max} to FS, symmetrical HPLC profile and preliminary composition data on this fraction may suggest that this preparation is pure enough for meaningful sequence analysis.

ACKNOWLEDGEMENTS

This project was carried out under Contract N01-HD-32826 with the Contraceptive Development Branch of NICHD.

REFERENCES

1. McCullagh DD (1932) Science 76:19
2. deJong FH (1979) Molecular and Cellular Endocrinology 13:1-10
3. Dobas M, Burger HG, Hearn MTW, Morgan, FJ (1983) Molecular and Cellular Endocrinology 31:187-198
4. Ramasharma K, Sairam MR, Seidah NH, Chretien M, Manjunath P, Schiller PW, Yamashiro D, Li CH (1984) Science 223:1199-1202
5. Vale W, Grant G, Amoss M, Blackwell R, Guillemin R (1972) Endocrinology 91:562-572
6. Vale W, Vaughan J, Smith M, Yamamoto G, Rivier J, Rivier C (1983) Endocrinology 113:1121-1131
7. Rivier J (1978) J Liquid Chromatography 1:343-367
8. Rivier J, Rivier C, Spiess J, Vale W (1983) Analytical Biochemistry 127:258-266
9. Rivier, J (1980) J Chromatography 202:221-222
10. Rivier J, McClintock R, Galyean R, Anderson H (1984) Journal of Chromatography 288:303-328
11. See abstracts and proceedings of the International Endocrine Society Meeting including Satellite Symposia held in Quebec, Canada, June 28 - July 7, 1984.

INDEX OF AUTHORS

SUBJECT INDEX

Prepared by Dr. E. A. van der Veen, Amsterdam